MEDICAL DISORDERS IN OBSTETRIC PRACTICE

Medical Disorders in Obstetric Practice

EDITED BY
Michael de Swiet
MD, FRCP
Academic Sub-Dean
Royal Postgraduate Medical School
Institute of Obstetrics and Gynaecology
Queen Charlotte's and Chelsea Hospital
London

THIRD EDITION

Blackwell
Science

Editorial Offices:
Osney Mead, Oxford OX2 0EL
25 John Street, London WC1N 2BL
23 Ainslie Place, Edinburgh EH3 6AJ
238 Main Street, Cambridge
Massachusetts 02142, USA
54 University Street, Carlton
Victoria 3053, Australia

Other Editorial Offices:
Arnette Blackwell SA
224, Boulevard Saint Germain
75007 Paris, France

Blackwell Wissenschafts-Verlag GmbH
Kurfürstendamm 57
10707 Berlin, Germany

Zehetnergasse 6
A-1140 Wien, Austria

First published 1984
Reprinted 1986
Second edition 1989
Reprinted 1992, 1993
Third edition 1995
Reprinted 1996

Set by Setrite Typesetters, Hong Kong
Printed and bound in Great Britain
at the University Press, Cambridge

DISTRIBUTORS
Marston Book Services Ltd
PO Box 269
Abingdon
Oxon OX14 4YN
(*Orders:* Tel: 01235 465500
Fax: 01235 465555)

USA
Blackwell Science, Inc.
238 Main Street
Cambridge, MA 02142
(*Orders:* Tel: 800 215-1000
617 876-7000
Fax: 617 492-5263)

Canada
Copp Clark, Ltd
2775 Matheson Blvd East
Mississauga, Ontario
Canada, L4W 4P7
(*Orders:* Tel: 800 263-4374
905 238-6074)

Australia
Blackwell Science Pty Ltd
54 University Street
Carlton, Victoria 3053
(*Orders:* Tel: 03 9347 0300
Fax: 03 9349 3016)

A catalogue record for this title
is available from the British Library

ISBN 0-632-03671-0

Library of Congress
Cataloging-in-publication Data

Medical disorders in obstetric practice/
edited by Michael de Swiet.
– 3rd ed.
p. cm.
Includes bibliographical references
and index.
ISBN 0-632-03671-0
1. Pregnancy – Complications.
I. De Swiet, Michael.
[DNLM: 1. Pregnancy Complications.
WQ 240 M4867 1995]
RG571.M426 1995
618.3 – dc20
DNLM/DLC
for Library of Congress

Contents

List of Contributors, vii

Preface to the Third Edition, ix

Preface to the First Edition, xi

1 Diseases of the Respiratory System, 1
Michael de Swiet

2 Blood Volume, Haematinics, Anaemia, 33
Elizabeth A. Letsky

3 Coagulation Defects, 71
Elizabeth A. Letsky

4 Thromboembolism, 116
Michael de Swiet

5 Heart Disease in Pregnancy, 143
Michael de Swiet

6 Hypertension in Pregnancy, 182
Christopher W.G. Redman

7 Renal Disease, 226
John Davison & Christine Baylis

8 Systemic Lupus Erythematosus and Other Connective Tissue Diseases, 306
Michael de Swiet

9 Disorders of the Liver, Biliary System and Pancreas, 321
Elizabeth A. Fagan

10 Disorders of the Gastrointestinal Tract, 379
Elizabeth A. Fagan

11 Diabetes, 423
Michael Maresh & Richard Beard

12 Thyroid Disease, 459
Ian Ramsay

13 Diseases of the Pituitary and Adrenal Gland, 483
Michael de Swiet

14 Bone Disease, Disease of the Parathyroid Glands and Some Other Metabolic Disorders, 505
Barry N.J. Walters & Michael de Swiet

15 Neurological Disorders, 535
James O. Donaldson

16 Fever and Infectious Diseases, 552
Dame Rosalinde Hurley

17 Pregnancy Outcome and Management in HIV Infected Women, 568
Frank D. Johnstone

18 Substance Abuse, 600
Michael de Swiet

19 Skin Diseases in Pregnancy, 610
Martin M. Black & Susan C. Mayou

20 Psychiatry in Pregnancy, 625
Peter F. Liddle

Index, 641

List of Contributors

Christine Baylis PhD, Professor of Physiology, West Virginia University, Charlottesville, West Virginia 22903, USA

Richard Beard MD FRCOG, Professor of Obstetrics and Gynaecology, Department of Obstetrics and Gynaecology, St Mary's Hospital Medical School, Praed Street, London W1 1PG, UK

Martin M. Black MD FRCP FRCPath, Chairman, Department of Dermatopathology, St John's Institute of Dermatology (UMDS), St Thomas' Hospital, Lambeth Palace Road, London SE1 7EH, UK

John Davison BSc MD MSc FRCOG, Consultant Obstetrician and Gynaecologist, Department of Obstetrics and Gynaecology, Royal Victoria Infirmary, Queen Victoria Road, Newcastle upon Tyne NE1 4LP, UK

Michael de Swiet MD FRCP, Academic Sub-Dean, Royal Postgraduate Medical School, Institute of Obstetrics and Gynaecology, Queen Charlotte's and Chelsea Hospital, Goldhawk Road, London W6 0XG, UK

James O. Donaldson MD, Professor of Neurology, University of Connecticut School of Medicine, Farmington, Connecticut 06030-1845, USA

Elizabeth A. Fagan MSc MD MRCP MRCPath, Senior Lecturer in Medicine, Royal Free Hospital, University College London Medical School, Rowland Hill Street, London NW3 2PF, UK

Dame Rosalinde Hurley DBE MD FRCPath, Professor of Microbiology, Royal Postgraduate Medical School, Institute of Obstetrics and Gynaecology, Queen Charlotte's and Chelsea Hospital, Goldhawk Road, London W6 0XG, UK

Frank D. Johnstone MD FRCOG, Senior Lecturer, Department of Obstetrics and Gynaecology, University of Edinburgh, 23 Chalmers Street, Edinburgh EH3 9EW, UK

Peter F. Liddle BMBCh MRCPsych, Senior Lecturer in Psychological Medicine, Royal Postgraduate Medical School, Hammersmith Hospital, DuCane Road, London W12 0HS, UK

Elizabeth A. Letsky MBBS FRCPath, Consultant Haematologist, Queen Charlotte's and Chelsea Hospital, Goldhawk Road, London W6 0XG, UK

Michael Maresh MD FRCOG, Consultant Obstetrician, St Mary's Hospital for Women and Children, Hathersage Road, Whitworth Park, Manchester M13 0JH, UK

Susan C. Mayou BSc MRCP, Consultant Dermatologist, Queen Mary's University Hospital, Roehampton and Westminster Children's Hospital, London SW15 5PN, UK

Ian Ramsay MD FRCP FRCPE, Consultant Physician, Department of Endocrinology, North Middlesex Hospital, Sterling Way, London N18 1QX, UK

Christopher W.G. Redman FRCP, Professor of Obstetric Medicine, Nuffield Department of Obstetrics and Gynaecology, John Radcliffe Hospital, Headington, Oxford OX3 9DU, UK

Barry N.J. Walters FRACP, Physician in Obstetric Medicine, Department of Obstetrics and Gynaecology, King Edward Memorial Hospital for Women, Perth, Western Australia 6000

Preface to the Third Edition

I am delighted by the continuing success of this book and wish to thank my co-authors for their enthusiastic hard work. All the chapters have been extensively revised for the third edition. There is a new chapter on psychiatric illness (an obvious omission from previous editions) by Peter Liddle and one on the relation of HIV infection to pregnancy by Frank Johnstone. AIDS is the most common cause of maternal mortality in some countries. The transmission of AIDS to the neonate and interventions that might reduce such transmission are some of the very important issues that are addressed in this chapter.

Finally, I wish to thank all my immediate and distant colleagues who have referred cases or discussed obstetric medical problems with me; and readers who have made helpful suggestions about the content of this book.

M. DE SWIET
Queen Charlotte's
Maternity Hospital
London

Preface to the First Edition

This book has been produced to replace *Medical Disorders in Obstetric Practice* which was written by my predecessor, as Consultant Physician at Queen Charlotte's Maternity Hospital, Cyril Barnes. In many ways Cyril Barnes established the subspecialty of obstetric medicine in Great Britain. Some would argue that obstetric medicine is not a subspecialty at all; that the already established subspecialties, such as cardiology and haematology, embrace a sufficient body of knowledge to deal adequately with all medical complications of pregnancy. I disagree. The physiology of the pregnant woman is so altered, and the constraint of the welfare of the fetus is so important, that subspecialists who can oversee the two widely different fields of obstetrics and medicine are needed.

Barnes' text was a model of clarity, and a tribute to his considerable clinical experience. I hope that with this book, we have been able to continue in the tradition of my predecessor. In particular, I hope that the obstetrician who may not always have optimal medical support, will find practical answers to his medical problems here. In addition, this is now a multi-author book, and we have tried to include the latest advances in a very rapidly progressing subject.

M. DE SWIET
Queen Charlotte's
Maternity Hospital,
London

1

Diseases of the Respiratory System

Michael de Swiet

Physiological adaptation to pregnancy, 1
Oxygen consumption, Pa_{O_2}, CO_2 production, P-50
Tidal volume
Ventilatory equivalent, Pa_{CO_2} and pH
The stimulus to hyperventilation
Vital capacity
Anatomical changes
Airways resistance
Gas transfer (pulmonary diffusing capacity)
Exercise, 4
Breathlessness in pregnancy, 5
General comments on disorders of the respiratory system in pregnancy, 5
Bronchial asthma, 6
The effect of pregnancy on asthma
The effect of asthma on pregnancy
Management of asthma in pregnancy
General measures
The management of labour
Anaesthesia and analgesia
Breast feeding
Genetic counselling
Tuberculosis, 12
Sarcoidosis and erythema nodosum, 14
Erythema nodosum
Wegener's granulomatosis, 15
Pulmonary lymphangioleio-myomatosis, 15
Pneumonia and other respiratory tract infections, 16
Upper respiratory tract
Pneumonia
Cystic fibrosis, 17
Chronic bronchitis, emphysema and bronchiectasis, 19
Kyphoscoliosis, 20
Adult respiratory distress syndrome, shock lung, 20
Pneumothorax and pneumomediastinum, 21
Pleural effusion, 22
Lung cancer, 22
Anaesthetic considerations, 22

Disorders of the lung severe enough to cause respiratory failure are rare in pregnancy [109] since the major causes, chronic bronchitis and emphysema, are more common in men or in women past their childbearing years. Nevertheless, respiratory failure may occur in bronchial asthma, in overwhelming infection, occasionally in connective tissue disorders and in neuromuscular problems such as Guillain–Barré syndrome or Charcot–Marie–Tooth disease [42]. It may be the cause of death in post-anaesthetic complications. Before considering these and other respiratory diseases in pregnancy, we should first review the physiological changes in the respiratory system that occur during pregnancy. For more detailed reviews of physiology see references [74,75,102,201].

Physiological adaptation to pregnancy

Oxygen consumption, Pa_{O_2}, CO_2 production, P-50

During pregnancy oxygen consumption rises by about 45 ml/min [4,112]. Since oxygen consumption at rest is approximately 300 ml/min [170,227] the increase is about 18 per cent. About one-third of the increased oxygen consumption is necessary for the metabolism of the fetus and placenta. The remainder is supplied for the extra metabolism of the mother, in particular the extra work of increased secretion and reabsorption by the kidney [75].

The majority of authors find little change in Pa_{O_2} during pregnancy. The normal value is about 13.6 kPa (103 mmHg) at the end of pregnancy [294].

Those authors such as Lucius *et al.* [185] that have

found a Pa_{O_2} reduced to 11.3 kPa (85 mmHg) in pregnancy have usually not specified the position of their patients. Pa_{O_2} may fall by up to 1.7 kPa (13 mmHg) on changing from the sitting to the supine position [10] probably due to a combination of haemodynamic alterations (e.g. reduction in cardiac output, Chapter 5) and changes in functional residual capacity and closing volume. These changes cause mismatching of ventilation and perfusion and subsequent hypoxaemia. Therefore arterial blood gas measurements should always be made in pregnancy in the sitting position if they are to be used for diagnostic purposes such as in suspected pulmonary embolism (see Chapter 4).

Although residence at extreme altitude is associated with decreased maternal Pa_{O_2} and intrauterine growth retardation, modern aircraft are pressurized to about 2500 m (8200 ft) and at these pressures Huch *et al.* [152] found no evidence of ill-effects on mother or fetus in 10 pregnancies studied during commercial flights.

The increase in oxygen consumption is associated with a corresponding increase in CO_2 output. Since respiratory quotient increases from 0.76 before pregnancy to 0.83 in late pregnancy, the increase in CO_2 production is proportionately greater than the increase in oxygen uptake [91,170]. This effect is likely to be due to an increase in the proportion of carbohydrate to fat metabolized during pregnancy.

P-50, an inverse measure of affinity of haemoglobin for oxygen, is progressively increased from 26 mmHg in the non-pregnant state to 30 mmHg at term [165]. This represents a decrease in affinity induced by pregnancy and would allow easier 'unloading' of oxygen from maternal blood to fetal blood in the placenta.

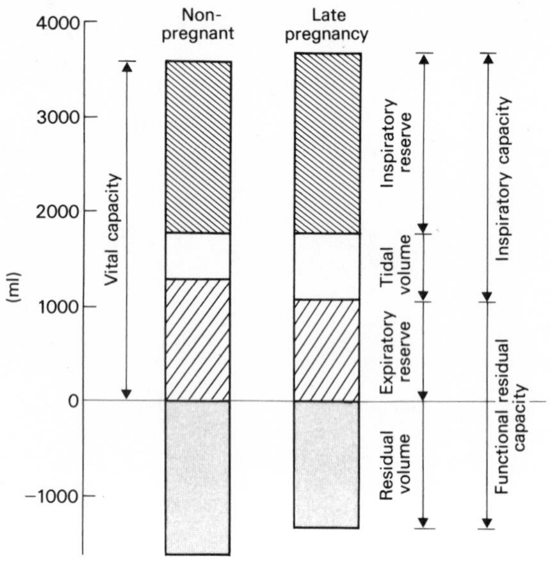

Fig. 1.1. Subdivisions of lung volume and their alterations in pregnancy. (From [67].)

Tidal volume

The increase in oxygen consumption is associated with a marked increased in ventilation of up to 40 per cent in pregnancy. This increase in ventilation is achieved efficiently by increasing tidal volume from 500 to 700 ml [68] rather than by any increase in respiratory rate [227] (Fig. 1.1). It occurs early in pregnancy [203]. Effective alveolar ventilation is further increased by a reduction of 20 per cent in residual volume — the volume of air in the lungs which remains at the end of expiration and with which the incoming air is diluted [4] (Fig. 1.2).

Ventilatory equivalent, Pa_{CO_2} and pH

The increase in ventilation of 40 per cent compared to the increase in oxygen consumption of 20 per cent causes a considerable increase in ventilatory equivalent — the minute volume divided by oxygen consumption — which rises from 3.2 l/min/100 ml oxygen consumed to 4.0 l/min/100 ml oxygen consumed. Therefore, the Pa_{CO_2} falls in pregnancy from non-pregnant levels of 4.7–5.3 kPa (35–40 mmHg) to about 4 kPa (30 mmHg) [92]. Most authors (e.g. Milne [201]) find the Pa_{CO_2} falls early in pregnancy in parallel with the change in ventilation, but Lucius *et al.* [185] and Bouterline-Young and Bouterline-Young [34] found a progressive fall in Pa_{CO_2}. The fall in Pa_{CO_2} is even greater at altitude where the mother is hyperventilating further in an attempt to maintain the Pa_{O_2} as high as possible. Hellegers *et al.* [145] found a Pa_{CO_2} of 3.7 kPa (28 mmHg) at 4400 m and Sobrevilla *et al.* [275] recorded a Pa_{CO_2} of 3.2 kPa (24 mmHg) at altitude.

The fall in Pa_{CO_2} is matched by an equivalent fall in plasma bicarbonate concentration and all the

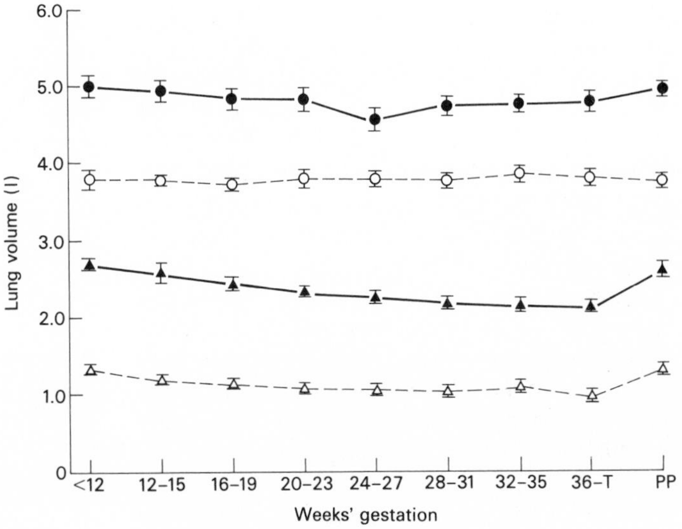

Fig. 1.2. Serial values of static lung volume during normal pregnancy and after delivery. (Values are mean ± SEM.) ● Total lung capacity; ○ vital capacity; ▲ functional residual capacity; △ residual volume.

evidence suggests that arterial pH is not altered from normal non-pregnant levels of about 7.40.

The stimulus to hyperventilation

The increase in ventilation and associated fall in $Pa\text{CO}_2$ occurring in pregnancy, is probably due to progesterone [81] which may act via a number of mechanisms. It lowers the threshold of the respiratory centre to CO_2 [317]. In addition, during pregnancy, the sensitivity of the respiratory centre increases [186] so that an increase in $Pa\text{CO}_2$ of 0.13 kPa (1 mmHg) increases ventilation by 5 l/min in pregnancy, compared to 1.5 l/min in the non-pregnant state [92,227,234]. It is also possible that progesterone acts as a primary stimulant to the respiratory centre independently of any change in CO_2 sensitivity or threshold [268]. Not only does progesterone stimulate ventilation, but it also increases the level of carbonic anhydrase B in the red cell [222,254]. An increase in carbonic anhydrase will facilitate carbon dioxide transfer, and also tend to decrease $Pa\text{CO}_2$ independently of any change in ventilation. The respiratory stimulant effect of progesterone has been used in the treatment of respiratory failure and emphysema with varying success [70,188,285]. A similar but smaller increase in ventilation is observed in the luteal phase of the menstrual cycle [93,204] and in patients taking some oral contraceptives [201].

Vital capacity

The vital capacity, the maximum volume of gas that can be expired after a maximum inspiration, probably does not change in pregnancy (Figs 1.1 & 1.2). Some have found that it increases [112,201], others have found that it decreases [92,242]; the majority have found no change [4,68,201]. Cugell *et al.* [68] found a transient fall in vital capacity in the puerperium. As the authors themselves noted, it is likely that this was due to maternal discomfort from, for example, episiotomy sutures preventing full cooperation.

Anatomical changes

The findings of no change in vital capacity with a reduction in residual volume are in keeping with the observed changes in the configuration of the chest during pregnancy. The level of the diaphragm rises by about 4 cm early in pregnancy even before it is under pressure from the enlarging uterus. This would account for the decrease in residual volume since the lungs would be relatively compressed at forced expiration.

Airways resistance

The work done in breathing may be partitioned into work done in overcoming the total airways resistance of the tracheobronchial tree — where the resistance of large airways (>2 mm in diameter) is much more important than small airways function [191] — and work done in expanding the lungs and chest wall, the compliance.

Measurements of forced expiratory volume in 1 second (FEV_1) and peak expiratory flow rate are indirect measurements that depend on both airways resistance and lung compliance. Neither measurement is affected by pregnancy [267], nor is airways conductance [203] nor lung compliance [113].

Bevan *et al.* [28] and Garrard *et al.* [111] found an increased closing volume in pregnancy with closure beginning during normal tidal volume in half their subjects. This would suggest that the calibre of small airways <2 mm in diameter decreases in pregnancy to the point where some airways close during respiration. However, others [16,66,244] have found no change in the point of airways closure during normal pregnancy, and Farebrother and McHardy [97] suggested that an increased closing volume was only a feature of complicated pregnancy. Certainly ventilation/perfusion imbalance occurs in severe pre-eclampsia [293]. More work is necessary in this field. If some airways do close during tidal breathing, this would lead to impairment of ventilation/perfusion ratio and a decreased efficiency of pulmonary gas exchange causing hypoxaemia.

Gas transfer (pulmonary diffusing capacity)

This factor is a measure of the ease with which carbon monoxide and therefore oxygen is transported across the pulmonary membrane. Earlier studies showed no change in transfer factor during pregnancy [22,173]. However, more recently, Milne *et al.* [205] showed a marked decrease in transfer factor early in pregnancy (Fig. 1.3). This could be related to the fall in haematocrit, but would be offset by the increase in cardiac output occurring early in pregnancy. A reduction in transfer factor would be one effect acting against the increase in ventilation to improve the efficiency of gas exchange in pregnancy.

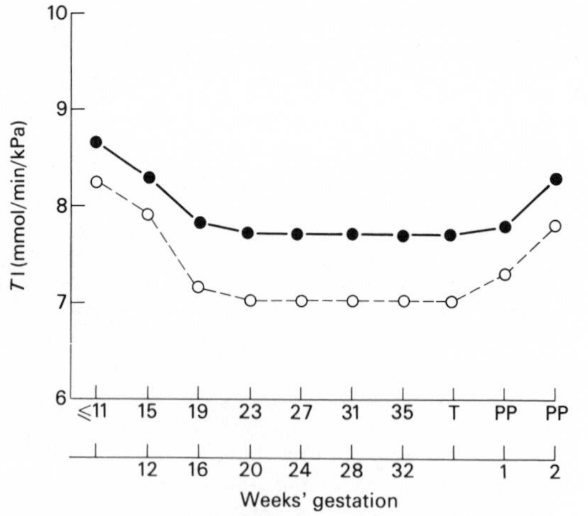

Fig. 1.3. Change in pulmonary transfer factor during normal pregnancy and after delivery (PP). ● Corrected for Hb and alveolar volume; ○ observed values. (After [204].)

In summary, the mother more than compensates for the increased oxygen consumption required by her and the fetus with a marked increase in tidal volume, leading to a considerable reduction in $Paco_2$. This is driven by progesterone, and respiratory efficiency is augmented by the decrease in residual volume. These effects could be offset by an increase in closing volume and a decrease in transfer factor.

Exercise

The interactions between pregnancy and exercise are of particular relevance in view of current obsessions with physical fitness. However, the capacity for exercise in pregnancy has not been fully tested [183]. This is because weight bearing exercise such as treadmill walking or step testing is heavily influenced by the change in weight associated with pregnancy. Sitting exercise (bicycle ergometry) should be less affected [89]. Also the capacity for maximum exercise depends on many other variables such as motivation which may themselves be altered by pregnancy. One question of interest is whether in pregnancy exercise costs more or is performed less efficiently. Artal *et al.* [12] found on treadmill testing in late pregnancy, that women could not increase oxygen consumption to such an extent as in the non-pregnant state and that the ventilatory equivalent increased with higher grades of exercise, i.e. ventilation was less efficient at extreme exercise.

Nevertheless, short-term exercise does not appear to affect the normal fetus, at least as measured in terms of fetal cardiac function assessed by M-mode echocardiography [276]. Longer exercise lasting more than 20 min does increase fetal heart rate although the mechanism is unknown [51]. Changes in uterine blood flow induced by maternal exercise may be compensated for by haemoconcentration (increasing oxygen carrying capacity) and increased oxygen extraction by the placenta [183]. In selected patients, participation in an exercise programme was associated with feeling good, improved American Pediatric Gross Assessment Record (APGAR) scores and a lower Caesarean section rate [136]. The consensus view is that moderate exercise improves the pregnancy outcome in women with no contraindication such as hypertension [153].

Breathlessness in pregnancy

Breathlessness is a subjective symptom and the degree to which patients are aware of the profound changes in ventilation occurring in pregnancy as breathlessness varies enormously between patients and in the same patient in different pregnancies.

The degree of breathlessness felt by women in pregnancy has been documented by Thomson and Cohen [298], Cugell *et al.* [68] and Milne *et al.* [202]. Milne *et al.* found that about 50 per cent of women were aware of breathlessness before 20 weeks' gestation. The maximum incidence of breathlessness at rest occurred between 28 and 31 weeks' gestation. However, the symptom of breathlessness cannot in general be correlated with any single parameter of respiratory function. Therefore, the reason for the maximum incidence of dyspnoea at 28–31 weeks' gestation remain unknown.

It is clearly important for the clinician to be aware that dyspnoea is a normal feature of pregnancy and does not necessarily represent cardiorespiratory disease. In the absence of any other symptoms of cardiorespiratory disease, normal findings on examination and a normal chest X-ray should be sufficient to exclude any serious pathology in the majority of women with breathlessness in pregnancy. Measurement of arterial blood gases and transfer factor should be reserved for those who are markedly breathless with particular relevance to pulmonary embolus and the possibility of diffuse infiltrative lung conditions, such as idiopathic pulmonary fibrosis.

One further test is to measure oxygen saturation transcutaneously and therefore non-invasively. The equipment to do this should be available in anaesthetic departments for monitoring oxygen saturation during general anaesthesia. The normal oxygen saturation is in excess of 95 per cent. A fall in saturation on exercise, e.g. climbing stairs, indicates cardiopulmonary disease and should be investigated further.

General comments on disorders of the respiratory system in pregnancy

Pregnancy stresses the respiratory system very little compared to its effect on the cardiovascular system. During pregnancy the minute ventilation increases by about 40 per cent from 7.5 to 10.5 l/min and oxygen consumption increases by about 18 per cent from about 250 to 300 ml/min. Yet, in exercise, minute ventilation can increase to 80 l/min [57], a 10-fold increase. Cardiac output also rises by approximately 40 per cent from 4.5 to 6 l/min in pregnancy (see Chapter 5), but in contrast, the maximum cardiac output achieved in exercise is probably no greater than 12 l/min, a threefold increase. Thus, although cardiac output and minute ventilation both increase by an equal fraction in pregnancy, the increase in cardiac output represents a far greater proportion of the maximum that the body is capable of, than does the increase in ventilation. Patients with respiratory disease are therefore less likely to deteriorate in pregnancy than those with cardiac disease since they have greater reserve.

Those chest diseases occurring frequently in pregnancy are described below. In addition, case reports suggest that fibrosing alveolitis may deteriorate in pregnancy [233] and that pulmonary fibrosis in association with systemic sclerosis is not affected [18].

Bronchial asthma

Asthma is a common condition affecting more than 3 per cent of women in their childbearing years [182] and the prevalence may well be increasing [44]. More recently, Hernandez *et al.* [148] reported that 1 per cent of 4529 pregnancies at Johns Hopkins Hospital were complicated by acute asthma: 0.15 per cent had severe attacks requiring hospitalization. It is therefore the most common respiratory disorder complicating pregnancy. For other general reviews see [102,124,125,148,277,280,301,310,311].

The effect of pregnancy on asthma

Asthma is a very variable condition. Its severity depends on the patient's exposure to allergens and the presence of respiratory infection, both also dependent on the season of the year. In addition, the patient's emotional state is important. If sufficient patients are studied to allow for these influences, pregnancy has no consistent effect on asthma. For example, White *et al.* [314] found that pregnancy improved asthma, whereas Gordon *et al.* [119] found that pregnancy was associated with a deterioration in bronchial asthma. Turner *et al.* [301] reviewed 1054 cases reported in nine different publications: 48 per cent showed no change in pregnancy, 29 per cent improved and 23 per cent deteriorated. Patients do not necessarily change in the same way during different pregnancies. Williams [318] found that 37 per cent of 63 patients with asthma reacted differently in different pregnancies; this difference did not depend on the sex of the fetus [318]. In a prospective study, Juniper *et al.* [164] followed airways responsiveness and treatment requirement (amongst other variables) in 16 patients from before conception and showed that both improved in a significant majority during pregnancy. When we followed measurements of FEV_1 serially through pregnancy in 27 patients with asthma, we were unable to find any consistent changes during pregnancy, or between pregnancy and the non-pregnant state [267]; this is in keeping with studies in non-asthmatic patients reviewed above.

If pregnancy does not cause any net change in airways resistance either in normal subjects or in those with asthma, this is likely to be the sum of several factors acting in opposing directions. The bronchodilator influences are increased progesterone secretion, which may cause bronchodilation directly and also by increasing β adrenergic activity [237], and increased free cortisol (see Chapter 13); the bronchoconstrictor influences are the reduced residual volume [36], reduced $Paco_2$ [216] and increased prostaglandin $F_{2\alpha}$ secretion [156]. Prostaglandin $F_{2\alpha}$ should therefore not be used in obstetric practice (therapeutic abortion, induction of labour) [103,104,156,172,271] unless there is a life-threatening emergency such as post-partum haemorrhage when it is injected directly into the uterus. Prostaglandin E is used more widely and is the preferred prostaglandin for use in asthmatic patients, although there is some controversy as to whether it may be a bronchoconstrictor or a bronchodilator [270].

The most common cause for asthma to deteriorate in pregnancy is because the patient has reduced treatment either because of her own or her attendants' mistaken belief that such treatment will harm the fetus.

The effect of asthma on pregnancy

Schatz *et al.* [250] found no excess risk to the fetus in 70 pregnancies of patients receiving corticosteroids for asthma, apart from a slight excess of prematurity; this risk was also noted by others [15,82]. However, Apter *et al.* [11] found no excess fetal morbidity in 21 adolescent patients with asthma even though these patients required aggressive treatment with multiple hospital admissions. By contrast it has been suggested that perinatal mortality is doubled over normals in patients with asthma in pregnancy, but this effect was largely confined to a black, presumably socially deprived, population [119]. We found no statistically significant extra risk to the fetus if the mother suffered from asthma in pregnancy, although there was a tendency towards growth retardation, particularly amongst fetuses of mothers taking oral steroid therapy [267]. These patients were more severely affected by asthma, and may have been intermittently hypoxic. The relation between growth retardation and impaired respiratory function has now been shown to be statistically significant in a group of 352 pregnant asthmatics [251]. Templeton [292] suggested that hypoxia was the cause of recurrent growth retardation that he noted in a patient with bronchiectasis. Alternatively, hyperventilation which may be associated with acute attacks of asthma, often causes hypocapnia, and this also has been related to fetal hypoxia [210,322]. Animal data would suggest that maternal respiratory alkalosis also causes fetal hypoxia [209] and both respiratory alkalosis and hypocapnia may act via a reduction in maternal placental perfusion [208,210].

A recent study [252] showed that transient tachypnoea was more common in the new-borns of asthmatic women (3.7 per cent) than in those of controls (0.3 per cent) but this did not affect their long-term outcome.

In summary, there is a slight increased risk to the fetus of the mother with asthma, but this effect is very small, and should not be exaggerated when counselling individual patients.

Management of asthma in pregnancy [96]

Pregnancy is a time when patients see their doctors frequently. This is a good opportunity to optimize the therapy of asthma, ideally in a combined medical or respiratory and obstetric clinic.

The diagnosis of bronchial asthma is made on the basis of the history of recurrent episodes of wheeze and breathlessness, often associated with trigger factors such as exposure to allergens (dust, pollen), infection or psychological factors. An arbitrary definition is a variation in peak expiratory flow rate or FEV_1 >20 per cent, either spontaneously or as a result of treatment. Some patients may present with a history of cough only. Patients with attacks only at night or on exercise may have a primary cardiac cause rather than bronchial asthma, but these usually have other signs of heart disease, or cardiomegaly on the chest radiograph. It is now possible to purchase inexpensive peak expiratory flow meters. Patients use these at home to record their peak flows throughout the day on diary cards. In patients with asthma these records show characteristic dips in peak flow at night or during the early morning. Respiratory function may deteriorate before the patient is aware of it. Home peak flow monitoring allows the patient to increase treatment (usually with inhaled or oral glucocorticoids) before her symptoms deteriorate.

In addition, pulmonary embolus may also rarely present as bronchospasm [320] and this should be remembered as a possibility in patients who have their first attack of 'asthma' in pregnancy [130] (see Chapter 4).

General measures

Asthma is by definition a variable condition which inevitably affects the patient's emotions. Also emotional upsets to which patients are particularly susceptible in pregnancy adversely affect asthma. It is therefore particularly important for the patient to develop a good relationship with an obstetrician and a physician whom she can trust.

Barbiturates and other sedative drugs should not be used because of the risk of respiratory depression; even diazepam is unsafe. The anxiety is much better treated by relief of symptoms with effective therapy. If the patient has any evidence of chest infection, as indicated by purulent sputum, this should be treated with an appropriate antibiotic (see below). However, eosinophilia may cause yellow sputum which looks purulent. Chest infection is probably overdiagnosed as a cause of exacerbation of asthma and such exacerbation should always be managed with an increase in bronchodilator therapy. In addition, it should be remembered that expectorants containing iodine should not be used in pregnancy, because the iodine may block thyroxine synthesis in the fetus making it hypothyroid or giving it a goitre [47,110]. Since iodine is preferentially excreted in breast milk [304], mothers who are breast feeding should also not use iodine-containing expectorants or cough medicine.

Those clinicians who use desensitization in the treatment of asthma [200] or penicillin allergy [312] have not found any problems specific to pregnancy [200], although the risk of desensitization (i.e. anaphylaxis) remains.

The use of bronchodilator drugs is considered below. However, a reasonable strategy in the patient presenting with asthma for the first time in pregnancy would be to give a selective β_2 sympathomimetic drug such as salbutamol or terbutaline by inhalation for the acute attack. If this is being used more than once a day, regular betamethasone inhalations, two puffs (100 μg) four times a day should be added. Because of concern that β sympathomimetics may be related to an increase in asthma deaths [45] current opinion favours inhaled glucocorticoids rather than β sympathomimetics as prophylactic therapy with β sympathomimetics used for breakthrough symptoms [132]. Oral slow-release aminophylline can also be used at this stage. If there is no improvement, a short course of oral prednisone should be given, starting at 60 mg/day, reducing the dose rapidly, and aiming to stop oral steroids completely within 10 days. Oral β sympathomimetics are now rarely used since they tend to cause tremor and anxiety, and they are not usually helpful. The British Thoracic Society guidelines for management of chronic persistent asthma [38] and acute severe asthma (see below) [38] should be followed in pregnancy as well as in the non-pregnant state.

If there is any difficulty in controlling asthma the patient should be admitted to hospital, particularly in pregnancy. Status asthmaticus is difficult to define and has been renamed acute severe asthma, but deteriorating asthma which fails to respond promptly to regular medication is a life-threatening condition [191] which has been shown to be particularly dangerous in pregnancy [119]. It is likely that this is because the condition is managed initially by those with an obstetric orientation. It is notoriously easy to underestimate the severity of attacks of asthma [189]. Therefore all patients with acute severe asthma in pregnancy should be managed in cooperation with a physician interested in respiratory disease, preferably in an intensive care unit. Ominous signs include a heart rate >110/min, respiratory rate >25/min, pulsus paradoxus of >18–20 mmHg, and peak expiratory flow <200 l/min in addition to dyspnoea, accessory muscle use and wheeze [101]. Be very worried about patients who cannot complete sentences in one breath!

The patient should be monitored with regular measurements of peak flow rate and blood gases. If this is done, there is no need for controlled oxygen therapy, and the patient can have oxygen, 10 l/min, given via a face mask. Because of the maternal risk, the patient should be managed as if she were not pregnant, giving optimal therapy for the respiratory condition. However, as outlined below, treatment with steroids, β sympathomimetics or theophyllines is unlikely to affect the fetus in any case. The only drug that should not be used is tetracycline (see below), but fortunately there are other, better, broad spectrum antibiotics available. Despite this, antibiotics should only be given if there is clear evidence of infection.

Ventilation is rarely necessary but should the patient require it, either because of exhaustion or rising $Paco_2$, it is clear that maternal $Paco_2$ should be maintained as near physiological levels as possible; indeed, this is the usual purpose of ventilation. As noted previously, Wulf *et al.* [322] showed that as maternal Po_2 fell from 12.1 to 6.3 kPa (91 to 47 mmHg), fetal umbilical vein Po_2 fell from 4.3 to 3.6 kPa (32 to 27 mmHg). However, hypocapnia (Pco_2 2.3 kPa, 17 mmHg) and alkalosis (pH > 7.6) should also be avoided, since these are associated with reduced fetal oxygenation, probably due to impaired placental transport [301,322]. If all therapy fails to improve the patient with acute severe asthma, termination of pregnancy may be life saving [114].

β sympathomimetic drugs (isoprenaline, salbutamol, terbutaline, fenoterol)

An inhaled β sympathomimetic is the first drug to use in treating patients who have occasional attacks of bronchospasm. It may be used prophylactically if the patient is particularly at risk, for example, from exercise-induced asthma. Although most of the β sympathomimetics such as salbutamol, terbutaline and fenoterol that are used for the treatment of asthma are relatively selective, stimulating β_2 rather than β_1 receptors, the dosage given is still limited by cardiac side-effects of tachycardia and irregularities of heart rhythm. In addition, patients may notice tremor and a feeling of anxiety or apprehension. These effects are more marked with non-selective β sympathomimetic drugs such as isoprenaline, which should not be used. There is little to choose between one selective β sympathomimetic drug and another. My own preference is to use salbutamol, which has been widely studied in pregnant and non-pregnant patients and to avoid fenoterol which may be less selective and is possibly marketed at too high a dose [321].

There is considerable experience of the use of β sympathomimetic agents in pregnancy, not only for the treatment of asthma, but also for preterm labour [180]. There is no evidence of teratogenicity and ephedrine in particular has been shown to be safe [144]. However, in the case of adrenaline when given in the first 4 months of pregnancy there was a small non-specific increased risk of teratogenicity (minor eye and ear abnormalities) found by the Perinatal Collaborative Project [144]; but it is possible that the acute condition for which adrenaline was given, rather than the drug itself, was the cause of the malformations.

The most worrying side-effects in pregnancy are pulmonary oedema and metabolic acidosis [76]. Although it is possible to demonstrate metabolic [186,305] and cardiovascular [76] side-effects after oral salbutamol, these serious complications are unlikely with normal therapy, providing the manufacturer's instructions are complied with. High dose intravenous therapy is much more likely to cause side-effects in patients receiving β sympathomimetics for preterm labour, rather than in the treatment of asthma where intravenous sympathomimetic drugs have only been used in the treatment of acute severe asthma and where more patients receive inhaled β sympathomimetics.

Oral β sympathomimetic therapy will cause hyperglycaemia in pregnant patients with diabetes [186]. Since control of blood glucose is so important in diabetic pregnancy (see Chapter 11), patients who have impaired glucose tolerance and develop asthma should either not be given oral β sympathomimetics or should have their blood glucose controlled particularly carefully.

Because β sympathomimetics are used in the treatment of preterm labour, their use for asthma might be expected to delay the onset or impede the progress of normal labour. The fact that this does not occur [267] is perhaps not surprising in view of doubts about their efficacy in preterm labour [146].

The newer long acting inhaled β_2 agonist salmeterol is likely to prove effective and popular [105,225]. Because very little inhaled salmeterol enters the maternal blood, it is unlikely that the fetus will be affected and there have not been any adverse reports in pregnancy yet. However, at present there are insufficient data to recommend the use of salmeterol in pregnancy.

Theophyllines

Aminophylline has been widely used and is safe in pregnancy [126]. It is available as a soluble preparation, a slow-release preparation or as rectal suppositories in varying dosages. The oral dose is up to 10 mg/kg/day. The slow-release preparation acts for up to 12 hours and should therefore be used in preference to suppositories for the control of nocturnal and early morning asthma [6]. Theophylline is also available as an elixir which is rapidly absorbed, giving therapeutic blood levels at 15 min [106]. Optimal treatment, particularly in acute severe asthma, is achieved by maintaining blood levels between 5 and 20 mg/ml [2,311]. The recommended infusion rate to achieve this in non-pregnant subjects is 0.7 mg/kg/hour for the first 12 hours after a 6 mg/kg bolus, followed by 0.5 mg/kg/hour thereafter. Earlier reports [286] suggested that theophylline pharmacokinetics do not change during pregnancy and the above regime could therefore be recommended for the pregnant state [192]. However, it may need to be modified according to the theophylline blood level particularly since a more recent study [243] suggests that clearance is increased in pregnancy (Fig. 1.4). In any case blood levels should always be checked in acute severe asthma. Aminophylline may cause nausea and also causes tachyarrhythmias, especially when given intravenously. The bolus dose should therefore be given slowly. Because aminophylline is also a pulmonary vasodilator, the patient should be receiving oxygen during intravenous administration to avoid hypoxaemia.

Aminophylline is assumed to cross the placenta [311] and is excreted in breast milk in small quantities [324] but this has not been shown to cause any long-term harm to the fetus [215]. The safety of theophyllines in pregnancy is also suggested by a recent study in which aminophylline was given to women at risk of preterm delivery. Therapy was associated with decreases in the incidence of neo-

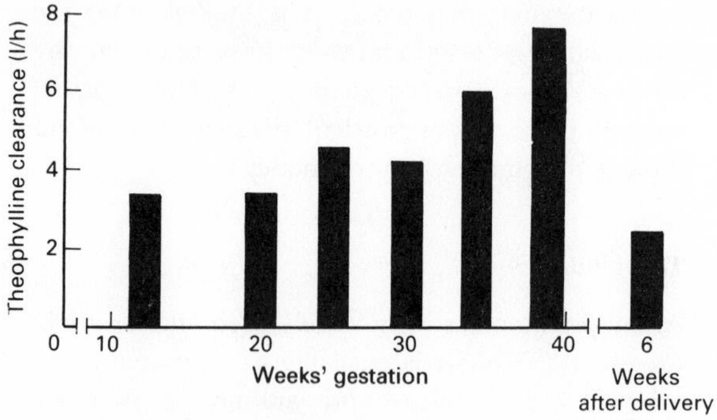

Fig. 1.4. Theophylline clearance calculated from steady state concentrations in a pregnant woman with asthma. Having been controlled before pregnancy on 250 mg every 12 hours, by the end of pregnancy this patient had subtherapeutic concentrations despite receiving 1500 mg/day. (From [242].)

natal respiratory distress syndrome and perinatal mortality. There were no adverse side-effects [134]. However, there are reports [13,323] of three newborn infants who showed theophylline toxicity (jitteriness, tachycardia, opisthotonos) after the mother had been given theophylline or aminophylline in late pregnancy. There were no long-term sequelae in any of these infants.

Disodium cromoglycate

Disodium cromoglycate is inhaled from a Spinhaler or conventional aerosols but the aerosols only deliver a small dose. It is used as a prophylactic to prevent the occurrence of asthma attacks. It appears to be safe for the fetus [88,310]. Since the drug is taken by inhalation the quantity entering the blood (8 per cent) is very small [88] and so little is transferred to the fetus. It occasionally causes bronchospasm at the time of inhalation and this can be avoided by using a combination preparation of disodium cromoglycate and isoprenaline.

Anticholinergic drugs, such as atropine or more recently ipratropium bromide given by aerosol, are also used in the prophylaxis of asthma [303]. Atropine has not been associated with any increased risk of teratogenesis [144], and fetal tachycardia is the only likely fetal side-effect.

Steroids

If patients cannot be managed with β adrenergic stimulants, inhaled steroids, theophylline preparations, disodium cromoglycate or anticholinergic drugs, an oral corticosteroid preparation should be used. The patient experiencing repeated severe attacks of asthma should receive steroids relatively early, before all other forms of treatment have been tried. An alternate day, oral steroid regime appears to reduce the side-effects of glucocorticoid therapy, although this has not been confirmed in pregnancy [1].

There is considerable debate concerning the use of steroids in pregnancy. Inhaled steroid therapy, e.g. beclomethasone, represents a considerable advance, since it permits the reduction or omission of oral therapy with prednisone. Inhaled beclomethasone acts locally on the bronchi, and is not absorbed if <1 mg (20 × 50 μg puffs of Becotide) is inhaled [139]. It has been used widely in pregnancy [126] and its safety is established [126]. The side-effects which occur with long-term use are monilial infections of the upper respiratory and gastrointestinal tracts, but these are not a specific risk of pregnancy and only a problem in 5 per cent of users. If patients are changed from *chronic* oral to inhaled steroid therapy, the dosage of oral steroid therapy should be reduced very slowly — no more rapidly than 1 mg reduction of prednisone per day every 4 weeks, if the dosage of prednisone is <10 mg/day. More rapid reduction has been associated with Addisonian collapse, a flare-up of other atopic manifestations such as allergic rhinitis, or just lethargy and non-specific malaise.

If patients require oral corticosteroid therapy for asthma, this should not be withheld because they are pregnant. Corticosteroids are said to cause cleft palate [107] but this risk appears to be confined to the rabbit [95]. Schatz *et al.* [250] did not find any excess of congenital malformations in 70 pregnancies complicated by asthma, treated with corticosteroids (average daily dose of prednisone, 8 mg) and this has been confirmed in other clinical studies [33,144,287] and reviewed by Turner *et al.* [301].

Steroid therapy will depress maternal adrenal activity. This can lead to a reduction in the adrenal and urinary secretion of oestriol if the dose is more than 30 mg of prednisone a day [83,207,307]. The effect, which is important if oestriol levels are used as an index of fetal well-being, may occur at dosages below 30 mg prednisone per day, but this has not been documented. In any case the urinary secretion of oestriol is now rarely used as an index of fetal well-being.

There is always concern that the hypothalamo-pituitary–adrenal axis of the fetus may be suppressed by maternal steroid therapy [308]; this would make the infant liable to collapse in the neonatal period. In practice this does not occur with prednisone, perhaps because little of this drug crosses the placenta. The maternal–fetal concentration of prednisone is 10 : 1 [23], in comparison to hydrocortisone 6 : 1 and betamethasone 3 : 1 [17]. Also the fetoplacental unit is relatively lacking in the enzymes to convert prednisone to its active metabolite prednisolone [17], and placental 11, β-ol-dehydrogenase is very efficient, deactivating 87 per cent of an injected dose of prednisone [122]. As indicated above, other glucocorticoids do cross the placenta and indeed have been given to the mother for treatment of the fetus, e.g. the use of betamethasone to 'mature' the pre-term fetal lung and dexamethasone to suppress the fetal adrenal gland in congenital adrenal hyperplasia (see Chapter 13).

The management of labour

It is unusual for labour to be complicated by attacks of asthma. Perhaps this is because of an even greater secretion of glucocorticoids from the adrenal cortex [163] and possibly also catecholamines from the adrenal medulla. Increased prostaglandin secretion during labour may also cause bronchodilatation. For attacks of asthma which do occur in labour, conventional treatment with inhaled β sympathomimetics should be used first, with earlier recourse to parenteral steroid therapy if the patient does not improve rapidly. Because of the risk of maternal suppression of the hypothalamopituitary–adrenal axis, it is conventional to give hydrocortisone 100 mg intramuscularly 6-hourly, to cover the period of labour, if the patient has taken continuous steroid therapy for any period of more than 2 weeks in the previous year; Addisonian collapse in labour is very rare. Prostaglandin $F_{2\alpha}$ should not be used because of its bronchoconstrictor action (see above); also syntocinon should be used rather than ergometrine because of concern that the latter may cause bronchospasm in patients with asthma [258,259].

Anaesthesia and analgesia

Epidural anaesthesia is preferable to general anaesthesia [193] because of the risk of atelectasis and subsequent chest infection following the latter. If a general anaesthetic cannot be avoided, halothane should be used because of its bronchodilating properties. Nebulized salbutamol can be given pre- and post-operatively. Opiates such as pethidine are best avoided because they cause bronchoconstriction and respiratory depression; but these remain relative rather than absolute contraindications and it would not be correct to deny a patient with asthma any effective analgesia at all if epidural anaesthesia were not available.

Breast feeding

Breast feeding should be encouraged. There is some, though conflicting, evidence that women with asthma in particular should breast feed because it may confer protection from food allergy in atopic individuals [160]. Turner *et al.* [301] have reviewed the secretion of drugs used in the treatment of asthma in breast milk. None of these drugs, including steroids, is likely to be secreted in sufficient quantities to harm the neonate, except tetracycline and iodides. In general, patients with asthma should therefore breast feed their infants.

Genetic counselling

The overall risk of any child having asthma is about 4 per cent. If one parent has asthma, the risk that the child will have asthma increases to 8–16 per cent, depending on whether the parent is also atopic. If both parents have asthma, and are also atopic, the risk may be as high as 30 per cent [264].

In conclusion, asthma is a common condition affecting many women who are pregnant. It is not usually a problem in pregnancy, either to the mother or the fetus. The major difficulties lie in realizing that the majority of drugs used in the treatment of pregnancy do not harm the fetus, and in maintaining the treatment of a potentially life-threatening illness despite the mother's pregnancy.

Tuberculosis

Pulmonary tuberculosis is now a rare complication of pregnancy in the general population of the UK, although some subgroups such as the Gujurati Indians and those with human immunodeficiency virus (HIV) infection (see Chapter 17) have an incidence that is up to 100 times greater than the national figure. At Queen Charlotte's Hospital we see one case every 2–3 years, delivering approximately 4500 patients per year. For this reason we and others [32,118,195] do not routinely perform chest X-rays in pregnancy, despite contrary recommendations [282]. In our population, routine chest radiographs are not worth the financial cost, or the very minimal extra risk to the fetus of irradiating the mother. Even in a population with 16 times the national average incidence of tuberculosis, a screening programme based on skin testing followed up by chest X-ray in positive cases, did not detect any cases in pregnancy that were not detected by clinical criteria (fever, cough or weight loss) [230]. Nevertheless, there should be no hesitation in performing chest X-rays if there is any clinical indication.

Before antituberculous drugs were available, the results of pregnancy complicated by tuberculosis were poor for both mother and fetus [53]; there was a particular tendency for patients to deteriorate in the puerperium [19,143]. However, Selikoff and Dormann [257] reported that pregnancy did not affect the 15–30 per cent of patients with untreated active tuberculosis, who deteriorated in the first 30 months after diagnosis. More recently, de March [73] was unable to find any deleterious effect of pregnancy in 100 patients with tuberculosis who had been pregnant, compared with 108 patients with pulmonary tuberculosis who had not been pregnant. Schaefer *et al.* [249] found that progression of pulmonary tuberculosis occurred in less than 1 per cent of patients managed during pregnancy at the New York Lying-In Hospital between 1957 and 1972. There is also no conclusive evidence that the outcome of pregnancy is adversely affected by tuberculosis [249,257]. However, Bjerkedal *et al.* [29] did notice an increased risk of abortion to 20 in 1000 patients with tuberculosis compared to two in 1000 controls. But two in 1000 is a very low incidence of abortion for the controls and these data should therefore be questioned. There is certainly no longer any justification for therapeutic abortion in maternal tuberculosis either for the sake of maternal health or because the fetus would otherwise be at such risk. Tuberculosis only very rarely affects the fetus by transplacental passage but, if the mother has open tuberculosis, the neonate is also at risk from infection after delivery. The criteria for congenital tuberculosis are:

1 the disease must be bacteriologically proven;
2 there must be a primary complex in the fetal or neonatal liver;
3 disease must appear early in the first days of life;
4 extrauterine infection must be excluded [24].

Infection may occur via the fetus swallowing infected amniotic fluid, or be blood-borne via the umbilical vein. If the diagnosis is made early, for which a high index of clinical suspicion is necessary, the outlook for the neonate is good. The mother may have tuberculosis infection of any severity from subclinical to miliary tuberculosis [274].

In pregnancy, pulmonary tuberculosis may present because of symptoms — cough, purulent sputum, haemoptysis, fever, weight loss, chest pain (tuberculous pleural effusion) — or as an incidental finding when a chest X-ray is taken for a different reason. The diagnosis is based on the chest X-ray appearance, sputum culture and examination of the pleural effusion, pleural biopsy, liver biopsy or by bone marrow aspiration. The Mantoux test will become positive within 4–12 weeks after the initial infection. Despite previous suggestions [100], Mantoux status is not affected by pregnancy itself [232].

The problem in managing a pregnant patient with tuberculosis is not her potential respiratory impairment, but the possible effects on the fetus of the chemotherapeutic drugs used. This subject has recently been extensively reviewed by Snider [272] and Snider *et al.* [274]. Overall, their findings were very encouraging, since 94 per cent of all pregnancies resulted in the delivery of apparently normal infants, and only 3 per cent of the infants exposed *in utero* were classified as having birth defects [274]. Before starting chemotherapy for tuberculosis, the obstetrician and/or general physician should consult a chest physician; since the general decline of tuberculosis in the community, chest physicians are the only specialists with sufficient experience of the varying regimes that are used.

The drugs for which there is considerable information are ethambutol, isoniazid, streptomycin and rifampicin. In addition, it is believed that ethionamide is teratogenic [231].

Ethambutol has replaced *para*-aminosalicylic acid (PAS) as a 'front-line' antituberculosis drug, because it is so much easier for the patient to take, though ethambutol has in term been replaced by pyrizinamide for non-pregnant patients. Although it may cause retrobulbar neuritis in adults in high doses [50], there is no evidence from abortion specimens [181] or the neonate [39] that the fetus is affected. Snider *et al.* [274] found only 14 infants or fetuses with abnormalities in 655 pregnancies treated with ethambutol and none had optic nerve abnormalities. The drug must therefore be considered safe in pregnancy.

The same is true of isoniazid. There have been 16 abnormal fetuses reported in a total of 1480 pregnancies [274]. This abnormality rate is lower than the normal hospital population. Monnet *et al.* [206] noted that four of five abnormal fetuses in their series of 125 patients treated with isoniazid, had central nervous system (CNS) abnormalities. Since isoniazid is known to cause peripheral neuritis, this is the potential difficulty in the use of isoniazid in pregnancy, but it must be emphasized that the high incidence of CNS abnormalities was only seen in one group of patients, all of whom had also received ethionamide [206]. In addition, the Collaborative Drug Project [144] found a small (twice excess) non-specific increase of congenital abnormalities in patients taking isoniazid. Because of the possible higher requirement of pyridoxine in pregnancy, all patients taking isoniazid in pregnancy should also take pyridoxine 50 mg/day [14] to reduce the risk of peripheral neuritis [41].

The real problems concern the use of streptomycin, rifampicin and pyrazinamide. Although at one time it was considered that streptomycin was relatively innocuous in pregnancy [60], this cannot be the current opinion. Conway and Birt [60] found no disabled children from 17 patients in whom the mother had been treated with streptomycin in pregnancy, but eight children had abnormal caloric tests and/or abnormal audiograms. Severe hearing loss was reported by Robinson and Cambon [240]. Snider *et al.* [274] found 34 cases of eighth nerve damage amongst the reports of 206 patients treated with streptomycin. This incidence of over 10 per cent appears excessive. Furthermore, the risk of eighth nerve damage will persist after the period of organogenesis, throughout gestation.

Although Scheinborn and Angelillo [253] initially suggested that rifampicin did not affect the fetus, Snider *et al.* [274] also found reports of 14 abnormal fetuses amongst 442 patients treated with rifampicin. The malformations were variable and severe. Nine of these cases have been reported in detail by the manufacturers [281]. There is one curious report of a nearly fivefold increase in the risk of deep vein thrombosis in patients treated with rifampicin for tuberculosis but this study was not performed in pregnant patients [314].

Pyrazinamide is increasingly used in antituberculous regimes because it rapidly renders the sputum negative for acid-fast bacilli and because 6 month rather than 9 month treatment periods are effective [56]. However, at present there is inadequate information concerning the safety of pyrazinamide in the first trimester and therefore it should be used with caution until after 14 weeks' gestation.

In summary, the patient presenting with tuberculosis in the first trimester of pregnancy should be treated with isoniazid and ethambutol in standard dosage unless the tuberculosis is widespread or deteriorating. After organogenesis is complete at 14 weeks' gestation it should be safe to use rifampicin and/or pyrizinamide. It may be necessary to admit the patient to establish the diagnosis, in which case she should be in a single room rather than have strict barrier nursing. The patient should also be in a single room when she is admitted for labour. However, now that antituberculosis therapy is so effective, the majority of treatment can be given as an outpatient. Nine months' treatment with isoniazid and rifampicin is considered sufficient for pulmonary tuberculosis or 6 months' treatment if the regime has included pyrazinamide.

Extrapulmonary tuberculosis is very rare in pregnancy because one of its principal manifestations, genital tract tuberculosis, is associated with infertility. Brooks and Stirrat [40] have recently reported a case of tuberculous peritonitis in pregnancy with a temporary Addisonian state which responded excellently to conventional antituberculous therapy. Tuberculous meningitis was a frequent terminal manifestation of women with tuberculosis in pregnancy [120,211] but is now very uncommon.

After birth, babies should only be isolated from their mothers if the mothers are still smear positive. Since modern antituberculosis regimes render the sputum sterile within 2 weeks and markedly reduce the number of organisms with 24 hours, this should not occur frequently. The neonate should be treated with prophylactic isoniazid for 3 months. After this period BCG vaccination is given in the UK although not in the USA [177]. It is not clear whether neonatal BCG vaccination adds any further protection to isoniaszid prophylaxis. It is not without risks: skin ulceration, osteitis and occasionally disseminated disease, particularly if the mother has an immunodeficiency state such as acquired immune deficiency syndrome (AIDS). As isoniazid therapy does not affect the immunogenicity of BCG vaccine, there is no longer any rationale for the use of isoniazid resistant BCG neonatal vaccination [177]. Mothers taking antituberculous therapy should be encouraged to breast feed since the infant will receive a maximum of 20 per cent of the normal infant dose by this route [273].

Sarcoidosis and erythema nodosum

Although sarcoid is common most in women aged 20–40 years, pulmonary sarcoid is rarely reported as a complication of pregnancy – perhaps 0.05 per cent of all pregnancies are affected by the condition [129]. Also, there have been few cases reported where there was any marked symptomatic impairment in respiratory function [129,142,238]. Nevertheless, specialist referral centres have experience of large numbers of patients with sarcoid in pregnancy [159]. The consensus of opinion is that sarcoidosis either does not change in pregnancy [3] or if it changes, improves, perhaps due to the increase in free as well as total cortisol (see Chapter 13); however, there is a tendency for the condition to relapse in the puerperium [310]. Nevertheless, the relapse is unlikely to be serious and should not be a contraindication to pregnancy, except in the rare patient who is severely affected. Apart from pulmonary complications of sarcoid, patients may occasionally have life-threatening heart, renal and neurological disease. Other risk factors are parenchymal lesions on chest X-ray, increasing maternal age and requirement for drugs other than steroids [142].

The usual presentation is with symmetrical bilateral hilar lymphadenopathy and mediastinal lymphadenopathy found on chest X-ray either by chance or in a patient with pyrexia or erythema nodosum. The patient may also have cervical lymphadenopathy. The differential diagnoses include lymphoma such as Hodgkin's disease [49] and tuberculosis. In tuberculosis and Hodgkin's disease the hilar lymphadenopathy is usually not symmetrical and tuberculosis is usually associated with parenchymal lung lesions in the acute attack in women of this age. The Kveim test is positive in the majority of women with sarcoid presenting with bilateral lymphadenopathy. If there is any doubt the patient should have fibre-optic bronchoscopy with transbronchial aspiration. If this is negative, mediastinotomy, mediastinoscopy or liver biopsy may be necessary to prove or disprove the diagnosis.

More advanced sarcoid is associated with diffuse lung infiltration, when the patient is more likely to be breathless and will frequently have a reduced transfer factor. Those patients that are symptomatic can be given alternate-day steroid therapy (see above), particularly if there is evidence of deteriorating pulmonary function. Since hilar lymphadenopathy may be absent, the differential diagnosis of diffuse lung infiltration is wide, ranging from hypersensitivity to drugs to connective tissue diseases and organic dust diseases. Lymphangioleiomyomatosis is a very rare cause of diffuse pulmonary infiltration that can occur in pregnancy but one that is specific to women in their childbearing years [197] (see below). In the absence of any clinical clues, transbronchial, fibre-optic lung biopsy is usually the definitive investigation. The late manifestations of sarcoid include lung fibrosis and cor pulmonale due to hypoxaemia. Steroid therapy rarely helps at this stage.

No special management is necessary for the average case in pregnancy. Angiotensin converting enzyme levels have been reported to fall [69] or to remain unchanged in normal pregnancy [94]. In addition they showed diurnal variation [69]. Also levels vary markedly in patients with sarcoid in pregnancy independent of apparent disease activity [94]. Thus converting enzyme levels may no longer be of value in monitoring patients with sarcoid who become pregnant [94].

Systemic steroids should not be withheld (see above) if they are indicated for the pulmonary condition. However, there is no evidence that steroid therapy influences the natural course of the disease. Sarcoid is not transmitted to the fetus [19], although sarcoid granulomata have been reported in the placenta in one patient [167] but not in others [238]. Since patients often take extra vitamins in pregnancy, they should be particularly warned not to take extra vitamin D, to which they may be very sensitive [159].

Erythema nodosum

This topic is included here because erythema nodosum frequently complicates sarcoid and tuberculosis. However, it may also complicate other infections (streptococcal, pertussis, measles, coccidiomycosis), drug therapy (particularly sulphonamides) and inflammatory bowel disease. For a general review of erythema nodosum in pregnancy see Bartelsmeyer and Petrie [21]. In many patients, the precipitating cause, if there is one, is not found. The rash consists of tender, pretibial red or purple nodules. New lesions appear while old ones are resolving, and each lesion lasts a few days to a few weeks. The whole illness may last several months, and be accompanied by fever and arthralgia.

Erythema nodosum occurs not infrequently in pregnancy. We see about one case in 1000 maternities at Queen Charlotte's Maternity Hospital. If the patient has none of the clinical conditions outlined above, a normal chest X-ray and a blood count that is normal for pregnancy, she may be reassured that the condition is most unlikely to have any sequelae and that her pregnancy will not be affected.

Salvatore and Lynch [246] reported 21 cases occurring in pregnancy, or in patients taking oral contraceptives. Since they could find no cause for 10 of these, they believed that pregnancy or oestrogen therapy could be precipitating factors. This remains unproven, since erythema nodosum occurs most frequently in women during their childbearing years.

Wegener's granulomatosis

This is a rare form of systemic vasculitis in which necrotizing granulomatous lesions affect the upper respiratory tract, (particularly the nose – causing perforation of the septum), lungs and kidneys. It presents with nasal symptoms, haemoptysis, general malaise or renal failure. Untreated, it is rapidly fatal but the condition is now being diagnosed more frequently in [213,288] or before [61] pregnancy as less severe cases are recognized and treated with prednisone and cyclophosphamide. The latter drug, an alkylating agent, is potentially teratogenic; at least three case reports have documented various abnormalities following first trimester use [52,122, 299]. Therefore, patients who conceived taking cyclophosphamide should be offered termination and patients who have Wegener's granulomatosis disease should wait until they are in remission so that cyclophosphamide can be stopped before pregnancy.

Cyclophosphamide has been used in the latter half of pregnancy in Wegener's granulomatosis [288] and other conditions [211]; the only fetal abnormality noted was leukopenia [313] but this is of concern in view of the potential for alkylating agents to induce leukaemia [48]. The titre of antineutrophil cytoplasmic antibody may be a guide to the necessity for restarting cyclophosphamide therapy [55] but this has not been evaluated in pregnancy. Furthermore, there is insufficient experience to comment whether the course of Wegener's granulomatosis is affected by pregnancy.

In a single case of pulmonary eosinophilic granuloma [179], respiratory function was not affected by pregnancy.

Pulmonary lymphangioleiomyomatosis

This is a very rare condition but it has attracted much interest and is of particular relevance since it occurs in young women during their childbearing years [64,266,291]. Pulmonary lymphangioleiomyomatosis is characterized by proliferation of smooth muscle in pulmonary mediastinal and retroperitineal lymphatics, in pulmonary vessels and in the smaller airways [64]. Patients present with breathlessness or with symptoms from pneumothorax or chylothorax.

Chest radiology may be normal initially or show interstitial thickening, pneumothorax or pleural effusion [266]. High resolution computed tomography (CT) scanning may be necessary to show the typical small cystic changes. Lung function tests show air flow obstruction and characteristically low gas transfer factor (though note that this is decreased in pregnancy, see above). The differential diagnosis of pulmonary infiltration includes eosinophilic granuloma, sarcoidosis and idiopathic pulmonary fibrosis. Diagnosis is usually confirmed by lung biopsy which can be performed safely in pregnancy.

Early reports [64] suggested that most patients died within 10 years of diagnosis. More recent studies, possibly in patients diagnosed earlier in the course of disease, are most optimistic. Taylor *et al*. [291] found that 78 per cent of patients were alive 8 years after diagnosis. The evidence that oestrogen [262] and pregnancy [154,212] cause the condition to deteriorate is anecdotal. Nevertheless, in the desire to give some form of active treatment for an otherwise fatal condition, patients have been offered oophorectomy with or without additional progesterone and tamoxifen therapies [291]. Lung transplantation has been performed for some patients [236].

Pre-pregnancy counselling and decisions about termination of pregnancy can only be based on a frank discussion of the uncertainty about the natural history of this fascinating condition.

Pneumonia and other respiratory tract infections

Upper respiratory tract

At least half of the infections of the upper respiratory tract are viral and due to adeno-, rhino- and parainfluenza viruses. In addition, acute bronchitis may be bacterial in origin due to organisms such as *Haemophilus influenzae*. Viral upper respiratory tract infections require no specific treatment. The condition is self-limiting and the patient improves with symptomatic therapy — analgesics and antipyretics (e.g. paracetamol) and bed rest. A high fluid intake is encouraged. If the patient has purulent sputum, a sample should be sent for culture and appropriate antibiotic therapy should be started. For acute bronchitis this should be broad spectrum therapy with ampicillin, amoxycillin or a cephalosporin. Erythromycin can be used in patients who are sensitive to penicillin. The safety of cotrimoxazole has not been established in pregnancy and tetracycline should definitely not be used because of the risks of abnormal bone formation and permanent discolouration of the child's teeth [90]. In addition, tetracycline therapy has been related to multiple congenital abnormalities [62], and parenteral tetracycline has caused pancreatitis and fatal liver failure in pregnancy [174]. Treatment for bronchitis should also include steam inhalation to liquefy secretions, but iodine-containing expectorants should not be used because of the adverse effects of iodine on the fetus (see Chapter 12). Bronchodilators to relieve bronchospasm may also be helpful (see above).

Pneumonia

This is associated with the clinical and radiological signs of lung consolidation. The patient presents with fever, cough, purulent sputum or chest pain. Patients frequently have a history of antecedent chest illness and the majority are smokers. No cause for the infection can be found in up to 52 per cent of cases [315]. The majority are bacterial in origin, due to *Streptococcus pneumoniae* (the pneumococcus) but many other organisms may be involved, particularly in epidemics. Hospital-acquired infection may be with *Haemophilus influenzae*, haemolytic streptococcus, *Staphylococcus aureus* or *Klebsiella pneumoniae* in the very debilitated. However, the influenza virus is an important cause of pneumonia during epidemics and chlamydia and mycoplasma may also cause pneumonia, although many cases previously thought to be due to mycoplasma may have been caused by *Legionella pneumophilia*.

Immunocompromised patients such as those with AIDS or those treated with immunosuppressive drugs are at risk of developing pneumonia due to atypical organisms; for example nocardiosis infection in a pregnant patient with sarcoid treated with high dose steroids [219] or *Pneumocystis carinii* infection in a patient with AIDS [161] (see also Chapter 17 for a discussion of pneumonia in pregnant patients with AIDS).

In patients who present with pneumonia outside hospital, therapy in the first instance should be with penicillin on the assumption that the patient has a *Strep. pneumoniae* infection. If the patient is sensitive to penicillin, she should receive erythromycin; this will also treat legionnaire's disease and mycoplasma infection. If the patient is thought to have a hospital-acquired infection she should also have a broad spectrum antibiotic (amoxycillin, cephalosporin, erythromycin) pending the results of sputum, blood culture and sensitivities tests, when further antibiotics may be necessary. Ampicillin dosage should be doubled in pregnancy [243] because of the increased drug clearance [229] due to increased renal blood flow. Patients should also receive paracetamol as an antipyretic and may require tepid sponging and full nursing care if they are very sick.

Pneumonia used to have a bad reputation in pregnancy with many patients aborting and a 20 per cent maternal mortality rate [221]. Now that effective antibiotics are available, this is no longer so, except for patients with HIV infection or those who are debilitated by drug abuse [25].

Preterm labour remains a definite risk, presumably related to pyrexia [221].

It is generally believed that viral pneumonia has a high mortality in pregnancy [123]; during influenza epidemics pneumonia may be responsible for half the cases of maternal mortality [108] and there have been isolated severe cases requiring ventilation associated with influenza and pneumonia [127,217]. However, such high maternal mortalities have not been reported recently, and the additional risk of influenza pneumonia due to pregnancy has probably been exaggerated [59]. In contrast 10 per cent of maternal varicella infections may be complicated by pneumonia and Parayani and Arvin [224] reported a series in which two patients required ventilation and one died. Not unreasonably, therefore Parayani and Arvin [224] suggested that pregnant women who have close exposure to varicella zoster virus and no antibody to varicella, should receive zoster immunoglobulin (ZIG) [224]. The effectiveness of ZIG in preventing fetal complications is not known [116]. Because of the high risk of infection in pregnancy, those patients who develop varicella should be treated with parenteral acyclovir 10–30 mg/kg daily in three divided doses for 5 days [35,65,117,133]. Parenteral acyclovir should be used with caution in pregnancy though it has been given without problem to large numbers of children with varicella from the age of 2 years [87].

Fungal lung infections are very uncommon in the UK (see Table 16.2). Cantanazaro [46] has reviewed the pulmonary mycoses which occur in pregnancy in North America. Cryptococcosis, blastomycosis and sporotrichosis are rare. However, coccidioidomycosis is more common and appears to be particularly dangerous in pregnancy possibly due to the stimulating effect of oestrogen and progesterone on coccidioides [85]. In 50 cases of coccidioidomycosis from North America, 22 became disseminated in pregnancy with a maternal mortality of nearly 100 per cent if untreated with amphotericin B [269].

There have been no reports of fetal toxicity from amphotericin B despite its use in the first trimester [46,158]. Flucytosine is also used in the treatment of fungal infections but such therapy is much more worrying since flucytosine is metabolized to the antimetabolite fluorouracil [46].

Cystic fibrosis

Cystic fibrosis is the most common important genetic disorder in Caucasians with a gene frequency of one in 20 [37]. Since heterozygotes are asymptomatic, homozygous patients who suffer from the condition are relatively common. The incidence is about one in 2500 live births [296]. Recently the mortality has improved markedly, so that many more women are surviving to become pregnant. The median age of survival for patients attending cystic fibrosis clinics is the USA in 1990 was 27.6 years [169]. In 1989 it was estimated that there were 1500 cystics over the age of 15 years in the UK [149] of whom about 500 would have been female.

Because of the large number of cystic fibrosis

mutations that have been identified (more than 150) only 80 per cent of all heterozygotes can be identified [306]. Nevertheless, cystic fibrosis carrier screening is a practical proposition in general practice [140]. In addition, first trimester prenatal diagnosis is possible on genetic material prepared from chorionic villi using linked DNA probes in at least two-thirds of couples presenting with one affected child; Super *et al.* [284] have described their experience with this technique in 96 families. The expected false negative and false positive rates of this procedure are 2 and 6 per cent, respectively [98]. Biochemical analysis of amniotic fluid is not sufficiently accurate at present to detect or exclude the affected fetus. The patient should also be aware that her child will be heterozygous for cystic fibrosis, even if it is not homozygous. This, in turn, is likely to increase the future genetic load in the community. An alternative approach is *in vitro* fertilization following preimplantation diagnostic testing to exclude the condition [138]. This technique consumes considerable resources and is likely to be applicable only in individual cases.

The improvement in mortality from cystic fibrosis has come from improved prophylactic bronchial toilet and widespread use of antibiotics, rather than any single therapeutic advance although the possibility of heart and lung transplantation is beginning to make a big difference to prognosis [256]. In addition, pancreatic enzymes and vitamins are added to a high protein and low fat diet. Carbohydrates are given as sugar to increase calorie intake.

For reviews of cystic fibrosis in pregnancy see [162,194,223,261]. The condition has been diagnosed in patients for the first time during pregnancy [162]. Such cases diagnosed later in life seem to have a better prognosis than those where the diagnosis is made in early childhood.

Phelan [228] reported only three successful pregnancies in 66 women aged more than 16 years, attending the Royal Children's Hospital, Melbourne. He comments that the low incidence of pregnancy was possibly due to fear of producing affected children, as well as possible infertility due to unfavourable cervical mucus and low lean body mass. (Most males with the condition are infertile due to atresia of the vas and epididymis [80].)

Cohen *et al.* [54] surveyed 119 centres in North America and reported the outcome in 129 patients delivered before 1975. Although 19 per cent of patients had therapeutic abortions, the incidence of spontaneous abortion (5 per cent) was not elevated. However, both the perinatal mortality (11 per cent) and the maternal mortality (12 per cent within 6 months of delivery) were considerably greater than that in the rest of the population. Although the maternal mortality is alarming it was not greater than reported for patients with cystic fibrosis who were not pregnant [72,309]. Corkey *et al.* [63] reported the outcome of 11 pregnancies in seven patients. Only one pregnancy required termination and these authors suggested that this prognosis is better when pancreatic function is maintained.

It has been reported that patients with cystic fibrosis show a decrease in residual volume as do normal women in pregnancy, but that they are unable to maintain vital capacity. Although they increase oxygen uptake, they do not show the 'hyperventilation' associated with normal pregnancy [217].

The judgement of individual physicians is likely to be influenced by their most recent experience of relatively few cases, and this would account for a wide diversity of clinical opinions regarding the advisability of pregnancy in patients with cystic fibrosis. Several indices have been suggested as a guide to the success of pregnancy, based on history, the nutritional status, the presence or absence of emphysema, cor pulmonale and such abnormalities in respiratory function as vital capacity less than 50 per cent predicted for height [223,290]. Although a vital capacity of less than 50 per cent than that predicted has been recommended as an indication for termination, many patients with a vital capacity of less than this in cystic fibrosis and other conditions such as kyphoscoliosis, have a normal pregnancy. Since patients die because of uncontrollable recurrent chest infection and cor pulmonale (which is in turn related to hypoxaemia) it is suggested that these should be the parameters considered when counselling patients.

Echocardiographic measurement of right ventricular cavity size at end diastole is a good estimate of clinical outcome [241,245] and this dimension is likely to be related to pulmonary artery pressure. If there is any doubt about the presence of hypoxaemia, the arterial blood gases should be measured. From the data of di Saint'Agnese and Davis [80], it would appear that an arterial Po_2 of <60 mmHg, when the patient is free from infection and breathing air, is associated with a National Institutes of Health (NIH) score of <50. This is the score at which pulmonary hypertension is present [263]. Pulmonary hypertension has a particularly poor outcome in pregnancy (see Chapter 5). In addition, if there is any doubt about the presence of pulmonary hypertension, the pulmonary artery pressure should be measured. When a flow-directed, Swan–Ganz catheter is used, X-ray screening should be unnecessary. If the pulmonary artery systolic pressure is <35 mmHg, the patient does not have cor pulmonale. This is a much more reliable measurement than inference from clinical signs, chest radiology or the electrocardiogram.

A recent study in a non-pregnant population [169] confirms the poor outcome if the Po_2 is <55 mmHg (2 year mortality > 50 per cent). Similar life expectancy was indicated by FEV_1 < 30 per cent predicted or PCo_2 > 50 mmHg.

Physicians should also be aware that patients with cystic fibrosis may have liver disease [235] and diabetes mellitus. However, the reported incidence of cirrhosis varies between 0.5 per cent [67] and 90 per cent [157] and this has not yet been reported to be a problem in pregnancy.

Apart from a high level of medical and obstetric care, paying particular attention to nutrition, there are no special measures which should be taken in the antenatal period once antenatal diagnosis of the fetus has been discussed. Because of the ototoxic and renal side-effects of the aminoglycosides reviewed above, intravenous and intramuscular use of these antibiotics should be avoided if possible in pregnancy, and the penicillins should be given instead. Nebulized gentamicin represents a real advantage here. However, it is reassuring that there were no congenital abnormalities amongst the 129 cases reviewed by Cohen *et al.* [54] of whom 26 received aminoglycosides during pregnancy.

During labour, particular care should be taken concerning fluid and electrolyte balance. Patients with cystic fibrosis lose large quantities of sodium in sweat and may easily become hypovolaemic. However, they will also be very intolerant of overhydration, if there is any degree of cor pulmonale. Oxygen may be freely administered if the $Paco_2$ is not elevated. Because of the risk of post-anaesthetic atelectasis, inhalation anaesthesia should be avoided and epidural or caudal anaesthesia substituted. Chest pain arising in labour should raise the suspicion of pneumothorax to which these patients are particularly predisposed. Forceps delivery should be performed if the second stage is at all prolonged.

Whitelaw and Butterfield [316] reported that the sodium content of breast milk from women with cystic fibrosis may be as high as 280 mmol/l, and suggested that this was a reason for these mothers not to breast feed. However, Alpert and Cormier [8] have found normal electrolyte content in milk from mothers with cystic fibrosis and believe that the sodium content found by Whitelaw and Butterfield was abnormally high because the milk was expressed from a woman who was not lactating freely. Such expressed milk was demonstrated to have abnormally high electrolyte content even if the mothers did not have cystic fibrosis. It would seem sensible to check the sodium content of breast milk from women with cystic fibrosis who are lactating, but it is unlikely that this will be a contra-indication to breast feeding.

Chronic bronchitis, emphysema and bronchiectasis

Since these conditions are now rarely important in patients during childbearing years, there is little information on their outcome in pregnancy. Although there have been reports of intrauterine growth retardation in patients with bronchiectasis [294,295], this does not regularly occur [151]. If pregnancy does occur in patients with bronchiectasis, they can be severely debilitated [295] and will need to be treated as high risk patients with regular supervision and attention to postural drainage and physiotherapy. Chest infection and airways obstruction should be managed as described earlier. As suggested by Lalli and Raju [175] a successful outcome to pregnancy may be limited by the presence of pulmonary hypertension and hypoxaemia (see above). In a single case report, emphysema due to α_1 antitrypsin deficiency did not affect the successful outcome of pregnancy [115] although another case was affected by severe pre-eclampsia [168]. This condition is now amenable to prenatal diagnosis by chorionic villus biopsy [131,176] and DNA polymorphism.

Kyphoscoliosis

The reported incidence of kyphoscoliosis is 0.1–0.7 per cent of pregnancies [171] but much depends on the definition in mild cases. Kopenhager [171] noted a marked increase in perinatal mortality to 102 in 1000, due to maternal hypoxia. In Mendelson's series [199] only one patient had a vital capacity of <1 l, and she was in heart failure during labour. However, we have successfully delivered two patients with kyphoscoliosis who had vital capacities of <1 l with no overt problems. Lao *et al.* [178] studied 10 pregnancies in eight patients in Hong Kong with severe kyphoscoliosis (average vital capacity approximately 1000 ml). There were no major maternal problems but four infants were delivered before 37 weeks and one died. In one case of kyphoscoliosis, very severe chronic maternal hypoxia (Pa_{O_2} = 5.9 kPa) has caused fetal brain damage [20]. Less severe kyphoscoliosis has a universally good outcome [265]. As in cystic fibrosis, the limiting factors are hypoxaemia, pulmonary hypertension and the presence of muscular weakness.

However, Sawicka *et al.* [248] on the basis of six cases with paralytic or early onset kyphoscoliosis suggest that patients with this form of the disease may be particularly at risk during pregnancy since four of their cases with vital capacities 1360 ml or less required long-term negative pressure ventilation in a tank-lung before and after delivery. Certainly those patients with idiopathic scoliosis who have a primary curve >25° may deteriorate in pregnancy [26]; lesser curves are not affected by pregnancy [26]. All these patients are more likely to require caesarean section, because of associated abnormalities of the bony pelvis and of abnormal presentations of the fetus [178]. Notwithstanding the spinal deformities, epidural anaesthetic is preferable to general anaesthesia.

Patients with achondroplasia and other chondrodystrophies may have similar though less severe respiratory and pelvic problems [7].

Adult respiratory distress syndrome, shock lung

This is the end point of several different types of obstetric disaster including inhalation of gastric contents during anaesthesia (see below). In addition, it may occur with disseminated intravascular coagulation (DIC) in pre-eclampsia, eclampsia, abruptio placentae, dead fetus syndrome and amniotic fluid embolism (see Chapter 3). The syndrome is also associated with hypovolaemic shock from postpartum haemorrhage with or without sepsis [9], with endotoxin shock [71] and with severe anaphylaxis. It is also found with metastatic cancer or, in pregnancy, with hydatidiform mole [220].

Adult respiratory distress syndrome in association with pyelonephritis in pregnancy seems to be a particular problem in the US [239,300]. Particular risk factors for the development of adult respiratory distress syndrome in a patient with pyelonephritis include maternal heart rate >110/min, pyrexia >39.4°C in patients with gestational age >20 weeks and the use of tocolytic agents.

In a group of 14 obstetric cases with adult respiratory distress syndrome 12 were caused by strictly obstetric factors such as pre-eclampsia or haemorrhage. The mortality was 43 per cent [271].

Changes in maternal physiology such as increased interstitial lung water [190] or activation of various pathways of arachidonic acid metabolism may be the reason for the apparent frequency of pregnancy as an underlying cause of adult respiratory distress in women. Alternatively, it may be that other secondary causes, such as anaesthesia, shock from haemorrhage and DIC (see Chapter 3) are more likely to be present in women in the pregnant than the non-pregnant state.

The patients are severely ill and should be managed in an intensive care unit. The clinical picture is of a patient who develops acute severe hypoxaemia despite a high inspired oxygen concentration, and shows diffuse infiltrates on the chest radiograph — where signs may take 24 hours to develop. It has been suggested that an acute fall in white cell count occurring after the initial insult may be of value in predicting those patients who will develop adult respiratory distress syndrome [297]. It is assumed that the primary problem is in the lung, where compliance and permeability are reduced due to extravasation of liquid, rather than in the heart. However, it may be necessary to prove that there is not a primary cardiac abnormality by demonstrating a normal (<14 mmHg) pulmonary artery wedge pressure, i.e. a normal left ventricular end diastolic pressure, using a flow-guided Swan–Ganz catheter [166]. Such a catheter (if left in place) can be of great assistance for management, since it can provide measurements of pulmonary artery pressure and cardiac output by green dye or thermodilution. Peripheral oedema, elevated jugular venous pressure and cardiomegaly are unusual and suggest cardiac, rather than pulmonary, pathology.

The therapeutic options available are correction of the underlying cause, artificial ventilation, membrane oxygenation and medication with diuretics, antibiotics, vasoactive drugs, inotropes and steroids.

Correction of the underlying cause is usually limited to reversal of DIC with fresh frozen plasma (followed by delivery of the dead fetus if present) and treatment of infection. Andersen *et al.* [9] suggest ventilation, preferably with an inspired oxygen concentration of <60 per cent, maintaining an end expiratory pressure of 5–35 cmH_2O to try to keep the arterial Po_2 >60 mmHg. The use of positive end expiratory pressure (PEEP) may help by thinning the layer of water in the alveolus and increasing alveolar area to improve gas exchange.

Fluid balance is crucial. If the patients are hypovolaemic, cardiac output and perfusion will decrease; hence infusion of albumin or blood (increasing oxygen carrying capacity) can be helpful, although there is a risk of further protein loss into the alveoli (see Chapter 3 for a further discussion of which fluid may be best in this situation). If they are hypervolaemic, there will be increased extravasation of fluid and increased preload, decreasing oxygenation and cardiac output. Diuretic therapy or dialysis will then be necessary. The necessity for manipulating blood volume and its effect, can be assessed by repeated measurement of pulmonary artery wedge pressure and cardiac output, using the Swan–Ganz catheter. Corticosteroids may reverse excess capillary permeability [319], but they may also increase susceptibility to infection [30] and a recent study suggests that they do not affect outcome [27].

Despite these measures, the mortality of adult respiratory distress syndrome is 50–60 per cent [260]. Nevertheless, every effort should be made in treating these patients since those who survive recover well. It is hoped, though not proven, that early aggressive treatment will reduce mortality of this condition [9].

Pneumothorax and pneumomediastinum

Both these conditions occur infrequently in pregnancy, but probably more commonly than in the non-pregnant state. They most commonly occur in susceptible individuals due to the expulsive efforts of labour [43,278], but pneumomediastinum in particular may occur at other times – for example in association with bronchial asthma [135] or ruptured oesophagus following vomiting [147]. Pneumothorax may occur in association with other chest conditions, such as emphysema, pulmonary tuberculosis or cystic fibrosis. In pneumomediastinum, which is more common in pregnancy than pneumothorax, a false passage is created between the airways and the mediastinal tissues. The condition usually, though not invariably [128] follows a strenuous labour. Air tracks through the mediastinum to the neck or pericardium (pneumopericardium) [184], and there may be widespread subcutaneous emphysema over the thorax or even the whole body. This produces a quite characteristic crackling sound and sensation on palpation, which does not occur in any other condition.

In addition, there may be a crunching noise (Hamman's sign [137]) synchronous with the heart beat at the left sternal edge.

In pneumothorax there is a false passage between the airways and the pleural cavity. Pneumothorax accompanies about one-third of the cases of pneumomediastinum that occur in pregnancy [282] but may also occur independently [99]. In both conditions, the patient complains of the sudden onset of chest pain and breathlessness and the diagnosis is confirmed by chest radiography. In tension pneumothorax the patient will become cyanosed and hypotensive due to the reduction in the venous return. A similar variant of pneumomediastinum 'malignant mediastinum' [121] also occurs but is much rarer.

Pneumomediastinum normally clears spontaneously and the treatment is therefore usually conservative, with oxygen and analgesics. Malignant mediastinum requires urgent relief either by multiple incisions over the subcutaneous tissue where air is trapped [121] or by splitting the sternum. Pneumothorax should be drained via an underwater seal if the lung is more than 25 per cent collapsed. Tension pneumothorax requires immediate relief by a large-bore needle inserted through the chest wall overlying the pneumothorax. If pneumothorax or pneumomediastinum has occurred in pregnancy, elective forceps delivery should be performed to minimize the chance of recurrence, caused by raised intrapulmonary pressure due to maternal straining.

Pleural effusion

Pleural effusion may arise in pregnancy secondary to conditions such as tuberculosis, pneumonia, pulmonary infarction and cardiac failure which also cause effusions in the non-pregnant state. Small pleural effusions are said to be a common finding in the first 24 hours post-partum [155]. Spring and Winston [279] found pleural effusions in a surprisingly high proportion (45–65 per cent of normal women) post-partum. This was not confirmed by Udeshi *et al.* [302] who used a sensitive ultrasound technique. They only found pleural effusions after delivery in women who had pre-eclampsia, an association that has been noted previously by Suonio *et al.* [283]. Perhaps the increased lung water of pregnancy [190] and/or the profound changes that must occur in the maternal circulation after delivery are the causes.

Lung cancer

This is an uncommon cancer in pregnancy (the most common are breast, cervix and haematopoietic); the incidence is likely to increase because of increased smoking amongst women. About 10 cases have been reported. Metastasis may occur in the pericardium and the placenta. There are insufficient data to state whether the natural history of lung cancer is affected by pregnancy.

Anaesthetic considerations

The two most recent confidential maternal mortality reports, which examined all maternal deaths occurring in the UK in the years 1985–90, indicates that there were three deaths due to inhalation of stomach contents, out of a total of 590 cases [78,79]. This represents a significant improvement over the previous series in which there were eight deaths from inhalation in England and Wales out of a total of 176 cases [77]. The management of adult respiratory distress syndrome has been discussed above. Further treatment of inhalation includes bronchoscopy for the patient who becomes acutely cyanotic following regurgitation of large particles of food which have obstructed major airways. It is also important to realize that pulmonary aspiration may occur without frank vomiting and regurgitation. The differential diagnosis of amniotic fluid embolism and aspiration is considered in Chapter 3 and Chapter 4.

Much of modern obstetric medical practice involves prevention of the complication of gastric aspiration. The increasing use of regional anaesthesia (epidural or spinal block) is one way of reducing the problem. It is also common practice to starve women during labour, but the stomach will continue to secrete fluid, even though in reduced quantities; also gastric emptying from meals taken before the onset of labour is much reduced. On the assumption that it is the acid component of gastric content that is harmful, patients in labour are often given up to 30 ml of antacid (magnesium trisilicate mixture) every 2 hours to maintain a pH >3.2 [226]. However, the Confidential Maternal Mortality series indicates that the number of deaths from aspiration during 1973–75, when antacid administration was widespread, was no less than the number occurring in 1970–72, before antacids were generally used [255]. Furthermore, Bond *et al.* [31] have described pulmonary aspiration syndrome after inhalation of stomach contents of pH 6.4, in a patient who had been given regular antacid therapy with magnesium and aluminium hydroxide. The one maternal death due to aspiration of stomach contents in the 1985–86 confidential enquiry [78] was in a woman who received adequate prophylaxis with ranitidine and sodium citrate. All this would suggest that the hydrogen ion concentration is not the only determinant of the pulmonary aspiration syndrome; either the antacid itself or other constituents of the gastric fluid must contribute. Although 0.3 mol/l sodium citrate solution may be a safer antacid [289], it is not so effective in reducing acidity [220]; both medicines increase the volume in the stomach which may be crucial. Alternative approaches are to use an H_2 antagonist such as cimetidine [86,196,198] which decreases acid secretion, or metoclopramide therapy which increases gastric emptying [150]. Large-scale comparative studies are necessary to determine which is the most effective.

Pending the results of such studies, a reasonable guide to prophylaxis is as follows [84].

1 Normal labour: starve patient; the place of additional antacid therapy is unclear.

2 High risk when general anaesthesia may be necessary: give oral antacid and H_2 receptor antagonist.

3 Elective caesarean section under general anaesthesia: oral H_2 receptor antagonist at least 90 min pre-operatively. Antacid 15 ml pre-operatively.

4 Emergency caesarean section under general anaesthetic. Antacid pre-operatively if none has been given recently. Metoclopramide 10 mg intravenously to promote gastric emptying. Ranitidine 50 mg intravenously pre-operatively to prevent any further acid formation. The best preventative measure would be to use epidural rather than general anaesthesia whenever possible.

Furthermore, in the patient who has respiratory impairment, general anaesthesia should be avoided because of the risk of intrapartum hypoxia, due to deteriorating ventilation perfusion imbalance, and the greater risk of postoperative atelectasis. In addition pain is a potent stimulant to hyperventilation which can increase oxygen consumption in labour as much as 100 per cent [5]. Therefore, the efficacy of regional anaesthesia as an analgesic, decreases oxygen consumption [247].

Because of the generalized muscular effort, labour is obviously a time when the patient with severe respiratory impairment is at risk of developing respiratory failure. But in addition, expulsive efforts specifically fatigue the diaphragm [214], exacerbating this risk. Epidural block can eliminate the desire to push, allowing forceps delivery at full dilation.

There are additional reasons for the use of epidural anaesthesia in any patient whose respiratory status is compromised. One caveat is that when used for caesarean section, even regional block is associated with reductions in FEV_1 of 19 per cent, FVC of 17 per cent and peak flow rate of 35 per cent [58]. Similar data have been reported by Harrop-Griffiths *et al.* [141]. Regional block is the best way to manage these patients but it does have some adverse effects.

References

1 Abramowicz M. Alternate-day corticosteroid therapy. *Medical Letters on Drugs and Therapeutics* 1975; **17**: 95.

2 Abramowicz M. Drugs for asthma. *Medical Letters on Drugs and Therapeutics* 1978; **20**: 69.

3 Agha FP, Vade A, Amendola MA & Cooper RF. Effects of pregnancy on sarcoidosis. *Surgery, Gynecology and Obstetrics* 1982; **155**: 817–22.

4 Alaily AB & Carrol KB. Pulmonary ventilation in pregnancy. *British Journal of Obstetrics and Gynaecology* 1978; **85**: 518–24.

5 Albright GA. *Anesthesia in Obstetrics, Maternal, Fetal and Neonatal Aspects*. Addison Wesley, Massachussetts, 1978.

6 Alkader AA & Cole RB. Effect of aminophylline on FEV_1 in patients with nocturnal asthma. *Thorax* 1978; **88**: 536–7.

7 Allanson JE & Hall JG. Obstetric and gynecologic problems in women with chondrodystrophies. *Obstetrics and Gynecology* 1986; **67**: 74–80.

8 Alpert SE & Cormier AD. Normal electrolyte and protein content in milk from mothers with cystic fibrosis: an explanation for the initial report of elevated milk sodium concentration. *Journal of Pediatrics* 1983; **102**: 77–80.

9 Andersen HF, Lynch JP & Johnson TRB. Adult respiratory distress syndrome in obstetrics and gynecology. *Obstetrics and Gynecology* 1980; **55**: 291–5.

10 Ang CK, Tan TH, Walters W & Wood C. Postural influence on maternal capillary oxygen and carbon dioxide tension. *British Medical Journal* 1969; **4**: 201.

11 Apter AJ, Greenberger PA & Patterson R. Outcomes of pregnancy in adolescents with severe asthma. *Archives of Internal Medicine* 1989; **149**: 2571–5.

12 Artal R, Wiswell R, Romen Y & Dorey F. Pulmonary responses to exercise in pregnancy. *American Journal of Obstetrics and Gynecology* 1986; **154**: 378–83.
13 Arwood LL, Dasta JF & Friedman C. Placental transfer of theophylline: two case reports. *Pediatrics* 1979; **63**: 844–6.
14 Atkins NA. Maternal plasma concentrations of pyridoxal phosphate during pregnancy: adequacy of vitamin B6 supplementation during isoniazid therapy. *American Review of Respiratory Medicine* 1982; **126**: 714–16.
15 Bahna SL & Bjerkedal T. The course and outcome of pregnancy in women with bronchial asthma. *Acta Allergolica* 1972; **27**: 397–400.
16 Baldwin GR, Moorthi S, Whelton JA & MacDoneal KF. New lung functions and pregnancy. *American Journal of Obstetrics and Gynecology* 1977; **127**: 235.
17 Ballard PL, Granberg P & Ballard RA. Glucocorticoid levels in maternal and cord serum after prenatal beclomethasone therapy to prevent respiratory distress syndrome. *Journal of Clinical Investigation* 1975; **56**: 1548–58.
18 Ballou SP, Morley JJ & Kushner I. Pregnancy and systemic sclerosis. *Arthritis and Rheumatology* 1984; **27**: 295–8.
19 Barnes CG. *Medical Disorders in Obstetric Practice*. Blackwell Scientific Publications, Oxford, 1974.
20 Barrett JFR, Dear PRF & Lilford RJ. Brain damage as a result of chronic intra-uterine hypoxia in a baby born of a severely kyphoscoliotic mother. *Journal of Obstetrics and Gynaecology* 1991; **11**: 260–1.
21 Bartelsmeyer JA & Petrie RH. Erythema nodosum, estrogens and pregnancy. *Clinical Obstetrics and Gynecology* 1990; **33**: 777–81.
22 Bedell GN & Adams RS. Pulmonary diffusing capacity during rest and exercise. A study of normal persons and persons with atrial septal defect, pregnancy and pulmonary disease. *Journal of Clinical Investigation* 1962; **41**: 1908.
23 Beitins R, Baynard F, Ances IG, Kowarsk A & Migeon CJ. The transplacental passage of prednisone and prednisolone in pregnancy near term. *Journal of Pediatrics* 1972; **81**: 936–45.
24 Beitzki NK. Uber die angioborne tuberkulase infektion. *Ergeb Tuberk Fortschr* 1935; **7**: 1–30.
25 Berkowitz K & LaSala A. Risk factors associated with the increasing prevalence of pneumonia during pregnancy. *American Journal of Obstetrics and Gynecology* 1990; **163**: 981–5.
26 Berman AT, Cohen DL & Schwentker EP. The effects of pregnancy on idiopathic scoliosis. *Spine* 1982; **7**: 76–7.
27 Bernard GR, Luce JM *et al*. High-dose corticosteroids in patients with adult respiratory distress syndrome. *New England Journal of Medicine* 1987; **317**: 1565–70.
28 Bevan DR, Holdcroft A *et al*. Closing volume and pregnancy. *British Medical Journal* 1974; **i**: 13–15.
29 Bjerkedal T, Bahna SL & Lehmann EH. Cause and outcome of women with pulmonary tuberculosis. *Scandinavian Journal of Respiratory Disease* 1975; **56**: 245–50.
30 Blaisdell FW & Schlobohm RM. The respiratory distress syndrome: A review. *Surgery* 1973; **74**: 251.
31 Bond VK, Stoetling RK & Gupta CD. Pulmonary aspiration syndrome after inhalation of gastric fluid containing antacids. *Anesthesiology* 1979; **51**: 452–3.
32 Bonebrake CR, Noller KL *et al*. Routine chest roentography in pregnancy. *Journal of the American Medical Association* 1978; **240**: 2747–8.
33 Bongionvanni AM & McPadden AJ. Steroids during pregnancy and possible fetal consequences. *Fertility and Sterility* 1960; **11**: 181–6.
34 Bouterline-Young H & Bouterline-Young E. Alveolar carbon dioxide levels in pregnant parturient and lactating subjects. *Journal of Obstetrics and Gynaecology of the British Empire* 1956; **63**: 509.
35 Boyd K & Walker E. Use of acyclovir to treat chickenpox in pregnancy. *British Medical Journal* 1988; **296**: 393–4.
36 Briscoe WA & Dubois AB. The relationship between airway resistance, airway conductance and lung volume in subjects of different age and body size. *Journal of Clinical Investigation* 1958; **37**: 1279.
37 *British Medical Journal* editorial. Cystic fibrosis in adults. *British Medical Journal* 1979; **2**: 626.
38 British Thoracic Society and others. Guidelines for the management of asthma: a summary. *British Medical Journal* 1993; **306**: 776–82.
39 Brobowitz ID. Ethambutol in pregnancy. *Chest* 1974; **66**: 20–4.
40 Brooks JM & Stirrat GM. Tuberculous peritonitis in pregnancy. Case report. *British Journal of Obstetrics and Gynaecology* 1986; **93**: 1009–10.
41 Brummer DL. Letter to the editor. *American Review of Respiratory Disease* 1972; **106**: 785.
42 Bryne DL, Chappatte OA, Spencer GT & Raju KS. Pregnancy complicated by Charcot–Marie–Tooth disease, requiring intermittent ventilation. *British Journal of Obstetrics and Gynaecology* 1992; **99**: 79–80.
43 Burgener L & Solmes JG. Spontaneous pneumothorax and pregnancy. *Canadian Medical Association Journal* 1979; **120**: 19.
44 Burney PG, Chinn S & Rona RJ. Has the prevalence of asthma increased in children? Evidence from national study of health and growth 1973–1986. *British Medical Journal* 1990; **300**: 1306–10.
45 Burrows B & Lebowitz MD. The beta-agonist dilemma. *New England Journal of Medicine* 1992; **326**: 560–1.
46 Cantanazaro A. Pulmonary mycosis in pregnant women. *Chest* 1984; **68**: 145–85.
47 Carswell F, Kerr MM & Hutchinson JH. Congenital goitre and hypothyroidism produced by maternal ingestion of iodides. *Lancet* 1970; **i**: 1241.

48 Casciato J. Leukaemia following cytotoxic therapy. *Medicine* 1979; **58**: 32–47.
49 Case BW & Benaroya S. Dyspnoea in a pregnant young woman. *Canadian Medical Association Journal* 1980; **122**: 890–6.
50 Citron K. Ethambutol: a review with special reference to ocular toxicity. *Tubercle* (suppl) 1969; **32**.
51 Clapp JF. Fetal heart rate response to running in mid-pregnancy and late pregnancy. *American Journal of Obstetrics and Gynecology* 1985; **153**: 251–2.
52 Coates A. Cyclophosphamide in pregnancy. *Australian and New Zealand Journal of Obstetrics and Gynaecology* 1970; **10**: 33–4.
53 Cohen JD, Patton EA & Badger TL. The tuberculous mother. *American Review of Tuberculosis* 1952; **65**: 1–23.
54 Cohen LF, di Saint'Agnese PA & Freidlander J. Cystic fibrosis and pregnancy. A national survey. *Lancet* 1980; **ii**: 842–4.
55 Cohen Tervaert JW, Huitema MG *et al*. Prevention of relapses in Wegener's granulomatosis by treatment based on antineutrophil cytoplasmic antibody titre. *Lancet* 1990; **336**: 709–11.
56 Cole RB. Modern management of pulmonary tuberculosis. *Prescribers Journal* 1985; **25**: 110–18.
57 Comroe JJ, Forster RE *et al*. *The Lung: Clinical Physiology and Pulmonary Function Tests*. Year Book Medical Publishers, Chicago, 1962.
58 Conn DA, Moffat AC, McCallum GDR & Thorburn J. Changes in pulmonary function test during spinal anaesthesia for caesarean section. *International Journal of Obstetric Anesthesia* 1993; **2**: 12–14.
59 *Contemporary Obstetrics and Gynecology* editorial. Pregnant patients and swine flu vaccine. *Contemporary Obstetrics and Gynecology* 1976; **8**: 74–5.
60 Conway N & Birt BD. Streptomycin in pregnancy: effect on the foetal ear. *British Medical Journal* 1965; **2**: 260–3.
61 Cooper K, Stafford J & Turner Warwick M. Wegener's granuloma complicating pregnancy. *British Journal of Obstetrics and Gynaecology* 1970; **77**: 1028–30.
62 Corcoran K & Castles JM. Tetracycline for acne vulgaris and possible teratogenesis. *British Medical Journal* 1977; **2**: 807–8.
63 Corkey CWB, Newth CJL, Corey M & Levison H. Pregnancy in cystic fibrosis: A better prognosis in patients with pancreatic function? *American Journal of Obstetrics and Gynecology* 1981; **140**: 737–42.
64 Corrin B, Liebow AA & Friedman PJ. Pulmonary lymphangiomyomatosis. A review. *American Journal of Pathology* 1975; **79**: 348–67.
65 Cox SM, Cunningham FG & Luby J. Management of varicella pneumonia complicating pregnancy. *American Journal of Perinatology* 1990; **7**: 300–1.
66 Craig DR & Toole MA. Airway closure in pregnancy. *Canadian Anaesthetics Society Journal* 1975; **22**: 665.
67 Crozier MD. Cystic fibrosis — a not-so-fatal disease. *Pediatric Clinics of North America* 1974; **21**: 935–7.
68 Cugell DW, Frank NR, Gaensler EA & Badger TL. Pulmonary function in pregnancy. I: Serial observations in normal women. *American Review of Tuberculosis* 1953; **67**: 568–97.
69 Cugini P, Letizia C *et al*. Circadian variation in serum angiotensin converting enzyme activity in normal and hypertensive pregnancy. *Journal of Obstetrics and Gynecology* 1989; **10**: 124.
70 Cullen JH, Brum VO & Reid TWH. The respiratory effects of progesterone in severe pulmonary emphysema. *American Journal of Medicine* 1959; **27**: 551–7.
71 Cunningham FG, Leveno KJ, Hawkins GDV & Whally PJ. Respiratory insufficiency associated with pyelonephritis during pregnancy. *Obstetrics and Gynecology* 1984; **63**: 121–5.
72 Cystic Fibrosis Foundation. *1974 Report on Survival of Patients with Cystic Fibrosis*. Cystic Fibrosis Foundation, Rockville, Maryland, 1976.
73 de March P. Tuberculosis and pregnancy. Five to ten year review of 215 patients in their fertile age. *Chest* 1975; **68**: 800–4.
74 de Swiet M. The respiratory system. In: Hytten F & Chamberlain G (eds), *Clinical Physiology in Obstetrics*, 2nd edn. Blackwell Scientific Publications, Oxford, 1990.
75 de Swiet M. Maternal pulmonary disorders. In: Creasy RK & Resnik R (eds), *Maternal Fetal Medicine: Principles and Practice*, 3rd edn. WB Saunders, Philadelphia, 1993.
76 de Swiet M & Fidler J. Heart disease in pregnancy: some controversies. *Journal of the Royal College of Physicians* 1981; **15**: 183–6.
77 Department of Health and Social Security. *Report on Confidental Enquiries into Maternal Deaths in England and Wales, 1979–1981*. HMSO, London, 1986.
78 Department of Health and Social Security. *Report on Confidential Enquiries into Maternal Deaths in England and Wales*. HMSO, London, 1991.
79 Department of Health. *Report on Confidential Enquiries into Maternal Deaths in the United Kingdom*, 1988–90. HMSO, London, 1994.
80 di Saint'Agnese PA & Davis PB. Cystic fibrosis in adults. *American Journal of Medicine* 1979; **66**: 121–32.
81 Doring GK & Loeschche HH. Atmung und Savre — Basengleichgewicht in der Schwangershaft Pflüger Archiv für die gesamte. *Physiologie des Menschen and der Terre* 1947; **249**: 437.
82 Dovcette JT & Bracken MB. Possible role of asthma in the risk of preterm labour and delivery. *Epidemiology* 1993; **4**: 143–50.
83 Driscoll AM. Urinary oestriol excretion in pregnant patients given large doses of prednisone. *British Medical Journal* 1969; **1**: 556–7.
84 Drug and Therapeutics Bulletin. Prophylaxis against Mendelson's syndrome. *Drug and Therapeutic Bulletin* 1986; **24**: 31–2.

85 Drutz DK, Muppert M, Sun SH & McGuire WL. Human sex hormones stimulate the growth and maturation of *Coccidioides immitis*. *Infections and Immunity* 1981; **32**: 897–907.

86 Dundee JW, Moore J, Johnston JF & McCaughey W. Cimetidine and obstetric anaesthesia. *Lancet* 1981; **ii**: 252.

87 Dunkle LM, Arvin AM *et al*. A controlled trial of acyclovir for chickenpox in normal children. *New England Journal of Medicine* 1991; **325**: 1539–44.

88 Dykes MHM. Evaluation of an anti-asthmatic agent cromolyn sodium (Aarare, Intal). *Journal of the American Medical Association* 1974; **227**: 1061–2.

89 Edwards MJ, Metcalfe J, Dunham MJ & Paul MS. Accelerated respiratory response to moderate exercise in late pregnancy. *Respiration Physiology* 1981; **45**: 229–41.

90 Elder HA, Santamarine BAG, Smith S & Kass EH. The natural history of asymptomatic bacteriuria during pregnancy: The effect of tetracycline on the clinical course and outcome of pregnancy. *American Journal of Obstetrics and Gynecology* 1971; **111**: 441–62.

91 Emerson K, Saxena BN & Poindexter EL. Caloric cost of normal pregnancy. *Obstetrics and Gynaecology* 1972; **49**: 786–94.

92 Eng M, Butler J & Bonich JJ. Respiratory function in pregnant obese women. *American Journal of Obstetrics and Gynecology* 1975; **123**: 241.

93 England SJ & Fahri LE. Fluctuations in alveolar CO_2 and in base excess during the menstrual cycle. *Respiration Physiology* 1976; **26**: 157.

94 Erskine KJ, Taylor KS & Agnew RAL. Serial estimation of serum angiotensin converting enzyme activity during and after pregnancy in a woman with sarcoidosis. *British Medical Journal* 1985; **290**: 269–70.

95 Fainstalt T. Cortisone-induced congenital cleft palate in rabbits. *Endocrinology* 1954; 55: 502.

96 Fan Chung K & Barnes PJ. Prescribing in pregnancy. Treatment of asthma. *British Medical Journal* 1987; **294**: 103–5.

97 Farebrother MJ & McHardy GJR. Closing volume and pregnancy. *British Medical Journal* 1974; **1**: 454.

98 Farrall M, Law H *et al*. First-trimester prenatal diagnosis of cystic fibrosis with linked DNA probes. *Lancet* 1986; **i**: 1402–5.

99 Farrell SJ. Spontaneous pneumothorax in pregnancy: a case report and review of the literature. *Obstetrics and Gynecology* 1983; **62**: 43S–45S.

100 Finn R, St Hill CA *et al*. Immunological responses in pregnancy and survival of fetal homograft. *British Medical Journal* 1972; **3**: 150–2.

101 Fischl MA, Pitchenick A & Gardner LB. An index predicting relapse and need for hospitalization in patients with acute bronchial asthma. *New England Journal of Medicine* 1981; **305**: 783–9.

102 Fishburne JI. Physiology and disease of the respiratory system in pregnancy. A review. *Journal of Reproductive Medicine* 1979; **22**: 177–89.

103 Fishburne JI, Brenner WE, Braaksma JT & Hendricks C. Bronchospasm complicating intravenous prostaglandin F2 for therapeutic abortion. *Obstetrics and Gynecology* 1972; **39**: 892–6.

104 Fishburne J, Brenner WE *et al*. Cardiovascular and respiratory responses to intravenous infusion of prostaglandin F2 in the pregnant woman. *American Journal of Obstetrics and Gynecology* 1972; **114**: 765–72.

105 Fitzpatrick M, Mackay T, Driver H & Douglas NJ. Salmeterol in nocturnal asthma: a double blind, placebo controlled trial of a long acting inhaled B_2 agonist. *British Medical Journal* 1990; **301**: 1365–8.

106 Fixley M, Shen DD & Azarnoff DL. Theophylline bioavailability. A comparison of the oral absorption of a theophylline elixir and two combination theophylline tablets to intravenous aminophylline. *American Review of Respiratory Disease* 1977; **115**: 955–62.

107 Francis HH & Smellie J. General disease in pregnancy. *British Medical Journal* 1964; **1**: 887–90.

108 Freeman DW & Barno A. Death with Asian influenza associated with pregnancy. *American Journal of Obstetrics and Gynecology* 1959; **78**: 1172–5.

109 Gaensler EA, Paton WE & Verstraeten JM. Pulmonary functions in pregnancy: III. Serial observations in patients with pulmonary insufficiency. *American Review of Tuberculosis* 1953; **67**: 779–97.

110 Galina MP, Avnet NL & Einhorn A. Iodides during pregnancy: Apparent cause of fetal death. *New England Journal of Medicine* 1962; **267**: 1124.

111 Garrard CG, Littler WAW & Redman CWG. Closing volume during normal pregnancy. *Thorax* 1978; **33**: 484.

112 Gazioglu K, Kaltreider NL, Rosen M & Yu PN. Pulmonary function during pregnancy in normal women and in patients with cardiopulmonary disease. *Thorax* 1970; **25**: 445–50.

113 Gee JBL, Packer BS, Millen JE & Robin ED. Pulmonary mechanics during pregnancy. *Journal of Clinical Investigation* 1967; **46**: 945–52.

114 Gelber M, Sidi Y *et al*. Uncontrollable life-threatening status asthmaticus — an indicator for termination of pregnancy by caesarean section. *Respiration* 1984; **46**: 320–2.

115 Giesler CF, Buehler JH & Depp R. Alpha-antitrypsin deficiency, severe obstructive lung disease and pregnancy. *Obstetrics and Gynecology* 1977; **49**: 31–4.

116 Gilbert GL. Chickenpox during pregnancy. *British Medical Journal* 1993; **306**: 1079–80.

117 Glaser JB, Loftus J *et al*. Varicella zoster infection in pregnancy. *New England Journal of Medicine* 1986; **315**: 1416.

118 Glass DD, Ginburgh FW & Boucot KK. Screening procedures for pulmonary disease in prenatal patients. *American Review of Respiratory Disease* 1960; **82**: 689.

119 Gordon M, Niswander KR *et al*. Fetal morbidity following potentially anoxigenic obstetric conditions. VII. Bronchial asthma. *American Journal of Obstetrics and Gynecology* 1970; **106**: 421–9.
120 Gordon-Nesbitt DC & Rajan G. Congenital TB successfully treated. *British Medical Journal* 1973; **i**: 233–4.
121 Gray JM & Hanson GC. Mediastinal emphysema: Aetiology, diagnosis and treatment. *Thorax* 1966; **21**: 325–31.
122 Greenberg LM & Tanaka KR. Congenital anomalies probably induced by cyclophosphamide. *Journal of the American Medical Association* 1964; **188**: 423–6.
123 Greenberg M, Jacobziner H, Paketer J & Weisel BAG. Maternal mortality in the epidemic of Asian influenza New York City 1957. *American Journal of Obstetrics and Gynecology* 1958; **76**: 897–902.
124 Greenberger PA & Patterson R. Betamethasone dipropionate for severe asthma in pregnancy. *Annals of Internal Medicine* 1983; **98**: 478–80.
125 Greenberger PA. Pregnancy and asthma. *Chest* 1985; **87**: 855–75.
126 Greenberger P & Patterson R. Safety of therapy for allergic symptoms during pregnancy. *Annals of Internal Medicine* 1978; **89**: 234–7.
127 Griffith ER. Viral pneumonia in pregnancy: Report of a case complicated by disseminated intravascular coagulation and acute renal failure. *American Journal of Obstetrics and Gynecology* 1974; **120**: 201–2.
128 Griffith HB & Barnes JC. Severe sarcoidosis in pregnancy. *Obstetrics and Gynecology* 1987; **7**: 272–3.
129 Grossman II JH & Littler MD. Severe sarcoidosis in pregnancy. *Obstetrics and Gynecology* 1976; **50** (suppl): 81S–84S.
130 Gurewich V, Sasahara AA & Stein M. In: Sasahara AA & Stein M (eds), *Pulmonary Embolic Disease*. Grune & Stratton, New York, 1965: 162.
131 Gustavii B, Edvall H *et al*. Acyclovir in prophylaxis and treatment of perinatal varicella. *Lancet* 1987; **i**: 161.
132 Haahtela T, Jarvinen M *et al*. Comparison of a B_2-agonist, terbutaline, with an inhaled corticosteroid, budesonide, in newly detected asthma. *New England Journal of Medicine* 1991; **325**: 388–92.
133 Haake DA, Zakowski PC, Haake DL & Bryson YJ. Early treatment with acyclovir for varicella pneumonia in otherwise healthy adults: retrospective controlled study and review. *Review of Infectious Diseases* 1990; **12**: 788–98.
134 Hadjigeogiou E, Kitsiou S *et al*. Antepartum aminophylline treatment for prevention of respiratory distress syndrome in premature infants. *American Journal of Obstetrics and Gynecology* 1979; **135**: 257–60.
135 Hague WM. Mediastinal and subcutaneous emphysema in a pregnant asthmatic. *British Journal of Obstetrics and Gynaecology* 1980; **87**: 440–3.
136 Hall DC & Kaufmann DA. Effects of aerobic and strength conditioning on pregnancy outcomes. *American Journal of Obstetrics and Gynecology* 1987; **157**: 1199–203.
137 Hamman L. Mediastinal emphysema. *Journal of the American Medical Association* 1945; **128**: 1.
138 Handyside AH, Lesko JG *et al*. Birth of a normal girl after *in vitro* fertilization and preimplantation diagnosis testing for cystic fibrosis. *New England Journal of Medicine* 1992; **327**: 905–9.
139 Harris DM. Some properties of beclomethasone dipropionate and related steriods in man. *Postgraduate Medical Journal* 1975; **51** (suppl 4): 20–5.
140 Harris H, Scotcher D *et al*. Cystic fibrosis carrier testing in early pregnancy by general practitioners. *British Medical Journal* 1993; **306**: 1580–3.
141 Harrop-Griffiths AW, Ravalia A, Browne DA & Robinson PN. Regional anaesthesia and cough effectiveness. A study of patients undergoing caesarean section. *Anaesthesia* 1991; **46**: 11–13.
142 Haynes de Regt R. Sarcoidosis and pregnancy. *Obstetrics and Gynecology* 1987; **70**: 369–72.
143 Hedvall E. Pregnancy and tuberculosis. *Acta Medica Scandinavica* 1953; **286** (suppl 147): 1–101.
144 Heinonen OP, Slone D & Shapiro S. *Birth Defects and Drugs in Pregnancy*. Publishing Sciences Group Inc., Massachusetts, 1977.
145 Hellegers A, Metcalfe J *et al*. The alveolar $P\text{CO}_2$ in pregnant and non-pregnant women at altitude. *Journal of Clinical Investigation* 1959; **38**: 1010.
146 Hemminki E & Starfield B. Prevention and treatment of premature labour by drugs: review of clinical trials. *British Journal of Obstetrics and Gynaecology* 1978; **85**: 411–17.
147 Henry RJW & Vadas RA. Spontaneous rupture of the oesophagus following severe vomiting in early pregnancy. Case report. *British Journal of Obstetrics and Gynecology* 1986; **93**: 392–4.
148 Hernandez E, Angel CS & Johnson JWC. Asthma in pregnancy: current concepts. *Obstetrics and Gynecology* 1980; **55**: 739–43.
149 Hodson ME. Managing adults with cystic fibrosis. *British Medical Journal* 1989; **298**: 471–2.
150 Howard FA & Sharp DS. Effect of metoclopramide on gastric emptying during labour. *British Medical Journal* 1973; **1**: 446–8.
151 Howie AD & Milne JA. Pregnancy in patients with bronchiectasis. *British Journal of Obstetrics and Gynaecology* 1978; **85**: 197–200.
152 Huch R, Baumann H *et al*. Physiologic changes in pregnant women and their fetuses during jet travel. *American Journal of Obstetrics and Gynecology* 1986; **154**: 996–1000.
153 Huch R & Erkkola R. Pregnancy and exercise — exercise and pregnancy. A short review. *British Journal of Obstetrics and Gynaecology* 1990; **97**: 208–14.
154 Hughes E & Hodder RV. Pulmonary lymphangiomyomatosis complicating pregnancy. A case report.

Journal of Reproductive Medicine 1987; **32**: 553–7.
155 Hughson WG, Friedman PJ *et al*. Postpartum pleural effusion: a common radiologic finding. *Annals of Internal Medicine* 1982; **97**: 856–8.
156 Hyman AL, Spannha KEEW & Kadowitz QJ. Prostaglandins and the lung: State of the art. *American Review of Respiratory Disease* 1978; **177**: 111–36.
157 Isenberg JN & L'Heureuse DR. Clinical observation on the biliary system in cystic fibrosis. *American Journal of Gastroenterology* 1976; **65**: 134–9.
158 Ismail MA & Lerner SA. Disseminated blastomycosis in a pregnant women. *American Review of Respiratory Disease* 1982; **128**: 350–3.
159 James DG. Sarcoidosis. *Disease-A-Month* 1970; **1**: 43.
160 Jellife DB & Jellife EFP. 'Breast is Best': modern meanings. *New England Journal of Medicine* 1977; **297**: 912–15.
161 Jensen LP, O'Sullivan MJ *et al*. Acquired immunodeficiency (AIDS) in pregnancy. *American Journal of Obstetrics and Gynecology* 1984; **148**: 1145–6.
162 Johnson SR, Varner MW, Yates SJ & Hanson R. Diagnosis of maternal cystic fibrosis during pregnancy. *Obstetrics and Gynecology* 1983; **61** (suppl): 2S–7S.
163 Jolivet A, Blanchier H, Gantray JP & Dhem N. Blood cortisol variations during late pregnancy and labour. *American Journal of Obstetrics and Gynecology* 1974; **119**: 775–83.
164 Juniper EF, Daniel EE *et al*. Improvement in airway responsiveness and asthma severity during pregnancy. *American Review of Respiratory Disease* 1989; **140**: 924–31.
165 Kambam JR, Handte RE, Brown WR & Smith BE. Effect of pregnancy on oxygen dissociation. *Anesthesiology* 1983; **59**: A395.
166 Keefer JR, Strauss RG, Givetta JM & Burke T. Noncardiogenic pulmonary edema and invasive cardiovascular monitoring. *Obstetrics and Gynecology* 1981; **58**: 46–51.
167 Keleman JT & Mandl L. Sarcoidose in der placenta. *Zentralblatt für Allgemeine Pathologie and Pathologische* 1969; **112**: 18.
168 Kennedy SH. A case of pre-eclampsia in a woman with homozygous Pizz-alpha-$_1$-antitrypsin deficiency. *British Journal of Obstetrics and Gynecology* 1987; **94**: 1103–4.
169 Kerem E, Reisman J *et al*. Prediction of mortality in patients with cystic fibrosis. *New England Journal of Medicine* 1992; **326**: 1187–91.
170 Knuttgen HG & Emerson K. Physiological response to pregnancy at rest and during exercise. *Journal of Applied Physiology* 1974; **36**: 549.
171 Kopenhager T. A review of 50 pregnant patients with kyphoscoliosis. *British Journal of Obstetrics and Gynaecology* 1977; **84**: 585.
172 Kreisman H, Van De Wiel N & Mitchell CA. Respiratory function during prostaglandin-induced labour. *American Review of Respiratory Disease* 1975; **111**: 564–6.
173 Krumholz RA, Echt CR & Ross JC. Pulmonary diffusing capacity, capillary blood volume, lung volumes and mechanics of ventilation in early and late pregnancy. *Journal of Laboratory and Clinical Medicine* 1964; **63**: 648.
174 Kunelis CT, Peters JL & Edmondson HA. Fatty liver of pregnancy and its relationship to tetracycline therapy. *American Journal of Medicine* 1965; **38**; 359–77.
175 Lalli CM & Raju L. Pregnancy and chronic obstructive pulmonary disease. *Chest* 1981; **80**: 759–61.
176 *Lancet* editorial. Alpha$_1$-antitrypsin deficiency and prenatal diagnosis. *Lancet* 1987; **i**: 421–2.
177 *Lancet* editorial. Perinatal prophylaxis of tuberculosis. *Lancet* 1990; **336**: 1479–80.
178 Lao TT, Yeung S & Leung BFH. Kyphoscoliosis and pregnancy. *Journal of Obstetrics and Gynaecology* 1986; **7**: 11–15.
179 Lavin JP & Miodovaik M. Pulmonary eosinophilic granuloma complicating pregnancy. *Obstetrics and Gynecology* 1981; **58**: 516–19.
180 Lewis PJ, de Swiet M, Boylan P & Bulpitt CJ. How obstetricians in the United Kingdom manage preterm labour. *British Journal of Obstetrics and Gynaecology* 1980; **87**: 574–7.
181 Lewitt T, Neibel L, Terracina S & Karman S. Ethambutol in pregnancy. Observations on embryogenesis. *Chest* 1974; **66**: 25–6.
182 Littlejohns P, Ebrahim S & Anderson R. Prevalence and diagnosis of chronic respiratory symptoms in adults. *British Medical Journal* 1989; **298**: 1556–60.
183 Lotgering FK, Gilbert RD & Longo L. The interactions of exercise and pregnancy: a review. *American Journal of Obstetrics and Gynecology* 1984; **149**: 560–8.
184 Luby BJ, Georgiev M, Warren SG & Capito R. Postpartum pneumopericardium. *Obstetrics and Gynaecology* 1978; **62**: 46S–50S.
185 Lucius H, Gahlenbeck H *et al*. Respiratory functions, buffer system and electrolyte concentrations of blood during human pregnancy. *Respiration Physiology* 1970; **9**: 311.
186 Lunell NO, Wager J, Fredholm BB & Person B. Metabolic effects of oral salbutamol in late pregnancy. *European Journal of Clinical Pharmacology* 1978; **14**: 95–9.
187 Lyons HA & Antonio R. The sensitivity of the respiratory centre in pregnancy and after the administration of progesterone. *Transactions of the Association of American Physicians* 1959; **72**: 173.
188 Lyons HA & Huang CT. Therapeutic use of progesterone in alveolar hypoventilation associated with obesity. *American Journal of Medicine* 1968; **44**: 881–8.
189 MacDonald JB, MacDonald ET, Seaton A & Williams DA. Asthma deaths in Cardiff 1963–1974: 53 deaths in hospital. *British Medical Journal* 1976; **2**: 721–3.
190 MacLennan FM. Maternal mortality from Mendelson's syndrome: an explanation. *Lancet* 1986; **i**: 587–9.
191 Maklem PT & Mead J. Resistance of central and peripheral airways measured by a retrograde catheter.

Journal of Applied Physiology 1967; **22**: 395.
192 Marx CM & Fraser DG. Treatment of asthma in pregnancy. *Obstetrics and Gynecology* 1981; **57**: 766–7.
193 Marx GF. Obstetric anesthesia in the presence of medical complications. *Clinics in Obstetrics and Gynecology* 1974; **17**: 165–81.
194 Matson JA & Capen CV. Pregnancy in the cystic fibrosis patient. *Journal of Reproductive Medicine* 1982; **27**: 373–5.
195 Mattox JH. The value of a routine prenatal chest X-ray. *Obstetrics and Gynaecology* 1973; **41**: 243–5.
196 McAvley DM, Halliday HL, Johnston JR & Dundee JW. Cimetidine in labour: absence of adverse effect on the high-risk fetus. *British Journal of Obstetrics and Gynaecology* 1985; **92**: 350–5.
197 McCarty KS, Mossler JA, McLelland R & Seiker HO. Pulmonary lymphangiomyomatosis responsive to progesterone. *New England Journal of Medicine* 1980; **303**: 1461–5.
198 McCaughey W, Howe JP, Moore J & Dundee JW. Cimetidine in elective Caesarean section: effect on gastric acidity. *Anaesthesia* 1981; **36**: 167–72.
199 Mendelson CL. Pregnancy and kyphoscoliotic heart disease. *American Journal of Obstetrics and Gynecology* 1958; **56**: 457.
200 Metzger WJ, Turner E & Patterson R. The safety of immunotherapy during pregnancy. *Journal of Allergy and Clinical Immunology* 1978; **61**: 268–72.
201 Milne JA. The respiratory response to pregnancy. *Postgraduate Medical Journal* 1979; **55**: 318–24.
202 Milne JA, Howie AD & Pack AI. Dyspnoea during normal pregnancy. *British Journal of Obstetrics and Gynaecology* 1978; **84**: 448.
203 Milne JA, Mills RJ, Howie AD & Pack AI. Large airways function during normal pregnancy. *British Journal of Obstetrics and Gynaecology* 1977; **84**: 448–51.
204 Milne JA, Pack AI & Coutts JRT. Gas exchange and acid–base status during ovulatory cycles and those regulated by oral contraceptives. *Proceedings of the Society of Endocrinology Journal of Endocrinology* 1977; **75**: 17P.
205 Milne JA, Pack AI & Coutts JRT. Maternal gas exchange and acid–base status during normal pregnancy. *Scottish Medical Journal* 1977; **22**: 108.
206 Monnet P, Kalb JC & Pujol M De. L'influence nocive de l'isoniazide sur le produit de conception. *Lyon Medical* 1967; **218**: 431–55.
207 Morrison J & Kilpatrick N. Low urinary oestriol excretion in pregnancy associated with oral prednisone therapy. *Journal of Obstetrics and Gynaecology of the British Commonwealth* 1969; **76**: 719–20.
208 Motoyama EK, Rivard G, Acheson F & Cook CD. Adverse effect of maternal hyperventilation of the fetus. *Lancet* 1966; **i**: 286–8.
209 Motoyama EK, Rivard G, Acheson F & Cook CD. The effect of changes in maternal pH and Pco_2 of fetal lambs. *Anesthesiology* 1967; **28**: 891–903.
210 Moya F, Morishima HO, Shnider SM & James LS. Influence of maternal hyperventilation on the new born infant. *American Journal of Obstetrics and Gynecology* 1975; **91**: 76–84.
211 Mucklow ES. Tuberculous meningitis in labour. *Journal of Obstetrics and Gynecology* 1987; **8**: 145.
212 Murata A, Takeda Y *et al*. A case of pulmonary lymphangiomyomatosis induced by pregnancy. *Nippon Kyobu Shikkan Gakkai Zasshi* 1989; **27**: 1106–11.
213 Murty GE, Davison JM & Cameron DS. Wegener's granulomatosis complicating pregnancy. *British Journal of Obstetrics and Gynaecology* 1990; **10**: 399–400.
214 Nava S, Zanotti E *et al*. Evidence of acute diaphragmatic fatigue in a 'natural' condition: the diaphragm during labour. *Annual Review of Respiratory Disease* 1992; **146**: 1226–30.
215 Nelson MM & Forfar JO. Associations between drugs administered during pregnancy and congenital abnormalities of the fetus. *British Medical Journal* 1971; **i**: 523–7.
216 Newhouse MT, Becklaile MR, Macklem PT & McGregor M. Effect of alterations in endtidal CO_2 on flow resistance. *Journal of Applied Physiology* 1964; **19**: 745.
217 Novy MJ, Tyler JM *et al*. Cystic fibrosis and pregnancy. *Obstetrics and Gynecology* 1967; **30**: 530–6.
218 Nyhan D, Bredin CP & Quigley C. Acute respiratory failure in pregnancy due to staphylococcal pneumonia. *Irish Medical Journal* 1982; **76**: 320–1.
219 Opsahl MS & O'Brien WF. Systemic nocardiosis in pregnancy. *Journal of Reproductive Medicine* 1983; **28**: 621–3.
220 O'Sullivan GM & Bullingham RES. The assessment of gastric acidity and antacid effect in pregnant women by a non-invasive radiotelemetry technique. *British Journal of Obstetrics and Gynaecology* 1984; **91**: 973–8.
221 Oxorn H. The changing aspects of pneumonia complicating pregnancy. *Obstetrics and Gynecology* 1955; **70**: 1057.
222 Paciorek J & Spencer N. An association between plasma progesterone and erythrocyte carbonic anhydrase 1 concentration in women. *Clinical Science* 1980; **58**: 161–4.
223 Palmer J, Dillon-Baker C *et al*. Pregnancy in patients with cystic fibrosis. *Annals of Internal Medicine* 1983; **99**: 596–600.
224 Parayani SG & Arvin AM. Intrauterine infection with varicella zoster after maternal varicella. *New England Journal of Medicine* 1986; **314**: 1542–6.
225 Pearlman DS, Chervinsky P *et al*. A comparison of salmeterol with albuterol in the treatment of mild to moderate asthma. *New England Journal of Medicine* 1992; **327**: 1420–5.
226 Pedersen H & Finster M. Anesthetic risk in the pregnant surgical patient. *Anesthesiology* 1979; **51**: 439–51.
227 Pernoll ML, Metcalfe J *et al*. Ventilation during rest and exercise in pregnancy and postpartum. *Respiration Physiology* 1975; **25**: 295.

228 Phelan D. Cystic fibrosis and pregnancy. *Medical Journal of Australia* 1981; **1**: 58.
229 Philipson A. Pharmacokinetics of ampicillin during pregnancy. *Journal of Infectious Diseases* 1977; **136**: 3070–6.
230 Plauche WC, Buechner HA & Diket AL. Tuberculosis prenatal screening and therapy during pregnancy. *Journal of Louisiana State Association* 1983; **135**: 13–15.
231 Potworoska M, Sianozeka E & Szufladowicz R. Ethionamide treatment in pregnancy. *Polish Medical Journal* 1966; **5**: 1152–8.
232 Present PA & Comstock GW. Tubercular sensitivity in pregnancy. *American Review of Respiratory Disease* 1975; **122**: 413–16.
233 Prichard MG & Musk AW. Adverse effect of pregnancy on familial fibrosing alveolitis. *Thorax* 1984; **39**: 319–20.
234 Prowse CM & Gaensler EA. Respiratory and acid–base changes during pregnancy. *Anesthesiology* 1965; **26**: 381.
235 Psacharopoulos HT, Howard ER *et al*. Hepatic complications of cystic fibrosis. *Lancet* 1981; **ii**: 78–80.
236 Raffin TA, Taylor JR, Ryu J & Colby TV. Treatment of lymphangiomyomatosis. *New England Journal of Medicine* 1991; **325**: 64.
237 Raz S, Zeigler M & Caine M. The effect of progesterone on the adrenergic receptors of the urethra. *British Journal of Urology* 1973; **45**: 131.
238 Reisfeld DR, Yahia C & Laurenz GA. Pregnancy and cardiorespiratory failure in Boeck's sarcoid. *Surgery, Gynecology and Obstetrics* 1969; **109**: 412–16.
239 Ridgway LF, Martin RW *et al*. Acute gestational pyelonephritis: the impact of colloid osmotic pressure, plasma fibronectin, and arterial oxygen saturation. *American Journal of Perinatology* 1991; **8**: 222–6.
240 Robinson GC & Cambon KG. Hearing loss in infants of tuberculous mothers treated with streptomycin during pregnancy. *New England Journal of Medicine* 1964; **271**: 949–51.
241 Rosenthal A, Tucker CR *et al*. Echocardiographic assessment of cor pulmonale in cystic fibrosis. *Pediatric Clinics in North America* 1976; **23**: 327–44.
242 Rubin A, Russo N & Goucher D. The effect of pregnancy upon pulmonary function in normal women. *American Journal of Obstetrics and Gynecology* **72**: 2963.
243 Rubin PC. Prescribing in pregnancy. General principles. *British Medical Journal* 1986; **293**: 1415–17.
244 Russell IF & Chambers WA. Closing volume in normal pregnancy. *British Journal of Anaesthesia* 1981; **53**: 1043–7.
245 Ryssing E. Assessment of cor pulmonale in cystic fibrosis by echocardiography. *Acta Paediatrica Scandinavica* 1977; **66**: 753–6.
246 Salvatore MA & Lynch PJ. Erythema nodosum, estrogens and pregnancy. *Archives of Dermatology* 1980; **116**: 557–8.
247 Sangoul F, Fox GS & Houle GL. Effect of regional analgesia on maternal oxygen consumption during the first stage of labour. *American Journal of Obstetrics and Gynecology* 1975; **121**: 1080.
248 Sawicka EH, Spencer GT & Branthwaite MA. Management of respiratory failure complicating pregnancy in severe kyphoscoliosis: a new use for an old technique? *British Journal of Diseases of the Chest* 1986; **80**: 191–6.
249 Schaefer G, Zervoudakis TA, Fuchs FF & David S. Pregnancy and pulmonary tuberculosis. *Obstetrics and Gynecology* 1975; **46**: 706–15.
250 Schatz M, Patterson R & Zeitz S. Corticosteroid therapy for the pregnant asthmatic patient. *Journal of the American Medical Association* 1975; **233**: 804–7.
251 Schatz M, Zeiger RS & Hoffman CP. Intrauterine growth is related to gestational pulmonary function in pregnant asthmatic women. Kaiser Permanent Asthma and Pregnancy Group. *Chest* 1990; **98**: 389–92.
252 Schatz M, Zeiger RS *et al*. Increased transient tachypnea of the newborn in infants of asthmatic mother. *American Journal of Diseases of Children* 1991; **145**: 156–8.
253 Scheinborn DJ & Angelillo VA. Antituberculous therapy in pregnancy: risks to the fetus. *Western Journal of Medicine* 1977; **127**: 195–8.
254 Schenker JG, Ben-Joseph Y & Shapira E. Erythrocyte carbonic anhydrase B levels during pregnancy and use of oral contraceptives. *Obstetrics and Gynecology* 1972; **39**: 237–40.
255 Scott DB. Mendelson's syndrome. *British Journal of Anaesthesia* 1978; **50**: 81–2.
256 Scott J, Higenbottam T *et al*. Heart–lung transplantation for cystic fibrosis. *Lancet* 1988; **ii**: 192–4.
257 Selikoff IJ & Dormann HL. Management of tuberculosis. In: *Medical, Surgical and Gynecologic Complications in Pregnancy*, 2nd edn. Williams & Wilkins, Baltimore, 1965.
258 Sellers WFS & Long DR. Bronchospasm following ergometrine. *Anaesthesia* 1979; **34**: 909.
259 Selwyn Crawford J. Bronchospasm following ergometrine. *Anaesthesia* 1980; **35**: 397–8.
260 Shanies HM. Non-cardiogenic pulmonary oedema. *Medical Clinics of North America* 1977; **61**: 1319.
261 Shaw LMA. Cystic fibrosis and reproductive function. *Journal of Obstetrics and Gynecology* 1985; **6**: 1–5.
262 Shen A, Iseman MD, Waldron JA & King TE. Exacerbation of pulmonary lymphangioleiomyomatosis by exogenous estrogens. *Chest* 1987; **91**: 782–5.
263 Siassi B, Moss AJ & Dooley RR. Clinical recognition of cor pulmonale in cystic fibrosis. *Journal of Pediatrics* 1971; **78**: 794.
264 Sibbald B. *A Family Study Approach to the Genetic Basis of Asthma*. University of London, PhD Thesis, 1981.
265 Siegler D & Zorab PA. Pregnancy in thoracic scoliosis. *British Journal of Disorders of the Chest* 1981; **75**: 367–700.

266 Silverstein EF, Ellis K, Wolff M & Jaretzki A. Pulmonary lymphangiomyomatosis. *American Roentgenology and Radium Therapy in Nuclear Medicine* 1974; **120**: 832–50.
267 Sims CD, Chamberlain GVP & de Swiet M. Lung function tests in bronchial asthma during and after pregnancy. *British Journal of Obstetrics and Gynaecology* 1976; **88**: 434–7.
268 Skatrud JB, Dempsey JA & Kaiser DG. Ventilatory response to the medroxy-progesterone acetate in normal subjects: time course and mechanism. *Journal of Applied Physiology Respiration Environmental and Exercise Physiology* 1978; **44**: 939–44.
269 Smale LE & Waechter KG. Dissemination of coccidiodomycosis. *American Journal of Obstetrics and Gynecology* 1976; **107**: 356–61.
270 Smith AP. The effects of intravenous infusion of graded doses of prostaglandins F2 and E2 on lung resistance in patients undergoing termination of pregnancy. *Clinical Science* 1973; **44**: 17–25.
271 Smith JL, Thomas F, Orme JF & Clemmer TP. Adult respiratory distress syndrome during pregnancy and immediately postpartum. *Western Journal of Medicine* 1990; **153**: 508–10.
272 Snider DE. Pregnancy and tuberculosis. *Chest* 1984; **86**: 10S–13S.
273 Snider DE. Should women taking antituberculous drugs breast feed? *Archives of Internal Medicine* 1984; **144**: 589–90.
274 Snider DE, Layde PM, Johnson NW & Lyle HA. Treatment of tuberculosis during pregnancy. *American Review of Respiratory Disease* 1980; **122**: 65–78.
275 Sobrevilla LA, Cassinelli MT, Carcelen A & Malaga JW. Human fetal and maternal oxygen tension, and acid–base status during delivery at high altitude. *American Journal of Obstetrics and Gynecology* 1971; **111**: 1111.
276 Sorensen KE & Borlum K. Fetal heart function in response to short-term maternal exercise. *British Journal of Obstetrics and Gynaecology* 1986; **93**: 310–13.
277 Spector SL. The treatment of the asthmatic mother during pregnancy and lactation. *Annals of Allergy* 1983; **51**: 173–8.
278 Spellacy WN & Prem KA. Subcutaneous emphysema and pregnancy. Report of three cases. *Obstetrics and Gynecology* 1963; **22**: 521–3.
279 Spring JE & Winston RML. Congenital lymphoedema and its complications in pregnancy and the puerperium. *Journal of Obstetrics and Gynaecology* 1985; **5**: 170–3.
280 Stablein JF & Lockey RF. Managing asthma during pregnancy. *Comprehensive Therapy* 1984; **10**: 45–52.
281 Steen JSM & Staintain-Ellis DM. Rifampicin in pregnancy. *Lancet* 1977; **ii**: 604–5.
282 Sulavik SB. Pulmonary disease. In: Burrow GN & Ferris TF (eds), *Medical Complications during Pregnancy*. WB Saunders, Philadelphia, 1975: 549.
283 Suonio S, Saaranen M & Saarikoski S. Left-sided hydrothorax in connection with severe pre-eclampsia: case reports. *International Journal of Gynaecology and Obstetrics* 1984; **22**: 357–61.
284 Super M, Ivinson A *et al*. Clinic experience of prenatal diagnosis of cystic fibrosis by use of linked DNA probes. *Lancet* 1987; **ii**: 782–4.
285 Sutton FD Jr, Zwillich CW *et al*. Progesterone for outpatient treatment of Pickwickian syndrome. *Annals of Internal Medicine* 1975; **83**: 476–9.
286 Sutton PL, Koup JR & Rose BS. The pharmacokinetics of theophylline in pregnancy. *Journal of Allergy and Clinical Immunology* 1978; **61**: 174.
287 Synder RD & Synder DL. Corticosteroids for asthma during pregnancy. *Annals of Allergy* 1978; **41**: 340–1.
288 Talbot SF, Main DM & Levinson AI. Wegener's granulomatosis: first report of a case with onset during pregnancy. *Arthritis and Rheumatology* 1984; **27**: 109–11.
289 Tatersall MP. Prescribing drugs in pregnancy. *British Journal of Hospital Medicine* 1983; **29**: 382.
290 Taussig LM, Kattwinkel J, Freidwald WT & di Saint' Agnese PA. A new prognostic score and clinical evaluation system for cystic fibrosis. *Journal of Pediatrics* 1973; **82**: 380–90.
291 Taylor RJ, Ryu J, Colby TV & Raffin TA. Lymphangiomyomatosis — clinical course in 32 patients. *New England Journal of Medicine* 1990; **323**: 1254–60.
292 Templeton A. Intrauterine growth retardation associated with hypoxia due to bronchiectasis. *British Journal of Obstetrics and Gynaecology* 1977; **84**: 389–90.
293 Templeton A & Kelman GR. Arterial blood gases in pre-eclampsia. *British Journal of Obstetrics and Gynaecology* 1977; **84**: 290–3.
294 Templeton A & Kelman GR. Maternal blood gases (PAo_2, Pao_2) physiological shunt and V_D/V_T in normal pregnancy. *British Journal of Anaesthesia* 1976; **48**: 1001–4.
295 Thaler I, Bronstein M & Rubin AE. The course and outcome of pregnancy associated with bronchiectasis. Case report. *British Journal of Obstetrics and Gynaecology* 1986; **93**: 1006–8.
296 The British Paediatric Working Party of Cystic Fibrosis. Cystic fibrosis in the United Kingdom 1977–85: an improving picture. *British Medical Journal* 1988; **297**: 1599–602.
297 Thommasen HV, Russell JA, Boyko WJ & Hogg JC. Transient leucopenia associated with adult respiratory distress syndrome. *Lancet* 1984; **i**: 809–12.
298 Thomson KJ & Cohen ME. Studies on the circulation in pregnancy. II: Vital capacity observations in normal pregnant women. *Surgery, Gynecology and Obstetrics* 1938; **66**: 591.
299 Toledo TM, Harper RC & Moser RH. Fetal effects during cyclophosphamide and radiation therapy. *Annals of Internal Medicine* 1971; **74**: 87–91.
300 Towers CV, Kaminskas CM *et al*. Pulmonary injury

associated with antepartum pyelonephritis: can patients at risk be identified? *American Journal of Obstetrics and Gynecology* 1991; **164**: 974–8.

301 Turner ES, Greenberger PA & Patterson R. Management of the pregnant asthmatic patient. *Annals of Internal Medicine* 1980; **6**: 905–18.

302 Udeshi UL, McHugo JM & Crawford JS. Postpartum pleural effusion. *British Journal of Obstetrics and Gynaecology* 1988; **95**: 894–7.

303 Van Arsdel PPJ & Paul GH. Drug therapy in the management of asthma. *Annals of Internal Medicine* 1977; **87**: 68–74.

304 Varheer H. Drug excretion in breast milk. *Postgraduate Medicine* 1974; **56**: 97–104.

305 Wager J, Fredholm BB, Lunell NO & Persson B. Metabolic and circulatory effects of oral salbutamol in the third trimester of pregnancy in diabetic and non-diabetic women. *British Journal of Obstetrics and Gynaecology* 1981; **88**: 352–61.

306 Wald NJ. Couple screening for cystic fibrosis. *Lancet* 1991; **338**: 1318–19.

307 Wallace SJ & Michie EA. A follow-up study of infants born to mothers with low oestriol excretion during pregnancy. *Lancet* 1966; **ii**: 560–63.

308 Warrell DW & Taylor R. Outcome for the fetus of mother receiving prednisolone during pregnancy. *Lancet* 1968; **i**: 117–18.

309 Warwick WJ, Progue RE, Gerber HM & Nesbitt CJ. Survival patterns in cystic fibrosis. *Journal of Chronic Diseases* 1975; **28**: 609–22.

310 Weinberger SE, Weiss ST *et al*. Pregnancy and the lung. *American Review of Respiratory Medicine* 1980; **121**: 559–81.

311 Weinstein AM, Dubin BD *et al*. Asthma and pregnancy. *Journal of the American Medical Association* 1980; **241**: 1161–4.

312 Wendel GD, Stark BJ *et al*. Penicillin allergy and desensitization in serious infection during pregnancy. *New England Journal of Medicine* 1985; **312**: 1229–32.

313 Wheeler GE. Cyclophosphamide associated leukaemia in Wegener's granulomatosis. *Annals of Internal Medicine* 1981; **94**: 161–2.

314 White RJ, Coutts II, Gibbs CJ & Macintyre C. A prospective study of asthma during pregnancy and the puerperium. *Obstetrical and Gynecological Survey* 1989; **83**: 240–1.

315 White RJ, Harrison KJ & Clarke SKR. Causes of pneumonia presenting to a district general hospital. *Thorax* 1981; **36**: 566–70.

316 Whitelaw A & Butterfield A. High breast milk sodium in cystic fibrosis. *Lancet* 1977; **ii**: 1288.

317 Wilbrand U, Porath Ch, Matthaes P & Jaster R. Der einfluss der Ovarialsteroide auf die Funktion des Atemzentrums. *Archiv für Gynakologie* 1952; **191**: 507.

318 Williams DA. Asthma and pregnancy. *Acta Allergolica* 1957; **22**: 311–23.

319 Wilson JW. Treatment or prevention of pulmonary cellular damage with pharmacological doses of corticosteroids. *Surgery, Gynecology and Obstetrics* 1972; **134**: 675.

320 Windebank WJ, Boyd G & Moran F. Pulmonary thromboembolism presenting as asthma. *British Medical Journal* 1973; **i**: 90.

321 Wong CS, Pavord ID *et al*. Bronchodilator, cardiovascular, and hypokalaemic effects of fenoterol, salbutamol, and terbutaline in asthma. *Lancet* 1990; **336**: 1396–7.

322 Wulf KH, Kunzel S & Lehman V. Clinical aspects of placental gas exchange. In: Longo LD & Bartels H (eds), *Respiratory Gas Exchange and Blood Flow in the Placenta*. US Department of Health, Education and Welfare, Bethesda, Maryland, 1972.

323 Yeh TF & Pildes RS. Transplacental aminophylline toxicity in a neonate. *Lancet* 1977; **i**: 910.

324 Yurchak AM & Jusko WJ. Theophylline secretion in breast milk. *Pediatrics* 1976; **75**: 518–20.

Further reading

de Swiet M. Respiration. In: Barnes JE & Newborn M (eds), *Scientific Foundations of Obstetrics and Gynaecology*, 4th edn. William Heinemann Medical, London, 1990.

Orr JW, Austin JM *et al*. Acute pulmonary edema associated with molar pregnancy: A high-risk factor for development of persistent trophoblastic disease. *American Journal of Obstetrics and Gynaecology* 1980; **136**: 412–14.

2

Blood Volume, Haematinics, Anaemia

Elizabeth A. Letsky

Blood volume, 33
Plasma volume
Red cell mass
Total haemoglobin
Iron metabolism
Iron absorption
Non-haematological effects of iron deficiency, 36
Haemoglobin concentration
Red cell indices
Serum iron and total iron binding capacity
Free erythrocyte protoporphyrin
Ferritin
Marrow iron
Management of iron deficiency, 39
The case for prophylactic iron therapy
Folic acid, 42
Folate metabolism
Plasma folate
Red cell folate
Excretion of formiminoglutamic acid
Folic acid post-partum
Interpretation of investigations
Megaloblastic anaemia, 43
Folic acid deficiency
Anticonvulsant drugs and pregnancy
Vitamin B_{12} deficiency
Haemoglobinopathies, 47
The thalassaemia syndromes, 47
α thalassaemia
β thalassaemia
Haemoglobin variants, 50
Sickle cell syndromes
Screening for haemoglobinopathy, 54
Prenatal diagnosis of haemoglobinopathies, 55
Fetal blood sampling
Globin gene analysis
Rationale for screening, 57
Implications for the future
Miscellaneous anaemias, 58
Aplastic anaemia
Autoimmune haemolytic anaemia and systemic lupus erythematosus
Polycythaemia rubra vera
Thrombocythaemia, thrombocytosis
Paroxysmal nocturnal haemoglobinuria
Leukaemia, 61
Hodgkin's disease, 62

Blood volume

Although the 'plethora' of pregnancy was recognized early in the nineteenth century and German work as far back as 1854 showed a rise of blood volume in pregnant laboratory animals, the evidence for plethora in pregnant women rested primarily on the demonstration of reduced concentration of solids and cells in the blood until the early 20th century [123]. The best estimate of total blood volume is obtained when plasma volume and red cell mass are measured simultaneously; however, the majority of published reports of blood volume in pregnancy are based on either measured plasma volume or total red cell mass, the fraction not directly estimated being calculated from body haematocrit.

Plasma volume

The measurement of plasma volume in pregnancy has a long history which was comprehensively reviewed by Hytten and Leitch [84], later summarized and updated [83]. Plasma volume rises progressively throughout pregnancy, with a tendency to plateau in the last 8 weeks [147]. The terminal fall in plasma volume described by almost all investigators previously, occurs only when measurements are made in the supine position. The underestimation in the supine position is due to the bulky uterus obstructing venous return from the lower limbs resulting in incomplete mixing of dye [28] — a similar condition to the reduction in cardiac output seen in patients in the supine position (see Chapter 5).

There is little doubt that the amount of increase

in plasma volume is correlated with obstetric outcome and the birthweight of the baby [84,129,147]. Since second and subsequent pregnancies tend to be more successful than the first, with bigger babies, a larger plasma volume increase in multigravidae would be expected; however, the evidence for this is not entirely satisfactory [84].

Women with multiple pregnancy have proportionately higher increments of plasma volume. The plasma volume at term was found to be approximately 1940 ml above control in eight women with twins and 2400 ml above control in two women with triplets [158]. One woman with a quadruplet pregnancy had raised her plasma volume by 2400 ml above her non-pregnant value by 34 weeks [55].

In contrast, women with poorly growing fetuses (particularly multigravidae with a history of poor reproductive performance) have a correspondingly poor plasma response [59].

In summary, healthy women in a normal first pregnancy increase their plasma volume from a non-pregnant level of almost 2600 ml by about 1250 ml. Most of the rise takes place before 32–34 weeks' gestation; thereafter there is relatively little change. In subsequent pregnancies, the increase is greater. The increase is related to the size of the fetus and there are particularly large increases in association with multiple pregnancy.

Red cell mass

The red cell 'mass' is a confusing term which expresses the total volume of red cells in the circulation. The more logical alternative of red cell volume cannot be used because of its specific meaning in haematology of the volume of a single erythrocyte.

There is less published information on red cell mass than plasma volume and the results are more variable. There is still disagreement as to how much the red cell mass increases in normal pregnancy. The extent of the increase is considerably influenced by iron medication which will cause the red cell mass to rise in apparently healthy women even if they have no clinical evidence of iron deficiency. The stimulus for increased red cell production is due in part to rising erythropoietin levels which are present from early pregnancy [70].

The early literature is summarized by Hytten and Leitch [84]. If one accepts a figure of about 1400 ml for the volume of red cells in average healthy women before pregnancy, then the rise in pregnancy for women not given iron supplements is about 240 ml (18 per cent) and for those given iron is 400 ml (30 per cent). The red cell mass increases steadily between the end of the first trimester and term. As with plasma volume, the extent of the increase is related to the size of the conceptus, particularly large increases being seen in association with multiple pregnancy [55,158].

The red cell mass falls immediately at delivery as a result of blood loss [105]. Non-pregnant blood volumes are reached around 3 weeks after delivery.

Changes in blood volume at parturition and during the puerperium

Acute blood loss causes dramatic changes in maternal blood volume at both vaginal delivery and caesarean section. If the blood loss at vaginal delivery is meticulously measured it is more than 500 ml of blood associated with singleton delivery and almost 1000 ml at delivery of twins. Caesarean section is associated with an average loss of 1000 ml.

In the normal pregnant female at term, hypervolaemia modifies the response to blood loss considerably. The blood volume drops following the acute loss at delivery but remains relatively stable unless the blood loss exceeds 25 per cent of the predelivery volume. There is no compensatory increase in blood volume and there is a gradual fall in plasma volume, due primarily to diuresis. The red cell mass increase during pregnancy not lost at delivery is slowly reduced as the red cells come to the end of their lifespan. The overall result is that the haematocrit gradually increases and the blood volume returns to non-pregnant levels.

In the first few days following delivery there are fluctuations in plasma volume and haematocrit due to individual responses to dehydration, pregnancy hypervolaemia and the rapidity of blood loss. The average blood loss which can be tolerated without causing a significant fall in haemoglobin concentration is around 1000 ml but this depends in turn on a healthy increase in blood volume prior to delivery. Almost all the blood loss occurs within the first hour following delivery under normal circumstances. In the following 72 hours only approximately 80 ml are lost vaginally. Patients with uterine atony, extended episiotomy or lacerations will, of course, lose much more. If the haematocrit or haemoglobin concentration at 5–7 days after delivery proves to be significantly less than before delivery, either there was pathological blood loss at delivery, or there was a poor increase in blood volume during pregnancy or both [143,179].

Benefits of hypervolaemia in pregnancy

The widely different responses in plasma volume and red cell mass should have an explanation that makes biological sense.

Hypervolaemia *per se* combats the hazard of haemorrhage for the mother at delivery, as described above. It also protects the mother from hypotension in the last trimester when sequestration occurs in the lower extremities on standing, sitting or lying supine (see Chapter 5).

The red cell mass should increase in line with the need for extra oxygen. It has been calculated that by the end of pregnancy the increase in oxygen requirement is around 15–16 per cent [83]. This is met adequately by the increase in red cell mass of 18–25 per cent [83].

The role of the much greater increase in plasma volume becomes clear when the distribution of the raised cardiac output is defined. Most of the extra cardiac output is directed to the skin and kidneys. Both serve as organs of excretion during pregnancy, the skin to allow for heat loss. For excretion they require plasma rather than the red cells. Also the decrease in viscosity caused by a low haematocrit causes decreased resistance to blood flow and allows an increase in cardiac output with relatively less increase in cardiac work. These factors make biological sense of what is often seen as a disproportionate increase in plasma volume.

Total haemoglobin

The haemoglobin concentration, haematocrit, and red cell count, fall during pregnancy because the expansion of the plasma volume is greater than that of the red cell mass. However, there is a rise in total circulating haemoglobin directly related to the increase in red cell mass. This in turn is dependent partly on the iron status of the individual. Published evidence for the rise in total haemoglobin is unsatisfactory and is confused by the varying iron status of the women studied. It is impossible to give physiological limits for the expected rise in total haemoglobin until better figures are available.

The lowest normal haemoglobin in the healthy adult *non-pregnant* woman living at sea level is defined as 12 g/dl [196]. In most published studies the mean minimum in pregnancy was between 11 and 12 g/dl. The lowest haemoglobin observed in a carefully studied iron-supplemented group was 10.44 g/dl [104]. The mean minimum acceptable to the World Health Organization (WHO) is 11 g/dl [196].

Iron metabolism

In pregnancy the demand for iron is increased to meet the needs of the expanding red cell mass and requirements of the developing fetus and placenta. By far the greatest single demand for iron is that for the expansion of the red cell mass. The fetus derives its iron from the maternal serum by active transport across the placenta mainly in the last 4 weeks of pregnancy [54]. The total requirement for iron is of the order of 700–1400 mg. Overall the requirement is 4 mg/day, but this rises to 6.6 mg/day in the last few weeks of pregnancy. This can be met only by mobilizing iron stores in addition to achieving maximum absorption of dietary iron, because a normal mixed diet supplies about 14 mg of iron each day of which only 1–2 mg (5–15 per cent) is absorbed.

Iron absorption is increased when there is erythroid hyperplasia — rapid iron turnover — and a high concentration of unsaturated transferrin, all of which are part of the physiological response in the healthy pregnant woman. There is evidence that absorption of dietary iron is enhanced in the latter half of pregnancy [5,84], but this would still not provide enough iron for the needs of pregnancy and the puerperium for a woman on a normal mixed diet.

Iron absorption

There are at least two distinct pathways for iron absorption: one for inorganic iron and one for iron attached to haem. The availability of dietary iron is quite variable. In most foods inorganic iron is in the 'ferric' form and has to be converted to the ferrous form before absorption can take place. In foods derived from grain, iron often forms a stable complex with phytates and only small amounts can be converted to a soluble form. The iron in eggs is poorly absorbed because of binding with phosphates present in the yolk. Milk, particularly cows' milk, is poor in iron content. Tea inhibits the absorption of iron. The traditional Scottish breakfast of porridge and eggs washed down with milky tea is rich in protein but provides very little, if any, absorbable iron!

The intestinal mucosal control in iron absorption is complex and incompletely understood; however, in general, absorption is enhanced in times of increased need and deficiency. Haem iron derived from the haemoglobin and myoglobin of animal origin is more effectively absorbed than non-haem iron. Factors interfering with or promoting the absorption of inorganic iron have no effect on the absorption of haem iron. This puts vegetarians at a disadvantage in terms of iron sufficiency. The amount of iron absorbed will depend very much on the extent of the iron stores, the content of the diet and whether or not iron supplements are given. It was found, in a carefully controlled study in Sweden [178], that absorption rates differed markedly between those pregnant women receiving 100 mg ferrous iron supplements daily and those receiving a placebo. Iron absorption increased steadily throughout pregnancy in the placebo group. In the supplemented group there was no increase between the 12th and 24th week of gestation and thereafter the increase was only 60 per cent of the placebo group. After delivery the mean absorption in the placebo group was markedly higher. These differences can be explained by the difference in storage iron between the two groups [178].

The commonest haematological problem in pregnancy is anaemia resulting from iron deficiency. The bulk of iron in the body is contained in the haemoglobin of the circulating red cells. Since many women enter pregnancy with depleted stores, it is not surprising that iron deficiency in pregnancy and the puerperium is so common when, in addition to the demands of the fetus and blood loss at delivery, the absolute red cell mass increases by approximately 25 per cent.

Over the years there have been many studies which have proved without doubt that iron supplements prevent the development of anaemia [23,29,56,113,114,127,176] and that even in women taking a good diet who are not apparently anaemic at booking, the mean haemoglobin level can be raised by oral iron therapy throughout pregnancy. The difference in favour of those so treated is most marked at term when the need for haemoglobin is maximal [104,127,143].

Non-haematological effects of iron deficiency

Overt symptoms of iron deficiency are generally not prominent. Defects in oxygen-carrying capacity are compensated for but the health implications of iron deficiency have been examined in a more detailed manner. Of particular interest are effects produced by impairment of the function of iron-dependent tissue enzymes. These are not the ultimate manifestation of severe untreated iron deficiency, but develop along with the fall in haemoglobin concentration [47].

It has been possible to demonstrate a marked decrease in work capacity in the iron-depleted but non-anaemic rat due to impaired mitochondrial function. There is also an impairment in temperature maintenance which has been shown in human subjects. Studies have suggested behavioural abnormalities in children with iron deficiency related to changes in concentration of chemical mediators in the brain. Iron deficiency in the absence of anaemia is also associated with poor performance on the Bayley Mental Development Index [139]. It has also been shown that children with iron-deficiency anaemia in infancy are at risk for long-lasting developmental disadvantage compared with their peers who have better iron status [112]. These developmental delays in iron-deficient infants can be reversed by treatment with iron [85].

Progress is being made in defining the biochemical abnormalities produced by iron deficiency in the central nervous system. It is well known that parenteral treatment of megaloblastic anaemia with appropriate haematinics, either folic acid or vitamin B_{12}, results in an immediate subjective feeling of improvement and well-being in the patient long before the haemoglobin level starts to rise. This is because of the non-haematological effects of depletion of these vitamins on various tissues. I have observed a similar immediate subjective feeling of well-being in those few patients under my care who have received a total dose infusion of iron, presumably for similar reasons (E.A. Letsky, personal observations). Tissue enzyme malfunction undoubtedly occurs even in the very first stages of iron deficiency. Effects of iron deficiency on neurovascular transmission may be responsible for anecdotal reports of increased blood loss at delivery in anaemic women given the importance of a well-contracted uterus to achieve haemostasis at the placental site post-partum. The various effects of iron deficiency may be responsible for the reported association between anaemia and pre-term birth [95,159]. It is obvious that the prevention of nutritional iron deficiency is a desirable objective, especially when there is maximal stress on the haemopoietic system in pregnancy.

Even more far-reaching effects of maternal iron deficiency during pregnancy have been suggested. A retrospective study of 8000 deliveries at a busy obstetric unit in Oxford showed a correlation between maternal iron deficiency, high placental weight and an increased ratio of placental to birthweight [63]. High blood pressure in adult life has been linked with lower birthweight and high placental/birthweight ratios. Prophylaxis of iron deficiency during pregnancy may therefore have important implications for the prevention of adult hypertension which appears to have its origin in fetal life [63].

Haemoglobin concentration

A reduction in concentration of circulating haemoglobin is a relatively late development in iron deficiency. This is preceded by a depletion of iron stores and then a reduction in serum iron before there is any detectable change in haemoglobin level. However, measurement of haemoglobin is the simplest, non-invasive practical test at our disposal and is the one investigation on which further action is usually taken.

The changes in blood volume and haemodilution are so variable that the normal range of haemoglobin concentration in healthy pregnancy at 30 weeks' gestation in women who have received parenteral iron is from 10 to 14.5 g/dl. However, haemoglobin values of <10.5 g/dl in the second and third trimesters are probably abnormal and require further investigation.

Red cell indices

The appearance of red cells on a stained film is a relatively insensitive gauge of iron status in pregnancy. The size of the red cell (MCV), its haemoglobin content (MCH) and haemoglobin concentration (MCHC) can be calculated from the red cell count (RBC), haemoglobin concentration and packed cell volume (PCV). A better guide to the diagnosis of iron deficiency in pregnancy is the examination of these red cell indices (Table 2.1, (see below).

The earliest effect of iron deficiency on the erythrocyte is a reduction in cell size (MCV) and with the dramatic changes in red cell mass and plasma volume of pregnancy this appears to be the most sensitive indicator of underlying established iron deficiency, but may still remain normal when stores first become depleted. Hypochromia and a fall in MCHC only appear with more severe degree of iron depletion.

Of course some women enter pregnancy with already established anaemia due to iron deficiency or with grossly depleted iron stores and they will quickly develop florid anaemia with reduced MCV, MCH and MCHC. These do not present any problems in diagnosis. It is those women who enter pregnancy in precarious iron balance with a normal haemoglobin who present the most difficult diagnostic problems.

Serum iron and total iron binding capacity (TIBC)

In health, the serum iron of adult non-pregnant

women lies between 13 and 27 μmol/l. It shows marked individual diurnal variation and fluctuates even from hour to hour. The total iron binding capacity in the non-pregnant state lies in the range 45–72 μmol/l. It is raised in association with iron deficiency and found to be low in chronic inflammatory states. In the non-anaemic the TIBC is approximately one-third saturated with iron.

Most workers report a fall in the serum iron and percentage saturation of the TIBC in pregnancy; the fall in serum iron can largely be prevented by iron supplements. Serum iron even in combination with TIBC is not a reliable indication of iron stores because it fluctuates so widely and is also affected by recent ingestion of iron and other factors such as infection not directly involved with iron metabolism. With these considerable reservations a serum iron of <12 μmol/l and a TIBC saturation of <15 per cent indicate deficiency of iron during pregnancy.

Free erythrocyte protoporphyrin (FEP)

Erythroblast protoporphyrin represents the substrate unused for haem synthesis and levels rise when there is defective iron supply for the developing red cell. This test takes 2–3 weeks to become abnormal once iron stores are depleted. Estimation may be of value in patients recently treated with iron because there is also a delay in values returning to normal. However, the use of this estimation is limited in that a misleading rise in FEP levels is observed in patients with chronic inflammatory disease, malignancy or infection.

Ferritin

Ferritin, a high molecular weight glycoprotein previously thought to be a totally intracellular iron storage compound, circulates in the plasma of healthy adults in amounts in the range of 15–300 μg/l [88]. It is stable, not affected by recent ingestion of iron, and appears to reflect the iron stores accurately and quantitatively — particularly in the lower range associated with iron deficiency which is so important in pregnancy [183]. A study of serum ferritin during the course of pregnancy in 154 women was carried out in Cardiff [45]. The patients were divided randomly into roughly equal groups, one of which received oral iron supplements. Although there was a rapid decrease in iron stores during early pregnancy in all women studied, the stores (as assessed by serum ferritin levels) were prevented from reaching iron-deficient levels during the latter half of pregnancy in the supplemented group. This pattern has been demonstrated previously in an examination of the stainable iron in bone marrow at term [104]. Interestingly, the concentration of ferritin in the cord blood was substantially greater than the maternal level at term in all cases; but the babies born to iron-deficient mothers had significantly decreased cord ferritin levels compared to the others.

This trend was apparent in the data of another study of maternal and infant iron stores [152], although the authors interpreted their data without reference to it. There is a reduction in the iron accumulated by the fetuses of mothers with depleted iron stores and this may have an important bearing on the iron stores of the child during the first year of life.

Serum ferritin is estimated by a sensitive immunoradiometric assay. Even if there is a delay in obtaining the result, it is valuable to have an accurate assessment of iron stores before therapy is started.

In ideal circumstances these measurements, together with the haemoglobin concentration, allow classification of iron-deficient individuals — those with depleted stores (decreased ferritin only), those with severe iron deficiency but as yet no anaemia (decreased ferritin and reduced TIBC saturation plus an increased FEP), and those with anaemia due to iron deficiency (reduced haemoglobin concentration and iron-deficient indices in addition to decreased ferritin, reduced TIBC saturation and increased FEP).

Marrow iron

The most rapid and reliable method of assessing iron stores in pregnancy is by examination of an appropriately stained preparation of a bone marrow sample. If properly performed, marrow aspiration need not result in any major discomfort — in skilful hands the procedure takes no more than 10 min. The iliac crest (anterior or posterior) should always be used as the aspiration site in preference to the sternum, for the benefit and comfort of the patient. In the absence of iron supplementation there is no detectable stainable iron in over 30 per cent of women at term [104]. A block of incorporation of iron into haemoglobin occurs in the course of chronic inflammation particularly of the urinary tract even if iron stores are replete. This problem will be revealed by examination of the marrow aspirate stained for iron.

Management of iron deficiency

In the UK the management of iron deficiency in pregnancy has largely become one of prevention by daily oral supplements. Oral supplementation of 60–80 mg elemental iron per day from early pregnancy maintains the haemoglobin in the recognized normal range for pregnancy but does not maintain or restore the iron stores [51,104]. WHO recommends that supplements of 30–60 mg/day be given to those pregnant women who have normal iron stores and 120–240 mg to those women with none. Whether all pregnant women need iron is controversial and is discussed below, but if it is accepted that iron is necessary, a bewildering number of preparations of varying expense are available for use. In those women to whom additional iron cannot be given by the oral route either because of non-compliance or because of unacceptable side-effects, intramuscular injection of 1000 mg iron more than ensures iron sufficiency for that pregnancy. The injections are painful and can stain the skin but in contrast to the rat there is no risk of incurring malignancy at the injection site in humans [119].

There is no haematological benefit in giving parenteral as opposed to oral iron, but some women will not take oral preparations. The sole advantage of parenteral therapy is that the physician can be sure that such patients have received adequate supplementation.

The side-effects of oral administration of iron have been shown to be related to the quantity administered [68]; if the daily dose is reduced to 100 mg they are rare with any preparation. Although some women do have gastric symptoms the most common complaint is constipation which is usually easily overcome by simple measures. Slow-release preparations, which are generally more expensive, are said to be relatively free of side-effects. This is only so because much of the iron is not released at all, is unabsorbed and excreted unchanged. This means that increased doses may have to be given to cover requirements, thereby further increasing expense. The majority of women tolerate the cheaper preparations with no significant side-effects and in the interests of economy these should be tried first. All the preparations used routinely in pregnancy are now combined with an appropriate dose of folic acid (see below). Prophylaxis of iron deficiency therefore depends partly on good antenatal care, but ultimately on regular attendance at the antenatal clinic and cooperation in taking the prescribed medication. In spite of evidence to the contrary, not all obstetricians are convinced of the value of prophylaxis with haematinics.

The management of iron-deficiency anaemia diagnosed late in pregnancy presents a particular challenge to the obstetrician because a satisfactory response must be obtained in a limited time. Parenteral iron is useful in this situation particularly if the woman cannot be relied upon to take oral medication. Iron sorbitol citrate can be given as a series of intramuscular injections but it is associated with toxic reactions such as headache, nausea and vomiting if given simultaneously with oral iron [161].

Iron dextran was an extensively used preparation and may be administered as a series of intramuscular injections. Unfortunately, this preparation is no longer supplied by the manufacturers for intravenous use in the UK. This preparation does not appear to be associated with toxicity if given simultaneously with oral iron [160,173].

In the absence of any other abnormality an increase in haemoglobin concentration of 1 g/dl/week in the non-pregnant state, 0.8 g/dl/week in pregnancy can be reasonably expected with adequate iron treatment, whether oral or parenteral. If there is not time to achieve a reasonable haemoglobin concentration before delivery, blood transfusion is indicated.

The case for prophylactic iron therapy

There is still considerable controversy about whether the fall in haemoglobin concentration which occurs in healthy women during pregnancy is an indication of iron deficiency and whether raising the haemoglobin with iron confers any benefit [3,9]. Many authors are not able to accept that the physiological requirements for iron in pregnancy are considerably higher than the usual intake of most healthy women with apparently good diets in industrialized countries. The arguments about policy among nutritionalists wishing to prevent iron deficiency are complicated by the problem of applying the same strategy in countries with differing standards of living. Paradoxically the greatest experience in prevention comes from those countries where iron deficiency is least common and least severe [89].

There is no doubt that in developing countries the incidence of anaemia and iron deficiency is high and many women enter pregnancy who are either anaemic or who have grossly depleted iron stores. A small but careful study of anaemia in pregnancy from Nigeria showed that once the major problems of malaria and the haemoglobinopathies were partially solved by giving antimalarials and folic acid routinely throughout pregnancy, iron deficiency was also present in many of the patients with pregnancy anaemia. The conclusion was that the deficiency was primarily due to poor iron content in the diet and routine iron supplementation was recommended. Another larger controlled trial from the Philippines [99] showed clearly that those women with normal haemoglobins given iron throughout pregnancy maintained their haemoglobin; anaemic women on a larger dose of iron raised their haemoglobins if compared to those taking placebo or ascorbic acid alone.

One of the earliest large studies in the UK came from Manchester [114]. Over 2000 women were studied during pregnancy. In those not taking iron a progressive drop in the haemoglobin was observed — the lowest level being reached at 32 weeks' gestation — but it took more than a year after delivery before the pre-pregnancy haemoglobin level was re-achieved. Those women who took iron had consistently higher haemoglobins and the effects persisted into the postnatal period — pre-pregnancy haemoglobin levels being much more rapidly re-achieved. However, the majority of the women, whether taking iron or not, were perfectly healthy and had no complaints. This raises the question of whether a haemoglobin level raised by iron therapy is in itself an advantage. There was no advantage in terms of subjective health conferred by iron treatment in another double-blind study [141] in Aberdeen.

In general there is no convincing evidence that the normal pregnant woman is at an advantage if she takes extra iron [84]. The fact that the fall of haemoglobin concentration in normal multigravidae is greater than in primigravidae has been interpreted as indirect evidence of depletion of iron concentration by repeated pregnancy; however, multigravidae have a greater rise of plasma volume than primigravidae and therefore a correspondingly lower haemoglobin is to be expected. All these findings emphasize the important principle that 'normality' in pregnancy cannot be judged by reference to non-pregnant standards. Fall in haemoglobin concentration due to haemodilution seems to cause anxiety in the mind of the obstetrician although a satisfactory level of haemoglobin concentration may indicate an unsatisfactory increase of plasma volume. The association of high maternal haemoglobin concentration with poor outcome of pregnancy in pre-eclampsia is, of course, due to inadequate plasma volume increase [129] and should not be taken as an argument against iron supplements. Plasma volume and red cell mass are under separate control (see above). Moreover the human female is not alone in reducing the concentration of her circulating red cell mass during pregnancy; this phenomenon is observed in other mammalian species as different as the dog, elephant and monkey.

Hemminki and Starfield [72] have reviewed controlled clinical trials of iron administration during pregnancy in developed Western countries. Seventeen trials were found which fulfilled their criteria. Their analysis showed that there was no beneficial effect in terms of birthweight, length of gestation, maternal and infant morbidity and mortality in those women receiving iron compared with controls. They maintain that while age, economic status and poor nutrition affect the outcome, pregnancy anaemia is not related and is simply associated with other risk factors. They did not take into account the withdrawal of anaemic patients from the trials they reviewed. Their analysis may be correct but anaemia remains a potential danger in pregnancy especially in the face of haemorrhage. The majority of women who do not receive iron supplements have no stores at all at the end of pregnancy [45,104]. Also offspring of non-anaemic women who have not received supplements have less iron stores than those of iron-replete women [45]. An analysis of factors leading to a 20 per cent reduction in iron deficiency in Swedish women of childbearing age in the 10-year period 1965–75 attributed this to greater prescribing of iron tablets (10 per cent) and fortification of food (7–8 per cent); oral contraception also played a part (2–3 per cent) [67].

The crucial information needed to interpret the physiological anaemia of pregnancy is whether or not the average young woman has sufficient storage iron. Svanberg [178] comments that the absence of iron stores in women of fertile age is not physiological and that the increased iron demand during pregnancy cannot be met by increased absorption. The conclusion is that, even with maximum iron content in the diet, the immediate demands of pregnancy cannot be covered by an increased absorption from the diet. From the evidence that is available, it would appear that a high proportion of women in their reproductive years do lack storage iron [45,104].

A study from South Africa [116a] reports the findings in Indian and black women attending antenatal clinics. Anaemia, by WHO standards, was found in 13 per cent of the Asian women in the first trimester, increasing to 28 and 47 per cent in the second and third trimesters respectively, but iron deficiency (serum ferritin <12 μg/l) was found to be far greater, i.e. 35 per cent in the first trimester rising to 86 per cent in the third.

The pregnant black women underwent similar investigations. Anaemia was detected in 19 per cent rising to 29 per cent. However, the proportion with iron deficiency was not so dramatically increased as in the Asian counterparts — 19 per cent rising to 40 per cent in the last trimester. This probably reflects the greater number of vegetarians among the Asian populations who therefore will not have sufficient reserves of storage iron to meet the needs of pregnancy.

The observations that oral iron supplements may reduce both the bioavailability of zinc [120] and maternal zinc levels during pregnancy [89] has led to speculation about the relationship of these observations. There have also been reports suggesting that maternal tissue zinc depletion is associated with fetal growth retardation [121]. The results of a study of serial changes in serum zinc and magnesium concentrations before conception, throughout pregnancy to 12 weeks post-partum, indicates that the decrease in concentrations of both elements is a normal physiological adjustment to pregnancy and that oral iron supplementation does not influence these changes [165].

It has been suggested that women at risk from iron-deficiency anaemia could be identified by estimating the serum ferritin concentration in the first trimester. A serum ferritin of <50 μg/l in early pregnancy is an indication for daily iron supplements. Women with serum ferritin concentrations of >80 μg/l are unlikely to require iron supplements. Unnecessary routine supplementation would thus be avoided in women enjoying good nutrition, and any risk to the pregnancy arising from severe maternal anaemia would be avoided by prophylaxis and prompt treatment [12].

A study carried out at Queen Charlotte's Maternity Hospital, London, is of interest in this respect. Serum ferritin levels were estimated in 669 consecutive women who booked at 16 weeks' gestation or earlier with a haemoglobin concentration of 11 g/dl or above. As many as 552 women (82 per cent) had serum ferritins of 50 μg/l or below, and would therefore qualify for routine daily iron supplements by the above criteria. These women were drawn from a cosmopolitan, largely well-nourished population; 12 per cent had serum ferritins of <12 μg/l and were therefore already iron deficient at booking in spite of having a haemoglobin of 11 g/dl or more. Only 51 (8 per cent) had ferritins of 80 μg/l or above [106].

In summary, negative iron balance throughout pregnancy, particularly in the latter half, may lead to iron-deficiency anaemia in the third trimester. This hazard — together with the increasing evidence of non-haematological effects of iron deficiency on exercise tolerance, cerebral function and temperature control — leads me to the conclusion that it is safer, more practical, and in the long term less expensive in terms of investigation, hospital admission and treatment, to give all women iron supplements from 16 weeks' gestation — especially as this would appear to do no harm [100,165].

Folic acid

Folate metabolism

Folic acid and iron are particularly important in nutrition during pregnancy. At a cellular level folic acid is reduced first to dihydrofolic (DHF) acid and then to tetrahydrofolic (THF) acid which forms the pivot of cellular folate metabolism since it is fundamental (through linkage with L-carbon fragments) both to cell growth and cell division. The more active a tissue is in reproduction and growth, the more dependent it will be on the efficient turnover and supply of folate co-enzymes. Bone marrow and epithelial linings are therefore particularly at risk.

Requirements for folate are increased in pregnancy to meet the needs of the fetus, the placenta, uterine hypertrophy and the expanded maternal red cell mass. They are increased still further by multiple pregnancy (see below). The placenta transports folate actively to the fetus even in the face of maternal deficiency, but maternal folate metabolism is altered early in pregnancy like many other maternal functions, before fetal demands act directly.

Plasma folate

With the exception of haemoglobin concentration and plasma iron, folic acid must be one of the most studied substances in maternal blood, but there are comparatively few serial data available. However, it is generally agreed that plasma folate levels fall as pregnancy advances so that at term they are about half the non-pregnant values [7,20,52,101]. Plasma clearance of folate by the kidneys is more than doubled by as early as the 8th week of gestation [49,101]. It has been suggested that urinary loss may be a major factor in the fall of serum folate. Although the glomerular filtration rate is raised (see Chapter 7), the marked contrast between the comparatively unchanging plasma levels and the wide variation in urinary loss suggests a change in tubular reabsorption. It is unlikely that this is a major drain on maternal resources and it cannot play more than a marginal role [101].

There have been conflicting reports about the part intestinal malabsorption may play in the aetiology of folate deficiency of pregnancy. Traditionally absorption has been assessed from plasma levels following an oral load. Earlier reports of decreased absorption [22] were probably due to the underestimation of the rapid clearance of folate following an oral dose. Placental and maternal tissues contribute from an early stage probably under the influence of oestrogens, as oral contraceptives also increase plasma clearance of folate [174]. There is no change in absorption of either folate monoglutamates or polyglutamates in healthy pregnancy [102,119], although there is a wide scatter of results. The incidence of abnormally low serum folates in late pregnancy varies with the population studied and presumably reflects the local nutritional standards.

Substantial day-to-day variation of plasma folate occurs and postprandial increases have been noted. This variability limits the diagnostic value of plasma folate estimation when occasional samples taken at a casual antenatal clinic visit are considered.

It could be argued that the changes noted in pregnancy are positively advantageous. There is no reason why reduced plasma levels of nutrients such as folate should necessarily indicate deficiency, particularly when the levels of other nutrients such as glucose and amino acids are disregarded. The reduced levels may aid conservation in the face of a raised glomerular filtration rate. It is possible that the placenta may be able to compete more effectively with maternal tissues for folate supplies at lower maternal plasma levels and compensate for its relatively small receptive area [101].

Red cell folate

The estimation of red cell folate may provide more useful information than plasma folate as it does not reflect the daily and other short-term variations of plasma folate. It is thought to give a better indication of overall body tissue levels, but the turnover of red blood cells is slow and there will be delay before significant reductions in the folate concentrations of the red cells, due to folate deficiency, are evident.

A number of investigations of erythrocyte folate in pregnancy have shown a slight downward trend even though, as would be expected, the fall is not so marked as that noted for plasma [6,24]. There is evidence that patients who have a low red cell folate at the beginning of pregnancy are more likely to develop megaloblastic anaemia in the third trimester [24].

Excretion of formiminoglutamic acid (FIGLU)

A loading dose of histidine leads to increased FIGLU excretion in the urine when there is folate deficiency (the FIGLU test). There is no longer much to recommend this as a screening test in pregnancy primarily because the metabolism of histidine is altered [20] and this results in increased FIGLU excretion in normal early pregnancy [175].

Folic acid post-partum

In the 6 weeks following delivery all indices of folate metabolism tend to return to non-pregnant values. However, should any deficiency of folate have developed and remained untreated in pregnancy, it may present clinically for the first time in the puerperium and its consequences may be detected for many months after delivery. Lactation provides an added folate stress. A folate content of 5 µg per 100 ml of human milk and a yield of 500 ml daily implies a loss of 25 µg folate daily in breast milk. In the Bantu, megaloblastic anaemia appears frequently in the year following pregnancy in association with lactation. Dietary folate intake is poor and it has been shown that folate deficiency becomes more apparent, as demonstrated by using FIGLU excretion, as lactation continues [164]. Red cell folate levels in lactating mothers are significantly lower than those of their infants during the first year of life [20]. In the UK, as early as 1919, Osler described the severe anaemias of pregnancy which had a high colour index and a striking incidence in the post-partum period [140].

Interpretation of investigations

The value of these various investigations in predicting megaloblastic anaemia and assessing subclinical folate deficiency has been the subject of numerous reports. Using these various tests it appears that folate 'deficiency' in pregnancy is not always accompanied by significant haematological change [164,175].

Even in the absence of any significant haematological changes in the peripheral blood, megaloblastic haemopoiesis should be suspected when the expected response to adequate iron therapy is not achieved. Evidence of megaloblastic haemopoiesis may become apparent only after iron therapy even though the rise in haemoglobin concentration appears adequate. No help can be expected from the use of tests of folate status. 'Abnormal' results are obtained with most of the tests but these are not significantly different from results in healthy pregnant women. The decline of serum folic acid levels from a mean of 6.0 µg/l in the non-pregnant to 3.4 µg/l at term should be viewed only as the physiological consequence of maternal tissue uptake, urinary loss and placental transfer — not of evidence of folate deficiency. The delay in fall of red cell folate makes this too impractical a test for folate deficiency in pregnancy. Therefore the diagnosis of folate deficiency in pregnancy has to be made ultimately on morphological grounds; this usually involves examinations of a suitably prepared marrow aspirate.

Megaloblastic anaemia

Folic acid deficiency

The cause of megaloblastic anaemia in pregnancy is nearly always folate deficiency. Vitamin B_{12} is only very rarely implicated (see below). A survey of reports from the UK over the past two decades suggest an incidence ranging from 0.2 to 5 per cent, but a considerably greater number of women have megaloblastic changes in their marrow which are not suspected on examination of the peripheral blood alone [20,111]. The incidence of megaloblastic anaemia in other parts of the world is considerably greater and is thought to reflect the nutritional standards of the population. Several workers have pointed to the poor socioeconomic status of their patients as the major aetiological factor contributing to anaemia [20,31], which may be further exacerbated by seasonal changes in the availability of stable foodstuffs. Food folates are only partially available and the amount of folate supplied in the diet is difficult to quantify. In the UK, analysis of daily folate intake in foodstuffs showed a range of 129–300 μg [19]. The folate content of 24-hour food collections in various studies in Sweden and Canada proved to be about 200 μg, with a range as great as 70–600 μg [20].

Foods that are very rich in folate include broccoli, spinach and brussel sprouts, but up to 90 per cent of their folate content is lost within the first few minutes, by boiling or steaming, and they are unlikely to be eaten raw. Asparagus, avocados and mushrooms also have a fairly high folate content but are expensive. Natural folates are protected from oxidation and degradation by the presence of reducing substances such as ascorbate. Analysis of the folate content of food will give very low results if ascorbate is not added to the assay system — as occurred in the very earliest studies [20]. Having established the content of folate in food, there is only indirect evidence about its absorption. Monoglutamates are almost completely absorbed. Polyglutamates from different sources are variably available, but in general are less well absorbed, so that total folate intake should be combined with information about the source of food folate to give a realistic appraisal of the available folate content. In general, dietary intake is likely to be greater, rather than smaller, during pregnancy, but obviously in certain areas of the world malnutrition is an essential aetiological factor in determining folate status.

The effects of dietary inadequacy may be further amplified by frequent childbirth and multiple pregnancy. An incidence of one in 11 in twin pregnancies compared with the expected incidence of one in 80 was noted in one survey of over 1000 patients with folate deficiency [20].

The normal dietary folate intake is inadequate to prevent megaloblastic changes in the bone marrow in approximately 25 per cent of pregnant women. The falls in serum and red cell folate levels could be a physiological phenomenon in pregnancy but the incidence of megaloblastic change in the bone marrow is reduced only when the blood folate levels are maintained in a steady state by adequate oral supplements. There is much controversy about the requirement for folate, particularly during pregnancy. WHO recommendations for daily folate intake are as high as 800 μg in the antenatal period, 600 μg during lactation and 400 μg in the non-pregnant adult [196]. There is an increased need of about 100 μg folic acid daily during pregnancy which, without supplements, must be found from natural folates in the diet [20]. The WHO recommended intakes clearly overestimate the needs. The daily amount of folate that has been given prophylactically in pregnancy varies from 30 to 500 μg and even to pharmacological doses of 5–15 mg [20]. Thirty micrograms daily was found to be too small to influence folate status appreciably [23] but supplements of 100 μg or more all reduced the frequency of megaloblastic changes in the marrow and eliminated megaloblastic anaemia as a clinical entity [19].

In order to meet the folate needs of those women with a dietary intake well below average, the daily supplement during pregnancy should be about 200–300 μg daily — still very much below the WHO recommended daily intake. The case for giving prophylactic folate throughout pregnancy is strong [20,60], particularly in countries where overt megaloblastic anaemia is frequent.

The main point at issue over recent years, however, is whether the apparently intrinsic folate deficiency of pregnancy can predispose the mother to a wide variety of other obstetric abnormalities and complications, in particular abortion, fetal malformations, prematurity and ante-partum haemorrhage [20,31,57,149]. The extensive literature would seem to be almost equally divided in its opinion, but there is virtually no evidence that the routine use of folic acid supplements *during* pregnancy has reduced the incidence of anything but megaloblastic anaemia [53,101] except in areas of malnutrition where an increase in birthweight has been noted [10] (see p. 46 for preconception prophylaxis).

Severe megaloblastic anaemia is now uncommon in the UK during pregnancy or the puerperium but may occasionally still occur. Two case histories of severe macrocytic anaemia presenting in the puerperium with pancytopenia have been published [116a]. In both cases leukaemia was considered because of the increase in promyelocytes in the bone marrow as well as florid megaloblastic change. Both responded completely to therapy with folic acid. Two similar cases have been seen at Queen Charlotte's Maternity Hospital, London, having been treated with intravenous iron alone for severe anaemia developing late in pregnancy, without additional parenteral folate supplementation.

An argument against routine folate supplementation in pregnancy is unrecognized vitamin B_{12} deficiency. Folate can aggravate the neuropathy due to vitamin B_{12} deficiency. The risk of adverse effects from folate administered to a pregnant women suffering from vitamin B_{12} deficiency is very small indeed (see below). In fact there is *no* report of this occurring amongst the many thousands of women who have received folate supplements in pregnancy [21].

Folic acid should never be given without supplemental iron. A wide variety of preparations supplying both iron and folate are available and, provided that the folate content is not less than 100 µg daily, all are satisfactory for prophylaxis in pregnancy.

Once megaloblastic haemopoiesis is established, treatment of folic acid deficiency becomes more difficult, presumably due to megaloblastic changes in the gastrointestinal tract resulting in impaired absorption. There is a small number of patients [60] who fail to respond to parenteral folate therapy and who only recover after delivery. It is far better to intervene before these difficulties arise and give routine prophylaxis throughout pregnancy.

Disorders which may affect folate requirement in pregnancy

Problems may be caused in pregnancy by disorders which are associated with an increased folate requirement in the non-pregnant state. Women with haemolytic anaemia, particularly hereditary haemolytic conditions such as haemoglobinopathies and hereditary spherocytosis, require extra supplements from early pregnancy if development of megaloblastic anaemia is to be avoided. The recommended supplement in this situation is 5–10 mg orally daily. The anaemia associated with thalassaemia trait is not strictly due to haemolysis but to ineffective erythropoiesis (see below). However, the increased, though abortive, marrow turnover still results in folate depletion and such women would probably benefit from the routine administration of oral folic acid 5 mg daily from early pregnancy.

Folate supplements are of particular importance in the management of sickle cell syndromes during pregnancy if aplastic crises and megaloblastic anaemia are to be avoided.

Anticonvulsant drugs and pregnancy

The additional demand for folate during pregnancy leads to a rapid fall in red cell folate and to a high incidence of megaloblastic anaemia in those women taking anticonvulsant drugs for control of epilepsy. This is not surprising because non-pregnant individuals taking anticonvulsants tend to become folate deficient [20].

The risk of interferring with the control of epilepsy by the regular administration of iron–folate preparations during pregnancy and the precipitation of status epilepticus [177] has been overestimated [74]. Anticonvulsant therapy during pregnancy is associated with an increased incidence of congenital abnormality [75], prematurity and low birthweight [14]. Therefore folate supplements should be given to all epileptic women taking anticonvulsants in pregnancy (see Chapter 15) as well as before conception (see below).

In addition, neonates born to women taking anticonvulsant drugs may have low prothrombin times and are at risk of bleeding. This risk appears to be preventable by giving the mothers vitamin K, 20 mg daily for 2 weeks before delivery [36].

The fetus and folate deficiency

There is an increased risk of megaloblastic anaemia occurring in the neonate of a folate-deficient mother, especially if delivery is pre-term.

The young infant's requirement for folate has been estimated at 20–50 μg/day (four to 10 times the adult requirement on a weight basis). Serum and red cell folate levels are consistently higher in cord than in maternal blood, but the pre-term infant is in severe negative folate balance because of high growth rate and reduced intake. The usual fall in serum and red cell folate in the term neonate is yet greater in the pre-term neonate and even in the absence of other complicating factors may result in megaloblastic anaemia. This can be prevented by giving supplements of folic acid 50 μg/day [71,138].

Data suggesting an association between periconceptional folic acid deficiency and harelip, cleft palate and most important of all, neural tube defects [103,168,169] which have been well reviewed in the past [58] have now been clarified by some important recent studies.

The association between periconceptional folate deficiency and recurrence of neural tube defects has been confirmed in a mass multicentre controlled trial of pre-pregnancy folate supplementation [128]. More recently, it has also been shown in a large randomized controlled trial in Hungary [32] that periconceptional supplement of 800 μg of folic acid in a combined vitamin preparation prevented the first occurrence of neural tube defects. The prevalence of harelip with or without cleft palate was not reduced by this supplementation.

Preconception prophylaxis

We do not yet understand the association between folic acid and neural tube closure — whether supplementation corrects a dietary deficiency, overcomes a defect in absorption or metabolism, or provides some extra benefit at supraphysiological doses. It is recommended that women contemplating pregnancy should take folate supplements of 400 μg daily [40,154]. This amount is currently marketed in the UK. A policy of targeted food fortification is under consideration both in the USA and UK.

Vitamin B_{12} deficiency

Muscle, red cell and serum vitamin B_{12} concentrations fall during pregnancy [7,20,39,181]. Non-pregnant serum levels of 205–1025 μg/l fall to 20–510 μg/l at term, with low levels in multiple pregnancy [181]. Women who smoke tend to have lower serum B_{12} levels [117], which may account for the positive correlation between birthweight and serum levels in non-deficient mothers.

Vitamin B_{12} absorption is unaltered in pregnancy [20,30]. It is possible that tissue uptake is increased by the action of oestrogens as oral contraceptives also cause a fall in serum vitamin B_{12} level. Cord blood serum vitamin B_{12} is higher than that of maternal blood. The fall in serum vitamin B_{12} in the mother is related to preferential transfer of absorbed B_{12} to the fetus at the expense of maintaining the maternal serum concentration [20], but the placenta does not transfer vitamin B_{12} with the same efficiency as it does folate. Low serum vitamin B_{12} levels in early pregnancy in vegetarian Hindus do not fall further while their infants often have subnormal concentrations. The vitamin B_{12} binding capacity of plasma increases in pregnancy analogous to the rise in iron binding capacity. The rise is confined to the liver-derived transcobalamin II concerned with transport rather than the leukocyte-derived transcobalamin I which is raised in other myeloproliferative conditions [50].

Pregnancy does not make a great impact on maternal vitamin B_{12} stores. Adult stores are of the order of 3000 μg or more and vitamin B_{12} stores in the newborn infant are about 50 μg [50].

Addisonian pernicious anaemia does not usually occur during the reproductive years. Vitamin B_{12} deficiency is associated with infertility and pregnancy is likely only if the deficiency is remedied [86]. Vitamin B_{12} deficiency in pregnancy may be associated with chronic tropical sprue. The megaloblastic anaemia which develops is due to long-standing vitamin B_{12} deficiency and superadded folate deficiency; the cord vitamin B_{12} levels remain above the maternal levels in these cases, but the concentration in the breast milk follows the maternal serum levels [20].

The recommended intake of vitamin B_{12} is 2 μg/day in the non-pregnant and 3 μg/day during pregnancy [196]. This will be met by almost any diet which contains animal products, however deficient in other essential substances. Strict vegans who do not eat animal-derived substances may have a deficient intake of vitamin B_{12} and their diet should be supplemented during pregnancy.

Haemoglobinopathies

Following the influx of immigrants from all parts of the world, obstetricians in the UK frequently encounter women with genetic defects of haemoglobin and its synthesis that are seldom seen in the indigenous population. It is important to recognize the specific defects early in pregnancy for the following reasons:

1 the clinical effects may complicate obstetric management and appropriate precautions can be taken;

2 it is now possible to offer prenatal diagnosis to those women carrying a fetus at risk of a serious defect of haemoglobin synthesis or structure at a time when termination of pregnancy is feasible [132,191].

The haemoglobinopathies are inherited defects of haemoglobin, resulting from impaired globin synthesis (thalassaemia syndromes) or from structural abnormality of globin (haemoglobin variants). Only some of these anomalies are of practical importance, so particular emphasis will be placed on those where adverse effects may be aggravated by pregnancy. A proper appreciation of these defects requires some understanding of the structure of normal haemoglobin.

The haemoglobin molecule consists of four globin chains each of which is associated with a haem complex. There are three normal haemoglobins in humans; HbA, HbA_2 and HbF — each of which contains two pairs of polypeptide globin chains. The synthesis and structure of the four globin chains α, β, γ and δ are under separate control (Fig. 2.1). The adult levels shown in Fig. 2.1 are those achieved by 6 months of age. It is obvious that only those conditions affecting the synthesis or structure of HbA ($\alpha_2 \beta_2$) which should comprise over 95 per cent of the total circulating haemoglobin in the adult, will be of significance for the mother during pregnancy. α chain production is under the control of four genes, two inherited from each parent; as can be seen the α chains are common to all three haemoglobins. β chain production, on the other hand, is under the control of only two genes — one inherited from each parent.

The thalassaemia syndromes

The thalassaemia syndromes are the commonest genetic disorders of the blood and constitute a vast public health problem in many parts of the world. The basic defect is a reduced rate of globin chain synthesis, the red cells being formed with an inadequate haemoglobin content. The syndromes are divided into two main groups, the α and the β thalassaemias depending on whether the α or the β globin chain synthesis of adult haemoglobin ($HbA\alpha_2 \beta_2$) is depressed.

α thalassaemia

Normal individuals have four functional α globin genes. α thalassaemia, unlike β thalassaemia, is

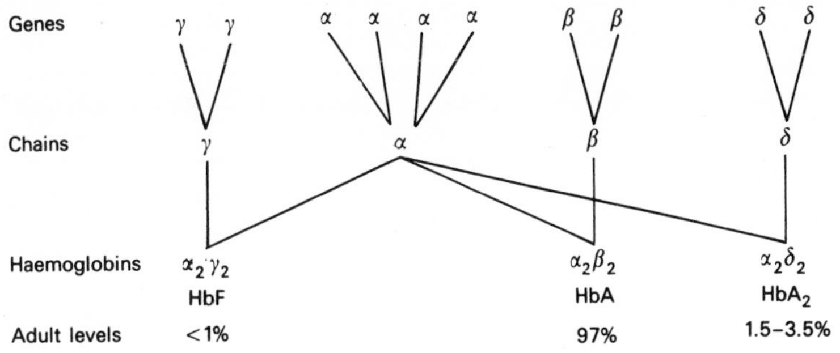

Fig. 2.1. Genetic control of globin synthesis. The adult levels shown are those reached by 6 months of age.

often, but not always, a gene deletion defect. There are two forms of α thalassaemia trait, the result of inheriting three or two normal α genes instead of the usual four. They are called α^+ and α^0 thalassaemia (Fig. 2.2). HbH disease is an intermediate form of α thalassaemia in which there is only one functional α gene and is the name given to the unstable haemoglobin formed by tetramers of the β chain (β_4), when there is a relative lack of α chains. α thalassaemia major in which there are no functional α genes (both parents having transmitted α^0 thalassaemia) is incompatible with life and pregnancy ends usually prematurely in a hydrops which will only survive a matter of hours if born alive. This is a common condition in South-East Asia. The name Hb Barts was given to tetramers of the γ chain of fetal haemoglobin (HbF$\alpha_2\gamma_2$). The tetramer (γ_4) forms *in utero* when no α chains are made and was first identified in a Chinese baby born at St Bartholomew's Hospital, London.

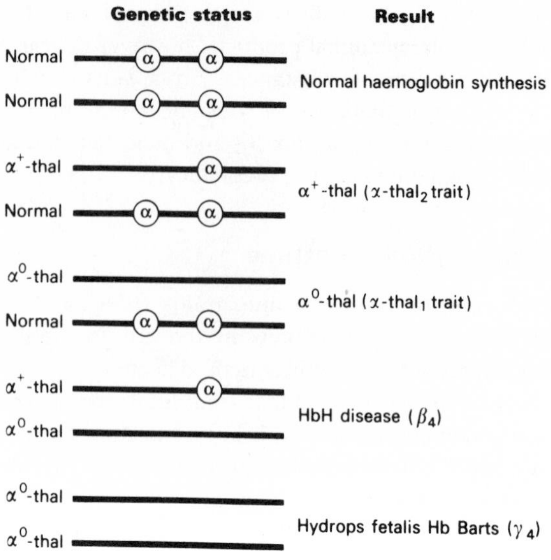

Fig. 2.2. Normal α gene status and the various changes observed in thalassaemia due to α gene deletion.

Management of α thalassaemia

During pregnancy, with its stress on the haemopoietic system, carriers of α thalassaemia, particularly those with α^0 thalassaemia (two deleted genes) may become very anaemic. They can be identified for further tests at booking, by finding abnormal red cell indices (Table 2.1). They have smaller red cells (MCV) and a reduced individual MCH, although the MCHC is usually within the normal range (Table 2.1). These changes are often minimal in α^+ thalassaemia (one deleted gene) (Fig. 2.2) but this condition is not so important as α^0 thalassaemia in terms of genetic counselling and prenatal diagnosis. This diagnosis can only be confirmed by globin chain synthesis studies or, in the case of gene deletion, by DNA analysis of nucleated cells. There is no abnormal haemoglobin made or excess or lack of one or other of the normal haemoglobins. These individuals need iron and folate oral supplements throughout the antenatal period. Sometimes intramuscular folic acid is helpful but parenteral iron should never be given (see below). If the haemoglobin level is not thought to be adequate for delivery at term, transfusion is indicated.

Patients with HbH disease have a chronic haemolytic anaemia and have 5–30 per cent HbH in their peripheral blood which can be identified by haemoglobin electrophoresis. They have a normal life expectancy but require daily oral folate supplements to cover the demands of increased marrow turnover. During pregnancy it is recommended to give 5.0 mg

Table 2.1. Red cell indices in thalassaemia and iron deficiency. PCV, packed cell volume; RBC, red cell count; Hb, haemoglobin; MCV, mean corpuscular volume; MCH, mean corpuscular haemoglobin; MCHC, mean corpuscular haemoglobin concentration

			Normal range	Iron deficiency	Thalassaemia
PCV/RBC	=	MCV	75–99 fl	↓	↓
Hb/RBC	=	MCH	27–31 pg	↓	↓
Hb/PCV	=	MCHC	32–36 g/dl	↓	→

folate daily to women with HbH disease. They will transmit either α^0 or α^+ thalassaemia to their offspring.

Pregnancy with an α thalassaemia hydropic fetus may be associated with severe, sometimes life-threatening pre-eclampsia in the mother (cf. severe rhesus haemolytic disease). Vaginal deliveries are associated with obstetric complication, due to the large fetus and very bulky placenta. It has been estimated in Thailand that in the absence of obstetric care up to 50 per cent of mothers carrying an hydropic fetus may suffer lethal complications [73]. If routine screening of the parents (see below) indicates that the mother is at risk of carrying such a child — both parents having α^0 thalassaemia — she should be referred for prenatal diagnosis (see below).

β thalassaemia

Thalassaemia major, homozygous thalassaemia resulting from the inheritance of a defective β globin gene from each parent was the first identified form of the thalassaemia syndromes. It was described in the 1920s by Cooley, a physician in practice in the USA. The first few cases were found in the children of Greek and Italian immigrants. The name thalassaemia was derived from the Greek *thalassa* meaning the sea, or in the classical sense the Mediterranean, because it was thought to be confined to individuals of Mediterranean origin; however, we know now that the distribution is virtually worldwide, although the defect is concentrated in a broad band which does not constitute a major health problem in the UK. However, in the UK there is a fair number of heterozygotes, particularly in the immigrant Cypriot and Asian populations. The child of parents who are both carriers of β thalassaemia has a one in four chance of inheriting thalassaemia major. The carrier rate in the UK is about one in 10 000 compared with one in seven in Cyprus. There are between 300 and 400 patients with thalassaemia major in the UK today but worldwide there are over 100 000 babies born each year with the condition.

Although the majority of the 360 or so cases currently living in England are still to be found in and around the Greater London area, there is an increasing proportion of cases in the Midlands, Manchester, Bradford and Leeds. This is not only due to the fact that there has been an influx of Asian immigrants to these areas but that the Cypriot population of Greater London is a homogeneous group who have taken advantage of the availability of prenatal diagnosis. Consequently there has been a dramatic reduction in the number of homozygotes born to Cypriot couples at risk.

The Asian immigrant population, unlike the Cypriot, is very heterogeneous, with incidence of thalassaemia varying markedly from group to group. They continue to have a high incidence of first cousin marriages. A large group of rural Indians and Pakistanis have settled in the industrial towns of the Midlands and North West. Few of this group make use of genetic counselling or fetal diagnosis and the birth of thalassaemic children in this group continues to rise.

Before the days of regular transfusion, a child born with homozygous β thalassaemia would die in the first few years of life from anaemia, congestive cardiac failure and intercurrent infection. Now that regular transfusion is routine where blood is freely available, survival is prolonged into the teens and early twenties. The management problem becomes one of iron overload derived mainly from the transfused red cells. This results in hepatic and endocrine dysfunction and, most important of all, myocardial damage — the cause of death being cardiac failure in the vast majority of cases. Puberty is delayed or incomplete. Successful pregnancy in a truly transfusion-dependent girl is very rare [65]. It remains to be seen how effective recently instituted intensive iron chelation programmes will be. The only way to cure this disease is to replace the defective gene with a healthy one. Bone marrow transplantation (BMT) is having increasing success and the question is no longer whether, but when to transplant the patient with a histocompatible donor. Strategies for stem cell transplantation and gene therapy are being developed. However, it is important that the current group of patients with thalassaemia major are maintained in optimal clinical status if they are to avail themselves of these developments in BMT and genetic engineering [146].

Management of β thalassaemia

Sometimes survival is possible without regular transfusion in thalassaemia major but this usually results in severe bone deformities due to massive expansion of marrow tissue, the site of the largely ineffective erythropoiesis. Although iron loading still occurs from excessive gastrointestinal absorption, stimulated by the accelerated marrow turnover, it is much slower than in those who are transfused and pregnancy may occur in this situation. Extra daily folate supplements should be given but iron in any form is contraindicated. The anaemia should be treated by transfusion during the antenatal period.

Perhaps the commonest problem associated with haemoglobinopathies and pregnancy in the UK today is the anaemia developing in the antenatal period in women who have thalassaemia minor, heterozygous β thalassaemia. They can be identified for further examination of the booking blood by finding, as in α thalassaemia, low MCV and MCH together with a normal MCHC (see Table 2.1). The level of haemoglobin at booking may be normal or slightly below the normal range. The diagnosis will be confirmed by finding a raised concentration of HbA_2 ($\alpha_2\delta_2$) with or without a raised HbF ($\alpha_2\gamma_2$), excess α chains combining with δ and γ chains because of the relative lack of β chains (see Fig. 2.1).

The women with β thalassaemia minor require the usual *oral* iron and folate supplements in the antenatal period. Oral iron for a limited period will not result in significant iron loading, even in the presence of replete iron stores, but parenteral iron should *never* be given. In our experience at Queen Charlotte's Maternity Hospital many women with thalassaemia minor enter pregnancy with depleted iron stores as do many women with normal haemoglobin synthesis. Those women with β thalassaemia trait particularly at risk of iron deficiency include Asian women on a traditional diet [8]. Iron deficiency has also been shown in non-pregnant women in the UK with thalassaemia minor in a study of serum ferritin levels [81]. If the anaemia does not respond to oral iron, and intramuscular folic acid has been tried, transfusion is indicated to achieve an adequate haemoglobin for delivery at term.

Haemoglobin variants

Over 250 structural variants of the globin chains of normal human haemoglobins have been described but the most important by far, both numerically and clinically, is sickle cell haemoglobin (HbS). This is a variant of the β globin chain where there is one amino acid substitution at the sixth position, a glutamine replacing a valine residue. HbS has the unique physical property that, despite being a soluble protein in its oxygenated form, in its reduced state the molecules become stacked on one another, forming tactoids, which distort the red cells to the characteristic shape which gives the haemoglobin its name. Because of their rigid structure these sickled cells tend to block small blood vessels. The sickling phenomenon occurs particularly in conditions of lowered oxygen tension but may also be favoured by acidosis or dehydration and cooling which cause stasis in small blood vessels (Fig. 2.3).

Sickle cell syndromes

The sickling disorders include the heterozygous state for sickle cell haemoglobin, sickle cell trait (HbAS), homozygous sickle cell disease (HbSS), compound heterozygotes of Hb variants, the most important of which is sickle cell/HbC disease (HbSC), and sickle cell thalassaemia. Although these disorders are more commonly seen in black people of African origin, they can be seen in Saudi Arabians, Indians and even in white Mediterraneans.

The characteristic feature of homozygous sickle cell anaemia (HbSS) is the occurrence of periods of health punctuated by periods of crisis. Between 3 and 6 months of age, when normal HbA production

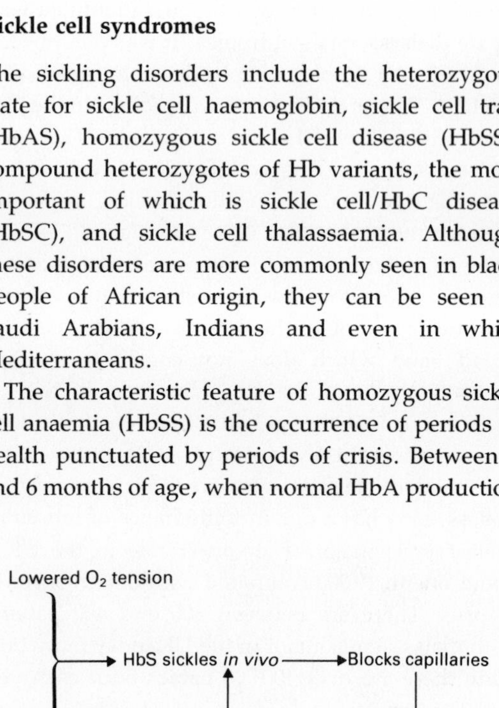

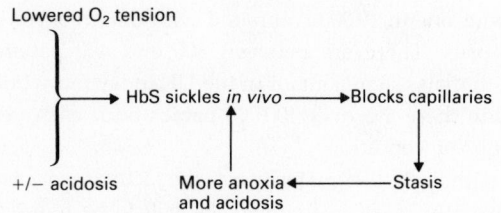

Fig. 2.3. Intravascular sickling.

usually becomes predominant, a chronic haemolytic anaemia develops — the haemoglobin level being between 6 and 9 g/dl. Even if the haemoglobin is in the lower part of the range, symptoms due to anaemia are surprisingly few; because of the low affinity of HbS for oxygen, oxygen delivery to the tissues is facilitated. The acute episodes due to intravascular sickling are of far greater practical importance since they cause vascular occlusion resulting in tissue infarction. The affected part is painful and the clinical manifestations are extremely variable, depending on the site at which sickling takes place. Sickling crises are often precipitated by infection and may be exacerbated by any accompanying dehydration. The majority of deaths are due to massive sickling following an acute infection. Prognosis depends in part on environmental factors such as availability of prompt treatment and prophylaxis of infection, but recent investigation of the variable clinical expression of sickle cell disease suggests that prognosis may largely be genetically determined [148]. Thirty per cent of young adults with sickle cell anaemia have a severe disorder which mimics the 70-year-old with generalized vasculopathy. This may be clinically expressed as glomerulosclerosis, restrictive lung disease, retinopathy and repeated strokes. Sixty per cent have moderate disease while 10 per cent run a benign course. Although high concentrations of fetal haemoglobin HbF inhibit polymerization of HbS they do not necessarily confer protection against all manifestations.

Polymorphisms of the DNA that flank the sickle gene in the promoter or suppressor region of the β^s gene cluster and interaction with α^+ thalassaemia appear to modify the polymerization kinetics of HbS in a more consistent manner.

The rate of progression of disease and development of end-stage vasculopathy are thus genetically controlled. The most severe clinical problems such as renal failure, cerebral infarction, chronic lung disease, retinopathy and leg ulcers are observed in those with the Central African Republic (CAR) haplotype although even this may be ameliorated by interaction with an α thalassaemia gene [148].

Sickle cell haemoglobin C disease (HbSC) is a milder variant of HbSS with normal or near normal levels of haemoglobin. One of the dangers of this condition is that, owing to its mildness, neither the woman nor her obstetrician may be aware of its presence. These women are at risk of massive, sometimes fatal, sickling crises during pregnancy and particularly in the puerperium. It is therefore vital that the abnormality is detected, preferably before pregnancy, so that the appropriate precautions can be taken. Clinical manifestations of the doubly heterozygous condition, sickle cell thalassaemia, are usually indistinguishable from HbSS; those who make detectable amounts of HbA are usually less severely affected but they are still at risk from sickling crises during pregnancy.

Sickle cell trait (HbAS) results in no detectable abnormality under normal circumstances although it is easily diagnosed by specific investigations including haemoglobin electrophoresis (see below). Affected subjects are not anaemic even under the additional stress of pregnancy, unless there are additional complications and sickling crises occur only in situations of extreme anoxia, dehydration and acidosis.

Management of sickle cell syndromes

At present there is no effective long-term method of reducing the liability of red cells to sickle *in vivo*. Once a crisis is established, there is no evidence that alkalis, hyperbaric oxygen, vasodilators, plasma expanders, urea or anticoagulants are of any value. Where beneficial effects have been reported they can usually be attributed to the meticulous care and supportive therapy received by the patient, rather than to the specific measures themselves. Adequate fluid administration alone probably accounts for most of the benefit.

CONTRACEPTION AND SICKLE CELL SYNDROMES

There is much more longitudinal experience in the US than there is as yet in the UK. Methods of contraception vary, but problems arise from the assumption that sicklers are at increased risk of thromboembolism if they use oral contraception. The patient's risk in taking the pill is less than that of pregnancy and there are almost no data to suggest that patients with sickle cell disease run a greater risk than any other patients using low oestrogen preparations [26]. The usual contraindications hold true of course and patients should be monitored carefully for alterations in blood pressure and liver function.

Since patients' response to pregnancy varies, there should not be 'blanket' recommendations for all patients with sickle cell disease.

SICKLE CELL DISEASE AND PREGNANCY

Women with sickle cell disease present special problems in pregnancy [27,144,185]. Fetal loss is high, presumably due to sickling infarcts in the placental circulation [4,26]. Abortion, pre-term labour and other complications are more common than in women with normal haemoglobin. Although many women with sickle cell disease have no complications, the outcome in any individual case is always in doubt. The only consistently successful way of reducing the incidence of these complications due to sickling is by regular blood transfusion at approximately 6-week intervals, to maintain the proportion of HbA at 60–70 per cent of the total [78]. Between 3 and 4 units of blood should be given at each transfusion. This regime has two effects: it dilutes the circulating sickle haemoglobin and, by raising the haemoglobin, reduces the stimulus to the bone marrow and therefore the amount of sickle haemoglobin produced.

Sickle cells have a shorter life than normal red cells and so the effect of each successive transfusion is more beneficial. If this regime has been instituted a general anaesthetic may be given with safety and sickling crises in the course of normal labour are much less likely. The management of sickle cell syndromes in pregnancy in the UK is a relatively recent problem and longitudinal data are lacking here. It is clear on review of the extensive US literature that although risks remain higher for pregnancy complicated by sickle cell disease, modern obstetric care alone, without transfusion, has reduced the maternal morbidity and mortality dramatically and also improved fetal outcome [27, 97,162]. Some obstetric centres still use prophylactic transfusion regimes but the real benefit of such regimes remains to be proven by a large trial with contemporary controls [184]. A small multicentre trial in the US suggests that the outcome is similar in women transfused prophylactically compared to those transfused only when indications arise [98].

These regular transfusion protocols are not without complications. Of course there is a risk of transmitting infection, particularly non A, non B hepatitis to which the pregnant woman with her altered immunity is especially susceptible.

Now that all blood donors are screened for exposure and response to the human immunodeficiency virus (HIV), the much publicized and feared hazard of HIV infection resulting from 1 unit blood donations (non-pooled blood products) is extremely small. The risk of infected blood being undetected has been calculated to be 0.7 per million donations and that is if high risk donors (homosexual men and drug addicts) are giving their blood. Such donors are asked not to give blood in the UK [1].

The most worrying complication of transfusion has been the development of atypical red cell antibodies [155], resulting from the fact that the donor populations differ in ethnic origin from the recipients and carry different minor red cell antigens. This has resulted in extreme difficulties in finding compatible blood [122,185] and even in haemolytic disease of the newborn [185]. There is a real danger that regular top-up transfusions or partial exchange transfusion regimes may become accepted therapy in pregnancy complicated by sickle cell disease before their true benefits and hazards have been properly evaluated. The consensus from the US is that until results of properly planned trials with contemporary controls are available, it would seem wise to give close obstetric supervision, and deliver women where there are special care baby units available. Transfusion should only be given in preparation for general anaesthesia or where there is evidence of maternal distress [26,27,97,98]. If the disorder presents late in pregnancy and there is more urgency because, for instance, the woman is profoundly anaemic or is suffering a crisis, exchange transfusion can be used.

The following suggested exchange transfusion regime for patients with sickle cell disease, has been used with success in a large number of patients (M. Brozović, personal communication).

EXCHANGE TRANSFUSION IN PATIENTS WITH SICKLE CELL DISEASE

1 Ensure free-flowing infusion in one arm. At least 1 l of fluid (dextrose, saline, FPP) should be given before the exchange is started.
2 Have cross-matched blood ready. (Preferably whole blood. Do not pack.)
3 Venesect 0.54 l (1 pint) from the other arm. Often a 50–100 cm^3 syringe must be used.
4 Give 0.54 l (1 pint) of blood.
5 Venesect another 0.54 l. If this is still very difficult and slow, venesection can be carried out at the same time as transfusion.
6 Continue 3, 4 and 5 above until 1 blood volume has been exchanged; estimate proportion of haemoglobin A to S. If S <40 per cent and Hb <8 g it is usually safe to 'top up' to approximately 13–14 g/dl.
7 It is often impossible to exchange more than 2 units on the first day. Venesection usually becomes easier after 2–3 units of exchange.
8 Do not give diuretics. Keep fluid balance chart, watch blood pressure, pulse, note any headache, drowsiness (central nervous system sludging), shortness of breath, etc.
9 Maintain an adequate fluid intake during exchange.
10 Give penicillin because of the probability of splenic infarction and possibility of overwhelming pneumococcal infection. Treat other infections as indicated.

It is obvious that it would be far better to prevent the emergency situation during pregnancy by identification of women before pregnancy and early booking for antenatal care. However, even after preparation with regular transfusion, tissue hypoxia, acidosis and dehydration should be avoided because they will make the patient's own remaining red cells more likely to sickle. Also, perhaps due to the anti-aldosterone actions of progesterone, hyperkalaemia has been reported in pregnant women with sickle cell disease at levels of renal dysfunction below those observed in non-pregnant individuals with HbSS disease [109]. Tourniquets should not be used. To minimize pulmonary infection, prophylactic antibiotics are desirable to cover all anaesthetics. Recurrent pulmonary sickling crises may lead to chronic lung disease. One such case during pregnancy has been reported with maternal death at 31 weeks' gestation [186]. Severe painful crises or vascular necrosis of bone may be followed by embolism of bone marrow with fatty globules which may be seen in lungs, eyes, brain and urine. Most cases have occurred during pregnancy and this complication is associated with a high mortality [163].

The worry concerning aspiration pneumonitis, hypoxia and other perioperative pulmonary problems may be avoided by using regional anaesthesia but substitutes the risk of hypotension and venous pooling in the vessels of the lower extremities. Wrapping the legs in elastic bandages and elevating them will reduce venous pooling and subsequent hypotension. Epidural is preferred to spinal anaesthesia because there is less risk of hypotension if proper pre-operative hydration regimes with left uterine displacement are adopted. Although a number of sicklers have been reported in the obstetric literature to have suffered pulmonary emboli [26,182], there is no good evidence to incriminate regional anaesthesia as a significant additional risk factor and indeed good physiological data to support it having a protective role. In an emergency both regional and general anaesthesia may have to be undertaken without ideal preparation. Good communication and cooperation between anaesthetist, obstetrician and haematologist, together with meticulous post-operative care are essential for a good outcome. Again as with the controversy over blood transfusion, it is simple lack of awareness of potential problem and relaxation of vigilance which change the outcome [26] rather than lack of knowledge of the details of the measures adopted to deal with the many and varied hazards of sickle haemoglobin in pregnancy.

No special preparation with blood transfusion is required in pregnancy for women with sickle cell trait (HbAS). However, as in patients with HbSS, it is essential that hypoxia and dehydration are avoided during anaesthesia and labour, particularly in the immediate post-delivery period. In fact the majority of unexpected deaths associated with HbS have occurred in patients with sickle cell trait in the immediate post-operative or post-partum period.

The single most important pregnancy precaution is for the woman's partner to be screened, so that the couple can be advised of the risk of a serious haemoglobin defect in their offspring.

DETECTION OF HbS

Any test designed to screen for the presence of HbS should detect not only sickle cell disease but also distinguish HbSC, HbS thalassaemia and sickle cell trait. The classic sickling test in which the red cell is suspended in a reducing agent is difficult to interpret and may occasionally give false negative results. Furthermore it is time-consuming and its usefulness is limited when diagnosis is urgent. A proprietary product (Sickledex) is available that overcomes these drawbacks: it detects HbS by precipitation of deoxygenated HbS. It is rapid, reliable, and does not give false negatives. Definitive diagnosis of the particular sickle cell syndrome involved, requires haemoglobin electrophoresis and sometimes, in the case of sickle cell thalassaemia, family studies. Screening early in pregnancy where there is no absolute urgency is probably better carried out by performing Hb electrophoresis. The sickling test will then only have to be carried out on blood from those women with an abnormal band in the S region. Electrophoresis on cellulose acetate in tris buffer at pH 8.9 will distinguish it from HbD which has similar mobility on conventional electrophoresis.

Screening for haemoglobinopathy

Unfortunately, at the moment, screening procedures are often not carried out until women are pregnant. In most cases this means that early prenatal diagnosis by DNA analysis of a chorion biopsy is not possible. Selection for screening in a busy antenatal clinic may be more time-consuming than it is worth and, to be efficient, should involve detailed documentation of a woman's heritage before excluding her from testing. For this reason, and because of the remote possibility of missing such a defect in the non-immigrant population, general screening for haemoglobinopathies is carried out routinely on every woman's blood during pregnancy at Queen Charlotte's Maternity Hospital, which serves a cosmopolitan population. This involves examination of red cell indices (see Table 2.1), haemoglobin electrophoresis and, where indicated, quantitation of HbA_2 and HbF on the booking sample of blood (Fig. 2.4). If a haemoglobin variant or thalassaemia is found, the partner is requested to attend so that his blood can also be examined. By this means we are able to assess the chances of a serious haemoglobin defect in the fetus early in pregnancy, to advise the parents of the potential hazard and to offer them prenatal diagnosis.

Although all cases of sickle cell disease and the vast majority of thalassaemia syndromes can be

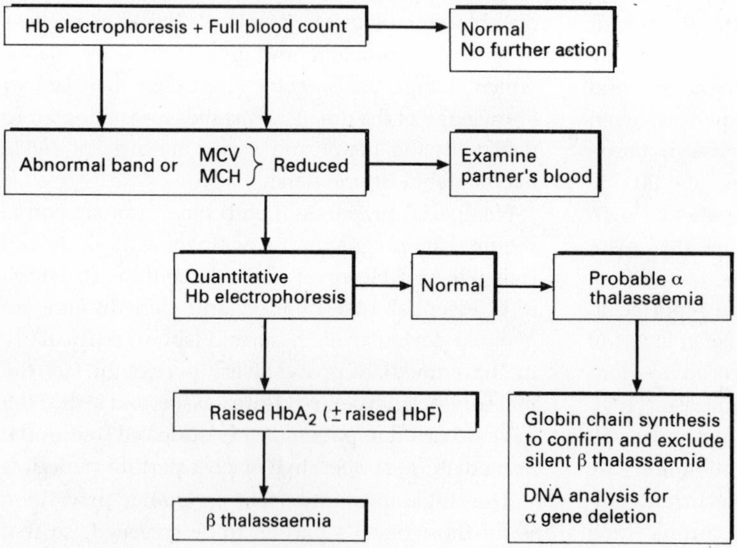

Fig. 2.4. Screening for haemoglobinopathy.

diagnosed by readily available DNA probes, the couples at risk would have to be identified before or within the first 8–10 weeks of fetal development for early prenatal diagnosis to be performed. With standard booking procedures this is unusual. We recognize that this inevitably results in late prenatal diagnosis and a painful, demoralizing, second trimester termination, if indicated; but unless couples at risk are identified *before* or during the first trimester of pregnancy, there is no other alternative.

Prenatal diagnosis of haemoglobinopathies

Fetal blood sampling

Until the mid-1970s the prenatal diagnosis of thalassaemia major and of sickle cell disease (also a β globin chain defect) was thought to be a relatively unrealistic goal for two reasons. Firstly, because information concerning β chain synthesis in the first and second trimesters of human pregnancy was lacking; and, secondly, because it was believed that any techniques necessary for acquisition of fetal blood would prove to be prohibitively dangerous with respect to the maintenance of the pregnancy.

Huehns *et al*. [79] at University College Hospital, showed that adult haemoglobin ($HbA\alpha_2\beta_2$) could be detected in the red cells of the fetus as early as 8–10 weeks' gestation (Fig. 2.5). Prenatal diagnosis of these haemoglobinopathies was accomplished for the first time in the 1970s by the use of globin chain synthesis studies of fetal blood obtained by fetoscopy or 'blind' placental aspiration [94] at 18–22 weeks' gestation. The fetal loss rates using these techniques could be as high as 12–15 per cent in those early days [2].

Since the mid 1980s pure fetal blood has been obtained from the fetal cord by means of an ultrasound-guided needle introduced through the maternal abdominal wall [133]. The risks to the ongoing pregnancy of this procedure are considerably less than those associated with previous methods. Currently fetal blood sampling overall carries a risk of fetal loss of 1–3 per cent [34,58,116]. However, fetal blood sampling for the prenatal diagnosis of the haemoglobinopathies, for which it was originally introduced, has now largely been superseded. It is now possible to detect genetic haemoglobin defects by DNA analysis of chorion villus samples and amniotic fluid fibroblasts. These samples can be obtained much earlier in gestation (see below) than fetal blood sampling.

Globin gene analysis

The last few years have seen remarkable advances in molecular biology and in particular the development of techniques for isolating and analysing DNA [192]. Normal globin genes have been examined using molecular hybridization and restriction endonuclease mapping techniques [134]. For the study of human genetic diseases, DNA is usually obtained

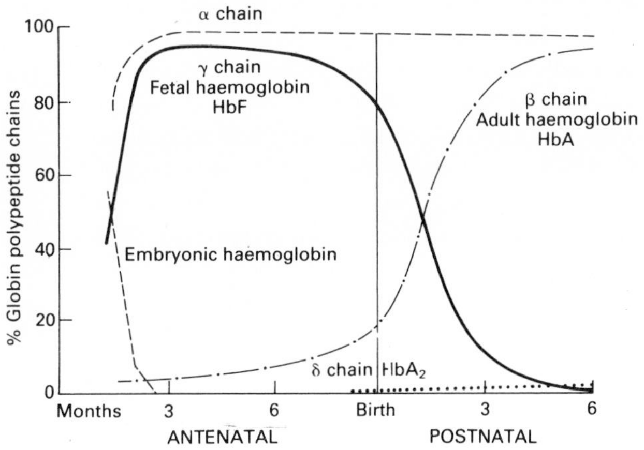

Fig. 2.5. The developmental changes in human haemoglobin (after [79]).

from the nuclei of white blood cells in a peripheral blood sample. However, in the prenatal diagnosis of haemoglobinopathies there are two possible alternative sources of DNA for diagnosis of fetal disease, namely amniotic fluid fibroblasts and trophoblast tissue obtained by a transcervical chorion biopsy technique [132,153,191]. The use of these techniques depends on being able to identify an abnormality of the DNA of the globin gene involved in the haemoglobinopathy or a closely linked polymorphism which is inherited with the relevant gene.

All cases of sickle cell disease can now be diagnosed prenatally by DNA analysis because of the identifiable base change in the β globin gene complex which synthesizes sickle haemoglobin. Most fetuses at risk for serious α thalassaemia syndromes can be identified because the abnormalities result from α gene deletion (see Fig. 2.2) [73,93]. Thalassaemias involving abnormal synthesis of both δ and β chains (δβ thalassaemias) are also diagnosable because they result from gene deletion [137]. A rapidly increasing number of cases of β thalassaemia have become identifiable by DNA analysis because of linked polymorphisms or partial gene deletions [18]. Unfortunately, however, in these cases, unless the couple has been identified and there is a large family available for study and plenty of time to perform the laboratory investigations required, the techniques have usually not been used until an affected child has been born.

A study of the Mediterranean population which of course, includes Cypriot immigrants to the UK, suggests that in the vast majority first pregnancies at risk for β thalassaemia, an affected fetus can be identified with oligonucleotide probes [191]. These are small, synthetic DNA fragments which are constructed specifically to detect single base changes in DNA. Although oligonucleotide probe technology is still being developed, it has already been possible to construct probes which identify the single base changes which cause human single gene disorders [191]. In those couples in which both partners carry a β thalassaemia determinant, β globin gene analysis is performed on amplified DNA in order to determine the molecular defect. The entire β globin gene is amplified by using the polymerase chain reaction (PCR) with appropriate primers. Known mutations may be detected by gel electrophoresis, restriction endonuclease analysis, dot blot analysis with allele-specific probes or primer-specific amplification [18].

It is now possible to identify the base change in the β globin gene complex which leads to the substitution of valine for glutamic acid and hence to the production of sickle haemoglobin. This means that all couples at risk of producing a child with sickle cell disease can have prenatal diagnosis using DNA analysis. The results of such analyses may be available on the same day that the fetal DNA is obtained [42].

Amniotic fluid fibroblasts

Amniocentesis is safer than fetal blood sampling and possibly safer than chorion villus sampling. Now that amplification of DNA is possible by PCR techniques, sufficient tissue is obtained for rapid prenatal diagnosis without the need for lengthy culturing procedures. Analysis of amniotic fluid fibroblast DNA for prenatal diagnosis of α thalassaemia hydrops has been used for more than a decade in the Far East but the recent improvements in detection and rapidity of tests have facilitated carrier detection and prenatal diagnosis of α thalassaemia syndromes considerably [77,96].

It may be asked why prenatal diagnosis for α thalassaemia should be attempted when the major form of the disease is incompatible with life, and HbH disease probably does not adversely affect life expectancy. One reason is that pregnancy with an α thalassaemia hydrops is associated with severe, sometimes life-threatening, pre-eclampsia in the mother. Also, vaginal deliveries are associated with obstetric complications due to the large size of the fetus and placenta associated with the haemoglobinopathy.

Chorion villus sampling

A report of 200 cases [136] of first trimester fetal diagnosis for haemoglobinopathies carried out in the UK using chorionic villus sampling (CVS) and DNA analysis suggested that provided CVS proves to be associated with an acceptably low fetal loss rate and that it has no significant long-term effects on fetal development, it will become the method of choice for fetal diagnosis of haemoglobinopathies and other single-gene disorders. The current CVS fetal loss rate is little more than 2 per cent which compares favourably with other methods used in prenatal diagnosis. However, limb reductions associated with this technique continue to give some cause for concern [16,48,80].

Initially transcervical villus sampling was carried out using an endoscope but this technique has largely been abandoned and biopsy specimens are obtained using a fine bore needle and cannula under ultrasound guidance. Even so the procedure still probably carries a risk of abortion at least two to three times greater than that of amniocentesis; there is also a maternal risk of endotoxic shock ascribed to penetration of a contaminated cervix. For these reasons, some workers have adopted the transabdominal approach [115]. They claim that this avoids the potentially infected endocervical canal and also that needle-guided transabdominal chorionic villus sampling is more easily learned than transcervical techniques. High abortion rates seemed to be associated with transcervical biopsy until the operator became skilled. In addition, the transabdominal method may be used over a wider gestational age range, i.e. 9–14 weeks as opposed to 9–12 weeks using the transcervical route. Maxwell *et al.* in 1986 [115] suggested that the technique should be widely evaluated in clinical practice possibly as part of a controlled trial comparing transabdominal with transcervical routes. There have now been two large randomized trials comparing the two techniques. In the USA [87] the safety of both techniques was found to be similar. In Denmark [167] the unintentional fetal loss rate was much higher using the transcervical route (7.7 per cent) compared with the transabdominal approach (3.7 per cent).

The vast majority of the limb anomalies described in association with CVS have been in fetuses sampled before 10 weeks' gestation [16,80] and are thought to have a vascular aetiology related to either decreased fetal perfusion or thrombosis of the sampling site [16]. In the UK each fetal medicine unit has its preferred technique but providing that the transcervical approach is avoided before 10 weeks' gestation (when there is an association with limb reduction) there appears to be no difference in outcome (N.M. Fisk, personal communication).

In summary, the prenatal diagnosis of the haemoglobinopathies originally performed by globin chain analysis of fetal blood samples taken in the second trimester has now largely been replaced by direct detection of the genetic defect by analysis of amplified DNA from fetal trophoblast or amniotic fluid cells obtained earlier in gestation.

Rationale for screening

The main reason why pre-pregnancy screening programmes for haemoglobinopathies should be set up, is the handicap associated with homozygous β thalassaemia. The management of homozygous β thalassaemia by regular blood transfusion and chelating agents is extremely expensive and puts a major burden on the health services particularly in the developing countries where the disease is so common. Undoubtedly, the most cost-effective approach to the problem of thalassaemia is the development of programmes for the pre-pregnancy screening of potential mothers and, in cases where they are found to be carriers, of their partners [193]. Where both parents are affected they should be offered the possibility of antenatal diagnosis by fetal blood or trophoblast sampling and of abortion of homozygous fetuses. This type of programme is now well established in many parts of the world, but screening usually takes place in the antenatal period when conception has already occurred. Even if the couple are known to be at risk, having already had an affected child, there may not be time for proper investigation, so that advantage can be taken of the more acceptable trophoblast sampling technique for DNA analysis of the fetus, if indicated.

Implications for the future

Now that first trimester fetal diagnosis has become possible for virtually all serious haemoglobinopathies and as the techniques become available in more centres over the world, screening should be extended beyond the antenatal clinic. It has been suggested [126] that education and counselling should be directed at three points in people's lives, namely at school, at marriage and at family planning clinics. The information given should include details of where blood testing can be carried out and advice on when this should be done, although it should probably be left to the individual in possession of the information to request the test. This will involve education of the communities at risk and also — a component which is often forgotten — education of the medical practitioners caring for these communities.

Miscellaneous anaemias

Many forms of anaemia, in particular the anaemia of renal failure, are made worse by pregnancy. However, supportive and prophylactic therapy for the various medical conditions concerned is improving and maternal risks for the most part have been reduced, as have the risks to the fetus. Each case has to be considered individually: there are no general rules that can be applied in terms of management.

Aplastic anaemia

There have been sporadic case reports of refractory hypoplastic anaemia, sometimes recurrent, developing in pregnancy and appearing to be related in some way to the pregnancy [180]. Occasionally pregnancy occurs when chronic acquired aplastic anaemia is present as an underlying disease. It has been generally considered that in both these situations pregnancy exacerbates the marrow depression, results in rapid deterioration, and should be terminated. It is true that many cases do remit spontaneously after termination [43], but there is no record of excessive haemorrhage at delivery despite profound thrombocytopenia. Supportive measures in this situation are improving and pregnancy should be maintained as long as the health of the mother is not seriously impaired [108].

There are a few cases in the literature of reversible pure red cell aplasia (associated with pregnancy) following delivery. One report describes the course of relapsing pure red cell aplasia during three pregnancies [145]. Anaemia can be profound and supportive red cell transfusions are necessary but the outcome is generally good if there are no other interacting complications. The whole subject has been recently reviewed [171].

Autoimmune haemolytic anaemia (AIHA) and systemic lupus erythematosus (SLE)

The rare combination of AIHA and pregnancy carries great risks to both the woman herself and the fetus. Very careful antenatal supervision and adjustment to steroid therapy is required [25].

Pregnancy may coincide with exacerbations of SLE although up to 50 per cent of women with this condition are reported to improve during pregnancy especially in the third trimester [38] (see also Chapter 8).

Haemolytic anaemia, leukopenia and thrombocytopenia (see Chapter 8) have all been observed in infants of women with active disease, presumably due to IgG antibody involved in the disease process crossing the placenta. There have been a number of reports in which women have been treated with steroids [130] and other immune suppressives throughout pregnancy for a variety of conditions including immune thrombocytopenic purpura (ITP), SLE, AIHA and some forms of malignancy. Possible effects of steroids are considered in Chapter 1. The problems of their use are essentially the same as those outside pregnancy but more frequent monitoring and adjustment are required due to the rapidly changing blood volume and changes in the circulating hormones during the antenatal and postnatal periods. There is also concern about the possible effects of azathioprine on the reproductive performance of female offspring (Chapter 8). A rare form of haemolytic anaemia appears to be specific to pregnancy. It remits after delivery but tends to recur in subsequent pregnancies in about half of the women affected. Although no autoantibody has been identified, the anaemia responds to steroids and immunoglobulin. The fetus may be affected in about 20 per cent of cases [66].

Polycythaemia rubra vera (PRV)

PRV is a myeloproliferative disease involving a pluripotent haemopoietic stem cell. It is an uncommon disorder with an estimated incidence of one in 50 000. It affects women less often than men and is usually seen after the 6th decade of life and is therefore only rarely encountered in pregnant women.

Reports in the literature are very sparse involving not many more than 15 pregnancies in nine women and were reviewed in 1983 [46].

Diagnosis of PRV depends on the demonstration of an increased red cell mass which distinguishes the condition from 'stress' erythrocytosis characterized by an increased haematocrit but a normal red cell mass. Differentiation from secondary polycythaemia is made by lack of increased erythropoietin levels in the urine. Also in PRV there is usually an absolute granulocytosis and thrombocytosis which is not found in secondary polycythaemia. The maternal outcome in the few reports available is usually good, but there is an increased incidence of pregnancy-induced hypertension and neonatal mortality is high due to frequent occurrence of abortion, still-birth and pre-term delivery.

Radioactive phosphorus ^{32}P has been the treatment of choice for older patients with PRV. Alkylating agents have been introduced more recently into treatment regimes. However, in younger patients these measures are usually avoided because of their leukaemogenic potential. During pregnancy the additional hazards of teratogenicity and other harm to the fetus precludes their use.

Control of haematological parameters is best achieved by repeated phlebotomy. The haematocrit should be maintained at a value of <50 per cent to reduce the associated hazards of abnormal bleeding, thrombosis and tissue hypoxia.

In PRV it has been recommended [46] that prophylactic antithrombotic measures should be taken during the intra and post-partum period because of the associated hypercoagulability in uncomplicated pregnancy (see Chapter 4). Low dose heparin appears to be the treatment of choice.

Surgery carries exceptional hazards of bleeding and thrombosis in the uncontrolled polycythaemic patient and emergency phlebotomy is indicated in the uncontrolled patient who needs an urgent caesarean section or other surgery.

Regional anaesthesia is the analgesic and anaesthetic of choice. During general anaesthesia alterations in pulmonary elasticity and ventilation perfusion defects could lead to respiratory acidosis. Long-term prognosis is difficult to predict for any individual. An erythrocytic phase is often followed by an inactive phase which may last as long as 25 years. As a rule survival is longer in patients who are younger at the time of diagnosis. Maternal survival in older patients has been estimated at 16 years. Myeloid metaplasia is seen as the duration of the disease increases, and death usually results from terminal development of acute leukaemia or myelofibrosis.

Thrombocythaemia, thrombocytosis

Essential and primary thrombocythaemia (thrombocytosis) usually affects subjects beyond the childbearing age. A myeloproliferative disorder, characterized by an isolated high platelet count, it is associated with both haemorrhagic and thromboembolic phenomena. Reports in the literature are sparse [11,92,170] and management strategies are therefore difficult to plan. If the thrombocythaemia is not accompanied by polycythaemia and there have been no previous complications then the treatment of choice should be aspirin (75 mg/day) to inhibit platelet aggregation and thrombosis. This should be instituted when the platelet count exceeds $600 \times 10^9/l$ [170]. Two asymptomatic women with platelet counts around $1000 \times 10^9/l$ at our hospital were managed throughout pregnancy with aspirin and no complications occurred in either mother or fetus. Recurrent late abortion associated with thrombocythaemia has been managed successfully with aspirin. Cytotoxic agents have been used in this disease [142] but should be avoided in gestation.

Interferon α may be given where complications have not been prevented by therapy with aspirin [142]. It has been used without ill-effect in human pregnancy.

Paroxysmal nocturnal haemoglobinuria (PNH)

This rare condition which occurs primarily in young adults is now known to be caused by a genetically determined somatic mutation in a haemopoietic stem cell giving rise to populations of defective red cells, granulocytes and platelets [76,125]. The intrinsic defect in the red cell makes it particularly sensitive to lysis by complement. The disease varies widely in severity; it usually begins insidiously and haemoglobinuria, as a presenting symptom, is found in only 25 per cent of all patients.

The laboratory diagnosis is made using a series of special tests which demonstrate the sensitivity of the patient's red cells to lysis by complement.

The main features of the disease are episodes of acute and chronic intravascular haemolysis with varying degrees of anaemia and haemoglobinuria. More important complications arise from the defective platelets and granulocytes produced by the abnormal clone of stem cells.

Thrombosis accounts for approximately 50 per cent of deaths in reported autopsies. The major morbidity also relates to venous thrombosis which has been reported in peripheral as well as in mesenteric, hepatic, portal and cerebral veins.

This hypercoagulable state has been attributed to the triggering effect of intravascular haemolysis and increased activity of coagulation factors, but the most relevant explanation for the enhanced thrombotic tendency is that the PNH platelets can bind much greater amounts of complement (C3) than normal platelets. Activation of the complement pathway triggers PNH platelets to undergo the release reaction and aggregate, thus initiating thrombosis [188]. Similarly poorly understood functional abnormalities of leukocyte function together with granulocytopenia are thought to contribute to the increased susceptibility to infection seen in patients with PNH.

As the disease progresses the abnormal clone of cells takes over and normal bone marrow becomes increasingly hypoplastic and ultimately aplastic [33,157].

The most serious complications associated with PNH are thrombosis, infection and ultimately, marrow aplasia.

The optimum treatment of PNH is replacement of the abnormal stem cell with cells producing normal cellular components by BMT, but this is not an option during pregnancy. Androgen therapy has been useful in suppressing haemolysis and increasing normal cell production in non-pregnant females and in males, but it has side-effects and its use is definitely contraindicated in pregnancy.

Prednisone in a dose of 1 mg/kg may be useful in reducing haemolysis; if the patient responds to prednisone, this may safely be used throughout pregnancy (Chapter 1).

Iron has been used to maintain the haematocrit and replace iron lost in the urine, but it has been shown in many studies to trigger acute haemolytic episodes and is therefore probably best avoided.

The fertility rate in this uncommon condition is thought to be low and experience of pregnancies associated with PNH is limited. To date less than 100 cases have been reported in the English literature. Awareness of the risks involved has led to the previous suggestion that conception should be avoided if possible. Although more recently there have been reports of successful maternal and fetal outcome of pregnancies associated with PNH [13,35,90], safe effective contraception needs to be considered. The hypercoagulable state in PNH rules out oral contraception and there has been a report of cerebral vein thrombosis in a woman with PNH associated with use of an oral contraceptive. The use of an intrauterine device is contraindicated in the presence of thrombocytopenia and granulocytopenia. If couples at risk wish to delay pregnancy, barrier methods should be recommended and if they decide against further reproduction, either tubal ligation or vasectomy should be advised.

If pregnancy is embarked upon, the main hazards appear to be spontaneous abortion, often following acute haemolytic episodes, and serious thrombotic events mainly in the puerperium.

Prophylactic transfusions with washed red cells, which are not a source of extrinsic complement, maintaining the haematocrit between 25 and 30 per cent, to suppress the production of abnormal cells, have been recommended in the first trimester [82]. The theory is that these transfusions will decrease the possibility of severe haemolytic episodes and therefore the risk of spontaneous abortion and the chance of a severe thrombotic episode early in pregnancy.

Hepatic vein thrombosis is the most common thrombotic complication, having a maximum incidence post-partum; antenatal pulmonary embolism has also been reported.

Low dose heparin has been shown to be ineffective prophylaxis in at least one case in the antenatal period [172]. The maximum risk period is still after delivery. It has been suggested therefore that full anticoagulation should be used to treat any thrombotic episode in the antenatal period and that full anticoagulation should be used prophylactically in the puerperium [82] (see Chapter 4).

'Nevertheless, despite the usual view that pregnancy is too hazardous in patients with PNH, a poor outlook may not be inevitable' [90].

Leukaemia

One in 1000 pregnancies is complicated by malignant disease [156,166]. The incidence of leukaemia in pregnancy should not exceed one in 75 000 pregnancies, but the information used to calculate this incidence is obtained from cases recorded in the literature — a method with serious limitations. Although peak incidence years for cancer do not coincide with the peak reproductive years, leukaemia was reported in 1969 as the second most common cause of death from malignant disease in females aged 15–34 in the USA. Several hundred cases of leukaemia in association with pregnancy have now been reported; most papers give an account of a specific case or cases and include a review of the published literature [e.g. 44,64,131] and some include management considerations [e.g. 118].

Adult leukaemia is almost invariably fatal and one of the reasons why acute leukaemia is seen so rarely in association with pregnancy is that, without the aggressive treatment with cytotoxic drugs instituted in the last decade, the disease is characterized by rapid deterioration and death within weeks of diagnosis.

There is no objective evidence that pregnancy has a deleterious effect on leukaemia [44,118]. Survival times in pregnant women with leukaemia do not differ statistically from those of non-pregnant women. The application of modern treatment can result in remission of the disease that is sometimes repeated, and more affected women may now have the opportunity to conceive or to survive until the fetus is viable.

The diagnosis during pregnancy is made most frequently in the second and third trimesters although the disease may have been present earlier. This is because the early symptoms are non-specific, the most common being fatigue, which is often attributed by the woman and her obstetrician to the pregnancy itself. This emphasizes the importance of carrying out proper investigations, including bone marrow examination of unexplained anaemia in pregnancy.

The occurrence of pregnancy in a woman suffering from or developing acute leukaemia creates special clinical problems which fall into two main groups — those arising from the disease process and those arising from its treatment. There are increased risks of infection, haemorrhage and abortion arising from the disease process itself and from the effects of chemotherapy [17]. Fetal loss occurs in approximately 14 per cent of women with chronic myeloid leukaemia and 33 per cent of women with acute leukaemia. Haemorrhage may result from thrombocytopenia due to bone marrow infiltration or from a consumption coagulopathy; this is a particularly common problem in acute myelomonocytic leukaemia. The powerful cytotoxic drugs which are often used to achieve remission in acute adult leukaemia include cytosine arabinoside, rubidomycin and thioguanine. Such agents have been shown to be toxic to fetal tissue in experimental animals. Malformations have occurred after treatment with cytotoxic drugs in the first trimester [131]. Methotrexate, a folic acid antagonist, is the most teratogenic drug known to man. Its administration early in pregnancy always results in either abortion or congenital malformation. Other published data have suggested that cytotoxic drugs might be given with safety in the second and third trimesters [64,131]. One more recently published study with follow-up of 43 children over a period of 3–19 years whose mothers had received chemotherapy for various malignancies including leukaemia, showed no adverse effect in the children. Nineteen of these mothers received treatment in the first trimester. A similar retrospective study also published in 1991 looked at 56 pregnancies in 48 women and found no increase in the incidence of complications during pregnancy compared with pregnancies in a healthy population [197]. Successful pregnancy has been reported in women receiving recombinant interferon α for management of chronic myeloid leukaemia [150].

It has been suggested [64] that a pregnant leukaemic woman should be treated with aggressive chemotherapy until a remission is achieved. The risk of a malformed fetus in a woman so treated in the first trimester is high and termination should be considered once she is in remission and this can be performed with safety. Termination of pregnancy when therapy is started in the second or third trimester is only indicated on moral and medicosocial grounds, as the fetus is likely to develop normally. Examination of chromosomes of fetal amniotic fluid cells and of fetal hair under the scanning electron microscope may provide evidence of fetal damage in those cases where treatment is started early in the second trimester [64]. An alternative approach later in the second trimester would be fetal blood sampling.

A more recent overview of leukaemia and lymphoma in pregnancy [107] tabulates published case reports of acute leukaemia since the comprehensive review of McLain [118]. Based on the combined data, the authors confirm the earlier conclusions that pregnancy itself has no adverse effect on the course of leukaemia unless specific chemotherapy is withheld for fear of damaging the fetus. However, the converse is not true. The greatest risks are maternal death before delivery and fetal damage or death related to maternal chemotherapy. Since 1989 there have been some reports of successful pregnancies in women who had prior allogeneic BMT, both in those whose conditioning therapy for BMT was by use of chemotherapy alone [124] and more recently in women who received total body irradiation [61].

Hodgkin's disease

The diagnosis of Hodgkin's disease depends upon the presence of the characteristic Reed–Sternberg cell in biopsy material. The various morphological subclasses of the Reed–Sternberg cell and the relative proportion of other cellular elements have no influence on the outcome of the disease unlike in the non-Hodgkin's lymphomata in which histology has a major influence on outcome [107,166, 189]. Prognosis depends on the staging of the disease at presentation.

Treatment for Hodgkin's disease involves adequate radiotherapy for patients with relatively localized disease. A cure rate of over 90 per cent can be expected in these cases. Combination chemotherapy regimes are used for those with wider spread disease and involvement both above and below the diaphragm. In those cases with no systemic symptoms such as unexplained weight loss, pyrexia or night sweats, chemotherapy alone will produce a complete remission in 80–100 per cent of patients with a probable cure in at least 50 per cent.

Widespread disease with systemic manifestations has a poorer prognosis and is treated with aggressive repeated courses of combination chemotherapy often combined with radiotherapy.

Because the choice of treatment requires precise staging of the disease, pregnancy should always be ruled out before undertaking diagnostic studies and therapy.

The incidence of Hodgkin's disease in pregnancy is low, so it is most unlikely that there will ever be prospective randomized studies to resolve which is the optimum management strategy for the various stages of the disease which may occur during the antenatal period. The largely American retrospective experience has been reviewed [107,189]. A recently published British retrospective study of 48 women who had Hodgkin's disease compared with non-pregnant women at similar stages of disease matched for age and therapy showed that the 20-year survival of those women with a pregnancy was no different from their matched controls [110].

A communication from Italy reports a retrospective analysis of 219 female patients presenting between 1971 and 1982 with Hodgkin's disease [62]. Twenty-one patients were pregnant at the time of presentation. One hundred and fifty-five patients aged 15–45 years when Hodgkin's disease was diagnosed were selected as controls. The authors concluded, as have others [107] that pregnancy does not influence the symptoms or presentation of the disease. The slightly higher proportion of advanced stages among the pregnant patients in the study may be explained by the masking of the early signs and symptoms by pregnancy itself. Pregnancy does not affect prognosis and the higher proportion of advanced stages has statistically negligible influence on survival. Pregnancy does not induce a higher relapse rate. A large proportion of treated patients whose menstruation is preserved are still fertile and can expect to produce apparently normal offspring especially in the younger age groups [62]. A more recent retrospective analysis of pregnancy outcome in 139 survivors of advanced Hodgkin's disease provided data on 302 pregnancies. There was an excess of low birthweights in women treated actively during the antenatal period but this was based on small numbers [91].

It would seem prudent to advise a patient to delay conception until 2 years after successful therapy has been completed because the risk of relapse falls off rapidly after that time. However, there is still concern about the long-term impact of ionizing radiation and chemotherapeutic agents on the ova and ultimately on the offspring of treated patients even if conception occurs well after therapy has been completed. It is known from animal studies that anomalies (induced in offspring) may not appear until later in life and it is even more difficult to evaluate the risk in the human.

Aborted fetuses, infants and children may not be adequately screened for defects. Applied therapy regimes differ from one treatment centre to another. Therapy-induced cases of mutagenesis tend to be emphasized in the literature making assessment of the true proportion of unfavourable outcome very difficult to estimate [15].

References

1 Acheson D. *Department of Health and Social Security, Press Release*, 87/5, 1987.

2 Alter BP. Prenatal diagnosis of haemoglobinopathies and other haematologic diseases. *Journal of Pediatrics* 1979; **95**: 501–13.

3 Anon. Do all pregnant women need iron? *British Medical Journal* 1978; **ii**: 1317.

4 Anyaegbunam A, Langer O *et al*. Third-trimester prediction of small-for-gestational-age infants in pregnant women with sickle cell disease. Development of the ultradop index. *Journal of Reproductive Medicine* 1991; **36**: 577–80.

5 Apte SV & Iyengar L. Absorption of dietary iron in pregnancy. *American Journal of Clinical Nutrition* 1970; **23**: 73–7.

6 Avery B & Ledger WJ. Folic acid metabolism in well nourished pregnant women. *Obstetrics and Gynecology* 1970; **35**: 616–24.

7 Ball EW & Giles C. Folic acid and vitamin B_{12} levels in pregnancy and their relation to megaloblastic anaemia. *Journal of Clinical Pathology* 1964; **17**: 165–74.

8 Bareford D. Thalassaemia in pregnancy (letter). *British Medical Journal* 1991; **303**: 120.

9 Barrett JFR, Whitaker PG, Williams JG & Lind T. Absorption of non-haem iron from food during normal, pregnancy. *British Medical Journal* 1994; **309**: 79–82.

10 Baumslag N, Edelstein T & Metz J. Reduction of incidence of prematurity by folic acid supplementation in pregnancy. *British Medical Journal* 1970; **i**: 16–17.

11 Beard J, Hillmen P *et al*. Primary thrombocythaemia in pregnancy. *British Journal of Haematology* 1991; **77**: 371–4.

12 Bentley DP. Iron metabolism and anaemia in pregnancy. In: Letsky EA (ed) *Haematological Disorders in Pregnancy. Clinics in Haematology* **14**. WB Saunders, Eastbourne, 1985: 613–28.

13 Beresford CH, Gudex DJ & Symmans WA. Paroxysmal nocturnal haemoglobinuria and pregnancy. *Lancet* 1986; **ii**: 1396–7.

14 Bjerkedal T & Bahna SL. The course and outcome of pregnancy in women with epilepsy. *Obstetrica et Gynaecologica Scandinavica* 1973; **52** (suppl): 245–8.

15 Blatt J, Mulvihill JJ *et al*. Pregnancy outcome following cancer chemotherapy. *American Journal of Medicine* 1980; **69**: 828.

16 Burton BK, Schulz CJ & Burd LI. Limb anomalies associated with chorionic villus sampling. *Obstetrics and Gynecology* 1992; **79**: 726–30.

17 Caligiuri MA & Mayer RJ. Pregnancy and leukemia. *Seminars in Oncology* 1989; **16**: 388–96.

18 Cao A & Rosatelli MC. Screening and prenatal diagnosis of the haemoglobinopathies. In: Higgs DR & Weatherall DJ (eds), *Baillière's Clinical Haematology, The Haemoglobinopathies*. Baillière Tindall, London, 1993: 263–86.

19 Chanarin I. The folate content of foodstuffs and the availability of different folate analogues for absorption. In: *Getting the Most out of Food*. Van den Bergh & Jurgens Ltd, London, 1975: 41.

20 Chanarin I. Megaloblastic anaemia of pregnancy. In: *The Megaloblastic Anaemias*, 2nd edn. Blackwell Scientific Publications, Oxford, 1979.

21 Chanarin I. Folate and cobalamin. In: Letsky EA (ed), *Haematological Disorders in Pregnancy. Clinics in*

Haematology **14**. WB Saunders, Eastbourne, 1985: 629–41.

22 Chanarin J, MacGibbon BM, O'Sullivan WJ & Mollin DL. Folic acid deficiency in pregnancy; the pathogenesis of megaloblastic anaemia of pregnancy. *Lancet* 1959; **ii**: 634–9.

23 Chanarin I, Rothman D & Berry V. Iron deficiency and its relation to folic acid status in pregnancy: Results of a clinical trial. *British Medical Journal* 1965; **i**: 480–5.

24 Chanarin I, Rothman D, Ward A & Perry J. Folate status and requirement in pregnancy. *British Medical Journal* 1968; **ii**: 390–4.

25 Chaplin H, Cohen R, Bloomberg G, Kaplan HJ, Moore J Aa. & Dorner I. Pregnancy and idiopathic autoimmune haemolytic anaemia. A prospective study during 6 months gestation and 3 months post-partum. *British Journal of Haematology* 1973; **24**: 219–29.

26 Charache S & Niebyl JR. Pregnancy in sickle cell disease. In: Letsky EA (ed) *Haematological Disorders in Pregnancy. Clinics in Haematology* **14**. WB Saunders, Eastbourne, 1985: 720–46.

27 Charache S, Scott J, Niebyl J & Bonds D. Management of sickle cell disease in pregnant patients. *Obstetrics and Gynecology* 1980; **55**: 407–10.

28 Chesley LC & Duffus GM. Posture and apparent plasma volume in late pregnancy. *Journal of Obstetrics and Gynaecology of the British Commonwealth* 1971; **78**: 406–12.

29 Chisholm J. A controlled clinical trial of prophylactic folic acid and iron in pregnancy. *Journal of Obstetrics and Gynaecology of the British Commonwealth* 1966; **73**: 191–6.

30 Cooper BA. Folate and vitamin B_{12} in pregnancy. *Clinics in Haematology* 1973; **2**: 461–76.

31 Coyle C & Geoghegan F. The problem of anaemia in a Dublin maternity hospital. *Proceedings of the Royal Society of Medicine* 1962; **55**: 764–6.

32 Czeizel AE & Dudás I. Prevention of the first occurrence of neural-tube defects by periconceptional vitamin supplementation. *New England Journal of Medicine* 1992; **327**: 1832–5.

33 Dacie JV & Lewis SM. Paroxysmal nocturnal haemoglobinuria: Clinical manifestations, haematology and nature of the disease. *Haematological Series* 1972; **5**: 3.

34 Daffos F, Capella-Pavlosky M & Forestier F. Fetal blood sampling during pregnancy with use of a needle guided by ultrasound: a study of 606 consecutive cases. *American Journal of Obstetrics and Gynecology* 1985; **153**: 655–60.

35 De Gramont A, Krulik M & Debray J. Paroxysmal noctural haemoglobinuria and pregnancy. *Lancet* 1987; **i**: 868.

36 Deblay MF, Vert P, Andre M & Marchal F. Transplacental vitamin K prevents haemorrhagic disease of infant of epileptic mother. *Lancet* 1982; **i**: 1247.

37 Desforges JF & Rutherford CJ. Hodgkin's disease. *New England Journal of Medicine* 1979; **301**: 1212.

38 Dubois EL. *Lupus Erythematosus*. McGraw Hill, New York, 1966.

39 Edelstein T & Metz J. The correlation between vitamin B_{12} concentration in serum and muscle in late pregnancy. *Journal of Obstetrics and Gynaecology of the British Commonwealth* 1969; **76**: 545–8.

40 Editorial. Folic acid and neural tube defects. *Lancet* 1991; **338**: 153–4.

41 Elwood JM. Can vitamins prevent neural tube defects? *Canadian Medical Association Journal* 1983; **129**: 1088–92.

42 Embury SH, Scharf SJ *et al*. Rapid prenatal diagnosis of sickle cell anaemia by a new method of DNA analysis. *New England Journal of Medicine* 1987; **316**: 656–61.

43 Evans IL. Aplastic anaemia in pregnancy remitting after abortion. *British Medical Journal* 1968; **iii**: 166–7.

44 Ewing PA & Whittaker JA. Acute leukaemia in pregnancy. *Obstetrics and Gynecology* 1973; **42**: 245–51.

45 Fenton V, Cavill I & Fisher J. Iron stores in pregnancy. *British Journal of Haematology* 1977; **37**: 145–9.

46 Ferguson JE, Ueland K & Aronson WJ. Polycythemia rubra vera and pregnancy. *Obstetrics and Gynecology* 1983; **62**: 16S–20S.

47 Finch CA & Huebers H. Perspectives in iron metabolism. *New England Journal of Medicine* 1982; **306**: 1520–8.

48 Firth HV, Boyd PA, Chamberlain P, MacKenzie IZ, Lindenbaum RH & Huson SM. Severe limb abnormalities after chorion villus sampling at 56–66 days gestation. *Lancet* 1991; **337**: 762–3.

49 Fleming AF. Urinary excretion of folate in pregnancy. *Journal of Obstetrics and Gynaecology of the British Commonwealth* 1972; **79**: 916–20.

50 Fleming AF. Haematological changes in pregnancy. *Clinics in Obstetrics and Gynaecology* 1975; **3**: 269–83.

51 Fleming AF, Martin JD, Hahnel R & Westlake AJ. Effects of iron and folic acid antenatal supplements on maternal haematology and fetal wellbeing. *Medical Journal of Australia* 1974; **ii**: 429–36.

52 Fleming AJ, Martin JD & Stenhouse NS. Pregnancy anaemia, iron and folate deficiency in Western Australia. *Medical Journal of Australia* 1974; **ii**: 479–84.

53 Fletcher J, Gurr A, Fellingham FR, Prankerd TAJ, Brant HA & Menzies DN. The value of folic acid supplements in pregnancy. *Journal of Obstetrics and Gynaecology of the British Commonwealth* 1971; **75**: 781–5.

54 Fletcher J & Suter PEN. The transport of iron by the human placenta. *Clinical Science* 1969; **36**: 209–20.

55 Fullerton WT, Hytten FE, Klopper AE & McKay E. Case of quadruplet pregnancy. *Journal of Obstetrics and Gynaecology of the British Commonwealth* 1965; **72**: 791–6.

56 Gatenby PBB. The anaemias of pregnancy in Dublin. *Proceedings of the Nutrition Society* 1956; **15**: 115–19.

57 Gatenby PBB & Little EW. Clinical analysis of 100 cases of severe megaloblastic anaemia of pregnancy. *British Medical Journal* 1960; **ii**: 1111–14.

58 Ghidini A, Sepulveda W, Lockwood CJ & Romero R. Complications of fetal blood sampling. *American Journal of Obstetrics and Gynecology* 1993; **168**: 1339–44.

59 Gibson HM. Plasma volume and glomerular filtration rate in pregnancy and their relation to differences in fetal growth. *Journal of Obstetrics and Gynaecology of the British Commonwealth* 1973; **80**: 1067–74.

60 Giles C. An account of 335 cases of megaloblastic anaemia of pregnancy and the puerperium. *Journal of Clinical Pathology* 1966; **19**: 1–11.

61 Giri N, Vowels MR, Barr AL & Mameghan H. Successful pregnancy after total body irradiation and bone marrow transplantation for acute leukaemia. *Bone Marrow Transplant* 1992; **10**: 93–5.

62 Gobbi PG, Attardo-Parrinello G *et al*. Hodgkin's disease in pregnancy. *Haematologica* 1984; **69**: 336–41.

63 Godfrey KM, Redman CW *et al*. The effect of maternal anaemia and iron deficiency on the ratio of fetal weight to placental weight. *British Journal of Obstetrics and Gynaecology* 1991; **98**: 886–91.

64 Gokal R, Durrant J, Baum JD & Bennett MJ. Successful pregnancy in acute monocyte leukaemia. *British Journal of Cancer* 1976; **34**: 299–302.

65 Goldfarb AW, Hochner-Celnikier D, Beller U, Menashe M, Dagan I & Palti Z. A successful pregnancy in transfusion dependent homozygous β-thalassaemia: a case report. *International Journal of Gynaecology and Obstetrics* 1982; **20**: 319–22.

66 Goodall HB, Ho Yen DO. Haemolytic anaemia of pregnancy. *Scandinavian Journal of Haematology* 1979; **22**: 185–91.

67 Hallberg L, Bengtsson C, Garby L, Lennartsson J, Rossander L. & Tibblin E. An analysis of factors leading to a reduction in iron deficiency in Swedish women. *Bulletin of the World Health Organization* 1979; **57**: 947–54.

68 Hallberg L, Ryttinger L & Solvell L. Side effects of oral iron therapy. *Acta Medica Scandinavica Supplement* 1966; **459**: 3–10.

69 Hambridge KM, Krebs NF, Jacobs MA, Guyette L & Ikle DN. Zinc nutritional status during pregnancy: a longitudinal study. *American Journal of Clinical Nutrition* 1983; **37**: 425–42.

70 Harstad TW, Mason RA & Cox SM. Serum erythropoietin quantitation in pregnancy using an enzyme-linked immunoassay. *American Journal of Perinatology* 1992; **9**: 233–5.

71 Haworth C & Evans DIK. Nutritional aspects of blood disorders in the newborn. *Journal of Human Nutrition* 1981; **35**: 323–34.

72 Hemminki E & Starfield B. Routine administration of iron and vitamins during pregnancy: Review of controlled clinical trials. *British Journal of Obstetrics and Gynaecology* 1978; **85**: 404–10.

73 Higgs DR. Alpha thalassaemia in haemoglobinopathies. In: Higgs DR & Weatherall DJ (eds), *Baillière's Clinical Haematology, The Haemoglobinopathies*. Baillière Tindall, London, 1993: 117–50.

74 Hiilesmaa VK, Teramo K, Granstrom M-L & Bardy AH. Serum folate concentration during pregnancy in women with epilepsy: relation to antiepileptic drug concentrations, number of seizures and fetal outcome. *British Medical Journal* 1983; **287**: 577–9.

75 Hill RM, Verniaud WM, Horning MG, McCulley LB & Morgan NF. Infants exposed in utero to anti-epileptic drugs. *American Journal of Diseases in Childhood* 1974; **127**: 645–53.

76 Hillmen P, Bessler M *et al*. Specific defect in *N*-acetylglucosamine incorporation in the biosynthesis of the glycosylphospatidylinositol anchor in cloned cell lines from patients with paroxysmal nocturnal hemoglobinuria. *Proceeding of the National Academy of Science USA* 1993; **90**: 5272–6.

77 Hsia YE. Detection and prevention of important alpha-thalassemia variants. *Seminars in Perinatology* 1991; **15** (suppl 1): 35–42.

78 Huehns ER. The structure and function of haemoglobin: clinical disorders due to abnormal haemoglobin structure. In: Hardisty RM & Weatherall DJ (eds), *Blood and Its Disorders*, 2nd edn. Blackwell Scientific Publications, Oxford, 1982: 365.

79 Huehns ER, Dance N, Beaven GH, Hecht F & Motulsky AG. Human embryonic haemoglobins. Cold Spring Harbor Symposium. *Quantitative Biology* 1964; **29**: 327–31.

80 Hurley PA & Rodeck CH. Fetal therapy. *Current Opinion in Obstetrics and Gynecology* 1992; **4**: 4–9.

81 Hussein SS, Hoffbrand AV, Laulicht M, Attock B & Letsky EA. Serum ferritin levels in beta thalassaemia trait. *British Medical Journal* 1975; **ii**: 920.

82 Hurd WH, Miodovnik M & Stys SJ. Pregnancy associated with paroxysmal noctural haemoglobinuria. *Obstetrics and Gynecology* 1982; **60**: 742–6.

83 Hytten F. Blood volume changes in normal pregnancy. In: Letsky EA (ed), *Haematological Disorders in Pregnancy. Clinics in Haematology* **14**. WB Saunders, Eastbourne, 1985: 601–12.

84 Hytten FE & Leitch I. The volume and composition of the blood. In: Hytten FE & Leitch I (eds) *The Physiology of Human Pregnancy*, 2nd edn. Blackwell Scientific Publications, Oxford, 1971: 1–68.

85 Idjradinata P & Pollitt E. Reversal of developmental delays in iron-deficient anaemic infants treated with iron. *Lancet* 1993; **341**: 1–4.

86 Jackson IMD, Doig WB & McDonald G. Pernicious anaemia as a cause of infertility, *Lancet* 1967; **ii**: 1159.

87 Jackson L, Zachary J *et al*. A randomized comparison of transcervical and transabdominal chorionic-villus sampling. *New England Journal of Medicine* 1992; **327**: 594–8.

88 Jacobs A, Miller F, Worwood M, Beamish MR & Wardrop CA. Ferritin in serum of normal subjects and patients with iron deficiency and iron overload. *British Medical Journal* 1972; **4**: 206–8.
89 Jacobs A & Worwood M. Iron metabolism, iron deficiency and iron overload. In: RM Hardisty & DJ Weatherall (eds), *Blood and Its Disorders*, 2nd edn. Blackwell Scientific Publications, Oxford, 1982.
90 Jacobs P & Wood L. Paroxysmal nocturnal haemoglobinuria and pregnancy. *Lancet* 1986; **ii**: 1099.
91 Janov AJ, Anderson J *et al*. Pregnancy outcome in survivors of advanced Hodgkin's disease. *Cancer* 1992; **70**: 688–92.
92 Kaibra M, Kobayashi T & Matsusmoto S. Idiopathic thrombocythemia and pregnancy: Report of a case. *Obstetrics and Gynecology Supplement* 1985; **65**: 185–6.
93 Kan YW, Golbus MS & Dozy AM. Prenatal diagnosis of thalassaemia: Clinical application of molecular hybridization. *New England Journal of Medicine* 1971; **295**: 1165–7.
94 Kan YW, Trecartin RF, Golbus MS & Filly RA. Prenatal diagnosis of thalassaemia and sickle cell anaemia. Experience with 24 cases. *Lancet* 1977; **i**: 269–71.
95 Klebanoff MA, Shiono PH *et al*. Anemia and spontaneous preterm birth. *American Journal of Obstetrics and Gynecology* 1991; **164**: 59–63.
96 Ko TM, Tseng LH *et al*. Carrier detection and prenatal diagnosis of alpha-thalassemia of south-east Asian deletion by polymerase chain reaction. *Human Genetics* 1992; **88**: 245–8.
97 Koshy M & Burd L. Management of pregnancy in sickle cell syndromes. *Hematology and Oncology Clinics of North America* 1991; **5**: 585–96.
98 Koshy M. Burd L *et al*. Prophylactic red cell transfusions in pregnant patients with sickle cell disease. *New England Journal of Medicine* 1988; **319**: 1447–52.
99 Kuizon MD, Platon TP, Ancheta LP, Angeles JC, Nunez CB & Macapinlac MP. Iron supplementation among pregnant women. *South East Asian Journal of Tropical Medicine* 1979; **10**: 520–7.
100 Kullander S & Kallen B. A prospective study of drugs and pregnancy. *Acta Obstetrica Gynecologica Scandinavica Supplement* 1976; **55**: 287–95.
101 Landon MJ. Folate metabolism in pregnancy. *Clinics in Obstetrics and Gynaecology* 1975; **2**: 413–30.
102 Landon MJ & Hytten FE. The excretion of folate in pregnancy. *Journal of Obstetrics and Gynaecology of the British Commonwealth* 1971; **78**: 769–75.
103 Laurence KM, James N, Miller MH, Tennant GB & Campbell H. Double-blind randomised controlled trial of folate treatment before conception to prevent recurrence of neural tube defects. *British Medical Journal* 1981; **282**: 1509–11.
104 Leeuw NKM de, Lowenstein L & Hsieh YS. Iron deficiency and hydremia in normal pregnancy. *Medicine, Baltimore* 1966; **45**: 291–315.
105 Leeuw NKM de, Lowenstein L, Tucker EC & Dayal S. Correlation of red cell loss at delivery with changes in red cell mass. *American Journal of Obstetrics and Gynecology* 1968; **100**: 1092–101.
106 Letsky EA. Anaemia in obstetrics. In: Studd J (ed), *Progress in Obstetrics and Gynaecology*, Volume 6. Churchill Livingstone, Edinburgh, 1987: 23–59.
107 Lewis BJ & Laros RK. Leukaemia and lymphoma, In: Laros RK (ed), *Blood Disorders in Pregnancy*. Lea & Febiger, Philadelphia, 1986: 85–101.
108 Lewis SM. Aplastic anaemia in pregnancy. In: Hardisty RM & Weatherall DJ (eds), *Blood and its Disorders*, 2nd edn. Blackwell Scientific Publications, Oxford, 1982.
109 Lindheimer MD, Richardson DA *et al*. Potassium homeostasis in pregnancy. *Journal of Reproductive Medicine* 1987; **32**: 517–26.
110 Lishner M, Zemlickis D, Degendorfer P, Panzarella T, Sutcliffe SB & Koren G. Maternal and foetal outcome following Hodgkin's disease in pregnancy. *British Journal of Cancer* 1992; **65**: 114–17.
111 Lowenstein L, Brunton L & Hsieh Y-S. Nutritional anaemia and megaloblastic anaemia of pregnancy. *Canadian Medical Association* 1966; **94**: 634–45.
112 Lozoff B, Jimenez E & Wolf AW. Long-term developmental outcome of infants with iron deficiency. *New England Journal of Medicine* 1991; **325**: 687–94.
113 Lund CJ. Studies on the iron deficiency anaemia of pregnancy including plasma volume, total hemoglobin, erythrocyte protoporphyrin in treated and untreated normal and anemic patients. *American Journal of Obstetrics and Gynecology* 1951; **62**: 947–61.
114 Magee HE & Milligan EHM. Haemoglobin levels before and after labour. *British Medical Journal* 1951; **ii**: 1307–10.
115 Maxwell D, Czepulkowski B, Clifford R, Heaton D & Coleman D. Transabdominal chorionic villus sampling. *Lancet* 1986; **i**: 123–6.
116 Maxwell DJ, Johnson P, Hurley P, Neales K, Allan L & Knott P. Fetal blood sampling and pregnancy loss in relation to indication. *British Journal of Obstetrics and Gynaecology* 1991; **98**: 892–7.
116a Mayet FGH. Anaemia of pregnancy. *South African Medical Journal* 1985; **67**: 804–9.
117 McGarry JM & Andrews J. Smoking in pregnancy and vitamin B_{12} metabolism. *British Medical Journal* 1972; **ii**: 74–7.
118 McLain CR. Leukemia in pregnancy. *Clinical Obstetrics and Gynecology* 1974; **17**: 185–94.
119 McLean FW, Heine MW, Held B & Streiff RR. Folic acid absorption in pregnancy: comparison of the pteroylpolyglutamate and pteroylmonoglutamate. *Blood* 1970; **36**: 628–31.
120 Meadows NJ, Grainger SL, Ruse W, Keeling PWN & Thompson RPH. Oral iron and the bioavailability of zinc. *British Medical Journal* 1983; **287**: 1013–14.
121 Meadows NJ, Ruse W *et al*. Zinc and small babies. *Lancet* 1981; **ii**: 1135–7.

122 Miller JM, Horger EO, Key TC & Walker EM. Management of sickle haemoglobinopathies in pregnant patients. *American Journal of Obstetrics and Gynecology* 1981; **141**: 237–41.
123 Miller JR, Keith NM & Rowntree LG. Plasma and blood volume in pregnancy. *Journal of the American Medical Association* 1915; **65**: 779–82.
124 Milliken S, Powles R *et al*. Successful pregnancy following bone marrow transplantation for leukaemia. *Bone Marrow Transplant* 1990; **5**: 135–7.
125 Miyata T, Takeda J *et al*. The cloning of PIG-A, a component in the early step of GPI-anchor biosynthesis. *Science* 1993; **259**: 1318–20.
126 Modell B. Prevention of haemoglobinopathies. *British Medical Bulletin* 1983; **39**: 386–91.
127 Morgan EH. Plasma iron and haemoglobin levels in pregnancy. The effect of oral iron. *Lancet* 1961; **i**: 9–12.
128 MRC Vitamin Study Research Group. Prevention of neural tube defects: Results of the Medical Research Council Vitamin Study. *Lancet* 1991; **338**: 131–7.
129 Murphy JF, O'Riordan J, Newcombe RG, Coles EC & Pearson JF. Relation of haemoglobin levels in first and second trimesters to outcome of pregnancy. *Lancet* 1986; **i**: 992–5.
130 Ng SC, Wong KK *et al*. Autoimmune haemolytic anaemia in pregnancy: a case report. *European Journal of Obstetrics Gynecology and Reproductive Biology* 1990; **37**: 83–85.
131 Nicholson HO. Leukaemia and pregnancy. *Journal of Obstetrics and Gynaecology of the British Commonwealth* 1968; **75**: 517–20.
132 Nicolaides KH, Rodeck CH & Mibashan RS. Obstetric management and diagnosis of haematological disease in the fetus. In: Letsky EA (ed), *Haematological Disorders in Pregnancy*. Clinics in Haematology **14**: WB Saunders, Eastbourne, 1985: 775–805.
133 Nicolaides KH, Soothill PW, Rodeck CH & Campbell S. Ultrasound-guided sampling of umbilical cord and placental blood to assess fetal wellbeing. *Lancet* 1986; **i**: 1065–7.
134 Old JM, Thein SL, Weatherall DJ, Cao A & Loukopoulos D. Prenatal diagnosis of the major haemoglobin disorders. *Molecular Biology and Medicine* 1989; **6**: 55–63.
135 Old JM, Ward RHT, Petrou M, Karagozlu F, Modell B & Weatherall DJ. First-trimester fetal diagnosis for haemoglobinopathies: three cases. *Lancet* 1982; **ii**: 1413–16.
136 Old JM, Fitches A *et al*. First-trimester fetal diagnosis for haemoglobinopathies. Report on 200 cases. *Lancet* 1986; **ii**: 763–7.
137 Orkin SH, Alter C *et al*. Application of endonuclease mapping to the analysis and prenatal diagnosis of thalassaemias caused by globin gene deletion. *New England Journal of Medicine* 1978; **299**: 166.
138 Oski FA. Nutritional anaemias. *Seminars in Perinatology* 1979; **3**: 381–95.
139 Oski FA. Iron deficiency — facts and fallacies. *Paediatric Clinics of North America* 1985; **32**: 493–7.
140 Osler W. Observations on the severe anaemias of pregnancy and the post-partum state. *British Medical Journal* 1919; **i**: 1–3.
141 Paintin DB, Thomson AM & Hytten FE. Iron and the haemoglobin level in pregnancy. *Journal of Obstetrics and Gynaecology of the British Commonwealth* 1966; **73**: 181–90.
142 Pearson TC. Clinical annotation — primary thrombocythaemia: diagnosis and management. *British Journal of Haematology* 1991; **78**: 145–8.
143 Peck TM & Arias F. Hematologic changes associated with pregnancy. *Clinical Obstetrics and Gynecology* 1979; **22**: 785–98.
144 Perry Jr KG & Morrison JC. The diagnosis and management of hemoglobinopathies during pregnancy. *Seminars in Perinatology* 1990; **14**: 90–102.
145 Picot C, Triadou P, Lacombe C, Casadevall N & Girot R. Relapsing pure red-cell aplasia during pregnancy. *New England Journal of Medicine* 1984; **311**: 196.
146 Piomelli S. Management of Cooley's anaemia. In: Higgs DR & Weatherall DJ (eds), *Baillière's Clinical Haematology, The Haemoglobinopathies*, Baillière Tindall, London, 1993: 287–98.
147 Pirani BBK, Campbell DM & Macgillivray I. Plasma volume in normal first pregnancy. *Journal of Obstetrics and Gynaecology of the British Commonwealth* 1973; **80**: 884–7.
148 Powars D, Chan LS & Schroeder WA. The variable expression of sickle cell disease is genetically determined. *Seminars in Hematology* 1990; **27**: 360–76.
149 Rae PG & Robb PM. Megaloblastic anaemia of pregnancy, a clinical and laboratory study with particular reference to the total and labile serum folate levels. *Journal of Clinical Pathology* 1970; **23**: 379–91.
150 Reichel RP, Linkesch W & Schetitska D. Therapy with recombinant interferon alpha-2c during unexpected pregnancy in a patient with chronic myeloid leukaemia. *British Journal of Haematology* 1992; **82**: 472–3.
151 Ring J & Messmer IL. Incidence and severity of anaphylactoid reactions to colloid volume substitutes. *Lancet* 1977; **i**: 466–9.
152 Rios ER, Lipschitz DA, Cook JD & Smith NJ, Relationship of maternal and infant iron stores as assessed by determination of plasma ferritin. *Paediatrics* 1975; **55**: 694–9.
153 Rodeck CH & Morsman JM. First trimester chorion biopsy. *British Medical Bulletin* 1983; **39**: 338–42.
154 Rosenberg IH. Folic acid and neural-tube defects — time for action? *New England Journal of Medicine* 1992; **327**: 1875–7.
155 Rosse WF, Gallagher D *et al*. Transfusion and alloimmunization in sickle cell disease. The Cooperative Study of Sickle Cell Disease. *Blood* 1990; **76**: 1431–7.

156 Rothman LA, Cohen CJ & Astarloa J. Placental and fetal involvement by maternal malignancy: A report of rectal carcinoma and review of the literature. *American Journal of Obstetrics and Gynecology* 1973; **116**: 1023–33.
157 Rotoli B & Luzzatto L. Paroxysmal nocturnal haemoglobinuria. *Baillière's Clinical Haematology* 1989; **2**: 113–38.
158 Rovinsky JJ & Jaffin H. Cardiovascular hemodynamics in pregnancy. I Blood and plasma volumes in multiple pregnancy. *American Journal of Obstetrics and Gynecology* 1965; **93**: 1–13.
159 Scholl TO, Hediger ML *et al*. Anemia vs. iron deficiency: increased risk of preterm delivery in a prospective study. *American Journal of Clinical Nutrition* 1992; **55**: 985–88.
160 Scott JM. Toxicity of iron sorbitol citrate. *British Medical Journal* 1962; **ii**: 480–1.
161 Scott JM. Iron sorbitol citrate in pregnancy anaemia. *British Medical Journal* 1963; **ii**: 354–7.
162 Serjeant GR. Sickle haemoglobin and pregnancy. *British Medical Journal* 1983; **287**: 628–30.
163 Serjeant GR. The clinical features of sickle cell disease. In: Higgs DR & Weatherall DJ (eds), *Baillière's Clinical Haematology, The Haemoglobinopathies*, Baillière Tindall, London, 1993: 93–115.
164 Shapiro J, Alberts HW, Welch P & Metz J. Folate and vitamin B_{12} deficiency associated with lactation. *British Journal of Haematology* 1965; **11**: 498–504.
165 Sheldon WL, Aspillaga MO, Smith PA & Lind T. The effects of oral iron supplementation on zinc and magnesium levels during pregnancy. *British Journal of Obstetrics and Gynaecology* 1985; **92**: 892–8.
166 Slade R & James DK. Pregnancy and maternal malignant haematological disorders. In: Turner TL (ed), *Perinatal Haematological Problems*. John Wiley & Sons, Chichester, 1991: 23–38.
167 Smidt-Jensen S, Permin M *et al*. Randomized comparison of amniocentesis and transabdominal and transcervical chorionic villus sampling. *Lancet* 1992; **340**: 1237–44.
168 Smithells RW, Sheppard S *et al*. Possible prevention of neural tube defects by periconceptional vitamin supplementation. *Lancet* 1980; **i**: 339–40.
169 Smithells RW, Nevin NC *et al*. Further experience of vitamin supplementation for prevention of neural tube defect recurrences. *Lancet* 1983; **i**: 1027–31.
170 Snethlage W & Tengate JW. Thrombocythaemia and recurrent late abortions. Normal outcome of pregnancies after anti-aggregatory treatment. *British Journal of Obstetrics and Gynaecology* 1986; **93**: 386–8.
171 Snyder TE, Lee LP & Lynch S. Pregnancy-associated hypoplastic anemia. a review. *Obstetrics and Gynecological Survey* 1991; **46**: 264–9.
172 Spencer JAD. Paroxysmal nocturnal haemoglobinuria in pregnancy. *British Journal of Obstetrics and Gynaecology* 1980; **87**: 246–8.
173 Stein ML, Gunston KD & May RM. Iron dextran in the treatment of iron-deficiency anaemia of pregnancy. Haematological response and incidence of side-effects. *South African Medical Journal* 1991; **79**: 195–6.
174 Stephens HEM, Craft I, Peters TJ & Hoffbrand AV. Oral contraceptives and folate metabolism. *Clinical Science* 1972; **42**: 405–14.
175 Stone ML, Luhby AL, Feldman R, Gordon M & Cooperman JM. Folic acid metabolism in pregnancy. *American Journal of Obstetrics and Gynecology* 1967; **90**: 638–48.
176 Stott G. Anaemia in Mauritius. *Bulletin of the World Health Organization 1960;* **23**: 781–91.
177 Strauss RG & Bernstein R. Folic acid and dilantin antagonism in pregnancy. *Obstetrics and Gynecology* 1974; **44**: 345–8.
178 Svanberg B. Absorption of iron in pregnancy. *Acta Obstetrica et Gynecologica Scandinavica Supplement* 1975; **48**: 107–8.
179 Taylor DJ, Mallen C, McDougall N & Lind T. Effect of iron supplementation on serum ferritin levels during and after pregnancy. *British Journal of Obstetrics and Gynaecology* 1982; **89**: 1011–17.
180 Taylor JJ, Studd JWW & Green ID. Primary refractory anaemia and pregnancy. *Journal of Obstetrics and Gynaecology of the British Commonwealth* 1968; **75**: 963–8.
181 Temperley IJ, Meehan MJM & Gattenby PBB. Serum vitamin B_{12} levels in pregnant women. *Journal of Obstetrics and Gynaecology of the British Commonwealth* 1968; **75**: 511–16.
182 Thomas AN, Pattison C & Serjeant GR. Causes of death in sickle-cell disease in Jamaica. *British Medical Journal* 1982; **285**: 633–5.
183 Thompson WG. Comparison of tests for diagnosis of iron depletion in pregnancy. *American Journal of Obstetrics and Gynecology* 1988; **159**: 1132–4.
184 Tuck SM, James CE, Brewster EM, Pearson TC & Studd JWW. Prophylactic blood transfusion in maternal sickle cell syndromes. *British Journal of Obstetrics and Gynaecology* 1987; **94**: 121–5.
185 Tuck SM, Studd JWW & White JM. Pregnancy in sickle cell disease in the United Kingdom. *British Journal of Obstetrics and Gynaecology* 1983; **90**: 112–17.
186 Van Enk A, Visschers G *et al*. Maternal death due to sickle cell chronic lung disease. *British Journal of Obstetrics and Gynaecology*. 1992; **99**: 162–3.
187 Van Leeuwen EF, Halmerhorst FM, Engelfriet CP & Von Dem Borne AEG Jr. Maternal autoimmune thrombocytopenia and the newborn. *British Medical Journal* 1981; **283**: 104.
188 Vermylen J, Blockmans D, Spitz B & Deckmyn H. Thrombosis and immune disorders. In: Chesterman N (ed), *Clinics in Haematology* **15**. WB Saunders, Eastbourne, 1986: 395.
189 Ward FT & Weiss RB. Lymphoma and pregnancy.

Seminars in Oncology 1989; **16**: 397–409.
190 Weatherall DJ. Prenatal diagnosis of thalassaemia. *British Medical Journal* 1984; **288**: 1321–2.
191 Weatherall DJ. Prenatal diagnosis of haematological disorders. In: Letsky EA, Hann IM & Gibson BES (eds), *Fetal and Neonatal Haematology*. Baillière Tindall, London, 1991: 285–314.
192 Weatherall DJ. *The New Genetics and Clinical Practice*, 3rd edn. Oxford University Press, Oxford, 1991.
193 Weatherall DJ & Letsky EA. Genetic haematological disorders. In: Wald NJ (ed), *Antenatal and Neonatal Screening*. Oxford University Press, Oxford, 1984.
194 Williamson R, Eskdale J, Coleman DV, Niazi M, Loeffler FE & Modell BM. Direct gene analysis of chorionic villi: a possible technique for first trimester antenatal diagnosis of haemoglobinopathies. *Lancet* 1981; **ii**: 1125–7.
195 Wood WG & Weatherall DJ. Haemoglobin synthesis during human fetal development. *Nature* 1973; **244**: 162–5.
196 World Health Organization. *Nutritional anaemias. Technical Report Series No. 503*. Geneva, 1972.
197 Zuazu J, Julia A *et al*. Pregnancy outcome in hematologic malignancies. *Cancer* 1991; **67**: 703–9.

Further reading

Alter BP. Prenatal diagnosis of haemoglobinopathies: a status report. *Lancet* 1981; **ii**: 1152–5.

Alter BP. Antenatal diagnosis using fetal blood. In: Weatherall DJ (ed) *The Thalassaemias*, Churchill Livingstone, Edinburgh, 1983: 114–33.

Alter BP, Modell CB *et al*. Prenatal diagnosis of haemoglobinopathy: a review of 15 cases. *New England Journal of Medicine* 1976; **295**: 1437–43.

Anon. Antenatal diagnosis of haemoglobin disorders. *Lancet* 1981; **ii**: 1147–8.

Anon. Molecular genetics for the clinician. *Lancet* 1984; **i**: 257–9.

Anon. Relapsing pure red cell aplasia during pregnancy. *New England Journal of Medicine* 1984; **311**: 196.

Apperley JF. Bone marrow transplant for the haemoglobinopathies: past, present and future. In: Higgs DR & Weatherall DJ (eds), *Baillière's Clinical Haematology, The Haemoglobinopathies*. Baillière Tindall, London, 1993: 299–325.

Aviles A, Diaz-Maqueo JC, Talavera A, Guzman R & Garcia EL. Growth and development of children of mothers treated with chemotherapy during pregnancy: current status of 43 children. *American Journal of Hematology* 1991; **36**: 243–8.

Boyer SH, Noyes AN & Boyer ML. Enrichment of erythrocytes of fetal origin from adult–fetal blood mixtures via selective haemolysis of adult blood cells: an aid to antenatal diagnosis of haemoglobinopathies. *Blood* 1976; **47**: 883–97.

Briggs M & Briggs M. Endocrine effect on serum vitamin B_{12}. *Lancet* 1972; **ii**: 1037.

Brozović M. Exchange transfusion in sickle cell crisis. Personal Communication. 1981.

Chan V, Ghosh A, Chan TK, Wong V & Todd D. Prenatal diagnosis of homozygous α-thalassaemia by direct DNA analysis of uncultured amniotic fluid cells. *British Medical Journal* 1984; **288**: 1327–9.

Chang H, Modell CB *et al*. Expression of the thalassaemia gene in the first trimester fetus. *Proceedings of the National Academy of Sciences, USA* 1975; **72**: 3633–7.

Chesley LC. Plasma and red cell volumes during pregnancy. *American Journal of Obstetrics and Gynecology* 1972; **112**: 440–50.

Clay B, Rosenberg B, Sampson N & Samuels SI. Reactions to total dose intravenous infusion of iron dextran (imferon). *British Medical Journal* 1965; **i**: 29–31.

Clegg JB, Naughton MA & Weatherall DJ. Abnormal human haemoglobins: separation and characterisation of the α and β chains by chromatography and the determination of two new variants Hb. Chesapeake and Hb.J (Bangkok). *Journal of Molecular Biology* 1966; **19**: 91–108.

de Swiet M. The respiratory system. In: Hytten FE & Chamberlain GVP (eds), *Clinical Physiology in Obstetrics*. Blackwell Scientific Publications, Oxford, 1980: 79–100.

de Swiet M. Prescribing in pregnancy — anti-coagulants. *British Medical Journal* 1987; **294**: 428–30.

Finch CA & Cook JD. Iron deficiency. *American Journal of Clinical Nutrition* 1984; **39**: 470–1.

Fisk NF & Bower S. Fetal blood sampling in retreat. *British Medical Journal* 1993; **307**: 143–4.

Fitzpatrick C. Birth control and paroxysmal noctural haemoglobinuria. *Lancet* 1987; **i**: 1260.

Hegde UM, Bowes A, Powell DK & Joyner MV. Detection of platelet bound and serum antibodies in thrombocytopenia by enzyme linked assay. *Vox Sanguinis* 1981; **41**: 306–12.

Herbert V. Biology of disease — megaloblastic anaemias. *Laboratory Investigations* 1985; **52**: 3–19.

Hobbins JC & Mahoney MJ. *In utero* diagnosis of haemoglobinopathies: Techniques for obtaining fetal blood. *New England Journal of Medicine* 1983; **290**: 1065–7.

Holmberg L, Bjorn C *et al*. Prenatal diagnosis of haemophilia by an immunoradiometric assay of Factor IX. *Blood* 1980; **56**: 397–401.

Homer LW, Lindsten J *et al*. Prenatal evaluation of fetus of risk for severe von Willebrand's disease. *Lancet* 1979; **ii**: 191–2.

Huehns ER, Davies SC & Brozović M. Fresh frozen plasma for vaso-occlusive crisis in sickle cell disease. *Lancet* 1981; **i**: 1310–11.

Hux PH, Wapner RJ, Chayen B, Rattan P, Jarrell B & Greenfield L. Use of the Greenfield filter for thromboembolic disease in pregnancy. *American Journal of Obstetrics and Gynaecology* 1986; **155**: 734–7.

Iyengar L. Folic acid requirements of Indian pregnant

women. *American Journal of Obstetrics and Gynecology* 1971; **111**: 13–16.

Kan YW & Dozy AM. Antenatal diagnosis of sickle cell anaemia by DNA analysis of amniotic fluid cells. *Lancet* 1978; **ii**: 810–12.

Kan YW, Nathan DG, Cividalli G & Crookston MC. Concentration of fetal red blood cells from a mixture of maternal and fetal blood anti-i serum: an aid to prenatal diagnosis of haemoglobinopathy. *Blood* 1974; **43**: 411–15.

Landon MJ & Hytten FE. Plasma folate levels following an oral load of folic acid during pregnancy. *Journal of Obstetrics and Gynaecology of the British Commonwealth* 1972; **79**: 577–83.

Lazarchick J & Hoyer LW. Immunoradiometric measurement of the Factor VIII procoagulant antigen. *Journal of Clinical Investigation* 1978; **62**: 1048–52.

Letsky EA. The haematological system. In: Hytten FE & Chamberlain GVP (eds), *Clinical Physiology in Obstetrics*, Blackwell Scientific Publications, Oxford 1980: 43–78.

Liang ST, Wong VCW, So WWK, Ma HK, Chan V & Todd D. Homozygous α-thalassaemia: clinical presentation, diagnosis and management. A review of 46 cases. *British Journal of Obstetrics and Gynaecology* 1985; **92**: 680–4.

MacKenzie IZ, Sayers L *et al*. Coagulation changes during second trimester abortion induced by intraamniotic prostaglandin E_2 and hypertonic solutions. *Lancet* 1975; **ii**: 1066–9.

Marengo Rowe AJ, Murff G, Leveson JE & Cook J. Haemophilia-like disease associated with pregnancy. *Obstetrics and Gynecology* 1972; **40**: 56.

McCann SR, Lawlor E, McGovern M & Temperley IJ. Severe megaloblastic anaemia of pregnancy. *Journal of the Irish Medical Association* 1980; **73**: 197–8.

McCollum C. Vena caval filters; keeping big clots down. *British Medical Journal* 1987; **294**: 1566.

McMillan R. Chronic idiopathic thrombocytopenic purpura. *New England Journal of Medicine* 1981; **304**: 1135–47.

O'Donnel D, Sevitz H, Seggie JL, Meyers AM, Botha JR & Myburgh JA. Pregnancy after renal transplantation. *Australian New Zealand Journal of Medicine* 1985; **15**: 320–5.

Ogunbode O, Akinyele IO & Hussain MA. Dietary iron intake of pregnant Nigerian women with anaemia. *International Journal of Gynaecology and Obstetrics* 1979; **17**: 290–3.

Okuyama T, Tawada T, Furuya H & Villee CA. The role of transferrin and ferritin in the fetal-maternal placental unit. *American Journal of Obstetrics and Gynecology* 1985; **152**: 344–50.

Paull JA. Prospective study of dextran-induced anaphylactoid reactions in 5745 patents. *Anaesthesia and Intensive Care* 1987; **15**: 163–7.

Pasteroke JG II & Saseiler B. Maternal death associated with sickle cell trait. *American Journal of Obstetrics and Gynecology* 1985; **151**: 295–7.

Reynolds EH. Anticonvulsants, folic acid and epilepsy. *Lancet* 1973; **i**: 1376–8.

Richards HG & Spiers AS. Chronic granulocytic leukaemia in pregnancy. *Journal of Clinical Pathology* 1974; **27**: 927.

Richmond HG. Induction of sarcoma in the rat by iron–dextran complex. *British Medical Journal* 1959; **1**: 947–9.

Roberts PD, James H, Petrie A, Morgan JO & Hoffbrand AV. Vitamin B_{12} status in pregnancy among immigrants to Britain. *British Medical Journal* 1973; **iii**: 67–72.

Rodeck CH & Nicolaides KH. Fetoscopy and fetal tissue sampling. *British Medical Bulletin* 1983; **39**: 332–7.

Sachs BP, Brown DAJ *et al*. Maternal mortality in Massachusetts. *New England Journal of Medicine* 1987; **316**: 667–72.

Samuels-Reid JH, Scott RB & Brown WE. Contraceptive practices and reproductive patterns in sickle cell disease. *Journal of the National Medical Association* 1984; **76**: 879–83.

Tuck SM. Sickle cell disease and pregnancy. *British Journal of Hospital Medicine* 1982; **28**: 125–7.

Van Besien K, Tricot G *et al*. Pregnancy-associated aplastic anemia – report of 3 cases. *European Journal of Haematology* 1991; **47**: 253–6.

Van Dinh T, Boor PJ & Garza JR. Massive pulmonary embolism following delivery of a patient with sickle cell trait. *American Journal of Obstetrics and Gynecology* 1982; **143**: 722–4.

3

Coagulation Defects

Elizabeth A. Letsky

Haemostasis and pregnancy, 71
Vascular integrity
Platelets
Arrest of bleeding after trauma
Local response
Coagulation system
The naturally occurring anticoagulants
Fibrinolysis
Summary of changes in haemostasis in pregnancy and delivery
Disseminated intravascular coagulation, 77
Haematological management of the bleeding obstetric patient
DIC in clinical conditions, 83
In vitro detection of low grade DIC
Abruptio placentae
Amniotic fluid embolism
Retention of dead fetus
Induced abortion
Intrauterine infection
Acute fatty liver of pregnancy
Conclusions
Acquired primary defects of haemostasis, 89
Thrombocytopenia
Pre-eclampsia and platelets
TTP and HUS
Factor VIII antibody
Inherited defects of haemostasis, 100
Hereditary platelet abnormalities
Hereditary coagulation disorders
Autoimmune thrombocytopenic purpura
Alloimmune thrombocytopenia

Haemostasis and pregnancy

Healthy haemostasis depends on normal vasculature, platelets, coagulation factors and fibrinolysis. These act together to confine the circulating blood to the vascular bed and arrest bleeding after trauma. Normal pregnancy is accompanied by dramatic changes in the coagulation and fibrinolytic systems [70,104,182] where there is a marked increase in some of the coagulation factors, particularly fibrinogen. Fibrin is laid down in the uteroplacental vessel walls and fibrinolysis is suppressed. These changes, together with the increased blood volume, help to combat the hazard of haemorrhage at placental separation, but play only a secondary role to the unique process of myometrial contraction which reduces the blood flow to the placental site. They also produce a vulnerable state for intravascular clotting, which is expressed as a whole spectrum of disorders in pregnancy ranging from thromboembolism (see Chapter 4) to bleeding due to disseminated intravascular coagulation (DIC) [102]. To make more understandable the pathophysiology and management of these disorders a short account follows of haemostasis during pregnancy and how it differs from that in the non-pregnant state.

Vascular integrity

It is not known how vascular integrity is normally maintained but it is clear that the platelets have a key role to play since conditions in which their number is depleted or their function is abnormal are characterized by widespread spontaneous capillary haemorrhages. It is thought that the platelets in health are constantly sealing microdefects of the vasculature, by forming mini fibrin clots, the unwanted fibrin being removed by a process of fibrinolysis. Generation of prostacyclin appears to be the physiological mechanism which protects the vessel wall from excess deposition of platelet aggregates, and explains the fact that contact of platelets with healthy vascular endothelium is not a stimulus for thrombus formation [131].

Prostacyclin (PGI_2) is an unstable prostaglandin first discovered in 1976. It is the principal prostanoid that blood vessels synthesize, a powerful vasodilator and a potent inhibitor of platelet aggregation. Moncada and Vane [131] have proposed that there is a balance between the production of prostacyclin by the vessel wall, and the production of the vasoconstrictor and powerful aggregating agent thromboxane by the platelet. Prostacyclin prevents aggregation at much lower concentrations than are needed to prevent adhesion, therefore vascular damage leads to platelet adhesion but not necessarily to aggregation and thrombus formation.

When injury is minor, small platelet thrombi form and are washed away by the circulation as described above, but the extent of the injury is an important determinant of the size of the thrombus — and whether or not platelet aggregation is stimulated (see below). Prostacyclin synthetase is abundant in the intima and progressively decreases in concentration from the intima to the adventitia, whereas the pro-aggregating elements increase in concentration from the subendothelium to the adventitia. It follows that severe vessel damage or physical detachment of the endothelium will lead to the development of a large thrombus as opposed to simple platelet adherence.

There are several conditions in which the production of prostacyclin could be impaired, thereby upsetting the normal balance. Deficiency of prostacyclin production has been suggested in platelet consumption syndromes such as haemolytic uraemic syndrome (HUS) and thrombotic thrombocytopenic purpura (TTP) [108]. Prostacyclin production has also been shown to be reduced in fetal and placental tissue from pre-eclamptic pregnancies, and the current role of prostacyclin in the pathogenesis of pre-eclampsia is undergoing active investigation.

However, the endothelium is now regarded as an extremely important component of the haemostatic system and endothelial cell injury leads to platelet activation and triggering of the coagulation system. It is possible that the changes in haemostatic components are purely a secondary response to underlying vascular disease.

Some studies have shown an increased oxygen free radical production in pre-eclampsia which will in turn decrease vascular prostacyclin and endothelial-dependent relaxing factor (i.e. nitric oxide, NO) release and increase thromboxane A_2 and endothelin release. The whole subject of endothelial function in pre-eclampsia has been well reviewed recently [204] (see also Chapter 6).

Platelets

Platelets are produced in the bone marrow by the megakaryocytes and have a lifespan of 9–12 days. At the end of their normal lifespan the effete cells are engulfed by cells of the reticulo-endothelial system and most damaged platelets are sequestered in the spleen.

There have been conflicting reports concerning the platelet count during normal pregnancy. A review of publications over 25 years [176] revealed a majority consensus (of six), suggesting a small fall in the platelet count towards term, during normal pregnancy — two publications suggesting that there is no change and one early, probably inaccurate, study documenting a rise. However, few of these studies obtained data on a longitudinal basis and in none of them was a within-patient analysis performed. Until recently platelet counts have been performed manually in a haemocytometer, calculating the number of platelets per cubic millimetre in anticoagulated blood samples. This is time-consuming and had to be performed as a separate investigation that was only requested in those patients giving concern. Now that automated platelet counting is available, platelet counts are part of the routine blood count and more information is available about the platelet count in normal, uncomplicated pregnancy. It is becoming clear that, if mean values for platelet concentration are analysed throughout pregnancy, there is a downward trend [67] even though the majority fall within the accepted non-pregnant range [15,69,176].

There is also conflicting evidence [155,197] of increased platelet turnover and low grade platelet activation as pregnancy advances resulting in a larger proportion of younger platelets with a greater mean platelet volume [67,176].

Most investigators agree that low grade chronic intravascular coagulation within the uteroplacental circulation is a part of the physiological response of all women to pregnancy. This is partially compensated and it is not surprising that the platelets should be involved either giving indices of increased turnover or in some cases a reduction in number.

A recent prospective study of 2263 healthy women delivering during 1 year at a Canadian obstetric centre [33] showed that 112 (8.3 per cent) had mild thrombocytopenia at term (platelet counts $97-150 \times 10^9/l$). The frequency of thrombocytopenia in their offspring was no greater than that of babies born to women with platelet counts in the normal accepted range and no infant had a platelet count $<100 \times 10^9/l$. An extension of this study to include 6715 deliveries substantiates these original findings [34].

In one study patients with a normal pregnancy were compared with non-pregnant controls. They were shown to have a significantly lower platelet count and an increase in circulating platelet aggregates. *In vitro* the platelets were shown to be hypo-aggregable. This was interpreted as suggesting platelet activation during pregnancy causing platelet aggregation and followed by exhaustion of platelets [144].

Earlier publications suggesting that there was no evidence of changes in platelet function or differences in platelet lifespan [155,162] between healthy non-pregnant and pregnant women have to be re-evaluated in the face of more recent investigations, but it is clear that *normal* pregnancy has little significant effect on the screening parameter that is usually measured, namely the platelet count.

The problem remains in defining completely normal pregnancy. Certain disease states specific to pregnancy have profound effects on platelet consumption, lifespan and function. For example, a decrease in platelet count [157] and changes in platelet function [2] have been observed in pregnancies with fetal growth retardation and the lifespan of platelets is shortened significantly even in mild pre-eclampsia [13,111].

Arrest of bleeding after trauma

An essential function of the haemostatic system is a rapid reaction to injury which remains confined to the area of damage. This requires a control mechanism which will stimulate coagulation after trauma, and also limit the extent of the response. The substances involved in the formation of the haemostatic plug normally circulate in an inert form, until activated at the site of injury, or by some other factor released into the circulation which will trigger intravascular coagulation.

Local response

Platelets adhere to collagen on the injured basement membrane, which triggers a series of changes in the platelets themselves, including shape change and release of adenosine diphosphate (ADP) and other substances. Release of ADP stimulates further aggregation of platelets, which triggers the coagulation cascade generating thrombin; which in turn leads to the formation of fibrin which converts the lone platelet plug into a firm, stable wound seal. The role of platelets is of less importance in injury involving large vessels, because platelet aggregates are of insufficient size and strength to breach the defect. The coagulation mechanism is of major importance here, together with vascular contraction.

Coagulation system

The end result of blood coagulation is the formation of an insoluble fibrin clot from the soluble precursor fibrinogen in the plasma. This involves a complex interaction of clotting factors, and a sequential activation of a series of pro-enzymes, the coagulation cascade (Fig. 3.1). When a blood vessel is injured, blood coagulation is initiated by activation of Factor XII by collagen (intrinsic mechanism) and activation of Factor VII by thromboplastin release (extrinsic mechanism) from the damaged tissues. Both the intrinsic and extrinsic mechanisms are activated by components of the vessel wall and both are required for normal haemostasis. Strict divisions between the two pathways do not exist and interactions between activated factors in both pathways have been shown. They share a common pathway following the activation of Factor X.

The intrinsic pathway (or contact system) proceeds spontaneously and is relatively slow, requiring 5–20 min for visible fibrin formation. All tissues contain a specific lipoprotein, thromboplastin (particularly concentrated in lung and brain), which markedly increases the rate at which blood clots. The placenta is also very rich in tissue factor (thromboplastin), which will produce fibrin formation within 12 seconds; the acceleration of coagulation is brought about by bypassing the reactions involving the contact (intrinsic) system (Fig. 3.1). Since blood coagulation is strictly confined to the site of tissue injury in normal circumstances, powerful control mechanisms must be at work to prevent dissemination of coagulation.

Normal pregnancy is accompanied by major changes in the coagulation system, with increases in levels of Factors VII, VIII and X, and a particularly marked increase in the level of plasma fibrinogen [26] (Fig. 3.1), which is probably the chief cause of the accelerated erythrocyte sedimentation rate observed during pregnancy. The effect of pregnancy on the coagulation factors can be detected from about the third month of gestation, and the amount of fibrinogen in late pregnancy is at least double that of the non-pregnant state [26].

The naturally occurring anticoagulants

Mechanisms that limit and localize the clotting process at sites of trauma are critically important to protect against generalized thrombosis — and also to prevent spontaneous activation of those powerful procoagulant factors which circulate in normal plasma.

The recent investigation of healthy haemostasis, switched emphasis from the factors which promote clotting to those that prevent generalized and spontaneous activation of these factors. It is not appropriate to give an account of the complex interactions and biochemistry of all of these factors here. Only those of major importance in haemostasis and their relevance to pregnancy will be mentioned — the balance of procoagulant and inhibitory factors is discussed elsewhere [98].

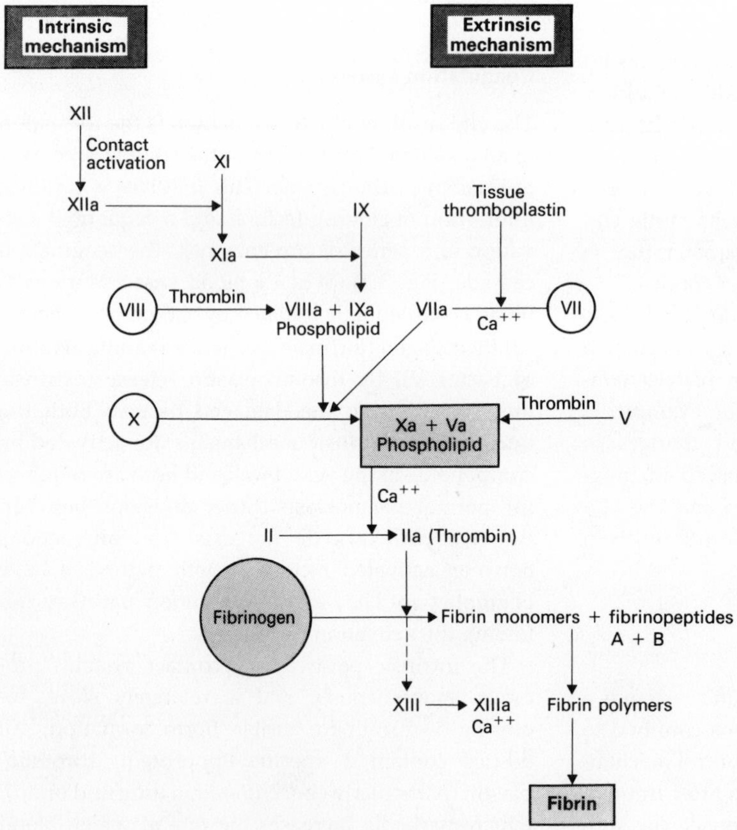

Fig. 3.1. The factors involved in blood coagulation and their interactions. The circled factors show significant increases in pregnancy.

Antithrombin III

Antithrombin III (ATIII) is considered to be the main physiological inhibitor of thrombin and Factor Xa. It is well known that heparin greatly enhances the reaction rate of enzyme ATIII interaction and this is the rationale for the use of low dose heparin as prophylaxis in patients at risk for thromboembolism post-operatively, in pregnancy and the puerperium. An inherited deficiency of ATIII is one of the conditions in which a familial tendency to thrombosis has been described (see Chapter 4).

ATIII is synthesized in the liver. Its activity is low in cirrhosis and other chronic diseases of the liver, as well as in protein-losing renal disease, DIC and hypercoagulable states. The commonest cause of a small reduction in ATIII is the use of oral contraceptives; this effect is related to the oestrogen content of the pill.

During pregnancy there is little change in ATIII level but there is some decrease at parturition and an increase in the puerperium [86]. However, there must be increased synthesis in the antenatal period to maintain normal concentrations in the face of an increasing plasma volume.

Protein C–thrombomodulin–protein S

Protein C inactivates Factors V and VIII in conjunction with its cofactors thrombomodulin and protein S. Protein C is a vitamin K dependent anticoagulant synthesized in the liver. To exert its effect it must be activated by an endothelial cell cofactor termed thrombomodulin. The importance of the protein C–thrombomodulin–protein S system is exemplified by the absence of thrombomodulin in the brain where the priority for haemostasis is higher than for anticoagulant.

Many kindreds with a deficiency or a functional deficit of protein C with associated recurrent thromboembolism have been described [20] (see Chapter 4). Purpura fulminans neonatalis is the homozygous expression of protein C deficiency with severe thrombosis and neonatal death [171].

Protein S, also a vitamin K dependent glycoprotein, acts as a cofactor for activated protein C by promoting its binding to lipid and platelet surface thus localizing the reaction.

Several families have been described with protein S deficiency and thromboembolic disease.

Data on protein C and protein S levels in healthy pregnancy are sparse. One study showed a significant reduction in functional protein S levels during pregnancy and the puerperium [51]. More recently, 14 patients followed longitudinally throughout gestation and post-partum, showed a rise of protein C within the normal non-pregnant range during the second trimester. In contrast free protein S fell from the second trimester onwards but remained within the confines of the normal range [199]. Another study supported these findings and extended their study to women using oral contraceptives in whom similar changes were found [119].

Although the investigation of natural anticoagulants has only just begun, the system has grown in complexity as our knowledge increases. There is little doubt that in the near future more components will be recognized as our ability to investigate objectively increases [3]. This will allow a better and more thorough understanding of the mechanisms underlying the control of the delicate balance between procoagulant and anticoagulant factors which results in a healthy haemostatic system [166] and enable us to manage these complex hypercoagulable states in pregnancy successfully [196].

For example, a further development is the recognition of Activated Protein C Resistance (APCR). Activated Protein C inactivates Factor V. Abnormal forms of Factor V resist such inactivation and may account for up to 25% of cases of thromboembolism in young people [183].

Fibrinolysis

Fibrinolytic activity is an essential part of the dynamic, interacting haemostatic mechanism, and is dependent on plasminogen activator in the blood (Fig. 3.2). Fibrin and fibrinogen are digested by plasmin, a pro-enzyme derived from an inactive plasma precursor plasminogen.

Increased amounts of activator are found in the plasma after strenuous exercise, emotional stress, surgical operations and other trauma. Tissue activator can be extracted from most human organs with the exception of the placenta. Tissues especially rich in activator include the uterus,

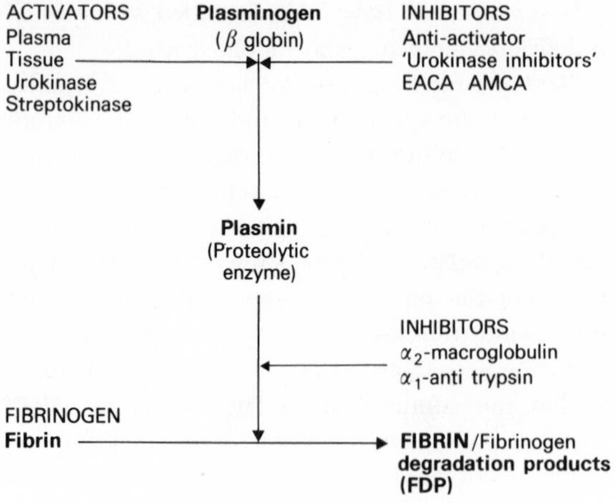

Fig. 3.2. Components of the fibrinolytic system.

ovaries, prostate, heart lungs, thyroid, adrenals and lymph nodes. Activity in tissues is concentrated mainly around blood vessels, veins showing greater activity than arteries.

The inhibitors of fibrinolytic activity are of two types — anti-activator (antiplasminogens) and the antiplasmins. Inhibitors of plasminogen include ε amino caproic acid (EACA) and tranexamic acid (AMCA). Aprotinin (Trasylol) is another antiplasminogen which is commercially prepared from bovine lung.

Platelets, plasma and serum exert a strong inhibitory action on plasmin. Normally, plasma antiplasmin levels exceed levels of plasminogen and hence the levels of potential plasmin; otherwise we would dissolve away our connecting cement! When fibrinogen or fibrin is broken down by plasmin, fibrin degradation products are formed; these comprise the high molecular weight split products X and Y, and smaller fragments, A, B, C, D and E (Fig. 3.3). When a fibrin clot is formed, 70 per cent of fragment X is retained in the clot, Y, D and E being retained to a somewhat lesser extent. Note that blood should be taken for estimation of fibrin degradation products (FDP) by clean venepuncture. The tourniquet should not be left on too long since venous stasis also stimulates fibrinolytic activity. The blood should be allowed to clot in the presence of an antifibrinolytic agent such as EACA to stop the process of fibrinolysis which would otherwise continue *in vitro*.

Plasma fibrinolytic activity is decreased during pregnancy, remains low during labour and delivery and returns to normal within 1 hour of delivery of the placenta [27]. This is thought to be due to the effect of placentally derived plasminogen activator inhibitor type 2 (PAI-2) which is present in abundance during pregnancy [28]. In addition the activity in the fibrinolytic system in response to stimulation has been found to be significantly reduced in pregnancy [12].

Summary of changes in haemostasis in pregnancy and delivery

The changes in the coagulation system in normal pregnancy are consistent with a continuing low

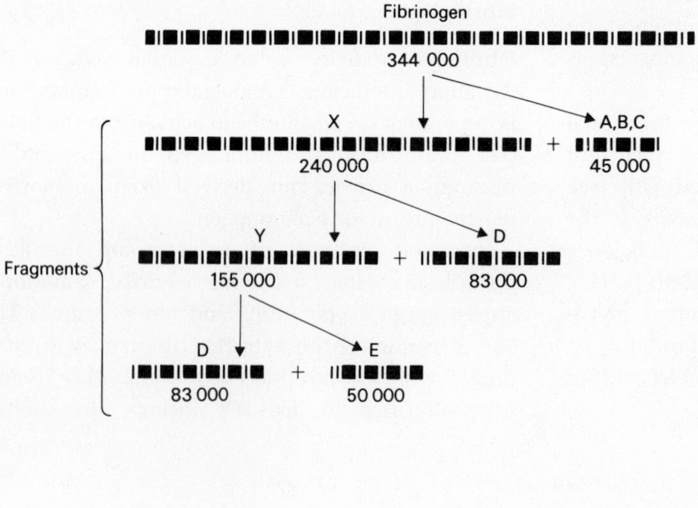

Fig. 3.3. Fibrin degradation products (FDPs) produced by action of plasma fibrinogen. The molecular weights are shown.

grade process of coagulant activity. Using electron microscopy, fibrin deposition can be demonstrated in the intervillous space of the placenta and in the walls of the spiral arteries supplying the placenta [173]. As pregnancy advances, the elastic lamina and smooth muscle of these spiral arteries are replaced by a matrix containing fibrin. This allows expansion of the lumen to accommodate an increasing blood flow and reduces the vascular resistance of the placenta. At placental separation during normal childbirth, a blood flow of 500–800 ml/min has to be staunched within seconds, or serious haemorrhage will occur. Myometrial contraction plays a vital role in securing haemostasis by reducing the blood flow to the placental site. Rapid closure of the terminal part of the spiral artery will be further facilitated by removal of the elastic lamina. The placental site is rapidly covered by a fibrin mesh following delivery. The increased levels of fibrinogen and other coagulation factors will be advantageous to meet the sudden demand for haemostatic components.

The changes also produce a vulnerable state for intravascular clotting and a whole spectrum of disorders involving coagulation which occur in pregnancy [102].

Disseminated intravascular coagulation (DIC)

The changes in the haemostatic system and the local activation of the clotting system during parturition carry with them a risk, not only of thromboembolism but also of DIC. This results in consumption of clotting factors and platelets, leading in some cases to severe, particularly uterine and sometimes generalized, bleeding [184].

The first problem with DIC is in its definition. It is never primary, but always secondary to some general stimulation of coagulation activity by release of procoagulant substances into the blood (Fig. 3.4). Hypothetical triggers of this process in pregnancy include the leaking of placental tissue fragments, amniotic fluid, incompatible red cells or bacterial products into the maternal circulation. There is a great spectrum of manifestations of the process of DIC (Table 3.1) ranging from a compensated state with no clinical manifestation but evidence of increased production and breakdown of coagulation factors, to the condition of massive uncontrollable haemorrhage with very low concentrations of plasma fibrinogen, pathological raised levels of FDP and variable degrees of thrombo-

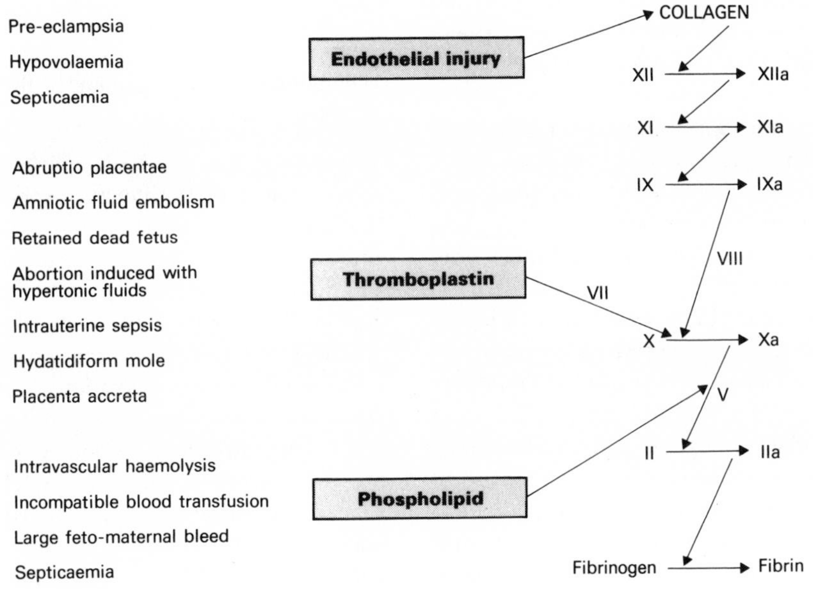

Fig. 3.4. Trigger mechanisms of DIC in pregnancy. Interactions of the trigger mechanisms occur in many of these obstetric complications.

Table 3.1. Spectrum of severity of DIC: its relationship to specific complications in obstetrics

	Severity of DIC	*In vitro* findings	Obstetric condition commonly associated
Stage 1	Low grade, compensated	FDPs increased Increased soluble fibrin complexes Increased ratio of von Willebrand factor to Factor VIIIC	Pre-eclampsia Retained dead fetus
Stage 2	Uncompensated but no haemostatic failure	As above, *plus* fibrinogen decreased platelets decreased Factors V and VIII decreased	Small abruption Severe pre-eclampsia
Stage 3	Rampant with haemostatic failure	Platelets marked decrease Gross depletion of coagulation factors, particularly fibrinogen FDPs elevated	Abruptio placentae Amniotic fluid embolism Eclampsia

Rapid progression from stage 1 to 3 is possible unless appropriate action is taken.

cytopenia. Further cause for confusion is that there appears to be a transitory state of intravascular coagulation during the whole of normal labour, maximal at the time of birth [74,182,198].

Fibrinolysis is stimulated by DIC, and the FDPs resulting from the process interfere with the formation of firm fibrin clots causing a vicious circle which results in further disastrous bleeding.

FDPs also interfere with myometrial function and possibly cardiac function and therefore in themselves aggravate both haemorrhage and shock (Fig. 3.5).

Obstetric conditions associated with DIC include abruptio placentae, amniotic fluid embolism, septic abortion and intrauterine infection, retained dead fetus, hydatidiform mole, placenta accreta, pre-eclampsia and eclampsia and prolonged shock from any cause (see Fig. 3.4).

Despite the advances in obstetric care and highly developed blood transfusion services, haemorrhage still constitutes a major factor in maternal mortality and morbidity [59,105]. For example, in the most recent Confidential Enquiry into Maternal Mortality, deaths from haemorrhage in the UK have doubled compared to the previous triennium [60].

There have been many reports concerning small series of patients or individual patients with coagulation failure during pregnancy. However, no significant controlled trials of the value of the many possible therapeutic measures have been carried out. This is mainly because no one person or unit is likely to see enough cases to randomize patients into groups in which the numbers would achieve statistical significance. Also the complex and variable nature of the conditions associated with DIC, which are often self-correcting and treated with a variety of measures, make it difficult to draw helpful conclusions from the published reports.

Haematological management of the bleeding obstetric patient

The management of the bleeding obstetric patient is an acute and frightening problem. Because of the urgency of the situation there should be a routine planned practice agreed by haematologist, physician, anaesthetist, obstetrician and nursing staff in all maternity units, to deal with this situation whenever it arises. Good, reliable, continuing communication between the various clinicians, nursing, paramedical and laboratory staff is essential.

It is imperative that the source of bleeding, often an unsuspected uterine or genital laceration, be located and dealt with. Prolonged hypovolaemic shock, or indeed shock from any cause, may also trigger DIC and this may lead to haemostatic failure and further prolonged haemorrhage.

The management of haemorrhage is virtually the

same whether the bleeding is caused or augmented by coagulation failure. The clinical condition usually demands urgent treatment and there is no time to wait for results of coagulation factor assays or sophisticated tests of the fibrinolytic system activity for precise definition of the extent of haemostatic failure. (Blood may be taken for this purpose and analysed later once the emergency is over.)

The simple rapid tests recommended below will establish the competence or otherwise of the haemostatic system. In the vast majority of obstetric patients, coagulation failure results from a sudden transitory episode of DIC triggered by a variety of conditions (see Figs 3.4 & 3.5).

As soon as there is any concern about a patient bleeding from any cause, venous blood should be taken and delivered into a set of bottles kept in an emergency pack with a set of laboratory request forms previously made out which only require the patient's name and identification number to be added to them.

In order to avoid testing artefacts it is essential that the blood is obtained by a quick, efficient, non-traumatic technique.

Thromboplastin release from damaged tissues may contaminate the specimen and alter the results. This is likely to occur if difficulty is encountered in finding the vein, if the vein is only partly canalized and the flow is slow, or if there is excessive squeezing of tissues and repeated attempts to obtain a specimen with the same needle. In such circumstances the specimen may clot in the tube in spite of the presence of anticoagulant, or the coagulation times of the various tests will be altered and not reflect the true situation *in vivo*. The platelets may aggregate in clumps and give a falsely low count, be it automated or manual.

Heparin characteristically prolongs the partial thromboplastin time and thrombin time out of proportion to the prothrombin time. As little as 0.05 units of heparin per millilitre will prolong the coagulation test times. It is customary, though not desirable, to take blood for coagulation tests from lines which have been washed through with fluids containing heparin to keep them patent. I believe that it is almost impossible to overcome the effect of such fluids on the blood passing through such a line however much blood is taken and discarded before obtaining a sample for investigation. I would strongly recommend taking blood from another site not previously contaminated with heparin.

Any blood taken into a glass tube without anticoagulant will clot within a few minutes and natural fibrinolysis will continue *in vitro*. Unless the blood is taken into a fibrinolytic inhibitor such as EACA, a falsely high level of FDPs will be found which bears no relationship to fibrinolysis *in vivo*. Similarly, leaving a tourniquet on too long before taking the specimen will stimulate local fibrinolytic activity *in vivo*.

Useful rapid screening tests for haemostatic failure include the platelet count, partial thromboplastin time, or accelerated whole-blood clotting time (which tests intrinsic coagulation), prothrombin time (which tests extrinsic coagulation), the thrombin time and estimation of fibrinogen (Fig. 3.6).

The measurement of FDPs provides an indirect test for fibrinolysis. In obstetric practice the measurement of FDPs is usually part of the investi-

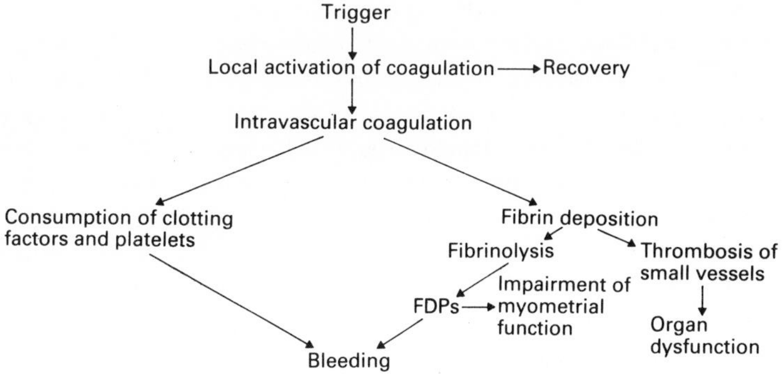

Fig. 3.5. Stimulation of coagulation activity and its possible consequences.

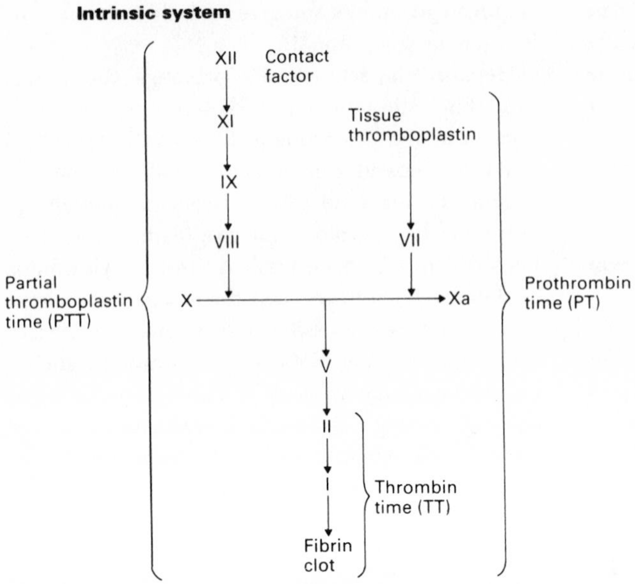

Fig. 3.6. *In vitro* screening tests of coagulation competence and their relationship to the system involved.

gation of suspected acute or chronic DIC. In the acute situation raised FDPs only confirm the presence of DIC, but are not diagnostic and once the specimen is taken the laboratory measurement should be delayed until after the emergency is over. In this way skilled laboratory workers can be performing a much more valuable service in providing results of coagulation screening tests and in providing blood and blood products suitable for transfusion. Of the tests of coagulation, probably the thrombin time, an estimation of the thrombin clottable fibrinogen in a citrated sample of plasma, is the most valuable overall rapid screen of haemostatic competence of coagulation factors. The thrombin time of normal plasma is adjusted in the laboratory to 10–15 seconds, and the fibrin clot formed is firm and stable. In the most severe forms of DIC there is no clottable fibrinogen in the sample, and no fibrin clot appears even after 2–3 min. Indication of severe DIC is obtained usually by a prolonged thrombin time with a friable clot which may dissolve on standing owing to fibrinolytic substances present in the plasma.

Prolongation of the thrombin time is observed not only with depleted fibrinogen but in conditions where FDPs are increased.

There is no point whatsoever in the obstetrician, anaesthetist or nursing staff wasting time trying to perform bedside whole-blood clotting tests. Whole-blood clotting normally takes up to 7 min and should be performed in clean tubes in a 37°C water bath with suitable controls. Bedside (or other) estimation of whole-blood clotting time furnishes little information of practical value and only creates more panic. The valuable hands at the bedside are of more use doing the things they are trained to do in this emergency situation rather than wasting time performing a test which is time consuming, of little value or significance unless performed under strictly controlled conditions, and will not contribute much, if anything, to management. The alerted laboratory worker will be able to provide helpful results on which the obstetrician can act within 30 min at the most of receiving the specimen in the laboratory.

The tests referred to above are straightforward and should be available from any routine haematology laboratory. It is not necessary to have a specialist coagulation laboratory to perform these simple screening tests to confirm or refute a diagnosis of DIC.

Treatment

Treatment of severe haemorrhage must include prompt and adequate fluid replacement in order to avoid renal shutdown. If effective circulation is restored without too much delay FDPs will be cleared from the blood mainly by the liver, which will further aid restoration of normal haemostasis. This is an aspect of management which is often not appropriately emphasized [153].

Plasma substitutes

There is much controversy around which plasma substitute to give to any bleeding patient. The remarks which follow relate to the supportive management of *acute haemorrhage from the placental site* and should not be taken to apply to those situations in which hypovolaemia may be associated with severe hypoproteinaemia such as occurs in septic peritonitis, burns and bowel infarction. The choice lies between simple crystalloids, such as Hartmann's solution or Ringer lactate, and artificial colloids, such as dextrans, hydroxyethyl starch and gelatin solution or the very expensive preparations of human albumin (Albuminoids). If crystalloids are used two to three times the volume of estimated blood loss should be administered because the crystalloid remains in the vascular compartment for a shorter time than colloids when renal function is maintained.

The infusion of plasma substitutes, i.e. plasma protein, dextran, gelatin and starch solutions may result in adverse reactions. Although the incidence of severe reactions is rare, they are diverse in nature, varying from allergic urticarial manifestations and mild fever to life-threatening anaphylactic reactions due to spasm of smooth muscle, with cardiac and respiratory arrest [62].

Dextrans adversely affect platelet function, may cause pseudo-agglutination and interfere with interpretation of subsequent blood grouping and crossmatching tests. They are, therefore, contraindicated in the pregnant woman who is bleeding since there is such a high chance of there being a serious haemostatic defect. Dextrans are also associated with allergic anaphylactoid reactions. The anaphylactoid reactions accompanying infusion of dextrans are probably related to IgG and IgM antidextran antibodies [161] which have subsequently been found in high concentrations in all patients with severe reactions.

Albuminoids are thought to be associated with fewer anaphylactoid reactions but they may be particularly harmful when transfused in the shocked patient by contributing to renal and particularly pulmonary failure, adversely affecting cardiac function and further impairing haemostasis [40].

Many studies suggested that the best way to deal with hypovolaemic shock initially is by transfusing simple balanced salt solutions (crystalloid) followed by red cells and fresh frozen plasma (FFP) [38,135,194]. More recent work [83] has challenged this approach and suggests that albumin-containing solutions are superior to crystalloids for volume replacement in post-operative shocked patients with respiratory insufficiency. This aspect of management of shocked patients with blood loss will remain controversial pending the results of further clinical trials. I advocate the use of a derivative of bovine gelatin — polygeline (Haemaccel) — as a first line fluid in resuscitation. It has a half-life of 8 years and can be stored at room temperature. It is iso-oncotic and does not interfere with platelet function or subsequent blood grouping or crossmatching. Renal function is improved when it is administered in hypovolaemic shock. Haemaccel is generally considered to be non-immunogenic and therefore does not trigger the production of antibodies in humans, even on repeated challenge. The reactions which occur related to Haemaccel infusion are thought to be due to histamine release [114], the incidence and severity of reactions being proportional to the extent of histamine release. There have been a few reports of severe reactions with bronchospasm and circulatory collapse, though rarely, but there has only been one report of a fatality [73]. Nevertheless, *whatever substitute is used, it is only a stop gap until suitable blood component therapy can be administered.*

The use of whole blood and component therapy

Whole blood may be the treatment of choice in coagulation failure associated with obstetric disorders [149], but whole fresh blood is no longer generally available in the UK, because there is insufficient time to complete hepatitis surface antigen, human immunodeficiency virus (HIV) antibody and blood grouping tests before it is released from the transfusion centre. To release it earlier than the usual 18–24 hours would increase the risk of transmitting hepatitis B, syphilis, HIV and of serologically incompatible transfusions. Cytomegalovirus (CMV) and Epstein–Barr virus (EBV) are examples of other infections not screened for which may be transmitted in fresh blood rather than stored blood. Their viability diminishes rapidly on storage at 4°C. These infections, particularly in immunosuppressed or pregnant patients can be particularly hazardous. Apart from the hazards of giving whole blood less than 6–24 hours old, the use of whole blood in the UK today represents a serious waste of vitally needed components required for patients with specific isolated deficiencies [30,105]. The use of FFP followed by bank red cells provides all the components, apart from platelets, present in whole fresh blood and allows the plasma from the freshly donated unit to be used to make the much needed blood components.

Plasma component therapy

FFP contains all the coagulation factors present in plasma obtained from whole blood within 6 hours of donation. Frozen rapidly and stored at −30°C, the factors are well preserved for at least 1 year. Although plasma protein fraction (albumin) does not contain coagulation factors, it does not carry the risk of transmitting infection. It can be of value in providing colloid in the management of haemorrhage. Concentrated fibrinogen which does not contain the labile clotting Factors V and VIII is no longer available and carried the hazard of transmitting infection. Moreover its use in the past was noted to result in a sharp fall of ATIII — suggesting that the concentrate may aggravate intravascular coagulation by adding 'fuel to the fire.'

Although cryoprecipitate is richer in fibrinogen than FFP it lacks ATIII which is rapidly consumed in obstetric bleeding associated with DIC. The use of cryoprecipitate also exposes the recipient to more donors and the potential associated hazards of infection.

Platelets, an essential haemostatic component, are not present in FFP and their functional activity rapidly deteriorates in stored blood. The platelet count reflects both the degree of intravascular coagulation and the amount of bank blood transfused. A patient with persistent bleeding and a very low platelet count ($<20 \times 10^9$/l), may be given concentrated platelets, although they are very seldom required in addition to FFP to achieve haemostasis. Indeed it has been suggested that platelet transfusions are more likely to do harm than good in this situation since most concentrates contain some damaged platelets which might in themselves provide a fresh trigger or mediator of DIC in the existing state [172]. A spontaneous recovery from the coagulation defect is to be expected once the uterus is empty and well contracted, provided that blood volume is maintained by adequate replacement monitored by central venous pressure and urinary output. Problems arise when the patient has a low haemoglobin before blood loss but this should be unusual at term in a well-managed obstetric patient (see Chapter 2).

Red cell transfusion

Crossmatched blood should be available within 40 min of the maternal specimen reaching the laboratory. If the patient has had all her antenatal care at the same hospital her blood group will be known and there is a good case for giving uncrossmatched blood of her same group should the situation warrant it, provided that blood has been properly processed at the transfusion centre. If the blood group is unknown, uncrossmatched group O, rhesus negative blood may be given if necessary. By the time this has been given, laboratory screening tests of haemostatic function should be available. If these prove to be normal, but vaginal bleeding continues, the cause is nearly always trauma or bleeding from the placental site due to failure of the myometrium to contract. It is imperative that the source of bleeding, often an unsuspected uterine or genital laceration, be located and dealt with. Prolonged hypovolaemic shock or indeed shock from any cause may also trigger DIC and this may lead to haemostatic failure and further prolonged haemorrhage.

Stored whole blood, even under optimal conditions, undergoes deleterious changes. The oxygen affinity of red cells increases inhibiting unloading of oxygen from haemoglobin in hypoxic tissues. Plasma ionic concentrations of potassium and hydrogen increase but these changes are not significant until after 4 days of shelf-life. Platelets deteriorate rapidly within the first 24 hours and after 72 hours they have lost all haemostatic function.

The activity of the labile coagulation Factors V and particularly Factor VIII decrease within the first 24 hours after donation. After 6 days' storage microaggregates of platelets, white cells and fibrin form.

If the blood loss is replaced only by stored bank blood which is deficient in the labile clotting Factors V and VIII and platelets, then the circulation will rapidly become depleted in these essential components of haemostasis even if there is no DIC initially as the cause of haemorrhage. It is advisable to transfuse 1 unit of FFP for every 6–8 units of bank red cells administered.

SAG-mannitol blood

The concept of removing all the plasma from a unit of blood and replacing it with a crystalloid solution has now become routine procedure in the UK in many regional blood transfusion centres so that the maximum use of a donated unit can be made.

The process involves centrifuging the anticoagulated unit of whole blood, removing all the plasma and resuspending the packed red cells in 100 ml of sodium chloride, adenine, glucose and mannitol (SAG-M). The resulting unit of packed red cells has better flow properties than plasma reduced blood and is very suitable for top-up transfusion, but contains practically no protein and no coagulation factors whatsoever. It is not recommended for transfusion in an obstetric emergency or any situation of massive rapid blood loss, but if this is all that is available on site at the time, then the following guidelines should be followed.

The regional transfusion centres do not recommend the use of more than 4 units of SAG-M blood, but in an emergency after the first 4 units of SAG-M red cells have been given, 1 unit of albumin should be given for every 2 further units of SAG-M blood in order to maintain plasma oncotic pressure. FFP should be considered after 8 units of SAG-M red cells have been transfused. In an obstetric emergency FFP should have been administered long before this. Most hospital blood banks are provided with a mixture of SAG-M and citrated whole blood or plasma reduced red cells.

Whole blood or plasma reduced red cells are always available on request to the regional transfusion centre.

Clinicians may be helped in the decision of which replacement fluid to give in an obstetric emergency by the knowledge that very few bleeding patients die from lack of circulating red cells, the oxygen-carrying moiety of the blood. Death in the majority of cases results from poor tissue perfusion due to hypovolaemia. Therefore every effort should be made to maintain a normal blood volume and restoration of red cell mass can be delayed until suitable compatibility tests have been performed and bleeding is at least partially controlled [121].

The single most important component of haemostasis at delivery is contraction of the myometrium stemming the flow from the placental site. Massive transfusion of all clotting factors and platelets will not stop haemorrhage if the uterus remains flabby. Vaginal delivery will make less severe demand on the haemostatic mechanism than delivery by caesarean section which requires the same haemostatic competence as any other major surgical procedure. Should DIC be established with the fetus *in utero*, rather than to embark on heroic surgical delivery, it is better to correct the DIC and wait for spontaneous delivery if possible, or stimulate vaginal delivery, avoiding soft tissue damage.

DIC in clinical conditions

In vitro detection of low grade DIC

Rampant uncompensated DIC results in severe haemorrhage with the characteristic laboratory findings described above. However, low grade DIC does not usually give rise to any clinical manifestations although the condition is a potentially hazardous one for both mother and fetus.

Many *in vitro* tests have been claimed to detect

low grade compensated DIC and space does not allow an account of all of these.

FDPs

Estimation of FDPs will give some indication of low grade DIC if these are significantly raised when fibrinogen, platelets and screening tests of haemostatic function appear to be within the normal range.

Soluble fibrin complexes

The action of thrombin on fibrinogen is crucial in DIC. Thrombin splits two molecules of fibrinopeptide A and two molecules of fibrinopeptide B from fibrinogen. The remaining molecule is called a fibrin monomer and polymerizes rapidly to fibrin (Fig. 3.7). Free fibrinopeptides in the blood are a specific measure of thrombin activity and high levels of fibrinopeptide A have been shown to be associated with compensated DIC in pregnancy [198].

Soluble fibrin complexes made up of fibrin–fibrinogen dimers are increased in conditions of low grade DIC [11]. These complexes are generated during the process of thrombin generation and the conversion of soluble fibrinogen to insoluble fibrin (Fig. 3.7). Levels of soluble fibrin complexes are increased in patients with severe pre-eclampsia and with a retained dead fetus [79].

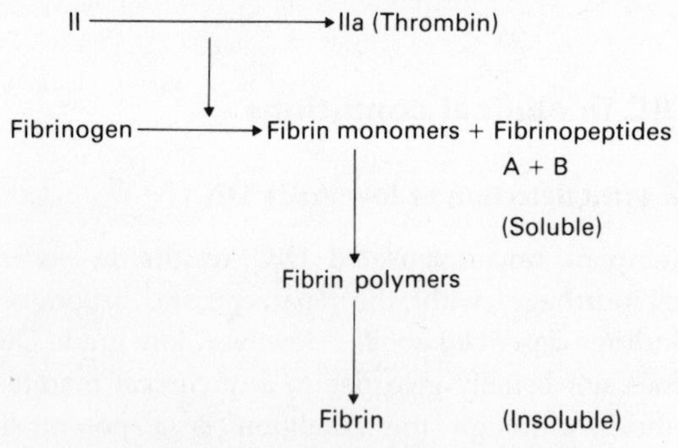

Fig. 3.7. Generation of soluble complexes during the conversion of fibrinogen to insoluble fibrin.

Factor VIII

During normal pregnancy the levels of both von Willebrand factor (vWF) and Factor VIII coagulation activity (VIIIC) rise in parallel [72,202]. An increase in the ratio of vWF to Factor VIIIC has been observed in conditions accompanied by low grade DIC whether associated with pregnancy or not.

The stages in the spectrum of severity of DIC (see Table 3.1) are not strictly delineated and there may be rapid progression from low grade compensated DIC as diagnosed by paracoagulation tests described above, to the rampant form with haemostatic failure.

There now follows an account of the obstetric conditions most commonly associated with DIC and the rationale for specific previous and current measures used to manage haemostatic failure optimally.

Abruptio placentae

Premature separation of the placenta or abruptio placentae is the most frequent obstetric cause of coagulation failure. Many of the problems which confront the attendant in this situation are common to other conditions associated with DIC in pregnancy so that abruption will be used as the central focus to discuss management controversies.

Abruptio placentae can occur in apparently healthy women with no clinical warning or in the context of established pre-eclampsia. It is possible that clinically silent placental infarcts may predispose to placental separation by causing low grade abnormalities of the haemostatic system such as increased Factor VIII consumption and raised FDPs [156].

There is a great spectrum in the severity of the haemostatic failure in this condition [75] which appears to be related to the degree of placental separation. Only 10 per cent of patients with abruptio placentae show significant coagulation abnormalities [138]. In some small abruptions there is a minor degree of failure of haemostatic processes and the fetus does not succumb (see Table 3.1). When the uterus is tense and tender and no fetal heart can be heard, the separation and retroplacental bleeding are extensive. No guide to the severity of the haemorrhage or coagulation failure will be given by the amount of vaginal bleeding. There may be no external vaginal blood loss, even when the placenta is completely separated, the fetus is dead, the circulating blood is incoagulable and there is up to 5 l of concealed blood loss resulting in hypovolaemic shock.

Haemostatic failure may be suspected if there is persistent oozing at the site of venepuncture or bleeding from the mucous membranes of the mouth or nose. Simple rapid screening tests, as described above and referred to below, will confirm the presence of DIC. There will be a low platelet count, greatly prolonged thrombin time, low fibrinogen, together with raised FDPs, due to secondary fibrinolysis stimulated by the intravascular deposition of fibrin [65]. The mainstay of treatment is to restore and maintain the circulating blood volume. This not only prevents renal shutdown and further haemostatic failure caused by hypovolaemic shock, but helps clearance of FDPs which in themselves act as potent anticoagulants. It has also been suggested that FDPs inhibit myometrial activity and serious post-partum haemorrhage in women with abruptio placentae was found to be associated with high levels of FDPs [14,174]. High levels of FDPs may also have a cardiotoxic effect resulting in low cardiac output and blood pressure despite a normal circulating blood volume.

If the fetus is dead the aim should be prompt vaginal delivery avoiding soft tissue damage, once correction of hypovolaemia is underway. There is no evidence that the use of oxytocic agents aggravates thromboplastin release from the uterus [25].

Following emptying of the uterus, myometrial contraction will greatly reduce bleeding from the placental site and spontaneous correction of the haemostatic defect usually occurs shortly after delivery, if the measures recommended above have been taken. However, post-partum haemorrhage is a not infrequent complication and is the commonest cause of death in abruptio placentae [59,60,61].

In cases where the abruption is small and the fetus is still alive, prompt caesarean section may save the baby, if vaginal delivery is not imminent. FFP, bank red cells and platelet concentrates should be available to correct the potentially severe maternal coagulation defect.

In rare situations where vaginal delivery cannot be stimulated and haemorrhage continues, caesarean section is indicated even in the presence of a dead fetus. In these circumstances normal haemostasis should be restored as far as possible by the administration of FFP and platelet concentrates if necessary, as well as transfusing red cells before surgery is undertaken.

Despite extravasation of blood throughout the uterine muscle, its function is not impaired and good contraction will follow removal of fetus, placenta and retroperitoneal clot. Regional anaesthesia or analgesia is contraindicated. Expansion of the lower limb vascular bed resulting from regional block can add to the problem of uncorrected hypovolaemia; in the presence of haemostatic failure there is the additional hazard of bleeding into the epidural space [26].

In recent years, heparin has been used to treat many cases of DIC, whatever their cause. There is, however, no objective evidence to demonstrate that its use in abruptio placentae decreased morbidity and mortality although anecdotal reports continue to suggest this [188]. Very good results have been achieved without the use of heparin [153]. Its use, with an intact circulation, would be sensible and logical to break the vicious circle of DIC, but in the presence of already defective haemostasis with a large bleeding placental site, it may prolong massive local and generalized haemorrhage [68].

Treatment with antifibrinolytic agents such as EACA or Trasylol (aprotinin) can result in blockage of small vessels of vital organs, such as the kidney or brain, with fibrin. Such agents are therefore contraindicated, although Bonnar [26] suggests that delayed severe and prolonged haemorrhage from the placental site several hours post-delivery may respond to their use if all other measures fail.

It has been suggested [174,175] that Trasylol may be helpful in the management of abruptio placentae particularly in those cases with uterine inertia associated with high levels of FDPs. There is a high incidence (1.5 per cent) of abruptio placentae in the obstetric admissions (18 000/annum) at the Groote Schuur Obstetric Unit, Cape Town, where the first study was carried out. The selection of Trasylol depended on its alleged anticoagulant activity in addition to its well-known antifibrinolytic properties [4]. There has been a resurgence of use of Trasylol recently, particularly in cardiac surgery [22] where significant reduction in blood loss has been shown following cardiac bypass operations. This is thought to be due predominantly to platelet sparing. It is doubtful whether Trasylol would have any advantage in management of obstetric DIC.

Obstetricians appear unconvinced of the benefits of Trasylol in the treatment of DIC and abruptio placentae. Prompt supportive measures alone, maintaining central venous pressure and replacing blood lost together with essential coagulation factors, will of course result in reduction in FDPs. This will improve myometrial function and contribute to the return of healthy haemostasis.

One patient with recurrent abruptio placentae successfully treated with the fibrinolytic inhibitor AMCA has been reported [6]; the compound is related to EACA. Investigations in this woman suggested abnormally increased fibrinolytic activity in the 26th week of her third pregnancy. The previous two pregnancies had been complicated by abruptio placentae associated with a neonatal death and a still-birth respectively. The intravenous administration of AMCA following a small vaginal bleed resulted in restoration of normal coagulation status and the bleeding stopped; oral administration was continued. Another small bleed occurred at 33 weeks' gestation, treated again with intravenous AMCA. The eventual successful outcome of this pregnancy was attributed by the authors to the use of this agent, but there may have been many other variables involved.

A recent report on reducing the frequency of severe abruption from Dallas, Texas [154] noted that the reduction in *fetal* death associated with abruption by 50 per cent over a period covering more than 30 years (1958–90) could be accounted for by the decrease in women of very high parity and an increase in the proportion of Latin-American as opposed to black women in the population served. Abruption in the latter part of the study recurred in 12 per cent of subsequent pregnancies and proved fatal to the fetus in 7 per cent, which was unchanged from earlier experience. With modern supportive measures, maternal death due directly to abruption is now extremely rare.

Amniotic fluid embolism [133]

This obstetric disaster usually occurs during or shortly after a vigorous labour with an intact amniotic sac, but can occur during a caesarean section. It is thought that amniotic fluid enters the maternal circulation via lacerations of membranes and placenta. Platelet fibrin thrombi are formed and trapped within the pulmonary blood vessels: profound shock follows, accompanied by respiratory distress and cyanosis. There is a high mortality at this stage from a combination of respiratory and cardiac failure [88]. If the mother survives long enough, massive intravascular coagulation with almost total consumption of coagulation factors invariably follows. There is bleeding from venepuncture sites and severe haemorrhage from the placental site after delivery.

Confirmation of diagnosis is usually made *post mortem* by finding histological evidence of amniotic fluid and fetal tissue within the substance of the maternal lungs; occasionally, similar material may be aspirated from a central venous pressure (CVP) catheter line — see below. It is, therefore, difficult to assess the value of therapeutic measures taken, in the few reports which have appeared, for the successful management of a clinical picture which can usually only be suggestive of amniotic fluid embolism [24,43,177].

The major differential diagnoses of amniotic fluid embolism in the collapsed patient are primary cardiovascular catastrophes such as pulmonary embolus or aspiration in the anaesthetized patient. Apart from the bleeding and evidence of DIC associated with amniotic fluid embolism, pulmonary embolus has specific features. These and other medical causes of shock in obstetric patients are considered in Table 4.1. Aspiration is usually associated with bronchospasm which is very rare in amniotic fluid embolus [133]. At any time, if there is doubt about the diagnosis, the rapid fluid infusion necessary for the treatment of amniotic fluid embolus should be controlled by careful assessment of the CVP. Such rapid fluid infusion would cause a marked rise in CVP in patients with pulmonary embolus, and could well lead to fatal fluid overload. In addition, the presence of the CVP line will allow aspiration of fetal material from the great veins, for confirmation of the diagnosis of amniotic fluid embolus [160]. Such material should also be sought in maternal sputum [189]. Since fetal material has been found in pulmonary arterial blood in some women who did not have amniotic fluid embolus [45] such a finding should not be considered pathognomonic for amniotic fluid embolus.

The object of the treatment is to sustain the circulation while the intravascular thrombin in the lungs is cleared by the fibrinolytic response of the endothelium of the pulmonary vessels. If bleeding from the placental site can be controlled by stimulation of uterine contraction, then the logical treatment is carefully monitored transfusion of FFP and packed red cells with heparin administration and, if necessary, ventilation.

Retention of dead fetus

The whole question of intrauterine fetal death and haemostatic failure has been reviewed [163]. There is a gradual depletion of maternal coagulation factors following intrauterine fetal death but the changes are not usually detectable *in vitro* until after 3–4 weeks [52,89]. Thromboplastic substances released from the dead tissues in the uterus into the maternal circulation are thought to be the trigger of DIC in this situation which occurs in about one-third of patients who retain the dead fetus for more than 4–5 weeks [152]. There is depletion of fibrinogen, Factor VIII and platelets, together with elevation of FDPs. Gross increase of soluble fibrin/fibrinogen complexes amounting to 25 per cent of the total fibrinogen in association with a dead fetus has been described [79]. About 80 per cent of pregnant women will go into spontaneous labour within 3 weeks of intrauterine fetal death. Problems arising from defective haemostasis are much less common with this situation in modern obstetric practice, because labour is induced promptly following diagnosis of fetal death before clinically significant coagulation changes have developed.

Rupture of the membranes is recommended once induced labour is established in such patients, as there is a risk of precipitate labour and amniotic fluid embolism has been known to occur [25].

If the screening tests previously described indicate that there is defective haemostasis the coagulation factors should be restored to normal before delivery is attempted. If the circulation is intact heparin is the logical treatment to interrupt the activation of the coagulation systems. Intravenous infusion of 1000 IU heparin hourly for up to 48 hours is usually sufficient to restore the platelet count, and the levels of fibrinogen and Factors V and VIII to normal [25]. The heparin should then be discontinued and the patient should be delivered. There should be a plentiful supply of compatible red cells and FFP standing by to treat promptly any haemorrhage at placental separation. Should the patient go into spontaneous labour while heparin is being administered the infusion should be stopped. It is not necessary to neutralize the heparin with protamine sulphate unless the patient is bleeding. There is no rational basis for the use of fibrinolytic inhibitors in the management of the patient with coagulation failure associated with a retained dead fetus. The increased fibrinolytic activity is secondary to DIC and the defective haemostasis will be corrected by the powerful anticoagulant effect of heparin in the presence of an intact circulation before the onset of labour.

Retained dead fetus and living twin

The occurrence of single fetal death in a pre-term multiple pregnancy poses unique therapeutic dilemmas. Prolongation of the pregnancy could result in life-threatening maternal haemostatic failure. Termination of the pregnancy for maternal indications would result in the birth of an immature infant. The incidence of this problem is unknown but is likely to be observed more frequently with the advent of widespread use of ultrasound in obstetrics. In addition, on occasion selective termination of the life of the affected twin is being offered in situations where only one fetus has been shown to be affected with a genetic disorder.

A report of the successful prolongation of pregnancy with the spontaneous death *in utero* of one of the twins at 26 weeks' gestation has recently been published [164]. The patient was treated with intravenous heparin and the reversal of the consumptive coagulopathy resulted in the uneventful prolongation of pregnancy for 8 weeks, at which time the fetus had achieved lung maturity.

Induced abortion

Changes in haemostatic components consistent with DIC have been demonstrated in patients undergoing abortion induced with hypertonic solutions of saline and urea [78,118,179,180,192]. This combination appears to be particularly hazardous [46] in comparison to the use of urea and prostaglandin or oxytocin [31]. The stimulus appears to be the release of tissue factor into the maternal circulation from the placenta which is damaged by the hypertonic solutions.

In later pregnancy DIC has been described with both dilatation and evacuation [57] and also with prostaglandin and oxytocin termination [168].

The haemorrhage resulting may be massive and has resulted in maternal deaths. Prompt restoration of the blood volume and transfusions with red cells and FFP as described above should resolve the situation which, once the uterus is empty, is self-limiting.

A unique case of DIC associated with chronic ectopic pregnancy has been reported [49].

Intrauterine infection [18]

Endotoxic shock associated with septic abortion and ante-partum or post-partum intrauterine infection can trigger DIC [77,181]. Infection is usually with Gram-negative organisms. Fibrin is deposited in the microvasculature owing to endothelial damage by the endotoxin, and secondary red cell intravascular haemolysis with characteristic fragmentation, so-called microangiopathic haemolysis, is characteristic of the condition.

The patient is usually alert and flushed with a rapid pulse and low blood pressure. Transfusion, has little or no effect on the hypotension in comparison to its benefit in the obstetric emergencies complicated by DIC. Elimination of the uterine infection remains the most important aspect of management; this is probably best performed by a short intensive period of antibiotic therapy followed by evacuation of the uterine contents. A few European centres have used heparinization in the management of septic abortion and have claimed a decrease in mortality [25]. If the uterus is empty and contracted, there is no undue risk of severe bleeding from the placental site. If there is evidence of a consumptive coagulopathy, heparin may be useful as part of the management of this hazardous emergency [46] but this remains controversial [18,19].

Purpura fulminans

This rare complication of infection sometimes occurs in the puerperium, precipitated by Gram-negative septicaemia.

Extensive haemorrhage occurs into the skin in association with DIC. The underlying mechanism is unknown but there appears to be an acute activation of the clotting system resulting in the deposition of fibrin thrombi within blood vessels of the skin and other organs [123]. The extremities and face are usually involved first, the purpuric patches having a jagged and erythematous border, which can be shown histologically to be the site of a leukocytoclastic vasculitis. Rapid enlargement of the lesions which become necrotic and gangrenous is associated with shock, tachycardia and fever. Without treatment the mortality rate is high and among those who survive, digit or limb amputation may be necessary. The laboratory findings are those of DIC with leukocytosis. In this situation treatment with heparin should be started as soon as the diagnosis is apparent. It will prevent further consumption of platelets and coagulation factors. It should always be remembered however that bleeding from any site in the presence of defective coagulation factors will be aggravated by the use of heparin. Survival in purpura fulminans is currently much improved because of better supportive treatment for the shocked patient and effective control of the triggering infection, together with heparin therapy.

Acute fatty liver of pregnancy (AFLP)

AFLP is a rare complication of pregnancy included in this section because it is often, if not always, associated with variable degrees of DIC which contributes significantly to its morbidity and mortality [68,99]. Only the haematological aspects will be discussed here. For a full account of the disorder the reader is referred to Chapter 9.

Early diagnosis and subsequent delivery are

essential for improving survival of both mother and child. Most patients have prodromal symptoms for at least 1 week before jaundice develops. The Royal Free series [32] draws attention to a characteristic blood picture of neutrophilia, thrombocytopenia and normoblasts. Some of the blood films available for review also showed basophilic stippling and giant platelets and the authors suggest that these appearances might help towards an early diagnosis of AFLP. However, these features are not specific to AFLP and may be seen in any condition of additional stress on a bone marrow already working to capacity in the last trimester of pregnancy.

DIC complicating severe liver failure is an extremely complex topic. In AFLP the haemostatic defect is frequently resistant probably owing to prolonged activation of coagulation combined with very low to undetectable ATIII levels [68,87,110]. The replacement of ATIII with plasma or ATIII concentrate to shorten the period of DIC and thereby decrease morbidity and mortality of AFLP has been suggested [68]. ATIII concentrate has also been used in the successful management of a patient with AFLP [100]. Heparin therapy can be very dangerous [76].

Conclusions

DIC is always a secondary phenomenon and the mainstay of management is therefore to remove the initiating stimulus if possible.

With rampant DIC and haemorrhage, recovery will usually follow delivery of the patient provided that the blood volume is maintained and shock due to hypovolaemia is prevented. An efficiently acting myometrium post-delivery will stem haemorrhage from the placental site. Measures taken to achieve a firm contracted uterus will obviously contribute one of the most important factors in preventing continuing massive blood loss from the placental site.

Acquired primary defects of haemostasis

Thrombocytopenia

The commonest platelet abnormality encountered in clinical practice is thrombocytopenia. During the hundred years since platelets were first described an increasing understanding of their role in haemostasis and thrombosis has taken place. At the same time there have been dramatic reductions in maternal and fetal mortality, but maternal thrombocytopenia remains a difficult management problem during pregnancy and can also have profound effects on fetal and neonatal well-being. The causes and management of maternal and fetal thrombocytopenia have recently been reviewed [50,150]. Emphasis here will be laid on those conditions which cause particular diagnostic and management problems in obstetric practice.

A low platelet count is seen most frequently in association with DIC (as already described). Sometimes severe megaloblastic anaemia of pregnancy is accompanied by thrombocytopenia, but the platelet count rapidly returns to normal after therapy with folic acid [26]. Toxic depression of bone marrow megakaryocytes in pregnancy can occur in association with infection, certain drugs and alcoholism. Neoplastic infiltration may also result in thrombocytopenia. Probably the single most important cause of isolated thrombocytopenia is autoimmune thrombocytopenic purpura (AITP) which is a disease primarily of young women in the reproductive years [124].

Autoimmune thrombocytopenic purpura (AITP)

AITP is common in women of childbearing age and has been found to have an incidence of one to two in 10 000 pregnancies [96]. Cases may present with skin bruising and platelet counts between 30 and $80 \times 10^9/l$ but it is rare to see severe bleeding associated with low platelet counts in the chronic form.

With the screening of pregnant women, very mild thrombocytopenia may be discovered as an incidental finding and is not associated with risk to the mother or infant [33,80]. It may be that incidental thrombocytopenia represents a very mild AITP but as it is not associated with adverse effects it must be distinguished from cases of AITP which can result in infants affected with severe thrombocytopenia and intracranial haemorrhage [94,95, 166]. There are no serological tests or clinical guidelines which reliably predict the hazard of thrombocytopenia in an individual fetus, the correlation between maternal and neonatal counts is poor [94, 167] and the risk has been overestimated [36]. It has been assumed that caesarean section delivery is less traumatic to the fetus than vaginal delivery and whilst that premise could be debated, recognizing and investigating the minority of pregnancies at risk of significant fetal thrombocytopenia would avoid many unnecessary fetal blood samples and caesarean sections.

Diagnosis of AITP

There have been a number of analyses of outcome of cases involving maternal AITP from the 1950s onwards. The findings may not be entirely applicable to current management because some of the documented poor fetal outcomes may have been associated with unrecognized maternal lupus, pre-eclampsia or alloimmune thrombocytopenia (AIT). Only symptomatic women and neonates were investigated because there was no general screening of the platelet count in healthy women. This resulted in an exaggerated incidence of both neonatal thrombocytopenia and the morbidity and mortality arising from it.

AITP is a diagnosis of exclusion with peripheral thrombocytopenia and normal or increased megakaryocytes in the bone marrow and the documented absence of other diseases. The red and white cells are essentially normal unless there is secondary anaemia. AITP requires the exclusion of systemic lupus erythematous (SLE), lupus anticoagulant and anticardiolipin antibody as they may coexist with thrombocytopenia (see Chapter 8).

The majority of thrombocytopenic patients are asymptomatic and tests to estimate the bleeding risk in these patients would obviously be helpful.

In chronic platelet consumption disorders, a population of younger larger platelets is established which have enhanced function. Measurement of the mean platelet volume (MPV) or, if not available, examination of the stained blood film will detect the presence of these large platelets. The risk of bleeding at any given platelet count is less in those patients with younger large platelets. The bleeding time which has recently been severely criticized [41,112] as a predictor of bleeding at surgery still has a place in this context according to some respected workers [35]. A bleeding time over 15 min indicates a greater risk than in those with a normal bleeding time.

The mechanism of immune destruction of platelets has been shown to be due to autoantibodies directed against platelet surface antigens. This has special relevance in pregnancy because the placenta has receptors for the constant fragment (Fc) of the IgG immunoglobulin molecule facilitating active transport of immunoglobulin across the placenta to the fetal circulation. The immunoglobulin passage increases with advancing pregnancy [142,186] and may result in fetal thrombocytopenia.

The role of circulating globulin in the pathogenesis of immune thrombocytopenia was first documented in the 1950s [66,82]. However, antibody on the platelet membrane and in the plasma, demonstrated by tests analogous to the direct and indirect Coombs' tests on red cells, have been slow to enter the routine repertoire of haematology laboratories because they have been fraught with technological difficulties such as the intrinsic reactivity of platelets and the presence of some platelet-associated immunoglobulin (PAIgG) in normal individuals.

Antibody from some cases of AITP demonstrates a specificity for the platelet glycoprotein IIb/IIIa [191] or for glycoprotein Ib. In one study, the minority of cases of AITP demonstrating this specificity fared less well in their responses to splenectomy [203].

Whilst some cases of AITP have normal or increased amounts of immunoglobulin on the platelets or in the plasma [44,136] 10–35 per cent of patients have no demonstrable (PAIgG). The presence of IgG rather than IgM antibodies [84] has relevance to the pregnant patient because only IgG antibodies can be transported across the placenta and cause thrombocytopenia in the fetus.

In a study of 162 consecutive pregnant patients with platelet counts $<150 \times 10^9/l$ gathered over 11 years, the absence of circulating IgG antiplatelet antibody at term, despite a history of thrombocytopenic purpura, was associated with minimal risk of thrombocytopenia in the fetus [167]. However, no currently available serological test can be used to reliably predict thrombocytopenia in the fetus [81].

The absence of a history of AITP prior to the

index pregnancy is a low risk indicator for neonatal thrombocytopenia [167]. In contrast, 18 neonates who were born with platelet counts $<50 \times 10^9$/l, out of a total of 178, were all born to mothers with a history of AITP prior to pregnancy. In addition, 40 per cent of mothers with a preceding history delivered infants with platelet counts $<100 \times 10^9$/l. Of 162 infants delivered in the index pregnancy, 10 had bleeding complications of which five were serious. Intracranial haemorrhage in infants born to women with a prior history of AITP and delivered vaginally, numbered two out of 17, whilst there were no cases of intracranial haemorrhage in women with similar histories who were delivered by caesarean section [167]. A more recent review of the literature of AITP in pregnancy [35] shows a neonatal mortality rate of six in 1000 AITP patients, about the same or better than the overall perinatal mortality rate. All the deaths in this survey occurred in babies delivered by caesarean section, unlike in other reports, and all events appeared more than 24–48 hours after delivery, the time of the platelet count nadir in the neonate.

Management of AITP in pregnancy

Management of AITP in pregnancy is directed at three aspects: (a) antenatal care of the mother; (b) management of the mother and fetus during delivery; and (c) the management of the neonate from the time of delivery.

The most important decision to make is whether the mother requires treatment at all. Many patients have significant thrombocytopenia (platelet count $<100 \times 10^9$/l) but no evidence of an *in vivo* haemostatic disorder. In general the platelet count must be $<50 \times 10^9$/l for capillary bleeding and purpura to occur.

There is no need to treat asymptomatic women with mild to moderate thrombocytopenia (count $>50 \times 10^9$/l) and a normal bleeding time. However, the maternal platelet count should be monitored at every clinical visit and signs of haemostatic impairment looked for. The platelet count will show a downward trend during pregnancy with a nadir in the third trimester and active treatment may have to be instituted to achieve a safe haemostatic concentration of platelets for delivery at term. The incidence of ante-partum haemorrhage is not increased in maternal AITP but there is a small increased risk of post-partum haemorrhagic complications not from the placental bed but from surgical incisions such as episiotomy and from soft tissue lacerations.

Intervention in the antenatal period is based on clinical manifestations of thrombocytopenia. The woman with bruising or petechiae requires measures to raise the platelet count but the woman with mucous membrane bleeding which may be life-threatening, requires urgent treatment with platelet transfusions and intravenous IgG, (see below) and occasionally emergency splenectomy.

The real dilemma in the pregnant woman with AITP is that nearly all patients have chronic disease. The long-term effects of treatment which is happily embarked on outside pregnancy have to be considered in the light of the possible complications on the progress of pregnancy in the mother and of any effects on the fetus. The hazard for the mother who is monitored carefully and where appropriate measures have been taken, is negligible but most of her management is orientated towards what are thought to be optimal conditions for the delivery of the fetus who in turn may or may not be thrombocytopenic (see below).

Corticosteroids are a satisfactory short-term therapy but are unacceptable as long-term support unless the maintenance dose is very small [39,124]. Side-effects for the mother include weight gain, subcutaneous fat redistribution, acne and hypertension, which are undesirable during pregnancy. In addition, the prevalence of gestational diabetes, post-partum psychosis and osteoporosis are all increased with the use of corticosteroids. Nevertheless, they are often used but should be reserved as short-term therapy for patients with obvious risk of bleeding or to raise the platelet count of an asymptomatic woman at term allowing her to have epidural or spinal analgesia for delivery if desired or indicated.

A suggestion in the older literature of an association between steroid administration and cleft lip or palate has been refuted by more recent studies. Suppression of fetal adrenal glands is a theoretical hazard but approximately 90 per cent of a dose of prednisolone or hydrocortisone is metabolized in the placenta and never reaches the fetus. This is in contrast to dexamethasone and betamethasone which cross the placenta freely (see also Chapter 1). It has been suggested [84] that high doses of corticosteroids given to elevate platelet counts at or near term should be avoided since they may increase the transplacental passage of IgG antibody and thus expose the fetus to greater risk of severe thrombocytopenia. In my experience this is a theoretical hazard not seen in practice.

INTRAVENOUS IgG

The recent introduction of a highly successful treatment for AITP has altered the management options dramatically. It is known that intravenous administration of monomeric polyvalent human IgG in doses greater than those produced endogenously prolongs the clearance time of immune complexes by the reticulo-endothelial system. It is thought that such a prolongation of clearance of IgG-coated platelets in AITP results in an increase in the number of circulating platelets but the mechanism is as yet unknown [63]. Used in the original recommended doses of 0.4 g/kg for 5 days by intravenous infusion, a persistent and predictable response was obtained in more than 80 per cent of reported cases. More recently, alternative dosage regimens of this very expensive treatment have been suggested which are just as effective, but easier to manage and use less total immunoglobulin [35]. A typical dose is 1 g/kg over 8 hours on 1 day. This dose will raise the platelet count to normal or safe levels in approximately half of patients. In those in whom the platelet count does not rise, a similar dose can be repeated 2 days later. The advantages of this treatment are that it is safe, has very few side-effects and that the response to therapy is more rapid than with corticosteroids. The response usually occurs within 48 hours and is maintained for 2–3 weeks. The main disadvantage is that it is very expensive and seldom produces a long-term cure of the AITP.

It has been suggested that IgG given intravenously can cross the placenta and should provoke an identical response in the fetus [134] at risk but this has never been proved. Indeed, analysis of more recent literature indicates that the postulated transplacental effect is unreliable [142,186] and that exogenous IgG may not cross the placenta [145]. The use of IgG has been recommended [84,85] in all pregnant patients with platelet counts $<75 \times 10^9$/l regardless of history or symptoms. There is no doubt about the value of IgG in selected cases of severe symptomatic thrombocytopenia where a rapid response is required but its indiscriminate use in all cases with significant thrombocytopenia would have to be shown to dramatically improve both maternal and fetal outcome to justify the high cost.

Splenectomy will produce a cure or long-term drug-free remission in 60–80 per cent of all patients with AITP. This is because the main site of antibody production is often the spleen and because many of the IgG-coated platelets are sequestered there. All patients should receive pneumovax before splenectomy and twice daily oral penicillin for life following surgery to protect against pneumococcal infection. Reviews of management of AITP have associated splenectomy during pregnancy with high fetal loss rates [39] and even an approximate 10 per cent maternal mortality rate in the past [16] but modern supportive measures and improved surgical practices have reduced the fetal loss rate considerably and the risk of maternal mortality is negligible [122]. In current practice, splenectomy is hardly ever indicated in the pregnant patient and should be avoided given the success of medical management. However, removal of the spleen remains an option if all other attempts to increase the platelet count fail. Splenectomy should be performed in the second trimester because surgery is best tolerated then and the size of the uterus will not make the operation technically difficult. The platelet count should be raised to safe levels for surgery if possible by intravenous IgG. Although transfused platelets will have a short life in the maternal circulation, they may help to achieve haemostasis at surgery. Platelet concentrates should be available but given only if abnormal bleeding occurs.

OTHER THERAPY

There are a number of other medications which have been used in AITP but most of them are contraindicated in pregnancy and only have moderate success rates. Danazol, an attenuated anabolic steroid, has been used with moderate success in a few patients, though it should not be used in pregnancy. Vincristine has a transient beneficial effect in many patients but it is not recommended in pregnancy and long-term associated neurotoxicity limits its usefulness.

Very occasionally immunosuppressives such as azothioprine and cyclophosphamide have to be used in severe intractable thrombocytopenia which does not respond to any other measures. Cyclophosphamide should be avoided in pregnancy if possible (though see Chapter 7 for an account of its use in renal transplant patients). Experience with relatively low doses of azathioprine in the increasing numbers of transplant patients who have now negotiated a subsequent pregnancy suggests that this drug is not associated with increased fetal or maternal morbidity. The most contentious issue in the management of AITP in pregnancy is the mode of delivery given that the fetus might be thrombocytopenic and may bleed from trauma during the birth process.

ASSESSMENT OF THE FETAL PLATELET COUNT

Hegde [84] analysed the reported cases in the literature from 1950 to 1983 which suggested an overall incidence of neonatal thrombocytopenia of 52 per cent with significant morbidity in 12 per cent of births. The incidence increases to 70 per cent of deliveries if maternal platelet counts were $<100 \times 10^9/l$ at term. The probability of fetal thrombocytopenia increased with the severity of maternal thrombocytopenia. As a result of this and other analyses many strategies were developed to predict the fetal platelet count and to determine the optimal mode of delivery since it was believed that elective caesarean section was the best option for an affected fetus at risk from trauma during a vaginal delivery.

We now know that the incidence in these retrospective analyses was distorted because only symptomatic women were likely to have been investigated and reported (see above). A recent report [167] studied the outcome of 162 consecutive pregnancies in women with presumed AITP presenting in the decade 1979–89. The overall incidence of thrombocytopenia (11 per cent) in the offspring of these women was much lower than the earlier reported analyses but two factors emerged of importance in predicting neonatal thrombocytopenia. In the absence of a history of AITP before pregnancy or in the absence of circulating platelet IgG antibodies in the index pregnancy in those with a history, the risk of severe thrombocytopenia in the fetus at term was negligible.

These findings are supported by other recent reports [34,36]. In Burrows and Kelton [34], 61 infants were born to 50 mothers with confirmed AITP. Only three (4.9 per cent) had a cord platelet count $<50 \times 10^9/l$. None of the infants had morbidity or mortality as a result of the thrombocytopenia. Two-thirds of the infants had a further fall in platelet count in the first 2 or 3 days after birth but in all the thrombocytopenia could easily be corrected. Some investigators have suggested that maternal splenectomy increases the probability of neonatal thrombocytopenia [39,190]. Closer scrutiny of published reports [35] shows that it is only in those women with splenectomy and persistent thrombocytopenia ($<100 \times 10^9/l$) that the risk of neonatal thrombocytopenia is increased. What has become clear over the years is that analysis of the older literature gave an exaggerated incidence of neonatal thrombocytopenia and of the morbidity and mortality arising from it. However, even with the benefit of accurate automated, easily repeated platelet counts, estimation of IgG platelet antibodies and taking into consideration splenectomy status, it is still impossible to predict the fetal platelet count in any individual case [93] and to plan the mode of delivery based on these maternal parameters is not logical or sensible.

FETAL BLOOD SAMPLING (FBS)

A method for direct measurement of the fetal platelet count in scalp blood obtained transcervically prior to or early in labour has been described [10, 170,185]. The authors recommend that caesarean section be performed in all cases where the fetal platelet count is $<50 \times 10^9/l$. This approach is more logical than a decision about the mode of delivery made on the basis of maternal platelet count, concentration of IgG or splenectomy status, but it is not without risk of significant haemorrhage in the truly thrombocytopenic fetus, often gives false positive results [35] and demands urgent action to be taken on the results. Also the cervix must be sufficiently dilated to allow the fetal scalp to be sampled and the uterine contraction to achieve this may have caused the fetus to descend so far in the birth canal that caesarean section is technically difficult and also traumatic for the fetus.

The only way a reliable fetal platelet count can be obtained so that a decision concerning the optimal mode of delivery can be taken is by a percutaneous transabdominal fetal cord blood sample taken before term [56,130,169]. This gives time for discussion with the obstetrician, paediatrician, haematologist, anaesthetist and anyone else involved concerning delivery. It should be performed at 37–38 weeks' gestation under ultrasound guidance as the transfer of IgG increases in the last weeks of pregnancy and an earlier sample may give a higher fetal platelet count than one taken nearer term. There is no need for sampling earlier in gestation because the fetus is not at risk from spontaneous intracranial haemorrhage *in utero* (cf. fetus with AIT).

There is a risk associated with the sampling but in skilled hands this is no more than 1 per cent [142]. A caesarean section may be precipitated because of fetal distress during the procedure even if the platelet count proves to be normal. This is another good reason for performing an FBS as late as possible in gestation if it is thought to be necessary. Given the low risk of identifying a problem and the risk of associated complications *in utero*, FBS cannot be justified in all AITP pregnancies.

NEONATAL PLATELET COUNT

After birth the platelet count will continue to fall for 2–5 days. If the cord platelet count shows severe thrombocytopenia and especially if there is evidence of skin or mucous membrane bleeding, measures can be taken to prevent this predicted fall. Intravenous hydrocortisone and platelet transfusion have been used with success but the recommended therapy nowadays should be intravenous IgG because of its relative safety and the rapidity with which a response is observed.

Mode of delivery in AITP

There is little risk to the mother whatever the mode of delivery. In most cases the maternal platelet count can be raised to haemostatic levels to cover the event. Even if the mother has to deliver in the face of a low platelet count, she is unlikely to bleed from the placental site once the uterus is empty but she is at risk of bleeding from any surgical incisions, soft tissue injuries or tears. Platelets should be available but not given prophylactically. It should be remembered that the unnecessary transfusion of platelet concentrates in the absence of haemostatic failure may stimulate more autoantibody formation synthesis and thus increase maternal thrombocytopenia. Most anaesthetists require that the platelet count is at least 80×10^9/l and preferably $>100 \times 10^9$/l before they will administer an epidural anaesthetic but there is no good evidence that counts $>50 \times 10^9$/l are not sufficient to achieve haemostasis in AITP [103].

The major risk at delivery is to the fetus with thrombocytopenia who as the result of birth trauma may suffer intracranial haemorrhage. If there is any question that a vaginal delivery will be difficult because of cephalopelvic disproportion, premature labour, previous history, etc., then elective caesarean section should be carried out.

For many centres the availability of planned or emergency transabdominal FBS is severely limited or non-existent and so decisions concerning the mode of delivery will have to be taken without knowing the fetal platelet count.

As discussed earlier, maternal platelet count, maternal PAIgG, history and splenectomy status show trends regarding the incidence of fetal and neonatal thrombocytopenia but can never be used to predict fetal thrombocytopenia with absolute confidence in an individual case. It does appear however that it is very unlikely for the fetus to have severe thrombocytopenia if the mother has no previous history of AITP before the index pregnancy and if she has no detectable free IgG platelet antibody [167].

Many of the options proposed in the literature presuppose that caesarean section is less traumatic than an uncomplicated vaginal delivery. There is no objective evidence to support this contention and there are undesirable associated complications of caesarean section *per se* for both mother and fetus. The only advantage is that there is more overall control of the delivery if it is by elective caesarean section and there are usually no unpredictable complications.

Based on an estimate of a 13–21 per cent perinatal mortality associated with AITP, it was proposed [137] that all patients should be delivered by caesarean section. The mortality rate quoted is a gross overestimate, probably for reasons previously stated of selection of severe symptomatic cases for the analysis. A recent review of the literature of AITP in pregnancy shows a neonatal mortality rate of six in 1000 AITP patients [35], about the same as or better than the overall perinatal mortality rate. All these deaths occurred in babies delivered by caesarean section and all events appeared more than 24–48 hours after delivery, the time of the platelet count nadir in the neonate.

The incidence of severe thrombocytopenia in the fetus of a woman with proven AITP is no more than 10 per cent. Even if caesarean section is the optimum mode of delivery for the thrombocytopenic fetus, this does not justify this mode of delivery for the nine out of 10 fetuses without thrombocytopenia.

It is not now thought to be optimum management to deliver all fetuses with potential or identified thrombocytopenia by caesarean section. If delivery by caesarean section is indicated for obstetric reasons there is no point in performing FBS to obtain the platelet count and elective caesarean section should be performed.

In our hospital there is considerable expertise in intrauterine FBS but we only recommend this procedure in the following circumstances:

1 where the women enters pregnancy with a history of AITP together with currently identifiable PAIgG antibodies; or

2 in those women who have to be treated for AITP during the index pregnancy.

Our obstetricians, like many others, prefer to deliver a fetus with significant thrombocytopenia (platelet count $<50 \times 10^9$/l) by caesarean section. However, individual units may need different policies depending on local expertise and practice.

Management of the neonate

An immediate cord platelet count should be performed following delivery in all neonates of mothers with AITP whenever or however diagnosed. The vast majority of babies will have platelet counts well above 50×10^9/l and will be symptom free. For those with low platelet counts, petechiae and purpura, steroids or preferably intravenous IgG should be administered. If there is mucous membrane bleeding, platelet concentrates should be administered also.

It should be remembered that the neonatal platelet count will fall further in the first few days of life and it is at the nadir that most complications occur, rather than at delivery. Measures should be taken to prevent the fall if the cord blood platelet count warrants this. The platelet count should be repeated daily for the first week in those neonates with thrombocytopenia at delivery.

The development of techniques to obtain fetal blood with relative safety to perform a fetal platelet count and the widely held concept that caesarean section is less traumatic for the fetus than a normal vaginal delivery has led to often unnecessary intervention with risks to both mother and fetus.

At the time of writing the emphasis of management is to return to a non-interventional policy [8] of sensible monitoring, supportive therapy, and a mode of delivery determined mainly by obstetric indications and not primarily on either the maternal or fetal platelet count.

AITP associated with HIV infection
(see also Chapter 17)

Thrombocytopenia is a well-recognized complication of HIV infection and may be due to drugs and severe infection. The subject has been reviewed [54]. However, patients with the immune deficiency syndromes may have thrombocytopenia otherwise indistinguishable from AITP. This may be due to immune platelet destruction resulting from cross-reaction between HIV and the platelet glycoproteins IIb/IIIa [21] which may explain acquired immune deficiency syndrome (AIDS) free, HIV-associated AITP. It has also been suggested that disturbances in the B cell subset, CD5, in HIV-infected patients may cause immunological changes correlating with the platelet count, and that non-specific deposition of complement and immune complexes on platelets leads to their removal from the circulation [92].

Whilst most HIV positive patients have so far been young men, it is possible that this complication will become commoner in young pregnant women although the degree of heterosexual spread of HIV is uncertain. Certainly, young pregnant women in a high risk group for HIV with thrombocytopenia should be considered for HIV testing.

Thrombocytopenia and SLE

SLE is frequently complicated by thrombocytopenia but this is seldom severe, less than 5 per cent of cases having platelet counts $<30 \times 10^9$/l during the course of the disease [92]. Thrombocytopenia is often the first presenting feature and may antedate any other manifestations by months or even years. Such patients are often labelled as suffering from AITP, unless appropriate additional tests are carried out. PAIgG is often found on testing but it is not clear whether this is due to antiplatelet antibody, immune complexes or both. The management of isolated thrombocytopenia associated with SLE in pregnancy does not differ substantially from that of AITP but immunosuppressive therapy should not be reduced or discontinued during pregnancy [193]. The main management problem of SLE and pregnancy is the complication of the variably present *in vitro* lupus anticoagulant and its paradoxical association with *in vivo* thromboembolism and recurrent fetal loss. For fuller discussion of these complications which have excited much current interest see Chapter 8.

Alloimmune thrombocytopenia (AIT) [107]

Fetal AIT is a syndrome that develops as a result of maternal sensitization to fetal platelet antigens. The antibody, usually HpA1 (formerly known as PlA1) is directed specifically against a paternally derived antigen which the mother lacks (cf. Rh(D) haemolytic disease).

The mother is not thrombocytopenic herself but the fetal platelets *in utero* have altered function. The platelet-specific antibody attaches to the membrane of the HpA1 binding site and interferes with the function of the glycoprotein IIb/IIIa ligand binding sites thus impairing platelet aggregation. The affected thrombocytopenic fetus is at risk of spontaneous intracranial haemorrhage from early in gestation unlike the fetus affected by maternal ITP.

It is obvious that the fetus at risk must be identified early in gestation if measures are to be taken to prevent intrauterine intracranial haemorrhage but this is not easy. In the vast majority of cases, a fetus at risk is identified because of a previously affected sibling. HpA1 is the most common antigen associated with AIT. The antigen is present in 97–98 per cent of the population. Two alleles are present HpA1 and HpA2 and 69 per cent of the population are homozygous for HpA1, the stronger sensitizing antigen. The immune response of the HpA1-negative mother seems to be determined in part by genes of the histocompatibility complex and antibody formation appears to be confined to those with HLA-B8 and HLA-DR3 anti- gens. First pregnancies may be affected (unlike Rh disease). Subsequent affected pregnancies will be of similar or increased severity and the recurrence rate is estimated to be between 75 and 90 per cent.

The monitoring of severity of the disease process also differs greatly from Rh haemolytic disease. The absence of antibodies does not guarantee a normal fetal platelet count although women with identifiable antibodies are at risk of producing a fetus with thrombocytopenia. Rises in titre and concentration of antibody do not correlate with severity.

To identify all women at risk of developing platelet alloantibodies by platelet (HpA1) grouping and HLA typing of all pregnant women is not cost-effective or feasible at the moment but the appropriate investigations should be carried out on all female relatives of women known to have had a baby affected by this disorder.

The incidence of neonatal AIT has been estimated to be one in 5000 births although more recent studies give a higher frequency of one in 2000–3000 births. Not all cases necessarily have severe manifestation. We have identified at least one symptomless case on routine screening of neonatal cord blood of an Rh(D) negative woman at delivery.

Management of AIT

All management protocols currently involve FBS early in gestation but preferably after 22 weeks' gestation when the risk of the procedure is reduced. In the identified affected fetus, subsequent management is controversial. Weekly maternal IgG infusion 1 g/kg with or without prednisone has been used in the successful management of pregnancies at risk of AIT [116]. This has not been the universal experience however. Others recommend weekly HpA1-negative platelet infusions until fetal lung maturity is achieved. All protocols involve frequent ultrasound examinations to check that no intracranial bleeds have occurred. Mode of delivery will be determined by maturity, fetal platelet count and obstetric indications.

The use of maternal platelet infusions to the fetus or neonate should be discouraged. Unless they are repeatedly washed the infused anti-HpA1 antibody has a much longer half-life than the platelets themselves. Repeated washing of platelets also reduces their function [150]. Moreover, suitably prepared platelets from accredited donors provided by the regional blood transfusion service are more effective and probably much safer. Post-delivery, the disease is usually self-limiting within a few weeks. If therapy is required, HpA compatible platelets are the treatment of choice. The aim of current antenatal management protocols, which are all controversial, is to deliver a relatively mature infant who has not suffered intracranial haemorrhage antenatally or during delivery.

AIT can be a devastating fetal disease and it should be excluded in all cases of fetal intracranial haemorrhage, unexplained porencephaly and neonatal thrombocytopenia.

Unlike ITP, because of the risk of spontaneous intrauterine fetal haemorrhage, early FBS is indicated and a mother with this potential problem should be referred early in pregnancy to an expert fetal medicine unit for investigation and management although delivery of a treated infant may still take place at the centre of referral.

At Queen Charlotte's Maternity Hospital we have successfully managed this condition with serial weekly fetal platelet transfusions starting as early as 22 weeks' gestation.

Preliminary encouraging reports of successful management with maternally administered intravenous IgG have not been borne out in other centres [94,142]. This may relate to the different preparations of immunoglobulin available and the effects of variable content of contaminating CD4 and CD8 molecules [23].

In conclusion, by contrast to AITP, FBS is both justified and indicated. Management of all cases should involve a fetal medicine unit skilled in intrauterine investigation and procedures.

Pre-eclampsia and platelets (see also Chapter 6)

There have been many reports showing that the circulating platelet count is reduced in pre-eclampsia and these have been recently reviewed [165]. It has also been shown that the platelet count can be used to monitor severity of the disease process and as an initial screening test if there is concern about significant coagulation abnormalities [101,157,178]. A fall in the platelet count precedes any detectable rise in serum fibrin(ogen) degradation products in women subsequently developing pre-eclampsia [157].

The combination of a reduced platelet lifespan and a fall in the platelet count without platelet-associated antibodies (see below) indicates a low grade coagulopathy. Platelets may either be consumed in thrombus formation or may suffer membrane damage from contact with abnormal surfaces and be prematurely removed from the circulation.

Rarely, in very severe pre-eclampsia the patient develops microangiopathic haemolytic anaemia. These patients have profound thrombocytopenia and this leads to confusion in the differential diagnosis between pre-eclampsia, thrombotic thrombocytopenic purpura (TTP) and haemolysis, elevated liver enzymes and low platelet (count) (HELLP) syndrome.

The activation of the haemostatic mechanisms in normal pregnancy has led to the view that the haematological manifestations of pre-eclampsia merely represent augmentation of the hypercoagulable state which accompanies normal pregnancy.

Many studies have been carried out on levels of individual coagulation factors. No clear pattern emerges but there appear to be some significant correlations of severity of the disease process with both the Factor VIII complex [158] and ATIII [201].

A readily available and sensitive indicator of activation of the coagulation system is assay of fibrinopeptide A concentration in the plasma. Although in mild pre-eclampsia patients may have a normal or only slight increase in fibrinopeptide A levels, marked increases occur in patients with severe pre-eclampsia [29,198].

Most studies in pre-eclampsia have shown increased levels of fibrinogen/fibrin degradation products in serum and urine. Plasma levels of soluble fibrinogen/fibrin complexes are also raised in pre-eclampsia compared with normal pregnancies [64,65]. Borok *et al.* [29] found that fibrinolytic activity is more pronounced than fibrin formation in patients with severe pre-eclampsia.

One study [187] estimated kaolin cephalin clotting time, prothrombin time, thrombin time, fibrinogen, englobulin clot lysis time, FDPs, platelet count, β thromboglobulin and platelet factor 4, and fibrinopeptide A in 400 women at 28 weeks' gestation. None of these tests proved predictive but once the disease process is established the most relevant coagulation abnormalities appear to be the platelet count, Factor VIII, and FDPs. Those women with the most marked abnormalities in these parameters suffer the greatest perinatal loss.

TTP and HUS

These conditions share so many features that they should probably be considered as one disease with pathologic effects confined largely to the kidney in HUS (see Chapter 7) and being more generalized in TTP. They are extremely rare and fewer than 100 cases have been reported in pregnancy [151]. These conditions are both due to the presence of platelet thrombin in the microcirculation which causes ischaemic dysfunction and microangiopathic haemolysis. In HUS, the brunt of the disease process is taken by the kidney particularly in the postnatal period. It has also been seen during pregnancy and in association with ectopic pregnancy [55]. It has been postulated that endothelial damage is mediated through neutrophil adhesion in association with infection and leads to the formation of platelet thrombin [71].

In TTP, the focus shifts to multisystem disease, often with neurological involvement and fever. It too has been associated with pregnancy and the post-partum period [200] and with use of the platelet anti-aggregating agent, ticlopidine [146]. It is associated with abnormal patterns of vWF multimers in the plasma [129]. Immunohistochemistry has shown the presence of vWF but not fibrinogen in the platelet aggregates in TTP [5]. It has been suggested that a calcium-dependent cysteine protease present in patient plasma may interact with vWF to render it highly reactive with platelets and thus contribute to the formation of platelet aggregates [132]. The underlying aetiology of TTP in pregnancy remains unknown and the various abnormalities which have been described may only be epiphenomena. It is feasible that there is a deficiency of prostacyclin activator or synthesis. The aetiology has been reviewed [7,117].

The pentad of fever, normal coagulation tests with low platelets, haemolytic anaemia, neurological disorders and renal dysfunction is virtually pathognomonic of TTP. The thrombocytopenia may range from 5 to 100×10^9/l. The clinical picture is severe with a high maternal mortality.

A crucial problem when dealing with TTP is to establish a correct diagnosis, because this condition can be confused with severe pre-eclampsia and placental abruption, especially if DIC is triggered (although DIC is uncommon in TTP).

Unlike in AFLP (see Chapter 9) there is no evidence that prompt delivery affects the course of HUS or TTP favourably. Most clinicians would recommend delivery if these conditions are present in late pregnancy so that the mother can be treated vigorously without fear of harming the fetus.

Empirical therapeutic strategies hinge on intensive plasma exchange or replacement. In a random allocation study of 102 non-pregnant patients with TTP, plasma exchange was found to be more effective than plasma infusion, with more than seven exchanges over 9 days. It has been suggested that plasma supplies a factor lacking in patients with TTP that stimulates the release of prostacyclin. Regimens may be supplemented with antiplatelet drugs such as low dose aspirin to prevent relapse [117] although their use has been contested by some authors [17]. Platelet infusions are contraindicated. Cryosupernatant has been shown to control the metabolism of unusually large vWF multimers [128] *in vivo*.

In one large series of 108 patients with HUS/TTP, of whom 9 per cent were pregnant, steroids alone were judged to be effective in mild cases, whilst there were eight deaths and 67 relapses in a group of 78 patients with complicated disease. They were treated with steroids and plasma exchange infusions. The overall survival was 91 per cent. Relapses occurred in 22 of 36 patients given maintenance plasma infusions. Of the nine pregnant patients, all were in the third trimester and all were delivered of normal infants. Five women went on to further normal pregnancies and deliveries [17].

In summary, it seems reasonable to treat all TTP patients with steroids. Severe cases will benefit from intensive plasma exchange but where that is difficult, intensive plasma infusion is indicated. Unresponsive cases may benefit from cryosupernatant infusions. The use of antiplatelet drugs is contested [128]. Plasma infusion should be tapered but continued until all objective signs have been reversed, in order to prevent recurrence.

Factor VIII antibody

An inhibitor of antihaemophilic factor is a rare cause of haemorrhage in previously healthy post-partum women [48,120,143,159,195]. There are less than 50 documented cases in the literature [159,195]. Women who may have had this type of haemorrhagic disorder were first reported in the late 1930s and the nature of the defect was first reported in 1946, when the plasma of two such patients was shown not only to resemble haemophilic plasma but to have an inhibitory effect on normal clotting. In the late 1960s it was demonstrated that these inhibitors of Factor VIII were immunoglobulins, as are the Factor VIII antibodies found in treated haemophiliacs [195]. Of the post-partum coagulation defects of this type reported, nearly all were found on *in vitro* testing to be directed against Factor VIII. Only two were found to be anti-Factor IX antibodies.

Aetiology

The aetiology of antibodies to Factor VIIIC is complex. The appearance of anti-VIII in non-haemophilic individuals is usually attributed to an autoimmune process, or in women post-partum to isoimmunization. However, no difference between maternal and fetal Factor VIII has been demonstrated and neutralization of both maternal and fetal Factor VIII by the antibody is similar.

At present there is no definite evidence that Factor VIII antigen allotypes exist. If the bleeding tendency is to be explained, the antibody formed by stimulation of the maternal immune system by fetal Factor VIII has to cross-react with maternal Factor VIII. One would expect such an antibody to reappear after some of the subsequent pregnancies (by analogy with rhesus sensitization), but relapses have not been reported. Assuming that these inhibitors are IgG antibodies, they are likely to cross the placenta and persist for several weeks in the neonate, as do antirhesus or antiviral antibodies. However, although Factor VIII antibody and reduced levels of Factor VIIIC have been found in neonates born to mothers with antibody there have been no case reports of haemorrhagic problems in their offspring. The variable nature of this disorder argues in favour of a more complex pathogenesis. There is an association between Factor VIII antibodies and autoimmune disorders such as rheumatoid arthritis and systemic lupus. There is also a well-known alteration of immune reactivity in normal pregnancy. These two observations suggest that a likely explanation of post-partum Factor VIII antibodies is that of a temporary breakdown in the mother's tolerance to her own Factor VIII (or Factor IX). This rare disorder does resemble other autoimmune states in its variable onset and duration, its varying severity and in the fact that its aetiology is still a mystery [195].

Clinical manifestations

The patient usually presents within 3 months of delivery with severe and sometimes life-threatening bleeding, extensive painful bruising, bleeding from the gastrointestinal and genitourinary tract, and occasional haemarthroses. The reported confirmed cases presented in a period of 3 days to 17 months post-partum. The diagnosis is established on the basis of characteristic laboratory findings. The prothrombin time and thrombin time are normal but the partial thromboplastin time is very long. The partial thromboplastin time is not corrected by the addition of normal plasma or Factor VIII.

Management

Any woman who develops such an antibody should be under the care of an expert coagulation unit. Treatment of the acute bleeding episode is difficult because conventional amounts of Factor VIII may just enhance antibody formation and fail to control the bleeding. Immunosuppressive agents in combination with corticosteroids have been used to reduce the antibody production [48].

In one reported case [159] after failure of therapy with Factor VIII concentrate and fresh plasma, improvement in the clinical status was achieved by administration of an anti-inhibitor coagulation complex (Autoplex), a preparation of pooled fresh plasma containing precursors and activated clotting factors. The mechanism of action of Autoplex is unknown. It does not suppress or destroy the inhibitor but seems to control the acute haemorrhagic diathesis [159].

The natural history is for the antibody to disappear gradually, usually within 2 years. Women should be advised to avoid further pregnancy until coagulation returns to normal, although in the one documented case where conception occurred in the presence of clinically active antibody, it disappeared during the course of the pregnancy [195].

Inherited defects of haemostasis

It is important to recognize these uncommon conditions not only because the morbidity and mortality they cause in the sufferer is almost completely preventable by correct diagnosis and treatment, but also because carriers of the most devastating of these conditions, particularly the X-linked haemophilias, can be identified and prenatal diagnosis offered if couples at risk so desire.

However, because of the profound changes in haemostasis during normal pregnancy, it is desirable to establish a correct diagnosis with appropriate family studies and DNA analysis where relevant before conception so that appropriate management and chorion villus sampling, in conditions where DNA prenatal diagnosis is feasible, can be planned in advance.

Severe congenital disorders of haemostasis are nearly always apparent early in life so that they will have been diagnosed before the obstetrician has to deal with the patient. Milder forms may go unrecognized until adult life and are more of a diagnostic challenge.

Patients with thrombocytopenia or platelet function abnormalities suffer primarily from mucosal bleeding, with epistaxes, gingival and gastrointestinal bleeding and menorrhagia. Bleeding occurs immediately after surgery or trauma and may not occur at all if primary haemostasis can be achieved with suturing.

In contrast, patients with coagulation disorders typically suffer deep muscle haematomata and haemarthroses. Bleeding after trauma or surgery may be immediate or delayed.

A history of previous vaginal deliveries without undue bleeding does not exclude a significant coagulopathy because of the increase in coagulation factors, particularly Factor VIII, during normal pregnancy and the fact that a healthy myometrium is the most important haemostatic factor at parturition.

It is not uncommon for adult patients to have significant bleeding after surgery because of previously undiagnosed inherited haemostatic disorders, due to the fact that surgery imposes a challenge on the haemostatic mechanisms which far exceeds anything encountered in everyday life.

Complete laboratory evaluation of a patient giving a history of 'easy bleeding or bruising' is time-consuming and expensive and a history of significant previous haemostatic challenges should be obtained. For example, a patient who has undergone tonsillectomy, without transfusion or special treatment and lived to tell the tale, cannot possibly have an inherited haemostatic disorder!

Of more relevance perhaps is any history of dental extractions where haemorrhage can occur with both platelet disorders and coagulopathies. If prolonged bleeding has occurred and particularly if blood transfusion has been required, then a high index of suspicion of a congenital haemorrhagic disorder is justified. In such cases, even if initial laboratory screening tests — partial thromboplastin time, prothrombin time, platelet count and bleeding time are normal, the diagnosis should be vigorously pursued in consultation with an expert haematologist.

The most common congenital coagulation disorders are von Willebrand's disease, Factor VIII deficiency (haemophilia A) and Factor IX deficiency (haemophilia B). Less common disorders include Factor XI deficiency, abnormal or deficient fibrinogen and deficiency of Factor XIII (fibrin stabilizing factor). All other coagulation factor disorders are extremely rare. The most frequent disorders of platelet function are von Willebrand's disease and storage pool disease [91].

Hereditary platelet abnormalities

Functional defects

Serious bleeding disorders due to inherited abnormalities of platelet function are rare, the inheritance being autosomal recessive. Clinically the signs and symptoms are similar to those of von Willebrand's disease (see below) with skin and mucosal haemorrhages. Spontaneous bruises are common but haemarthroses are not. Although these disorders can lead to life-threatening haemorrhage, particularly after surgery or trauma, the bleeding tendency is usually mild. The essential defect is intrinsic to the platelet. Bleeding time is prolonged and platelet function tests are abnormal, showing reduced aggregation and/or adhesion. In thrombasthenia (Glanzmann's disease), the platelets appear morphologically normal but they fail to aggregate with collagen, ADP or ristocetin. In the very rare Bernard–Soulier syndrome the aggregation defect is similar but the platelets have a characteristically abnormal giant appearance. Serious bleeding episodes are treated with fresh platelet concentrate infusions and plasmapheresis [147]. Families who have one or other of these rare defects may seek termination of pregnancy because of the severity of symptoms or the difficulties arising from management. It is theoretically possible to diagnose the condition prenatally from a pure FBS, since specific membrane glycoprotein defects have been identified in both syndromes. A sensitive monoclonal immunoassay applicable to small volumes of whole fetal blood, without the necessity of separating the platelets, greatly facilitates prenatal diagnoses in these conditions (see [126]).

Thrombocytopenia

Genetically determined thrombocytopenia may be associated with aplastic anaemia or isolated megakaryocytic aplasia. The syndrome of absent radii with thrombocytopenia is known as the TAR syndrome: these are thought to be autosomal recessive defects and have been successfully diagnosed prenatally by examination of fetal blood samples [9,56,141].

Patients with May–Heggelin anomaly, an autosomal dominant condition with variable thrombocytopenia and giant platelets, may receive platelet concentrates to achieve haemostasis at delivery and can be offered prenatal diagnosis [50].

Another X-linked symptom complex is the Wiskott–Aldrich syndrome comprising severe immune deficiency with thrombocytopenia. It presents in the neonatal period but is probably expressed *in utero* and therefore susceptible to diagnosis prenatally. The five pregnancies at risk reported so far have been female and were not examined further [126]. Fanconi's anaemia, a familial autosomal recessively inherited condition, is a syndrome of aplastic anaemia with varying skeletal and other physical anomalies. Although thrombocytopenia is the earliest and dominant feature of marrow aplasia, presentation is usually delayed until at least 3 or 4 years of age, so that intrauterine diagnosis by detecting thrombocytopenia in fetal blood is precluded. However, the diagnosis has been made on the basis of excessive chromosomal breaks in chemically treated amniotic fluid fibroblast cultures [9]. A more rapid result could be obtained by using percutaneous transabdominal FBS for culture of fetal cells [126].

Hereditary coagulation disorders

Von Willebrand's disease

Von Willebrand's disease [90] is the most frequent of all inherited haemostatic disorders with an incidence of overt disease of more than one in 10 000, similar to that of haemophilia A; but because subclinical forms of the disorder are common the total incidence of von Willebrand's disease is greater than that of haemophilia.

In contrast to haemophilia (an X-linked condition) von Willebrand's disease has an autosomal inheritance and equal incidence in males and females and therefore is the most frequent genetic haemostatic disorder encountered in obstetric practice.

NATURE OF THE DEFECT

Von Willebrand's disease is a disorder of the vWF portion of the human Factor VIII complex.

Factor VIII circulates as a complex of two proteins of unequal size (Table 3.2). There is a low molecular weight portion VIIIC (290 000) which promotes coagulation linked to a large multimer known as both vWF (VIIIWF) and VIIIRAg (VIII-related antigen). Factor VIII circulates as polymers ranging in size from 800 000 to more than 10 000 000 daltons. The biosynthesis of Factor VIIIC coded for by the X chromosome is reduced or abnormal in haemophilia A. The larger VIIIWF which serves as a 'carrier' for VIIIC is under separate autosomal control and is unaffected in haemophilia. vWF appears to stabilize the small coagulant protein or perhaps protect it from proteolytic digestion. Reduction in VIIIWF usually leads to comparable decrease in VIIIC activity.

vWF is the major protein in plasma that promotes platelet adhesion forming a bridge between the subendothelial collagen and a specific receptor on the platelet membrane. The large multimeric forms of VIIIWF appear to have the greatest physiological effect in promoting this adhesion, which is the first step in coagulation *in vivo*, followed by platelet aggregation. However, *in vitro* tests of platelet aggregation will be entirely normal in von Willebrand's disease because the initial step is bypassed and different platelet receptors are activated when they are exposed to collagen, ADP or thrombin in standard laboratory conditions. The platelet abnormality in von Willebrand's disease can be studied *in vitro* using the antibiotic ristocetin which takes advantage of the fact that it will agglutinate platelets by a mechanism involving VIIIWF. The most sensitive test for detection of von Willebrand's disease is ristocetin cofactor assay — a functional assay for vWF. The ability of patients' plasma to agglutinate normal platelets in the presence of ristocetin is assessed in this test. Ristocetin cofactor levels are normal in less than 10 per cent of patients with von Willebrand's disease, and this test shows the best correlation with clinical manifestations of the disease. If the patient's own platelet-rich plasma is used in this test system the ristocetin aggregation is normal in more than one-third. However, the direct

Table 3.2. Factor VIII molecular complex

VIII	Molecular complex	Molecular weight $>1 \times 10^6$
VIIIC	Procoagulant in plasma (detected in bioassay)	Molecular weight 293 000 X chromosome
VIIICAg	Antigen detectable by human antibody to VIIIC Immunoradiometric assay (IRMA)	
VIIIWF	von Willebrand factor Measured by bleeding time Ristocetin aggregation of platelets	Molecular weight (Polymers × 220 000) Chromosome 12
VIIIRAg	Antigen detectable by heterologous antibody raised in rabbit to human factor VIII (IRMA)	

ristocetin platelet aggregation test may be useful in the diagnosis of one of the variants of von Willebrand's disease type IIb (see below).

Clinical manifestations are primarily those of a platelet defect, namely spontaneous mucous membrane and skin bleeding, with prolonged bleeding following trauma or surgery. In addition there is a variable secondary defect of Factor VIII coagulant activity and if this is severely depressed there may be clinical manifestations of a coagulation disorder. The most frequent problem encountered in the non-pregnant female is menorrhagia which may be quite severe at times.

Patients with mild abnormalities may be asymptomatic and picked up only after excessive haemorrhage following trauma or related to surgery.

The severity of the disorder does not run true within families and fluctuates from time to time in the same individual.

SUBTYPES OF VON WILLEBRAND'S DISEASE

The most common type of von Willebrand's disease accounting for 80 per cent of all cases is type I. It is inherited as an autosomal dominant trait. The protein is quantitatively normal but there is a reduction in Factor VIII activity, both coagulation activity and platelet function being affected in roughly equal proportion. The manifestations result from a quantitative deficiency of a normal protein. The condition is usually mild.

A rare, apparently autosomal recessive form of the disorder is described in which there is absent *in vitro* Factor VIIIC, Factor VIIIRAg and ristocetin cofactor activity, which is accompanied by a severe bleeding disorder. It is in these cases that couples at risk may seek prenatal diagnosis (see below).

Type II von Willebrand's disease is characterized by an absence of large multimers of vWF which seem to be essential for normal platelet function. In type IIa the large and intermediate size multimers are absent from both plasma and platelets and it accounts for less than 10 per cent of all cases.

Approximately 5 per cent of cases belong to the subtype IIb in which the large multimers are absent in the plasma but present in the platelets. Types IIc and IId and pseudo von Willebrand's disease have also been described on the basis of multimeric pattern and distribution of VIIIWF. It must be obvious from the discussion so far that any woman who is contemplating or has entered pregnancy with von Willebrand's disease or a history suggestive of this complex disorder must be managed by a unit which has access to expert haemostatic advice. The subtype must be correctly identified because this has serious implications in terms of the optimum management (see below).

TREATMENT

There are several forms of treatment of von Willebrand's disease in current use. In any given case the choice depends on the severity and type of the disease and also the clinical setting. The aim is to correct the platelet and coagulation disorder by achieving normal levels of Factor VIII coagulant activity and a bleeding time within the normal range. The key feature in treatment is substitution with plasma concentrates containing functional vWF and VIIIC. In less severe cases the vasopressin analogue L-diamino-8-arginine-vasopressin (DDAVP) has been used with success. Contraceptive hormones have been used with success in treatment of menorrhagia in von Willebrand's disease [90]. It is extremely important that aspirin and related anti-inflammatory drugs should not be used in von Willebrand's disease. They will further compromise platelet function and aspirin has been shown to prolong the bleeding time markedly in patients with platelet/coagulation disorders.

SUBSTITUTION THERAPY

The main treatment in von Willebrand's disease used to be replacement therapy with cryoprecipitate or FFP. The latter is efficient, but large volumes may be required to secure haemostasis. In obstetric practice, however, this did not cause any problems when covering delivery. Cryoprecipitate used to be the product of choice to cover cold surgery. Factor VIII concentrates were not used in the management of von Willebrand's disease because in commercial preparations, the factor promoting platelet adhesion may be lost and because of the increased risk of transmitting infection. However, the newer preparations of Factor VIII concentrate are now the treatment of choice. They retain some platelet promoting activity and have the added advantage of being heat-treated and therefore sterile. They now no longer carry the hazard of transmitting HIV and other viral infections. The use of cryoprecipitate and FFP is now contraindicated and cannot be recommended.

DDAVP

This vasopressin analogue has been shown to cause release of vWF from endothelial cells where it is synthesized and stored. This results in increased plasma levels of both ristocetin cofactor and of Factor VIIIC. It is therefore of benefit to patients with von Willebrand's disease and haemophilia A. It is particularly effective in mildly affected patients and may in some cases replace the use or need for blood products in patients undergoing surgery. Toxicity associated with use of this product has been trivial. Occasional patients experience flushing and dizziness [58,90]. The theoretical risk of water intoxication and hyponatraemia due to the vasopressive effect has not been observed using the current dosage schedules. The recommended dose is an intravenous infusion of 0.3 μg/kg of DDAVP given over 30 min with a total dose of 15–25 μg. This may be repeated every 12–24 hours [113]. Patients with mild type I von Willebrand's disease would be expected to derive maximal benefit from this mode of treatment. VIIIC levels are dramatically increased provided that the baseline level is more than 10 per cent. The effect of the use of DDAVP on the bleeding time is controversial but the overall consensus is that *in vitro* ristocetin co-factor levels increase and there is an overall reduction in clinical bleeding.

In patients with severe type I von Willebrand's disease, DDAVP will have no effect and replacement therapy must be used.

In type IIB von Willebrand's disease the use of DDAVP is contraindicated. *In vivo* platelet aggregation and severe thrombocytopenia will follow the infusion although it does transiently improve the plasma multimeric pattern.

Von Willebrand's disease and pregnancy

A rise in both Factor VIIIC and vWF is observed in normal pregnancy. Patients with all but the severest forms of von Willebrand's disease show a similar but variable rise in both these factors, although there may not be a reduction in the bleeding time [37,42,53,91].

After delivery, normal women maintain an elevated Factor VIIIC level for at least 5 days. This is followed by a slow fall to baseline levels over 4–6 weeks. The duration of Factor VIII activity post-partum in women with von Willebrand's disease seems to be related to the severity of the disorder. Those women with severer forms of the condition may have a rapid fall in Factor VIII procoagulant and platelet haemostatic activity. They are then at risk of quite severe secondary post-partum haemorrhage.

What is the haemorrhagic risk during pregnancy and delivery for women with von Willebrand's disease? An analysis of published reports of 33 pregnancies in 22 women showed abnormal bleeding in 27 per cent of pregnancies at the time of abortion, delivery or post-partum [53].

The vast majority of women will have increased their Factor VIIIC production to within the normal range (50–150 per cent) by late gestation and although Factor VIII concentrate should be standing by at delivery it will probably not be needed to achieve haemostasis [125].

There is virtually no place for DDAVP in obstetric practice except perhaps in the puerperium because if a rise in Factor VIII is possible under the influence of DDAVP (milder cases) then it will have been achieved during the stimulus of pregnancy itself. However, DDAVP has an obvious valuable place in the management of women with von Willebrand's disease undergoing gynaecological surgery.

The haemophilias

The haemophilias are inherited disorders associated with reduced or absent coagulation Factors VIII or IX with an incidence of about one in 10 000 in developed countries [93]. The most common is haemophilia A which is associated with deficiency of Factor VIII: about one-sixth of the 3000–4000 cases in the UK today have a condition known as Christmas disease due to a lack of coagulation Factor IX (haemophilia B). Clinical manifestations of the two conditions are indistinguishable, the symptoms and signs being variable and depending on the degree of lack of the coagulation factors concerned. Severe disease with frequent spontaneous bleeding (particularly haemarthroses) are associated with clotting factor levels of 0–1 per cent. Less severe disease is found in subjects with clotting factors of 1–4 per cent. Spontaneous bleeding and severe bleeding after minor trauma are rare in cases with coagulation factor levels between 5 and 30 per cent; the danger is that the condition may be clinically silent but during the course of major surgery or following trauma, such subjects behave as if they have the very severest forms of haemophilia. Unless the defect is recognized and the lacking coagulation factor is replaced, such patients will continue to bleed. The inheritance of both haemophilias is X-linked recessive, being expressed in the male and carried by the female.

The risks in pregnancy for a female carrier of haemophilia are twofold:

1 she may, by process of lyonization, have a very low Factor VIII or IX level which puts her at risk of excessive bleeding, particularly following a traumatic or surgical delivery;

2 fifty per cent of her male offspring will inherit haemophilia and 50 per cent of her daughters will be carriers like herself.

This has important implications now that prenatal diagnosis of these conditions is possible (see below).

MANAGEMENT OF HAEMOPHILIA IN PREGNANCY

Female carriers of haemophilia do not usually have clinical manifestations but in rare individuals in whom the Factor VIIIC or IX levels are unusually low (10–30 per cent of normal) abnormal bleeding may occur after trauma or surgery [115]. It is important to identify carriers prior to pregnancy, not only to provide genetic counselling (see below) but so that appropriate provision can be made for those cases with pathologically low coagulation factor activities. Fortunately the level of the deficient factor tends to increase during the course of pregnancy as it does in normal women. There have been anecdotal reports of female homozygotes for haemophilia A who have negotiated pregnancy successfully [115]. Haemorrhage post-partum does not appear to be a consistent feature, particularly if delivery is by the vaginal route at term with little or no soft tissue damage. The effect of pregnancy on Factor VIIIC levels in these rare cases has not been studied.

If the Factor VIII level remains low in carriers of haemophilia A, cryoprecipitate should be given to cover delivery and continued for 3–4 days post-partum following a normal vaginal delivery, such that Factor VIII levels are maintained above 50 per cent. This cover will have to be maintained for a longer period if delivery is by caesarean section or there has been extensive soft tissue damage. Factor VIII concentrates should be avoided because they expose the woman unnecessarily to the hazards of multiple donations.

DDAVP has been shown to be of benefit in patients with mild haemophilia as with von Willebrand's disease (see above). However, the storage pools of Factor VIII released during treatment may become exhausted and tachyphylaxis does occur [113]. There are no controlled studies concerning the use of DDAVP for bleeding disorders during pregnancy although it appears to be safe in the treatment of diabetes insipidus (see Chapter 13).

However, as indicated previously if the stimulus of pregnancy has not raised the level of Factor VIII as an expected physiological response in mild haemophilia, it is unlikely that DDAVP will do so.

A clinical problem is more likely in carriers of Factor IX deficiency (Christmas disease) than in those women who carry Factor VIII deficiency [106].

In the exceptionally rare situations where Factor IX level is very low and remains low during pregnancy, the patient should be managed with high purity Factor IX concentrates to cover delivery and for 3–4 days post-partum. Low purity factor IX concentrates (prothrombin concentrate) contains Factors II, VII and X, as well as Factor IX, and therefore carry a much greater thrombogenic hazard adding to the innate risk of thromboembolism in pregnancy. FFP will carry the very remote hazard (in the UK) of transmitting HIV infection [1]. The product of choice is therefore high purity Factor IX concentrate. These patients should be managed in a unit with access to expert advice, 24-hour laboratory coagulation service and immediate access to the appropriate plasma components required for replacement therapy.

PRENATAL DIAGNOSIS OF THE HAEMOPHILIAS

Haemophilia is a relatively uncommon disease. In the UK there are between 3000 and 4000 cases and one in 25000 of the population has the disease in a severe form. The ratio of haemophilia A to Christmas disease is in the region of 5:1. Affected males within the same family have similar residual levels of coagulation factor activity (<1 per cent severe, 1–5 per cent moderate, >6 per cent mild).

Antenatal screening for these conditions will be largely restricted to families in which there is a history of the disease. It is usually indicated if a woman wishes to undergo prenatal diagnosis to determine whether her male fetus has the disease. Approximately one-third of cases have no family history and are presumed to result from spontaneous mutations.

Obligate carriers [127] are:

1 all daughters of a haemophiliac father;

2 a woman with more than one haemophiliac son;

3 a woman with one haemophiliac son and a proven haemophiliac relative in her own family or her mother's;

4 the relative of a haemophiliac sufferer, the male fetus of whom is found to be haemophiliac on prenatal testing.

Putative carriers are daughters of a known haemophiliac carrier who have a 50:50 chance of inheriting the abnormal X chromosome as do their brothers. The homozygous male is easily identified, but the heterozygous female may have to be content with a statistical estimate of her genotype by discriminant analysis utilizing family data and haematological investigation (see below).

A further aid to carrier detection in a few females was the demonstration of a linkage between haemophilia A and a G6PD variant, another X-linked genetic marker. It cannot be overemphasized that the clarification of carrier status goes hand in hand with prenatal diagnosis. This is particularly so when using direct DNA analysis (see below) [148].

Although it has proved possible to diagnose carrier status during pregnancy [126] the need to make early plans for fetal sexing and to take the required blood samples means that the status should be established before pregnancy whenever practicable.

Female carriers of haemophilia have on average 50 per cent of the normal mean level of the coagulation factor involved, but because of the wide range of normal and variability of lyonization of the X chromosome, carriers often have levels within the normal range. As far as haemophilia A is concerned it is sometimes possible to improve discrimination by measuring the level of vWF, the autosomally coded carrier protein for Factor VIII. Carriers, unlike the normal population, have lower levels of VIIIC than vWF (reduced VIIIC:vWF ratio)—but firm diagnosis of carrier status is still not possible in about 15 per cent of cases.

In recent years specialist centres managing these diseases are turning to DNA technology for diagnosis. The Factor VIII and IX genes have been isolated and sequenced and many of the mutations that underlie haemophilia and Christmas disease have been determined. They may result from point mutations or deletions involving these genes. In addition, many restriction fragment length polymorphisms (RFLPs) have been found both within and in the flanking regions of these genes.

The specialist studies involved can be undertaken by the regional haemophilia centre in collaboration with the regional genetics centre.

For identified female carriers, prenatal diagnosis can be carried out in the majority of cases by DNA analysis of chorion villus samples. In the few families where DNA analysis is not currently informative, assay of plasma Factor VIIIC or IXC in a fetal blood sample taken from 18 weeks' gestation onwards will provide an accurate but undesirable late prenatal diagnosis.

Factor XI deficiency (plasma thromboplastin antecedent (PTA) deficiency)

This is a rare coagulation disorder less common than the haemophilias but more common than the very rare inherited deficiencies of the remaining coagulation factors. It is inherited as an autosomal recessive, predominantly in Ashkenazi Jews and both men and women may be affected. Usually only the homozygotes have clinical evidence of a coagulation disorder though occasionally carriers may have a bleeding tendency. It is a mild condition in which spontaneous haemorrhages and haemarthroses are rare but the danger lies in the fact that profuse bleeding may follow major trauma or surgery if no prophylactic Factor XI concentrate is given. Indeed it is often diagnosed late in life following surgery in an individual who was unaware of a serious haemostatic defect. The diagnosis is made by finding a prolonged partial thromboplastin time, with a low Factor XI level in a coagulation assay system in which all other coagulation tests are normal. Management consists of replacement with Factor XI concentrates as prophylaxis for surgery or to treat bleeding and to cover operative delivery.

The effective haemostatic level of Factor XI has a half-life of around 2 days. To cover surgery or delivery, women can be treated with one infusion of Factor XI concentrate to raise the level to 80–100 per cent and until primary healing is established.

Fortunately the condition rarely causes problems either during pregnancy and labour or in the child: in particular prolonged bleeding at ritual circumcision is not usual. There is therefore, no justification in screening routinely for this condition either in the mother, fetus or neonate.

Genetic disorders of fibrinogen (Factor I)

Fibrinogen is synthesized in the liver, has a molecular weight of 340 000 and circulates in plasma at a concentration of 300 mg/dl. Both quantitative and qualitative genetic abnormalities are described.

AFIBRINOGENAEMIA OR HYPOFIBRINOGENAEMIA

These are rare autosomal recessive disorders resulting from reduced fibrinogen synthesis. Most patients with hypofibrinogenaemia are heterozygous.

Afibrinogenaemia is characterized by a lifelong bleeding tendency of variable severity. Prolonged bleeding after minor injury and easy bruising are frequent symptoms. Menorrhagia can be very severe. Spontaneous deep tissue bleeding and haemarthroses are rare, but severe bleeding can occur after trauma or surgery and several patients have suffered intracerebral haemorrhages.

In afibrinogenaemia all screening tests of coagulation are prolonged, but corrected by addition of normal plasma or fibrinogen. A prolonged bleeding time may be present. The final diagnosis is made by quantitating the concentration of circulating fibrinogen.

There are no fibrinogen concentrates available and plasma or cryoprecipitate have to be used as replacement therapy to treat bleeding, or to cover surgery or delivery. The *in vivo* half-life of fibrinogen is between 3 and 5 days. Initial replacement should be achieved with 25 ml plasma/kg and daily maintenance with 5–10 ml/kg for 7 days.

Congenital hypofibrinogenaemia has been associated with recurrent early miscarriages and with recurrent placental abruption [139].

DYSFIBRINOGENAEMIA

Congenital dysfibrinogenaemia is an autosomal dominant disorder. In contrast to patients with afibrinogenaemia, patients with this disorder are often symptom free. Some have a bleeding tendency; others have been shown to have thromboembolic disease. The diagnosis is made by demonstrating a prolonged thrombin time with a normal immunological fibrinogen level.

Affected women, like those with hypofibrinogenaemia, may have recurrent spontaneous abortion or repeated placental abruption [139].

Factor XIII deficiency (fibrin stabilizing factor deficiency)

This is an autosomal recessive disorder classically characterized by bleeding from the umbilical cord during the first few days of life and later by ecchymoses, prolonged post-traumatic haemorrhage and poor wound healing. Bleeding is usually delayed and characteristically of a slow oozing nature. Intracranial haemorrhage has been described in a significant proportion of reported cases. Spontaneous recurrent abortion with excessive bleeding occurs in association with Factor XIII deficiency [97]. All standard coagulation tests are normal. Diagnosis of severe Factor XIII deficiency is made by the clot solubility test. Normal fibrin clots will not dissolve when incubated overnight in 5 mol/l urea solutions, whereas the unstable clots formed in the absence of Factor XIII will be dissolved.

Factor XIII has a half-life of 6 days to 2 weeks and only 5 per cent of normal Factor XIII levels are needed for effective haemostasis; therefore patients can be treated with FFP in doses of 5 ml/kg, which can be repeated every 3 weeks. Using this therapy, pregnancy has progressed safely to term in a woman who had previously suffered repeated abortions. Because of the high incidence of intracranial haemorrhage, replacement therapy should be recommended for all individuals who are known to have Factor XIII deficiency [97].

OTHER PLASMA FACTOR DISORDERS

Congenital deficiencies of Factors II, V, VII and X are extremely rare and the reader is referred to a more detailed review of hereditary coagulopathies in pregnancy for an account of their diagnosis and special management problems [37].

References

1 Acheson D. *Department of Health and Social Security Press Release* 87/5. HMSO, London, 1987.

2 Ahmed Y, Sullivan MH *et al*. Changes in platelet function in pregnancies complicated by fetal growth retardation. *European Journal of Obstetrics, Gynecology and Reproductive Biology* 1991; **42**: 171–5.

3 Alving BM & Comp PC. Recent advances in understanding clotting and evaluating patients with recurrent thrombosis. *American Journal of Obstetrics and Gynecology* 1992; **167**: 1184–91.

4 Amris CJ & Hilden M. Anticoagulant effects of Trasylol: *in vitro* and *in vivo* studies. *Annals of the New York Academy of Sciences* 1968; **146**: 612–94.

5 Asada Y, Sumiyoshi A *et al*. Immunohistochemistry of vascular lesion in TTP with special reference to factor VIII related antigen. *Thrombosis Research* 1985; **38**: 469–79.

6 Astedt B & Nilsson IM. Recurrent abruptio placentae treated with the fibrinolytic inhibitor tranexamic acid. *British Medical Journal* 1978; **i**: 756–7.

7 Aster RH. Plasma therapy for thrombotic thrombocytopenic purpura. *New England Journal of Medicine* 1985; **312**: 985–7.

8 Aster RH. 'Gestational' thrombocytopenia: A plea for conservative management. *New England Journal of Medicine* 1990; **323**: 264–6.

9 Auerbach AD, Adler B & Chaganti RSK. Prenatal and postnatal diagnosis and carrier detection of Fanconi anaemia by a cytogenetic method. *Paediatrics* 1981; **67**: 128–35.

10 Ayromlooi J. A new approach to the management of immunologic thrombocytopenia purpura in pregnancy. *American Journal of Obstetrics and Gynecology* 1978; **130**: 235–6.

11 Aznar J, Gilabert J, Estelles A, Fernandex MA, Villa P & Aznar JA. Evaluation of the soluble fibrin monomer complexes and other coagulation parameters in obstetric patients. *Thrombosis Research* 1982; **27**: 691–701.

12 Ballegeer VC, Mombaerts P *et al*. Fibrinolytic response to venous occlusion and fibrin fragment D-dimer levels in normal and complicated pregnancy. *Thrombosis and Haemostatis* 1987; **58**: 1030–2.

13 Ballegeer VC, Spitz B *et al*. Platelet activation and vascular damage in gestational hypertension. *American Journal of Obstetrics and Gynecology* 1992; **166**: 629–33.

14 Basu HK. Fibrinolysis and abruptio placentae. *Journal of Obstetrics and Gynaecology of the British Commonwealth* 1969; **76**: 481–96.

15 Beal DW & de Masi AD. Role of the platelet count in the management of the high-risk obstetric patient. *Journal of American Osteopathic Association* 1985; **85**: 252–5.

16 Bell WR. Hematologic abnormalities in pregnancy. *Medical Clinics of North America* 1977; **61**: 1–165.

17 Bell WR, Braine HG *et al*. Improved survival in thrombotic thrombocytopenic purpura-hemolytic uremic syndrome. *New England Journal of Medicine* 1991; **325**: 398–403.

18 Beller FK. Sepsis and coagulation. *Clinical Obstetrics and Gynecology* 1985; **28**: 46–52.

19 Beller FK & Uszynski M. Disseminated intravascular coagulation in pregnancy. *Clinical Obstetrics and Gynecology* 1974; **17**: 264–78.

20 Bertina RM, Briet E *et al*. Protein C deficiency and the risk of venous thrombosis. *New England Journal of Medicine* 1988; **318**: 930–1.

21 Bettaieb A, Fromont P *et al*. Presence of cross-reactive antibody between human immunodeficiency virus (HIV) and platelet glycoproteins in HIV-related immune thrombocytopenic purpura. *Blood* 1992; **80**: 162–9.

22 Bidstrup BP, Royston D *et al*. Reduction in blood loss and blood use after cardiopulmonary bypass with high dose aprotinin (Trasylol). *Journal of Thoracic and Cardiovascular Surgery* 1989; **97**: 364–72.

23 Blasczyk R, Westhoff U & Grosse-Wilde H. Soluble CD4, CD8, and HLA molecules in commercial immunoglobulin preparations. *Lancet* 1993; **341**: 789–90.

24 Bonnar J. Blood coagulation and fibrinolysis in obstetrics. *Clinics in Haematology* 1973; **2**: 213–33.

25 Bonnar J. Haemorrhagic disorders during pregnancy.

In: Hathaway WE & Bonnar J (eds), *Perinatal Coagulation Monographs in Neonatology*. Grune & Stratton, New York, 1978.

26 Bonnar J. Haemostasis and coagulation disorders in pregnancy. In: Bloom AL & Thomas DP (eds), *Haemostasis and Thrombosis* 2nd edn. Churchill Livingstone, Edinburgh, 1987: 570–84.

27 Bonnar J, Prentice CRM, McNicol GP & Douglas AS. Haemostatic mechanism in uterine circulation during placental separation. *British Medical Journal* 1971; **ii**: 564–7.

28 Booth NA, Reith A & Bennett B. A plasminogen activator inhibitor (PA1-2) circulates in two molecular forms during pregnancy. *Thrombosis and Haemostasis* 1988; **59**: 77–9.

29 Borok Z, Weitz J *et al*. Fibrinogen proteolysis and platelet α-granule release in pre-eclampsia/eclampsia. *Blood* 1984; **63**: 525–31.

30 Boulton FE & Letsky E. Obstetric haemorrhage: causes and management. In: *Clinics in Haematology* **14** (3). WB Saunders, London, 1985: 683–728.

31 Burkman RT, Bell WR, Atizenza MF & King TM. Coagulopathy with midtrimester induced abortion. Association with hyperosmolar urea administration. *American Journal of Obstetrics and Gynecology* 1977; **127**: 533–6.

32 Burroughs AK, Seong NG, Dojcinoov DM, Scheuer PJ & Sherlock SVP. Idiopathic acute fatty liver of pregnancy in 12 patients. *Quarterly Journal of Medicine* 1982; **51**: 481–97.

33 Burrows RF & Kelton JG. Incidentally detected thrombocytopenia in healthy mothers and their infants. *New England Journal of Medicine* 1988; **319**: 142.

34 Burrows RF & Kelton JG. Thrombocytopenia at delivery: A prospective survey of 6715 deliveries. *American Journal of Obstetrics and Gynecology* 1990; **162**: 731–4.

35 Burrows RF & Kelton JG. Thrombocytopenia during pregnancy. In: Greer IA, Turpie AG & Forbes CD (eds), *Haemostasis and Thrombosis in Obstetrics and Gynaecology*. Chapman & Hall, London, 1992: 407–29.

36 Burrows RF, Kelton JG. Fetal thrombocytopenia and its relation to maternal thrombocytopenia. *New England Journal of Medicine* 1993; **329**: 1463–6.

37 Caldwell DC, Williamson RA & Goldsmith JC. Hereditary coagulopathies in pregnancy. *Clinical Obstetrics and Gynecology* 1985; **28**: 53–72.

38 Carey LC, Cloutier CT & Lowery BD. The use of balanced electrolyte solution for resuscitation. In: Fox CL & Nahas GG (eds), *Body Fluid Replacement in the Surgical Patient*. Grune & Stratton, New York, 1970.

39 Carloss HW, McMillan R & Crosby WH. Management of pregnancy in women with immune thrombocytopenic purpura. *Journal of the American Medical Association* 1980; **244**: 2756–8.

40 Cash J. Blood replacement therapy. In: Bloom AL & Thomas DP (eds), *Haemostasis and Thrombosis*, 2nd edn. Churchill Livingstone, Edinburgh, 1987: 585–606.

41 Channing Rodgers RP & Levin J. A critical reappraisal of the bleeding time. In: *Seminars in Thrombosis and Hemostasis*. Thieme Medical Publishers, 1990: **16**: 1–19.

42 Chediak JR, Alban GM & Maxey B. Von Willebrand's disease and pregnancy: management during delivery and outcome of off-spring. *American Journal of Obstetrics and Gynecology* 1986; **155**: 618–24.

43 Chung AF & Merkatz IR. Survival following amniotic fluid embolism with early heparinisation. *Obstetrics and Gynecology* 1973; **42**: 809–14.

44 Cines DB, Dusak B, Tomaski A, Mennuti M & Schreiber AD. Immune thrombocytopenic purpura and pregnancy. *New England Journal of Medicine* 1982; **306**: 826–31.

45 Clark SL, Pavlova Z, Greenspoon J, Hortenstein J & Phelan JP. Squamous cells in the maternal pulmonary circulation. *American Journal of Obstetrics and Gynecology* 1986; **154**: 104–6.

46 Clarkson AR, Sage RE & Lawrence JR. Consumption coagulopathy and acute renal failure due to Gram negative septicaemia after abortion. Complete recovery with heparin therapy. *Annals of Internal Medicine* 1969; **70**: 1191–9.

47 Cohen E & Ballard CA. Consumptive coagulopathy associated with intra-amniotic saline instillation and the effect of intravenous oxytocin. *Obstetrics and Gynecology* 1974; **43**: 300–3.

48 Coller BS, Hultin MB, Homer LW, Miller F, Dobbs JV, Dosik MH & Berger ER. Normal pregnancy in a patient with a prior post-partum Factor VIII inhibitor: With observations on pathogenesis and prognosis. *Blood* 1981; **58**: 619–24.

49 Collier CB & Birrell WRS. Chronic ectopic pregnancy complicated by shock and disseminated intravascular coagulation. *Anaesthesia in Intensive Care* 1983; **11**: 246–8.

50 Colvin BT. Thrombocytopenia. In: Letsky EA (ed), *Haematological Disorders in Pregnancy, Clinics in Haematology* **14**, WB Saunders, London, 1985: 661–81.

51 Comp PC, Thurnau GR, Welsh J & Esmon CT. Functional and immunologic Protein S levels are decreased during pregnancy. *Blood* 1986; **68**: 881–5.

52 Constantine G & Menor V. Coagulation studies in cases of intrauterine death: overkill? *British Medical Journal* 1987; **294**: 678.

53 Conti M, Mari D, Conti E, Muggiasca ML & Mannuci PM. Pregnancy in women with different types of von Willebrand disease. *Obstetrics and Gynecology* 1986; **68**: 282–5.

54 Costello C. Haematological abnormalities in human immunodeficiency virus (HIV) disease. *Journal of Clinical Pathology* 1988; **41**: 711–15.

55 Creasy GW & Morgan J. Haemolytic uremic syndrome after ectopic pregnancy: post ectopic nephrosclerosis. *Obstetrics ad Gynecology* 1987; **69**: 448–9.

56 Daffos F, Forestier F *et al*. Prenatal diagnosis and management of bleeding disorders with fetal blood sampling. *American Journal of Obstetrics and Gynecology* 1988; **158**: 939–46.
57 Davis G. Midtrimester abortion. Late dilation and evacuation and DIC. *Lancet* 1972; **ii**: 1026.
58 Davison JM, Sheills EA *et al*. Metabolic clearance of vasopressin and an analogue resistant to vasopressinase in human pregnancy. *American Journal of Physiology* 1993; **264**: F348–53.
59 Department of Health. *Report on Confidential Enquiries into Maternal Deaths in the United Kingdom 1985–1987*. HMSO, London, 1991: 37–45.
60 Department of Health. Report on Confidential Enquiries into Maternal Deaths in the United Kingdom 1988–1990. HMSO, London, 1994: 34–42.
61 Department of Health and Social Security. *Report on Health and Social Subjects 26: Report on Confidential Enquiries into Maternal Deaths in England and Wales 1976–78*. HMSO, London, 1982.
62 Doenicke A, Grote B & Lorenz W. Blood and blood substitutes in management of the injured patient. *British Journal of Anaesthesia* 1977: **49**: 681–8.
63 Dwyer JM. Manipulating the immune system with immune globulin. *New England Journal of Medicine* 1992; **326**: 107–16.
64 Edgar W, McKillop C & Howie PW. Composition of soluble fibrin complexes in pre-eclampsia. *Thrombosis Research* 1977; **10**: 567–74.
65 Estelles A, Gilabert J *et al*. Fibrinolysis in pre-eclampsia. *Fibrinolysis* 1987; **1**: 209–14.
66 Evans RS, Takahashi K *et al*. Primary thrombocytopenic purpura and acquired hemolytic anemia: evidence for a common etiology. *Archives of Internal Medicine* 1951; **87**: 48–65.
67 Fay RA, Hughes AO & Farron NT. Platelets in pregnancy: hyperdestruction in pregnancy. *Obstetrics and Gynecology* 1983; **61**: 238–40.
68 Feinstein DI. Diagnosis and management of disseminated intravascular coagulation: the role of heparin therapy. *Blood* 1982; **60**: 284–7.
69 Fenton V, Saunders K & Cavill I. The platelet count in pregnancy. *Journal of Clinical Pathology* 1977; **30**: 68–9.
70 Forbes CD & Greer IA. Physiology of haemostasis and the effect of pregnancy. In: Greer IA, Turpie AGG & Forbes CD (eds), *Haemostasis and Thrombosis in Obstetrics and Gynaecology*. Chapman & Hall, London, 1992: 1–25.
71 Forsyth KD, Simpson AC *et al*. Neutrophil mediated endothelial injury in HUS. *Lancet* 1989; **2**: 411–14.
72 Fournie A, Monrozies M, Pontonnier G, Boneu B & Bierne R. Factor VIII complex in normal pregnancy, pre-eclampsia and fetal growth retardation. *British Journal of Obstetrics and Gynaecology* 1981; **88**: 250–4.
73 Freeman M. Fatal reaction to haemaccel. *Anaesthesia* 1979; **34**: 341–3.
74 Gilabert J, Aznar J, Parilla J, Reganon E, Vila V & Estelles A. Alteration in the coagulation and fibrinolysis system in pregnancy, labour and puerperium, with special reference to a possible transitory state of intravascular coagulation during labour. *Thrombosis and Haemostasis* 1978, **40**: 387–96.
75 Gilabert J, Estelles A, Aznar J & Galbis M. Abruptio placentae and disseminated intravascular coagulation. *Acta Obstetrica et Gynecologica Scandinavica* 1985; **64**: 35–9.
76 Goodlin RC. Acute fatty liver of pregnancy. *Acta Obstetrica et Gynaecologica Scandinavica* 1984; **63**: 379–80.
77 Graeff H, Ernst E & Bocaz JA. Evaluation of hypercoagulability in septic abortion. *Haemostasis* 1976; **5**: 285–94.
78 Grundy MFB & Craven ER. Consumption coagulopathy after intra-amniotic urea. *British Medical Journal* 1976; **ii**: 677–8.
79 Hafter R & Graeff H. Molecular aspects of defibrination in a reptilase treated case of 'dead fetus syndrome'. *Thrombosis Research* 1975; **7**: 391–9.
80 Hart D, Dunetz C *et al*. An epidemic of maternal thrombocytopenia associated with elevated antiplatelet antibody: platelet count and antiplatelet antibody in 116 consecutive pregnancies: relationship to neonatal platelet count. *American Journal of Obstetrics and Gynecology* 1986; **154**: 878–83.
81 Harrington WJ. Are platelet-antibody tests worthwhile? *New England Journal of Medicine* 1987; **316**: 211–12.
82 Harrington WJ, Sprague CC *et al*. Immunologic mechanisms in idiopathic and neonatal thrombocytopenic purpura. *Annals of Internal Medicine* 1953; **38**: 433–69.
83 Hauser CJ, Shoemaker WC, Turpin I & Goldberg SJ. Oxygen transport responses to colloids and crystalloids in critically ill surgical patients. *Surgica Gynecologica Obstetrica* 1980; **159**: 181–6.
84 Hegde UM. Immune thrombocytopenia in pregnancy and the newborn. *British Journal of Obstetrics and Gynaecology* 1985; **92**: 657–9.
85 Hegde UM. Immune thrombocytopenia in pregnancy and the newborn: a review. *Journal of Infection* 1987; **15**: 55–8.
86 Hellgren M & Blomback M. Blood coagulation and fibrinolysis in pregnancy, during delivery and in the puerperium. *Gynecologic Obstetric Investigation* 1981; **12**: 141–54.
87 Hellgren M, Hagnevik K, Robbe H, Bjork O, Blomback M & Eklund J. Severe acquired antithrombin III deficiency in relation to hepatic and renal insufficiency and intrauterine fetal death in late pregnancy. *Gynecologic Obstetric Investigation* 1983; **16**: 107–8.
88 Herbert WNP. Complications of the immediate puerperium. *Clinical Obstetrics and Gynecology* 1982; **25**: 219–32.
89 Hodgkinson CR, Thompson RJ & Hodari AA. Dead fetus syndrome. *Clinics in Obstetrics and Gynaecology*

1964; **7**: 349–58.

90 Holmberg L & Nilsson IM. Von Willebrand disease. In: Ruggeri AM (ed), *Coagulation Disorders Clinics in Haematology*, **14**. WB Saunders, London, 1985: 461–88.

91 How HY, Bergmann F *et al*. Quantitative and qualitative platelet abnormalities during pregnancy. *American Journal of Obstetrics and Gynecology* 1991; **164**: 92–8.

92 Hughes GRV. Systemic lupus erythematosus. In: Hughes GRV (ed), *Connective Tissue Diseases*, 3rd edn. Blackwell Scientific Publications, Oxford, 1987: 3–71.

93 Jones P. Developments and problems in the management of haemophilia. *Seminars in Haematology* 1977; **14**: 375–90.

94 Kaplan C, Daffos F *et al*. Fetal platelet counts in thrombocytopenic pregnancy. *Lancet* 1991; **336**: 979–82.

95 Kelton JC. Management of the pregnant patient with idiopathic thrombocytopenic purpura. *Annals of Internal Medicine* 1983; **99**: 796–800.

96 Kessler I, Lancet M *et al*. The obstetrical management of patients with immunologic thrombocytopenic purpura. *International Journal of Gynecology and Obstetrics* 1982; **20**: 23–8.

97 Kitchens CS & Newcomb TF. Factor XIII. *Medicine* 1979; **658**: 413–29.

98 Lammle B & Griffin JH. Formation of the fibrin clot: The balance of procoagulant and inhibitory factors. In: Ruggeri ZM (ed), *Coagulation Disorders. Clinics in Haematology*, **14**. WB Saunders, London, 1985: 281–342.

99 Laursen B, Frost L, Mortensen JZ, Hansen KB & Paulsen SM. Acute fatty liver of pregnancy with complicating disseminated intravascular coagulation. *Acta Obstetrica et Gynecologica Scandinavica* 1983; **62**: 403–7.

100 Laursen B, Mortensen JZ, Frost L & Hansen KB. Disseminated intravascular coagulation in hepatic failure treated with antithrombin III. *Thrombosis Research* 1981; **22**: 701–4.

101 Leduc L, Wheeler JM *et al*. Coagulation profile in severe pre-eclampsia. *Obstetrics and Gynecology* 1992; **79**: 14–18.

102 Letsky EA. Coagulation problems during pregnancy. *Current Reviews in Obstetrics and Gynaecology* 1985; **10**.

103 Letsky EA. Haemostasis and epidural anaesthesia. *International Journal of Obstetrics and Anesthesia* 1991; **1**: 51–4.

104 Letsky EA. Mechanisms of coagulation and the changes induced by pregnancy. *Current Obstetrics and Gynaecology* 1991; **1**: 203–9.

105 Letsky EA. Management of massive haemorrhage — the haematologists role. In: Patel N (ed), *Maternal Mortality — The Way Forward*. Royal College of Obstetrics and Gynaecologists, London, 1992: 63–71.

106 Levin J. Disorders of blood coagulation and platelets. In: Barrow GN & Ferris TF (eds), *Medical Complications During Pregnancy*, 2nd edn. WB Saunders, London, 1982: 70–3.

107 Levine AB & Berkowitz RL. Neonatal alloimmune thrombocytopenia. *Seminars in Perinatology* 1991; **15**: 35–40.

108 Lewis PJ. The role of prostacyclin in pre-eclampsia. *British Journal of Hospital Medicine* 1982; **62**: 1048–52.

109 Lewis PJ, Boylan P, Friedman LA, Hensman CN & Downing I. Prostacyclin in pregnancy. *British Medical Journal* 1980; **280**: 1581–2.

110 Liebman HA, McGehee WG, Patch MJ & Feinstein DI. Severe depression of anti-thrombin III associated with disseminated intravascular coagulation in women with fatty liver of pregnancy. *Annals of Internal Medicine* 1983; **98**: 330–3.

111 Lin KC, Chou TC *et al*. The role of aggregation of platelets in pregnancy-induced hypertension: a comprehensive and longitudinal study. *International Journal of Cardiology* 1991; **33**: 125–31.

112 Lind SE. The bleeding time does not predict surgical bleeding. *Blood* 1991; **77**: 2547–52.

113 Linkler CA. Congenital disorders of haemostasis. In: Laros RK (ed), *Blood Disorders in Pregnancy*. Lea & Febiger, Philadelphia, 1986: 160.

114 Lorenz W, Doenicke A *et al*. Histamine release in human subjects by modified gelatin (Haemaccel) and dextran: An explanation for anaphylactoid reactions observed under clinical conditions. *British Journal of Anaesthesia* 1976; **48**: 151–65.

115 Luscher JM & McMillan CW. Severe Factor VIII and IX deficiency in females. *American Journal of Medicine* 1978; **65**: 637.

116 Lynch L, Bussel JB, McFarland JG, Chitkara U & Berkowitz RL. Antenatal treatment of alloimmune thrombocytopenia. *Obstetrics and Gynecology* 1992; **8**: 67–71.

117 Machin SJ. Thrombotic thrombocytopenic purpura. *British Journal of Haematology* 1984; **56**: 191–7.

118 MacKenzie IZ, Sayers L *et al*. Coagulation changes during second trimester abortion induced by intra-amniotic prostaglandin E_{2+} and hypertonic solutions. *Lancet* 1975; **ii**: 1066–9.

119 Malm J, Laurell M & Dahlback B. Changes in the plasma levels of vitamin K-dependent proteins C and S and of C4b-binding protein during pregnancy and oral contraception. *British Journal of Haematology* 1988; **68**: 437–43.

120 Marengo-Rowe AJ, Murff G, Leveson JE & Cook J. Haemophilia-like disease associated with pregnancy. *Obstetrics and Gynecology* 1972; **40**: 56–64.

121 Marshall M & Bird T. *Blood Loss and Replacement*. Edward Arnold, London, 1983.

122 Martin JN, Morrison JC & Files JC. Autoimmune thrombocytopenia purpura: current concepts and recommended practices. *American Journal of Obstetrics and Gynecology* 1984; **150**: 86–96.

123 McGibbon DH. Dermatological purpura. In: Ingram GIC, Brozovic M & Slater NGP (eds), *Bleeding Dis-*

orders — Investigation and Management, 2nd edn. Blackwell Scientific Publications, Oxford, 1982: 220–42.
124 McMillan R. Chronic idiopathic thrombocytopenic purpura. *New England Journal of Medicine* 1981; **304**: 1135–47.
125 Milaskiewicz RM, Holdcroft A & Letsky EA. Epidural anaesthesia and von Willebrand's disease. *Anaesthesia* 1990; **45**: 462–4.
126 Mibashan RS & Millar DA. Fetal haemophilia and allied bleeding disorders. *British Medical Bulletin* 1983; **39**: 392–8.
127 Mibashan RS, Rodeck CH *et al*. Dual diagnosis of prenatal haemophilia A by measurement of fetal Factor VIIIC and VIIIC antigen (VIIICAg). *Lancet* 1980; **ii**: 994–7.
128 Moake JL. TTP — Desperation, empiricism, progress. *New England Journal of Medicine* 1991; **325**: 426–8.
129 Moake JL, Rudy CK *et al*. Unusually large plasma factor VIII: vWF multimers in chronic relapsing TTP. *New England Journal of Medicine* 1982; **307**: 1432–5.
130 Moise KJ, Carpenter RJ *et al*. Percutaneous umbilical cord sampling in the evaluation of fetal platelet counts in pregnant patients with autoimmune thrombocytopenia purpura. *Obstetrics and Gynecology* 1988; **72**: 346–50.
131 Moncada MD & Vane JR. Arachidonic acid metabolites and the interactions between platelets and blood-vessel walls. *New England Journal of Medicine* 1979; **300**: 1142–7.
132 Moore JC, Murphy WG & Kelton JG. Calpain proteolysis of vWF enhances its binding to platelet membrane glycoprotein IIbIIIa: an explanation for platelet aggregation in TTP. *British Journal of Haematology* 1990; **74**: 457–64.
133 Morgan M. Amniotic fluid embolism. *Anaesthesia* 1979; **34**: 20–32.
134 Morgenstern GR, Measday B & Hegde UM. Autoimmune thrombocytopenia in pregnancy. New approach to management. *British Medical Journal* 1983; **287**: 584.
135 Moss G. An argument in favour of electrolyte solutions for early resuscitation. *Surgical Clinics in North America* 1972; **52**: 3–17.
136 Mueller-Ekhardt C, Kayser W *et al*. The clinical significance of platelet-associated IgG: a study on 298 patients with various disorders. *British Journal of Haematology* 1980; **46**: 123–31.
137 Murray JM & Harris RE. The management of the pregnant patient with idiopathic thrombocytopenic purpura. *American Journal of Obstetrics and Gynecology* 1976; **126**: 449–51.
138 Naumann RO & Weinstein L. Disseminated intravascular coagulation — the clinician's dilemma. *Obstetrical and Gynecological Survey* 1985; **40**: 487–92.
139 Ness PM, Budzynski AZ *et al*. Congenital hypofibrinogenemia and recurrent placental abruption. *Obstetrics and Gynecology* 1983; **61**: 519–23.
140 Newland AC, Boots MA & Patterson KG. Intravenous IgG for autoimmune thrombocytopenia in pregnancy. *New England Journal of Medicine* 1984; **310**: 261–2.
141 Nicolaides KH, Rodeck CH & Mibashan RS. Obstetric management and diagnosis of haematological disease in the fetus. In: Letsky E (ed), *Haematological Disorders in Pregnancy Clinics in Haematology* **14**. WB Saunders, London, 1985: 775–804.
142 Nicolini U, Tannirandorn Y *et al*. Continuing controversy in alloimmune thrombocytopenia; fetal hypergammaglobulinemia fails to prevent thrombocytopenia. *American Journal of Obstetrics and Gynecology* 1990; **163**: 1144–6.
143 O'Brien JR. An acquired coagulation defect in a woman. *Journal of Clinical Pathology* 1954; **7**: 22–5.
144 O'Brien WF, Saba HI, Knuppel RA, Scerbo JC & Cohen GR. Alterations in platelet concentration and aggregation in normal pregnancy and pre-eclampsia. *American Journal of Obstetrics and Gynecology* 1986; **155**: 486–90.
145 Pappas C. Placental transfer of immunoglobulins in immune thrombocytopenic purpura. *Lancet* 1986; **1**: 389.
146 Page Y, Tardy B *et al*. Thrombotic thrombocytopenic purpura related to ticlopidine. *Lancet* 1991; **337**: 774–6.
147 Peaceman AM, Katz AR & Laville M. Bernard–Soulier syndrome complicating pregnancy. A case report. *Obstetrics and Gynecology* 1989; **73**: 457–9.
148 Pembury ME & Mibashan RS. Prenatal diagnosis of haemophilia A. In: Seghatchian MJ & Savidge VF (eds), *Factor VIII Von Willebrand Factor*. CRC Press, Boca Raton Florida, 1987.
149 Phillips LP. Transfusion support in acquired coagulation disorders. *Clinics in Haematology* 1984; **13**: 137–50.
150 Pillai M. Platelets and pregnancy. *British Journal of Obstetrics and Gynaecology* 1993; **100**: 201–4.
151 Pinette MG, Vintzileos AM & Ingardia CJ. Thrombotic thrombocytopenia purpura as a cause of thrombocytopenia in pregnancy: Literature review. *American Journal of Perinatology* 1989; **6**: 55–7.
152 Pritchard JA. Fetal death *in utero*. *Obstetrics and Gynecology* 1959; **14**: 573–80.
153 Pritchard JA. Haematological problems associated with delivery, placental abruption, retained dead fetus and amniotic fluid embolism. *Clinics in Haematology* 1973; **2**: 563–80.
154 Pritchard JA, Cunningham FG *et al*. On reducing the frequency of severe abruptio placentae. *American Journal of Obstetrics and Gynecology* 1991; **165**: 1345–51.
155 Rakoczi I, Tallian F, Bagdan YS & Gati I. Platelet lifespan in normal pregnancy and pre-eclampsia as determined by a non-radioisotope technique. *Thrombosis Research* 1979; **15**: 553–6.
156 Redman CWG. Coagulation problems in human pregnancy. *Postgraduate Medical Journal* 1979; **55**:

367–71.
157 Redman CWG, Bonnar J & Bellin C. Early platelet consumption in pre-eclampsia. *British Medical Journal* 1978; **1**: 467–9.
158 Redman CWG, Denson KW *et al*. Factor VIII consumption in pre-eclampsia. *Lancet* 1977; **ii**: 1249–59.
159 Reece EA, Fox HE & Rapoport F. Factor VII inhibitor: a cause of severe postpartum haemorrhage. *American Journal of Obstetrics and Gynecology* 1982; **144**: 985–7.
160 Resnik R, Swartz WH, Plumer MH, Bernirske K & Stratthaus ME. Amniotic fluid embolism with survival. *Obstetrics and Gynecology* 1976; **47**: 395–8.
161 Richter AW & Hedin HI. Dextran hypersensitivity. *Immunology Today* 1982; **3**: 132–8.
162 Romero R & Duffy TP. Platelet disorders in pregnancy. *Clinics in Perinatology* 1980; **7**: 327–48.
163 Romero R, Copel JA & Hobbins JC. Intrauterine fetal demise and hemostatic failure: the fetal death syndrome. *Clinical Obstetrics and Gynecology* 1985; **28**: 24–31.
164 Romero R, Duffy T, Berkowitz RL, Change E & Hobbins JC. Prolongation of a preterm pregnancy complicated by death of a single twin *in utero* and disseminated intravascular coagulation. *New England Journal of Medicine* 1986; **310**: 772–4.
165 Romero R, Mazor M *et al*. Clinical significance, prevalence and natural history of thrombocytopenia in pregnancy-induced hypertension. *American Journal of Perinatology* 1989; **6**: 32–8.
166 Salem HH. The natural anticoagulants. In: Chesterman CN (ed), *Thrombosis and The Vessel Wall. Clinics in Haematology* **15**. WB Saunders, London, 1986: 371–91.
167 Samuels P, Bussel JB *et al*. Estimation of the risk of thrombocytopenia in the offspring of pregnant women with presumed immune thrombocytopenic purpura. *New England Journal of Medicine* 1990; **323**: 229–35.
168 Savage W. Abortion: methods and sequelae. *British Journal of Hospital Medicine* 1982; **27**: 364–84.
169 Scioscia AL, Grannum PAT *et al*. The use of percutaneous umbilical blood sampling in immune thrombocytopenia purpura. *American Journal of Obstetrics and Gynecology* 1988; **159**: 1066–8.
170 Scott JR, Cruickshank DP, Kochenou RMD, Pitkin RM & Warenski JC. Fetal platelet counts in the obstetric management of immunologic thrombocytopenia purpura. *American Journal of Obstetrics and Gynecology* 1980; **136**: 495–9.
171 Seligsohn U, Berger A *et al*. Homozygous protein C deficiency manifested by massive venous thrombosis in the newborn. *New England Journal of Medicine* 1984; **310**: 559–62.
172 Sharp AA. Diagnosis and management of disseminated intra-vascular coagulation. *British Medical Bulletin* 1977; **33**: 265–72.
173 Sheppard BL & Bonnar J. The ultrastructure of the arterial supply of the human placenta in early and late pregnancy. *Journal of Obstetrics and Gynaecology of the British Commonwealth* 1974; **81**: 497–511.
174 Sher G. Pathogenesis and management of uterine inertia complicating abruptio placentae with consumption coagulopathy. *American Journal of Obstetrics and Gynecology* 1977; **129**: 164–70.
175 Sher G & Statland BE. Abruptio placentae with coagulopathy: A rational basis for management. *Clinical Obstetrics and Gynecology* 1985; **28**: 15–23.
176 Sill PR, Lind T & Walker W. Platelet values during normal pregnancy. *British Journal of Obstetrics and Gynaecology* 1985; **92**: 480–3.
177 Skjodt P. Amniotic fluid embolism — a case investigated by coagulation and fibrinolysis studies. *Acta Obstetrica et Gynecologica Scandinavica* 1965; **44**: 437–57.
178 Spencer JA, Smith MJ *et al*. Influence of pre-eclampsia on concentrations of haemostatic factors in mothers and infants. *Archives of Diseases in Children* 1983; **58**: 739–41.
179 Spivak JL, Sprangler DB & Bell WR. Defibrination after intra-amniotic injection of hypertonic saline. *New England Journal of Medicine* 1972; **287**: 321–3.
180 Stander RW, Flessa HC *et al*. Changes in maternal coagulation factors after intraamniotic injection of hypertonic saline. *Obstetrics and Gynecology* 1971; **37**: 321–3.
181 Steichele DF & Herschlein HJ. Intravascular coagulation in bacterial shock. Consumption coagulopathy and fibrinolysis after febrile abortion. *Medizinische Welt* 1968; **1**: 24–30.
182 Stirling Y, Woolf L, North WRS, Seghatchian MJ & Meade TW. Haemostasis and normal pregnancy. *Thrombosis and Haemostasis* 1984; **52**: 176.
183 Svensson PS & Dahlbäck B. Resistance to activated Protein C as a basis for venous thrombosis. *New England Journal of Medicine* 1994; **330**: 517–22.
184 Talbert IM & Blatt PM. Disseminated intravascular coagulation in obstetrics. *Clinics in Obstetrics and Gynecology* 1979; **22**: 889–900.
185 Tchernia G. Immune thrombocytopenic purpura and pregnancy. *Current Studies in Hematology and Blood Transfusion* 1988; **55**: 81–9.
186 Tchernia G, Dreyfus M, Laurian Y, Derycke M, Merica C & Kerbrat G. Management of immune thrombocytopenia in pregnancy: Response of infusions of immunoglobulins. *American Journal of Obstetrics and Gynecology* 1984; **148**: 225–6.
187 Thornton JG, Molloy BJ *et al*. A prospective study of haemostatic tests at 28 weeks gestation as predictors of pre-eclampsia and growth retardation. *Thrombosis and Haemostasis* 1989; **61**: 243–5.
188 Thragarajah S, Wheby MS, Jarn R, May HV, Bourgeois J & Kitchin JD. Disseminated intravascular coagulation in pregnancy. The role of heparin therapy. *Journal of Reproductive Medicine* 1981; **26**: 17–24.
189 Tuck CS. Amniotic fluid embolus. *Proceedings of the Royal Society of Medicine* 1972; **65**: 94–5.

190 Van Leeuwen EF, Helmerhorst FM, Engelfriet CP & Von Dem Borne AEG. Maternal autoimmune thrombocytopenia and the newborn. *British Medical Journal* 1981; **283**: 104.

191 Van Leeuwen EF, Van der Ven JTM *et al*. Specificity of autoantibodies in autoimmune thrombocytopenia. *Blood* 1982; **59**: 23–6.

192 Van Royen EA. *Haemostasis in Human Pregnancy and Delivery*. MD Thesis, University of Amsterdam, 1974.

193 Varner MW, Meehan RT, Syrop CH, Strottmann MP & Goplerud CP. Pregnancy in patients with systemic lupus erythematosus. *American Journal of Obstetrics and Gynecology* 1983; **145**: 1025–37.

194 Virgilio RWK, Rice CL *et al*. Crystalloid versus colloid resuscitation: is one better? *Surgery* 1979; **85**: 129–39.

195 Voke J & Letsky E. Pregnancy and antibody to Factor VIII. *Journal of Clinical Pathology* 1977; **30**: 928–32.

196 Walker ID. Management of thrombophilia in pregnancy. *Blood Review* 1991; **5**: 227–33.

197 Wallenberg HCS & Van Kessel PH. Platelet lifespan in normal pregnancy as determined by a non-radioisotopic technique. *British Journal of Obstetrics and Gynaecology* 1978; **85**: 33–6.

198 Wallmo L, Karlsonn K & Teger-Nilsson A-C. Fibrinopeptide and intravascular coagulation in normotensive and hypertensive pregnancy and parturition. *Acta Obstetricia et Gynecologica Scandinavica* 1984; **63**; 637–40.

199 Warwick R, Hutton RA, Goff L, Letsky E & Heard M. Changes in Protein C and free Protein S during pregnancy and following hysterectomy. *Journal of Royal Society of Medicine* 1989; **82**: 591–4.

200 Weiner CP. Thrombotic microangiopathy in pregnancy and the postpartum period. *Seminars in Haematology* 1987; **2**: 119–29.

201 Weiner CP, Kwaan HC *et al*. Antithrombin III activity in women with hypertension during pregnancy. *Obstetrics and Gynecology* 1985; **65**: 301–6.

202 Whigham KAE, Howie PW, Shaf MM & Prentice CRM. Factor VIII related antigen and coagulant activity in intrauterine growth retardation. *Thrombosis Research* 1979; **16**: 629–38.

203 Woods VL Jr & McMillan R. Platelet autoantigens in chronic ITP. *British Journal of Haematology* 1984; **57**: 1–4.

204 Zeeman GG, Dekker GA, vanGeisn HP & Krayenbrink AA Endothelial function in normal and pre-eclamptic pregnancy: a hypothesis. *European Journal of Obstetrics, Gynecology and Reproductive Biology* 1992; **43**: 113–22.

Further reading

Atlas M, Barkai G, Menczer J, Houlu N & Lieberman P. Thrombotic thrombocytopenic purpura in pregnancy. *British Journal of Obstetrics and Gynaecology* 1982; **89**: 476–9.

Bukowski RM. Thrombotic thrombocytopenic purpura. *Progress in Haematology and Thrombosis* 1982; **6**: 287–337.

Bussel JB, Berkowitz RL, McFarland JG, Lynch L & Chitkara U. Antenatal treatment of neonatal alloimmune thrombocytopenia *New England Journal of Medicine* 1988; **319**: 1374–8.

Caires D, Arocha-Pinango CL, Rodriguez S & Linares J. Factor VIII R:Ag/Factor VIII:C and their ratios in obstetrical cases. *Acta Obstetrica et Gynecologica Scandinavica* 1984; **63**: 411–16.

Daffos F, Forest ER *et al*. Prenatal treatment of allo-immune thrombocytopenia. *Lancet* 1984; **ii**: 632.

Davies GE. Thrombotic thrombocytopenia in pregnancy with maternal survival. *British Journal of Obstetrics and Gynaecology* 1984; **91**: 396–8.

Davies SV, Murray JA, Gee H & Giles H McC. Transplacental effect of high-dose immunoglobulin in idiopathic thrombocytopenia (ITP). *Lancet* 1986; **i**: 1098–9.

de Swiet M. Some rare medical complications of pregnancy. *British Medical Journal* 1985; **290**: 2–4.

De Vries LS, Connell J *et al*. Recurrent intracranial haemorrhages *in utero* in an infant with allo-immune thrombocytopenia. *British Journal of Obstetrics and Gynaecology* 1988; **95**: 299–302.

Dolyniuk M, Oriel E, Vania H, Karlman R & Tomich P. Rapid diagnosis of amniotic fluid embolism. *Obstetrics and Gynecology* 1983; **61**: 28S–30S.

Epstein RD, Longer EL & Conbey JT. Congenital thrombocytopenic purpura. Purpura haemorrhage in pregnancy and the newborn. *American Journal of Medicine* 1950; **9**: 44–56.

Firschein SI, Hoyer LW *et al*. Prenatal diagnosis of classic haemophilia. *New England Journal of Medicine* 1979; **300**: 937–41.

Giannelli F, Choo KH, Rees DJG, Boyd Y, Rizza CR & Brownlee DG. Gene deletions in patients with haemophilia B and antifactor IX antibodies. *Nature* 1983; **303**: 181–2.

Ginsburg D, Handin RI *et al*. Human Von Willebrand factor (VWF) isolation and complementary DNA (CDNA) clones and chromosome localisation. *Science* 1985; **228**: 1401–6.

Gitschier J, Drayna D, Tuddenham EGD, White RC & Lawn RM. Genetic mapping and diagnosis of haemophilia A achieved through a polymorphism in the Factor VIII gene. *Nature* 1984; **314**: 738–40.

Graham JB, Barrow ES, Flyer P, Dawson DN & Elston RC. Identifying carriers of mild haemophilia. *British Journal of Haematology* 1980; **44**: 671–8.

Graham JB, Rizza CR *et al*. Carrier detection in haemophilia A: a cooperative international study I. The carrier phenotype. *Blood* 1986; **67**: 1444–9.

Hegde UM, Bowes A, Powell DK & Joyner MV. Detection of platelet bound and serum antibodies in thrombocytopenia by enzyme linked assay. *Vox Sanguinis* 1981; **41**: 306–12.

Hegde UM, Gordon-Smith EC & Worrlledge SM. Platelet

antibodies in thrombocytopenic patients. *British Journal of Haematology* 1977; **56**: 191–7.

Holmberg L, Bjorn C *et al*. Prenatal diagnosis of haemophilia β by an immunoradiometric assay of Factor IX. *Blood* 1980; **56**: 397–401.

Ingram GIC, Brozović M & Slater NGP. Thrombotic thrombocytopenic purpura and the haemolytic uraemic syndrome. In: *Bleeding Disorders — Investigation and Management*, 3rd edn. Blackwell Scientific Publications, Oxford, 1982: 131–5.

Kelton JC, Inwood MJ *et al*. The prenatal prediction of thrombocytopenia in mothers with clinically diagnosed immune thrombocytopenia. *American Journal of Obstetrics and Gynecology* 1982; **144**: 449–54.

Kelton JC, Blanchette VS & William EW. Neonatal thrombocytopenia due to passive immunisation. Prenatal diagnosis and distinction between maternal platelet alloantibodies and autoantibodies. *New England Journal of Medicine* 1980; **302**: 1401–3.

Kouri YH, Basch RS & Karpatkin S. B-cell subsets and platelet counts in HIV-1 seropositive subjects. *Lancet* 1992; **339**: 1445–6.

Lavery JP, Koontz WL, Liu YK & Howell R. Immunologic thrombocytopenia in pregnancy: use of antenatal immunoglobulin therapy: Case report and review. *Obstetrics and Gynecology* 1985; **66**: S41–3.

Lazarchick J & Hoyer LW. Immunoradiometric measurement of the Factor VIII pro-coagulant antigen. *Journal of Clinical Investigation* 1978; **62**: 1048–52.

Lian EC, Harkness DR, Byrnes JJ, Wallach H & Nunez R. Presence of a platelet aggregating factor in the plasma of patients with thrombotic thrombocytopenic purpura (TTP) and its inhibition by normal plasma. *Blood* 1979; **53**: 333–8.

Machin SJ, Defrey NG, Vermylen J & Willoughby MLN. Prostacyclin deficiency in thrombotic thrombocytopenic purpura (TTP) and the haemolytic uraemic syndrome (HUS). *British Journal of Haematology* 1981; **49**: 141–2.

Mant MJ & King EG. Severe acute disseminated intravascular coagulation. A reappraisal of its pathophysiology, clinical significance and therapy, based on 47 patients. *American Journal of Medicine* 1979; **67**: 557–63.

Moake JL, Byrnes JJ *et al*. Effects of fresh-frozen plasma and its cryosupernatant fraction on von Willebrand factor multimeric forms in chronic relapsing thrombotic thrombocytopenic purpura. *Blood* 1985; **65**: 1232–6.

Nicolaides KH, Soothill PW, Rodeck CH & Campbell S. Ultrasound-guided sampling of umbilical cord and placental blood to assess fetal well-being. *Lancet* 1986; **i**: 1065–7.

Peake IR & Bloom AL. Immunoradiometric measurement of procoagulation Factor VIII antigen in plasma and serum and its reduction in haemophilia. *Lancet* 1978; **i**: 473–5.

Peake IR, Lilleycrap DP *et al*. Report of a joint WHO/WFH meeting on the control of haemophilia: carrier detection and prenatal diagnosis. *Blood Coagulation and Fibrinolysis* 1993; **4**: 313–44.

Peake IR, Newcombe RG, Davies BL, Furlong RA, Ludlam CA & Bloom AL. Carrier detection in haemophilia A by immunological measurement of factor VIII related antigen (VIIIRAg) and factor VIII clotting antigen VIIICAg. *British Journal of Haematology* 1981; **48**: 651–60.

Pritchard JA & Brekken AL. Clinical and laboratory studies on severe abruptio placentae. *American Journal of Obstetrics and Gynecology* 1967; **57**: 681–95.

Remuzzi G, Misiani R *et al*. Haemolytic-uraemic syndrome. Deficiency of plasma factor(s) regulating prostacyclin activity? *Lancet* 1978; **ii**: 871–2.

Rock GA, Shumack KH *et al*. Canadian Apheresis Study Group. Comparison of plasma exchange with plasma infusion in the treatment of thrombotic thrombocytopenic purpura. *New England Journal of Medicine* 1991; **325**: 393–7.

Rodeck CH & Campbell S. Sampling pure fetal blood by fetoscopy in second trimester of pregnancy. *British Medical Journal* 1978; **11**: 728–30.

Rodeck CH & Morsmen J. First trimester chorion biopsy. *British Medical Bulletin* 1983; **39**: 338–42.

Shaper AG, Kear J, MacIntosh DM, Kyobe J & Njama D. The platelet count, platelet adhesiveness and aggregation and the mechanism of fibrinolytic inhibition in pregnancy and the puerperium. *Journal of Obstetrics and Gynaecology of the British Commonwealth* 1968; **75**: 433–41.

Smith BT & Torday JS. Steroid administration in pregnant women with autoimmune thrombocytopenia. *New England Journal of Medicine* 1982; **306**: 744–5.

Stratta P, Canavese CK, Bussolino P, Mansueto MG, Gagliardi G & Vercellone A. Haemolytic anaemic syndrome. *Lancet* 1983; **ii**: 424–5.

Suraínder SY, Bellar B, Choudry A, Chilis TJ & Rao S. Isoimmune thrombocytopenia: coordinated management of mother and infant. *Obstetrics and Gynecology* 1981; **57**: 124–8.

Terao T Oilne J *et al*. Pregnancy complication by idiopathic thrombocytopenic purpura. *Journal of Obstetrics and Gynecology* 1981; **2**: 1–10.

Territo M, Finkelstein J & Oh O. Management of autoimmune thrombocytopenia in pregnancy and the neonate. *Obstetrics and Gynecology* 1973; **41**: 579–82.

Tygart SG, McRoyan DK, Spinnato JA, McRoyan CJ & Kitay DZ. Longitudinal study of platelet indices during normal pregnancy. *American Journal of Obstetrics and Gynecology* 1986; **154**: 883.

Weatherall DJ. *The New Genetics and Clinical Practice*, 2nd edn. Oxford University Press, Oxford, 1985.

Webster J, Rees AJ, Lewis PJ & Hensby CN. Prostacyclin deficiency in haemolytic uraemic syndrome. *British Medical Journal* 1980; **281**: 271.

Zulneraitis EL, Young RSK & Krishanmoorthy KS. Intracranial haemorrhage *in utero* as a complication of isoimmune thrombocytopenia. *Journal of Pediatrics* 1979; **95**: 611–14.

4

Thromboembolism

Michael de Swiet

Incidence and significance, 116
Risk factors, 117
Clotting factors
Venous stasis
Bed rest
Operative delivery
Other factors
Diagnosis of thromboembolism, 119
Deep vein thrombosis
Pulmonary embolus
Treatment, 121
Acute phase
Chronic phase
Recurrent thromboembolism
Prophylaxis of thromboembolism, 129
Thrombophilia, 132
Antithrombin III deficiency
Protein C and S deficiencies
Septic pelvic thrombophlebitis, 134

In this chapter we will consider deep vein thrombosis and pulmonary embolus complicating pregnancy, and inherited abnormalities of the clotting and fibrinolytic systems such as antithrombin III deficiency. For other general reviews see de Swiet [67–69], Letsky and de Swiet [156] and Letsky [154].

The importance of pulmonary embolus is as a cause of maternal mortality. If the patient does not die, she usually recovers completely, although a few patients subsequently have symptomatic pulmonary hypertension and rather more than might be expected have abnormal lung function tests [218]. Deep vein thrombosis is important because it predisposes to pulmonary embolus. Also, only 22 per cent of patients with deep vein thrombosis are symptom free when followed up 11 years after having had deep vein thrombosis and 4 per cent even have skin ulceration [22].

Cerebral vein thrombosis is described in Chapter 15 and systemic thromboembolism arising from mitral valve disease and artificial heart valves is considered in Chapter 5. See Chapter 8 for the association between lupus anticoagulant and thromboembolism and Chapter 3 for the physiology of the clotting system.

Incidence and significance

Pulmonary embolism together with hypertension is currently the most frequent cause of maternal mortality in the UK and is responsible for the deaths of about 9 women per year before or immediately after delivery (12 in every million maternities) [80]. We can be reasonably confident of these data because death from pulmonary embolus is relatively easy to diagnose. Also, 99 per cent of all maternal deaths in the UK were analysed in a recent report [79]. In addition pulmonary embolus was the second cause of maternal death in Massachusetts, USA between 1982 and 1985 (mortality rate 12 per million) [206]. However, pulmonary embolism and deep vein thrombosis are not easy to diagnose in non-fatal cases and particularly in pregnancy (see below). It is therefore difficult to obtain accurate data for the incidences of non-fatal deep vein thrombosis and pulmonary embolism.

It appears that pregnancy increases the risk of thromboembolism sixfold [205] and the overall incidence varies between 0.3 [234] and 1.2 per cent of all pregnancies [116] with between one-fifth and one-half occurring antenatally [118,143,234]. The incidence of pulmonary embolism in pregnancy is between 0.3 [96] and 1.2 per cent [240]. The incidence of deep vein thrombosis is between 0.5 and 0.7 per cent [2,23,96] and this increases to 1.4 per cent if superficial thrombophlebitis is included [1]. Lower incidences are found in later studies where in general the diagnosis has been made objectively (see below). Treffers *et al.* [234] have found that the incidence of post-partum (but not antenatal) thromboembolism is declining and during the period 1973–79 was half that in the period 1952–72. Changing patterns of obstetric care and changes in the population becoming pregnant (few elderly grandmultiparae) are likely causes.

Risk factors

Clotting factors (see also Chapter 3)

Any alteration in the balance between thrombosis due to activated clotting factors, and clot lysis due to fibrinolytic mechanisms and/or thrombin inhibitors, can precipitate blood clotting. During pregnancy, each of these systems is altered to change the balance towards clotting. After the first trimester, levels of Factors I (fibrinogen), II (prothrombin), VII, VIII, IX and X are increased [28,97] and a further increase in the levels of Factors V, VII and X occurs in the first few days after delivery, even in normal pregnancy [28]; this further postnatal rise could account for the extra risk of thromboembolism at this time. Yoshimura *et al.* [251] confirm these data by showing increased levels of fibrinopeptide A and thrombin–antithrombin III complexes (indicating increased blood clotting) at the time of placental separation; however, this effect is balanced by increased thrombolysis (raised tissue plasminogen activator and α_2 plasmin inhibitor–plasmin complexes) which starts during the first stage of labour.

Dalaker [61] has shown that Factor VII levels rise to about 250 per cent of non-pregnant values from 17 weeks' gestation due to the formation of phospholipid–Factor VII complex. This complex is possibly induced by the placenta, since its level falls very rapidly after delivery. He documented an increase of Factors II and X to 136 and 171 per cent respectively [61]. Weiner *et al.* [243] suggest that an extra 400 mg of fibrinogen are consumed each day at the end of normal pregnancy on the basis of elevated levels of fibrinopeptide A, the first peptide split from fibrinogen during thrombin-mediated fibrin formation. The effect of an increase in clotting factors is added to by a decrease in the activity of some components of the fibrinolytic system [97]. For example the globulin lysis time decreases in pregnancy [127] as does the level of tissue plasminogen activator [238]. But other fibrinolytic indices such as plasminogen α_2–antiplasmin increase [238]. On balance it seems likely that both thrombosis and fibrinolysis increase in pregnancy. Certainly both thrombosis and fibrinolysis are under endocrine control at a cellular level [100] and deep vein thrombosis has been reported in association with ovarian hyperstimulation [141]. However, although studies demonstrate an increased tendency of blood to clot in pregnancy it is difficult to define which patients are at risk of thrombosis on the basis of test of coagulation [66]. For example, one study of clotting factors estimated 6–12 months after delivery in 43 patients who had had thromboembolism in pregnancy, showed no excess clotting activity compared to controls and only a slight decrease in fibrinolysis [24].

Venous stasis

Although the overall circulation time is reduced by the hyperdynamic circulation of pregnancy, venous return from the lower limbs is reduced because the pregnant uterus obstructs the inferior vena cava [47,250]. A decrease in venous tone [93,170] may be another factor promoting venous stasis and thus increasing the risk of deep vein thrombosis. Since women are particularly at risk from venous thromboembolism in association with air travel [174,212] pregnant patients should be careful to keep mobile in any plane journey lasting >3 hours [174].

Bed rest

Venous stasis is the presumed mechanism whereby bed rest is associated with an increase in the risk of thromboembolism. This was noted in pregnancy by the Confidential Maternal Mortality reports [77] which also drew attention to the particular risk in patients with severe pre-eclamptic toxaemia who are first rested in bed and then delivered by caesarean section [78].

Operative delivery

The 1979–81 maternal mortality series [78] suggested

that the risk of fatal thromboembolism following caesarean section was markedly increased compared to that after vaginal delivery. In the 1976–78 series, there were nine deaths following caesarean section, compared to 22 following vaginal delivery. The overall caesarean section rate was likely to have been between 5 and 10 per cent; therefore the extra mortality risk associated with caesarean section was between four- and eightfold in the patients of the confidential series. Finnerty and MacKay [92] found that caesarean section increases the overall risk of thromboembolism to 0.66 in 100 deliveries compared to 0.26 in 100 deliveries for vaginal delivery. Hiilesma [119] showed a similar increase from 1.1 to 2.2 per cent. Bergqvist *et al.* [21] performed strain gauge plethysmography on 169 women following caesarean section and showed that the incidence of deep vein thrombosis was 1.8 per cent. However, in a series of over 1000 patients delivered by caesarean section the incidence of thromboembolism detected clinically was <1 per cent [186]. It is likely that the increased risk of operative delivery is not specific to caesarean section, since Aaro and Juergens [1] found that 25 per cent of cases of thromboembolism occurred in complications of pregnancy which included difficult forceps deliveries and prolonged labour, as well as caesarean section, pre-eclamptic toxaemia and haemorrhage.

Other factors

Other risk factors include age and parity, which operate independently of each other. The risk of fatal thromboembolism is 20 times greater in women over the age of 40 having their fifth or more pregnancy, compared with women of 20 in their first pregnancy [76]. Oestrogen treatment to suppress lactation was shown to increase the risk of thromboembolism by Daniel *et al.* [65] and Jeffcoate *et al.* [139]; if any drug treatment is necessary for suppression of lactation, bromocriptine should be used rather than oestrogen. Sickle cell anaemia is probably a risk factor for pulmonary embolus, since a high proportion of mortalities, due to sickle cell disease, have been reported to occur in pregnancy, usually due to pulmonary embolus [231]. Van Dinh *et al.* [237] have also reported massive pulmonary embolus in a patient with sickle cell trait.

The current Confidential Maternal Mortality report demonstrates the importance of obesity [80]. Congestive heart failure, dehydration, cancer [82] and anaemia are all said to increase the risk of thromboembolism [151] and probably do; but in general these risks have not been documented in obstetric practice. Similar risk factors have been demonstrated by Kimball *et al.* [144] for deaths caused by pulmonary embolus following legally induced abortion.

The risk of repeated thromboembolism in pregnancy in patients who have had thromboembolism in the past is considered below.

The presence of blood group O is associated with a decreased incidence of thromboembolism. To have a blood group other than O is therefore a positive risk factor [140]. This too is confirmed in the Confidential Maternal Mortality series from 1963 to 1975: the expected frequency of blood group O in the general population in England and Wales is 46 per cent, but only 38 per cent of those with pulmonary emboli had blood group O [76].

Venous thromboembolism is very rare in Africa and the Far East. The mechanism is unknown, but it is so uncommon that the cause is unlikely to be due to lack of ascertainment. For example in a series of 438 maternal deaths in Hong Kong from 1961–85, pulmonary embolism was not a major cause of mortality [83]. It has been suggested that the rise in protein C level (see below) at the end of pregnancy in Chinese women accounts for this low prevalence of thromboembolism [150]. However, the apparent difference between Western and Chinese women in this respect may represent methodological differences only.

The presence of lupus anticoagulant or cardiolipin antibodies is clearly a risk for both venous and arterial thromboembolism (see Chapter 8) and patients with lupus anticoagulant may have venous thromboembolism in atypical sites such as the arm and portal vessels. But thromboembolism in such sites also occasionally occurs in pregnancy in the absence of lupus anticoagulant [136].

Patients with homocystinuria are also at increased risk from arterial and venous thromboembolism [181]. This risk has been demonstrated in pregnancy [53,145]. The mechanism of increased risk is unknown [66]. Pyridoxine therapy may be beneficial in those patients where the metabolic defect responds to such treatment [53] (see Chapter 14 for further details on homocystinuria in pregnancy).

Antithrombin III deficiency and other inherited abnormalities of fibrinolysis are considered below. There is also increased risk of thromboembolism in paroxysmal nocturnal haemoglobinuria (see Chapter 2).

Diagnosis of thromboembolism

Deep vein thrombosis

In pregnancy, possibly due to the way in which the uterus lies, deep vein thrombosis is much more common in the left femoral vein and its tributaries than in the right. The ratio is approximately 8:1 [23,24]. The history and physical signs of this condition are well described in the standard textbooks.

It is probable that women who do not have a typical history are unlikely to have a deep vein thrombosis, and asymptomatic deep vein thrombosis is probably much rarer in pregnancy than other gynaecological surgery. This is supported by the study of Bergqvist *et al.* [21] who showed by occlusion plethysmography that the incidence of deep vein thrombosis was only 1.8 per cent even after caesarean section in comparison to the 10–20 per cent found after major gynaecological surgery [31,96]. It is clear that it is very difficult to make an accurate diagnosis based on physical signs alone [224], since perhaps 50 per cent of patients who have an acutely tender swollen calf do not have deep vein thrombosis. If an objective test such as ultrasound, plethysmography or venography is not used for the diagnosis of deep vein thrombosis, one to two patients are treated unnecessarily for every one treated correctly [203,211]. Therefore, some form of investigation(s) must be performed to support a clinical diagnosis.

The non-invasive investigations available are based on the demonstration of blood clotting by β thromboglobulin elevation [159], the measurement of blood flow and most recently by imaging of the blood clot by ultrasound [244]. Simple measurement of C reactive protein has been shown to have a sensitivity of 100 per cent in a small series of non-pregnant patients [232], i.e. a normal C reactive protein excluded deep vein thrombosis in this study. The C reactive protein level is not affected by pregnancy and this study should be repeated in a series of pregnant patients.

Reduced blood flow in the affected limb may be shown by Doppler flow studies [198], impedance plethysmography [129] and thermography [210]. Using liquid crystal thermography to document the increased warmth of the affected leg, Sandler and Martin [210] showed that the technique had a sensitivity of 97 per cent but rather low specificity (62 per cent) in non-pregnant patients. The predictive value of a negative thermogram was helpful (96 per cent). The technique could be improved by using ^{99m}Tc venoscanning in positive cases but this would need to be evaluated in pregnancy. Radioactive iodine should not be used in pregnancy. In the antenatal period it is trapped by the fetal thyroid and may cause hypothyroidism [88] or subsequent carcinoma. It is also secreted in high concentration in breast milk and the same risks apply to the breast-fed infant. Because of the problems of treatment in the index and future pregnancies (see below), an objective form of diagnosis is recommended in all patients who are considered to have deep vein thrombosis in pregnancy, unless the clinical diagnosis seems overwhelmingly certain. This occurs in severe proximal iliac vein thrombosis where the whole limb is markedly swollen.

The three techniques that are most appropriate for use in pregnancy are plethysmography, ultrasound and venography. Because of the radiation involved and the pain of the procedure, venography should now be reserved for use in those centres where plethysmography or ultrasound cannot be used, when there are technical difficulties with these procedures or to confirm a positive plethysmograph test.

Plethysmography has been very carefully evaluated in non-pregnant subjects [128,131]. Studies should be performed in the left lateral position before delivery in order to reduce the reduction in venous return caused by the obstruction of the gravid uterus. Since blood flow from the leg is reduced in pregnancy [47], a normal (by non-pregnant standards) plethysmograph probably excludes significant deep vein thrombosis. A normal plethysmograph repeated over a 10-day period would also exclude a calf vein thrombosis extending to the thigh and therefore becoming clinically significant. This approach has been vindicated in pregnancy by withholding anticoagulant therapy from 139 patients clinically suspected of having deep vein thrombosis but who had negative plethysmograph studies. None had symptomatic pulmonary embolus or recurrent venous thrombosis [132]. However, we do not yet know what constitutes a positive plethysmograph in pregnancy and positive tests should therefore be confirmed by ultrasound or venography.

In the future, light reflection rheography may be a simpler, cheaper substitute for plethysmography [182].

Ultrasound has been shown to be highly effective in the diagnosis of symptomatic proximal deep vein thrombosis by comparison with venography (though in non-pregnant patients). The veins may be identified by Doppler and then imaged. If a clot is present, the vein is incompressible and it also does not dilate when venous pressure is raised during a Valsalva manoeuvre. The clot itself may also be imaged. The sensitivity and specificity of this technique have been reported to be over 97 per cent for proximal vein thrombosis [153], but a formal comparison of ultrasound and venography has not been made in pregnancy. However, studies performed in pregnancy have been encouraging [103,195] and there is no reason to believe that ultrasonography would be any less accurate in pregnancy than in the non-pregnant state.

Neither ultrasound nor impedance plethysmography is suitable for diagnosis of calf vein thrombosis but since calf vein thrombi very rarely cause pulmonary emboli and since the tests being non-invasive can be repeated in worrying cases, this is not a problem. By contrast with plethysmography, ultrasound cannot be used for diagnosis of isolated thrombosis above the inguinal ligament. However, such thrombi are very rare in symptomatic patients [130]. At present ultrasound is the initial diagnostic technique of choice for pregnancy: it does not require the particular expertise and equipment of plethysmography and the apparatus should be available in all major obstetric centres.

Venography of the femoral and more distal veins can be performed in pregnancy. With adequate shielding of the uterus, the direct radiation dose is very small, and less than in pelvimetry [151], although there will be some additional scattered radiation. The use of less irritant, water-soluble, non-ionic contrast media makes it much less likely that venography itself will provoke thromboembolism [233].

Pulmonary embolus

Patients with major pulmonary emboli collapse with hypotension, chest pain, breathlessness and cyanosis. Occasionally they may present with abdominal pain only, due presumably to irritation of the diaphragm [183]. On further examination, they are also found to have a third heart sound, parasternal heave and elevated jugular venous pressure. It is the latter that helps to distinguish them from most of the other relatively common causes of collapse in pregnancy, where the diagnosis is not obvious, as it is in ante- and post-partum haemorrhage or ruptured or inverted uterus. These causes of collapse and some differentiating features are shown in Table 4.1. Most of the other causes are also considered elsewhere: pulmonary aspiration in Chapter 1, amniotic fluid embolus in Chapter 3, myocardial infarction in Chapter 5 and Gram-negative septicaemia in Chapters 3, 7 and 16.

The diagnosis of major pulmonary embolus is rarely in doubt. However, pulmonary embolus is often preceded by smaller emboli, and a high index of clinical suspicion is essential to diagnose these. Warning signs and symptoms of small pulmonary emboli that are often ignored are unexplained pyrexia, syncope, cough, chest pain and breathlessness. Unless the patient has a high temperature or is producing quantities of purulent sputum, pleurisy should not be considered to be due to infection until pulmonary embolism has been excluded. It may be necessary to treat the patient with both antibiotics and anticoagulants until diagnosis becomes clear.

Chest radiograph, electrocardiogram and blood gases

In considering the diagnosis of pulmonary embolus, it should be emphasized that the chest radiography may be normal and that the electrocardiogram may be normal or may show features such as a deep S wave in lead I and Q wave and inverted T wave in lead III that can be caused by pregnancy alone. Blood gas measurement can be helpful, although false positive and false negative results may occur [204]. If the patient is hypoxaemic, with Pa_{O_2} <70 mmHg and Pa_{CO_2} normal or reduced, it is likely that pulmonary embolus is the cause of chest symptoms, providing there is no radiological evidence of diffuse pulmonary disease or any other cause of reduced cardiac output. Such arterial samples should always be taken with the patient sitting, not supine (see Chapter 1).

Lung scans

Since it is so important to make an accurate diagnosis of thromboembolism in pregnancy, lung scans should be obtained, preferably with ventilation/perfusion imaging in all suspicious cases. The isotopes used in these scans, krypton 81 m for ventilation and technetium 99 m for perfusion, have very short half-lives. The radiation to the fetus is therefore minimal, about 0.5 Sv (50 mrem) or one-tenth of the maximum gestational exposure recommended to radiation workers in the USA [165]. Even if the mother is breast feeding the quantities of technetium secreted in milk after the injection of technetium 99 m macro-aggregated albumen are negligible [235]. The lung scan is particularly helpful in cases where the chest X-ray is normal. A normal lung scan then excludes a pulmonary embolus since false negative results are very rare [132]. Anticoagulants were withheld from 515 patients with suspected pulmonary embolus and negative lung scan unless they had deep vein thrombosis. Only one had symptomatic pulmonary embolus on follow-up [132]. Although false positives may occur, a large perfusion defect in the presence of a normal chest X-ray is likely to be due to pulmonary embolus. If the chest X-ray is abnormal, ventilation scanning is helpful. A reduction in perfusion with maintenance of ventilation indicates pulmonary embolus. If ventilation is reduced as well as perfusion, the condition is likely to be infective if the X-ray changes are acute. If the lung scan is equivocal it is helpful to examine the legs for deep vein thrombosis [177] by any of the techniques described above. If there is no evidence of deep vein thrombosis, the chance of subsequent or future clinical pulmonary emboli is small [177].

Treatment

Patients with massive pulmonary embolus present with a catastrophic reduction in cardiac output and the immediate treatment should be the standard cardiac arrest procedure. If it is thought likely that the cause of the arrest is pulmonary embolus, intravenous heparin 20 000 units should be given to reverse the bronchoconstriction and vasoconstriction caused by the release of serotonin from platelets [135]. In addition, prolonged cardiac massage is advisable since this may break up the original clot, permitting an increase in pulmonary blood flow [114]. After emergency resuscitation for pulmonary embolus, the treatment of both deep vein thrombosis and pulmonary embolus may be divided into an initial acute phase which lasts for up to a week and a subsequent chronic phase lasting for several months, where the aim of therapy is to prevent further incidents of thromboembolism.

Uncontrolled studies by Villasanta [240] indicate that the maternal mortality associated with pulmonary embolus and deep vein thrombosis in pregnancy is reduced from 13 to 1 per cent by anticoagulant therapy. A similar mortality (one in 113 patients) was found by Moseley and Kerstein [180] in a literature search of anticoagulant-treated patients. It is generally accepted that anticoagulation is the treatment of choice in pulmonary embolism without shock [178] and that it is highly efficacious [99]. Therefore it would now be unethical to compare an anticoagulant and placebo treatment in thromboembolism, whether associated with pregnancy or not. The only controlled trial of anticoagulant versus placebo therapy in pulmonary embolus was abandoned because of the high mortality in the placebo group [17].

Treatments used in the acute phase are heparin, surgery and thrombolytic agents such as streptokinase [160]. Treatment in the chronic phase is with warfarin or heparin.

Table 4.1. Features of some 'occult' causes of collapse in pregnancy. This table excludes more obvious causes, such as ante- or post-partum haemorrhage, and ruptured or inverted uterus

	Predisposing circumstances	Common presenting features	Helpful diagnostic features in *acute* stage*	
			Clinical	Investigations
Amniotic fluid embolism (Chapter 3)	Labour, not necessarily precipitate	Respiratory distress, cyanosis		Squames in SVC or sputum
Pulmonary embolus (Chapter 4)	Increasing age, multiparity, thromboembolism, operative delivery, bed rest, oestrogens, haemoglobinopathy	Respiratory distress, cyanosis, chest pain	JVP+; third heart sound, parasternal heave	ECG, chest X-ray, lung scan, blood gas, pulmonary angiography
Myocardial infarction (Chapter 5)	Increasing age	Chest pain, respiratory distress, cyanosis	Pain character, JVP+; crepitations	ECG
Dysrrhythmia (Chapter 5)	Pre-existing heart disease	Tachycardia/bradycardia	Pulse	ECG
Aspiration of gastric contents (Chapter 1)	Anaesthesia, not necessarily with vomiting	Respiratory distress, cyanosis	Bronchospasm	

Pneumothorax and pneumomediastinum	Previous history, labour	Chest pain	Chest signs	Chest X-ray
Intra-abdominal bleeding	Labour, though may occur spontaneously	Abdominal pain	JVP not+; signs in abdomen, laparotomy, paracentesis, culdocentesis	
Septicaemia (Chapters 3,7,16)	Previous infection (not necessarily)	Fever, rigors	Fever, rigors	Gram stain on blood sample. Blood culture positive
Intracerebral catastrophe	Pre-eclampsia/eclampsia A-V malformation	Seizures	CNS signs, neck stiffness	CT scan
Hypoglycaemia	Diabetes mellitus Addison's disease Hypopituitarism Hypothyroidism	Sweating, loss of consciousness		Blood glucose
Hyperglycaemia	Diabetes mellitus	Hyperventilation		Blood glucose, blood gas

* These features are not absolute. For example, it is possible to have pulmonary crepitations in patients with pulmonary embolus, and septicaemia without fever or rigors.

Acute phase

Heparin

The majority of cases of venous thromboembolism are treated initially with heparin. Heparin, because it is so strongly polar, has particular advantages in pregnancy, since it does not cross the placenta [122] for which lipid solubility is necessary. The object of heparin therapy in the initial phase of treatment of venous thromboembolism is to prevent further, possibly fatal, episodes. It is not believed that heparin increases the re-absorption of the original thrombus. In order to prevent further clot formation, relatively high blood levels of heparin must be achieved; it has been suggested that particularly large doses are necessary in the presence of a large initial thrombus [29]. Although up to 40 000 units/day of heparin have been given subcutaneously [30], this is not usually practical because of bruising and irregular absorption, and the initial treatment should be with intravenous heparin: initially a 5000 unit bolus followed by 40 000 units/day (approximately 1600 units/hour) by continuous infusion, aiming to achieve a level of 0.6–1.0 unit/ml as assayed by the protamine sulphate neutralization test [58]. Although most haematology laboratories and other authorities [151] suggest monitoring heparin treatment by the partial thromboplastin test, the protamine sulphate neutralization test appears to be more useful in our hands; a control sample taken from the patient before treatment is not necessary, and the test seems to reflect the patient's risk of bleeding more accurately than does the partial thromboplastin time. Furthermore, when the partial thromboplastin or kaolin cephalin clotting times [89] are used for control of heparin infusion, the results are often ignored if outside the therapeutic range (1.5–2.5 times control for kaolin cephalin clotting time) [89]. Also, clinicians should be aware that such assays have a 45 per cent between-occasion variability even in patients on a continuous and steady infusion of heparin. This variation may be diurnal in nature, higher values occurring at night [74]. In addition, infusion pumps may not run steadily and the partial thromboplastin time also varies depending on the time between testing and drawing blood [90].

In the acute phase, the heparin should be given by intravenous infusion [208]. Heparin is not stable in dextrose and should therefore be given in saline [137] preferably made up in a small volume of 10–20 ml and very slowly infused with a constant infusion pump. If this is not practical, the same total dose of heparin may be given by repeated intravenous injections, but no less frequently than every 3 hours. The half-life of heparin is only about 1.5 hours [87] and if the drug is given by large, infrequent intravenous injections, this produces unacceptable swings between hyper- and hypocoagulability [214]. The only side-effect of acute heparin administration is bleeding (see below for side-effects of prolonged therapy), although its preservative, cholorbutol, may cause hypotension [32].

If it is necessary to reverse heparin therapy, cessation of infusion alone will be sufficient for most patients given intravenous heparin. There will be undetectable levels in the blood 6 hours after therapy has stopped. In the more urgent situation the patient can be given protamine 1 mg per 1090 units of administered heparin. When using a continuous infusion of heparin, twice the quantity of protamine should be given to neutralize the hourly dose. No more than 50 mg of protamine should be given in a 10-min period, since protamine itself can cause bleeding [151]. A better alternative is to calculate the quantity of protamine needed from the protamine sulphate neutralization test [58]. The neutralizing dose of protamine sulphate may be calculated as follows [154]:

$$\begin{array}{l}\text{protamine}\\ \text{sulphate}\\ \text{required (mg)}\\ \text{to neutralize}\\ \text{heparin}\end{array} = \begin{array}{l}\text{plasma heparin}\\ \text{concentration}\\ \text{IU/ml}\end{array} \times \begin{array}{c}\text{plasma}\\ \text{volume}\end{array} \times 0.01.$$

Plasma volume in pregnancy is 50 ml/kg bodyweight; so for example a 70-kg woman with plasma heparin concentration 1.2 IU/ml would require $1.2 \times (70 \times 50) \times 0.01 = 42$ mg protamine sulphate. If there is any doubt about the efficacy or desirability of protamine reversal, fresh frozen plasma should restore blood clotting to normal.

Because of the risk of haematoma formation in patients who are fully anticoagulated, other injections such as antibiotics should be given intravenously rather than intramuscularly. Arterial blood sampling should be from an intra-aterial cannula or by needling a superficial artery, such as the radial artery rather than the deeper femoral artery.

Initial phase, high dose intravenous heparin therapy is continued for an arbitrary period of 3–7 days; the length of treatment depends on the severity of the initial episode of venous thromboembolism and whether there is any evidence of recurrence. Studies using intravenous heparin for only 5 days [134] have not been performed in pregnancy and have only been performed in the non-pregnant state in patients with deep vein thrombosis, not pulmonary embolus.

Promising studies have also reported using fixed dose subcutaneous low molecular weight heparin (logiparin [133], fraxiparin [196]) in the initial phase of treatment of non-pregnant patients with deep vein thrombosis [132,196]. In the study of Hull *et al.* [133] not only were there the obvious advantages of subcutaneous fixed dose versus adjusted dose intravenous therapy but there was less bleeding in the acute phase and fewer recurrences. Although we have some experience using a different low molecular weight heparin (enoxparine) for thromboembolism prophylaxis [228] (see below), low molecular weight heparins have not yet been evaluated for thromboembolism treatment in pregnancy. They could represent a major advance in treatment.

The alternatives to heparin in the initial phase of treatment are surgery and thrombolytic therapy. Both these alternatives have the advantage of therapy directed towards removing the initial clot. Both should be considered in the non-pregnant state for initial treatment in patients with major pulmonary embolus or massive iliofemoral deep vein thrombosis.

Thrombolytic therapy

Thrombolytic agents are probably underused in the non-pregnant state since there is evidence that patients who have had a deep vein thrombosis are much less likely to develop post-phlebitic leg symptoms after being given thrombolytic therapy than after conventional treatment with heparin and warfarin [86]. Browse [40] also suggests that thrombolytic therapy is preferable to conventional anticoagulation to minimize the risk of massive pulmonary embolus in patients with extensive iliofemoral thrombosis where the proximal end of the clot is floating free; but this has not been proven.

Comparison of medical therapies

In a comparison of heparin and oral anticoagulants with urokinase in the treatment of pulmonary embolus in the non-pregnant state, urokinase therapy was associated with earlier resolution as shown by pulmonary angiography [236]. A recent review [147] suggests that there should be trials of streptokinase not only in (non-pregnant) patients with major pulmonary embolus, but also in those with minor emboli.

It has also been shown that, after a pulmonary embolus, the pulmonary capillary blood volume and pulmonary diffusing capacity are normal in patients treated with thrombolytic therapy, whereas they usually remain abnormal in patients treated with heparin and warfarin, even if they are asymptomatic at follow-up 1 year later [218].

Pfeiffer [194] claimed successful treatment of deep vein thrombosis in 12 pregnant patients with streptokinase given as a loading dose (250 000 units by intravenous infusion over 20 min) followed by an infusion of 160 000 units/hour for 4 hours, with subsequent alteration of the infusion rate depending on the plasma thrombin time. Bell and Meek [20] discount the necessity for adjusting the dosage schedule and would recommend a maintenance therapy of 100 000 IU/hour for 24–72 hours after the initial loading dose. Although Pfeiffer [193] suggests that very little streptokinase crosses the human placenta, pregnancy is considered a minor contraindication to the use of thrombolytic therapy, and subsequent delivery within 10 days is a major contraindication to thrombolytic therapy [184]. Since it is possible that thrombolytic therapy may precipitate premature labour by causing an increase in circulating plasminogen levels [8], there is a risk that the relatively minor contraindication will become a major contraindication. However, it has also been suggested that streptokinase therapy will cause relative uterine atony because of the interference of fibrin degradation products with uterine contraction [111].

If it is necessary to reverse thrombolytic therapy in pregnancy, aprotinin, which has large molecules and does not cross the placenta, should be used rather than aminocaproic acid. However, apart from the 12 patients treated in pregnancy by Pfeiffer [194], other studies are only case reports [8,111,171] and therefore there is really still not sufficient experience to recommend the use of thrombolytic agents in pregnancy except in exceptional circumstances [94] such as life-threatening pulmonary embolus (see below).

Surgery

Surgical removal of the thrombus (thrombectomy) may be indicated in massive iliofemoral deep vein thrombosis because of the suggestion that this too reduces the incidence of post-phlebitic leg symptoms [169]; however, this has not been substantiated in follow-up studies [148] and thrombectomy is a technically difficult operation involving considerable blood loss. Thrombectomy had been advocated where limb swelling is so great as to cause venous gangrene [108,216]. In pregnancy such patients should be delivered because the reduction of additional obstruction by the enlarged uterus often reduces limb swelling. Surgery (venous plication or insertion of a vena caval umbrella) has also been advocated to prevent pulmonary embolus in cases of iliofemoral thrombosis [216]. With adequate anticoagulation this is rarely necessary [223] and in any case devices to filter large clots in the inferior vena cava are now usually placed percutaneously via the other patent femoral vein or via the jugular vein rather than at open surgery [16]. This is discussed below under recurrent thromboembolism.

In cases of pulmonary embolus, patients who are shocked at the time of the initial event have traditionally been considered for pulmonary embolectomy using cardiopulmonary bypass [82,101], as have those with any of the following features 1 hour later: (a) systolic blood pressure <90 mmHg; (b) Pao_2 <60 mmHg; or (c) urine output <20 ml/hour [214]. The decision whether to operate would usually be supported by pulmonary angiography which is also necessary to localize the embolus. At pulmonary angiography it may be possible to fragment the clot using a guideline wire to advance the catheter through the clot [33]. This may obviate the necessity for pulmonary embolectomy.

However, it is currently believed that surgery for pulmonary embolus in non-pregnant patients should be reserved for those who deteriorate following thrombolytic therapy or who present with such haemodynamic compromise that the thrombolytic therapy is not justifiable [102]. The risks of thrombolytic therapy that are specific to pregnancy are the initiation of incoordinate pre-term labour and subsequent post-partum haemorrhage. I think it reasonable to accept these risks in life-threatening massive pulmonary embolus. In the severely compromised patient, I would therefore suggest pulmonary angiography, an attempt to disperse the clot once it has been demonstrated, thrombolytic therapy if this fails or does not improve the haemodynamic status of the patient and then possibly surgery according to the criteria described above [102].

Chronic phase

Warfarin

It is established that there is a definite, though low, incidence of teratogenesis associated with the use of warfarin in the first trimester of pregnancy [5,19,142,192]. The most common syndrome is chondrodysplasia punctata, in which cartilage and bone formation is abnormal [19,219], although warfarin is not the only cause of this abnormality [221] which may also be inherited [57]. The asplenia syndrome [54] and diaphragmatic herniae have also been reported [187]. It has also been recognized that the use of warfarin in late pregnancy after 36 weeks' gestation is associated with serious retroplacental and intracerebral fetal bleeding [240] since, unlike heparin, warfarin does cross the placenta. As premature infants have low levels of Factors XI and XII [10], it is likely that the fetus has low levels of clotting factors; therefore the fetus will be excessively anticoagulated if the mother's prothrombin time is within the normal therapeutic range. For these reasons Hirsh *et al*. [122] used to recommend that after the initial period of heparinization in the acute attack, heparin should continue to be used for the first trimester, followed by warfarin between 13 and 36 weeks, reverting to heparin for the last weeks of pregnancy. These recommendations were widely followed at one time [36,70,118,199,229] and indeed in 1980, 73 per cent of practising obstetricians would have followed them [70]. However, by 1993 only 35% of obstetricians in the UK used warfarin for thromboprophylaxis [104] and the question has arisen as to whether oral anticoagulants should be used even after the first trimester [36] because of the risk of fetal malformation. Sherman and Hall [222] described a case of microcephaly in a patient who had taken warfarin for the last 6 months of pregnancy, and this stimulated further reports [109,110], including one by Holzgreve *et al.* [124] in which five cases of microcephaly occurring in California were described. It has been suggested that warfarin causes repeated small intracerebral haemorrhages and that these are the causes of the optic atrophy, microcephaly and mental retardation that have been described [220]. Gross subdural haemorrhage may also occur in the fetus before 36 weeks' gestation [225].

These teratogenic risks may not be so great as anecdotal reports would suggest. Chen *et al.* [42] studied the outcome of 22 pregnancies, where the mother had taken warfarin in the first trimester, and 20 pregnancies where warfarin had been taken between 13 and 36 weeks. Warfarin was being used in the management of artificial heart valves. Although the spontaneous abortion rate was high (36 per cent in those taking warfarin) there were no cases of chondrodysplasia punctata or microcephaly. In another study in which we compared the infants of 20 patients who had taken warfarin in the second and third trimesters with those of well-matched controls, there was no difference in intellectual attainment at a mean age of 4 years [44]. Microcephaly is therefore unlikely to be common in the children of women taking warfarin. It may relate to the method of control used for warfarin therapy and therefore to the amount of warfarin taken. Central nervous system (CNS) malformations do seem more common in those taking higher doses of warfarin.

Bleeding also appears to be more of a problem in pregnant women treated with warfarin than in those treated with heparin, even if the patients have prothrombin times within the normal therapeutic range [73]. Even if patients are not anticoagulated, they are at risk from ante- and post-partum haemorrhages in pregnancy, and this risk seems to be increased by warfarin therapy. Fetomaternal haemorrhage has also been reported [157].

For all the above reasons I, and others [151], believe that warfarin should not be used in the chronic phase of treatment of venous thromboembolism in pregnancy, or in the first week of the puerperium. The only situation where warfarin therapy is recommended in pregnancy is in the management of some patients with artificial heart valves or mitral valve disease (see Chapter 5). The risk of genital tract bleeding is much less by 7 days after delivery, and it is therefore reasonable to use warfarin at that time as an alternative to subcutaneous heparin.

Patients may continue to breast feed [34] since there is no detectable secretion of warfarin in breast milk [189]. This is not so for phenindione where maternal therapy has caused severe haemorrhage in a breast-fed infant [84]. However, phenindione may not be so teratogenic as warfarin [188]; unfortunately there is not sufficient experience to confirm this.

Heparin

Subcutaneous, self-administered heparin is the preferred chronic phase treatment for venous thromboembolism in pregnancy [121], since it does not have the risks of warfarin. (The possible complications of long-term heparin therapy are described below.)

The half-life of heparin injected subcutaneously is about 18 hours in comparison to intravenous heparin which has a half-life of 1.5 hours. The majority of patients are given acute phase high dose intravenous heparin therapy for 3–7 days though some with massive deep vein thrombosis or severe pulmonary embolus may benefit from intravenous heparin for up to 14 days. The patients are then given subcutaneous heparin, initially 10 000 units twice daily. This is monitored by the heparin assay which is based on heparin's anti-Xa activity

[75]. The small dose of heparin used in chronic therapy does not affect the whole blood-clotting system, and is below the limits of detection of more conventional tests, such as the partial thromboplastin time or protamine sulphate neutralization test. Provided there is detectable heparin activity, the dose of heparin is not increased above 10 000 units every 12 hours. If the heparin assay exceeds 0.2 units/ml, the dose is reduced, since such levels are associated with excessive bleeding [29]. Heparin levels are stable in patients who are taking subcutaneous heparin, but because of pregnancy-induced changes in blood volume and renal handling of heparin, and because treatment with heparin may continue for up to 6 months, repeated heparin assays should be made. We usually perform these as frequently as the patient attends for normal antenatal visits. In addition we have found that the onset of pre-eclamptic toxaemia may be preceded by a decrease in heparin requirements, possibly due to impaired renal excretion of heparin [29] but this suggestion is only based on isolated clinical observations.

The anti-Xa heparin assay is quite difficult to perform and not widely available. An acceptable alternative is to measure the thrombin time. By contrast this test is widely available as part of the normal clotting screen. It is very sensitive to heparin and patients who are taking more than prophylactic levels of heparin show a marked prolongation of the thrombin time. Therefore the risk of bleeding in patients taking subcutaneous heparin can be assessed with the thrombin time: if it is not prolonged, the patients will not bleed. The thrombin time cannot be used to assess the efficacy of subcutaneous heparin prophylaxis but since it is not our practice to increase the dose of heparin in the chronic phase of treatment above 10 000 units twice daily, and since the optimal level of heparin for prophylaxis is not known, this is not really relevant.

Although patients often show initial reluctance, the majority can be taught to give themselves subcutaneous heparin and can therefore be discharged home. Patients should use the concentrated heparin solution of 50 000 units/ml. We have not found any difference in bruising between sodium and calcium heparins. The heparin should be drawn up in a tuberculin syringe because of the small volumes used, and injected subcutaneously though a short (16 mm) 25 gauge needle. The injections should be made perpendicular to the skin surface to minimize the risk of trauma to skin blood vessels. Possible sites are the thighs and abdominal wall.

Because of the high incidence of thromboembolism in the days following labour and delivery [77], subcutaneous heparin administration should be continued through labour. The heparin assay or thrombin time can be checked in the week preceding delivery, since patients attend the hospital weekly at this time in pregnancy. There is no increased risk of intra- or post-partum haemorrhage in these patients [72,120], although those patients who inadvertently take too much heparin are at risk of bleeding [9]. Providing that the thrombin time is normal, it is now believed the epidural block is not contraindicated [155] although formerly it was thought that there was an excessive risk of epidural haematoma [56].

After delivery, the dose of subcutaneous heparin is empirically reduced to 7500 units twice daily because of the contraction in circulating blood volume and because the clotting factors return to normal levels during the puerperium. The heparin assay is checked at least once after delivery if the patient continues to take subcutaneous heparin for the recommended 6 weeks post-partum. Alternatively 1 week after delivery, when the risk of secondary post-partum haemorrhage is much less, the patient may take warfarin rather than heparin. In either case breast feeding is safe. Heparin is not secreted in breast milk and would not be absorbed from the infant's stomach. Warfarin is not excreted in breast milk [189]. The option as to whether to continue heparin or to switch to warfarin depends on which the patient finds less inconvenient. Heparin has the disadvantage of multiple injections but does not require laboratory control after the first week. Warfarin therapy has the disadvantage of needing repeated prothrombin estimations but is given orally.

If the patient does opt to switch to warfarin the drug is given daily; the first two doses should be 10 mg each; the international normalized ratio (INR) is checked before giving the third dose: and dosing then depends on the value of the INR. The target INR for the treatment of deep vein thrombosis is 2–3 [37]. Treatment with heparin should be continued until the target level is achieved (or exceeded). Heparin treatment does not interfere with estimation of the INR, providing that the activated partial thromboplastin time ratio is <2.5 or heparin level is <1.5 units/ml.

Therapy with heparin initiated in pregnancy or warfarin if introduced after 7 days post-partum, is continued for an arbitrary period of 6 weeks post-partum, at which time the extra risk of thromboembolism associated with pregnancy is considered to have passed. Patients who develop venous thromboembolism in the puerperium should be treated as above, except that, after the acute phase, warfarin may be used alone in chronic phase treatment if it is not given for the first 7 days after delivery. The total length of anticoagulant treatment should be at least 6 weeks.

Alternative methods of heparin administration for those intolerant of twice daily subcutaneous injection are by continuous subcutaneous infusion using pumps such as are used for infusion of insulin [108,201], or by continuous intravenous infusion (see above).

Recurrent thromboembolism

Patients who have a history of recurrent thromboembolism particularly arterial or in atypical sites or if associated with a poor obstetric history should be screened for lupus anticoagulant and the presence of cardiolipin antibodies (see Chapter 8). In addition, if they have recurrent thromboembolism or if there is a family history they should be screened as far as is possible for inherited abnormalities that affect blood clotting; these are homocystinuria (see Chapter 14), antithrombin III deficiency, protein C deficiency, activated protein C resistance, protein S deficiency and abnormal forms of fibrinogen (see below). Such a screen is particularly important in patients seen for pre-pregnancy counselling so that an estimate of the risks of thromboembolism and efficacy of prophylaxis may be given.

In patients who develop recurrent thromboembolism during acute or chronic phase treatment, the diagnosis should again be established by objective criteria. The adequacy of anticoagulant treatment up to the time of recurrence should be reviewed. Patients should be screened for causes of recurrent thromboembolism as described above, although the diagnosis may be difficult in patients who are already taking anticoagulants. If there really has been recurrent thromboembolism despite adequate anticoagulation, the patient should receive long-term intravenous heparin [50] preferably by a Hickman line [185]; the dose should be adjusted to achieve a heparin level (protamine sulphate neutralization test, see above) of 0.8–1.0 units/ml. This dose will need to be reduced at the time of delivery in the same way as for patients with artificial heart valves (see Chapter 5). If the source appears to be in the legs or pelvic veins surgical interruption of the inferior vena cava or iliac veins with a sieve or Greenfield filter [16,32,123] could be considered.

Prophylaxis of thromboembolism

There are two groups of patients in whom prophylaxis might be considered: (a) those who are at high risk because of age, parity, obesity or operative delivery [77,80]; and (b) those who have had thromboembolism in the past [14]. With regard to the former group, it is generally believed (although not proven) that the risk of thromboembolism is greatest in the puerperium and therefore that any prophylaxis need only be used during this period and to cover labour. The Confidential Maternal Mortality series very clearly shows that the risks of thromboembolism are increased markedly with high parity and increasing age, and that these risks are partly independent of each other [76]. Applying these and other data, there is a case for using some form of prophylaxis in all patients who have had bed rest for at least 1 week before delivery, the obese, those undergoing operative delivery over the age of 30 years, and also in those over the age of 35 or in their fourth pregnancy (excluding abortion), even if they have a spontaneous vaginal delivery [158]. Dextran given during labour or caesarean section could be used. At present I would favour heparin because of the risks of anaphylaxis [190] in patients taking dextran and also because of the difficulty of cross-matching patients who have been given dextran. Although there has been no systemic evaluation of the efficacy and risks of either form of treatment in pregnancy; Bergqvist *et al.* [21] found no cases of deep vein thrombosis when they screened 32 patients given Dextran 70 during caesarean section, whereas three out of 150 patients who did not have dextran did have deep vein thrombosis following caesarean section.

The second group of patients are those who have had thromboembolism in the past; they are considered to be at risk throughout pregnancy. Badaracco and Vessey [14] in a retrospective study estimated that there was about a 12 per cent risk of developing pulmonary embolism of deep vein thrombosis in pregnancy if a patient had had thromboembolism in the past. The risk was not affected by the circumstances of the original event, i.e. whether it was associated with the contraceptive pill or not. The risk is likely to be exaggerated (see below): the study was based on a postal survey, and information is not available as to how the thromboembolism was diagnosed in pregnancy. If a patient has had thromboembolism in the past, there is a particularly strong tendency to diagnose it again on rather flimsy evidence.

In a previous survey, most British obstetricians (88 per cent) would have used prophylactic anticoagulants for such patients if the index thromboembolism had previously occurred during pregnancy. Some (73 per cent) would have used prophylaxis if the thromboembolism had occurred when taking the pill, and fewer (50 per cent) would have used prophylaxis if the original thromboembolism had occurred 10 years previously when the patients were neither taking the pill nor were pregnant [70]. These figures were not substantially changed in a later survey in 1993 [104].

The majority of obstetricians no longer use the modified Hirsh regime of warfarin [122] until 36 weeks' gestation for venous thromboembolism prophylaxis [104], and this now seems unacceptable because of the maternal and fetal complications of warfarin therapy outlined above. The alternative is to use subcutaneous heparin throughout pregnancy. However, since these patients are asymptomatic at the beginning of treatment and because the treatment is only being used prophylactically, the safety of such therapy for mother and fetus must be established even more rigorously than in the treatment of established venous thromboembolism.

Hall *et al*. [110] performed a retrospective study of the outcome of pregnancies associated with anticoagulant therapy, based on literature reports. Such a study is likely to be biased towards the reporting of complications, but they found that of 135 fetuses, 13 per cent were still-born, 14 per cent were born prematurely and 7 per cent died in the neonatal period. A comparative study performed at Queen Charlotte's Maternity Hospital of antenatal heparin prophylaxis compared to no antenatal prophylaxis did not show such a high perinatal mortality [126].

The most obvious maternal complication is bruising at the injection site. This can be reduced by good injection technique but rarely eliminated. Although this is undoubtedly an inconvenience, and at times painful, most mothers tolerate a degree of bruising. A further maternal complication of prolonged heparin therapy is a form of bone demineralization described as osteopenia [13,138,227]. This occurred in one of our patients, and presented as severe backache which was much worse in the puerperium [248]. Radiography in the puerperium showed that the patient had three collapsed vertebrae. Griffith *et al*. [105] reported that heparin-induced osteopenia only occurs in patients receiving more than 15 000 units/day for at least 6 months but bone demineralization has been reported following the administration of only 10 000 units of heparin per day in pregnancy for 19 weeks [106]. The incidence of symptomatic bone demineralization in those receiving heparin thromboprophylaxis has been estimated to be about 2% in a series of 184 pregnant women [62]. The cause of the osteopenia is unknown. It had been attributed to a deficiency of 1,25−dihydroxytachysterol [3,4] but this has not been confirmed in subsequent studies. Since heparin-induced osteopenia is much more common in pregnancy, it is likely that the enhanced bone turnover of pregnancy [60] and the fetal demand for calcium [175] are contributing factors. A follow-up study of those patients who are taking subcutaneous heparin suggests that even those patients who are asymptomatic may have some degree of bone demineralization [71]. This is particularly worrying because of fears that the osteoporosis will progress further at the menopause. Fortunately a follow-up study from Sweden based on radiological assessment of the spine suggests that heparin-induced osteopenia does regress once heparin treatment has been stopped [63]. Also Ginsberg *et al.* [98] studied 61 patients, 2 years after stopping long-term heparin treatment and found no difference in bone density when they were compared with controls. Both of these studies suggest that heparin-induced osteoporosis regresses on cessation of therapy.

It has also been reported that heparin may cause thrombocytopenia [112] with subsequent bleeding [45] or thrombotic complications [41,43]. It may also cause alopecia and allergic reactions. Thrombocytopenia either presents acutely as a result of platelet aggregation or occurs 7–10 days after treatment starts because of an interaction between platelets, heparin and a specific IgG autoantibody [46,249]. However, these additional complications have not been problems in our experience.

The risk of heparin-induced thrombocytopenia seems to be reduced but not eliminated [85,152] by the use of low molecular weight heparins.

Because of the possible fetal and definite maternal complications of prolonged subcutaneous heparin therapy, I believe that it should no longer be used as a routine for prophylaxis throughout pregnancy in all patients who have had thromboembolism in the past. Since there are even more problems with warfarin therapy, there is no form of prophylaxis that can be considered harmless and effective.

Our present approach [149] is to counsel patients about the relative risks of prophylactic therapy and recurrence of thromboembolism in the antenatal period. We only use subcutaneous heparin before labour in those patients who are considered particularly at risk, having had thromboembolism more than once in the past or having inherited abnormalities of the clotting or thrombolytic systems such as antithrombin III deficiency (see below) or having the lupus/anticardiolipin syndrome and a single episode of thromboembolism in the past. Subcutaneous heparin is also used in those patients who themselves are particularly concerned about the risk of repeated thromboembolism. In addition we use subcutaneous heparin in low risk patients who have only had a single episode of thromboembolism at times when they are most at risk, such as during admission to hospital for surgery or bed rest.

High risk patients who will take heparin throughout pregnancy start taking heparin 10 000 units subcutaneously twice daily as described above regarding chronic phase therapy for the management of established thromboembolism in pregnancy. They are monitored haematologically in the same way. The dose is reduced to 7500 units delivered subcutaneously twice daily during labour also as described above. After delivery the patients receive subcutaneous heparin 7500 units twice daily for at least 1 week and either subcutaneous heparin or warfarin for a further 5 weeks making a total of 6 weeks' postnatal treatment. The choice between warfarin and heparin again depends on which treatment the patient finds less inconvenient (see above). As in the treatment of an established case of thromboembolism in pregnancy (see above) the length of time for which prophylaxis is continued after delivery is arbitrary. Breast feeding is safe in patients taking warfarin [189].

Patients who have only had a single episode of thromboembolism in the past, no matter what the associated circumstances, are considered at low risk of recurrence in pregnancy. These patients enter the above schedule when they present in labour or at elective delivery. They are given subcutaneous heparin 7500 units twice daily. They are then managed in the same way as the high risk patients.

Although this regime for low risk patients is a compromise since it does not provide any cover during the antenatal period before labour, we have not observed any cases of antenatal or postnatal thromboembolism in over 60 patients treated in Queen Charlotte's Maternity Hospital in this way. They had all been treated for at least 6 weeks for an episode of deep vein thrombosis or pulmonary embolism before the index pregnancy. It therefore seems likely that the study of Badaracco and Vessey [14] which suggests a 12 per cent risk of thromboembolism in patients who have had deep vein thrombosis or pulmonary embolism in the past, very much over-estimates the risk of antenatal thromboembolism; the risk appears to be of the order of 2 per cent or less.

Other options would be to use antiplatelet agents, such as aspirin or to use low molecular weight heparin. Although adjusting the dose of conventional heparin to maintain a specific heparin level (0.08–0.15 unit/ml) is attractive since it allows lower heparin doses [59] there is no evidence this it is beneficial. The incidence of heparin-induced osteoporosis is independent of the doses that have been used [63]; we have found heparin prophylaxis is effective with a fixed dose regime and there would be a lot more inconvenience for the patient and potential error adjusting the dose of heparin on the basis of frequent anti-Xa heparin assays.

Antiplatelet drugs such as aspirin and dipyridamole have not yet been evaluated in pregnancy for thromboprophylaxis. However, there are promising data concerning their efficacy from meta-analysis of trials in general medical and surgical patients [11].

A further alternative for management of the antenatal period would be to develop more accurate models to determine precisely which patients are at risk of repeat thromboembolism. Although it is difficult to define the prethrombotic state on the basis of coagulation tests (see above), Clayton *et al.* [48,55] were able to correctly identify 95 per cent of gynaecological patients who had postoperative deep vein thrombosis on the basis of four items of clinical information and measurement of fibrin degradation products and plasminogen activator activity. Hellgren [115] has used discriminant analysis and shown that a combination of fibrinopeptide A, fibrinogen, Factor VIIIC, antithrombin III and plasmin activator estimation will help detect women at risk of thromboembolism in pregnancy. But these techniques are time-consuming and also do not predict the individual risk with sufficient precision.

Like conventional heparin, low molecular heparin does not cross the placenta [95,207] and it is hoped that it may interact with platelets and thrombin less than conventional heparin, thus causing less bleeding while maintaining heparin's antithrombin III activity and continuing to reduce the risk of blood clotting [207]. Certainly our initial impression at Queen Charlotte's Hospital using enoxparine, a low molecular weight heparin, has been that it is effective when given once daily for thromboprophylaxis [228]. However, the numbers that we have treated (27 pregnancies as of 1994) are still too small for meaningful comparison of efficacy with unfractionated heparin.

Undoubtedly patients prefer once daily injections. Unfortunately low molecular weight heparin is more expensive than unfractionated heparin. Low molecular weight heparin might cause less bone demineralization but this has not yet been evaluated in humans. Preliminary studies are not encouraging: when given to both men and women with deep vein thrombosis unfractionated and fractionated heparins caused similar degrees of bone demineralization [176] and in rats, low molecular weight heparin causes similar changes in bone density to those caused by unfractionated heparin [168].

Thrombophilia

Thrombophilia is the term applied to the condition in which patients have defects or abnormalities which alter the physiological haemostatic balance in favour of fibrin formation or persistence and hence which increase the risk of thrombosis [230]. Such abnormalities may be inherited (antithrombin III, protein C and protein S deficiencies, abnormalities of fibrinolysis — see [197] and Chapter 14) or acquired (lupus anticoagulant/cardiolipin syndrome — see Chapter 8). But many patients with the laboratory abnormalities of thrombophilia do not suffer with thromboses and many patients who from their histories appear to have a familial tendency to thrombosis, have no demonstrable haematological abnormality. In general the risk of thrombosis increases with age and exposure to risk factors such as pregnancy and oestrogen. The management of thrombophilia in pregnancy has been reviewed by Walker [241].

Antithrombin III deficiency

Antithrombin III is a naturally occurring substance produced by the liver which inhibits the actions of thrombin and other clotting factors [146]. Since thrombin promotes blood clotting by forming fibrin from fibrinogen, antithrombin III decreases the tendency of blood to clot. Antithrombin III deficiency, where the level of antithrombin III activity is 25–70 per cent of normal, is therefore associated with an increased risk of blood clotting. Antithrombin III activity can be measured in laboratories that take a particular interest in blood clotting. The condition is inherited as a Mendelian dominant trait [161] in the 40 or so families that have been described [35]. It is rare; Bergqvist [24] has not found a single case in over 500 patients screened for antithrombin III deficiency following severe thrombotic disease. Only three cases were found in a Dutch study of 277 patients with deep vein thrombosis [113]. In the Dutch study the overall prevalence of inherited thrombophilia (antithrombin III deficiency, protein C, protein S and plasminogen deficiencies) was 8.3 per cent and recurrent thromboembolism, juvenile thromboembolism and a positive family history had very low predictive values (9–16 per cent) [113].

In some families the condition is due to gene deletion [200]. Antithrombin III deficiency may either be expressed as a quantitative deficiency of a qualitatively normal molecule or the molecule itself may be abnormal [213]. It is clear that antithrombin III deficiency is quite heterogeneous since some abnormal forms of antithrombin III have been described which are also inherited in Mendelian dominant fashion and where coagulation studies are normal [64]. Characterization of the form of antithrombin III deficiency may be important in defining the risk of thromboembolism [91]. Note that antithrombin III levels are also reduced in liver disease and in all forms of consumption coagulopathy including pre-eclampsia (see Chapter 6).

In common with other forms of thrombophilia, antithrombin III deficiency often presents for the first time after oestrogen exposure either taking the contraceptive pill or in pregnancy, where the risk of thromboembolism is about 70 per cent (32 of 47 pregnancies), if no prophylaxis is used [117]. Winter *et al.* [247] found an even higher risk in three Scottish families (thrombosis in 15 of 16 pregnancies) though more recent studies suggest that the risk is nearer 40 per cent [52]. Nevertheless the risk is so great that some form of prophylaxis must be considered. These patients are usually treated for life with warfarin because of the risk of fatal pulmonary embolism [239]. However, for the reasons given above, warfarin should be avoided in pregnancy. Although subcutaneous heparin treatment may be associated with a paradoxical decrease in antithrombin III levels [164], Hellgren *et al.* [117] have shown that only one of seven patients adequately treated with subcutaneous heparin and antithrombin III concentrate in pregnancy had an episode of thromboembolism; this must therefore be the treatment of choice and heparin should be started instead of warfarin as soon as the patient knows that she is pregnant. The patient should have been counselled about the risk of bone demineralization from long-term heparin therapy before she became pregnant.

Hellgren used high dose heparin, 20 000–45 000 units every 24 hours to give a 5–10 second prolongation of the activated partial thromboplastin time, equivalent to 0.8–1.0 units of heparin/ml of plasma. In addition she gave antithrombin III concentrate at the time of labour [115] when heparin levels should be reduced to avoid the risk of bleeding. A similar approach was suggested by Brandt and Stenbjerg [35] and by Samson *et al.* [209]. Although it appears more elegant to perform a dose finding exercise in order to give the correct dose of antithrombin III to normalize antithrombin III levels at the time of delivery, this is quite difficult to achieve in practice. It is not easy for busy laboratories to perform repeat assays of antithrombin III over a period of days. We successfully managed one patient with antithrombin III deficiency by empirically giving her an infusion of 50 units/kg of antithrombin III on the day of delivery having stopped subcutaneous heparin on the previous day. After delivery heparin levels should be increased again to give the same degree of anticoagulation as was recommended for the antenatal period. One week after delivery, the patient could be fully warfarinized as in the non-pregnant state. Fresh frozen plasma may be a suitable alternative source of antithrombin III rather than antithrombin III concentrate [252].

Thrombosis is a recognized complication of venography to which patients with antithrombin III deficiency are particularly susceptible [245]. Such patients should either not have venography or, as Winter *et al.* [245] recommended, have venography using the less thrombogenic though more expensive contrast medium, metrizamide [7] washed through with heparin.

If thrombosis does occur in patients with antithrombin III deficiency they should be treated with heparin and antithrombin III concentrate [172,246]. Thrombolytic therapy has also been used in pregnancy in these circumstances [18].

Since thrombosis has occurred in the neonatal period [27] antithrombin III should be assayed in the neonate in at risk cases. Parents will also be anxious to know the status of their child. However, neonatal antithrombin levels in normals are about 50 per cent those of the adult level [191]. If the antithrombin III level is less than 30 per cent, antithrombin III concentrate should be given in the neonatal period because of the risk of thrombosis [209]. However, antithrombin III should be re-assayed when the child is at least 6 months before finalizing the diagnosis.

Protein C and S deficiencies

Protein C is another protein which after activation to protein Ca selectively inhibits Factors V and VIII [49]. Therefore a deficiency of protein C increases the risk of thromboembolism particularly in pregnancy [179].

Protein C deficiency is probably more common than antithrombin III deficiency, being present in 8 per cent of patients with a first episode of thromboembolism before age 40 and 7 per cent of patients with recurrent episodes [125]. In an unselected group of patients with deep vein thrombosis the prevalence was 3 per cent [113]. There is less experience than there is with antithrombin III deficiency concerning prophylaxis in pregnancy. Pregnancy was an associated factor in seven of 14 female cases of thromboembolism associated with protein C deficiency [125]. It has recently been suggested that protein C deficiency is associated with a bad obstetric outcome such as severe growth retardation or fulminating pre-eclampsia [25] in the same way as in the cardiolipin syndrome (see Chapter 8). Both protein C deficiency and the cardiolipin syndrome may adversely affect pregnancy by causing placental infarction.

Protein C deficiency may be inherited either as an autosomal dominant [39] or as a recessive [217] and functional abnormalities as well as deficiencies have been described [167]. The levels of both functional and immunological protein C do not change in pregnancy [242].

Heparin treatment is effective in the acute phase of thromboembolism and therefore subcutaneous heparin may provide adequate prophylaxis. Care should be taken with warfarin therapy since this has caused skin necrosis [38]. Assay of protein C is only available in specialist laboratories. Protein C concentrate is now available for the treatment of purpura fulminans (see below) [81]. It could in theory be used for the treatment of thrombotic episodes and the management of labour.

Protein C deficiency is amenable to perinatal diagnosis by fetal blood sampling in the second trimester [173].

Protein S is a cofactor for protein C. It exists in both free and bound forms. The level of free protein S is thought to be more important. By contrast with protein C, the level of free protein S falls by about 20 per cent by the end of the third trimester [150,242]. Families that are deficient in this protein have been described [51] and they have an increased risk of thromboembolism. However, their risk (if any) of developing thromboembolism in pregnancy has not been evaluated. The status of families with aberrant forms of fibrinogen [6,26] and plasminogen [12,226] is similar.

In an unselected group of patients with deep vein thrombosis the prevalence of protein S deficiency was 2 per cent [113]. Skin necrosis may also occur with warfarin treatment in protein S deficiency [107] but it is less common than in protein C deficiency. The neonate with protein C deficiency [166] and with homozygous protein S deficiency [162] is also at risk of massive bleeding into the skin, purpura fulminans.

A recent development is the discovery of Activated Protein C Resistance (APCR) [228a]. Activated Protein C inactivates Factor V. Patients with APCR inherit an abnormal form of Factor V which is resistant to activated Protein C. It is claimed that APCR may account for 25% of all cases of venous thromboembolism and we have detected such cases in pregnancy at Queen Charlotte's Hospital; but it would be premature to discuss the interaction between APCR and pregnancy.

Septic pelvic thrombophlebitis

This is a diagnosis made by exclusion. The patient has fever, usually following caesarean section, for which no cause can be found and which does not remit with appropriate antibiotic therapy. The more diligently the cause of a fever is sought, and the better the judgment in choice of antibiotic, the lower the incidence of 'septic pelvic thrombophlebitis'. Malkamy [163] found 11 patients in 1263 caesarean deliveries (0.9 per cent) over a 2.5-year period. In those cases where a laparotomy or venography has been performed, the thrombosis is often seen to start in the ovarian vein(s) and may extend into the inferior vena cava [202] and renal vein [15]. In these circumstances computed tomographic scanning to demonstrate clot in the inferior vena cava and renal vein may be helpful diagnostically [15].

References

1 Aaro KA & Juergens JL. Thrombophlebitis and pulmonary embolism as a complication of pregnancy. *Medical Clinics of North America* 1974; **58**: 829.

2 Aaro LA, Johnson TR & Juergens JL. Acute deep vein thrombosis associated with pregnancy. *Obstetrics and Gynecology* 1966; **28**: 553–8.

3 Aarskog D, Aksnes L & Lehmann V. Low 1, 25-dihydoroxyvitamin D in heparin-induced osteopenia. *Lancet* 1980; **ii**: 650–1.

4 Aarskog D, Aksnes L, Markestad T, Ulstein M & Sagen N. Heparin-induced inhibition of 1,25 dihydroxyvitamin D formation. *American Journal of Obstetrics and Gynecology* 1984; **148**: 1141–2.

5 Abbott A, Sibert JR & Weaver JB. Chondrodysplasia punctata and maternal warfarin treatment. *British Medical Journal* 1977; **i**: 1639–40.

6 Al-Mondhiry HAB, Bilezikian SB & Nossel HL. Fibrinogen — 'New York' — an abnormal fibrinogen association with thromboembolism: functional evaluation. *Blood* 1975; **45**: 607–19.

7 Albrechtsson U & Olsson CG. Thrombosis after phlebography: a comparison of two contrast media. *Cardiovascular Radiology* 1979; **2**: 9–18.

8 Amias AG. Streptokinase, cerebral vascular disease — and triplets. *British Medical Journal* 1977; **i**: 1414–15.

9 Anderson DR, Ginsberg JS, Burrows R & Brill-Edwards P. Subcutaneous heparin therapy during pregnancy: a need for concern at the time of delivery. *Thrombosis and Haemostasis* 1991; **65**: 248–50.

10 Andrew M, Bhogal M & Karpatkin M. Factors XI and XII and prekallikrein in sick and healthy premature infants. *New England Journal of Medicine* 1981; **305**: 1130–3.

11 Antiplatelet Trialists' Collaboration. Collaborative overview of randomised trials of antiplatelet therapy-III: Reduction in venous thrombosis and pulmonary embolism by antiplatelet prophylaxis among surgical and medical patients. *British Medical Journal* 1994; **308**: 235–46.

12 Aoki N, Moroi M, Sakata Y & Yoshida N. Abnormal plasminogen. A hereditary molecular abnormality found in a patient with recurrent thrombosis. *Journal of Clinical Investigation* 1978; **61**: 1186–95.

13 Avioli LV. Heparin-induced osteopenia: an appraisal. *Advances in Experimental Medicine and Biology* 1975; **52**: 375–87.

14 Badaracco MA & Vessey M. Recurrence of venous thromboembolism disease and use of oral contraceptives. *British Medical Journal* 1974; **i**: 215–17.

15 Bahnson RR, Wendel EF & Vogelzang RL. Renal vein thrombosis following puerperal ovarian vein thrombophlebitis. *American Journal of Obstetrics and Gynecology* 1985; **1**: 152–290.

16 Banfield PJ, Pittam M & Marwood R. Recurrent pulmonary embolism in pregnancy managed with the Greenfield vena caval filter. *International Journal of Gynecology and Obstetrics* 1990; **33**: 275–8.

17 Barritt DW & Jordan SC. Anticoagulant drugs in the treatment of pulmonary embolism: A controlled trial. *Lancet* 1960; **i**: 1309–12.

18 Baudo F, Caimi TM *et al*. Emergency treatment by recombinant tissue plasminogen activator of pulmonary embolism in a pregnant woman with antithrombin III deficiency. *American Journal of Obstetrics and Gynecology* 1990; **163**: 1274–5.

19 Becker MH, Genieser NB & Feingold M. Chondrodysplasia punctata: is maternal warfarin therapy a factor? *American Journal of Disease in Childhood* 1975; **129**: 356–7.

20 Bell WR & Meek AG. Guidelines for the use of thrombolytic agents. *New England Journal of Medicine* 1979; **301**: 1266–70.

21 Bergqvist A, Bergqvist D & Hallbrook T. Acute deep vein thrombosis (DVT) after Caesarean section. *Acta Obstetricia et Gynecologica Scandinavica* 1979; **58**: 473–6.

22 Bergqvist A, Bergqvist D, Lindhagen A & Matzsch T. Late symptoms after pregnancy-related deep vein thrombosis. *British Journal of Obstetrics and Gynaecology* 1990; **97**: 338–41.

23 Bergqvist D, Bergqvist D & Hallbrook T. Deep vein thrombosis during pregnancy. A prospective study. *Acta Obstetrica et Gynecologica Scandinavica* 1983; **62**: 443–8.

24 Bergqvist D & Hedner U. Pregnancy and venous thromboembolism. *Acta Obstetrica et Gynecologica Scandinavica* 1983; **62**: 449–53.

25 Bertault D, Mandelbrot L, Tchobroutsky C & Sultan Y. Unfavourable pregnancy outcome associated with congenital protein C deficiency. Case report. *British Journal of Obstetrics and Gynaecology* 1991; **98**: 934–6.

26 Bithell TC. Hereditary dysfibrinogenaemia — the first 25 years. *Acta Haematologica* 1984; **71**: 145–49.

27 Bjarte B, Herin P & Blomback M. Neonatal aortic thrombosis, a possible clinical manifestation of congenital antithrombin III deficiency. *Acta Paediatrica Scandinavica* 1974; **63**: 247–301.

28 Bonnar J. The blood coagulation and fibrinolytic systems in the newborn and the mother at birth. *British*

Journal of Obstetrics and Gynaecology 1971; **78**: 355.

29 Bonnar J. Thromboembolism in obstetric and gynaecological patients. In: AN Nicolaides (ed), *Thromboembolism Aetiology, Advances in Prevention and Management*. MTP Press, Lancaster, 1975: 311–34.

30 Bonnar J. Long-term self-administered heparin therapy for prevention and treatment of thromboembolic complications in pregnancy. In: Kakkar VV & Thomas DP (eds), *Heparin Chemistry and Clinical Usage*. Academic Press, London, 1976.

31 Bonnar J & Walsh J. Prevention of thrombosis after pelvic surgery by British dextran 70. *Lancet* 1972; **ii**: 614.

32 Bowler GMR, Galloway DW, Meiklejohn BH & Macintyre CCA. Sharp fall in blood pressure after injection of heparin containing chlorbutol. *Lancet* 1986; **i**: 848–9.

33 Brady AJB, Crake T & Oakley CM. Percutaneous catheter fragmentation and distal dispersion of proximal pulmonary embolus. *Lancet* 1991; **338**: 1186–9.

34 Brambel CE & Hunter RE. Effect of dicoumarol on the nursing infant. *American Journal of Obstetrics and Gynecology* 1950; **59**: 1153–9.

35 Brandt P & Stenbjerg A. Subcutaneous heparin for thrombosis in pregnant women with hereditary antithrombin deficiency. *Lancet* 1979; **i**: 100–1.

36 *British Medical Journal* Editorial. Venous thromboembolism and anticoagulants in pregnancy. *British Medical Journal* 1975; **ii**: 421–2.

37 British Society for Haematology. British Committee for standards of Haematology, Haemostasis and Thrombosis Task F. Guidelines on oral anticoagulation: second edition. *Journal of Clinical Pathology* 1990; **43**: 177–83.

38 Broekmans AW, Bertina RM, Loeliger EA, Hoffman V & Klingeman HG. Protein C and the development of skin necrosis during anticoagulant therapy. *Thrombosis and Haemostasis* 1983; **49**: 251.

39 Broekmans AW, Veltkamp JJ & Bertina RM. Congenital protein C deficiency and venous thromboembolism. A study of three Dutch families. *New England Journal of Medicine* 1983; **309**: 340–4.

40 Browse N. Diagnosis of deep vein thrombosis. *British Medical Bulletin* 1978; **34**: 163–67.

41 Calhoun BC & Hesser JW. Heparin-associated antibody with pregnancy: Discussion of two cases. *American Journal of Obstetrics and Gynecology* 1987; **156**: 964–6.

42 Chen WWC, Chan CS, Lee PR, Wang RYR & Wong VCW. Pregnancy in patients with prosthetic heart valves: An experience with 45 pregnancies. *Quarterly Journal of Medicine* 1982; **51**: 358–65.

43 Chong BH, Pitney WR & Castaldi PA. Heparin-induced thrombocytopenia: association of thrombotic complications with heparin-independent IgG antibody that induces thromboxane synthesis and platelet aggregation. *Lancet* 1982; **ii**: 1246–8.

44 Chong MKB, Harvey D & de Swiet M. Follow-up study of children whose mothers were treated with warfarin during pregnancy. *British Journal of Obstetrics and Gynaecology* 1984; **91**: 1070–3.

45 Cines DB, Kaywin P, Bina M, Tomaski A & Schreiber AD. Heparin-associated thrombocytopenia. *New England Journal of Medicine* 1980; **303**: 788–95.

46 Cines DB, Tomaski A & Tannenbaum S. Immune endothelial-cell injury in heparin-associated thrombocytopenia. *New England Journal of Medicine* 1987; **316**: 581–9.

47 Clarke Pearson DL & Jelovsek FR. Alternatives of occlusion cuff impedance plethysmography in the obstetric patient. *Surgery* 1981; **89**: 594–8.

48 Clayton JK, Anderson JA & McNicol GP. Preoperative prediction of postoperative deep vein thrombosis. *British Medical Journal* 1976; **ii**: 910–12.

49 Clouse LH & Comp RC. The regulation of hemostasis: the protein C system. *New England Journal of Medicine* 1986; **314**: 1298–304.

50 Cohen AW, Gabbe SG & Mennuti MT. Adjusted-dose heparin therapy by continuous intravenous infusion for recurrent pulmonary embolism during pregnancy. *American Journal of Obstetrics and Gynecology* 1983; **146**: 463–4.

51 Comp PC & Esmon CT. Recurrent venous thromboembolism in patients with a partial deficiency of protein S. *New England Journal of Medicine* 1984; **311**: 1525–8

52 Conard J, Horellou MH, van Dreden P, LeCompte T & Samama M. Thrombosis and pregnancy in congenital deficiencies in ATIII, protein C or protein S: Study of 78 women. *Thrombosis and Haemostasis* 1990; **63**: 319–20.

53 Constantine G & Green A. Untreated homocystinuria: a maternal death in a woman with four pregnancies. *British Journal of Obstetrics and Gynaecology* 1987; **94**: 803–6.

54 Cox DR, Martin L. & Hall BD. Asplenia syndrome after fetal exposure to warfarin. *Lancet* 1977; **ii**: 1134.

55 Crandon AJ, Peel KR, Anderson JA, Thompson V & McNicol GP. Postoperative deep vein thrombosis: identifying high-risk patients. *British Medical Journal* 1980; **281**: 343–4.

56 Crawford JS. *Principles and Practice of Obstetric Anaesthesia*, 4th edn. Blackwell Scientific Publications, Oxford, 1978: 182–3.

57 Curry CJR, Magenis RE *et al*. Inherited chondrodysplasia punctata due to a deletion of the terminal short arm of X chromosome. *New England Journal of Medicine* 1984; **311**: 1010–15.

58 Dacie J. *Practical Haematology*. Churchill Livingstone, Edinburgh, 1975: 413–14.

59 Dahlman TC, Hellgren MSE & Blomback M. Thrombosis prophylaxis in pregnancy with use of subcutaneous heparin adjusted by monitoring heparin concentration in plasma. *American Journal of Obstetrics and Gynecology* 1989; **161**: 420–5.

60 Dahlman T, Sjoberg HE, Hellgren M & Bucht E. Cal-

cium homeostasis in pregnancy during long-term heparin treatment. *British Journal of Obstetrics and Gynaecology* 1992; **99**: 412–16.

61 Dalaker K. Clotting factor VII during pregnancy, delivery and puerperium. *British Journal of Obstetrics and Gynaecology* 1986; **93**: 17–21.

62 Dahlmann TC. Osteoporotic fractures and the recurrence of thromboembolism during pregnancy and the puerperium in 184 women undergoing thromboprophylaxis with heparin. *American Journal of Obstetrics and Gynecology* 1993; **168**: 1265–70.

63 Dalhman T, Lindvall N & Hellgren M. Osteopenia in pregnancy during long-term heparin treatment: A radiological study post partum. *British Journal of Obstetrics and Gynaecology* 1990; **97**: 221–8.

64 Daly M, O'Meara A & Hallinan F. Characterisation of a novel mutant form of antithrombin III (antithrombin 'Dubin'). *Clinical Science* 1986; **71**: 84P.

65 Daniel DG, Campbell H & Turnbull AC. Puerperal thromboembolism and suppression of lactation. *Lancet* 1967; **ii**: 287.

66 Davies JA. The pre-thrombotic state. *Clinical Science* 1985; **69**: 641–6.

67 de Swiet M. Thromboembolism in obstetrics. *Current Obstetrics and Gynaecology* 1991; **1**: 191–5.

68 de Swiet M. Thromboembolism in pregnancy. In James DK, Steer PJ, Weiner CP & Gonik B (eds), *High Risk Pregnancy*. WB Saunders, London, 1992.

69 de Swiet M. Thromboembolism in pregnancy. In: Ledingham JGG, Warrell DA & Weatherall D. *Oxford Textbook of Medicine*, 3rd edn. Oxford University Press, Oxford, 1995.

70 de Swiet M, Bulpitt CJ & Lewis PJ. How obstetricians use anticoagulants in the prophylaxis of thromboembolism. *Journal of Obstetrics and Gynaecology* 1980; **1**: 29–32.

71 de Swiet M, Dorrington Ward P *et al*. Prolonged heparin therapy in pregnancy causes bone demineralisation (heparin induced-osteopenia). *British Journal of Obstetrics and Gynaecology* 1983; **90**: 1129–34.

72 de Swiet M, Fidler J, Howell R & Letsky E. Thromboembolism in pregnancy. In: Jewell DP (ed), *Advanced Medicine* **17**. Pitman Medical, London, 1981: 309–17.

73 de Swiet M, Letsky E & Mellows H. Drug treatment and prophylaxis of thromboembolism in pregnancy. In: Lewis PJ (ed), *Therapeutic Problems in Pregnancy*. MTP Press, Lancaster, 1977: 81–9.

74 Decousus HA, Croze M *et al*. Circadian changes in anticoagulant effect of heparin infused at a constant rate. *British Medical Journal* 1985; **290**: 341–4.

75 Denson KWE & Bonnar J. The measurement of heparin: a method based on the potentiation of anti-factor Xa. *Thrombosis et Diathesis Haemorrhagica* 1973; **30**: 471.

76 Department of Health and Social Security. *Report on Confidential Enquiries into Maternal Deaths in England and Wales, 1973–1975*. HMSO, London, 1979.

77 Department of Health and Social Security. *Report on Confidential Enquiries into Maternal Deaths in England and Wales, 1975–1978*. HMSO, London, 1982.

78 Department of Health and Social Security. *Report on Confidential Enquiries into Maternal Deaths in England and Wales 1979–1981*. HMSO, London, 1986.

79 Department of Health. *Report on Confidential Enquiries into Maternal Deaths in the United Kingdom 1985–87*. HMSO, London, 1991.

80 Department of Health. *Report on Confidential Enquiries into Maternal Deaths in the United Kingdom 1988–1990*. HMSO, London, 1994.

81 Dreyfus M, Magny JF *et al*. Treatment of homozygous protein C deficiency and neonatal purpura fulminans with a purified protein C concentrate. *New England Journal of Medicine* 1991; **325**: 1565–8.

82 Duff P & Greene VP. Pregnancy complicated by solid-papillary epithelial tumour of the pancreas, pulmonary embolism and pulmonary embolectomy. *American Journal of Obstetrics and Gynecology* 1985; **1**: 152–80.

83 Duthie SJ, Ghosh A & Ma HK. Maternal mortality in Hong Kong 1961–1985. *British Journal of Obstetrics and Gynaecology* 1989; **96**: 4–8.

84 Eckstein H & Jack B. Breast feeding and anticoagulant therapy. *Lancet* 1970; **i**: 672–3.

85 Eichinger S, Kyrle PA *et al*. Thrombocytopenia associated with low-molecular-weight heparin. *Lancet* 1991; **337**: 1425–6.

86 Elliot MS, Immelman EJ *et al*. A comparative trial of heparin versus streptokinase in the treatment of acute proximal venous thrombosis: an interim report of a prospective trial. *British Journal of Surgery* 1979; **66**: 838–43.

87 Estes JW. Kinetics of the anticoagulation effect of heparin. *Journal of the American Medical Association* 1970; **212**: 1492.

88 Excess R & Graeme B. Congenital athyroidism in the newborn infant from intrauterine radioactive iodine. *Biology of the Neonate* 1974; **24**: 289–91.

89 Fennerty A, Campbell IA & Routledge PA. Anticoagulants in venous thromboembolism. *British Medical Journal* 1988; **297**: 1285–7.

90 Fennerty AG & Levine MN. Non-biological factors in day to day variation of heparin requirements. *British Medical Journal* 1989; **299**: 1009–13.

91 Finazzi C, Caccia R & Barboi T. Different prevalence of thromboembolism in the subtypes of congenital antithrombin III deficiency: Review of 404 cases. *Thrombosis and Haemostasis* 1987; **58**: 1094.

92 Finnerty JJ & MacKay BR. Antepartum thrombophlebitis and pulmonary embolism. *Obstetrics and Gynecology* 1962; **19**: 405.

93 Flessa HC, Glueck HI & Dritshilo A. Thromboembolic disorders in pregnancy. *Clinical Obstetrics and Gynaecology* 1974; **17**: 195.

94 Flute PT. Thrombolytic therapy. *British Journal of Hospital Medicine* 1976; **16**: 135–42.

95 Forestier F, Daffos F & Capella-Pavlovsky M. Low molecular weight heparin (PK 10169) does not cross the placenta during the second trimester of pregnancy: study by direct fetal blood sampling under ultrasound. *Thrombosis Research* 1984; **34**: 557–60.

96 Friend JR & Kakkar VV. Deep vein thrombosis in obstetric and gynaecological patients. In: Kakkar W & AJ (eds) *Thromboembolism, Diagnosis and Treatment*. Churchill Livingstone, London, 1972: 131–8.

97 Gallus AS. Venous thromboembolism; incidence and clinical risk factors. In: Madden JL & Hume M (eds), *Venous Thromboembolism*. Appleton-Century-Crofts, New York, 1976.

98 Ginsberg JS, Kowah Chuk G *et al*. Heparin effect on bone density. *Thrombosis and Haemostasis* 1990; **64**: 286–9.

99 Girard P, Mathieu M *et al*. Recurrence of pulmonary embolism during anticoagulant treatment: a prospective study. *Thorax* 1987; **42**: 481–6.

100 Grant PJ & Medcalf RL. Hormonal regulation of haemostasis and the molecular biology of the fibrinolytic system. *Clinical Science* 1990; **78**: 3–11.

101 Gray HH & Miller GAH. Pulmonary embolectomy is still appropriate for a minority of patients with acute massive pulmonary embolism. *British Journal of Hospital Medicine* 1989; **41**: 467–8.

102 Gray HH, Miller GAH & Paneth M. Pulmonary embolectomy: Its place in the management of pulmonary embolism. *Lancet* 1988; **i**: 1441–4.

103 Greer IA, Barry J, Mackon N & Allan PL. Diagnosis of deep venous thrombosis in pregnancy: a new role for diagnostic ultrasound. *British Journal of Obstetrics and Gynaecology* 1990; **97**: 53–7.

104 Greer IA & de Swiet M. Thrombosis prophylaxis in Obstetrics and Gynaecology. *British Journal of Obstetrics and Gynaecology* 1993; **100**: 37–9.

105 Griffith GC, Nichols G, Asher JD & Hanagan B. Heparin osteoporosis. *Journal of the American Medical Association* 1965; **193**: 91–4.

106 Griffiths HT & Liu DTY. Severe heparin osteoporosis in pregnancy. *Postgraduate Medical Journal* 1984; **60**: 424–5.

107 Grimaudo V, Gueissaz F, Hauert J, Sarraj A, Kruithof EKO & Bachman F. Necrosis of skin induced by coumarin in a patient deficient in protein S. *British Medical Journal* 1989; **298**: 233–4.

108 Gurll W, Helfand Z, Salzman EF & Silen W. Peripheral venous thrombophlebitis during pregnancy. *American Journal of Surgery* 1971; **121**: 449–53.

109 Hall JG. Warfarin and fetal abnormality. *Lancet* 1976; **i**: 1127.

110 Hall JG, Pauli RM & Wilson KM. Maternal and fetal sequelae of anticoagulation during pregnancy. *American Journal of Medicine* 1980; **68**: 122–40.

111 Hall RJC, Young C, Sutton GC & Cambell S. Treatment of acute massive pulmonary embolism by streptokinase during labour and delivery. *British Medical Journal* 1972; **iv**: 647–9.

112 Hatjis CG. Heparin-induced thrombocytopenia in pregnancy. A case report. *Journal of Reproductive Medicine* 1984; **29**: 337–8.

113 Heijboer H, Brandjes DPM, Buller HR, Sturk A & ten Cate WJ. Deficiencies of coagulation-inhibiting and fibrinolytic proteins in outpatients with deep-vein thrombosis. *New England Journal of Medicine* 1990; **323**: 1512–16.

114 Heimbecker RO, Keon WJ & Richards KU. Massive pulmonary embolism: a new look at surgical management. *Archives of Surgery* 1973; **107**: 740–6.

115 Hellgren M. *Thromboembolism and Pregnancy*. MD Thesis, Karolinska Institute, Stockholm, 1981.

116 Hellgren M & Nygards EB. Long term therapy with subcutaneous heparin during pregnancy. *Gynecological and Obstetric Investigation* 1981; **13**: 76–89.

117 Hellgren M, Tengborn L & Abildgaard U. Pregnancy in women with congenital antithrombin III deficiency: Experience of treatment with heparin and antithrombin. *Gynecological and Obstetric Investigation* 1982; **14**: 127–41.

118 Henderson SR, Lund CJ & Creasman WT. Antepartum pulmonary embolism. *American Journal of Obstetrics and Gynecology* 1972; **112**: 476–86.

119 Hiilesma VK. Occurrence and anticoagulant treatment of thromboembolism in gravidas, parturients and gynecologic patients. *Acta Obstetrica et Gynecologica Scandinavica* 1960; **39**: 5.

120 Hill NCW, Hill JG, Sargent JM, Taylor CG & Bush PV. Effect of low dose heparin on blood loss at caesarean section. *British Medical Journal* 1988; **296**: 1505–6.

121 Hirsh J. Heparin. *New England Journal of Medicine* 1991; **324**: 1565–74.

122 Hirsh J, Cade JF & O'Sullivan EF. Clinical experience with anticoagulant therapy during pregnancy. *British Medical Journal* 1970; **i**: 270–3.

123 Hix CH, Wapner RJ, Chayen B, Ratten P, Jarrell B & Greenfield L. Use of the Greenfield filter for thromboembolic disease in pregnancy. *American Journal of Obstetrics and Gynecology* 1986; **155**: 734–7.

124 Holzgreve W, Carey JC & Hall BD. Warfarin-induced fetal abnormalities. *Lancet* 1976; **ii**: 914–15.

125 Horellou MH, Conard J, Bertina RM & Samana M. Congenital protein C deficiency and thrombotic disease in nine French families. *British Medical Journal* 1984; **289**: 1285–7.

126 Howell R, Fidler J, Letsky E & de Swiet M. The risks of antenatal subcutaneous heparin prophylaxis: a controlled trial. *British Journal of Obstetrics and Gynaecology* 1983; **90**: 1124–8.

127 Howie PW. Blood clotting and fibrinolysis in pregnancy. *Postgraduate Medical Journal* 1979; **55**: 362–6.

128 Huisman MY, Buller HR, ten Cate JW & Vreeken J. Serial impedance plethysmography for suspected deep vein thrombosis in patients. The Amsterdam Research Practitioners Study. *New England Journal of Medicine* 1986; **314**: 823–8.

129 Hull R, Hirsh J & Sackett DL. Combined use of leg

scanning and impedance plethysmography in suspected venous thrombosis. An alternative to venography. *New England Journal of Medicine* 1977; **296**: 1497–500.

130 Hull R, Hirsh J *et al*. Replacement of venography in suspected venous thrombosis by impedance plethysmography and 125I-fibrinogen leg scanning: a less invasive approach. *Annals of Internal Medicine* 1981; **94**: 12–15.

131 Hull RD, Hirsh J *et al*. Diagnostic efficacy of impedance plethysmography of clinically suspected deep-vein thrombosis. *Annals of Internal Medicine* 1985; **102**: 21–8.

132 Hull RD, Raskob GE, Coates G & Panju AA. Clinical validity of a normal perfusion lung scan in patients with suspected pulmonary embolism. *Chest* 1990; **91**: 23–6.

133 Hull RD, Raskob GE *et al*. Subcutaneous low-molecular-weight heparin compared with continuous intravenous heparin in the treatment of proximal-vein thrombosis. *New England Journal of Medicine* 1992; **326**: 975–82.

134 Hull RD, Raskob GE *et al*. Heparin for 5 days as compared with 10 days in the initial treatment of proximal venous thrombosis. *New England Journal of Medicine* 1990; **322**: 1260–4.

135 Hume M, Sevitt S & Thomas DP. *Thrombosis and Pulmonary Embolism*. Harvard University Press, Cambridge, Massachusetts, 1970.

136 Islam T. Portal vein thrombosis in pregnancy. *Journal of Obstetrics and Gynaecology* 1984; **4**: 242.

137 Jacobs J, Kletter I, Superstine E, Hill KR, Lynn B & Webb RA. Intravenous infusions of heparin and penicillins. *Journal of Clinical Pathology* 1973; **26**: 742–6.

138 Jaffe MD & Willis PW. Multiple fractures associated with long-term sodium heparin therapy. *Journal of the American Medical Association* 1965; **193**: 152–4.

139 Jeffcoate TNA, Miller J, Ros RF & Tindall VR. Puerpural thromboembolism in relation to the inhibition of lactation by oestrogen therapy. *British Medical Journal* 1968; **iv**: 19.

140 Jick H, Slone D *et al*. Venous thromboembolic disease and ABO blood group. A cooperative study. *Lancet* 1969; **i**: 539–42.

141 Kaaja R, Seigberg R, Titinen A & Koskimies A. Severe ovarian hyperstimulation syndrome and deep venous thrombosis. *Lancet* 1989; **ii**: 1043.

142 Kerber IJ, Warr OS III & Richardson C. Pregnancy in a patient with a prosthetic mitral valve associated with a fetal anomaly attributed to warfarin sodium. *Journal of the American Medical Association* 1968; **203**: 223–5.

143 Kierkegaard A. Incidence and diagnosis of deep vein thrombosis associated with pregnancy. *Acta Obstetrica et Gynecologica Scandinavica* 1983; **62**: 239–43.

144 Kimball AM, Hallum AV & Cates W. Deaths caused by pulmonary thromboembolism after legally induced abortion. *American Journal of Obstetrics and Gynecology* 1978; **132**: 169–74.

145 Lamon JM, Lenke RR, Levy HL, Schulmann JD & Shih VE. Selected metabolic diseases. In: Schulmann JD & Simpson JL (eds), *Genetic Diseases in Pregnancy*. Academic Press, New York, 1980: 6–8.

146 *Lancet* editorial. Familial antithrombin III deficiency. *Lancet* 1983; **i**: 1021–2.

147 *Lancet* editorial. Thrombolysis for pulmonary embolism. *Lancet* 1992; **340**: 21–2.

148 Lansing AM & Davies WM. Five year follow-up study of ilio femoral venous thromboectomy. *Annals of Surgery* 1968; **168**: 620–8.

149 Lao TT, de Swiet M, Letsky E & Walters BNJ. Prophylaxis of thromboembolism in pregnancy: an alternative. *British Journal of Obstetrics and Gynaecology* 1985; **92**: 202–6.

150 Lao TT, Yuen PMP & Yin JA. Protein S and protein C levels in Chinese women during pregnancy, delivery and the puerperium. *British Journal of Obstetrics and Gynaecology* 1989; **96**: 167–70.

151 Laros RK & Alger LS. Thromboembolism and pregnancy. *Clinical Obstetrics and Gynecology* 1979; **22**: 871–88.

152 LeCompte T, Luo SK, Stieltjes N, Lecrubier C & Samama MM. Thrombocytopenia associated with low-molecular-weight heparin. *Lancet* 1991; **338**: 1217.

153 Lensing AWA, Prandoni P *et al*. Detection of deep-vein thrombosis by real-time B-mode ultrasonography. *New England Journal of Medicine* 1989; **320**: 342–5.

154 Letsky EA. *Coagulation Problems during Pregnancy* Churchill Livingstone, Edinburgh, 1985.

155 Letsky EA. Haemostasis and epidural anaesthesia. *International Journal of Obstetric Anesthesia* 1991; **1**: 51–4.

156 Letsky E & de Swiet M. Maternal haemostasis. Coagulation problems of pregnancy. In: Loscalzo J & Schafer AI (eds), *Thrombosis and Haemorrhage*. Blackwell Scientific Publications, Oxford, 1992.

157 Li TC, Smith ARB & Duncan SLB. Feto-maternal haemorrhage complicating warfarin therapy during pregnancy. *Journal of Obstetrics and Gynaecology* 1990; **10**: 401–2.

158 Lowe GDO, Cooke T *et al*. Thromboembolic risk factors (THRIFT) risks of and prophylaxis for venous thromboembolism in hospital patients. *British Medical Journal* 1992; **305**: 567–74.

159 Ludlam CA, Bolton AE, Moore S & Cash JD. New rapid method of diagnosis of deep vein thrombosis. *Lancet* 1975; **ii**: 259–60.

160 Ludwig H. Results of streptokinase therapy in deep vein thrombosis during pregnancy. *Postgraduate Medical Journal* 1973; **49** (suppl. 5): 65–7.

161 Mackie M, Bennett B, Ogston D & Douglas A. Familial thrombosis: inherited deficiency of antithrombin III. *British Medical Journal* 1978; **i**: 136–8.

162 Mahasandana C, Suvatte V *et al*. Neonatal purpura fulminans associated with homozygous protein S deficiency. *Lancet* 1990; **335**: 61–2.
163 Malkamy H. Heparin therapy in post Caesarean septic pelvic thrombophlebitis. *International Journal of Gynaecology and Obstetrics* 1980; **17**: 564–6.
164 Marciniak E & Gockerman JP. Heparin-induced decrease in circulating antithrombin III. *Lancet* 1977; **ii**: 581–4.
165 Marcus CS, Mason GR, Kuperus JH & Mena I. Pulmonary imaging in pregnancy maternal risk and fetal dosimetry. *Clinical Nuclear Medicine* 1985; **10**: 1–4.
166 Marciniak E, Wilson HD & Marlar RA. Neonatal purpura fulminans: a genetic disorder related to the absence of Protein C in blood. *Blood* 1950; **65**: 15–20 (abstract).
167 Matsuda M, Sugo T *et al*. A thrombotic state due to an abnormal protein C. *New England Journal of Medicine* 1988; **319**: 1265–8.
168 Matzsch T, Bergqvist D, Hedner V, Nildson B & Ostergaard P. Effects of low molecular weight heparin and unfractionated heparin on induction of osteoporosis in rats. *Thrombosis and Haemostasis* 1990; **63**: 505–9.
169 Mayor GE. Deep vein thrombosis — surgical management. *British Medical Journal* 1969; **iv**: 680–2.
170 McCausland AM, Hyman C, Winsor T & Trotter AD. Venous distensibility during pregnancy. *American Journal of Obstetrics and Gynecology* 1961; **81**: 472–9.
171 McTaggart DR & Engram TC. Massive pulmonary embolism during pregnancy treated with streptokinase. *Medical Journal of Australia* 1977; **1**: 18–20.
172 Megha A, Finzi G, Poli T, Manotti C & Dettori AG. Bilateral deep vein thrombosis in a pregnant woman with antithrombin III deficiency: treatment of acute episodes and preparation for delivery with replacement treatment. *Journal of Obstetrics and Gynaecology* 1990; **10**: 220–1.
173 Mibashan RS, Millar DS, Rodeck CJ, Nicolaides KH, Berger A & Seigsohn U. Prenatal diagnosis of hereditary protein C deficiency. *New England Journal of Medicine* 1985; **313**: 1607.
174 Milne R. Venous thromboembolism and travel: is there an association? *Journal of the Royal College of Physicians of London* 1992; **26**: 47–9.
175 Misra R & Anderson DC. Providing the fetus with calcium. *British Medical Journal* 1991; **300**: 1220–1.
176 Monreal M, Olive A, Lafoz & Del Rio L. Heparins, coumarin, and bone density. *Lancet* 1991; **338**: 706.
177 Morrell NW & Seed WA. Diagnosing pulmonary embolism. *British Medical Journal* 1992; **304**: 1126–7.
178 Morris GK & Mitchell JRA. Clinical management of venous thromboembolism. *British Medical Bulletin* 1978; **34**: 169–75.
179 Morrison AE, Walker ID & Black WP. Protein C deficiency presenting as deep venous thrombosis in pregnancy. Case report. *British Journal of Obstetrics and Gynaecology* 1988; **95**: 1077–80.
180 Moseley P & Kerstein MD. Pregnancy and thrombophlebitis. *Surgery, Gynecology and Obstetrics* 1980; **150**: 593–7.
181 Mudd SH, Skovby F *et al*. The natural history of homocystinemia due to cystathionine β-synthatase deficiency. *American Journal of Human Genetics* 1985; **37**: 1–31.
182 Mukherjee D, Anderson CA, Sado AS & Bertoglio MC. Use of light reflection rheography for diagnosis of axillary or subclavian venous thrombosis. *American Journal of Surgery* 1991; **161**: 651–6.
183 Mussein IY & Critchey HOD. An unusual presentation of pulmonary thromboembolism in late pregnancy. Case report. *British Journal of Obstetrics and Gynaecology* 1986; **93**: 1161–2.
184 National Institute of Health. Consensus Conference Thrombolytic Therapy in Treatment of Pulmonary Embolus. *British Medical Journal* 1980; **280**: 1585–7.
185 Nelson DM, Stempel LE, Fabri PJ & Talbert M. Hickman catheter use in a pregnant patient requiring therapeutic heparin anticoagulation. *American Journal of Obstetrics and Gynecology* 1984; **149**: 461–2.
186 Nielsen TF & Hokegard K-H. Postoperative caesarean section morbidity. A prospective study. *American Journal of Obstetrics and Gynecology* 1983; **146**: 911–16.
187 O'Donnel D, Sevitz H, Seggie JL, Meyers AM, Botha JR & Myburgh JA. Pregnancy after renal transplantation. *Australian and New Zealand Journal of Medicine* 1985; **15**: 320–5.
188 Oakley CM & Hawkins DF. Pregnancy in patients with prosthetic heart valves. *British Medical Journal* 1983; **287**: 358.
189 Orme ML'E, Lewis PJ *et al*. May mothers given warfarin breast-feed their infants? *British Medical Journal* 1977; **i**: 1564–5.
190 Paull JA. Retrospective study of dextran-induced anaphylactoid reactions in 5745 patients. *Anaesthesia and Intensive Care* 1987; **15**: 163–7.
191 Peters M, Jansen E, ten Cate JW, Kahle LH, Ockleford P & Brederveld D. Neonatal antithrombin III. *British Journal of Haematology* 1984; **58**: 579–87.
192 Pettifor JM & Benson R. Congenital malformations associated with the administration of oral anticoagulants during pregnancy. *Journal of Pediatrics* 1975; **86**: 459–62.
193 Pfeiffer GW. Distribution and placental transfer of ^{141}I streptokinase. *Australasian Annals of Medicine* 1970; (suppl) 17–18.
194 Pfeiffer GW. The use of thrombolytic therapy in obstetrics and gynaecology. *Australasian Annals of Medicine* 1970; (suppl): 28–31.
195 Polak JF & Wilkinson DL. Ultrasonographic diagnosis of symptomatic deep vein venous thrombosis in pregnancy. *American Journal of Obstetrics and Gynecology* 1991; **165**: 625–9.
196 Prandoni P, Lensing AWA *et al*. Comparison of subcutaneous low-molecular-weight with intravenous standard heparin in proximal deep-vein thrombosis. *Lancet* 1992; **339**: 441–5.

197 Preissner KT. Biological relevance of the protein C system and laboratory diagnosis of protein C and protein S deficiencies. *Clinical Science* 1990; **78**: 351–64.
198 Preston Flanigan D, Goodreau JJ, Burnham SJ, Bergan JJ & Yao JST. Vascular laboratory diagnosis of clinically suspected acute deep vein thrombosis. *Lancet* 1978; **i**: 331–4.
199 Pridmore BR, Murray KH & McAllen PM. The management of anticoagulant therapy during and after pregnancy. *British Journal of Obstetrics and Gynaecology* 1975; **82**: 740–4.
200 Prochownik EV, Antonarakis S, Bauer KA, Rosenberg RD, Fearon ER & Orkin SH. Molecular heterogenicity of inherited anti-thrombin III deficiency. *New England Journal of Medicine* 1983; **308**: 1549–52.
201 Rabinovici J, Mani A, Barkai G, Hod H, Frenkel Y & Mashiach S. Long term ambulatory anticoagulation by constant subcutaneous heparin infusion in pregnancy. *British Journal of Obstetrics and Gynaecology* 1987; **94**: 89–91
202 Raja Rao AK, Zucker M & Sacks D. Right ovarian vein thrombosis with extension to the inferior vena cava. *British Journal of Radiology* 1980; **53**: 160–1.
203 Ramsay LE. Impact of venography on the diagnosis and management of deep vein thrombosis. *British Medical Journal* 1983; **286**: 698–9.
204 Robin ED. Overdiagnosis and overtreatment of pulmonary embolism: The emperor may have no clothes. *Annals of Internal Medicine* 1977; **87**: 775–81.
205 Royal College of General Practitioners. Oral contraception and thrombo-embolic disease. *Journal of the Royal College of General Practitioners* 1967; **13**: 267–9.
206 Sachs BP, Brown DAJ *et al*. Maternal mortality in Massachusetts. Trends and prevention. *New England Journal of Medicine* 1987; **316**: 667–72.
207 Salzman EW. Low-molecular-weight heparin. Is small beautiful? *New England Journal of Medicine* 1986; **315**: 957–9.
208 Salzman EW, Deykin D, Shapiro RM & Rosenberg R. Management of heparin therapy — controlled prospective trial. *New England Journal of Medicine* 1975; **292**: 1046–50.
209 Samson D, Stirling Y, Wolf L, Howarth D, Seghatchian MJ & de Chazel R. Management of planned pregnancy in a patient with congenital antithrombin III deficiency. *British Journal of Haematology* 1984; **56**: 243–9.
210 Sandler DA & Martin JF. Liquid crystal thermography as a screening test for deep-vein thrombosis. *Lancet* 1985; **i**: 665–8.
211 Sandler DA, Martin JF *et al*. Diagnosis of deep-vein thrombosis: comparison of clinical evaluation, ultrasound, plethysmograph and venoscan with X-ray venogram. *Lancet* 1984; **ii**: 716–19.
212 Sarvesranan R. Sudden natural deaths associated with commercial air-travel. *Medicine, Science and the Law* 1986; **26**: 35–8.
213 Sas G, Blasko G, Banhegy D, Jake L & Palos LA. Abnormal antithrombin III (antithrombin III 'Budapest') as a cause of familial thrombophilia. *Thrombosis et Diathesis Haemorrhagica* 1974; **32**: 105–15.
214 Sasahara AA. Therapy for pulmonary embolism. *Journal of the American Medical Association* 1974; **229**: 1795.
215 Sasahara AA & Barsamian EM. Another look at pulmonary embolectomy. *Annals of Thoracic Surgery* 1973; **16**: 317–20.
216 Sautter RD. In: Fratantoni J & Wessler S (eds), *Prophylactic Therapy of Deep Vein Thrombosis and Pulmonary Embolism*. National Institutes of Health, Betheseda, 1975: 137–42.
217 Seligsohn U, Berger A *et al*. Homozygous protein C deficiency manifested by massive venous thrombosis in the new born. *New England Journal of Medicine* 1984; **310**: 559–62.
218 Sharma GVRK, Burlesco VA & Sasahara AA. Effect of thrombolytic therapy on pulmonary capillary blood volume in patients with pulmonary embolism. *New England Journal of Medicine* 1980; **303**: 842–5.
219 Shaul WL, Emery H & Hall JG. Chondrodysplasia punctata and maternal warfarin use during pregnancy. *American Journal of Diseases in Children* 1975; **129**: 360–2.
220 Shaul WL & Hall JG. Multiple congenital anomalies associated with anticoagulants. *American Journal of Obstetrics and Gynecology* 1977; **127**: 191–8.
221 Sheffield LJ, Danks DM, Mayne V & Hutchinson LA. Chondrodysplasia punctata — 23 cases of mild and relatively common variety. *Journal of Pediatrics* 1976; **89**: 916–23.
222 Sherman S & Hall BD. Warfarin and fetal abnormality. *Lancet* 1976; **i**: 692.
223 Silver D & Sabiston DC. The role of vena caval interruption in the management of pulmonary embolism. *Surgery* 1975; **77**: 3–10.
224 Simpson FG, Robinson PJ, Bark M & Losowsky MS. Prospective study of thrombophlebitis and pseudo thrombophlebitis. *Lancet* 1980; **i**: 331–3.
225 Smith MF & Cameron MD. Warfarin as teratogen. *Lancet* 1979; **i**: 727.
226 Sorin J, Soria C, Bertrand O, Dunn F, Drovet L & Caen JP. Plasminogen Paris 1: congenital abnormal plasminogen and its incidence in thrombosis. *Thrombosis Research* 1983; **32**: 229–38.
227 Squires JW & Pinch LW. Heparin induced spinal fractures. *Journal of the American Medical Association* 1979; **241**: 2417–18.
228 Sturridge F, Letsky E & de Swiet M. The use of low molecular weight heparin for thromboprophylaxis. *British Journal of Obstetrics and Gynaecology* 1994; **101**: 69–71.
228a Svensson PJ & Dahlbäck B. Resistance to activated Protein C as a basis for venous thrombosis. *New England Journal of Medicine* 1994; **330**: 517–22.

229 Szekely P, Turner R & Snaith L. Pregnancy and the changing pattern of rheumatic heart disease. *British Heart Journal* 1973; **35**: 1293–303.

230 The British Committee for Standards of Haematology. Guidelines on the investigation and management of thrombophilia. *Journal of Clinical Pathology* 1990; **43**: 703–9.

231 Thomas AN, Pattison C & Serjeant GR. Causes of death in sickle-cell disease in Jamaica. *British Medical Journal* 1982; **285**: 633–5.

232 Thomas EA, Cobby MJD, Rhys Davies E, Jeans WD & Whicher JT. Liquid crystal thermography and C reactive protein in the detection of deep venous thrombosis. *British Medical Journal* 1989; **299**: 951–2.

233 Thomas ML, Keeling FP, Piaggio RB & Treweeke PS. Constrast agent induced thrombophlebitis following leg phlebography: iopamidol versus meglumine iothalamate. *British Journal of Radiology* 1984; **57**: 205–7.

234 Treffers PE, Huidekoper BL, Weenik GH & Kloosterman GJ. Epidemiological observations of thrombo-embolic disease during pregnancy and in the puerperium in 56 022 women. *International Journal of Gynaecology and Obstetrics* 1983; **21**: 327–31.

235 Tribukait B & Swedjemark GA. Secretion of 99TcM in breast milk after intravenous injection of marked macroaggregated albumin. *Acta Radiologica Oncology* 1978; **17**: 379–82.

236 Urokinase Pulmonary Embolism Trial Study Group. Urokinase pulmonary embolism trial: Phase 1. *Journal of the American Medical Association* 1970; **214**: 2163–72.

237 Van Dinh T, Boor PJ & Garza JR. Massive pulmonary embolism following delivery of a patient with sickle cell trait. *American Journal of Obstetrics and Gynecology* 1982; **143**: 722–4.

238 van Wersch JWJ & Ubacks JMH. Blood coagulation and fibrinolysis during normal pregnancy. *European Journal of Clinical Chemistry and Biochemistry* 1991; **29**: 45–50.

239 Vellenga E, van Imhoff GW & Aarnoudse JG. Effective prophylaxis with oral anticoagulants and low-dose heparin during pregnancy in an antithrombin III deficient woman. *Lancet* 1983; **ii**: 224.

240 Villasanta U. Thromboembolic disease in pregnancy. *American Journal of Obstetrics and Gynecology* 1965; **93**: 142–60.

241 Walker ID. Management of thrombophilia in pregnancy. *Blood Reviews* 1991; **5**: 1–7.

242 Warwick R, Hutton RA, Goff L, Letsky E & Heard M. Changes in protein C and free protein S during pregnancy and following hysterectomy. *Journal of the Royal Society of Medicine* 1989; **82**: 591–4.

243 Weiner CP, Kwaan H, Hauck WW, Duboe FJ, Paul M & Wallemark CB. Fibrin generation in normal pregnancy. *Obstetrics and Gynecology* 1984; **64**: 46–8.

244 Whitehouse G. Radiological diagnosis of deep vein thrombosis. *British Medical Journal* 1987; **295**: 801–2.

245 Winter JH, Fenech A, Bennett B & Douglas AS. Thrombosis after venography in familial antithrombin III deficiency. *British Medical Journal* 1981; **283**: 1436–7.

246 Winter JH, Fenech A, Mackie M, Bennett B & Douglas AS. Treatment of venous thrombosis in antithrombin III deficient patients with concentrates of antithrombin III. *Clinical and Laboratory Haematology* 1982; **4**: 101–8.

247 Winter JH, Fenech A *et al*. Familial antithrombin III deficiency. *Quarterly Journal of Medicine* 1982; **204**: 373–95.

248 Wise PH & Hall AJ. Heparin induced osteopenia in pregnancy. *British Medical Journal* 1980; **281**: 110–11.

249 Wolf H & Wick G. Antibodies interacting with, and corresponding binding site for heparin on human thrombocytes. *Lancet* 1986; **ii**: 222–3.

250 Wright HP, Osborn SB & Edmund DG. Changes in the rate of flow of venous blood in the leg during pregnancy, measured with radioactive sodium. *Surgery, Gynecology and Obstetrics* 1950; **90**: 481–5.

251 Yoshimura T, Ito M, Nakamura T & Okamura H. The influence of labour on thrombotic and fibrinolytic systems. *European Journal of Obstetrics and Reproductive Biology* 1992; **44**: 195–9.

252 Zucker ML, Comperts ED & Marcus RG. Prophylactic and therapeutic use of anticoagulants in inherited antithrombin III deficiency. *South African Medical Journal* 1976; **50**: 1743–8.

5

Heart Disease in Pregnancy

Michael de Swiet

General considerations, 143
Physiology
Natural history
Incidence
Maternal mortality
Management
History
Physical signs
Investigations
Clinical management and surgery
Treatment of heart failure and dysrhythmias
Anticoagulant therapy
Labour
Endocarditis and its prevention
Pulmonary oedema and other cardiovascular side-effects of β sympathomimetic drugs
Specific conditions occurring during pregnancy, 160
Acquired heart disease
Chronic rheumatic heart disease
Acute rheumatic fever
Pregnancy in patients with artificial heart valves, tissue valves or prostheses
Myocardial infarction
Cardiomyopathy
Endomyocardial fibrosis
Pericardial disease
Congenital heart disease
Eisenmenger's syndrome and other causes of pulmonary vascular disease
Coarctation of the aorta
Marfan's syndrome
Congenital heart block
Tricuspid atresia and the Fontan procedure
Miscellaneous

Heart disease is a worrying problem to the obstetrician. As we shall see, it is uncommon, with an overall incidence of <1 per cent of all pregnancies; thus any one obstetrician is unlikely to acquire much experience in the management of heart disease in pregnancy. But heart disease is important, since it causes about 7 maternal deaths per year in the UK, making it, with haemorrhage, about third to hypertension and pulmonary embolism as a cause of maternal mortality [80]. However, although the overall incidence is <1 per cent, symptoms such as breathlessness or signs such as an ejection systolic murmur that are suggestive of heart disease, may be present in up to 90 per cent of the pregnant population as a consequence of the physiological changes induced by pregnancy itself. There is the problem of diagnosis, therefore, as well as that of management of a relatively rare condition. In this chapter, we review first the physiological changes that occur in pregnancy, then consider the incidence, effects and management of heart disease in general. Sections follow, where relevant, on specific congenital and acquired conditions. For other reviews see [88,233,289,310,313,314].

General considerations

Physiology

In normal individuals, pregnancy is associated with a rise in cardiac output of approximately 40 per cent, i.e. from about 3.5 to 6.0 l/min when at rest [9]. Such data derived from the cardiac catheter laboratory must be viewed with objectivity, and too much reliability must not be placed on individual measurements. There is considerable variation between individuals, and the experimental conditions under which investigations have been made are not always relevant to the situations of clinical importance, such as labour or other forms of exercise. The time of this rise in cardiac output is also open to discussion. However, those investigators that have measured cardiac output early in pregnancy find that it is already markedly elevated in the first trimester.

What has been disputed is whether the cardiac output falls at the end of pregnancy and, if so by how much. It was originally thought that falls in cardiac output demonstrated in late pregnancy were spurious and associated with measurements made in the supine position [68]. However, the fall of cardiac output associated with lying in the supine position is very variable and may be no more than 3 per cent [211].

More recently some non-invasive studies [322] using electrical impedence cardiography [68,202] and Doppler estimation of aortic velocity [143] have also suggested that cardiac output falls to non-pregnant levels at term. Both these techniques are subject to criticism, the former [85] because of changes that may occur in pregnancy in the pulmonary blood vessels [75] that lead to underestimation of the cardiac output [199] and the latter because the aorta dilates in pregnancy [121]. However, Doppler studies that have also measured the cross-sectional area through which the blood is flowing at the pulmonary [264,266], aortic [266] or mitral [266] valves or at the ascending aorta [82] are much more reliable and have shown a high correlation with cardiac output measured by thermodilution. The cardiac output is elevated at the onset of labour (mean 7 l/min), rising further within labour. A recent serial study performed by this technique has confirmed the early rise in cardiac output with no fall at the end of pregnancy [267]. Within the first 2 weeks after delivery cardiac output falls considerably [264] and at 24 weeks after delivery, the cardiac output has fallen further to 5 l/min [266] which is approximately normal for a non-pregnant woman.

The increase in cardiac output is caused partly by an increase in heart rate [49] and partly by an increase in stroke volume. Since blood pressure does not rise in pregnancy, and usually falls, the increase in cardiac output is associated with a marked fall in peripheral vascular resistance. Indeed, it is likely that the fall in peripheral resistance is one if not the major factor that causes the rise in cardiac output [240,285]. Only part of the change in peripheral vascular resistance can be accounted for by blood flow through the low resistance shunt of the pregnant uterus since cardiac output is elevated during the first trimester, at a time when there is very little change in uterine blood flow.

Oestrogens [280], prostaglandins, including prostacyclin and other locally produced vasoactive substance such as nitric oxide, are likely mediators of the alterations in haemodynamics caused by pregnancy. Calcitonin gene-related peptide also increases in concentration in pregnancy and may contribute to the increase in cardiac output [301]; so too may relaxin which has positive chronotropic and inotropic effects [151] and rises in concentration in the first trimester in particular. (For further reviews of these changes see [69,71]).

In contrast to the considerable volume of studies of the haemodynamics of pregnancy in normal individuals, there is little information concerning patients with heart disease. Ueland *et al.* showed that patients with asymptomatic mitral valve disease are unable to increase their cardiac output on exercise in pregnancy to the same level as normal patients at rest [324]. More recently the application of Swan–Ganz catheterization to obstetric patients [52] has begun to yield further information. The usual indication has been the critically ill patient either with very severe pre-eclampsia [326] or septic shock [167]. This technique involves the placing of a catheter, usually via the jugular or subclavian vein, without X-ray screening, in the pulmonary artery and wedged pulmonary artery positions, the latter for the indirect measurement of left atrial pressure. Injection of cold saline in the right atrium and subsequent measurement of temperature in the pulmonary artery allows measurement of cardiac output by the 'dye' dilution technique. This technique should only be performed by those skilled in its use since there are many complications such as pneumothorax. As an example of the benefits of this technique, Clarke *et al.* [52] demonstrated a sharp (10 mmHg) rise in left atrial pressure in patients with mitral stenosis immediately after delivery. These authors found that data from Swan–Ganz catheterizations were particularly helpful in the management of labour in such patients. Similar data have been published in a patient in labour following myocardial infarction in pregnancy [124].

Natural history

Incidence

The prevalence and incidence of all heart disease in pregnancy varies between 0.3 [181] and 3.5 per cent [194]. Other studies include those of Etheridge [94] who found a prevalence of 0.5 per cent in Australia, Rush *et al.* [275] of 0.8 per cent in South Africa, Buemann and Kragelund [35] of 0.9 per cent in Scandinavia, and de Swiet and Fidler [74] of 0.5–1.8 per cent in London. These figures probably do vary because of a genuine difference in the prevalence of heart disease in different communities. For example, the incidence of rheumatic fever varies considerably between countries, and is strongly and inversely related to their relative affluence. In addition, diagnostic criteria change with time and with the different referral populations of different hospitals.

Nevertheless, it is likely that we will see a genuine change in the pattern of congenital heart disease in pregnancy following the increase in paediatric cardiac surgery which occurred between 1965 and 1975. These patients will start to become pregnant in significant numbers from the age of 18 years onwards so the change should be obvious by the end of the millennium.

In all series, the dominant lesion in rheumatic heart disease has been mitral stenosis [93,94,111, 112,307,313]. In 1048 patients with rheumatic heart disease reported in Newcastle, Szekely *et al.* [313] found dominant mitral stenosis in 90 per cent, mitral regurgitation in 6.6 per cent, aortic regurgitation in 2.5 per cent, and aortic stenosis in 1 per cent.

At present, the experience of congenital heart disease in pregnancy is still limited to relatively simple defects which have usually not been corrected. Five representative series are shown in Table 5.1. Although the total numbers in each series are different, the overall pattern is similar [242]. The most common lesions are patent ductus arteriosus, atrial septal defect and ventricular septal defect, together accounting for about 60 per cent of cases; followed by pulmonary stenosis, Fallot's tetralogy and coarctation of the aorta, which, together, contribute another 24 per cent. Isolated lesions such as aortic and mitral valve disease account for the remainder [55,206,229,307]. It is likely that these data reflect no more than the incidence of congenital heart disease in the general female population. However, three of the series are quite old, dating from 1963–75. In the more recent series from Dublin (1981) [307] and Leicester (1985) [181] we see the effect of surgery and more cases of patent ductus arteriosus have been corrected.

Other conditions, such as coronary artery disease or symptomatic arrhythmias, are so rarely associated with pregnancy that it is difficult to give a true incidence. However, Rush *et al.* [275] reported coronary artery disease in 0.4 per cent of 697 patients with heart disease in pregnancy. The same authors found an incidence of 17 cases of arrhythmia in 679 patients with heart disease in pregnancy. Szekely *et al.* [313] found that 69 of 1048 cases of rheumatic heart disease are complicated by atrial fibrillation. The incidence of cardiomyopathy of pregnancy is discussed later in the chapter.

Table 5.1. The prevalence (percentage) of various forms of congenital heart disease in pregnancy

	Ohio[1] ($n = 125$)	Queensland[2] ($n = 93$)	Dublin[3] ($n = 74$)	Connecticut[4]† ($n = 482$)	Leicester[5] ($n = 73$)	Total ($n = 847$)
Patent ductus arteriosus	24	27	9	22	11	21
Atrial septal defect	29	26	38	14	22	20
Pulmonary stenosis	4	12	6	10*	11	9
Ventricular septal defect	22	14	13	20	16	19
Tetralogy of Fallot	4	4	13	8	8	8
Coarctation of the aorta	10	6	6		7	7
Aortic valve disease	3	4	6	12	7	5
Mitral valve disease				7	14	5
Other	2	2		7	4	5
Unclassified	5	5				4

[1] [55]; [2] [206]; [3] [307]; [4] [337]; [5] [181].
* Includes all pregnancies where mother had obstruction to right ventricular outflow.
† Expressed as percentage of all 233 mothers who became pregnant (some had more than one pregnancy).

Maternal mortality

As we have seen above, heart disease is now the third most common cause of maternal mortality in the UK. Although sporadic fatalities will be seen in all forms of heart disease in pregnancy maternal mortality is most likely in those conditions where pulmonary blood flow cannot be increased [146]. Note that in normal pregnancy the pulmonary blood flow has to increase *pari passu* with systemic flow and the pulmonary vascular resistance also falls [267]. The failure to increase pulmonary blood flow occurs because of obstruction, either within the pulmonary blood vessels or at the mitral valve. The situation is documented clearly in Eisenmenger's syndrome, where up to now there has been no effective treatment and where the maternal mortality is between 30 and 50 per cent [112,201,206, 243]. The Confidential Enquiries into Maternal Mortality in England and Wales [79,80] indicate that Eisenmenger's syndrome was the most frequent form of congenital heart disease associated with maternal mortality and was responsible for 17 of the 47 cases of death due to congenital heart disease between 1961 and 1975 [78]. In the 1985–1987 report three of the 10 deaths due to congenital heart disease were in patients with Eisenmenger's syndrome and a further four were in patients with other causes of pulmonary hypertension [133]. Only Batson [14] has reported a series of 23 pregnancies with no maternal deaths; the reason for this unusual success is not clear. Elevations in pulmonary vascular resistance are also found in pregnancy in cor pulmonale [275], patients with single ventricle [302], pulmonary veno-occlusive disease [194] and in primary pulmonary hypertension. In the latter condition the maternal mortality is about 50 per cent [1,186,201,293].

In contrast, in Fallot's tetralogy where the pulmonary vascular resistance is normal, the reported maternal mortality varies between 4 and 20 per cent [141,195,201]. Furthermore, the figure of 20 per cent is only based on one maternal death in five pregnancies in the study of Jacoby [141]. Espino Vela and Alvarado [92] have reported a series of 105 patients with atrial septal defect (confirmed by catheter in 41 patients) who had up to 10 or more pregnancies with no maternal mortality.

The Connecticut series [337] shows how good the results can be with obsessional care, since in 482 pregnancies from 233 women, including eight mothers with Eisenmenger's syndrome, there were no maternal deaths.

In Ehlers–Danlos syndrome the arterial and classic forms have also been associated with high mortality, due to arterial dissection and bleeding [11,235,236]. More recently the Ehlers–Danlos syndrome has been characterized on the basis of the specific collagen defect [295] and in Ehlers–Danlos syndrome type IV, the maternal mortality is said to be as high as 25 per cent in North America [274]. This high mortality which is largely due to haemorrhage from major blood vessels has been disputed by Pope and Nicholls [245] in a different series from the UK implying a different referral population or genetic heterogeneity. (There is also a high fetal loss rate attributable to premature rupture of the membrane if either father or mother has Ehlers–Danlos syndrome [172]. This is presumably due to a collagen defect in the fetal membranes.)

In rheumatic heart disease maternal mortality can now be very low although rheumatic heart disease is still a major cause of mortality in developing countries [88]. Szekely *et al.* [313] reported 26 mortalities in 2856 pregnancies (about 1 per cent) complicated by rheumatic heart disease between 1942 and 1969. Half of the deaths were due to pulmonary oedema, which became less common once mitral valvotomy was freely available. These authors reported no maternal deaths in about 1000 pregnancies occurring in 1960. Rush *et al.* [275] also reported a maternal mortality of 0.7 per cent in 450 mothers with rheumatic heart disease in South Africa.

Although prognosis is good in patients with rheumatic heart disease in pregnancy, many clinicians still believe that '... every pregnancy was so many nails of a coffin of a woman with heart disease' [334]. Chesley [46] has reported a group of 38 patients with 51 pregnancies occurring after they were diagnosed as having severe heart disease. These were compared with a group of 96 women with equally severe rheumatic heart disease who did not have any pregnancies after diagnosis. The mean survival time (14 years) was no less and, in fact, was greater in the group who did have further pregnancies compared to the group that did not (12 years). I would agree with Chesley [46] that pregnancy does not affect the long-term survival of a woman with rheumatic heart disease, providing that she survives pregnancy itself.

Fetal outcome

The fetal outcome in rheumatic heart disease in pregnancy is usually good, and little different from that in patients who do not have heart disease [181,275,307]. However, the babies are likely to be lighter [323], by about 200 g in the study of Ho *et al.* [130].

In the five series of patients with congenital heart disease in pregnancy cited in Table 5.1, there was no excess fetal mortality except in the group with cyanotic congenital heart disease, whether associated with pulmonary hypertension or not. Here the babies are generally growth retarded [14,284,337], and the fetal loss including abortion may be as high as 45 per cent [14,55,111,337]. Even in the tetralogy of Fallot, which does not have a particularly high maternal mortality, the fetal loss rate may be as high as 57 per cent [55] and the majority of the babies are growth retarded [141]. This is hardly surprising, in view of the mechanisms of placental exchange which cannot compensate for the maternal systemic hypoxaemia. It is likely that the fetus dies because of inadequate oxygen supply or because of prematurity [111] which may be iatrogenic due to elective pre-term delivery. In contrast, the fetal results in 40 pregnancies following 27 cases of total correction of Fallot's tetralogy were excellent [292].

Uncorrected coarctation of the aorta has been associated with a 13 per cent fetal loss rate [39] and intrauterine growth retardation [24], presumably because of inadequate placental perfusion. This has also been demonstrated by Doppler ultrasound in Takayasu's arteritis [106]. However, severe aortic occlusion requiring axillofemoral grafting may be compatible with a normally grown fetus [298].

Women or men who themselves have congenital heart disease are naturally concerned that their children may be similarly afflicted. Earlier studies suggested that for most forms of congenital heart disease the risk to the fetus was 2–4 per cent if either parent was affected [214], at least double

Table 5.2. Risk of recurrence in the fetus of women with congenital heart disease. The number of women studied is given in parenthesis. From [215,216]

Lesion	%	Total
Aortic stenosis	18	(95)
A-V canal defect	14	(36)
Ventricular septal defect	9	(347)
Pulmonary stenosis	6	(248)
Atrial septal defect	5	(783)
Coarctation	4	(146)
Patent ductus arteriosus	4	(828)
Fallot's tetralogy	3	(196)

the risk in the normal population. However, recent studies by Nora and Nora [215,216] (Table 5.2) indicate that the risk depends on the nature of the lesion varying from 3 per cent (Fallot's tetralogy) to 18 per cent (aortic stenosis). The defect is usually concordent, i.e. of the same nature as that of the mother [90]. Surprisingly the risk to the fetus is much greater if the mother is affected than if the father is affected [215] suggesting the possibility of cytoplasmic inheritance [215] or some form of genomic imprinting.

However, congenital heart disease in the mother may have arisen because of environmental exposure when she herself was a fetus *in utero*. An obvious example is the maternal rubella syndrome. If the maternal abnormality can be shown to be due to an environmental factor, then the fetus probably has the same risk as that of a normal woman without congenital heart disease [38].

All women who have congenital heart disease themselves or who have already borne a child with congenital heart disease should have detailed fetal abnormality ultrasound scans in pregnancy: the precision of these scans will improve with increasing experience and better equipment [287]. In the majority of cases the mothers' anxiety about having an abnormal baby will be allayed; in the minority who do have affected fetuses management of the infant including surgery can be planned; termination can also be considered in the exceptional very severely affected fetus [59].

Management

All pregnant patients with heart disease should be

managed in a combined obstetric/cardiac clinic by one obstetrician and one cardiologist. In this way, the number of visits that the patient makes to the hospital is kept to a minimum, and the obstetrician and cardiologist obtain the maximum experience in the management of these relatively rare conditions.

History

As in all forms of medicine, the history is of paramount importance in the assessment of patients with heart disease. In the UK, most patients with heart disease know that they have it, or that they have a heart murmur. It is now rare to make a diagnosis of heart disease *de novo* in pregnancy. In all developed countries, women have frequent medical examinations from the time that they are babies, and attend infant welfare clinics, to when they visit family planning clinics or attend for examination prior to employment. The exceptions are recent immigrants and patients from deprived social classes.

The most frequent symptom of heart disease in pregnancy is breathlessness. This is difficult to assess because it is a variable feature of normal pregnancy [198].

Some patients are aware of increasing their ventilation; others are not. Breathlessness arising in pregnancy does not therefore necessarily indicate heart disease, and it is important to consider whether the patients were breathless before they became pregnant. The New York Heart Association (NYHA) classification of heart disease is largely based on limitation of physical activity and associated symptoms of heart disease and is shown below.

Class 1 — no resulting limitation of physical activity. Ordinary physical activity does not cause undue fatigue, palpitation, dyspnoea or anginal pain.

Class 2 — slight limitation of physical activity. Patients are comfortable at rest. Ordinary physical activity results in fatigue, palpitation, dyspnoea or anginal pain.

Class 3 — marked limitation of physical activity. Patients are comfortable at rest. Less than ordinary activity causes fatigue, palpitation, dyspnoea or anginal pain.

Class 4 — inability to carry on any physical activity without discomfort. Symptoms of cardiac insufficiency or of anginal syndrome may be present even at rest. If any physical activity is undertaken, discomfort is increased [195].

However, such a classification is only of value if it indicates the severity of the condition at the time of classification, and if it is reliable in predicting the outcome of pregnancy. Both these criteria may not be met with regard to the NYHA classification. We have seen that symptoms of breathlessness are unreliable in pregnancy, and it is also well recognized that patients with mitral stenosis may have no symptoms at the beginning of pregnancy (class 1) and yet have pulmonary oedema by the end of pregnancy (class 4) [132,313]. Indeed, Sugrue *et al.* [307] reported that 39 per cent of 38 patients with rheumatic heart disease, who developed heart failure in pregnancy, were originally classified as class 1; Szekely *et al.* reported that the majority of maternal deaths occurred in women who were initially in NYHA class I or II [313]. Therefore a precise anatomical diagnosis supported by a pathophysiological assessment of the severity of the condition is preferable.

Syncope is also a very common feature of normal pregnancy, particularly in the middle trimester. Presumably in these patients, peripheral vascular resistance transiently decreases more than cardiac ouput increases. However, syncope may also occur rarely in severe aortic stenosis, hypertrophic obstructive cardiomyopathy (HOCM, subaortic stenosis), Fallot's tetralogy and Eisenmenger's syndrome. Syncope, like chest pain, can occur because of dysrhythmias. The patient may also be aware of the dysrhythmia as a feeling of palpitation.

Chest pain is usually a feature of ischaemic disease, which is uncommon in pregnancy (see below) but chest pain may also occur in severe aortic stenosis or, more commonly in pregnancy, in HOCM.

Physical signs

The hyperdynamic circulation of pregnancy causes alterations in the cardiovascular system which mimic heart disease. Thus 20 per cent of patients originally thought in pregnancy to have rheumatic heart disease may have none at all, following a reassessment performed up to 30 years later [112].

Premature atrial and ventricular ectopic beats are common in pregnancy [307] and the peripheral pulse is increased in volume, suggesting aortic valve disease to the unwary. The neck veins pulsate more vigorously in pregnancy, but the mean right atrial pressure is unchanged (10 mmHg [120]) and therefore the height of the jugular venous pressure is also unchanged. The heart apex beat is more forceful and because of the increase in cardiac output may suggest cardiomegaly in normal patients. However, if the apex heart beat is >2 cm outside the midclavicular line, this should be considered definitely abnormal.

Oedema is a non-specific sign of heart disease, even in non-pregnant patients. In pregnancy, oedema is a very common finding particularly in the lower limbs where obstruction to the venous return by the enlarging uterus is presumably an important factor. The fall in intravascular colloid osmotic pressure is another cause of oedema. This may be exacerbated by injudicious administration of crystalloid solutions [113,114], but it is offset by a concomitant fall in interstitial colloid osmotic pressure [225]. Oedema is so normal in pregnancy that by itself it should not be considered a sign of raised right atrial pressure and therefore of heart disease.

The auscultatory changes in normal pregnancy have been well documented in a phonocardiographic study by Cutford and MacDonald [63]. The first heart sound is loud and a third heart sound is audible in 84 per cent of patients. This is the single greatest cause of confusion, since the third heart sound is interpreted as a diastolic murmur or opening snap. An ejection systolic sound can be heard in 96 per cent of apparently normal pregnant women [63]. The murmur is widely conducted, and can even be heard over the back. Recent Doppler studies suggest that this murmur may often be due to tricuspid regurgitation [19]. Although it is said that a diastolic murmur may be present in normal patients, due to blood flow across the tricuspid valve [63], this should be a diagnosis based on exclusion after echocardiography. In addition murmurs may be heard over the right and left second intercostal space, about 2 cm from the sternal edge. They may be systolic or continuous, and can be modified by pressure of the stethoscope. They are thought to be due to blood flow in mammary vessels [63]. Venous hums — continuous murmurs usually audible in the neck and modified by posture — may also be heard in pregnancy as in the non-pregnant state.

Any other murmurs or additional heart sounds should be considered significant. Particular difficulty occurs with systolic murmurs since they are so common in normal pregnancy. Those that are significant are:

1 pansystolic murmurs (ventricular septal defect, mitral regurgitation, tricuspid regurgitation);

2 late systolic murmurs (mitral regurgitation, mitral valve prolapse);

3 ejection systolic murmurs that are louder than grade 3/6 (aortic stenosis), or vary with respiration (pulmonary stenosis), or are associated with other abnormalities, e.g. ejection clicks (valvar pulmonary and aortic stenosis).

The clinical signs of heart disease are briefly discussed in some individual conditions below, but an assessment of the patient's cardiac status should also include the signs of heart failure, whether the patient is cyanosed or has finger clubbing, the presence of pulse deficits and other peripheral signs of endocarditis such as splinter haemorrhages.

Investigations

CHEST RADIOGRAPHY

The increase in cardiac output and pulmonary blood volume causes slight cardiomegaly, increased pulmonary vascular markings and distension of the pulmonary veins. These return to normal after delivery, and they do not necessarily indicate that the patient has heart disease. The chest radiograph is unhelpful in the diagnosis of minor degrees of heart disease but will, of course, show typical changes in those who have haemodynamically significant heart disease.

ELECTROCARDIOGRAPHY

Oram and Holt [230], reported innocent depression of the S–T segment and flattening of the T wave in the left-sided precordial leads in 14 per cent of normal pregnant women. They state that such changes would normally lead one to suspect cardiomyopathy. Boyle and Lloyd-Jones [32] disputed these findings, but most physicians would accept that even T wave inversion and Q waves in lead III [42], which would normally be considered pathologic, may be seen in healthy pregnant women. Although a change in the electrical axis of the heart during pregnancy may be part of the explanation [43], it does not account for all these findings. Indeed, pregnancy itself does not account for all the findings, and there may be more variability in the electrocardiogram of healthy non-pregnant women than had previously been realized [230]. As a consequence, in pregnancy the electrocardiogram is more helpful in the diagnosis of dysrhythmias and of rare cases of cardiomyopathy than in the demonstration of a structural abnormality of the heart.

ECHOCARDIOGRAPHY

Studies in non-pregnant individuals have shown that the majority of structural cardiac abnormalities can be detected by echocardiography [300], and this is the technique of choice in pregnancy, since there is no radiation hazard, and because of the detailed information available in skilled hands. Certain abnormalities such as the presence of bacterial vegetations [91] or prosthetic valve dysfunction [154] are better demonstrated by transoesophageal echocardiography where the transducer is mounted on a flexible endoscope passed into the oesophagus at the level of the mediastinum.

Rubler *et al.* [273], in an echocardiographic study designed to look at changes in cardiac output, also established normal values for chamber size in pregnancy.

To establish the place of routine echocardiography in pregnancy, Northcoate *et al.* [217] studied 50 consecutive patients referred to a cardiac clinic because of murmurs in pregnancy. They found that echocardiography did not contribute anything further if the clinical assessment and electrocardiogram were normal. A similar study in 103 patients by Mishra *et al.* [200] had an identical outcome. Therefore, it is not necessary to perform echocardiography in patients who present to cardiologists in pregnancy with heart murmurs and where the cardiologist thinks the heart is normal.

Doppler may also be used to study flow patterns. In a study of 107 apparently normal women, Robson *et al.* [269] showed regurgitant flow across the tricuspid, mitral and pulmonary valves in 41–90 per cent depending on the valve and gestational age. The prevalence of regurgitant flow across the right heart valves was significantly greater in normal women in pregnancy than in the non-pregnant state. These findings need to be considered when using Doppler to assess abnormal heart valves in pregnancy.

Clinical management and surgery

Patients should be seen in the combined clinic and the nature and severity of their heart lesion assessed. Many patients will have no evidence of any lesion at all, and no further follow-up will be required. Some may only have a mild lesion with no haemodynamic problems, such as congenital mitral valve prolapse which has an excellent prognosis [252]. Again, no further follow-up is necessary although, in my opinion, they should receive antibiotic prophylaxis in labour (see below). The remainder do have a condition with real or potential haemodynamic implications. They must first be assessed as to the need for termination, if seen early enough in pregnancy, and secondly as to the need for surgery. In patients with well-managed heart disease, these decisions should have been made before the patient becomes pregnant [45,242], but inevitably some patients present for the first time in pregnancy or have been lost to follow-up before pregnancy.

Because of the mortality statistics indicated above, only Eisenmenger's syndrome, primary pulmonary hypertension and pulmonary veno-occlusive disease are absolute indications for termination of pregnancy. Termination may also be indicated very rarely in patients with such severe pulmonary disease that they have pulmonary hypertension. Under these circumstances, pulmonary artery pressure, if not known, should be measured directly by Swan–Ganz catheter (see Chapter 1). In all other cases, the decision whether the pregnancy should continue, depends on an individual assessment of the risk of pregnancy compared to the patient's desire to have children.

In general, the indications for surgery in pregnancy are similar to those in the non-pregnant state: failure of medical treatment with either intractable heart failure or intolerable symptoms. However, because of the bad reputation of severe mitral stenosis in pregnancy, closed mitral valvotomy [73] or valvuloplasty is performed relatively commonly in patients with suitable heart valves, whereas open heart surgery is done with reluctance because of worries about the fetus. Szekely *et al.* [313] reported 69 mitral valvotomies during pregnancy after 1951, although only five were performed between 1966 and 1969; presumably after 1966 the majority of patients with mitral stenosis had their valvotomies performed before pregnancy. The indications for valvotomy are pulmonary congestion not responding rapidly to drugs, any episode of pulmonary oedema before pregnancy (likely to recur in pregnancy) and profuse haemoptysis. In patients considered for closed valvotomy or valvuloplasty, there should be no significant mitral regurgitation, the mitral valve should not be calcified, and there should be no other significant valve involvement. The operation is usually performed in the middle trimester, but may be done at any time in pregnancy. Szekely *et al.* [313] reported only two operative deaths with good fetal results (though there were two spontaneous abortions and six perinatal deaths) in 69 valvotomies in pregnancy. In a series of 110 closed mitral valvotomies from Sri Lanka there were no maternal deaths and only three fetal losses, all due to abortion [169]. Similar studies have been reported from South Africa (41 valvotomies) [328] and India (126 valvotomies) [234]. Nevertheless, mitral valvotomy has become a rare procedure in the UK. Only one has been performed in a patient referred to Queen Charlotte's Maternity Hospital in the last 10 years, and Sugrue *et al.* reported only three cases from Dublin in 387 pregnancies complicated by rheumatic heart disease. Since very few cardiac surgeons now perform closed mitral valvotomies, preferring the improved control offered by open heart surgery, this trend will continue. Furthermore percutaneous balloon mitral valvuloplasty is now an accepted non-surgical technique for relieving mitral stenosis [52,118] and this treatment could and should be used in many patients who previously would have had closed mitral valvotomies, i.e. those with pliable valves who do not have major mitral regurgitation. The only potential problems in pregnancy are the extra radiation (which may be minimized by careful planning) and the need for the patient to remain supine for up to 1 hour. The technique has been used successfully in pregnancy [183] and is likely to supersede closed mitral valvotomy.

In addition aortic valvuloplasty has also been performed in pregnancy [6,192] and may avoid the problems of open heart surgery in pregnancy (see below). The contraindications are again heavy valve calcification and significant regurgitation flow. Aortic valvuloplasty should probably be considered more of a palliative procedure than is mitral valvuloplasty and these patients are likely to require aortic valve replacement after delivery.

A review of open heart surgery during pregnancy by Zitnik *et al.* [343] indicated that, although maternal results are reasonable (5 per cent mortality in a group of 22 women with severely affected hearts), the fetal results are not, with a perinatal mortality of 33 per cent. There has been speculation that these poor figures are due to inadequate perfusion of the placenta during cardiopulmonary bypass, either because of relative hypotension or because of lack of pulsatile pumping [232]. (Even though the pump may be non-pulsatile, blood flow in the uterine vessels does pulsate.) These speculations have been supported by several recent reports of lack of beat-to-beat variation and bradycardia recorded by external cardiotachography during cardiopulmonary bypass [10,87,160,173,343]. Alternatively, some of these cardiotachographic findings may be accounted for by the artificially induced hypothermia occurring during cardiopulmonary bypass. It is likely that the fetus whose placental circulation is already compromised by maternal pre-eclampsia or growth retardation, will be particularly susceptible to the further insults of cardiopulmonary bypass [140]. The earlier reports summarized by Zitnik *et al.* [343] were all of surgery performed early in pregnancy with a high abortion rate. More recently, Eilen *et al.* [87] have reviewed the literature and found no fetal losses in patients operated on after the first trimester. Becker [17] found only one per cent maternal and 20 per cent fetal loss in 68 patients operated on at all stages of pregnancy. Nevertheless, the indication for open heart surgery in pregnancy is usually life-threatening pulmonary oedema that cannot be managed medically.

Although the first case of open heart surgery in pregnancy involved a woman with Fallot's tetralogy [82] cardiac surgery in pregnancy is rarely considered in congenital heart disease. In coarctation of the aorta, the risk of dissection in pregnancy has probably been exaggerated (see below). Repair would therefore not be advised unless hypertension could not be controlled medically. Valve replacement with an additional aortic prosthesis might be considered in some cases of Marfan's syndrome; the risks would be those already discussed of open heart surgery.

ANTENATAL CARE

After initial assessment of the patient, the remainder of medical management during pregnancy is associated with avoiding, if possible, those factors which increase the risk of heart failure, and treating heart failure vigorously if it occurs. Risk factors for heart failure include infections (particularly urinary tract infection in pregnancy), hypertension (both pregnancy-associated and pregnancy-induced), obesity, multiple pregnancy, anaemia, the development of arrhythmias and, very rarely, the development of hyperthyroidism. The increase in cardiac output in twin pregnancy which is about 30 per cent greater than in singleton pregnancy, is made by increasing heart rate and contractility rather than by increasing venous return. This suggests that cardiac reserve is particularly compromised in multiple pregnancy [324].

Obstetric management before labour includes early ultrasound examination of the conceptus to confirm gestational age and in women with congenital heart disease (see above) second trimester examination of the fetal heart by ultrasound to exclude congenital malformations. In experienced hands this technique will diagnose or exclude all major congenital malformations by 18 weeks' gestation [3] allowing termination in selected cases, planning of paediatric care in less severely affected fetuses and reassurance of the mother in the majority.

Those women who do not have haemodynamically significant heart disease require no special obstetric antenatal management. However, if there is haemodynamically significant heart disease and particularly if maternal arterial Po_2 is reduced as in cyanotic congenital heart disease, the fetus should be monitored for growth retardation and intrauterine asphyxia. This would currently entail assessment of fetal growth and amniotic fluid volume clinically and by ultrasound, measurements of abnormalities in fetal heart rate by ultrasound (cardiotocography), measurement of fetal and maternal placental blood flow indices by Doppler ultrasound and possibly fetal blood sampling for direct assessment of fetal hypoxia.

ADMISSION FOR BED REST

One cannot make recommendations that all patients with a certain degree of heart disease should be admitted at a certain gestation. Each patient must be considered individually. For some, particularly those with other children, the emotional stress of separation from the rest of their families may cause more harm than the rest does good. Other patients will benefit, and the gain may be more to the fetus at risk from intrauterine growth retardation than to its mother. All patients with heart failure must be treated in hospital, and few can be discharged for long before delivery.

Treatment of heart failure and dysrhythmias

The principles of treatment of heart failure in pregnancy are the same as in the non-pregnant state.

DIGOXIN

The indications for the use of digoxin are to control the heart rate in atrial fibrillation and some other supraventricular tachycardias, and to increase the force of contraction when given acutely in heart failure. If patients do develop atrial fibrillation in pregnancy, consideration should be given to anticoagulation with warfarin (see below) because of the risk of systemic embolism [312]. Supraventricular tachycardia in the fetus arising *in utero* has also been managed by maternal digoxin therapy both successfully [119] and unsuccessfully [182,210,341]. Propranolol [155,316], procainamide [83], amiodarone, flecainide [182] and verapamil [258] have also been given to the mother for this purpose.

Dosage requirements for digoxin are believed to be the same in pregnancy as in the non-pregnant state [54]. Both digoxin [276] and digitoxin [227] cross the placenta, and produce similar drug levels in the fetus to those seen in the mother [270,276]. Digoxin enters the umbilical circulation within 5 min of intravenous administration to the mother [276]. In general, these is no evidence that therapeutic maternal drug levels of digoxin affect the neonatal electrocardiogram [195,270] or cause harm to the fetus. However, Szekely and Snaith [312] reported one case of transient junctional rhythm in the newborn infant of one of a series of mothers who had been digitalized in pregnancy. Although therapeutic maternal drug levels do not harm the fetus, toxic levels do, as was shown in one case of maternal digitoxin poisoning where electrocardiographic changes of digitalis toxicity were demonstrated in the neonate which died aged 3 days [288].

The demonstration of the production of digoxin-like immunoreactive substance by the feto-placental unit [318,340] particularly in hypertensive pregnancy [246] questions the validity of some the above statements. In addition digoxin may not cross the placenta so rapidly if fetal placental blood flow is impaired as in the hydropic fetus with congestive cardiac failure *in utero* [341].

Digoxin is also secreted in breast milk, but since the total daily excretion in the mother with therapeutic blood levels would not exceed 2 μg [174] this too is unlikely to cause any harm to the neonate unless it has any other predisposing causes of digitalis toxicity such as hypokalaemia.

Weaver and Pearson [333] have reported that the shorter labours generally believed to occur in patients with heart disease were confined to those patients who took digoxin and they postulated a direct stimulating effect of digoxin on the myometrium. But the babies born to the digoxin-treated mothers were small and born more prematurely and these factors may have been the cause of the more rapid labours.

There may be a place for prophylactic digoxin therapy in selective patients who are not in heart failure. This is most likely to be of value to those patients who are at risk from developing atrial fibrillation, i.e. those with rheumatic mitral valve disease who have an enlarged left atrium, and possibly those who have paroxysmal atrial fibrillation or frequent atrial ectopic beats. But this form of treatment had not been subjected to formal clinical trial, and there is certainly no case for digitalization of all patients with heart disease in pregnancy.

DIURETIC THERAPY

Frusemide is the most commonly used and rapidly acting loop diuretic for the treatment of pulmonary oedema. Ethacrynic acid has also been used successfully in the management of pulmonary oedema associated with mitral stenosis in labour. In congestive cardiac failure where speed of action is not so important, oral thiazides are usually used in the first instance, although the extra potency of the loop diuretics may be necessary in a minority of cases. Anderson [4] showed that the use of thiazide in late pregnancy was not associated with any significant salt or water depletion in the neonate.

There are no risks to the use of diuretics in the treatment of heart failure that are specific to pregnancy, but, as in the non-pregnant state, hypokalaemia is an important complication in a patient who may also be taking digoxin.

Treatment of pulmonary oedema should also include opiates such as morphine, which reduce anxiety and decrease venous return by causing venodilation, and also aminophylline if there is associated bronchospasm. If the patient does not respond to these measures, vasodilating drugs should be used to unload the left ventricle. These include nitrates (cause venous dilatation and reduce preload) and angiotensin-converting enzyme inhibitors such as captopril or enalapril and hydrazaline (cause arteriolar dilatation and reduce afterload). In this desperate situation the risks to the fetus of captopril (see Chapter 6) and nitrates (which decrease fetal heart variability [58] are not so important as the maternal risk. Life-threatening pulmonary oedema that does not respond to drug therapy may be helped by mechanical ventilation. If this is successful and in other cases which do not respond to medical treatment, cardiac surgery should be considered, if the patient has a potentially operable lesion.

DYSRHYTHMIAS

In general, most haemodynamically significant dysrhythmias are due to ischaemic heart disease which usually presents in women after their childbearing years, and is rare in pregnancy [109,136]. Therefore, there is limited experience in the treatment of dysrhythmias during pregnancy. Nevertheless, the problem does exist, particularly in patients who have non-ischaemic abnormalities of cardiac conducting tissue, such as occur in the Wolff–Parkinson–White and Lown–Ganong–Levine syndromes.

In addition paroxysmal atrial tachycardia is said to occur more frequently in pregnancy than in the non-pregnant state [311] and also persistent atrial tachycardia may be specific to pregnancy [133,259]. In cases of supraventricular tachycardia, hyperthyroidism should always be excluded. The long QT syndrome which predisposes to ventricular dysrhythmias has been managed by pre-pregnancy removal of the left stellate ganglion [34]. Propranolol has also been used for the long QT syndrome in twin pregnancy [338].

The successful management of pregnancy in a patient with autosomal dominant ventricular dysrhythmia has been reported by Sachs and Van Idekinge [278].

The antidysrhythmic drugs that have been used most frequently in pregnancy are digoxin (discussed above), quinidine and β adrenergic blocking agents, in particular propranolol, atenolol and oxprenolol. The indications for use of these drugs are unaltered by pregnancy. Although there are isolated case reports of intrauterine growth retardation, acute fetal distress in labour and hypoglycaemia in the neonate, in patients taking β adrenergic blocking agents [57,110,116] these have not been confirmed in clinical trials of oxprenolol [97,104], when used for hypertension in pregnancy (see Chapter 6). It would seem reasonable, therefore, to use propranolol or oxprenolol in both acute and long-term treatment of supraventricular and ventricular tachycardia in pregnancy. There is concern that antenolol may cause growth retardation, particularly when taken in the first half of pregnancy [272] though not when used in later pregnancy [272]. Therefore it is best to avoid atenolol if β blockers are needed for control of tachyrhythmia in pregnancy. The dose of oxprenolol received by infants breast fed by mothers taking oxprenolol is very small (0.1 mg/kg/24 hours) [96]. The concentrations of verapamil [138] and the calcium blocking agent diltiazem [226] are approximately the same in breast milk as in maternal blood. The dose transferred to the infant would therefore be small and breast feeding should be encouraged in these circumstances [70].

Quinidine is used to maintain or induce sinus rhythm in patients either after DC conversion or when taking digoxin. It is well tolerated in pregnancy [322] and has only minimal oxytocic effect [194]. However, caution is necessary should the patient require succinylcholine for anaesthesia; pseudocholinesterase levels are depressed in pregnancy and quinidine reduces the enzyme activity still further [153]. Although there is little documentary evidence of the safety of verapamil in pregnancy, it has been widely used and should be considered safe in short-term therapy. There is much less experience of other antidysrhythmic drugs such as bretylium tosylate, disopyramide or amiodarone.

A case report has suggested that mexiletine is safe in pregnancy for the treatment of ventricular dysrhythmias and shown that mexiletine levels in cord blood are similar to those in maternal plasma [317]. However, mexiletine is secreted in fairly high proportions in breast milk where the concentration may be more than four times that in maternal plasma [179] so caution is necessary concerning breast feeding. The use of disopyramide has been associated with hypertonic uterine activity on one occasion [171] but not in others [99]; therefore disopyramide should be used in pregnancy with caution. The long-term risks of phenytoin are well known, and are described in Chapters 2 and 15; however, this drug is only likely to be used in acute treatment of dysrhythmias, particularly those induced by digitalis intoxication. Szekely and Snaith

[312] have also used procainamide successfully to abolish atrial fibrillation in pregnancy.

The use of amiodarone has been reviewed in at least 30 pregnancies [13,103]. There is no evidence of teratogenicity in the relatively few pregnancies reported [241]. Amiodarone contains large quantities of iodine, is known to affect the maternal thyroid and might affect the fetal thyroid, producing hypo- or hyperthyroidism. Although neonatal hypothyroidism has been noted in one poorly documented case [117] other abnormalities have been mild and transient [237,262]. In addition, neonatal bradycardia and prolongation of QT intervals in the infant have also been found [187,237]. These abnormalities have also been transient and do not seem to have caused any harm. Amiodarone is a potentially dangerous drug but on the basis of these reports, it would seem reasonable to use amiodarone in arrhythmias resistant to all other therapy in late pregnancy. Patients should not breast feed when they are taking amiodarone.

Adenosine has become the agent of choice for the acute management of tachyarrythmias in preference to verapamil [40]. There is very little published experience with this drug in pregnancy but it is most unlikely to affect the fetus adversely since it has such a short plasma half-life, <2 seconds [40].

DC conversion for tachyarrhythmias is safe in pregnancy and does not harm the fetus [98].

The difficulty arises in considering long-term prophylactic treatment with antidysrhythmic drugs which have not been extensively used in pregnancy. Here each case must be considered on its own merits, paying particular attention to the frequency and severity of the attacks of the dysrhythmia. A single short episode of supraventricular tachycardia associated with no other symptoms does not require prophylactic treatment. Frequent attacks of ventricular tachycardia associated with syncope would require prophylaxis — whatever the outcome for the fetus.

Cardiopulmonary arrest occurring in pregnancy should be managed initially in the same way as in the non-pregnant state with intubation, ventilation, external cardiac massage and treatment of dysrythmia.

However, very early consideration must be given to immediate delivery by caesarean section for both fetal and maternal reasons. The fetus is relatively resistant to maternal hypoxia and healthy babies have been delivered up to 15 min after their mothers died [224,335]. In addition it can be difficult to perform effective external cardiac massage because of inadequate venous return due to obstruction of the inferior vena cava by the gravid uterus. Although this could in theory be overcome by placing the patient in the left lateral position, most maternity units do not have firm wedges which allow cardiopulmonary resuscitation in the left lateral position. Caesarean section is a more practical way of relieving the obstruction [224] and as indicated above may be of benefit for the fetus who would otherwise certainly have died.

Anticoagulant therapy (see also section on artificial heart valves, below and Chapter 4)

This is a major problem in the management of patients with heart disease in pregnancy. Anticoagulant therapy may be necessary in patients with congenital heart disease who have pulmonary hypertension due to pulmonary vascular disease, those who have artificial valve replacements, and those with atrial fibrillation. Limet and Crondin [176] have reported two patients with embolic problems following artificial valve replacement when the patients were either not anticoagulated or anticoagulated inadequately during pregnancy. They calculated from their own series that the risk of a woman having an embolic episode if she had an artificial valve and did not take anticoagulants was one in every 100 months of exposure. Their literature search suggested that the risk of thromboembolism in such patients is higher (25 per cent per pregnancy, one in 40 months) and that this risk can be reduced to 5 per cent, if the patient takes anticoagulants.

For conditions such as pulmonary embolus, subcutaneous heparin is safer than warfarin (see Chapter 4). There appears to be less maternal bleeding and no fetal risk of congenital abnormalities, such as chondrodysplasia punctata or optic atrophy. However, where there is a risk of systemic thromboembolism as in heart disease, subcutaneous heparin treatment does not seem to be adequate. Indeed there are reports of Starr–Edwards aortic and Bjork–Shiley mitral prosthetic valves that thrombosed during pregnancy when the mothers were either managed with subcutaneous heparin [23,188] or were not anticoagulated [45]. Such disasters have been managed by emergency cardiopulmonary bypass and caesarean section (assuming fetal maturity) followed by prosthetic valve replacement [22].

Ahmad *et al*. [2] and Biale *et al*. [25] have reported one and four cases respectively, where patients with artificial heart valves have been treated with dipyridamole alone during pregnancy. There were no incidents of thromboembolism, but since the data of Limet and Crondin [176] suggest that risk is only between one in four and one in 10 pregnancies if no anticoagulants are used, larger series are necessary to establish the effectiveness of this form of treatment.

There is no ideal solution to the problem. Even though the risk of fetal malformations such as optic atrophy may persist after 16 weeks' gestation [279], I believe that warfarin should be used until about 37 weeks' gestation because subcutaneous heparin does not give adequate protection. Furthermore even subcutaneous heparin therapy has the risk of bone demineralization (Chapter 4) and the risks of warfarin have probably been overestimated because of overdosing in previous series (see also Chapter 4). In the series by Javares of 42 pregnancies in patients receiving warfarin throughout pregnancy until 34–36 weeks for artificial heart valves, there was the expected high abortion rate (29 per cent); but there were only two other fetal losses (one still-birth and one pre-term), one case of cerebral haemorrhage, one case of nasal hypoplasia and three growth retarded fetuses [144]. Similar data have been described in other series [20,137,180,327]. The data of the series by Javares suggest that patients with mitral valve replacement where cardiac function remains more impaired than in aortic valve replacement, may be particularly at risk from abortion. Also use of the minimum dose of warfarin maintaining an international normalized ratio (INR) no greater than 3 may decrease the teratogenic and abortion risks of warfarin [144] without any increase in the risk of thromboembolism [283].

It is also possible that the teratogenic effect of dindevan may be less than that of warfarin [99] but there are not the data to prove this; since there is more experience in general with warfarin, I would suggest that this drug should be used in preference.

At 37 weeks when the risk of bleeding in the warfarinized fetus in association with labour seems to be too great, the patient should be admitted to hospital and given continuous intravenous heparin. The aim should be to achieve a heparin level as assayed by protamine sulphate neutralization [64] or anti-Xa assay of 0.5–1.0 unit/ml [64]. Heparin does not cross the placenta [101] and therefore will not cause bleeding in the fetus. It is believed that the clotting system of the fetus will return to normal after warfarin has been withheld for about 1 week. At that time, maternal heparin therapy should be reduced to give a heparin level of <0.2 units/ml, and/or a thrombin time that is not prolonged and labour should be induced. If the patient inadvertently goes into labour taking warfarin, she should be given vitamin K to reverse the action of warfarin in the fetus and started on heparin therapy as above. In extreme cases, vitamin K has been given intramuscularly to the fetus *in utero* by transamniotic injection [165]. It could now be given by cordocentesis.

After delivery, because of the risk of maternal post-partum haemorrhage, the patient should continue to receive heparin for about 7 days; then warfarin may be recommenced. This is not a contraindication to breast feeding, since insignificant quantities of warfarin are secreted in breast milk [231]. However, dindevan is excreted in breast milk [86] and patients taking dindevan should not breast feed.

An alternative approach to anticoagulation in the early part of pregnancy was that of Iturbe-Alessio *et al*. [139] in Mexico. They discontinued warfarin in 35 women as soon as they reported in pregnancy and substituted subcutaneous heparin 5000 units twice daily until the end of the 12th week. At this stage warfarin was recommenced to be replaced by heparin at the end of pregnancy. The results were compared with those in 37 controls who continued warfarin throughout the early part of pregnancy. In the control group there was an extraordinarily high rate of embryopathy (30 per cent) mostly diagnosed on the basis of minor abnormalities of the face. There were no cases of embryopathy and only two abortions in 23 women who discontinued warfarin before 7 weeks; there were two cases of embryopathy in eight continuing pregnancies where warfarin was discontinued between 7 and 12 weeks. The price to pay for this form of treatment was two massive valve thromboses in the heparin-treated group. Although the diagnosis of warfarin embryopathy must be questioned because of its very high incidence in the control group, it does appear that it may be prevented by withholding warfarin between 7 and 12 weeks. Ten thousand units of heparin per day is a very low dose in pregnancy and a more aggressive policy [250], possibly with an adjusted dose continuous intravenous infusion [208], or adjusted dose subcutaneous treatment might reduce the incidence of embolism. For example Lee *et al.* [166] performed a similar study in 18 pregnancies substituting subcutaneous heparin for warfarin from as soon as pregnancy was confirmed until 13 weeks. Their target was to achieve a partial thromboplastin time 1.5 times the control value. This is a relatively low level of anticoagulation. Fortunately there were no thrombotic episodes and no abnormal live born infants. However, by contrast with the study of Iturbe-Alessio [138], the abortion rate was 50 per cent. These forms of management have not been fully evaluated yet.

Our suggestion would be to substitute heparin for warfarin from 7–12 weeks, giving it intravenously by Hickman line and aiming for a heparin level of 1 unit/ml, or doubling the partial thromboplastin time.

Labour

Labour should not be induced because of heart disease; indeed, the risks of failed induction and of possible sepsis are relative contraindications. Nevertheless, these risks are slight, and induction should not be withheld if it is necessary for obstetric reasons. Furthermore, induction near term may be justified to plan delivery in daylight hours, in complicated cases requiring optimal medical support. A note of caution is necessary concerning the use of prostaglandin E_2 for the induction of labour in cardiac patients. Prostaglandin E_2 is a potent vasodilator and causes a marked rise in cardiac output [339]. In very high dosage when used for post-partum haemorrhage [170] and for termination of pregnancy [152] prostaglandin E has caused cardiac arrest in patients with normal hearts. Although there need not be a moratorium on the use of prostaglandin E for induction of labour in cardiac patients, the minimum dose should be used and prolonged treatment should not be attempted.

Patients with heart disease, particularly those with restrictive heart disease such as mitral stenosis are at risk during labour because of the increase in cardiac output that occurs at this time [264]. This occurs for a number of reasons: physical exertion, pain and the contractile effect of the uterus which expels blood and has been shown to cause an increase in left atrial pressure [142]. In addition many women in labour are given copious quantities of intravenous crystalloid fluids. If they have normal hearts, they can cope with the resultant increase in circulating blood volume and decrease in colloid osmotic pressure [114]. Patients with heart disease cannot and may easily develop pulmonary oedema.

Patients with heart disease are also particularly sensitive to aortocaval compression by the gravid uterus in the supine position, causing marked hypotension with maternal and fetal distress. The risk of this is even greater after epidural anaesthesia [321]. Wedges to maintain the patient in the left lateral position can be helpful [254].

Some centres are gaining increasing experience in the use of elective central catheterization (Swan–Ganz technique) to measure the right atrial pressure, wedge pressure (indirect left atrial pressure) and the cardiac output in labour in patients with heart disease (see above). There is no doubt that this technique allows a much more rational use of fluid therapy, diuretics and inotropic agents. Preliminary results would also suggest that measurement of central venous pressure alone is so misleading as an index of left ventricular filling pressure that it should not be used for this purpose (although it is still invaluable in patients with bleeding problems). However, the technique of Swan–Ganz catheterization is quite difficult and it has a significant morbidity. Therefore, it should only be used in centres where there is sufficient experience.

Most patients with heart disease do have quite rapid uncomplicated labours, particularly if they are taking digoxin [333]. In the majority, analgesia is best given by epidural anaesthesia which is a highly effective form of analgesic treatment. The effects of epidural block are complex and have not been fully evaluated. In normal patients having elective caesarean section where the cardiac output has not increased because of labour, epidural block in the left lateral position does not decrease cardiac output even though the systemic arterial pressure falls [265]. (By contrast spinal anaesthesia causes a marked fall in cardiac output [263].) But in the labouring woman epidural block has the capacity to reduce the elevated cardiac output because of its efficacy as an analgesic and because of venodilation and reduction of preload. But the effects of caval occlusion may be exaggerated by epidural block which can also inhibit compensatory mechanisms for blood loss [162]. And in some specific cardiac conditions such as Eisenmenger's syndrome and hypertrophic cardiomyopathy there is concern about the use of epidural block because of the reduction of afterload and preload. Also if epidural block is used rather than general anaesthesia for caesarean section, patients who are breathless may not be able to lie flat enough when awake.

However, in most cases regional block is now preferred to general anaesthesia for maternal and fetal reasons in uncomplicated pregnancy and there are therefore *a priori* reasons for preferring regional block in patients with heart disease. But in the end the decision concerning the use of epidural block in patients with heart disease must be made jointly by the anaesthetist, obstetrician, cardiologist and the patient.

It would seem sensible to keep the second stage of labour short in order to decrease maternal effort in patients with heart disease, but there is obviously no advantage in performing a forceps delivery in a woman who is going to push the baby out easily herself.

The use of oxytocic drugs in the third stage of labour is debated. The theoretical disadvantage is that ergometrine and Syntocinon will cause a tonic contraction of the uterus, expressing about 500 ml of blood into a circulation whose capacitance has also been made smaller by associated venoconstriction. In patients with heart disease, left atrial pressure may rise by 10 mmHg at the third stage of labour. This is particularly obvious in patients with mitral stenosis (Fig. 5.1) [50]. However, the management of post-partum haemorrhage in a patient with heart disease is not easy. I would suggest using Syntocinon in all patients in the third stage, unless they are in heart failure when oxytocics should be withheld altogether. Syntocinon has less effect on blood vessels than ergometrine and can be given by infusion. This infusion can be accompanied by intravenous frusemide.

Endocarditis and its prevention

The Confidential Enquiries into Maternal Death in England and Wales show that five of the 23 cardiac deaths in the UK between 1985 and 1987 were in association with endocarditis [79]. In the majority of the 124 cases that have been reported in obstetric and gynaecological practice, the organism was a streptococcus [286]. However, the case for antibiotic prophylaxis in labour has not been proven. There are several large series of patients with heart disease in pregnancy where no antibiotics have been given, and where no endocarditis has been observed [100,296,307]. It is difficult to document bacteraemia in labour [39,255]. Several authors have argued persuasively against antibiotic prophylaxis [104,313,

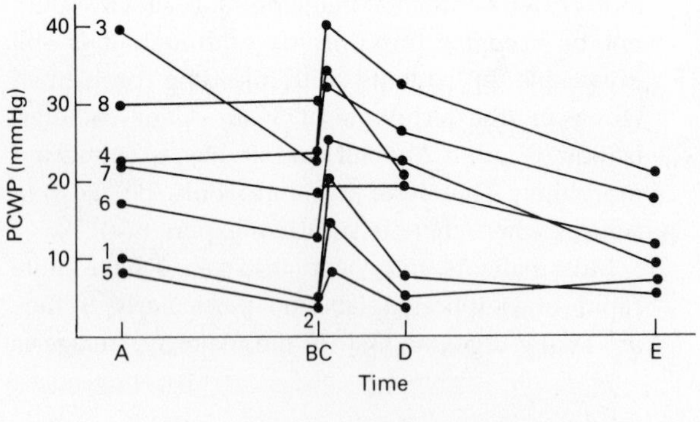

Fig. 5.1. Intra-partum alterations in pulmonary capillary wedge pressure (PCWP) in eight patients with mitral stenosis. A, first stage labour; B, second stage labour, 15–30 min before delivery; C, 5–15 min post-partum; D, 4–6 hours post-partum; E, 18–25 hours post-partum [45].

314]. A British working party recommended antibiotic prophylaxis in labour only in women with artificial heart valves, who are a particularly high risk group if they do contract endocarditis [257].

Yet, from the data of the Confidential Maternal Mortality series, it would seem that women are at increased risk from endocarditis in pregnancy. What is not clear from some of these reports is whether endocarditis was contracted during labour, and was potentially preventable by peripartum antibiotic prophylaxis, or whether it arose at some other time. One case that is described in detail in the 1973–75 report [78] did appear to develop endocarditis during a normal delivery, and other similar non-fatal cases have been reported [72], in one associated with premature rupture of membranes as a possible source of sepsis [134]. Until more details are available, I will continue to advise antibiotic prophylaxis in all patients with structural heart disease except mitral valve prolapse without a systolic murmur where there appears to be no risk of endocarditis [65]. The antibiotics that we use are intramuscular ampicillin 500 mg and intramuscular gentamicin 80 mg; three injections are given every 8 hours at the onset or induction of labour [84]. The patient who is penicillin sensitive receives one intravenous injection of vancomycin 1 g [84,105] followed by intravenous gentamicin 120 mg [253]. Vancomycin should be given over 60 minutes [291] because of the risk of idiosyncratic hypotensive reactions [129]. Because of these risks, intravenous teicoplanin 400 mg has been suggested as an alternative to vancomycin and gentamicin [290].

A compromise is to use prophylactic antibiotics only in those cases at high risk, i.e. those with previous endocarditis, valve replacement, instrumental delivery or delivery following prolonged rupture of membranes.

Pulmonary oedema and other cardiovascular side-effects of β sympathomimetic drugs

Those obstetricians and physicians who practise in Western communities are more likely to see pulmonary oedema related to treatment of other conditions in pregnancy such as pre-term labour and pre-eclampsia (see Chapter 6) or even malaria [210] than to structural heart disease. For example in over 6000 obstetric admissions in Hamilton, Ontario, there were 12 cases of pulmonary oedema of which seven were related to parenteral tocolytic therapy. The incidence of pulmonary oedema in patients treated with isoxsuprine was 0.5 per cent [212]. Although adverse cardiovascular side-effects of salbutamol and other β sympathomimetic agents given in premature labour have been reported, there is still a general lack of awareness of their importance. Whitehead *et al.* [336] reported the occurrence of chest pain and ischaemic electrocardiogram changes in one patient treated for 5 hours with intravenous salbutamol (4.2 mg) and subsequently reported pulmonary oedema in another patient given salbutamol 2.2 mg intravenously over 6 hours [329]. They suggested that vasodilation caused by concurrent administration of hydralazine and methyldopa for hypertension might be an additional factor in increasing circulating blood volume, and cited one similar maternal death reported to the Committee of Safety of Medicine after use of salbutamol and methyldopa. Davies and Robertson [67] reported another case of pulmonary oedema after the use of higher infusion rates of salbutamol (20 μg/min) over a longer period (56 hours). In this case, betamethasone was used, and this may also have increased the circulating blood volume. These authors suggested that ergometrine given after delivery may have decreased the venous capacitance and thus contributed to the development of pulmonary oedema.

In North America, terbutaline (Bricanyl) is used to treat pre-term labour. It has the advantage that it can be given subcutaneously. Stubblefield [306] reported one case of pulmonary oedema in which dexamethasone administration was an additional risk factor. Rogge *et al* [271] reported three similar cases and cited knowledge of six other cases occurring in California. Pulmonary oedema has also been reported with the use of fenoterol [159] and ritodrine [89,91].

β sympathomimetics are widely used for the treatment of premature labour [175] even though there are contradictory reports concerning their efficacy [127]. They cause tachycardia both directly and reflexly because of associated vasodilation. Both the tachycardia and the increased blood volume associated with vasodilation may contribute to the risk of pulmonary oedema, particularly if the vascular capacitance is suddenly reduced by ergometrine after delivery [67]. In addition, β sympathomimetic agents have metabolic effects. They cause a rise in blood glucose by increasing glycogenolysis and decreasing glucose uptake. Free fatty acid and lactate concentrations increase, and hypokalaemia has also been reported [122]. These factors may further impair myocardial function in a situation which is already haemodynamically unfavourable. Although it has been suggested that tachycardia alone [244] and/or circulatory overload [67,102] are the real causes of pulmonary oedema in these patients, this seems unlikely. Pulmonary oedema is a rare complication of modern obstetrics, and its occurrence on so many occasions with the use of β sympathomimetics suggests that there is specific interaction.

Since there is no universal belief in the efficacy of long-term β sympathomimetics, and because of the maternal risk, the following guidelines are suggested concerning their use for the treatment of pre-term labour. β sympathomimetic infusions should not be given for more than 24 hours, except in exceptional circumstances. The risk of cardiovascular side-effects increases in infusions given for more than 24 hours. A delay in delivery of 24 hours should allow glucocorticoids to enhance fetal lung maturation. β sympathomimetic drugs should be given with great care to patients with pre-existing heart disease. They may even unmask previously asymptomatic peripartum cardiomyopathy [28]. The nature and severity of the heart disease are obviously critical (e.g. there would probably be no additional risk of giving salbutamol to a patient with mild mitral regurgitation, whereas such therapy could be fatal in a patient with severe mitral stenosis). β sympathomimetics should not be used in conditions that predispose to supraventricular tachycardia such as Wolff–Parkinson–White and Lown–Ganong–Levine syndromes [41]. β sympathomimetic drugs should be stopped if any arrhythmias develop, if the heart rate exceeds 120/min or if the patient develops chest pain or breathlessness. However, non-specific electrocardiogram changes, ST depression, T wave inversion and prolonged QT interval occur in about 75 per cent [21,128] of patients given ritodrine. Similar data have been obtained in patients taking fenoterol [331]. Therefore if β sympathomimetics are used, these electrocardiogram changes occurring on their own, should not be criteria for stopping therapy.

Auscultation of the lung basis should be performed regularly in patients given parental β sympathomimetics to detect early signs of pulmonary oedema. But this is a relatively insensitive technique. Transcutaneous monitoring of oxygen saturation is now widely available and will almost certainly detect hypoxaemia due to pulmonary oedema before any abnormalities can be found in the lungs. Therefore continuous monitoring of oxygen saturation should be employed in all patients receiving β sympathomimetics for tocolysis [332] if the equipment is available. The critical level appears to be an oxygen saturation of 94 per cent corresponding to a Po_2 of 10 kPa (75 mmHg). Above this level there is no threat to the mother (or fetus) [313].

If β sympathomimetic drugs are used, the obstetrician should also be aware of the risk of other therapies. Glucocorticoids will exacerbate hyperglycaemia as well as causing an increase in circulating blood volume due to associated mineralocorticoid activity. This will be exacerbated by vasodilator drugs, so scrupulous attention must be paid to fluid balance and the maternal heart rate.

Specific conditions occurring during pregnancy

Many specific conditions have already been mentioned. However, some give particular management problems and are considered below.

Acquired heart disease

Chronic rheumatic heart disease

This form of heart disease has been commonest in pregnancy in the UK and still is in many parts of the world. Szekeley *et al.* have given exhaustive accounts from Newcastle of rheumatic heart disease in pregnancy [312,313]. By far the most important lesion is mitral stenosis, which may be the only lesion or the dominant abnormality amongst several others. Women with mitral stenosis are particularly likely to develop pulmonary oedema in pregnancy because of the increase in cardiac output, the increase in heart rate preventing ventricular filling and the increase in pulmonary blood volume [39]. Mitral stenosis is the lesion that is most likely to require treatment for pulmonary oedema or heart failure (see above) and also to require surgery during pregnancy. Open and closed heart surgery and also mitral valvuloplasty have already been discussed above (see above). The haemodynamic changes associated with labour in patients with mitral stenosis have been documented by Swan–Ganz catheterization. Patients entering labour with a wedge pressure (indirect left atrial pressure) <14 mmHg are unlikely to develop pulmonary oedema [51] (see Fig. 5.1).

Mitral regurgitation puts a volume load on the left atrium and left ventricle, but it does not cause pulmonary hypertension until late in the condition, and heart failure is rare in pregnancy; it usually occurs in older women. Endocarditis is more common in patients with mitral regurgitation, particularly if they are in sinus rhythm. It is now realized that many patients who were thought to have rheumatic mitral regurgitation do in fact have congenital abnormalities of the mitral valve. Although such abnormalities may be associated with arrhythmias and endocarditis, this is uncommon, particularly in pregnancy. For practical purposes (i.e. endocarditis prophylaxis) patients with mitral valve prolapse are only at risk of endocarditis if they have mitral regurgitation.

Pregnancy may be associated with rupture of the chordae tendineae of the mitral valve [44] and the subsequent deterioration in cardiac function. This may occur in normal mitral valves or in those affected by rheumatic carditis or other disease (e.g. systemic lupus erythematosus) [228]. Very rarely, obstruction in the left atrium may be due to left atrial myxoma which has been reported in pregnancy [184]. The echocardiogram is pathognomonic and the tumour should be removed surgically.

Rheumatic aortic valve disease is much less common in women than in men, and much less common than mitral valve disease in pregnancy. Severe aortic regurgitation causes pulmonary oedema; aortic stenosis may be associated with chest pain, syncope and sudden death; although both conditions are usually not severe enough to be a problem in pregnancy, critical aortic stenosis may cause maternal death and should be relieved by aortic valve surgery or valvuoplasty (see above).

Disease of the tricuspid valve almost never occurs in isolation. Also, tricuspid valve disease rarely requires specific treatment; the patient improves when the rheumatic disease of the other valves is treated, either medically or surgically. Although there are case reports of successful pregnancy following triple valve replacement (aortic, mitral and tricuspid) it is unusual for such surgery to be necessary for patients within the reproductive age group [204].

Acute rheumatic fever

In general there has been a steady decline in the incidence of rheumatic fever though there was a resurgence in the USA between 1985 and 1988 [26]. Acute rheumatic fever is now very uncommon in pregnancy. The diagnosis may often be missed in patients who only complain of non-specific malaise and joint pains, and who on investigation, only have fever and anaemia that does not respond to haematinics. The more florid signs of swollen joints, rheumatic nodules and skin rashes do not necessarily occur in adults. The diagnosis may be made on the basis of a history of previous sore throat, elevated ASO titre, and electrocardiogram evidence of prolonged PR and QT intervals. The erythrocyte sedimentation rate (ESR) should be elevated to >80 mm/hour, since levels of 40 mm/hour are common in pregnancy. The level of C reactive protein is also elevated and this is not affected by pregnancy.

If rheumatic fever does develop in pregnancy, it is likely to be severe with a high risk of heart failure due to myocarditis, which is part of the triad of pericarditis and endocarditis. Treatment should be bed rest, salicylates, steroids and penicillin (for any residual streptococcal infection). The patient should then receive a prolonged period of prophylactic penicillin therapy. Chorea, another manifestation of the rheumatic process, is described in Chapter 15.

Pregnancy in patients with artificial heart valves, tissue valves or prostheses

As described earlier, anticoagulation is the major problem in these patients and the maternal need for a high level of anticoagulation has been stressed. Those patients who have successful isolated aortic or mitral valve replacement usually have near normal cardiac functioon and do not incur haemodynamic problems in pregnancy [221]. Even those patients with multiple valve replacements usually have sufficient cardiac reserve for a successful pregnancy [5].

The fetal problem of anticoagulation is shown in four series from the Hammersmith Hospital, London [222], the National Maternity Hospital, Dublin [220], from Hong Kong [45] and from Barcelona [144] (Table 5.3). In the Dublin series of 18 pregnancies, all the patients were anticoagulated and there were eight fetal losses and one case of warfarin embryopathy. In the Hammersmith series, 24 pregnancies not treated with anticoagulants (usually because they had biological valves) resulted in 23 normal babies. Fifteen pregnancies treated with oral anticoagulants resulted in only seven healthy babies. In the Hong Kong series there were 10 fetal losses in 30 pregnancies treated with anticoagulants but only one fetal loss in the group not treated with anticoagulants. In a mixed series of 98 pregnancies Vitali *et al*. [327] confirmed that the risk of warfarin is increased fetal loss, particularly abortion. The risk of withholding warfarin and substituting any other form of anticoagulation except full heparinization is maternal thromboembolism.

With regard to the use of tissue heart valves rather than mechanical prostheses a recent *Lancet* editorial [163] commented on the Edinburgh series in which Bjork–Shiley valves were compared with porcine xenographs in a long-term controlled trial outwith pregnancy [29]: 'patients undergoing mitral valve replacement should have a mechanical prosthesis, unless anticoagulation cannot be undertaken for pressing reasons'. The reasons for this conclusion were increased mortality and a greater need for reoperation in the porcine tissue valve group because of failure and calcification [280]. For the fetal reasons given above some have considered pregnancy to be a pressing reason why anticoagulation cannot be undertaken. They have therefore suggested that women contemplating pregnancy should have a tissue valve implanted in the knowledge that this will need to be replaced within 10 years when hopefully the patient's family will be completed. However, it has recently been found that pregnancy is likely to be associated with accelerated calcification and therefore the failure of tissue

Table 5.3. Fetal outcome of oral anticoagulation in pregnancy in mothers with artificial heart valves

	Hammersmith[1]	Dublin[2]	Hong Kong[3]	Barcelona[4]
Number of pregnancies	39	18	41	46
Number anticoagulated and fetal mortality and morbidity (% of those anticoagulated)	15 (53)	18 (50)	30 (40)	42 (31–38)*
Causes of fetal mortality and morbidity (% of those anticoagulated)				
Abortion	3 (20)	8 (44)	10 (33)	12 (21–29)*
Perinatal deaths	4 (27)	0 (0)	0 (0)	2 (0–5) *
Fetal malformation	1 (7)	1 (5)	2 (7)	2 (0–4) *
Number not anticoagulated and fetal mortality and morbidity (% of those not anticoagulated)	24 (4)	0 (0)	11 (9)	3†

[1] [222]; [2] [220]; [3] [45]; [4] [144].
* Not stated which of the fetal losses etc. were in the anticoagulated group so possible range is given.
† Fetal mortality and morbidity not known in the group who were not anticoagulated.

xenographs [8]. This may be a feature of using tissue valves in young patients [280] rather than an effect of pregnancy [8] but on this basis elective tissue valve replacement can no longer be advised for women who want to become pregnant. In conclusion they should have an artificial valve and accept the fetal hazards of warfarin therapy for the majority of pregnancy which can be minimized by substituting intravenous heparin over the period of organogenesis (see above).

Myocardial infarction

Myocardial infarction is rare in pregnancy and in young women in general. Only 1 per cent of admissions for myocardial infarction occur in women younger than 45 years [239]. In 1988, Trouton *et al.* [319] cited only 77 cases of myocardial infarction in pregnancy in the literature since 1922. Most of these cases were in women aged 30–40 years. However, the increasing incidence of myocardial infarction in women and the increasing age at which women become pregnant may result in an increased incidence of myocardial infarction in pregnancy.

The immediate mortality from myocardial infarction in pregnancy is 26 per cent; some women die up to 4 years after the original event, making the overall mortality 32 per cent [56]. The overall mortality from myocardial infarction rises during pregnancy from nil in the first trimester to 50 per cent in the puerperium; surprisingly younger patients are more likely to have myocardial infarction in the puerperium and therefore have a higher mortality [108]. Pregnancies in these younger patients have frequently been complicated by pre-eclampsia [16].

The precise mechanism of myocardial infarction is open to speculation in all patients and in particular in pregnancy. Women have a high incidence of coronary spasm, and atypical mechanisms seem to be common in pregnancy. Beary *et al.* [16] suggest that the group of patients with myocardial infarction occurring in the puerperium includes those that are most likely to have spasm or coronary artery thrombosis unassociated with atherosclerotic narrowing as described by Ciraulo and Markovitz [48]. The syndrome of myocardial infarction with normal coronary arteries occurring in young women is well documented [299]. In the non-pregnant state the prognosis is good if they survive the initial episode [106]. Primary dissection of the coronary arteries is another cause of myocardial infarction particularly peri-partum [36,145] when some cases have been associated with β sympathomimetic tocolysis [125]. Coronary artery dissection in general is rare but more than 70 per cent of cases occur in women and 25 per cent of these cases have occurred at the end of or immediately after pregnancy [325]. This is presumably another example of the tendency for any fault in arteries such as coronary, splenic, adrenal or even aorta [297] to predispose to rupture in pregnancy (see section on coarctation of the aorta, below). For this reason caution is necessary concerning angioplasty immediately following myocardial infarction in pregnancy [109] or even concerning coronary arteriography which itself may precipitate dissection [203].

Anomalous origin of the coronary arteries [156] and arteritis due to systemic lupus or Kawasaki's disease [213] are other rare causes of myocardial infarction in pregnancy.

Left ventricular aneurysm formation may complicate myocardial infarction but is not an absolute contraindication to further pregnancies since a successful case has been reported [260]. Successful pregnancy is also possible following severe myocardial infarction which may include cardiac arrest [303]. Termination of pregnancy is therefore not mandatory under these circumstances.

The diagnosis of myocardial infarction in pregnancy will be made on the basis of chest pain, with possible pericardial friction rub and fever. Only serial electrocardiographic changes are meaningful, because of the electrocardiographic changes induced by pregnancy itself (see above); also regional anaesthesia (spinal or epidural block) is associated with 'ischaemic' electrocardiographic changes (ST depression) in about 60 per cent of cases [189]. Moderate elevations of the white cell count and ESR are seen in normal pregnancy, when the level of lactic acid dehydrogenase may also be raised [304]. However, elevations of serum glutamic acid transaminase and creatinine phosphokinase levels would indicate myocardial infarction in the appropriate clinical setting [304]. During the puerperium interpretation of these enzymes levels must be cautious, because they are liberated by the associated tissue destruction of the involuting uterus. However the MB isoenzyme of creatinine phosphokinase is specific to cardiac muscle. The differential diagnosis of other occult causes of collapse in pregnancy is considered in p. 120 and in Table 4.1.

It is difficult to be confident about management, since there is little experience and the pathology may be diverse. It would be sensible to treat the initial episode in a coronary care unit, with conventional opiate analgesics and medication for complications such as dysrhythmias. Because of the possibility of coronary spasm, nitroglycerine or other vasodilators should be used early in patients with continuing pain. Once the patient has been delivered (again in an intensive care environment), there is a good case for coronary arteriography to delineate the pathology which may be atypical (though note the caution above about the possibility of coronary artery dissection) [203]. The angiographic demonstration of coronary embolus would be an indication for anticoagulation, but otherwise, the benefits of anticoagulation in myocardial infarction unassociated with pregnancy do not seem enough to justify the considerable extra risks imposed on the pregnancy. Similarly thrombolytic therapy, though it improves mortality in non-pregnant patients should not be used (except in early pregnancy) because of the possibility of precipitating pre-term delivery and the bleeding hazards of delivery if it does occur (see Chapter 4). However, there is increasing experience in the use of aspirin in pregnancy for the prophylaxis of pre-eclampsia; this drug has also been shown to decrease mortality in myocardial infarction and patients with myocardial infarction should therefore be given aspirin 300 mg at presentation and 150 mg daily thereafter unless there are any of the usual contraindications to aspirin therapy.

Patients should be allowed a spontaneous vaginal delivery, preferably with epidural anaesthesia, unless there are good obstetric reasons for interfering. However, as in other cases of heart disease, the second stage should be limited by forceps delivery. Syntocinon infusion should be used rather than ergometrine in the third stage, since ergometrine is more likely to cause coronary artery spasm.

There is no evidence that pregnancy predisposes to myocardial infarction. Unless it is thought that the patient has had a coronary embolus, pregnancy should not be discouraged in patients who have had myocardial infarction in the past.

Cardiomyopathy

HYPERTROPHIC OBSTRUCTIVE CARDIOMYOPATHY (HOCM)

Cardiomyopathy may arise *de novo* during pregnancy, and there is probably at least one form of cardiomyopathy (puerperal cardiomyopathy, see below) that is specific to pregnancy. Alternatively, any form of cardiomyopathy due to other causes may complicate pregnancy [149]. By far the most common of these other causes is HOCM (subaortic stenosis) and even this condition is relatively rare. The cause is unknown, but the pathological features are hypertrophy and disorganization of cardiac muscle, particularly that of the left ventricular outflow tract. The patient presents with chest pain, syncope, arrhythmias, or the symptoms of heart failure; alternatively HOCM may be a chance finding at echocardiography performed because of a heart murmur in pregnancy. Some cases are familial and there is a lot of work being done to establish the genetic basis of the disease. The diagnosis can usually be made by echocardiography which shows abnormally thickened and disorganized cardiac muscle.

Extensive experience of the management of this condition in pregnancy has been reported by Oakley *et al.* from the Hammersmith Hospital [223]. These authors originally advocated β adrenergic blockade in all cases to reduce the risk of syncope, due to obstruction of the left ventricular outflow tract [200]; this is now reserved for symptomatic patients only. Patients should not be allowed to become hypovolaemic, since this too increases the risk of obstruction of the left ventricular outflow tract. They should not lie supine because of the risk of caval obstruction and subsequent decrease in venous return. Particular care should be taken to give adequate fluid replacement if there is ante-partum haemorrhage and also to avoid post-partum haemorrhage. During labour, patients with HOCM should be given epidural anaesthesia with caution, since this causes relative hypovolaemia by increasing venous capacitance in the lower limbs.

PUERPERAL CARDIOMYOPATHY (PERIPARTUM CARDIOMYOPATHY, PREGNANCY CARDIOMYOPATHY)

This condition was first described by Hull and Hafkesbring [135] and was extensively reviewed by Stuart [305], Meadows [190] and others [131,149,201] whose papers should be consulted for further references. The incidence in the UK is probably < one in 5000. The condition usually arises in the puerperium (Fig. 5.2). There is no other predisposing cause for the heart failure and the heart is grossly dilated. Although patients have been described as usually multiparous, black, relatively elderly and of poor social class this does not seem to be so in sporadic cases seen in the UK. Pregnancy has often been complicated by hypertension. Multiple pregnancy is another risk factor [77]. Pulmonary, peripheral and particularly cerebral embolization is a major cause of morbidity and mortality, which is 25–50 per cent [131]. The majority of deaths occur around the time of presentation but some women have protracted illnesses and die up to 8 years later. However, if the patient recovers fully from the initial episode, the long-term prognosis is good. The condition is likely to recur in future pregnancies [77] which are therefore contraindicated in view of the overall poor prognosis. For this reason any patient who develops pulmonary oedema peri-partum should be investigated thoroughly in case the diagnosis of peripartum cardiomyopathy is made unjustifiably.

On investigation, the chest X-ray is not specific, showing pulmonary venous congestion and a large heart. The electrocardiogram may be normal or there may be widespread abnormalities. Rhythm disturbances are also common. The diagnosis of cardiomyopathy is confirmed by echocardiography which also excludes other subtle causes of raised left and/or right atrial blood pressure such as mitral valve disease, left atrial myxoma [184] and pericardial disease (see below). The distinction of puerperal cardiomyopathy from other forms of cardiomyopathy depends on the history and clinical features; the diagnosis is based on the exclusion of other known causes of cardiomyopathy. Apart from conventional antifailure treatment which now includes angiotensin-converting inhibitors, these patients should also receive anticoagulant therapy until the heart size has returned to normal, and until they have no further dysrhythmias.

The place of immunosuppressive therapy with either prednisone or azathioprine is unclear. These have been used successfully in cases associated with acute myocarditis demonstrated by endomyocardial biopsy [92,196] but such treatment cannot be routinely recommended [7].

Those few patients who present before delivery

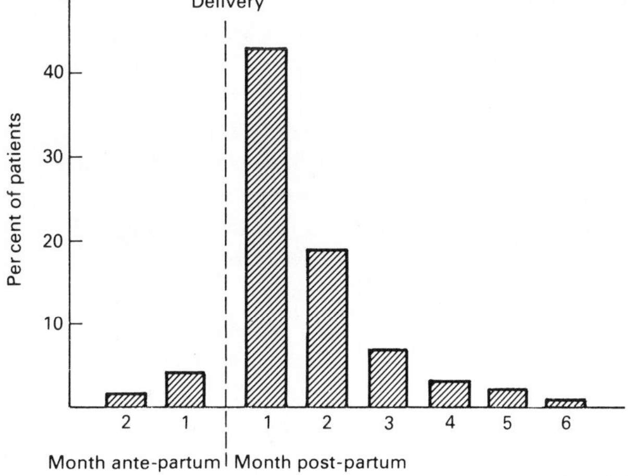

Fig. 5.2. Onset of peri-partum cardiomyopathy in relation to time of delivery. Total number of patients was 347 [111]. (Reproduced with permission of the Editor, *New England Journal of Medicine*.)

(Fig. 5.2) should be electively delivered since in the long term, the demand on their hearts will decrease after pregnancy. If the cervix is favourable vaginal delivery should be chosen; if not, the patients should be delivered by caesarean section. Skilled epidural anaesthesia is preferred for both routes of delivery. There is no evidence that breast feeding influences the course of puerperal cardiomyopathy.

Because of the poor prognosis of puerperal cardiomyopathy, the patients' young age and their social responsibilities having just been delivered, they should receive early consideration and high priority for cardiac transplantation [7]. The indication for transplantation is intractable pump failure despite optimal medical therapy.

The pathogenesis of this condition is unknown [131]; therefore some authors have denied that puerperal cardiomyopathy is a specific entity [33] and considered the condition to be another form of congestive cardiomyopathy caused by hypertension [22]. Rand *et al.* [251] on the basis of antibodies to heart muscle present in cord blood and serum from the mother in a case of pregnancy cardiomyopathy, postulate an immunological cause. Alternatively, the combination of multiparity and low social class has suggested that the condition is due to an undefined nutritional defect. Melvin *et al.* [191] described three cases of puerperal cardiomyopathy due to myocarditis, proven by endomyocardial biopsy at cardiac catheterization, and these authors propose that infection may be an important cause. Cunningham *et al.* [62] reviewed 28 cases of obscure cardiomyopathy occurring in 106 000 pregnancies in Texas. In only seven cases was the condition really idiopathic, emphasizing the rarity of the condition, but these patients fared very badly. Four were dead within 8 years.

Davidson and Parry [66] have described a specific form of puerperal cardiac failure occurring in the Hausa tribe in Northern Nigeria. They were able to document 224 cases and claimed that in the peak season (summer) half the female medical beds in Zaria are occupied by patients with this condition. The peak incidence is 4 weeks post-partum. During this period, for up to 40 days after delivery, the Hausa woman spends 18 hours/day lying on a mud bed, heated so that the ambient temperature reaches 40°C. She also increases her sodium intake to 450 mmol/day by eating kanwa salt from Lake Chad. Many of the patients are hypertensive, but the condition regresses rapidly with diuretic and digoxin therapy, which causes a weight loss of 29 per cent in 15 days. Echocardiographic studies do not support ventricular dysfunction in this condition [282]. The contribution of hypertension to the heart failure is debated [281] but this would seem an extreme example of the instability of the cardiovascular system in the first weeks of the puerperium interacting with the particular susceptibility of West Africans to dilated cardiomyopathy [161]. In all normal women, blood volume and cardiac output must fall while peripheral resistance rises after delivery. The practices of the Hausa tribe will cause a marked rise in circulating blood volume, which could be sufficient to produce clinical cardiac failure.

The high incidence of heart failure in the Hausa tribe demonstrates the vulnerability of the cardiovascular system in the puerperium and perhaps explains why so many of Stuart's cases presented at this time. In addition if peripheral vascular resistance rises very rapidly, before cardiac output falls, systemic hypertension will ensue, as is not infrequently seen in normal patients in the UK who have no history of antecedent hypertension in pregnancy before delivery [331].

Endomyocardial fibrosis

In this uncommon condition, the endocardium is thickened and replaced by fibrous tissue. Haemodynamically the condition behaves like constrictive pericarditis (see below) since the heart cannot relax in diastole. Although the condition is more common in tropical climates there have been three patients described in pregnancy. The most recent [219] developed congestive cardiac failure during pregnancy and died despite subsequent cardiac transplantation.

Pericardial disease

This is a rare complication of pregnancy but should be considered because of its specific haemodynamic problems [27]. Acute pericarditis is normally not of any haemodynamic consequence and is only of importance because it must be considered in patients presenting with chest pain and because of the necessity to diagnose the underlying cause. However, patients with significant pericardial effusion or more commonly with calcific pericarditis suffer because they cannot increase ventricular filling above the limit restricted by the pericardium. Therefore they can only increase cardiac output by increasing heart rate and they are dependent on maintaining both venous filling and heart rate in pregnancy.

Patients usually present with oedema, hepatomegaly, ascites and raised jugular venous pressure. Symptoms and signs of pulmonary oedema are a late finding. The diagnosis is often suggested by seeing calcification in the pericardium on X-ray and confirmed by echocardiography.

Patients should be treated with diuretics only if they develop pulmonary oedema or if peripheral oedema is a major problem. Digoxin is only indicated for atrial tachyarrhythmias. β adrenergic blocking agents should not be used. Patients should not become hypovolaemic. The condition improves when circulating blood volume decreases after delivery. Definitive treatment is pericardiectomy which can usually be deferred until after delivery [282]. Tuberculosis is an important cause of constrictive pericarditis.

Congenital heart disease

Eisenmenger's syndrome and other causes of pulmonary vascular disease

(see Maternal mortality above)

As indicated above, Eisenmenger's syndrome has a very high maternal mortality. Only recently has there been any form of surgical treatment and this, heart and lung transplantation, must be considered experimental [256]. A recent series of 28 cases of heart–lung transplantation had a perioperative mortality of 29 per cent mainly due to obliterative bronchiolitis which was also a problem of the survivors [37].

Most patients with Eisenmenger's syndrome who die in pregnancy, do so in the puerperium. Although deaths are occasionally sudden, due to thromboembolism, this is not usually so. More frequently, these patients die due to a slowly falling systemic $Pa\text{O}_2$ with associated decrease in cardiac output. A consideration of the haemodynamics involved (Fig. 5.3) suggests how this might occur and how it could be managed. In a defect, such as a large ventricular septal defect, the blood is freely mixed in the right and left ventricles and the ratio of blood flow in the pulmonary circuit (Q_p) to that in the systemic circuit (Q_s) is inversely proportional to the ratio of the pulmonary resistance (R_p) to the systemic resistance (R_s), i.e.

$$Q_p/Q_s \propto R_s/R_p. \qquad (5.1)$$

Pulmonary blood flow is also proportional to cardiac output (CO) so

$$Q_p \propto \text{CO} \times R_s/R_p. \qquad (5.2)$$

Thus any fall in the ratio $R_s : R_p$ or in the cardiac output will cause a fall in pulmonary blood flow. For example, in pre-eclampsia, the pulmonary vascular resistance increases and the cardiac output falls [178]. These factors would therefore decrease pulmonary blood flow and this could account for the observed deterioration in Eisenmenger's syndrome, associated with hypertensive pregnancy [201].

What can be offered to the pregnant patient with Eisenmenger's syndrome? Unfortunately, abortion would appear to be the answer. The maternal mortality associated with abortion is only 7 per cent in comparison to 30 per cent for continuing pregnancy [112]. However, if the patient decides to continue with pregnancy, prophylactic anticoagulation, probably with subcutaneous heparin, should be offered, because of the risk of thromboembolism, both systemic and pulmonary. Labour should not be induced unless there are good obstetric reasons. Induced labour carries a higher risk of caesarean section which is associated with a particularly high maternal mortality in Eisenmenger's syndrome [112].

There is controversy concerning the place of epidural anaesthesia for the management of labour. Although epidural anaesthesia should decrease the $Q_p : Q_s$ ratio by decreasing the systemic vascular resistance, this may not occur, at least it did not in the one case studied by Midwall *et al.* [197]. On balance, a carefully administered elective epidural

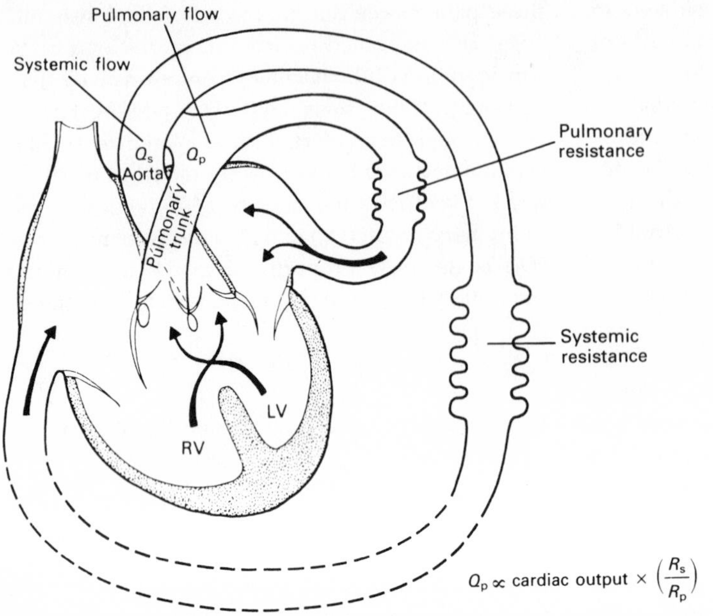

Fig. 5.3. Pulmonary and systemic blood flows and resistances in Eisenmenger's syndrome associated with ventricular septal defect [65] (see text). (Courtesy of the Editor, *Journal of the Royal College of Physicians.*)

anaesthetic at the beginning of labour is probably preferable to emergency epidural or general anaesthesia if it is suddenly decided that instrumental delivery is necessary [60,112].

If the patient does become hypotensive with increasing cyanosis and decreasing cardiac output, it has been shown that high inspired oxygen concentrations can decrease pulmonary vascular resistance, increase the $Q_p : Q_s$ ratio and increase peripheral oxygen saturation [197]. In addition, α sympathomimetic agents, such as phenylephrine, methoxamine and noradrenaline, will increase R_s and thus increase pulmonary blood flow [81]. However, drugs such as tolazline, phentolamine, nitroprusside and isoprenaline, which have been used to decrease pulmonary vascular resistance in other clinical situations, probably should not be given, since they will also decrease the systemic vascular resistance [81]. If R_s decreases more than R_p, pulmonary blood flow will decrease rather than increase. The same problem occurs with dopamine and β sympathomimetric drugs which have been given to increase cardiac output. They too will decrease R_s and if R_s decreases more than the cardiac output increases, pulmonary blood flow will fall. Two other pulmonary vasodilators deserve mention. There is evidence of thromboxane/prostacyclin imbalance in primary pulmonary hypertension with too much thromboxane production and too little prostacyclin production [47]. In these circumstances prostacyclin infusion may act as a relatively selective pulmonary vasodilator [148]. The drug is expensive and has to be given by intravenous infusion, but it might just tip the balance in the deteriorating Eisenmenger patient to allow improved pulmonary blood flow and better myocardial oxygenation. Also, nitric oxide has now been identified as the endothelium-derived relaxing factor which in turn is a very powerful vasodilator. When inhaled it could be a relatively selective pulmonary vasodilator and it has been shown to be effective both in the neonate [261] and in adults [238] with pulmonary hypertension. However, both these forms of therapy are somewhat experimental. In summary, the management of the deteriorating patient with Eisenmenger's syndrome depends on giving oxygen and α sympathomimetic amines.

COR PULMONALE, PULMONARY VENO-OCCLUSIVE DISEASE, PRIMARY PULMONARY HYPERTENSION

In cor pulmonale, pulmonary veno-occlusive disease and primary pulmonary hypertension where there is pulmonary hypertension and vascular disease in small blood vessels, the maternal mortality is still high and termination of pregnancy is still the management of choice [30]. Two successful cases would suggest that peripheral pulmonary stenosis like pulmonary valvular stenosis and Fallot's tetralogy where the small pulmonary blood vessels are not affected should have a more successful outcome [164,318]. The problem in these conditions still appears to be one of maintaining adequate pulmonary blood flow for adequate oxygenation. Even though blood cannot be shunted directly from the pulmonary to the systemic circuit as in Eisenmenger's syndrome, excessive vasodilation in the systemic circulation during epidural anaesthesia could still decrease preload to the right ventricle and therefore further decrease pulmonary blood flow. Unfortunately as in Eisenmenger's syndrome selective pulmonary vasodilators are not available. The options include nitroprusside [207] and oxygen and the effects of prostacyclin infusion and nitric oxide inhalation are being investigated. In addition, manoeuvres which suddenly increase venous return (ergometrine injection, movement from supine to left lateral position) should be avoided as should those which increase vagal tone (e.g. bladder catheterization). Several patients with primary pulmonary hypertension have died in association with bradycardia and atrioventricular block which suggest vagally mediated mechanisms. These patients should be delivered in an intensive care environment with elective insertion of a Swan–Ganz catheter (not withstanding the risk in patients with pulmonary hypertension) and facilities for pacing [207]. If circumstances permit, there are strong arguments for elective testing of various potential pulmonary vasodilators on the day before delivery to see which (if any) will work in the event that the patient deteriorates [294]. To maintain haemodynamic stability Abboud *et al.* [1] used intrathecal morphine as an analgesic in labour in a patient with primary pulmonary hypertension. Intrathecal morphine gives very effective analgesia with little change in maternal haemodynamics and little transfer to the fetus. The most common side-effects are pruritus and late respiratory depression. The immediate results in this case were excellent as judged clinically and by Swan–Ganz monitoring. Unfortunately the patient died 7 days later from acute right ventricular strain. The theoretical advantage of epidural morphine over epidural anaesthesia is the lack of haemodynamic effects. Yet conventional epidural anaesthesia when skillfully applied can be very beneficial in primary pulmonary hypertension [294] and fentanyl (an opiate) and bupivacaine have been combined with success for delivery in primary pulmonary hypertension [329]. The anaesthetist's experience is likely to dictate which is the more suitable form of anaesthesia in these difficult and very uncommon situations.

Coarctation of the aorta

In both coarctation of the aorta and Marfan's syndrome (see below), the maternal risk is dissection of the aorta associated with the hyperdynamic circulation of pregnancy and possibly with an increased risk of medial degeneration due to the hormonal environment of pregnancy [157]. These mechanisms could also explain the well-known pregnancy associated risks in all patients, of rupture of aneurysms in the splenic, adrenal, renal, cerebral, coronary and ovarian arteries. Patients with coarctation also have the specific risk of cerebral haemorrhage due to ruptured berry aneurysm. The maternal mortality in coarctation has been stated as to be as high as 17 per cent [193]. It has therefore been suggested that all patients with coarctation presenting in pregnancy should either be aborted or have the defect repaired before delivery. However, Mendelson's series [193] dates from 1858 to 1939, and there have only been 14 maternal deaths reported in the whole of the literature, none of which occurred in the 83 patients studied since 1960 [76]. The risk of dissection has therefore probably been exaggerated and good obstetric care and effective antihypertensive therapy would decrease the risk still further. It is probable that we no longer see the patients similar to those of Mendelson's series, since most patients with severe coarctation are operated on in infancy. Only those patients who already have evidence of dissection should have the coarctation repaired in pregnancy. Any upper limb hypertension should be treated aggressively with antihypertensive drugs [24]. If there is gross widening of the ascending aorta suggesting intrinsic disease of the aorta, the patient should be delivered by elective caesarean section to reduce the risk of dissection associated with labour.

Marfan's syndrome (see also Chapter 14 for non-cardiological aspects)

Some authors consider the risk of dissection to be so high in Marfan's syndrome that they advise avoidance of pregnancy or termination if there is any degree of aortic dilation [248]. Again, this seems an extreme attitude, which Pyeritz had modified to suggest that dilation of the aorta to >40 mm (as determined echocardiographically) should be the limit at which pregnancy is contraindicated [247]. Some patients and families with Marfan's syndrome have formes frustes of the condition where there may be arachnodactyly, a high arch palate, lens abnormalities and long patella tendons with no evidence of disease of the aorta or aortic valve; there may only be minor mitral valve abnormalities, if there is any cardiac disease at all. The families tend to 'breed true' and pregnancy would confer no extra risk. Therefore, there cannot be an overall condemnation of pregnancy in all cases of Marfan's syndrome [18]. Pyeritz *et al.* [247] have recently reported a series of pregnancies in 26 women with Marfan's syndrome. There was only one fatality and that patient died from endocarditis.

As in coarctation of the aorta, any associated hypertension should be treated aggressively with β blockade to decrease the haemodynamic load on the ascending aorta. β blocking drugs (propranolol) should also be used even in the absence of hypertension, if there is any dilation of the aorta. Delivery should be by caesarean section if there is evidence of aortic disease.

Dissection of the aorta, even in labour [99] and of the iliac artery [12] have been successfully managed with cardiopulmonary bypass in pregnancy. The treatment is surgical, either as an isolated procedure if the fetus is not yet viable [53] or following caesarian section if the fetus is viable [95,185].

Spontaneous uterine inversion has been reported in one case of Marfan's syndrome in pregnancy, possibly due to a generalized abnormality of connective tissue [249].

Once the aorta has dilated to 6 cm, elective replacement of the ascending aorta and aortic valve with a Bentall composite graft is a practical procedure [115] and pregnancy might be considered after this has been performed.

It has recently been shown that Marfan's syndrome is due to a defect in fibrillin synthesis. In Marfan's syndrome (but not in some other marfanoid conditions such as contractural arachnodactyly) this defect is due to mutations of a fibrillin gene on chromosome 15 [320]. Definitive diagnosis in the index case and prenatal diagnosis in fetuses of patients with Marfan's disease is now possible in many families.

Congenital heart block

Congenital heart block is usually no problem in pregnancy. Although part of the normal response to pregnancy includes an increase in heart rate to increase the cardiac output, this is not obligatory. There are many records of successful pregnancy in patients with heart block, both paced [107] and not paced [311]. Presumably, patients are able to increase stroke volume sufficiently to cope with the increased demands of pregnancy. A few patients are unable to increase cardiac output sufficiently at the end of pregnancy or during labour [31]. Therefore, patients with heart block who are not paced, or those where there is any question of pacemaker failure, should be managed in obstetric units where there is access to pacing facilities.

Tricuspid atresia and the Fontan procedure

In tricuspid atresia there is no communication between the right atrium and the right ventricle. If the child or fetus survives blood exits the right atrium via an atrial septal defect and perfuses the lungs via a ventricular septal defect. In the Fontan procedure the right atrium is connected directly to the pulmonary artery to improve pulmonary blood flow and the atrial and ventricular septal defects are closed. There have been a number of reports of pregnancy in patients with tricuspid atresia, both corrected and uncorrected [53,123,218]. In general the maternal outcome depends on her state of health at the beginning of pregnancy and the fetal outcome on the degree of maternal cyanosis. But in addition these patients have a high thromboembolic risk. In part this is due to the polycythaemia of cyanosis but in addition the Fontan procedure is associated with an acquired thrombotic state due in part to protein C, antithrombin III and protein S deficiencies (see Chapter 4) [61]. It is likely that these deficiencies are due to impaired liver function possibly due to the high venous pressure resulting from the Fontan procedure. Protein C, antithrombin III and protein S should be estimated in all patients following the Fontan procedure, particularly if they are contemplating pregnancy and suitable thromboprophylaxis should be used if there are significant abnormalities. Subcutaneous heparin would be the obvious choice in pregnancy.

Miscellaneous

Pregnancy has been described in a number of patients with univentricular hearts, with or without transposition and usually after a surgical procedure [15,147,169,174,330,342]. The maternal outcome depends on the degree of pulmonary vascular disease, her symptoms, whether she has been in congestive cardiac failure and the nature of other abnormalities. The fetal outcome depends on the degree of maternal cyanosis.

There is a single report of pregnancy following the Mustard operation for transposition of the great arteries. The patient was delivered at 37 weeks when she developed pulmonary oedema due to atrial flutter but the pregnancy was otherwise uneventful [209]. In Ebstein's malformation, the tricuspid valve is displaced into the right ventricle. The malformation which can be diagnosed by echocardiography is associated with maternal lithium therapy. The major risks are right-sided heart failure and arrhythmias but successful pregnancies have been reported [150,177].

Experience is increasing with pregnancy following heart transplantation. Guidelines for management have been published [158] and there has even been a successful case of twin pregnancy [126]. In general the problems are not haemodynamic but those of managing immunosuppressive therapy and for these we can draw on the much greater experience of renal transplants (see Chapter 7). However, since a significant proportion of heart transplant patients are performed in young women because of puerperal cardiomyopathy [7] and since puerperal cardiomyopathy tends to reoccur in successive pregnancies there is the theoretical risk that some of the transplanted patients may have a reoccurrence of puerperal cardiomyopathy if they embark on further pregnancies.

References

1 Abboud TK, Raya J, Noueihed R & Daniel J. Intrathecal morphine for relief of labour pain in a parturient with severe pulmonary hypertension. *Anaesthesiology* 1983; **59**: 477–9.

2 Ahmad R, Rajah SM, Mearns AJ & Deverall PB. Dipyridamole in successful management of pregnant women with prosthetic heart valve. *Lancet* 1976; **ii**: 1414–15.

3 Allan LD, Crawford DC, Chita SK, Anderson RM & Tynan M. Familial recurrence of congenital heart disease in the prospective series of mothers referred for fetal echocardiography. *American Journal of Cardiology* 1986; **58**: 334–7.

4 Anderson JB. The effect of diuretics in late pregnancy on the new born infant. *Acta Paediatrica Scandinavica* 1970; **59**: 659–63.

5 Andrinopoulos GC & Arias F. Triple heart valve prosthesis and pregnancy. *Obstetrics and Gynecology* 1980; **55**: 762–4.

6 Angel JL, Chapman C *et al*. Percutaneous balloon aortic valvulopasty in pregnancy. *Obstetrics and Gynecology* 1988; **72**: 438–40.

7 Aravot DJ, Banner NR *et al*. Heart transplantation for peripartum cardiomyopathy. *Lancet* 1987; **ii**: 1024.

8 Badduke BR, Jamieson WR *et al*. Pregnancy and childbearing in a population with biologic valvular prostheses. *Journal of Thoracic Cardiovascular Surgery* 1991; **102**: 179–86.

9 Bader RA, Bader ME, Rose DJ & Braunwald E. Haemodynamics at rest and during exercise in normal pregnancy as studied by cardiac catheterization. *Journal of Clinical Investigation* 1955; **34**: 1524–36.

10 Bahary CM, Ninio A, Gorodesky IG & Weri A. Tococardiography in pregnancy during extra corporeal bypass for mitral valve replacement. *Israel Journal of Medical Science* 1980; **16**: 395–7.

11 Barabas AP. Heterogeneity of the Ehlers–Danlos syndrome: description of three clinical types and a hypothesis to explain the basic defect(s). *British Medical Journal* 1967; **ii**: 612–13.

12 Barker SG & Burnand KG. Retrograde iliac artery dissection in Marfan's syndrome. A case report. *Journal of Cardiovascular Surgery Torino* 1989; **30**: 953–4.

13 Barrett PA & Penn IM. Amiodarone in pregnancy. *Clinical Progress in Electrophysiology* 1986; **4**: 158–9.

14 Batson GA. Cyanotic congenital heart disease and pregnancy. *British Journal of Obstetrics and Gynaecology* 1974; **81**: 549–53.
15 Baumann H, Schneider H, Drack G, Alon E & Huch A. Pregnancy and delivery by Caesarean section in a patient with transposition of the great arteries and single ventricle. Case report. *British Journal of Obstetrics and Gynaecology* 1987; **94**: 704–8.
16 Beary JF, Summer WR & Bulkley BH. Postpartum acute myocardial infarction: a rare occurrence of uncertain etiology. *American Journal of Cardiology* 1979; **43**: 158–60.
17 Becker RM. Intracardiac surgery in pregnant women. *Annals of Thoracic Surgery* 1983; **36**: 453–8.
18 Beighton P. Pregnancy in the Marfan syndrome. *British Medical Journal* 1982; **285**: 464.
19 Bell WR & Meek AG. Guidelines for the use of thrombolytic agents. *New England Journal of Medicine* 1979; **301**: 1266–70.
20 Ben Ismail M, Abid F, Travelsi S, Taktar M & Fekih M. Cardiac valve prosthesis anticoagulation and pregnancy. *British Heart Journal* 1986; **55**: 101–5.
21 Ben-Shlomo I, Zohar S, Marmore A, Blondheim DS & Sharir T. Myocardial ischaemia during intravenous ritodrine treatment: is it so rare? *Lancet* 1986; **ii**: 917–18.
22 Benchimol AB, Carneiro RD & Schlesinger P. Postpartum heart disease. *British Heart Journal* 1959; **21**: 89.
23 Bennett GG & Oakley CM. Pregnancy in a patient with a mitral valve prosthesis. *Lancet* 1968; **i**: 616–19.
24 Benny PS, Prasao J & MacVicar J. Pregnancy and coarctation of the aorta. Case report. *British Journal of Obstetrics and Gynaecology* 1980; **87**: 1159–61.
25 Biale Y, Cantor A, Lewen Thal H & Gueron M. The course of pregnancy in patients with artificial heart valves treated with dipyridamole. *International Journal of Obstetrics and Gynaecology* 1980; **18**: 128–32.
26 Bisno AL. Group A streptococcal infections and acute rheumatic fever. *New England Journal of Medicine* 1991; **325**: 783–93.
27 Blake S, Bonar F *et al*. Pregnancy with constrictive pericarditis. *British Journal of Obstetrics and Gynaecology* 1984; **91**: 404–6.
28 Blickstein I, Zalel Y, Katz Z & Lancet M. Ritodrine-induced pulmonary edema unmasking underlying peripartum cardiomyopathy. *American Journal of Obstetrics and Gynecology* 1988; **159**: 332–3.
29 Bloomfield P, Wheatley DJ, Prescott RJ & Miller HC. Twelve-year comparison of a Bjork–Shiley mechanical heart valve with porcine hioprathesis. *New England Journal of Medicine* 1991; **324**: 373–9.
30 Bowers C, Devine PA & Chervenak FA. Dilation and evacuation during the second trimester of pregnancy in a woman with primary pulmonary hypertension. *Journal of Reproductive Medicine* 1988; **33**: 787–8.
31 Bowman PR & Millar-Craig MW. Congenital heart block and pregnancy: a further case report. *Journal of Obstetrics and Gynaecology* 1980; **1**: 98–9.
32 Boyle DMcC & Lloyd-Jones RL. The electrocardiographic S-T segment in pregnancy. *Journal of Obstetrics and Gynaecology of the British Commonwealth* 1966; **73**: 986–7.
33 Brown AK, Doukas N, Riding WD & Wyn Jones E. Cardiomyopathy and pregnancy. *British Heart Journal* 1967; **29**: 387–93.
34 Bruner JP, Barry MJ & Elliott JP. Pregnancy in a patient with idiopathic long QT syndrome. *American Journal of Obstetrics and Gynecology* 1984; **149**: 690–1.
35 Buemann B & Kragelund E. Clinical assessment of heart disease during pregnancy. *Acta Obstetrica et Gynecologica Scandinavica* 1962; **41**: 57.
36 Bulkley BH & Roberts WC. Dissecting aneurysm (haematoma) limited to coronary artery. *American Journal of Medicine* 1973; **55**: 747–56.
37 Burke CM, Theodore J *et al*. Twenty-eight cases of human heart–lung transplantation. *Lancet* 1986; **i**: 517–19.
38 Burn J. The next lady has a heart defect. *British Journal of Obstetrics and Gynaecology* 1987; **94**: 97–9.
39 Burwell CS & Metcalfe J. *Heart Disease and Pregnancy; Physiology and Management*. Little, Brown, Boston, Massachussetts, 1973.
40 Camm AJ & Garratt CJ. Adenosine and supraventricular tachycardia. *New England Journal of Medicine* 1991; **325**: 1621–9.
41 Carpenter RJ & Decuir P. Cardiovascular collapse associated with oral terbutaline tocolytic therapy. *American Journal of Obstetrics and Gynecology* 1984; **148**: 821–3.
42 Carr FB, Hamilton BE & Palmer RS. The significance of large Q in lead III of the electrocardiogram during pregnancy. *American Heart Journal* 1933; **8**: 519.
43 Carruth SE, Mirvis SB, Brogan DR & Wenger NK. The electrocardiogram in normal pregnancy. *American Heart Journal* 1981; **102**: 1075–8.
44 Caves PK & Paneth M. Acute mitral regurgitation in pregnancy due to ruptured chordae tendinae. *British Heart Journal* 1972; **34**: 541–4.
45 Chen WWC, Chan CS, Lee PR, Wang RYR & Wong VCW. Pregnancy in patients with prosthetic heart vales: An experience with 45 pregnancies. *Quarterly Journal of Medicine* 1982; **51**: 358–65.
46 Chesley LC. Severe rheumatic cardiac disease and pregnancy: the ultimate prognosis. *American Journal of Obstetrics and Gynecology* 1980; **136**: 552–8.
47 Christman BW, McPherson CD *et al*. An imbalance between the excretion of thromboxane and prostacyclin metabolites in pulmonary hypertension. *New England Journal of Medicine* 1992; **327**: 70–5.
48 Ciraulo DA & Markovitz A. Myocardial infarction in pregnancy associated with a coronary artery thrombosis. *Archives of Internal Medicine* 1979; **139**: 1046–7.

49 Clapp JF III. Maternal heart rate in pregnancy. *American Journal of Obstetrics and Gynecology* 1985; **152**: 659–60.

50 Clark SL, Morenstein JM, Phelan JP, Montag TW & Paul RH. Experience with pulmonary artery catheter. *Obstetrics and Gynecology* 1985; **152**: 374–80.

51 Clark SL, Phelan JP, Greenspoon J, Aldahl D & Mortenstein J. Labour and delivery in the presence of mitral stenosis: Central hemodynamic observations. *American Journal of Obstetrics and Gynecology* 1985; **8**: 984–8.

52 Cohen DJ, Kuntz RE *et al*. Predictors of long-term outcome after percutaneous balloon mitral valvuloplasty. *New England Journal of Medicine* 1992; **327**: 1329–35.

53 Coln LM & Lavin JP Sr. Pregnancy complicated by Marfan's syndrome with aortic arch dissection, subsequent aortic arch replacement and triple coronary artery bypass grafts. *Journal of Reproductive Medicine* 1985; **30**: 685–8.

54 Conradsson TB & Werko L. Management of heart disease in pregnancy. *Progress in Cardiovascular Disease* 1974; **16**: 407–19.

55 Copeland WE, Wooley CF, Ryan JM, Runco V & Levin HS. Pregnancy and congenital heart disease. *American Journal of Obstetrics and Gynecology* 1963; **86**: 107–10.

56 Cortis BS, Freese E, Luisada AA, Motto S & Zummo B. Precordial pain and myocardial infarction in pregnancy. *Gionale Italiano Cardiologica* 1979; **9**: 532–4.

57 Cotrill CM, McAllister RG Jr, Gettes J & Noonan JA. Propranolol therapy during pregnancy, labour and delivery: evidence for transplacental drug transfer and impaired neonatal drug disposition. *Journal of Pediatrics* 1977; **91**: 812–14.

58 Cotton DB, Longmire S, Jones MM, Dorman KF, Tessem J & Joyce TH. Cardiovascular alterations in severe pregnancy-induced hypertension: effects of intravenous nitroglycerin coupled with blood volume expansion. *American Journal of Obstetrics and Gynecology* 1986; **145**: 1053–9.

59 Crawford DC, Chita SK & Allan LD. Prenatal detection of congenital heart disease: Factors affecting obstetric management and survival. *American Journal of Obstetrics and Gynecology* 1988; **159**: 352–6.

60 Crawford JS, Mills WG & Pentecost BL. A pregnant patient with Eisenmenger syndrome. *British Journal of Anaesthesia* 1971; **43**: 1091–4.

61 Cromme-Dijkhuis AH, Henkens CMA *et al*. Coagulation factor abnormalities as possible thrombotic risk factors after Fontan operations. *Lancet* 1990; **336**: 1087–90.

62 Cunningham FG, Pritchard JA, Hankins GDV, Anderson PL, Lucas MJ & Armstrong KF. Peripartum heart failure: Idiopathic cardiomyopathy of compounding cardiovascular events. *Obstetrics and Gynecology* 1986; **67**: 157–68.

63 Cutforth R & MacDonald CB. Heart sounds and murmurs in pregnancy. *American Heart Journal* 1966; **71**: 741–7.

64 Dacie J. *Practical Haematology*. Churchill Livingstone, Edinburgh, 1975: 413–14.

65 Danchia N, Brinncon S *et al*. Mitral valve prolapse as a risk factor for infective endocarditis. *Lancet* 1989; **i**: 743–5.

66 Davidson NMcD & Parry EHO. Peri-partum cardiac failure. *Quarterly Journal of Medicine* 1978; **47**: 431–61.

67 Davies AE & Robertson MJS. Pulmonary oedema after the administration of intravenous salbutamol and ergometrine. *British Journal of Obstetrics and Gynaecology* 1980; **87**: 529–41.

68 Davies P, Francis RI, Docker MF, Watt JM & Crawford JS. Analysis of impedance cardiography longitudinally applied in pregnancy. *British Journal of Obstetrics and Gynaecology* 1986; **93**: 717–20.

69 de Swiet M. The cardiovascular system. In: Hytten F & Chamberlain GVP (eds), *Clinical Physiology in Obstetrics*. Blackwell Scientific Publications, Oxford, 1980.

70 de Swiet M. Excretion of verapamil in human milk. *British Medical Journal* 1984; **288**: 644–5.

71 de Swiet M. The physiology of normal pregnancy. In: Rubin PC (ed), *Hypertension in Pregnancy*, Volume 12, *Handbook of Hypertension*. Elsevier, Amsterdam, 1988.

72 de Swiet M, de Louvois J & Hurley R. Failure of cephalosporins to prevent bacterial endocarditis during labour. *Lancet* 1975; **ii**: 186.

73 de Swiet M & Deverall PB. Pregnancy — still an indication for closed mitral valvotomy. *International Journal of Cardiology* 1990; **27**: 323–4.

74 de Swiet M & Fidler J. Heart disease in pregnancy: some controversies. *Journal of the Royal College of Physicians* 1981; **15**: 183–6.

75 de Swiet M & Talbert DG. The measurement of cardiac output by electrical impedance plethysmography in pregnancy. Are the assumptions valid? *British Journal of Obstetrics and Gynaecology* 1986; **93**: 721–6.

76 Deal K & Wooley CF. Coarctation of the aorta and pregnancy. *Annals of Internal Medicine* 1973; **78**: 706–10.

77 Demarkis JG, Rahimtoola SM *et al*. Natural course of peri-partium cardiomyopathy. *Circulation* 1971; **44**: 1053–61.

78 Department of Health and Social Security. *Report on Confidential Enquires into Maternal Deaths in United Kingdom, 1975–1978*. HMSO, London, 1982.

79 Department of Health and Social Security. *Report on Confidential Enquiries into Maternal Deaths in the United Kingdom 1985–87*. HMSO, London, 1991.

80 Department of Health and Social Security. *Report on Confidential Enquiries into Maternal Deaths in the United Kingdom 1988–90*. HMSO, London, 1994.

81 Devitt JH & Noble WH. Eisenmenger's syndrome and pregnancy. *New England Journal of Medicine* 1980; **302**: 751.

82 Dubourg G. Correction complete d'une triade de Fallot

en circulation extra-corporelle chez une femme enceinte. *Archives des Maladies du Coeur* 1959; **52**: 1389–91.

83 Dumesic DA, Silverman NH, Tobias D & Golbus MS. Transplacental cardioversion of fetal supraventricular tachycardia with procainamide. *New England Journal of Medicine* 1982; **307**: 1128–31.

84 Durack DT. Current practice in prevention of bacterial endocarditis. *British Heart Journal* 1975; **37**: 478–81.

85 Easterling TR, Benedetti TJ, Carlson KL & Watts DH. Measurement of cardiac output in pregnancy by thermodilution and impedance techniques. *British Journal of Obstetrics and Gynaecology* 1989; **96**: 67–9.

86 Eckstein H & Jack B. Breast feeding and anticoagulant therapy. *Lancet* 1970; **i**: 672–3.

87 Eilen B, Kaiser IH, Becker RM & Cohen MN. Aortic valve replacement in the third trimester of pregnancy: case report and review of literature. *Obstetrics and Gynecology* 1981; **57**: 119–21.

88 Elkayam U & Gleicher N. *Cardiac Problems in Pregnancy. Diagnosis and Management of Maternal and Fetal Disease*. Alan R Liss, New York, 1982.

89 Elliott HR, Abdulla U & Hayes PJ. Pulmonary oedema associated with ritodrine infusion and betamethasone administration in premature labour. *British Medical Journal* 1978; **ii**: 799–800.

90 Emmanuel R, Somervill J, Inns A & Withers R. Evidence of congenital heart disease in the offspring of parents with atrioventricular defects. *British Heart Journal* 1983; **49**: 144–7.

91 Erbel R, Rohmann S *et al*. Improved diagnostic value of echocardiography in patients with infective endocarditis by transesophageal approach: a prospective study. *European Heart Journal* 1988; **9**: 43–53.

92 Espino Vela J & Alvarado-Toro A. Natural history of atrial septal defect. *Cardiovascular Clinics* 1971; **2**: 104–25.

93 Etheridge MJ. Heart disease and pregnancy. *Medical Journal of Australia* 1966; **2**: 1172.

94 Etheridge MJ. Heart disease and pregnancy. *Australian and New Zealand Journal of Obstetrics and Gynaecology* 1969; **9**: 7–11.

95 Ferguson JE, Veland K, Stinson EB & Maly RP. Marfan's syndrome: acute aortic dissection during labor, resulting in fetal distress and cesarean section, followed by successful surgical repair. *American Journal of Obstetrics and Gynecology* 1983; **147**: 759–62.

96 Fidler J, Smith V & de Swiet M. The excretion of oxprenolol and timolol in breast milk. *British Journal of Obstetrics and Gynaecology* 1983; **90**: 961–5.

97 Fidler J, Smith V, Fayers P & de Swiet M. Randomised controlled comparative study of methyldopa and oxprenolol for the treatment of hypertension in pregnancy. *British Medical Journal* 1983; **286**: 1927–30.

98 Finlay AY & Edmunds V. DC cardioversion in pregnancy. *British Journal of Clinical Practice* 1979; **33**: 88–94.

99 Finnerty JJ & MacKay BR. Antepartum thrombophlebitis and pulmonary embolism. *Obstetrics and Gynecology* 1962; **19**: 405.

100 Fleming HA. Antibiotic prophylaxis against infective endocarditis after delivery. *Lancet* 1977; **i**: 144–5.

101 Flessa HC, Kapstrom AB, Glueck MI & Will JJ. Placental transport of heparin. *American Journal of Obstetrics and Gynecology* 1965; **93**: 570–3.

102 Fogarty AJ. Cardiac failure in a hypertensive woman receiving salbutamol for premature labour. *British Medical Journal* 1980; **281**: 226.

103 Foster CJ & Love HG. Amiodarone in pregnancy. Case report and review of literature. *International Journal of Cardiology* 1988; **20**: 307–16.

104 Gallery EDM, Saunders DM, Hunyor SN & Gyory AZ. Improvement in fetal growth with treatment of maternal hypertension in pregnancy. *Clinical Science and Molecular Medicine* 1978; **55**: 359–61.

105 Garrod JP & Waterworth PM. The risks of dental extraction during penicillin treatment. *British Heart Journal* 1962; **24**: 39–46.

106 Giles WB, Young AA, Howlin KJ, Cook CM & Trudinger BJ. Doppler ultrasound features of stenosis of the aorta in a pregnancy complicated by Takayasu's arteritis. *British Journal of Obstetrics and Gynaecology* 1987; **94**: 902–9.

107 Ginns HM & Holinrake K. Complete heart block in pregnancy treated with an internal cardiac pacemaker. *Journal of Obstetrics and Gynaecology of the British Commonwealth* 1970; **77**: 719.

108 Ginz B. Myocardial infarction in pregnancy. *Journal of Obstetrics and Gynaecology of the British Commonwealth* 1970; **77**: 610.

109 Giudici MC, Artis AK, Webel RR & Alpert MA. Postpartum myocardial infarction treated with percutaneous transluminal coronary angioplasty. *American Heart Journal* 1989; **118**: 614–16.

110 Gladstone GR, Hordof A & Gersony WM. Propranolol administration during pregnancy: effects on the fetus. *Journal of Pediatrics* 1975; **86**: 962–4.

111 Gleicher N, Knutzen VK, Elkayam U, Loew S & Kerenyi TB. Rheumatic heart disease diagnosed during pregnancy. A 30-year follow-up. *International Journal of Obstetrics and Gynaecology* 1979; **17**: 51–7.

112 Gleicher N, Midwall J, Hockberger D & Jaffin H. Eisenmenger's syndrome and pregnancy. *Obstetrical and Gynaecological Survey* 1979; **34**: 721–41.

113 Gonik B & Cotton DB. Peripartum colloid osmotic pressure changes: Influence of intravenous hydration. *American Journal of Obstetrics and Gynecology* 1982; **150**: 99–100.

114 Gonik B, Cotton D, Spillman T, Abouleish E & Zavisca F. Peripartum colloid osmotic pressure changes: effects of controlled fluid management. *American Journal of Obstetrics and Gynecology* 1985; **151**: 812–15.

115 Gott VL, Pyeritz RE, Magovern GJ Jr, Cameron DE & McKusick VA. Surgical treatment of aneurysms of the

ascending aorta in the Marfan syndrome. Results of composite graft repair in 50 patients. *New England Journal of Medicine* 1986; **314**: 1070–4.

116 Habib A & McArthy JS. Effects on the neonate of propranolol administered during pregnancy. *Journal of Pediatrics* 1977; **91**: 808–11.

117 Haffeje E. In discussion – amiodarone pharmacokinetics. *American Heart Journal* 1983; **106**: 847.

118 Hall R & Kirk R. Balloon dilatation of heart valves. *British Medical Journal* 1992; **305**: 487–8.

119 Harrigan JT, Kangos JJ *et al*. Successful treatment of fetal congestive heart failure secondary to tachycardia. *New England Journal of Medicine* 1981; **304**: 1527–9.

120 Hart CW & Nauton RF. The ototoxicity of chloroquine phosphate. *Archives of Otolaryngology* 1964; **80**: 407.

121 Hart MV, Morton MJ, Hosenpud JD & Metcalf J. Aortic function during normal pregnancy. *American Journal of Obstetrics and Gynecology* 1986; **154**: 887–91.

122 Hastwell G & Lambert BE. The effect of oral salbutamol on serum potassium and blood sugar. *British Journal of Obstetrics and Gynaecology* 1978; **85**: 767–9.

123 Hatjis CG, Gibson M *et al*. Pregnancy in a patient with tricuspid atresia. *American Journal of Obstetrics and Gynecology* 1983; **145**: 114–15.

124 Hawkins GDV, Wendel GD, Leveno KJ & Stoneham J. Myocardial infarction during pregnancy: a review. *Obstetrics and Gynecology* 1985; **65**: 139–47.

125 Hayden J, Mort T & Rintel T. Acute coronary artery dissection during pregnancy. Case report. *International Journal of Obstetric Anesthesia* 1991; **1**: 43–5.

126 Hedon B, Montoya F & Cabrol A. Twin pregnancy and vaginal birth after heart transplantation. *Lancet* 1990; **335**: 476–7.

127 Hemminki E & Starfield B. Prevention and treatment of premature labour by drugs: review of clinical trials. *British Journal of Obstetrics and Gynaecology* 1978; **85**: 411–17.

128 Hendricks SK, Keroes J & Katz M. Electrocardiographic changes associated with ritodrine-induced maternal tachycardia and hypokalemia. *American Journal of Obstetrics and Gynecology* 1986; **154**: 921–3.

129 Hill LM. Fetal distress secondary to vancomycin-induced maternal hypotension. *American Journal of Obstetrics and Gynecology* 1985; **153**: 74–5.

130 Ho PC, Chen TY & Wong V. The effect of maternal cardiac disease and digoxin administration on labour, fetal weight and maturity at birth. *Australian and New Zealand Journal of Obstetrics and Gynaecology* 1980; **20**: 24–7.

131 Homans DC. Peripartum cardiomyopathy. *New England Journal of Medicine* 1985; **312**: 1432–7.

132 Howitt G. Heart disease and pregnancy. *Practitioner* 1971; **206**: 765–72.

133 Hubbard WN, Jenkins BAG & Ward DE. Persistent atrial tachycardia in pregnancy. *British Medical Journal* 1983; **287**: 327.

134 Hughes LO, McFadyen IR & Raftery EB. Acute bacterial endocarditis on a normal aortic valve following vaginal delivery. *International Journal of Cardiology* 1988; **18**: 261–2.

135 Hull E & Hafkesbring E. 'Toxic' postpartal heart disease. *New Orleans Medical and Surgical Journal* 1937; **89**: 550.

136 Husaini MH. Myocardial infarction during pregnancy: report of two cases and review of the literature. *Postgraduate Medical Journal* 1971; **47**: 660.

137 Ibarra-Perez C, Arevalo-Toledo N, Alvarez-De Lacadena O & Noriega-Guerra L. The course of pregnancy in patients with artificial heart valves. *American Journal of Medicine* 1976; **61**: 504–12.

138 Inoue M, Unno N *et al*. Excretion of verapamil in breast milk. *British Medical Journal* 1983; **287**: 1596.

139 Iturbe-Alessio I, Fonseca M, Mutchinik O, Santos MA, Zajartas A & Salazar E. Risks of anticoagulant therapy in pregnant women with artificial heart valves. *New England Journal of Medicine* 1986; **315**: 1390–3.

140 Izquierdo LA, Kushnir O *et al*. Effect of mitral valve prosthetic surgery on the outcome of a growth-retarded fetus. A case report. *American Journal of Obstetrics and Gynecology* 1990; **163**: 584–6.

141 Jacoby WJ. Pregnancy with tetralogy and pentalogy of Fallot. *American Journal of Cardiology* 1964; **14**: 866–73.

142 Jakobi P, Adler Z, Zimmer EZ & Milo S. Effect of uterine contractions on left atrial pressure in a pregnant woman with mitral stenosis. *British Medical Journal* 1989; **298**: 27.

143 James CF, Banner T, Levelle P & Caton D. Noninvasive determination of cardiac output throughout pregnancy. *Anaesthesiology* 1985; **63**: A434.

144 Javares T, Coto EC, Maiques V, Rincon A, Such M & Caffarena JM. Pregnancy after heart valve replacement. *International Journal of Cardiology* 1985; **5**: 731–9.

145 Jewett JF. Two dissecting coronary artery aneurysms post partum. *New England Journal of Medicine* 1978; **278**: 1255–6.

146 Jewett JF. Pulmonary hypertension and pre-eclampsia. *New England Journal of Medicine* 1979; **301**: 1063–4.

147 Johnston TA & De Bono D. Single ventricle and pulmonary hypertension. A successful pregnancy. Case report. *British Journal of Obstetrics and Gynaecology* 1989; **96**: 731–4.

148 Jones K, Higenbottam T & Wallwork J. Pulmonary vasodilation with prostacyclin in primary and secondary hypertension. *Chest* 1989; **96**: 748–89.

149 Julian DG & Szekely P. Peripartum cardiomyopathy. *Progress in Cardiovascular Diseases* 1985; **27**: 223–40.

150 Kahler RL. Cardiac disease. In: Burrow GN & Ferris (eds) *Medical Complications during Pregnancy*. WB Saunders, Philadelphia, 1975: 105–45.

151 Kakouris H, Eddie LW & Summers RJ. Cardiac effects of relaxin in rats. *Lancet* 1992; **339**: 1076–8.

152 Kalra PA, Litherland D *et al*. Cardiac standstill induced by prostaglandin pessaries. *Lancet* 1989; **i**: 1460–1.
153 Kambam JR, Franks JJ & Smith BE. Inhibitory effect of quinidine on plasma pseudocholinesterase activity in pregnant women. *American Journal of Obstetrics and Gynecology* 1987; **157**: 897–9.
154 Khanderia BK, Seward JB *et al*. Value and limitations of transesophageal echocardiography in assessment of mitral valve prostheses. *Circulation* 1991; **83**: 1956–68.
155 Klein AM, Holzman IR & Austin EM. Fetal tachycardia prior to the development of hydrops — attempted pharmacological cardioversion: Case report. *American Journal of Obstetrics and Gynecology* 1979; **134**: 347–8.
156 Klein VR, Repke JT, Marquette GP & Niebyl JR. The Bland–White–Garland syndrome in pregnancy. *American Journal of Obstetrics and Gynecology* 1984; **150**: 106–7.
157 Konishi Y, Tatsuta N *et al*. Dissecting aneurysm during pregnancy and the puerperium. *Japanese Circulation Journal* 1980; **44**: 726–32.
158 Kossoy LR, Herbert CM & Wentz AC. Management of heart transplant recipients: Guidelines for the obstetrician-gynecologist. *American Journal of Obstetrics and Gynecology* 1988; **159**: 490–9.
159 Kubli F. Proceedings of the fifth study group of the Royal College of Obstetricians and Gynaecologists. In: Anderson A, Beard R, Brudenell M & Dunn PM (eds), *Preterm Labour*. Royal College of Obstetricians and Gynaecologists, London, 1977: 218–20.
160 Lamb MP, Ross K, Johnstone AM & Manners JM. Fetal heart monitoring during open heart surgery. *British Journal of Obstetrics and Gynaecology* 1981; **88**: 669–74.
161 *Lancet* Editorial. Dilated cardiomyopathy in Africa. *Lancet* 1985; **i**: 557–8.
162 *Lancet* Editorial. Epidural block for caesarean section and circulatory changes. *Lancet* 1989; **ii**: 1076–8.
163 *Lancet* Editorial. Which heart valve? *Lancet* 1991; **337**: 705–6.
164 Landsberger EJ & Grossman II JH. Muitiple peripheral pulmonic stenosis in pregnancy. *American Journal of Obstetrics and Gynecology* 1986; **154**: 152–3.
165 Larsen JF, Jacobsen B, Holm HH, Pedersen JF & Mantoni M. Intrauterine injection of vitamin K before delivery during anticoagulant treatment of the mother. *Acta Obstetrica et Gynecologica Scandinavica* 1978; **57**: 227–30.
166 Lee P-K, Wang RYC *et al*. Combined use of warfarin and adjusted subcutaneous heparin during pregnancy in patients with an artificial heart valve. *Journal of the American College of Cardiology* 1986; **8**: 221–4.
167 Lee W, Clark SL *et al*. Septic shock during pregnancy. *American Journal of Obstetrics and Gynecology* 1988; **159**: 410–16.
168 Lees MM, Scott DB, Kerr MG & Taylor SH. The circulatory effects of recumbent postural change in late pregnancy. *Clinical Science* 1967; **32**: 453–563.
169 Leibbrand G, Muench U & Gander M. Two successful pregnancies in a patient with single ventricle and transposition of the great arteries. *International Journal of Cardiology* 1982; **1**: 257–62.
170 Lennox CE & Martin J. Cardiac arrest following intramyometrial prostaglandin E2. *Journal of Obstetrics and Gynaecology* 1991; **11**: 263–4.
171 Leonard RF, Braun TE & Levy AM. Initiation of uterine contractions by disopyramide during pregnancy. *New England Journal of Medicine* 1978; **299**: 84.
172 Levick K. Pregnancy loss and fathers with Ehlers–Danlos syndrome. *Lancet* 1989; **ii**: 1151.
173 Levy DL, Warringer RA & Burgess GE. Fetal response to cardiopulmonary bypass. *Obstetrics and Gynecology* 1980; **56**: 112–15.
174 Levy M, Grait L & Laufer N. Excretion of drugs in human milk. *New England Journal of Medicine* 1977; **297**: 789.
175 Lewis PJ, de Swiet M, Boylan P & Bulpitt CJ. How obstetricians in the United Kingdom manage preterm labour. *British Journal of Obstetrics and Gynaecology* 1980; **87**: 574–7.
176 Limet R & Crondin CM. Cardiac valve prosthesis, anticoagulation and pregnancy. *Annals of Thoracic Surgery* 1977; **23**: 337–431.
177 Littler WA. Successful pregnancy in a patient with Ebstein's anomaly. *British Heart Journal* 1970; **32**: 711–13.
178 Littler WA, Redman CWG, Bonnar J, Berkin LS & Lee G de J. Reduced pulmonary arterial compliance in hypertensive pregnancy. *Lancet* 1973; **i**: 1274–8.
179 Lownes HE & Ives TJ. Mexiletine use in pregnancy and lactation. *American Journal of Obstetrics and Gynecology* 1987; **157**: 446–7.
180 Lutz DJ, Noller KL, Spittell JA, Danielson GK & Fish CR. Pregnancy and its complications following cardiac valve prosthesis. *American Journal of Obstetrics and Gynecology* 1978; **131**: 460–8.
181 MacNab G & MacAfee CAJ. A changing pattern of heart disease associated with pregnancy. *Journal of Obstetrics and Gynaecology* 1985; **5**: 139–42.
182 Macphail S & Walkinshaw SA. Fetal supraventricular tachycardia: detection by routine auscultation and successful in-utero management. Case report. *British Journal of Obstetrics and Gynaecology* 1988; **95**: 1073–6.
183 Mangione JA, Zuliani MF *et al*. Percutaneous double balloon mitral valvuloplasty in pregnant women. *American Journal of Cardiology* 1989; **64**: 99–102.
184 Mann MS, Gossham PS, Baker JL & Hurley PA. Left atrial myxoma in the second trimester of pregnancy. Case report. *British Journal of Obstetrics and Gynaecology* 1987; **94**: 592–3.
185 Maruyama Y, Oguma F, Kosuge T, Yokosawa T & Eguchi S. Successful repair of an acute type A dissection during pregnancy. *Nippon Kyoha Geka Gakkai Zasshi* 1990; **38**: 2296–9.

186 McCaffrey RM & Dunn LJ. Primary pulmonary hypertension and pregnancy. *Obstetrical and Gynaecological Survey* 1964; **19**: 567–91.
187 McKenna WJ, Harris L, Rowland E, Whitelaw A, Storey G & Holt D. Amiodarone therapy during pregnancy. *American Journal of Cardiology* 1983; **51**: 1231–3.
188 McLeod AA, Jennings KP & Townsend ER. Near fatal puerperal thrombosis on Bjork–Shiley mitral valve prosthesis. *British Heart Journal* 1978; **40**: 934–7.
189 McLintic AJ, Lilley S *et al.* Electrocardiographic changes during caesarean section under regional anaesthesia. *International Journal of Obstetric Anesthesia* 1991; **1**: 55–7.
190 Meadows WR. Myocardial failure in the last trimester of pregnancy and the puerperium. *Circulation* 1957; **15**: 903–14.
191 Melvin KR, Richardson PJ, Olsen EGJ, Daly K & Jackson G. Peripartum cardiomyopathy due to myocarditis. *New England Journal of Medicine* 1982; **307**: 731–4.
192 Melvor RA. Percutaneous balloon aortic valvuloplasty during pregnancy. *International Journal of Cardiology* 1991; **32**: 1–4.
193 Mendelson CL. Pregnancy and coarctation of the aorta. *American Journal of Obstetrics and Gynecology* 1940; **39**: 1014–42.
194 Mendelson CL. Disorders of the heart beat during pregnancy. *American Journal of Obstetrics and Gynecology* 1956; **72**: 1268.
195 Mendelson CL. *Cardiac Disease in Pregnancy.* EA Davis, Philadelphia, 1960.
196 Midei MG, DeMent SH *et al.* Peripartum myocarditis and cardiomyopathy. *Circulation* 1990; **81**: 922–8.
197 Millwall J, Jaffin H, Herman MV & Kuper Smith J. Shunt flow and pulmonary haemodynamics during labour and delivery in the Eisenmenger syndrome. *American Journal of Cardiology* 1978; **42**: 299–303.
198 Milne JA, Mowie AD & Pack AI. Dyspnoea during normal pregnancy. *British Journal of Obstetrics and Gynaecology* 1978; **85**: 260–3.
199 Milsom I, Forssman L, Sivertsson R & Dottori O. Measurement of cardiac stroke volume by impedance cardiography in the last trimester of pregnancy. *Acta Obstetrica et Gynecologica Scandinavica* 1983; **62**: 473–9.
200 Mishra M, Chambers JB & Jackson G. Murmurs in pregnancy: an audit of echocardiography. *British Medical Journal* 1992; **304**: 1413–14.
201 Morgan Jones A & Howitt G. Eisenmenger syndrome in pregnancy. *British Medical Journal* 1965; **i**: 1627–31.
202 Morton MJ, Paul MS, Campos GR, Hart MV & Metcalf J. Exercise dynamics in late gestation: effects of physical training. *American Journal of Obstetrics and Gynecology* 1985; **152**: 91–7.
203 Movsesian AM & Wray RB. Postpartum myocardial infarction. *British Heart Journal* 1989; **62**: 154–6.
204 Nagorney DM & Field CS. Successful pregnancy 10 years after triple cardiac valve replacement. *Obstetrics and Gynecology* 1981; **57**: 386–8.
205 Nathwani D, Currie PF *et al. Plasmodium falciparum* malaria in pregnancy: a review. *British Journal of Obstetrics and Gynaecology* 1992; **99**: 118–21.
206 Neilson G, Galea EG & Blunt A. Congenital heart disease and pregnancy. *Medical Journal of Australia* 1970; **1**: 1086–8.
207 Nelson DM, Main E, Crafford W & Ahumada GG. Peripartum heart failure due to primary pulmonary hypertension. *Obstetrics and Gynecology* 1983; **62**: 58S–63S.
208 Nelson DM, Stempel LE, Fabri PJ & Talbert M. Hickman catheter use in a pregnant patient requiring therapeutic heparin anticoagulation. *American Journal of Obstetrics and Gynecology* 1984; **149**: 461–2.
209 Neukermans K, Sullivan TJ & Pitlick PT. Successful pregnancy after the Mustard operation for transposition of the great arteries. *American Journal of Cardiology* 1988; **62**: 838–9.
210 Newburger JW & Keane JF. Intrauterine supraventricular tachycardia. *Journal of Pediatrics* 1979; **95**: 780–6.
211 Newman B, Derrington C & Sore C. Cardiac output and the recumbent position in late pregnancy. *Anaesthesia* 1983; **38**: 332–5.
212 Nimrod C, Rambihar V, Fallen E, Effer S & Cairns J. Pulmonary edema associated with isoxsuprine therapy. *American Journal of Obstetrics and Gynecology* 1984; **148**: 625–9.
213 Nolan TE & Savage RW. Peripartum myocardial infarction from presumed Kawasaki's disease. *Southern Medical Journal* 1990; **83**: 1360–1.
214 Nora JJ & Nora AH. The evolution of specific genetic and environmental counselling in congenital heart diseases. *Circulation* 1978; **57**: 205–13.
215 Nora JJ & Nora AH. Maternal transmission of congenital heart diseases: New recurrent risk figures and the question of cytoplasmic inheritance and vulnerability to teratogens. *American Journal of Cardiology* 1987; **59**: 459–63.
216 Nora JJ & Nora AH. Update on counselling the family with a first degree retative with a congenital heart defect. *American Journal of Medical Genetics* 1988; **29**: 137–42.
217 Northcote RJ, Knight PV & Ballantyne D. Systolic mumurs in pregnancy: Value of echocardiographic assessment. *Clinical Cardiology* 1985; **8**: 327–8.
218 Novy MJ, Peterson EN & Metcalfe J. Respiratory characteristics of maternal and fetal blood in cyanotic congenital heart disease. *American Journal of Obstetrics and Gynecology* 1968; **100**: 821.
219 Nysenbaum AM. Pregnancy in a patient with endocardial fibroelastosis. *Journal of Obstetrics and Gynaecology* 1986; **7**: 121–2.
220 O'Neill H, Blake S, Sugrue D & MacDonald D. Problems in the management of patients with artificial

heart valves during pregnancy. *British Journal of Obstetrics and Gynaecology* 1982; **89**: 940–3.
221 Oakley CM. Pregnancy in patients with prosthetic heart valves. *British Medical Journal* 1983; **286**: 1680–2.
222 Oakley CM & Doherty P. Pregnancy in patients with valve replacement. *British Heart Journal* 1976; **38**: 1040–8.
223 Oakley GDG, McGarry K, Limb DG & Oakley CM. Management of pregnancy in patients with hypertrophic cardiomyopathy. *British Medical Journal* 1979; **i**: 1749–50.
224 Oates S, Williams GL & Rees GAD. Cardiopulmonary resuscitation in late pregnancy. *British Medical Journal* 1988; **297**: 404–5.
225 Oian P, Malthau JM, Noddeland H & Fadnes HO. Oedema-preventing mechanisms in subcutaneous tissue of normal pregnant women. *British Journal of Obstetrics and Gynaecology* 1985; **92**: 113–19.
226 Okada M, Inoue H, Nakamura Y, Kishimoto M & Suzuki T. Excretion of diltiazem in human milk. *New England Journal of Medicine* 1985; **312**: 922–3.
227 Okita GT, Poltz EJ & Davis ME. Placental transfer of radioactive digitoxin in pregnant woman and its fetal distribution. *Circulation Research* 1956; **4**: 376–80.
228 Olivera DBG, Dawkins KD, Kay PH & Paneth M. Chordal rupture 1: Aetiology and natural history. *British Heart Journal* 1983; **50**: 312–17.
229 Ong HC & Puraviappan AP. Congenital heart disease and pregnancy in the tropics. *Australia and New Zealand Journal of Obstetrics and Gynaecology* 1975; **15**: 99–103.
230 Oram HC & Holt M. Innocent depression of the ST segment and flattening of the T-wave during pregnancy. *Journal of Obstetrics and Gynaecology of the British Commonwealth* 1961; **68**: 765–70.
231 Orme ML'E, Lewis PJ *et al*. May mothers given warfarin breast-feed their infants? *British Medical Journal* 1977; **i**: 1564–5.
232 Page PA & Toung TA. A new probe for measurement of muscle PO_2 and its use during cardiopulmonary bypass. *Surgery, Gynecology and Obstetrics* 1975; **141**: 579–81.
233 Patton DE, Lee W *et al*. Cyanotic maternal heart disease in pregnancy. *Obstetric and Gynaecological Survey* 1990; **45**: 594–600.
234 Pavankumar P, Venugopal P *et al*. Closed mitral valvotomy during pregnancy. *Scandinavian Journal of Thoracic and Cardiovascular Surgery* 1988; **22**: 11–15.
235 Peaceman AM & Cruikshank DP. Ehlers–Danlos syndrome and pregnancy: association of type IV disease with maternal death. *Obstetrics and Gynecology* 1987; **69**: 428–31.
236 Pearl W & Spicer M. Ehlers–Danlos syndrome. *Southern Medical Journal* 1981; **74**: 80–1.
237 Penn IM, Barrett PA, Pannikote V, Barnaby PF, Campbell JB & Lyons NR. Amiodarone in pregnancy. *American Journal of Cardiology* 1985; **56**: 196–7.
238 Pepke-Zaba J, Higenbottam TW *et al*. Inhaled nitric oxide as a cause of selective pulmonary vasodilatation in pulmonary hypertension. *Lancet* 1991; **338**: 1173–4.
239 Peterson DR, Thompson DJ & Chinn N. Ischaemic heart disease prognosis. A community-made assessment (1966–1969). *Journal of the American Medical Association* 1972; **219**: 1423–7.
240 Phippard AF, Horvath JS *et al*. Circulatory adaptation to pregnancy — serial studies of haemodynamics, blood volume, renin and aldosterone in the baboon (*Papio harmadryas*). *Journal of Hypertension* 1986; **4**: 773–9.
241 Pitcher D, Leather HM, Storey GCA & Holt DW. Amiodarone in pregnancy. *Lancet* 1983; **i**: 597–8.
242 Pitkin RM, Perloff JK, Koos BJ & Beall MH. Pregnancy and congenital heart disease. *Annals of Internal Medicine* 1990; **112**: 445–54.
243 Pitts JA, Crosby WM & Basta LC. Eisenmenger's syndrome in pregnancy. *American Heart Journal* 1977; **93**: 321–6.
244 Poole Wilson PA. Cardiac failure in hypertensive woman receiving salbutamol for premature labour. *British Medical Journal* 1980; **281**: 226.
245 Pope FM & Nicholls AC. Pregnancy and Ehlers–Danlos syndrome type IV. *Lancet* 1983; **i**: 249–50.
246 Poston L, Morris JF, Wolfe CD & Hilton PJ. Serum digoxin-like substances in pregnancy-induced hypertension. *Clinical Science* 1989; **77**: 189–94.
247 Pyeritz RE. Maternal and fetal complication of pregnancy in the Marfan syndrome. *American Journal of Medicine* 1981; **71**: 784–90.
248 Pyeritz RE & McKuisick VA. The Marfan syndrome: diagnosis and management. *New England Journal of Medicine* 1979; **300**: 772–7.
249 Quinn RJ & Mukerjee B. Spontaneous uterine inversion in association with Marfan's syndrome. *Australia and New Zealand Journal of Obstetrics and Gynaecology* 1982; **22**: 163–4.
250 Rabinovici J, Mani A, Barkai G, Hod H, Frenkel Y & Mashiach S. Long term ambulatory anticoagulation by constant subcutaneous heparin infusion in pregnancy. *British Journal of Obstetrics and Gynaecology* 1987; **94**: 89–91.
251 Rand RH, Jenkins DM & Scott DG. Maternal cardiomyopathy in pregnancy causing stillbirth. *British Journal of Obstetrics and Gynaecology* 1975; **82**: 172–5.
252 Rayburn WF & Fontana ME. Mitral valve prolapse and pregnancy. *American Journal of Obstetrics and Gynecology* 1981; **141**: 9–11.
253 Recommendations from the Endocarditis Working Party of the British Society for Antimicrobial Chemotherapy. Antibiotic prophylaxis of infective endocarditis. *Lancet* 1990; **335**: 88–9.
254 Redick LF. An inflatable wedge for prevention of aortocaval compression during pregnancy. *American Journal of Obstetrics and Gynecology* 1979; **133**: 458–9.
255 Redleaf PD & Farell EJ. Bacteremia during partur-

ition – prevention of subacute bacterial endocarditis. *Journal of the American Medical Association* 1959; **169**: 1284–5.

256 Reitz BA, Wallwork JL *et al*. Heart–lung transplantation. Successful therapy with pulmonary vascular disease. *New England Journal of Medicine* 1982; **306**: 557–64.

257 Report of a Working Party of the British Society for Antimicrobial Chemotherapy. The antibiotic prophylaxis of infective endocarditis. *Lancet* 1982; **ii**: 1323–6.

258 Rey E, Duperron L, Gauthier R, Lemay M, Grignon A & LeLorier J. Transplacental treatment of tachycardia – induced fetal heart failure with verapamil and amiodarone: a case report. *American Journal of Obstetrics and Gynecology* 1985; **153**: 311–12.

259 Robards GJ, Saunders DM & Donnelly GL. Refractory supraventricular tachycardia complicating pregnancy. *Medical Journal of Australia* 1973; **2**: 278–80.

260 Roberts ADG, Low RAL, Rae AP & Hillis WS. Left ventricular aneurysm complicating myocardial infarction occurring during pregnancy. Case report. *British Journal of Obstetrics and Gynaecology* 1983; **90**: 969–70.

261 Roberts JD, Polaner DM, Lang D & Zapol WM. Inhaled nitric oxide in persistent pulmonary hypertension of the newborn. *Lancet* 1992; **340**: 818–19.

262 Robson DJ, Raj MVJ, Storey GCA & Holt DW. Use of amiodarone in pregnancy. *Postgraduate Medical Journal* 1985; **61**: 75–7.

263 Robson SC, Boys R, Rodeck C & Morgan B. Haemodynamic changes during epidural and spinal anaesthesia for elective caesarean section: correlation with umbilical artery pH. *Clinical Science* 1991; **11**: 301.

264 Robson SC, Dunlop W, Boys RJ & Hunter S. Cardiac output during labour. *British Medical Journal* 1987; **295**: 1169–72.

265 Robson SC, Dunlop W *et al*. Haemodynamic changes associated with caesarean section under epidural anaesthesia. *British Journal of Obstetrics and Gynaecology* 1989; **96**: 642–7.

266 Robson SC, Hunter S, Boys RJ & Dunlop W. Serial study of factors influencing changes in cardiac output during human pregnancy. *American Journal of Physiology* 1989; **256**: H1060–5.

267 Robson SC, Hunter S, Boys RJ & Dunlop W. Serial changes in pulmonary haemodynamics during human pregnancy: a non-invasive study using Doppler echocardiography. *Clinical Science* 1991; **80**: 113–17.

268 Robson SC, Hunter S, Moore M & Dunlop W. Haemodynamic changes during the puerperium; a Doppler and M-mode echocardiographic study. *British Journal of Obstetrics and Gynaecology* 1987; **94**: 1028–39.

269 Robson SC, Richley D, Boys RJ & Hunter S. Incidence of Doppler regurgitant flow velocities during normal pregnancy. *European Heart Journal* 1992; **13**: 84–7.

270 Rogers ME, Willerson JT, Goldblatt A & Smith TW. Serum digoxin concentrations in the human fetus, neonate and infant. *New England Journal of Medicine* 1972; **287**: 1010–13.

271 Rogge P, Young S & Goodlin R. Post-partum pulmonary oedema associated with preventive therapy for premature labour. *Lancet* 1979; **i**: 1026–7.

272 Rubin PC, Butters L *et al*. Placebo-controlled trial of atenolol in treatment of pregnancy associated hypertension. *Lancet* 1983; **i**: 431–4.

273 Rubler S, Damani PM & Pinto ER. Cardiac size and performance during pregnancy estimated with echocardiography. *American Journal of Cardiology* 1977; **40**: 534–40.

274 Rudd NL, Nimrod C, Holbrook KA & Byers PH. Pregnancy complications in type IV Ehlers–Danlos syndrome. *Lancet* 1983; **i**: 50–3.

275 Rush RW, Verjans M & Spracklen FHN. Incidence of heart disease in pregnancy. A study done at Penisular Maternity Services Hospital. *South African Medical Journal* 1979; **55**: 808–10.

276 Saarikoski S. Placental transfer and fetal uptake of 3H-digoxin in humans. *British Journal of Obstetrics and Gynaecology* 1976; **83**: 879–84.

277 Sachs BP, Lorell BH, Mehrez M & Damien M. Constrictive pericarditis and pregnancy. *American Journal of Obstetrics and Gynecology* 1986; **154**: 156–7.

278 Sachs BT & Van Idekinge B. Successful pregnancy in a patient with autosomal diurnal ventricular dysrhythmia. *American Journal of Obstetrics and Gynecology* 1979; **133**: 932–3.

279 Sahul WL & Hall JG. Multiple congenital anomalies associated with oral anticoagulants. *American Journal of Obstetrics and Gynecology* 1977; **127**: 191–8.

280 Sanders SP, Levy RJ, Freed MD, Norwood WI & Castaneda AR. Use of Hancock porcine xenografts in children and adolescents. *American Journal of Cardiology* 1980; **46**: 429–38.

281 Sanderson JE. Oedema and heart failure in the tropics. *Lancet* 1977; **ii**: 1159–61.

282 Sanderson JF, Adesanya CO, Anjorin FI & Parry EHO. Post partum cardiac failure – heart failure due to volume overload. *American Heart Journal* 1979; **97**: 613–21.

283 Saour JN, Sieck JO, Mamo LA & Gallus AS. Trial of different intensities of anticoagulation in patients with prosthetic heart valves. *New England Journal of Medicine* 1990; **322**: 428–32.

284 Schaefer G, Arditi LI, Solomon HA & Ringland JE. Congenital heart disease and pregnancy. *Clinical Obstetrics and Gynecology* 1968; **11**: 1048–63.

285 Schrier RW. A unifying hypothesis of body fluid volume regulation. *Journal of the Royal College of Physicians in London* 1992; **26**: 295–306.

286 Seaworth BJ & Durack DT. Infective endocarditis in obstetric and gynecologic practice. *American Journal of Obstetrics and Gynecology* 1986; **154**: 180–8.

287 Sharland GK & Allan LD. Screening for congenital heart disease prenatally. Results of a 2.5 year study

in the South East Thames Region. *British Journal of Obstetrics and Gynaecology* 1992; **99**: 220–5.
288 Sherman JL & Locke RV. Transplacental neonatal digitalis intoxication. *American Journal of Cardiology* 1960; **6**: 834.
289 Shine J, Mocarski EJM *et al*. Congenital heart disease in pregnancy: Short- and long-term implications. *American Journal of Obstetrics and Gynecology* 1987; **156**: 313–22.
290 Simmons NA, Ball AP *et al*. Antibiotic prophylaxis and infective endocarditis. *Lancet* 1992; **339**: 1292–3.
291 Simmons NA, Cawson RA *et al*. Prophylaxis of infective endocarditis. *Lancet* 1986; **i**: 1267.
292 Singh H, Bolton PJ & Oakley CM. Pregnancy after surgical correction of tetralogy of Fallot. *British Medical Journal* 1982; **285**: 168–70.
293 Sinnenberg RJ. Pulmonary hypertension in pregnancy. *Southern Medical Journal* 1980; **73**: 1529–31.
294 Slomka F, Salmeron S *et al*. Primary pulmonary hypertension and pregnancy: Anesthetic management of delivery. *Anesthesiology* 1988; **69**: 959–61.
295 Smith R. The molecular genetics of collagen disorders. *Clinical Science* 1986; **17**: 129–35.
296 Smith RH, Radford DJ, Clark RA & Julian DG. Infective endocarditis: a summary of cases in the South-East region of Scotland 1969–72. *Thorax* 1976; **31**: 373–9.
297 Snir E, Levinsky L, Salomon J, Findler M, Levy MJ & Vidne BA. Dissecting aortic aneurysm in pregnant women without Marfan disease. *Surgical Gynecology and Obstetrics* 1988; **167**: 463–5.
298 Socol ML, Conn J & Frederiksen MC. Pregnancy associated with partial aortic occlusion. *American Journal of Obstetrics and Gynecology* 1981; **139**: 965–7.
299 Sonel A, Erol C *et al*. Acute myocardial infarction and normal coronary arteries in a pregnant woman. *Cardiology* 1988; **75**: 218–20.
300 St John Sutton MG, St John Sutton M *et al*. Valve replacement without preoperative cardiac catheterization. *New England Journal of Medicine* 1981; **305**: 1233–8.
301 Stevenson JC, MacDonald DWR, Warren RC, Booker MW & Whitehead MI. Increased concentration of circulating calcitonin gene related peptide during normal human pregnancy. *British Medical Journal* 1986; **293**: 1329–30.
302 Stiller RJ, Vintzileos AM, Nochimson DJ, Clement D, Campbell WA & Leach CN. Single ventricle in pregnancy: Case report and review of the literature. *Obstetrics and Gynecology* 1984; **64** (suppl. 3): 19S–20S.
303 Stokes IM, Evans J & Stone M. Myocardial infarction and cardiac output in the second trimester followed by assisted vaginal delivery under epidural anaesthesia at 38 weeks gestation. Case report. *British Journal of Obstetrics and Gynaecology* 1984; **91**: 197–8.
304 Stone ML, Lending M, Slobody LB & Mestern J. Glutamine oxalacetic transaminase and lactic dehydrogenase in pregnancy. *American Journal of Obstetrics and Gynecology* 1960; **80**: 104.
305 Stuart KL. Cardiomyopathy of pregnancy and the puerperium. *Quarterly Journal of Medicine* 1968; **37**: 463–78.
306 Stubblefield PG. Pulmonary edema occurring after therapy with dexamethasone and terbutaline for premature labour. A case report. *American Journal of Obstetrics and Gynecology* 1978; **132**: 341–2.
307 Sugrue D, Blake S & MacDonald D. Pregnancy complicated by maternal heart disease at the National Maternity Hospital, Dublin, Ireland 1969 to 1978. *American Journal of Obstetrics and Gynecology* 1981; **139**: 1–6.
308 Sugrue D, Blake S & MacDonald D. Infective endocarditis during pregnancy. *Journal of Obstetrics and Gynaecology* 1982; **2**: 210–14.
309 Sugrue D, Blake S, Troy P & MacDonald D. Antibiotic prophylaxis against infective endocarditis after normal delivery — is it necessary? *British Heart Journal* 1980; **44**: 499–502.
310 Sullivan JM & Ramanathan KB. Management of medical problems in pregnancy — severe cardiac disease. *New England Journal of Medicine* 1985; **313**: 304–9.
311 Szekely P & Snaith L. Paroxysmal tachycardia in pregnancy. *British Heart Journal* 1953; **15**: 195.
312 Szekely P & Snaith L. *Heart Disease and Pregnancy*. Churchill Livingstone, Edinburgh, 1974.
313 Szekely P, Turner R & Snaith L. Pregnancy and the changing pattern of rheumatic heart disease. *British Heart Journal* 1973; **35**: 1293–303.
314 Tamari I, Eldar M, Rabinowitz B & Neufeld HN. Medical treatment of cardiovascular disorders during pregnancy. *American Heart Journal* 1982; **104**: 1357–63.
315 Taylor MB & Whitwam JG. The current status of pulse oximetry. *Anaesthesia* 1986; **41**: 943–9.
316 Teuscher A, Bossi E, Imhof P, Erb E, Stocker FP & Weber JW. Effect of propranolol on fetal tachycardia in diabetic pregnancy. *American Journal of Cardiology* 1978; **42**: 304–7.
317 Timmis A'D, Jackson G & Holt OW. Mexiletine for control of ventricular dysrhythmias in pregnancy. *Lancet* 1980; **ii**: 647–8.
318 Togo T, Sugishita A *et al*. Uneventful pregnancy and delivery in a case of multiple peripheral pulmonary stenosis. *Acta Cardiologica* 1983; **38**: 143.
319 Trouton TG, Sidhu H & Adgey A. Myocardial infarction in pregnancy. *International Journal of Cardiology* 1988; **18**: 35–9.
320 Tsipouras P, Del Mastro R *et al*. Genetic linkage of the Marfan syndrome, ectopia lentis and congenital contractural arachnodactyly to the fibrillin genes on chromosomes 15 and 5. *New England Journal of Medicine* 1992; **326**: 905–90.
321 Ueland K, Gills R & Hanson JM. Maternal cardiovascular dynamics. 1. Caesarean section under subarachnoid block anesthesia. *American Journal of Obstetrics and Gynecology* 1968; **100**: 42–53.
322 Ueland K, McAnulty JH, Ueland FR & Metcalfe J.

Special considerations in the use of cardiovascular drugs. *Clinical Obstetrics and Gynecology* 1981; **24**: 809–23.
323 Ueland K, Novy MJ & Metcalfe S. Hemodynamic responses of patients with heart disease to pregnancy and exercise. *American Journal of Obstetrics and Gynecology* 1972; **113**: 47–59.
324 Veille JC, Morton MJ & Burry KJ. Maternal cardiovascular adaptations to twin pregnancy. *American Journal of Obstetrics and Gynecology* 1985; **153**: 261–3.
325 Vicari R, Eybel C & Monson D. Survival following spontaneous coronary artery dissection: Surgical repair by extrusion of intramural haematoma. *American Heart Journal* 1986; **111**: 593–4.
326 Visser W & Wallenburg HCS. Central haemodynamic observations in untreated pre-eclamptic toxaemia. *Hypertension* 1991; **17**: 1072–7.
327 Vitali E, Donatelli F *et al*. Pregnancy in patients with mechanical prosthetic heart valves. *Journal of Cardiovascular Surgery* 1986; **27**: 221–7.
328 Vosloo S & Reichart B. The feasibility of closed mitral valvotomy in pregnancy. *Journal of Thoracic Cardiovascular Surgery* 1987; **93**: 675–9.
329 Voto LS, Agranatti D *et al*. Successful maternal and fetal outcome in a pregnant woman with primary pulmonary hypertension. *Current Obstetrics and Gynaecology* 1992; **2**: 177–9.
330 Walsh T, Savage R & Bakersmith Hess D. Successful pregnancy in a patient with a double inlet left ventricle treated with a septation procedure. *Southern Medical Journal* 1990; **83**: 358–9.
331 Walters BWJ, Thompson ME, Lee A & de Swiet M. Blood pressure in the puerperium. *Clinical Science* 1986; **71**: 589–94.
332 Watson NA & Morgan B. Pulmonary oedema and salbutamol in preterm labour. Case report and literature review. *British Journal of Obstetrics and Gynaecology* 1989; **96**: 1445–8.
333 Weaver JB & Pearson JF. Influence of time of onset and duration of labour in women with cardiac disease. *British Medical Journal* 1973; **ii**: 519.
334 Webster JC. The conduct of pregnancy and labour in acute and chronic affections of the heart. *Transactions of the American Gynecology Society* 1913; **38**: 223.
335 Weil AM & Graber VR. The management of the near-term pregnant patient who dies undelivered. *American Journal of Obstetrics and Gynecology* 1957; **73**: 754–8.
336 Whitehead MI, Mander AM, Hertogs K & Rothman MT. Myocardial ischaemia after withdrawal of salbutamol for pre-term labour. *Lancet* 1979; **ii**: 904.
337 Whittemore R, Hobbins JC & Engle MA. Pregnancy and its outcome in women with and without surgical treatment of congenital heart disease. *American Journal of Cardiology* 1982; **50**: 641–51.
338 Wilkinson C, Gyaneshwar R & McCusker C. Twin pregnancy in a patient with idiopathic long QT syndrome. Case report. *British Journal of Obstetrics and Gynaecology* 1991; **98**: 1300–2.
339 Willis DC, Caton D, Levelle JP & Banner T. Cardiac output response to prostaglandin E2-induced abortion in the second trimester. *American Journal of Obstetrics and Gynecology* 1987; **156**: 170–3.
340 Wolfe CAD, Petruckevitch A *et al*. The rate of rise of corticotrophin releasing factor and endogenous digoxin-like immunoreactivity in normal and abnormal pregnancy. *British Journal of Obstetrics and Gynaecology* 1990; **97**: 832–7.
341 Younis JS & Granat M. Insufficient transplacental digoxin transfer in severe hydrops fetalis. *American Journal of Obstetrics and Gynecology* 1987; **157**: 1268–9.
342 Yuzpe AA, Sanghvi VR, Johson FL & Robinson JG. Successful pregnancy in a patient with single ventricle and other congenital cardiac anomalies. *Canadian Medical Association Journal* 1970; **108**: 1073–5.
343 Zitnik RS, Brandenburg RO, Sheldon R & Wallace RB. Pregnancy and open heart surgery. *Circulation* 1969; **39** (suppl.): 257.

Further reading

Collins ML, Leal J & Thompson NJ. Tricuspid atresia and pregnancy. *Obstetrics and Gynecology* 1977; **50**: 72–3.

Department of Health and Social Security. *Report on Confidential Enquiries into Maternal Deaths in England and Wales, 1979–1981*. HMSO, London, 1986.

Easterling TR, Carlson KL *et al*. Measurement of cardiac output in pregnancy by Doppler technique. *American of Journal of Perinatology* 1990; **7**: 220–2.

El Kady AA, Saleh S *et al*. Obstetric deaths in Menoufia Governorate, Egypt. *British Journal of Obstetrics and Gynaecology* 1989; **96**: 9–14.

Weiner CP, Landas S & Persoon TJ. Digoxin-like immunoreactive substance in fetuses with and without cardiac pathology. *American Journal of Obstetrics and Gynecology* 1987; **157**: 368–71.

Whitehead MI, Mander AM, Hertogs K, Williams RM & Pettingale KW. Acute congestive cardiac failure in a hypertensive woman receiving salbutamol for premature labour. *British Medical Journal* 1980; **i**: 1221–2.

Wiest W, Hiltman WD *et al*. Einfluss von Partusisten und Isoptin auf das Mutterliche EKG und herzspezifische Serumenzyme. *Archives of Gynecologie* 1979; **134**: 228.

Williams G. Cardiac output — the Doppler approach. *Current Opinions in Cardiology* 1986; **1**: 250–2.

Young BK & Haft JI. Treatment of pulmonary edema with ethacrynic acid during labour. *American Journal of Obstetrics and Gynecology* 1970; **107**: 330–1.

6

Hypertension in Pregnancy

Christopher W.G. Redman

Cardiovascular changes in pregnancy, 182
Factors influencing blood pressure in normal pregnancy, 183
Errors in the measurement of blood pressure
Can a pregnant woman be categorized by her blood pressure?
What is hypertension in pregnancy?
Summary of the definition of hypertension in pregnancy
Terminology, 187
Clinical presentation and incidence of pre-eclampsia, 187
Involvement of the maternal cardiovascular system, 188
Complications of hypertension
Maternal renal system and fluid retention, 189
Plasma volume, colloid osmotic pressure and oedema
Complications of fluid retention and renal impairment
Involvement of the maternal coagulation system, 190
Involvement of the liver, 191
Involvement of the nervous system, 192
The pathogenesis of eclamptic convulsions
Underlying pathology of the maternal syndrome, 193
Primary pathology and the fetal syndrome, 194
Summary of the features of pre-eclampsia, 194
Diagnosis of pre-eclampsia, 194
Principles of diagnosis
Hypertension as a diagnostic sign
Diagnostic value of oedema and changes in renal function
Diagnostic value of changes in the coagulation system
Maternal risk factors, 198
Management of pre-eclamptic hypertension and associated problems, 198
Antihypertensive drugs
Treatment of extreme pre-eclamptic hypertension
Conservative management of severe pre-eclampsia (BP > 170/110)
Longer term control of severe pre-eclamptic hypertension
Escape from blood pressure control
Prevention and treatment of eclamptic fits, 202
Use of anticonvulsants
Diazepam
Phenytoin
Magnesium sulphate
Other measures for the treatment of pre-eclampsia and its complications, 204
Sedatives
Salt restriction, diuretics and plasma volume expansion
Treatment of the coagulation disturbances
Prevention of pre-eclampsia, 205
Antihypertensive treatment and the prevention of pre-eclampsia
Dietary factors
Antiplatelet agents
Management of labour and delivery, 207
Analgesia and anaesthesia for labour and delivery
Post-partum hypertension, 208
Summary of treatment of pre-eclampsia, 208
Chronic hypertension in pregnancy, 208
Treatment of CHT in pregnancy
Antihypertensive agents that are used in CHT
β adrenergic blocking agents (β blockers)
Other drugs
Unusual causes of hypertension in pregnancy, 211
Phaeochromocytoma
Coarctation of the aorta
Cushing's syndrome
Conn's syndrome
Long-term sequelae of hypertension in pregnancy, 212
Contraception, 212
Conclusions, 212

Cardiovascular changes in pregnancy

(see also Chapter 5)

Cardiac output increases by about 40 per cent during the first trimester. According to some investigators it declines during the third trimester [14,366,382], partly because, in the supine position, the venous return to the heart is obstructed by the gravid uterus. This reduces cardiac output acutely by 20 per cent or more [192]. However, measurements in

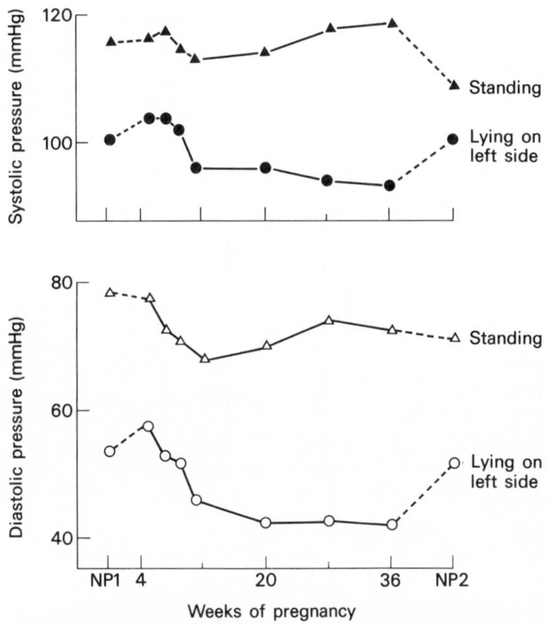

Fig. 6.1. The arterial pressures of 10 women were measured using a London School of Hygiene sphygomanometer to reduce observer bias. Readings were taken in the right arm and phase IV of the Korotkoff sounds defined the diastolic pressures. Pressures taken before conception (NP1), during pregnancy, and 6 weeks after delivery (NP2) are shown, both standing (▲, △) and supine on the left side (●, ○). The fall in both systolic and diastolic pressures in the first trimester is clearly seen (C.W.G. Redman, unpublished observations).

the lateral position show either little or no fall in the cardiac output during the third trimester [193,366].

Arterial pressure falls during pregnancy (Fig. 6.1), beginning in the first trimester, when the cardiac output is already rising, and reaching a nadir in mid-pregnancy [216]. Arterial pressure is determined by total peripheral resistance and cardiac output; so there must be a fall in arterial resistance in the first trimester [14], which cannot be caused by the uteroplacental circulation which is too small at this time to affect the peripheral resistance. During the third trimester both systolic and diastolic readings slowly rise to about the pre-pregnant levels [216]. However, the measurements depend on posture. In the supine position, with vena caval compression and reduced venous return, arterial pressure is maintained by reflex vasoconstriction [192], which causes a narrowing of the pulse pressure [150]. The systolic pressure may fall nevertheless, by more than 30 per cent in 10 per cent of cases [150]. Signs and symptoms of 'supine hypotension' may then occur including restlessness, faintness, hyperpnoea and pallor. There may also be aortic compression in the supine position [34], which can mimic a minor degree of aortic coarctation causing higher arterial pressures in the arm than in the leg. At least some cases of late gestational hypertension may be caused by this change alone [314].

The reduced peripheral resistance of normal pregnancy is associated with relative arterial refractoriness to the constrictor actions of exogenous angiotensin II (AII) but not noradrenaline [118,271]. Reduced reactivity to AII is already detectable at 8 weeks gestation and maximal at mid-pregnancy [118]. The mechanism of this blunted responsiveness has not been elucidated but it may be prostaglandin dependent. An alternative is that the reduced responsiveness may relate to changes in AII receptors on vascular smooth muscle. Whereas direct measurements have not been made in blood vessels, those on platelets (which may reflect those on vascular smooth muscle) are downregulated early in normal pregnancy as the pressor responses to AII diminish [17].

Factors influencing blood pressure in normal pregnancy

In non-pregnant individuals, blood pressure levels are influenced by age, sex, race, build and many other factors particularly the circumstances under which the measurement is taken. Pregnant women are predominantly young and usually fit. The range of blood pressures is therefore narrower than in the general population and distributed around mean levels which change at different stages of gestation but which in mid-pregnancy are lower than in a comparable non-pregnant population.

The term 'hypertension in pregnancy' carries three implications: (a) that it is possible to measure blood pressure accurately; (b) that a gravid woman's status can be characterized by one or more blood pressure readings; and (c) that there is a sensible threshold above which an abnormal blood pressure can be recognized.

Errors in the measurement of blood pressure

The indirect method of measuring blood pressure gives an approximate estimate of the true intra-arterial pressure. There is no agreement as to the cause or magnitude of the discrepancies between direct and indirect measurements in non-pregnant subjects [257]. In two studies of simultaneous measurements in pregnant women the direct readings differed on average by −6/−15 and +5/−7 mmHg respectively from indirect readings [126, 272]. The discrepancies were not related to the level of blood pressure, arm skinfold thickness or arm circumference [272]. It is generally agreed that hypertension in obese individuals is overdiagnosed if the cuff is too small in relation to the arm circumference. When the latter exceeds 35 cm either a larger arm cuff (15 × 33 cm) or even a thigh cuff (18 × 36 cm) should be used rather than a regular cuff (12 × 23 cm) [220].

The mean arm circumference of chronically hypertensive pregnant women is 27.5 cm, exceeding 35 cm in <5 per cent of this group, so the problem of a large arm is not a common one. The effect of bodyweight on the booking blood pressure in pregnant women is shown in Fig. 6.2.

Indirect blood pressure measurements should be made with the cuff at the level of the heart. If it is above or below this position the pressure in the brachial artery will fall or rise because of hydrostatic forces. Thus a pressure in the right (uppermost) arm with the patient lying on her left side will seem to be lower than the same reading when she lies flat on her back (Fig. 6.3). This is relevant when the lateral position is used in the third trimester to avoid the 'supine hypotension syndrome'. If the patient sits or stands peripheral resistance increases, by vasoconstriction in the lower extremities to maintain systolic pressure, with the effect of increasing diastolic pressure (Fig. 6.3). Thus standardization of posture and arm position is crucial. The problem can be resolved by taking blood pressures in the sitting patient as recommended in the recent consensus report from the US [241].

Another problem is the interpretation of the Korotkoff sounds. Phase I of the Korotkoff sounds defines the systolic pressure. In non-pregnant individuals phase V (extinction of Korotkoff sounds) is recommended as the diastolic end point rather than phase IV (muffling) [178]. In some pregnant women, the Korotkoff sounds are heard at zero cuff pressure. In these, phase IV has to be used as the diastolic end point even though phase V, when present, is slightly better correlated with the directly measured diastolic pressure [272]. Previously it was rec-

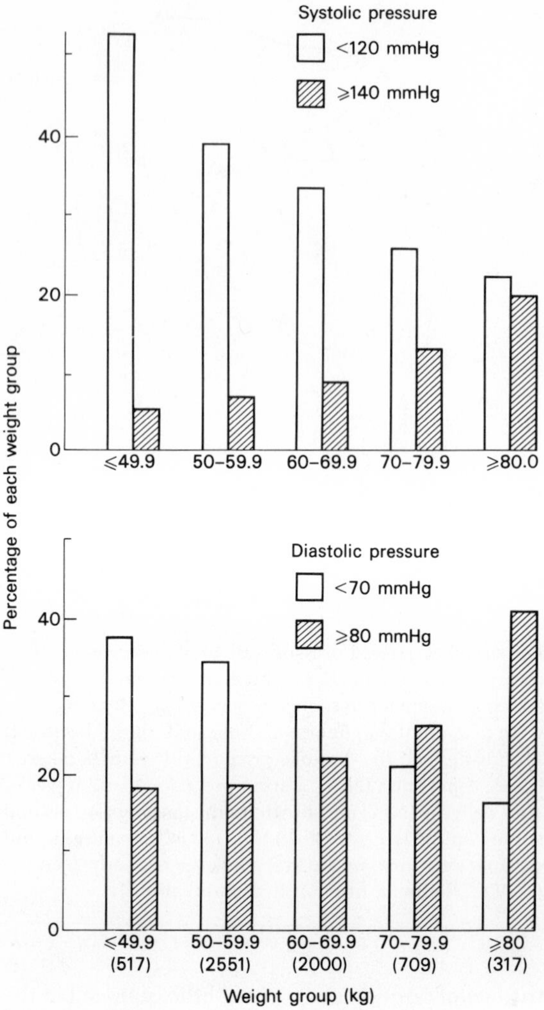

Fig. 6.2. The arterial pressures of 6094 women who booked for antenatal care at 10–20 weeks have been studied. The effect of maternal weight is shown in terms of the preponderance of small women with low pressures, and heavy women with high pressures. The numbers in parentheses are the totals for each weight group (C.W.G. Redman, unpublished observations).

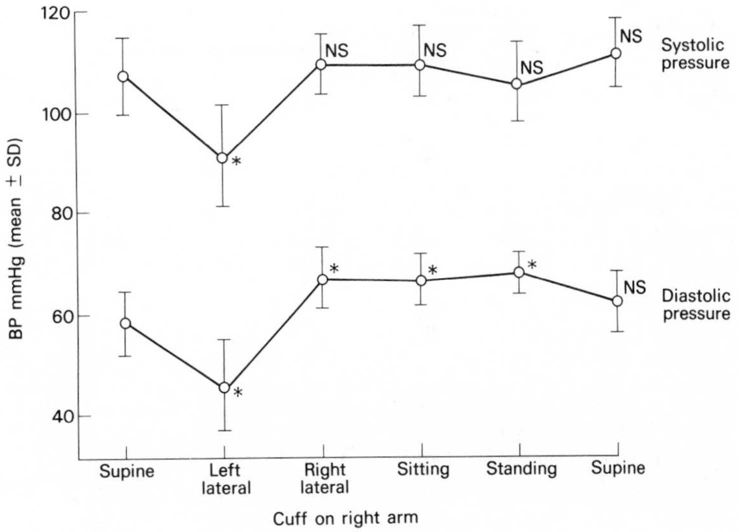

Fig. 6.3. Twenty normal women were studied in mid-pregnancy. Their arterial pressures were taken in the right arm using a London School of Hygiene sphygomanometer. The diastolic pressures were taken at phase IV of the Korotkoff sounds. The effect of different positions is clearly shown, particularly the reduced pressure in the uppermost arm when the subject lies on her left side. (Difference from supine position: NS, not significant; * $P < 0.05$) (C.W.G. Redman, unpublished observations).

ommended that diastolic pressure measurements in pregnancy were based on phase IV readings but now phase V is preferred, to be consistent with practice in other branches of medicine [241]. In pregnant women the median difference between phase IV and V readings is 2.7 mmHg [253] compared with 0.7 mmHg in non-pregnant control subjects; in 5 per cent the differences exceed 10 mmHg but in this survey the investigators did not find, as reported previously [216], that Korotkoff sounds at zero cuff pressure are a problem.

The Korotkoff sounds are produced by vibrations in the arterial wall [393]. They are less distinct if the arterial wall is rigid — for example in shock [76] or eclampsia [322] — when the indirect readings may grossly underestimate the arterial pressure.

Can a pregnant woman be categorized by her blood pressure?

Figure 6.4 shows a 24-hour blood pressure record of a hospitalized woman in the third trimester classified by conventional clinical criteria as having mild chronic hypertension. Her blood pressure varies from 130/85 to 70/40. As in non-pregnant individuals the major change occurs in sleep [282]. However, even whilst awake the patient's blood pressure fluctuates from 100/50 to 130/85. This well-known variability of blood pressure means that any one reading, however carefully and accurately taken, may deviate significantly from what is typical for an individual. In other words there are large sampling errors, which are distinct from the possible technical errors of measurement. These can be reduced by averaging a large number of readings taken under standard conditions. In clinical practice, and in most clinical investigations, this ideal is never approached, although it may be in the future as more use is made of non-invasive 24-hour ambulatory monitoring [329]. Comparisons are made between individuals based on unstandardized and frequently restricted samples of their blood pressure measurements. Furthermore these unsatisfactory readings are used to define 'normotension' and 'hypertension' giving an illusion of precision where none exists.

What is hypertension in pregnancy?

Many years ago Pickering emphasized that high blood pressure is a 'sign not a disease'; that arterial pressure is 'distributed continuously in the population at large'; and that the dividing line between normotension and hypertension is 'nothing more than an artefact' [255]. These observations are as true for pregnant women as for the general population. Hypertension in pregnancy is an artificial concept. An arbitrary threshold is used which

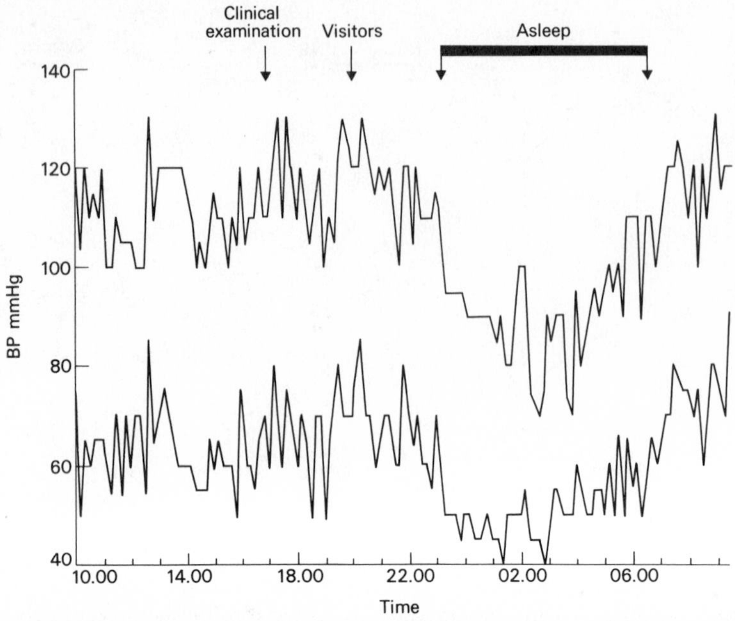

Fig. 6.4. The circadian pattern of the arterial pressure of a pregnant woman at rest in bed during the third trimester is shown. The major change in the levels is the normal fall which occurs during sleep (C.W.G. Redman, unpublished observations).

divides the population quantitatively but not qualitatively – an important but frequently forgotten distinction. A very high blood pressure may be unusual, but not necessarily abnormal.

The average blood pressure of over 6000 women booking before 20 weeks for delivery in Oxford was 120/70. Two and three standard deviations above this mean were 144/87 and 156/95 respectively. The actual distribution of the readings is shown in Table 6.1. Later in pregnancy the blood pressure rises. A maximum antenatal reading (excluding those taken in labour) of 140/90 or more was found in 21.6 per cent of all women; of 170/110 or more in 1.2 per cent. A maximum reading is a biased statistic. The greater the number of available readings the greater the chance of an 'atypical' freak level. Nevertheless these data describe the blood pressures observed in a unit serving an unselected obstetric population. By convention the threshold for 'diagnosing' hypertension in pregnancy is 140/90 mmHg. In the first half of pregnancy this identifies a small group (<2 per cent) of hypertensive individuals. In the second half, a much greater proportion (21.6 per cent) exceeds this limit at least once. So although 140/90 is an appropriate limit to begin with, in the second half of pregnancy it would be better to use a cut-off of 170/110 (maximum antenatal reading) to identify the extreme end of the distribution in populations which resemble the Oxford population.

Summary of the definition of hypertension in pregnancy

Blood pressure should be measured in the sitting position with a cuff which is large enough for the patient's arm. Phases I and V of the Korotkoff

Table 6.1. Blood pressures in 6790 women in pregnancy. Cumulative frequency distributions

Blood pressure (mmHg)	At booking <20 weeks (%)	Maximum antenatal (%)
≥170/110	0.0	1.2
≥160/100	0.1	3.7
≥150/95	0.4	8.7
≥140/90	2.0	21.5
≥130/85	5.0	38.7
≥120/80	21.0	76.7
Total	100	100

sound identify the systolic and diastolic pressures respectively. A single reading cannot characterize an individual's blood pressure status accurately. Hypertension is not a disease but one end of the continuous distribution of all individuals' blood pressures. 140/90 is the conventional dividing line for obstetric hypertension. In the first half of pregnancy this is appropriate. In the second half of pregnancy a maximum reading of 170/110 or more would be better for defining a small hypertensive group. All classifications of individuals as normotensive and hypertensive are crude and to some extent arbitrary simplifications.

Terminology

In this chapter the term 'hypertension' is used to describe a blood pressure deemed to be higher than average. Hypertension in pregnancy has three possible aetiologies either singly or in combination: it may be caused by the pregnancy itself; it may be a long-term problem present before the pregnancy began; or much more rarely, it may be a new medical problem, by chance coinciding with pregnancy.

Pre-eclampsia, pre-eclamptic toxaemia (PET) or gestosis are roughly synonymous terms describing a common syndrome which becomes detectable in the *second half* of pregnancy (although the origins may lie in the first half) and which is defined in terms of the new development of hypertension and proteinuria. Toxaemia is an obsolete expression, previously used to describe any hypertension or proteinuria in pregnancy, whether pregnancy-induced or not, so the term pre-eclampsia is to be preferred.

The syndrome of pre-eclampsia has been defined in terms of pregnancy-induced hypertension and proteinuria in various different ways [85,288]. Because fluid retention is a common (but not invariable) symptom, easily detected, it has also featured in some of the older definitions (reviewed in [278]).

Pregnancy-induced hypertension (PIH), transient hypertension of pregnancy, or gestational hypertension are terms used to describe new hypertension which appears after mid-term (20 weeks) and resolves after delivery. They describe one of the components of the pre-eclampsia syndrome. For reasons that are historical and, to some extent arbitrary rather than logical, PIH is deemed to be a mandatory part of the syndrome. But a syndrome requires at least two specific features before it can be recognized. Thus PIH on its own (a common clinical presentation) is not pre-eclampsia; at least one more sign is required. It is to be regretted that many clinicians and investigators fail to appreciate this fact and use PIH and pre-eclampsia interchangeably so muddling an already muddled subject.

A syndrome is a cluster of clinical features, no more and no less. The cluster is chosen for convenience, describes outward appearances and embodies no special truth about the underlying disease or diseases. When a syndrome such as pre-eclampsia is 'defined', rules are set that bring consistency to what is being discussed. The rules may be sensible or not but their validity cannot be tested because there is no standard to which to refer. All the definitions of pre-eclampsia suffer from these limitations; nor will there be progress until the disease or diseases that contribute to the syndrome are defined in precise pathological terms.

'Chronic hypertension' is used to describe the condition of long-term high blood pressure. The usual cause is 'essential hypertension', meaning an inherited condition with no underlying pathology. There are other rarer causes — discussed later. Superimposed pre-eclampsia describes a mixed syndrome comprising pre-eclampsia in an individual with pre-existing or chronic hypertension.

Clinical presentation and incidence of pre-eclampsia

The syndrome of pre-eclampsia develops in the second half of pregnancy, during labour or in the immediate puerperium, but always resolves more remotely after delivery. It is common, dangerous to both mother and baby, and of unknown cause.

The incidence of pre-eclampsia depends on how it is defined and how assiduously the signs are sought. Thus it is possible only to estimate the size of the problem rather than obtain exact measurements. Just as the classification of hypertension has many observational problems so does that of proteinuria which is the key second defining feature of the syndrome. Urine testing is more often omitted than blood pressure measurements particularly during labour or the early puerperium when significant pre-eclampsia may present for the first time; or, if the test is done, a positive result may be discounted because it was not confirmed in a 24-hour urine collection (for which, in all the worst presentations, there is never time) or a urine infection was not excluded.

In Aberdeen about 5 per cent of primigravidae are affected [212,242]. Lower incidences of 3.1 and 0.7 per cent were documented in the British and Greek national perinatal surveys of 1970 [55] and 1983 [365] respectively. In the USA (1979–86) there was an incidence of 2.3 per cent, using somewhat broader diagnostic criteria [309]. The incidences will be affected by the proportion of primigravidae in the different populations but in addition there may be true regional differences superimposed. The incidence of proteinuric pre-eclampsia in the UK is therefore of the order of one in 20–30 maternities.

The commonly used definitions of pre-eclampsia have been devised primarily for use in epidemiological studies [57,242,297]. They are not so useful to the clinician who has to make individual diagnoses. In different ways they emphasize three features — hypertension, oedema and proteinuria — not because these are known to be the most important but because, historically, they were the first to be defined and happened to be easily accessible signs. Pre-eclampsia is a disorder of the second half of pregnancy which regresses after delivery. Its cause is not yet known but must lie within the gravid uterus. Hence although pre-eclampsia is conventionally defined by hypertension it is not primarily a hypertensive disease. The raised blood pressure and other maternal signs by which it is recognized are secondary features, reflections of an intrauterine problem. Because pre-eclampsia is a disorder of pregnancy and not simply a maternal problem, the fetus is invariably involved and may suffer its own morbidity or mortality. The signs of pre-eclampsia are therefore best considered as secondary to a uteroplacental disorder, affecting specific maternal target systems. The targets include the maternal cardiovascular, renal, coagulation and hepatic systems. The widespread systemic nature of the maternal disturbances is all too often not recognized. Many clinicians wrongly conceive of pre-eclampsia as only the aggregate of its conventionally defined signs of hypertension, oedema and proteinuria.

Pre-eclampsia, once established is relentlessly progressive until delivery. Throughout almost all its course the patient is symptomless — a critical feature where diagnosis and management are concerned. Terminally the patient feels ill with headaches, visual disturbances, nausea, vomiting, epigastric pain and neurological irritability — including clonus and shaking. At this point convulsions may occur and the illness has progressed to its end point of eclampsia.

Involvement of the maternal cardiovascular system

The hypertension of pre-eclampsia is an early feature, not associated with a single haemodynamic pattern. Some investigators find increased cardiac output [31,96,211] others the converse [138,181,187, 373]. Some of the differences between studies may reflect drug use — for example, treatment with vasodilators stimulates cardiac output by reducing afterload [138]. However, in a serial study, with Doppler ultrasound measurements, those who developed pre-eclampsia had higher estimates of cardiac output before, during and after the episode of pre-eclampsia unrelated to treatment [96].

The blood pressure is typically unstable at rest [58], possibly owing to reduced baroceptor sensitivity [385]. Circadian variation is altered with, first, a loss of the normal fall in blood pressure at night [322] then, in the worst cases, a reversed pattern with the highest readings during sleep [282].

Arterial reactivity to exogenous vasopressor substances such as catecholamines [351] and AII [118] is increased in pre-eclampsia, the last having been demonstrated both *in vivo* [118] and *ex vivo* using omental vessels taken at caesarean section [1].

The increased responsiveness may relate to changes in AII receptors on vascular smooth muscle. Again direct measurements have not been made, but those on platelets follow the expected pattern, being downregulated early in normal pregnancy [17] but significantly increased in the third trimester in pre-eclampsia [18].

The hypertension is important for two reasons: (a) it is a key early diagnostic sign; and (b) if extreme, it can cause direct arterial injury.

Complications of hypertension

In general, a sudden increase of blood pressure above a critical threshold causes acute arterial damage and loss of vascular autoregulation. This has been demonstrated both experimentally, for example in rats [129] and clinically [165]. The central nervous system appears to be particularly sensitive to hypertensive pathology including cerebral haemorrhage which antihypertensive treatment helps to prevent giving further proof of the aetiology [259].

Pre-eclampsia may cause blood pressures which are well above the level (i.e. a mean arterial pressure of about 140 mmHg) at which arterial and arteriolar damage would be expected. It is not surprising that the most common cause of maternal death from pre-eclampsia and eclampsia is cerebral haemorrhage, the pathology of which is similar to that seen in other hypertensive states [328]. In England and Wales maternal death from hypertensive and other cerebral injury exceeds the sum of all other causes of death from pre-eclampsia and eclampsia [291, 292,293,294,295 and Table 6.2]. Similar findings have been reported from Australia [240].

In summary, hypertension is an early secondary sign of pre-eclampsia. Severe hypertension is the main cause of maternal death from this disorder.

Maternal renal system and fluid retention (see also Chapter 7)

Proteinuria is the conventionally recognized but late sign of renal involvement in pre-eclampsia. Once present it indicates a poorer prognosis for both mother and baby than when it is absent [46,239,354]. On average it appears about 3 weeks before intrauterine death or mandatory delivery [281]. It is moderately selective in terms of the molecular size of the filtered proteins [229,340], and may be heavy (>5 g/day). Overall, pre-eclampsia is the commonest cause of nephrotic syndrome in pregnancy [107].

Proteinuria is one of several signs of involvement of the renal glomerulus in pre-eclampsia. Renal biopsy has shown a characteristic non-inflammatory lesion, primarily of swelling of the glomerular endothelial cells, which encroach on and occlude the capillary lumina — 'glomerular endotheliosis'. The epithelial cells are also swollen but the foot processes are intact [262]. It should be noted that renal biopsy is never indicated to resolve the differential diagnosis of pre-eclampsia, however atypical or difficult the presentation. The investigation is reserved for those who continue to have significant proteinuria and/or renal impairment at a remote time after delivery. It has been claimed [343] and denied [106] that the glomerular lesions are pathognomonic. The former view makes pre-eclampsia a primary renal disease, whereas renal involvement must always be secondary to the utero-placental problem. Normal renal histology has been found in some cases of eclampsia [89] so does not exclude the diagnosis.

Renal function is also impaired. The changes are biphasic involving first tubular function and later glomerular function. An early feature of pre-eclampsia is a reduced uric acid clearance, reflecting altered tubular function [67], and causing a reciprocal rise in plasma urate. Later, at about the time that proteinuria develops, glomerular filtration becomes impaired. A rising plasma urate is thus an early sign of pre-eclampsia which precedes a later rise in

Table 6.2. Maternal deaths from hypertensive disease England and Wales 1973–84 and UK 1985–90

Cause of death	1973–75	1976–78	1979–81	1982–84	1985–87	1988–90	Total
Cerebral haemorrhage	17 (44%)	17 (59%)	9 (25%)	13 (52%)	11 (41%)	12 (44%)	79
Other CNS pathology	6 (15%)	4 (14%)	8 (22%)	8 (32%)	11 (41%)	2 (44%)	39
Hepatic pathology	4	1	8	1	1	1	16
Pulmonary pathology	1	1	2	3	12	10	29

Figures derived from: [291,292,293,294,295,296].

plasma creatinine or urea [281]. It is also the biochemical change which best correlates with the renal biopsy appearances of pre-eclampsia [262].

Another relatively early change in renal function is hypocalciuria [311,353] which is not a feature of pregnant women with other forms of hypertension. It is associated with significantly decreased concentrations of serum 1,25-dihydroxyvitamin D [11,321]. Increased serum concentrations of 1,25-dihydroxyvitamin D are characteristic of normal pregnancy [122], probably because 1α-hydroxylation of 25-hydroxyvitamin D, usually confined to the kidney, occurs in the decidua and placenta [390]. That 1,25-dihydroxyvitamin D is reduced in pre-eclampsia may be a manifestation of the fact that it is primarily a placental disorder.

Plasma volume, colloid osmotic pressure and oedema

Maternal plasma volume normally increases during the second and third trimesters of pregnancy [158, 260]. The extent of the increase depends on the size of the conceptus, being higher in women with multiple pregnancy [112,305], and least in those with fetuses which are small for gestational age [94,158,260]. Maternal plasma volume is reduced in pre-eclampsia in relation to normal pregnancy [110, 117,214]. Pre-eclampsia is frequently associated with fetal growth retardation which accounts for some of the observed change in plasma volume. But whether the plasma volume is further decreased, even given fetal size, has not been determined. Hypertension itself may be a factor, because it is associated with reduced plasma volumes in non-pregnant subjects [35]. More important may be the hypoalbuminaemia characteristic of the disorder [152,348] which causes a lower colloid osmotic pressure [30,400]. This alters the Starling forces governing fluid transport across the capillaries, so that the vascular system in pre-eclampsia becomes 'leaky', with a maldistribution of fluid: too much in the interstitial spaces (oedema) and too little in the vascular compartment (hypovolaemia).

Of women with proteinuric pre-eclampsia, 85 per cent have oedema [358]. However, pre-eclampsia without oedema — 'dry pre-eclampsia' — has long been recognized as a particularly dangerous variant [97], for example the perinatal mortality is higher than if oedema is present [59]. The oedema fluid is an ultrafiltrate of plasma.

The fluid retention of pre-eclampsia is associated with renal retention of both sodium and potassium. The pre-eclamptic woman excretes a sodium load more slowly than normal pregnant women. In part, this is because the filtered load of sodium is reduced by the lower glomerular filtration rate; in part because net tubular re-absorption of sodium tends to be increased [66]. It is likely but not proven that the renal changes are secondary to the oedema-forming process.

Complications of fluid retention and renal impairment

Ascites is not uncommon, for example affecting 13 of 99 women seen personally with severe pre-eclampsia. Pulmonary oedema is a rare but life-threatening complication presenting before or after delivery [346,350]. Laryngeal oedema may cause respiratory obstruction as well as difficulties if a general anaesthetic is required [169]. Acute renal failure with tubular, partial cortical or total cortical necrosis are terminal complications, more common previously than in current medical practice. The latter two events are more likely in the context of an abruptio placentae complicating pre-eclampsia or eclampsia [342].

Involvement of the maternal coagulation system (see also Chapter 3)

The coagulation system is a target for the pre-eclamptic process. Normal pregnancy is a 'hyper-coagulable' state, meaning that the blood response to clotting stimuli is brisker and that the natural turnover of the system is enhanced. The latter change is detected by the increased circulating levels of soluble fibrin monomer complexes in the third trimester [29]. The turnover is further exaggerated in early pre-eclampsia.

At this time the platelet count may be moderately reduced [286] owing to increased consumption with a reduced platelet lifespan [40,274]. Platelet activation has been confirmed by the higher circulating levels of the platelet-specific proteins, β thromboglobulin [19,92,280] and platelet factor 4 [12], which are products of the platelet release reaction; and by the loss of the platelet content of 5-hydroxytryptamine [391]. The platelets are relatively unresponsive to various aggregating agents [7,391], that is they are desensitized as a result of activation *in vivo*. The platelets tend to be larger (that is, probably younger) [125], even in the absence of thrombocytopenia [347]. If the platelet count is reduced it usually recovers within 4 days of delivery [174]. Thrombocytopenia is an inconsistent part of the syndrome, for example affecting only 29 per cent of one series of eclamptic women, when thrombocytopenia was defined as having platelet counts $\leqslant 150 \times 10^9$/l [265].

There is also increased intravascular thrombin generation shown by higher circulating levels of D-dimer [362] — a specific fibrin degradation product, fibrinopeptide A [92] — a product of the action of thrombin on fibrinogen, and thrombin–antithrombin III complexes [87,290].

In the earlier stages this is a chronic, fully compensated process which cannot be labelled as a pathological disseminated intravascular coagulation (DIC) which is, however, the end stage of the process. The inhibitors of the coagulation pathway — antithrombin III [87,388] and protein C — [13,87] are reduced.

DIC is a late and inconsistent feature of pre-ictal pre-eclampsia and eclampsia, first demonstrated at autopsy [227]. It is particularly severe if there is concomitant hepatic involvement [176]. Consumption of coagulation factors — fibrinogen, factors VII and VIII — and elevated serum fibrin/fibrinogen degradation products, is associated with the severe systemic disturbances of failure of the microcirculation. Thus the problems affecting the coagulation system proceed through two phases: (a) an early abnormal but fully compensated activation; and (b) a later decompensation when the fibrinolytic system is overwhelmed by widespread fibrin deposition. Specific lesions include renal cortical necrosis, adrenal and pituitary haemorrhage and necrosis, and periportal hepatic necrosis. Microangiopathic haemolysis is one complication associated with haemoglobinaemia, a sudden fall in the haemoglobin concentration, a reduced haptoglobin level (because the haptoglobin binds to the free haemoglobin and is rapidly cleared) and fragmented or distorted red cells in the peripheral blood film [270,370,389].

Involvement of the liver

(see also Chapter 9)

Liver dysfunction is a feature of pre-eclampsia detected by elevations of circulating hepatic enzymes [332], which may progress to jaundice and severe hepatic impairment [86,176,203]. Epigastric pain and vomiting are the typical symptoms associated with liver involvement but are not always present [325]. Unless evidence for hepatic derangement is sought in all cases of proteinuric pre-eclampsia, dangerous presentations will be missed. About two-thirds of women dying from eclampsia have specific lesions in the liver [324] which are periportal 'lake' haemorrhages and various grades of ischaemic damage, including complete infarction [327]. The haemorrhages arise from the arteries and arterioles of the portal tract, which show diffuse mural damage [326]. In addition there are thromboses in the portal tract vessels which may extend into the tributaries of the portal vein. Most of this pathology has been defined post-mortem although it has been confirmed in biopsy studies. In mild cases of pre-eclampsia, without thrombocytopenia or disturbances of the plasma liver enzymes, there is fibrin/fibrinogen deposition in the hepatic sinusoids [9]. This may merely be a sign of clearance of an increased burden of intravascular fibrin by the reticuloendothelial system of the liver.

Liver damage is particularly associated with DIC in pre-eclampsia. If this occurs together with microangiopathic haemolysis the acronym HELLP syndrome has been used to label the concurrence of haemolysis, elevated liver enzymes and low platelet counts [333,389]. This is merely a convenient way of bringing the presentation — which has been documented, albeit incompletely, for many years [176,270] — into focus. It is a dangerous complication that is often not associated with marked hypertension [389]. Indeed liver damage and low platelet counts have been demonstrated in primigravidae, without hypertension or proteinuria, but with the typical hepatic histology of pre-eclampsia including fibrin deposition in the sinusoids [2].

The fulminant condition presents very suddenly, often in the immediate post-partum period and may be associated with eclampsia and acute renal failure. Recovery from the primary problem may take up to 11 days [217] and be complicated by rebound hypercoagulability which can cause fatal thrombosis [173].

In certain severe cases, typically of multiparae rather than primiparae, there may be bleeding under the liver capsule. Subsequently this may rupture to cause massive haemoperitoneum, shock and (usually) maternal death [36]. There may well be an overlap between the liver involvement in pre-eclampsia and in acute fatty liver of pregnancy [184].

Involvement of the nervous system

(see also Chapter 15)

By definition eclampsia is the end point of pre-eclampsia, although it is still unclear if the prodromal disorder is always evident before convulsions begin. Even at the time of eclampsia, up to 41 per cent of cases have been reported to have little or no proteinuria [97,263,337] and only a minority (30 per cent) are thrombocytopenic [265]. Eclampsia with an apparently normal blood pressure may arise from errors in sphygmomanometry; nevertheless, as far as it is known, extreme hypertension is not a necessary (or indeed sufficient) predisposing factor. This said, eclampsia occurs seven to eight times more commonly in the context of proteinuric than of non-proteinuric pre-eclampsia [242] and the average blood pressures of women with eclampsia are higher than those with severe pre-eclampsia [337].

The incidence of eclampsia is now modified by obstetric practice, particularly that of ending pregnancies by induction or caesarean section. The incidence in the UK is not measured but is probably <0.1 per cent. Eclampsia usually occurs in the second half of pregnancy, occurring more commonly towards term [356], but has been observed as early as 16 weeks of pregnancy [198]. In about half the cases convulsions begin before labour [33,97,263]. Most post-partum fits occur within 24 hours of delivery [263], but have been described up to 23 days post-partum [310]. Perhaps as many as half the cases of post-partum eclampsia occur more than 48 hours after delivery [387].

The pathogenesis of eclamptic convulsions

The question as to what causes eclamptic convulsions remains unresolved. It is not likely that they result directly from sudden increases in blood pressure. However, eclampsia *is* a form of hypertensive encephalopathy, an acute or subacute syndrome of diffuse rather than focal cerebral dysfunction, not ascribable to uraemia. Hypertensive encephalopathy is a rare complication of malignant hypertension [72], but more frequently occurs in the context of acute nephritis.

Hypertensive encephalopathy in non-pregnant individuals has many features in common with eclampsia. Headaches, nausea and vomiting are typical associated symptoms [69]. It can occur at relatively low blood pressure levels. Gross papilloedema or retinopathy are rare but cortical blindness is a complication [164], as it is with severe pre-eclampsia or eclampsia [137,194].

The cerebral pathology of eclampsia resembles that of other hypertensive encephalopathies and comprises thrombosis, fibrinoid necrosis of the cerebral arterioles, diffuse microinfarcts and petechial haemorrhages [69,328]. These changes are not found in malignant hypertension. Whether or not cerebral oedema is a consistent feature of eclampsia is not clear. It is said to be the cause of death in about 20 per cent of those dying from pre-eclampsia or eclampsia [148]. But whereas it was the only cerebral pathology documented in 20 per cent of one series of deaths [205] it was not demonstrated at all in another [328]. Primary and secondary pathology cannot be readily distinguished after death, but diffuse and focal cerebral oedema has been documented by computed tomography (CT) [24,177] but not when the scans are done immediately after the convulsions [230]. Other lesions include haemorrhages [23,230] and infarcts [113] which have also been demonstrated by CT. Likewise focal areas of oedema in the white matter have been observed with CT scans in cases of hypertensive encephalopathy [273] even though oedema is not a consistent feature at autopsy [69]. Magnetic resonance imaging (MRI) of the brains of eclamptic women reveals reversible focal changes characteristic of ischaemia [312,318].

The pressure of the cerebrospinal fluid (CSF) of

eclamptic women is increased compared to that of pregnant women with convulsions from other causes [105]; similarly CSF pressure is usually but not invariably raised in non-pregnant individuals with hypertensive encephalopathy [164]. Focal cerebral oedema can be induced experimentally by extreme hypertension [48], but the cause of the cerebral dysfunction in hypertensive encephalopathy is still not fully defined. One view is that the problem is of ischaemia secondary to intense vasoconstriction [328]. However, the vasoconstriction is an essential, protective response to extremes of arterial pressure [165], which prevents an uncontrolled increase in tissue perfusion and damage to the microcirculation distal to the arterioles. In normal individuals, arterial constriction ensures that cerebral perfusion remains constant, at mean arterial pressures between 60 and 150 mmHg [345] (autoregulation).

At very high arterial pressures autoregulation is lost because the arterial smooth musche is not strong enough to sustain protective constriction and pressure-forced dilation begins, allowing uncontrolled increases in cerebral blood flow. Then high pressure perfusion begins to rupture the more delicate distal microcirculation. The dilatation is associated with damage to the vessel wall, allowing insudation of plasma (infiltration of plasma proteins into the vessel wall); abnormal permeability is confined to the dilated segments [123,129]. To what extent this may contribute to hypertensive encephalopathy is not known; the occurrence of eclampsia at relatively low arterial blood pressures makes it unlikely.

Recovery from the medical condition is associated with control of the blood pressure, so that a cause and effect relationship has been imputed. However, this is not justified by the available evidence and certainly there is no direct evidence that eclampsia is caused by sudden increases in blood pressure or prevented by adequate blood pressure control.

Severe pre-eclampsia or eclampsia share some clinical features, (proteinuria, renal impairment and DIC) but not others (retinopathy, renal vascular pathology), with malignant hypertension [199]. Therefore, according to the usual terminology, most cases of severe pre-eclampsia or eclampsia cannot be classified as malignant hypertension.

Underlying pathology of the maternal syndrome

The maternal syndrome is surprisingly variable, in the time of onset, speed of progression and the extent to which it involves different systems. Until recently it was impossible to explain a condition that could present not only with hypertension but also convulsions, jaundice, abdominal pain or normotensive proteinuria (amongst others) by a single underlying pathological process; certainly hypertension could not account for all these features.

But the concept that the maternal endothelium is the target organ for the pre-eclampsia process has resolved this difficulty [298]. In short the maternal syndrome can be explained if it is seen, not as a hypertensive problem, but as the sum of the consequences of diffuse endothelial dysfunction.

There is both structural and functional evidence for endothelial dysfunction in pre-eclampsia. One example is the renal lesion of glomerular endotheliosis [262]. Endothelial swelling is also seen in uterine venules [323] and myocardial vessels [20]. There is one report that desquamated endothelial cells can be detected in blood samples from pre-eclamptic women [128] as they can in some other medical conditions [313].

Together these reports comprise the case for endothelial injury in pre-eclampsia. There is preliminary evidence for circulating factors that are toxic to endothelium in pre-eclamptic women [303,363] or that alter their lipid metabolism and ability to release prostacyclin [206]. It has been proposed that these factors might include products of free radical activity (lipid peroxides) perhaps derived from hypoxic placental tissue [156].

When endothelium is injured, or activated, it releases certain products including cellular fibronectin, the von Willebrand factor and type 1 plasminogen activator inhibitor. All are increased in the plasma of pre-eclamptic women [124,287,355]. So these findings are consistent with the hypothesis.

If the maternal endothelial system is the principal site of pathology in pre-eclampsia what is the trigger? There is considerable evidence that it is the placenta and that ultimately pre-eclampsia is not a maternal hypertensive disorder but a primary placental problem.

Primary pathology and the fetal syndrome

The primary problem is in the placenta [279]. It is obvious that pre-eclampsia is a specific disorder of pregnancy; but it also complicates some cases of hydatidiform mole [320] where the uterus contains only disordered placental tissue. Thus a fetus is not necessary, only the placenta. The illness always ultimately regresses when the uterus is emptied of placental tissue, which confirms that the placenta is the cause of pre-eclampsia and justifies the standard and only effective treatment which is delivery.

The problem in the placenta seems to be a relative insufficiency of the uteroplacental circulation.

The maternal uteroplacental circulation in the human is unlike any other in the adult. It lacks a microcirculation; there are no arterioles, capillaries or venules. Instead more than 100 spiral arteries deliver the 500 ml/min of blood normally required by full term directly into the intervillous space. In pre-eclampsia they may be affected by two lesions. The first is a relative lack of the physiological adaptations between weeks 8 and 18, during placentation [301], when there is major remodelling which dilates the arteries so that they can transmit the expanded uteroplacental blood flow of the second half of the pregnancy. The problem develops at a time when there is no clinical disease. The inference is that poor placentation is the primary pathology of pre-eclampsia. The problem is not specific to pre-eclampsia; it is also found in some cases of intrauterine growth retardation without a maternal syndrome [330].

The second lesion in the spiral arteries is 'acute atherosis' — aggregates of fibrin, platelets and lipid-loaded macrophages (lipophages) which partially or completely block the arteries [300,399]. The time course of their development is obscure, but it is likely that they are a late pathological feature. The cause is not known. The lesions are not the consequence of hypertensive injury. The pathology is endothelial so acute atherosis may represent one aspect of the generalized maternal endothelial disturbances of pre-eclampsia.

Acute atherosis and the associated thromboses are the cause of placental infarctions [42,378] which are more common in pre-eclampsia [202]. The two spiral artery pathologies also can explain the reduced uteroplacental blood flow of pre-eclampsia [166,223] and the desaturation of intervillous blood [153] in the disorder; also why some placental functions are impaired [119]. All these changes are consistent with an underlying placental ischaemia, but provide largely indirect evidence that placental ischaemia is a fundamental part of the pathological process of pre-eclampsia.

It is probable that the maternal signs of pre-eclampsia are also secondary to placental ischaemia. Experimental models of pre-eclampsia in baboons, dogs, rabbits or rats all depend on procedures which reduce placental blood flow [5,53,91,384,396].

Impairment of the uteroplacental circulation affects the placental functions that sustain the fetus. Pre-eclampsia is conventionally considered to be a maternal disorder in which the fetus is an incidental participant. A more complete perception is that pre-eclampsia is a placental disorder causing both maternal and fetal syndromes. The balance of the two syndromes varies: in some cases there is a major fetal problem whereas the maternal features are relatively trivial; in others the converse picture may be seen.

Summary of the features of pre-eclampsia

Pre-eclampsia is a primary placental disorder which causes secondary changes in different maternal target systems by which the disease is recognized. Hypertension is one of many aspects of pre-eclampsia. It is neither its primary feature nor its only significant sign. A list of some of the maternal complications of pre-eclampsia is given in Box 6.1.

Diagnosis of pre-eclampsia

Principles of diagnosis

Diseases can be diagnosed but syndromes can only be recognized. Identifying, or screening for, a syndrome is, at best, imprecise and always, in terms of logic, unsatisfactory. The false positive and negative rates of the various diagnostic criteria cannot be measured properly because, without a specific diagnostic test, there is no sensible standard to

Box 6.1. Complications of pre-eclampsia

- Central nervous system
  - Eclamptic convulsions
  - Cerebral haemorrhage
  - Cerebral oedema
  - Cortical blindness
  - Retinal oedema
  - Retinal detachment
- Renal system
  - Renal cortical necrosis
  - Renal tubular necrosis
- Respiratory system
  - Laryngeal oedema
  - Pulmonary oedema
- Liver
  - Jaundice
  - Hepatic infarction
  - HELLP syndrome
  - Hepatic rupture
- Coagulation system
  - Disseminated intravascular coagulation
  - Microangiopathic haemolysis
  - HELLP syndrome
- Placenta
  - Placental infarction
  - Retroplacental bleeding and abruptio placentae

which to refer. Of many possible features of the pre-eclampsia syndrome PIH and pregnancy-induced proteinuria are, by convention, emphasized more because they are easy to detect in practice than because they are the central to the progression of the disorder. Abnormal fluid retention is used less now than formerly, because it is assessed subjectively and easy to confuse with the physiological oedema that most pregnant women have.

As we have seen, there are many possible features of the syndrome for example hyperuricaemia, thrombocytopenia, abnormal liver enzymes or haemoconcentration (arising from a reduced plasma volume); and the fetal syndrome yields its own signs of which smallness for gestational age is the most obvious. But none is consistently present and so although the signs can be used to recognize pre-eclampsia their absence never excludes the condition. Eclampsia can occur without proteinuria [337]. Even hypertension seems not to be an essential component [319]. Until we understand the causes of whatever disease or diseases underlie the pre-eclampsia syndrome we cannot diagnose but merely recognize potentially sinister clusters of signs and we should not be too rigid in demanding that one or other *must* be present before there is the need for concern. Nor should the clinician limit the range of his or her search for signs of pre-eclampsia simply because they do not feature in one or other of the 'definitions' of the syndrome. Possible signs that may be considered are listed in Box 6.2. For diagnostic purposes all the secondary features of the disorder should be considered as possible components. Hypertension and hyperuricaemia are early signs. Proteinuria, major coagulation disturbances, significant hepatic dysfunction and placental impairment are late signs.

If it is accepted that the condition of pre-eclampsia, as it is perceived clinically, is a secondary maternal adaptation to a primary uteroplacental

Box 6.2. Recognition of the pre-eclampsia syndrome

- Signs of the maternal syndrome
  - Pregnancy-induced hypertension
  - Excessive weight gain (>1 kg/week)
  - Generalized oedema
  - Ascites
  - Hyperuricaemia
  - Proteinuria
  - Hypocalciuria
  - Raised plasma concentration of von Willebrand factor
  - Raised plasma concentration of cellular fibronectin
  - Reduced plasma concentration of antithrombin III
  - Thrombocytopenia
  - Increased haematocrit
  - Increased blood concentrations of liver enzymes
- Signs of the fetal syndrome
  - Intrauterine growth retardation
  - Intrauterine hypoxaemia

problem, then large variability in presentation must be expected, reflecting individual differences in the susceptibility of maternal target-organ systems. So, pre-eclampsia cannot be stereotyped. Its different components vary from one case to the next so that one woman may have severe hypertension but little renal involvement, another severe renal involvement but little hypertension, and a third predominantly hepatic involvement.

One consequence of these considerations is that it is impossible to diagnose pre-eclampsia before the onset of proteinuria without resorting to laboratory investigations — it cannot be detected by observing changes in the blood pressure alone. The diagnosis of mild pre-eclampsia at term is always uncertain because delivery prevents the appearance of the corroborative signs of more advanced disease.

Hypertension as a diagnostic sign

The hypertension of pre-eclampsia is detected by a rise in the blood pressure during the second half of pregnancy which is abnormal in magnitude relative to the time of pregnancy at which it occurs. Thus a diastolic rise of about 10 mmHg is normal for the last 12 weeks of pregnancy [216] (Fig. 6.5) but a rise of only 5 mmHg between weeks 20 and 30 is associated with significantly higher rates of maternal proteinuria, prematurity and perinatal death [213]. Hence to identify pre-eclampsia in terms of blood pressure readings it is necessary to refer to a change from a baseline rather than an absolute level: for example that the systolic and diastolic pressures increase by at least 30 and 15 mmHg respectively [241].

A high blood pressure reading by itself does not necessarily signify pre-eclampsia. Before 20 weeks it indicates hypertension which preceded pregnancy. After 20 weeks it may represent a continuation of chronic hypertension or a *de novo* (i.e. pre-eclamptic) problem. Given the technical and sampling errors of blood pressure measurement, small increases of pre-eclamptic origin are difficult to detect. Diagnostic accuracy may be improved by rigid standardization of the methods of measurement [116].

A normal blood pressure in the first half of pregnancy does not necessarily mean long-term normotension because the fall in blood pressure induced in early pregnancy may be exaggerated in some women; many with relatively severe hypertension may have normal blood pressures by 12 weeks, without treatment. In other words some women enjoy the benefits of pregnancy-induced normo-

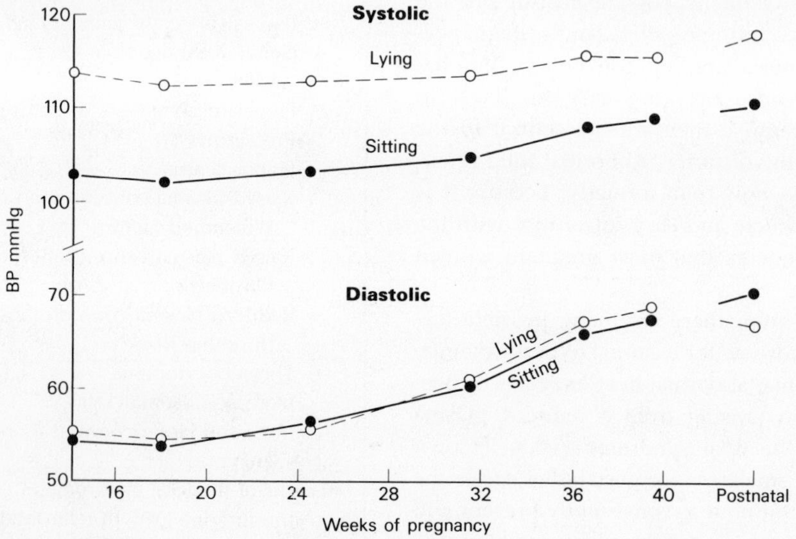

Fig. 6.5. Serial arterial pressures in 226 primigravidae taken both lying and sitting [216]. Reproduced by permission.

tension just as others suffer the disadvantages of PIH. Pregnancy-induced normotension tends to be lost in the third trimester. If the pre-pregnancy blood pressures are unknown then this development may be misinterpreted as PIH. In one extreme case, a woman had pre-pregnancy readings of 224–280/140–180 mmHg; during pregnancy the pressure fell, without treatment, which was not available at that time, to normal levels of 110–130/60–80 mmHg [64]. During the third trimester extreme hypertension developed as the woman's normal cardiovascular status re-appeared. This case report demonstrates clearly how chronic hypertension can masquerade as PIH — a common problem in clinical practice, although its exact extent has never been assessed.

Diagnostic value of oedema and changes in renal function

The pathological oedema of pre-eclampsia is easily confused with the physiological oedema found in 80 per cent of normal pregnant women [299]. Physiological oedema has not been shown to be the precursor of pathological oedema, but will appear to be so, if definitions of pre-eclampsia are used which emphasize oedema even in the absence of hypertension (such as those of the American Committee on Maternal Welfare). In the best prospective study, pregnant women with no oedema, or early or late onset oedema, all had a similar incidence of hypertension [299]. For all these reasons the detection of oedema is not useful clinically, nor should oedema be included in the definition of pre-eclampsia [374].

Development of oedema is associated with a higher rate of weight gain, hence the numerous reports associating excessive weight gain with the development of pre-eclampsia [4].

An elevated plasma uric acid is usually a useful diagnostic feature of early pre-eclampsia [79,186, 228]. It precedes the development of proteinuria and is a simple investigation which can confirm the diagnosis in non-proteinuric pre-eclampsia. Two standard deviations above the mean of the plasma concentrations at 16, 28, 32 and 36 weeks are 0.28, 0.29, 0.34 and 0.39 mmol respectively (C.W.G. Redman, unpublished data). Levels above these values in the third trimester are suggestive of pre-eclampsia. However, as with all other signs of pre-eclampsia, hyperuricaemia is both non-specific and, to some extent, variable in its time course in relation to other features. It may also result from long-term renal impairment, diuretic use, or merely reflect a long-term constitutional characteristic of the gravid woman. Women with chronic hypertension without pre-eclampsia have normal plasma urate levels [281]. Thus an elevated plasma urate should distinguish pre-eclamptic hypertension, with a poor fetal outcome, from chronic hypertension with a normal fetal outcome. This has been demonstrated [285]: for a given blood pressure level a plasma urate >0.35 mmol identifies a subgroup with a 10-fold increase in perinatal mortality. A raised plasma creatinine (≥90 μmol/l) or blood urea (≥6-mmol/l) is usual only with proteinuric pre-eclampsia. In this situation these measurements are essential not for diagnosis but to anticipate increasing renal impairment which might precede acute renal failure.

Diagnostic value of changes in the coagulation system

Although a declining platelet count may be an early feature of pre-eclampsia [286], it has limited diagnostic value because of the large variability between individuals in normal pregnancy. Prospective serial counts in selected high risk patients are more useful when the patient's own baseline is established early in pregnancy. An alternative technique is to monitor for falling plasma concentrations of anti-thrombin III [388]. Markers of endothelial cell activation may be increased early in the disease: for example von Willebrand factor [287] or fibronectin [355]. But there are no definitive studies that demonstrate the benefits or limitations of these measurements.

It is probably still true that, in early disease it is easier to detect the renal changes rather than the clotting disturbances [95].

The clotting disturbances of advanced pre-eclampsia are more readily observed, correlate with an adverse outcome and can be used to monitor the course of the disease [154]. A diminished platelet count and raised fibrin/fibrinogen degradation products are the most easily detected changes. In severe pre-eclampsia it is essential to know the degree of the clotting disturbance because if DIC is present it indicates a much more serious situation.

Maternal risk factors

Diagnosis must be made in symptomless women by screening. Given that pre-eclampsia can begin at any time after 20 weeks gestation and progress to a dangerous extent within a 2-week period or even less, how often should a mother be screened for this condition? Current routines of care for primigravidae consist of monthly visits to 28 weeks, fortnightly visits to 36 weeks and weekly visits thereafter. The infrequent checks between 20 and 28 weeks make this a vulnerable period during which pre-eclampsia can easily progress undetected. Antenatal screening should therefore be more intensive if the mother is known to have a high risk of developing pre-eclampsia. Hence the assessment of risk is an important part of management.

Primigravidae are 15 times more likely to develop proteinuric pre-eclampsia than parous women [212]. Even secundiparae with an affected first pregnancy have a lower overall incidence, which nevertheless is 10–15 times higher than for secundiparae with a previously normal pregnancy [50]. The risk increases slightly with age but is not affected by social class [16]. The predisposition to pre-eclampsia may be inherited [65,201] so that a positive family history is a risk factor: the daughters of eclamptic women are eight times more likely to have pre-eclampsia than would be expected [62]. However, there is poor concordance between identical twin sisters [360].

It is widely believed that overweight women are more susceptible to the disorder [213,344]. Unless stringent criteria are used, a population of pre-eclamptic women will include some chronically hypertensive individuals who tend to be heavier than average [257]. This bias was recognized by Lowe [207], who found that by applying more specific diagnostic criteria for 'toxaemia' the association with increased maternal weight disappeared. Instead, the affected women were, if anything, lighter than average. Likewise, women who have suffered eclampsia tend to be underweight, not obese [61]. Pre-eclamptic women also tend to be shorter than average [16]. However, even when appropriate diagnostic criteria are used, heaviness is associated with pre-eclampsia in some studies [96,99]. This issue is still unresolved.

Chronically hypertensive women are three to seven times more likely to develop higher blood pressure combined with proteinuria or 'superimposed pre-eclampsia' than are normotensive women [46,64,142,381]. If hypertension is combined with renal disease then the risk is particularly high [101]. Although maternal smoking is associated with other major perinatal problems, nearly all authors agree that gravidae who smoke have a lower incidence of pre-eclampsia [93,368,397].

Predisposing fetal factors include multiple pregnancy [212] hydatidiform mole [71], hydrops fetalis with or without rhesus isoimmunization [163], fetal triploidy [251] and fetal trisomy 13 [41]. Most of these are associated with an abnormally large placental mass, which leads to the concept of 'hyperplacentosis' [163] in which, it is presumed, there is a mismatch between placental demand and maternal blood supply.

It is not known whether all these risk factors can be formally combined to give clinically useful predictions of the onset of pre-eclampsia.

Management of pre-eclamptic hypertension and associated problems

Pre-eclampsia is probably the most common cause of secondary hypertension in clinical practice; delivery always reverses the problem because it removes the causative organ — the placenta. The principles of management are: screening of the symptomless patient, diagnosis, and well-timed delivery. Interposed between diagnosis and delivery is the need for hospital admission. This achieves two objectives: bed rest and close monitoring of the mother's condition.

The evidence that bed rest is beneficial is not reliable [185], and is derived circumstantially from the dramatic improvements in outcome when early admission to hospital was introduced in an uncontrolled way for the management of pre-eclampsia [140]. Only two controlled trials of bed rest have been conducted: both of them were small, thus rendering the results difficult to interpret. Bed rest was beneficial in pregnancies complicated by severe albuminuric hypertension with hyperuricaemia and a fetus grossly small for dates [219]. In a controlled trial of bed rest for non-albuminuric hypertension, there was no evidence of benefit [218].

If the value of bed rest can be questioned, nevertheless, as pre-eclampsia develops, admission to hospital becomes essential for the correct timing and management of pre-emptive delivery. What is in question is not if but when the pre-eclamptic patient should be admitted. Once the diagnosis has been made, decisions about management critically depend on an assessment of the speed with which the condition is progressing. In hospital, it is possible to keep track of this dangerous, unpredictable and changeable condition; at home it is not. In general, symptomatic pre-eclampsia (symptoms, hypertension and proteinuria) justifies an emergency admission. Symptomless proteinuric pre-eclampsia demands urgent admission on the day of diagnosis. Pre-eclampsia without proteinuria which has been confirmed by biochemical testing (e.g. hyperuricaemia) is usually best managed in a day assessment unit where frequent detailed checks are routine. Mild hypertension with no other complicating factor can be managed conservatively from routine clinics.

Antihypertensive drugs

Antihypertensive treatment will prevent only those problems directly caused by maternal hypertension. From the preceding discussion it will be apparent that pre-eclamptic hypertension is a secondary or peripheral feature of a more fundamental problem; that extreme pre-eclamptic hypertension causes direct arterial injury and the cerebral haemorrhages which make pre-eclampsia a potentially lethal disorder. Hence pre-eclamptic women must be managed to avoid hypertension of a degree which can cause arterial injury. The threshold at which this occurs is at about a mean arterial pressure of 140 mmHg (180–190/120–130). Definitive treatment is delivery, but antihypertensive agents may be needed to protect the mother before, during and after parturition. Our aim is to keep all blood pressure readings below 170/110; hence treatment is started if maximum blood pressures repeatedly reach these limits in any period. Other centres have slightly different thresholds; the exact levels are less important than the understanding of the principles which determine the need for treatment.

Treatment of extreme pre-eclamptic hypertension

The vasospasm responds best to the drugs that directly relax vascular smooth muscle. A smooth and sustained reduction is to be preferred to sudden short-term changes. A number of vasodilating agents given parenterally have been used, including hydralazine, labetalol, diazoxide, nitroglycerine or sodium nitroprusside. In addition, oral calcium channel blocking agents are increasingly administered for this purpose.

Hydralazine

Hydralazine has been the preferred antihypertensive agent for the treatment of acute severe pre-eclampsia [54,196,267]. It may be given intravenously by either continuous infusion [172] or intermittent boluses [267], or by intramuscular or subcutaneous injections [277]. After intravenous administration there is a significant delay in the onset of action of 20–30 min. Hydralazine directly inhibits the contractile activity of smooth muscle [162]. In the cerebral circulation it first dilates the capacitance vessels causing an increase in the intracranial pressure [248] which probably accounts for the common side-effect of severe headaches. This is an undesirable action, particularly in the context of actual or impending eclampsia where intracranial pressure may already be increased. Subsequently the resistance vessels dilate and cerebrovascular flow increases [221,248]. Cardiac output increases [10,111] because of the increased venous return. A marked tachycardia nearly always occurs. Originally this was thought to result from stimulation of baroceptor reflexes. But hydralazine also causes a prolonged release of noradrenaline [195] which correlates closely with the tachycardia, and could also explain the anxiety, restlessness and hyperreflexia which are common side-effects. These symptoms and signs, together with headaches, may affect 50 per cent of women [10] and simulate the features of impending eclampsia. Then the symptoms of the disease cannot be disentangled from those caused by the treatment.

It is relevant that hydralazine stimulates the release of noradrenaline which is a potent vasoconstrictor of the uteroplacental circulation in sheep [182], guinea-pigs [127] and rhesus monkeys [377], and therefore probably in humans. Thus although it increases cardiac output, hydralazine fails to improve indices of uteroplacental perfusion in pre-eclamptic women [171,209,349]. Signs of fetal distress (heart rate decelerations) have been noted after its use [371,372].

Thus hydrazaline is not an ideal drug. It is easier to use if the sympathetic nervous system is already inhibited by methyldopa or adrenergic blocking agents. A continuous infusion is not a rational way to achieve control of the blood pressure for more than 4–6 hours, for which purpose either methyldopa or labetalol should be given orally. Our own practice has been to give intermittent intramuscular hydrazaline (10 mg) combined with an oral loading dose of methyldopa (500–1000 mg). The hydralazine can be repeated every 2 or 3 hours until the action of methyldopa begins 6–8 hours later. Monitoring of the fetus is essential but in our experience fetal distress is rare, and more related to the severity of the pre-eclampsia than the administration of the hydralazine.

Other drugs for the acute control of hypertension

Labetalol is a combined α and β adrenergic blocking agent which can be given intravenously. It lowers the blood pressure smoothly but rapidly without the tachycardia characteristic of treatment with hydralazine although collapse with atrioventricular tachcycardia has been reported with post-partum use [246]. A typical regimen starts with 20 mg/hour, which is doubled every 30 min until control has been gained [120]. In that α adrenergic stimulation is thought to constrict the uteroplacental circulation labetalol would be expected to enhance flow; in fact no effect, good or bad, has been observed [210]. A fetal death associated with a sudden response in the blood pressure after labetalol has been reported [245]. Single case reports may be misleading and there are no adequate trials of its parenteral use in pregnancy to show how it might affect perinatal outcome.

Diazoxide is a powerful and rapid vasodilator; an intravenous bolus dose may cause severe hypotension, cerebral ischaemia or death from cerebral infarction [191]. A maternal death in this setting has been reported [146]. It should therefore be used, *only* with extreme caution.

Other vasodilators include sodium nitroprusside [331] and nitroglycerine [81], given intravenously to severely hypertensive pregnant women. Neither is to be recommended except in extreme circumstances of specialist intensive care. Sodium nitroprusside is potentially toxic to the fetus but normal fetal survival has been associated with its use [130]. Nitroglycerine has been used to attenuate the pressor response to endolaryngeal intubation during caesarean section [204].

The calcium channel blocking agent, nifedipine, is an effective vasodilator which acts rapidly when given by mouth. Two oral preparations are available: nifedipine capsules act within 10–15 min; nifedipine in slow-release tablets has a slower onset of action (about 60 min) but a more prolonged effect. The experience of nifedipine in pregnancy is limited, but so far nifedipine appears to be at least as safe as hydralazine [C.W.G. Redman, unpublished observations, 379] and, in some aspects of neonatal complications of prematurity with severe pre-eclampsia, possibly superior [102]. Tachycardia occurs but is less of a problem than with hydralazine. As with some other drugs the half-life is shorter than that in non-pregnant individuals [21] so that regimens need to be adjusted accordingly. In theory there could be a problem if parenteral magnesium sulphate were also used for the prophylaxis or treatment of eclampsia because of the separate effect of the magnesium ion on calcium channel functions [160]; and indeed there has been a report of two cases of profound hypotension in this context [375]. The advantage of nifedipine over hydralazine is its ease of administration; like hydralazine it can cause severe headaches. Reports of the effects of nifedipine on the fetal or uteroplacental circulations (assessed by Doppler ultrasonography) are so far reassuring (many reports, for example [141]). An inhibitory effect of nifedipine on platelet function [307] could be an advantage, as could a possible anticonvulsant action [188]. An antitocolytic effect on uterine muscle [367] might predispose to post-partum haemorrhage although this complication has not been reported. Nimodipine, another calcium channel blocker, with a selective effect on the cerebral circulation, has been used to treat cerebral ischaemia in an eclamptic woman [151].

Lowering the blood pressure and placental perfusion

How perfusion of the human placenta is controlled is poorly understood because of the obvious ethical problems of measurement and experimentation. Whether or not acute hypotensive treatment causes reduced placental perfusion cannot be answered directly. Nor do clinical studies of fetal morbidity or mortality after treatment provide useful information, because there are no controlled observations. Blood flow in a vascular bed depends on resistance as well as arterial pressure, therefore a lowered blood pressure does not necessarily mean a reduction of flow. One set of uncontrolled observations indicates that hypotensive treatment of severely pre-eclamptic gravidae with hydralazine was associated with changes in fetal heart rate patterns suggesting aggravation of fetal compromise [372]. If perfusion of the pre-eclamptic placenta can only be maintained by a blood pressure that directly threatens maternal well-being, then urgent delivery is the main priority. In practice this is a rare circumstance.

Conservative management of severe pre-eclampsia (blood pressure > 170/110)

There have to be compelling special reasons to leave women with proteinuric pre-eclampsia undelivered beyond 36 weeks. Indeed, after 34 weeks it becomes increasingly more difficult to justify conservative management. The same arguments can be transposed to women with definite non-proteinuric pre-eclampsia at 38–40 weeks.

The most difficult problems arise with proteinuric pre-eclampsia, without symptoms, presenting between 26 and 34 weeks of pregnancy. Although delivery is desirable it is not essential. If it can be deferred for 2 weeks or longer significant maturation of the fetus may be achieved to reduce the problems of immaturity after birth. Conservative management of proteinuric pre-eclampsia can only be undertaken by an experienced team offering continuous monitoring and care. It is not easy, and sometimes impossible, for this to be achieved in understaffed busy units with heavy routine commitments. It is thus desirable that such patients are moved at an early stage to specialized regional centres.

The conservative approach needs to be used with discretion and in the knowledge that in some patients it will achieve little or no gain in time. To defer delivery safely it is essential to know how all the maternal systems are affected by the disorder. The fetal state must also be reviewed continually. Delivery is necessary if: (a) the maternal blood pressure cannot be controlled; (b) the platelet count is $<50 \times 10^9$/l; (c) the plasma creatinine has risen from normal levels to >120 μmol; (d) there is evidence of liver damage. In some cases, increasing fetal problems may make extra-uterine life safer. Any of these developments can happen unpredictably and suddenly, and will be missed unless the monitoring and care is maintained at a high level.

Of 122 cases of symptomless proteinuric pre-eclampsia presenting before 32 weeks in Oxford in 1980–85 conservative management extended the life of the pregnancy beyond the onset of proteinuria by an average time of 15 days. Thirty-one per cent were delivered because of maternal problems, 48 per cent because of fetal problems and 7 per cent because of both. The remainder were delivered non-urgently because adequate maturation had been achieved, or because they went into spontaneous labour. Five infants all weighing <1000 g and who were all but one at <28 weeks died *in utero*. A small trial comparing conservative management with immediate delivery has confirmed the potential advantages of a cautiously expectant approach [244]. However, the experience of others has been less favourable, particularly with respect to maternal complications [338].

Longer term control of severe pre-eclamptic hypertension

Parenteral therapy is inappropriate if conservative management is being attempted, and oral agents need to be used. Methyldopa is the first choice.

The safety of methyldopa in pregnancy has been established by case control studies [190,283,284]. No serious adverse fetal effects have yet been documented. Methyldopa crosses the placenta and accumulates in relatively high concentrations in amniotic fluid [167]. Neonatal blood pressure is transiently reduced for a short period after delivery [392]. None of these effects is clinically important. Its use not only relieves the patient of the problems of parenteral therapy, but if, at a later time, hydralazine or another vasodilator is needed, their action is potentiated.

Oral administration can achieve an adequate therapeutic response within 12 hours provided a large initial loading dose of 750–1000 mg is used. This can be followed by 1–2 g/day which is rapidly adjusted to 3–4 g/day as needed. A satisfactory drop in blood pressure tends to provoke transient oliguria, which may cause anxiety about renal failure — a complication discounted by measuring the plasma urea and creatinine. Despite good blood pressure control, the other changes of pre-eclampsia (abnormalities of renal, coagulation and placental function) remain unchanged. Thus, hypotensive treatment is merely suppressing one dangerous manifestation of this disorder. The treatment regimen of hypertension in pre-eclampsia may need to anticipate nocturnal hypertension [282] by a variable schedule with the largest doses at night.

The β adrenergic antagonists (β blockers) have the advantage of causing fewer subjective side-effects but their safety in pregnancy has not been so exhaustively investigated. A preparation such as atenolol has a slow onset of action and a flat dose response curve which make the day to day titration of blood pressure control almost impossible. However, its short-term safety for the fetus and neonate has been adequately demonstrated [306]. Oxprenolol and labetalol are faster acting alternatives, labetalol being the antihypertensive agent most used in current British obstetric practice [157]. Claims that oxprenolol enhanced fetal growth [115] have not been substantiated [104]. Which agent is preferred probably matters less than the clinician's familiarity with its use (see also below for further comments on the long-term use of β blockers for the treatment of hypertension in pregnancy).

Escape from blood pressure control

While pregnancy continues, pre-eclampsia is a relentlessly progressive disorder, so that sooner or later escape from blood pressure control can be expected. In general, the maternal and fetal condition deteriorate together and it is not difficult to see when the limits of conservative management have been reached and delivery is indicated. Oral vasodilators, however, may be usefully added to the medical regimen to prevent loss of blood pressure control. Oral hydralazine which on its own is a weak hypotensive agent, effectively augments methyldopa given at doses of 25–75 mg every 6 hours. An alternative, is slow release nifedipine, at doses of 10–30 mg up to four times/day.

Antihypertensive treatment would be expected to help prevent cerebral haemorrhages but not eclampsia (see section on convulsions above). For this purpose other measures are needed.

Prevention and treatment of eclamptic fits

Eclampsia is now rare and few obstetricians have extensive experience of its presentation and management. There is no consensus about the best ways of either treating or preventing the condition. Given that the aim of good care is to prevent fits, it is disappointing that in the majority of cases the first eclamptic convulsion occurs after admission to hospital [121,337,356]. This indicates that either the women who are likely to have convulsions are not identified accurately or that the treatment that is given is ineffective.

It is not the grand mal convulsions themselves that are the dangerous feature of eclampsia so much as the severity of the underlying disturbances such as cerebral microinfarcts, oedema or haemorrhages. The aim of management is to protect the maternal airway, control convulsions, control extreme hypertension and expedite delivery.

Use of anticonvulsants

If a patient needs anticonvulsant medication she also needs urgent delivery. The treatment is a short-term 'holding' measure whilst the underlying cause of the problem — the pregnancy — is ended. In the UK intravenous diazepam has been preferred [157]. This is the agent of choice to stop convulsions, but is inappropriate for longer term prevention. In the US parenteral magnesium sulphate is used. This is not a good agent to stop seizures, but appears to be effective for preventing them. Although it is not routine obstetric practice it is better to consider the problems of stopping and preventing convulsions as separate. Then diazepam becomes the preferred treatment to stop fits; whereas for prevention either magnesium sulphate or phenytoin should be considered.

With respect to prophylaxis it is difficult to identify accurately which women are likely to have fits. The level of the blood pressure, the degree of proteinuria or fluid retention are not helpful signs. In many units the problem is side-stepped by treating all women with advanced pre-eclampsia with anticonvulsants. This is undesirable because it greatly increases the number of treated women, and therefore the risks of major side-effects. We have suggested that treatment and prophylaxis could be reserved for those who have had their first convulsion [70] and reported the good outcome of operating that policy. However, this approach may be inappropriate in different populations who receive less antenatal care than our own.

Diazepam

The anticonvulsant action is achieved only by intravenous administration but is short-lived and is correlated with the period of overt sedation. Slow intravenous injection of 10 mg can be repeated intermittently as necessary with each new convulsion to a total of 50 mg. The continuous infusion of 10 mg/hour [189] should not be necessary except in the most intractable cases and is illogical in view of the drug's very long half-life (18 hours). Diazepam impairs consciousness and in high doses may depress respiration. It crosses the placenta rapidly to cause loss of fetal heart rate variation within 2 min of administration [316]. When maternal doses exceed 30 mg neonatal side-effects become prominent including low Apgar scores, respiratory depression, poor feeding and hypothermia [83]. For these reasons diazepam should be used only to stop fits, not to maintain anticonvulsant treatment thereafter. The effects of diazepam can be reversed by flumazenil, a specific benzodiazepine antagonist.

Phenytoin

Phenytoin has been little used in obstetrics [341], although in medical practice there is an extensive experience of its administration. It has a long half-life so that after loading it needs to be given only once or twice a day. It is absorbed slowly, variably and sometimes incompletely from the gut. To prevent fits acutely, 15 mg/kg is given intravenously at the rate of not more than 50 mg/min, with an onset of action after 20 min; followed by 5 mg/kg 2 hours later [308]. If it is given too quickly cardiovascular collapse or central nervous system depression may occur. Electrocardiogram monitoring is desirable in any case. The intravenous preparation is very alkaline, irritant to veins, but should not be diluted to avoid precipitation. The major advantage of phenytoin is that the patient remains alert. A possible disadvantage is that what little evidence there is demonstrates a lower efficacy than that of magnesium sulphate [90].

Magnesium sulphate

In the US the prevention of eclampsia has long been based on the use of parenteral magnesium sulphate, administered intramuscularly or intravenously to achieve therapeutic plasma concentrations of 4–7 mmol/l. It does not cause depression of the central nervous system of either mother or neonate [234]. Although its efficacy has been extolled [266] the rationale for its use has not been clear, since magnesium sulphate is not an anticonvulsant. But it does relax vascular smooth muscle [84], although *in vivo* the effect of magnesium administration on the hypertension of pre-eclampsia is transient and slight [264]. However, extreme hypermagnesaemia has been associated with refractory hypotension in a non-pregnant patient [233]. Cardiac and uterine muscle contractility are also impaired: a side-effect of an overdose is cardiac arrest [224]; and parenteral magnesium sulphate can also be used as a tocolytic agent.

It is therefore likely that magnesium sulphate acts by reversing cerebral vasoconstriction [25], making it more logical treatment for eclampsia than drugs that are given to suppress dysfunctional neurones.

Although in skilled hands it is clearly a safe and effective preparation, at high concentrations it causes a relative blockade at neuromuscular junctions which can lead to a loss of deep tendon reflexes or respiratory depression [269]. Its other side-effects include failure to control fits [269, 337], maternal death from overdosage [147], hypocalcaemic tetany [98] and neonatal hypermagnesaemia associated with hyporeflexia and respiratory depression [200].

At the moment few obstetricians in the UK use magnesium sulphate, preferring diazepam or chlormethiazole [157]; but it is expected that this will change over the next few years. There has been a marked reluctance to test different managements for eclampsia by properly randomized trials. The multicentre trial now in progress (in 1993), organized by the World Health Organization, therefore represents a landmark in the development of rational therapies for eclampsia.

Other measures for the treatment of pre-eclampsia and its complications

Sedatives

The purpose of the medical treatment of severe pre-eclampsia or eclampsia is to prevent or control convulsions, not to 'sedate' the patient. In obstetric practice anticonvulsants and sedatives have been curiously confused, and the fact that not all sedatives are anticonvulsants, nor anticonvulsants sedatives, has been ignored. It has also been assumed that acute sedation of the pre-ictal patient should be extended to chronic sedation of the milder cases of pre-eclampsia. Thus it used to be not uncommon to find domiciliary patients treated with phenobarbitone. This is illogical: if the patient is at immediate risk of fitting she needs to be in hospital; if she is well enough to stay at home, she does not need phenobarbitone. As a final point, it is still believed by some that the hypertension of pre-eclampsia is a direct consequence of anxiety, and so can be relieved by sedation. In this respect sedatives are occupying 'a time honoured place among the magical drugs used in the treatment of hypertension' [258], despite well-designed trials which have shown them to be useless [68,80]. The hypertension of pre-eclampsia responds to delivery, not relief of anxiety. To make a patient feel that her anxiety is compounding her problems is both unkind and unnecessary.

Salt restriction, diuretics and plasma volume expansion

Oedema, the symptom of pre-eclampsia, has been extensively treated by both salt restriction and the use of diuretics. Salt restriction is still an important part of the management of hypertension in non-pregnant patients and is widely used for the treatment of pre-eclampsia in some countries, although not in the UK. Salt restriction in pregnancy has been tested in only one controlled trial [302]. Perinatal mortality in the salt restricted group was significantly increased by nearly twofold, and was associated with more 'toxaemia', both in nulliparous and parous patients. Salt restriction is not without hazards. It may aggravate renal impairment [236] and contribute to a puerperal shock syndrome which used to be seen in severely pre-eclamptic patients [352]. The evidence establishes no case for salt restriction in the prophylaxis or management of pre-eclampsia.

After their introduction, the thiazide diuretics were prescribed widely for the prevention and treatment of pre-eclampsia. Nearly 7000 women were randomized in 11 controlled trials of varying size and quality. In the pooled data the incidence of still-birth was reduced by one-third, a difference which is not statistically significant [78]. Otherwise there was no evidence of benefit. A number of serious side-effects have been associated with the use of thiazide diuretics. In addition they may cause hyperuricaemia, which obscures one of the more useful signs of early pre-eclampsia. For these reasons diuretics should not now be used in the management of pre-eclampsia, except for treating the rare complication of pulmonary oedema.

Pre-eclampsia is associated with hypovolaemia which, some believe, is enough to cause a latent or actual state of shock [73]. It has been claimed that plasma volume expansion is beneficial [131,235] to correct poor renal and placental function. The evidence in favour of plasma volume expansion is circumstantial, unvalidated and inconsistent. For example some [114] but not others [26,386] find that plasma protein infusions lower blood pressure in pre-eclamptic women. The postulated improvement in uteroplacental circulation has not been demonstrated [170]. The possibility that it could cause circulatory overload and pulmonary oedema makes the treatment potentially dangerous. It cannot therefore be considered to be a part of routine management.

Treatment of the coagulation disturbances

In general the only remedy for DIC is to correct the underlying problem. In pre-eclampsia this means delivery. With the knowledge that abnormal coagulation probably mediates at least some of the terminal complications of the disorder, various regimens of anticoagulation have been tried. Heparinization failed to modify the course of severe pre-eclampsia [155]. Prostacyclin infusion corrected the hypertension in one case, but not the underlying fetal problems which necessitated premature delivery [103]. Successful prophylactic anticoagulation with warfarin has been reported twice [317,369]. The dangers of anticoagulation in patients at risk of cerebral haemorrhage needs to be emphasized. Overall, in routine clinical practice, anticoagulation should not be used either prophylactically or therapeutically.

The poor haemostasis of individuals recovering from severe DIC post-partum can, in rare circumstances, cause intractable haemorrhage. Transfusions of platelets and fresh frozen plasma may be needed in addition to the replacement of whole blood as supportive treatment.

Prevention of pre-eclampsia

All the evidence is that, once pre-eclampsia becomes overt, it cannot be reversed except by delivery. So to resolve this severe and common problem preventive strategies are paramount.

As discussed in previous sections salt restriction is deleterious, increasing the incidence of pre-eclampsia [302], and diuretics confer no benefit [78].

Antihypertensive treatment and the prevention of pre-eclampsia

There are two issues to be considered: (a) can antihypertensive treatment attenuate the progression of early pre-eclampsia; and (b) can it prevent superimposition of pre-eclampsia in chronically hypertensive women, who otherwise are more susceptible to the disorder? The questions should not be considered in isolation but related to known or possible mechanisms of disease progression. There is no obvious reason why uteroplacental circulatory insufficiency (the probable primary cause of pre-eclampsia) should be prevented by antihypertensive treatment; indeed by reducing perfusing pressure it might aggravate the problem. If treatment reduced the endothelial dysfunction that is thought to underlie the maternal syndrome, then it would be conferring benefit: not by its antihypertensive effects, but some other mechanism. Either way there is no convincing rationale for antihypertensive treatment for prevention.

Undoubtedly treatment can lower the blood pressure in early pre-eclampsia; by so doing it can modify the medical interventions that are triggered when hypertension of a particular severity is observed. Some of the benefits claimed, for example less hospital admissions [306], or fewer caesarean sections [261], may reflect this fact rather than genuine alterations in disease severity. If the interventions are, in reality, unnecessary then all that the drug treatment achieves is to protect the patient from her doctors. An exception is where the hypertension is so severe that delivery is essential to preserve maternal safety. At early gestational ages antihypertensive treatment can allow prolongation of pregnancy in this context. The benefit is not from prevention but palliation. The extent of the presumed benefit has not been measured because severe hypertension is a reason for exclusion from randomized trials of treatment.

Treatment has been associated with a reduced incidence of proteinuria in two trials [38,306]. Had the pre-eclamptic processes truly been prevented then perinatal outcome should have been improved. But it was not: in one of the trials there was no difference [306] and in the other there was significantly more intrauterine growth retardation [38].

Most trials are not associated with an improved perinatal outcome, which has been reported only once [284]; in this study the excess of fetal losses in the control group, which included several mid-pregnancy losses, could not be ascribed to pre-eclampsia-related pathology. In general anti-hypertensive treatment does not seem to modify the pre-eclamptic process. The evidence, in many regards imperfect, is most reliable with respect to the inability of treatment to prevent superimposed pre-eclampsia in women with chronic hypertension [277,336].

Dietary factors

It is still widely believed that dietary restriction of weight gain will prevent the onset of pre-eclampsia despite the absence of a rationale for this regimen and any evidence that it is effective. The best investigation has been a randomized controlled trial of calorie restriction in primigravidae with excessive weight gain [49]. Dieting did not alter the incidence of pre-eclampsia, but did cause a significant reduction in the birthweights. A partial follow up on the children at 4–6 years of age showed that the diet-treated cases were less well-grown than the controls [39].

Although weight restriction is not useful, indeed may be harmful, some specific dietary supplements, for example calcium, appear to be more effective. It has been postulated that calcium deficiency predisposes to pre-eclampsia and PIH [27]. Just as calcium supplements reduce the blood pressure in men and non-pregnant women [222] so they lessen the incidence of PIH [28] and diminish arterial sensitivity of pregnant women to infused AII [175].

Other dietary components may also be important — for example vitamin E, of which the blood concentration is significantly reduced in pre-eclampsia [383]. As an antioxidant it may help prevent the formation of free radicals which could initiate endothelial or other forms of tissue damage [156]. The largest randomized controlled trial of dietary supplements did show a modest but significant reduction in the incidence of pre-eclampsia in a pre-war London population [252]. The supplements comprised minerals and vitamins only, the latter including halibut liver oil to provide vitamins A and D. But fish oil, such as halibut liver oil, is also a source of long chain, ω-3 unsaturated fatty acids that yield eicosapentaenoic acid for the synthesis of thromboxane A3 (TXA3) and prostacyclin I3 (PGI3) instead of TXA2 and PGI2 derived from arachidonic acid. These shift the balance of platelet reactivity towards inhibition of aggregation: in effect fish oil supplements are an alternative to antiplatelet drugs (see below). It is possible that the benefit seen in this trial was derived from the fatty acid content of the halibut liver oil rather than the extra vitamins and minerals [247].

Antiplatelet agents

The only drug-based intervention that appears to be promising is the use of antiplatelet agents, in particular low doses of aspirin. Given that the maternal syndrome of pre-eclampsia appears to originate from diffuse systemic endothelial dysfunction and given that it is associated, from an early stage, with platelet disturbances [286], it could be supposed that platelet activation might either amplify or even cause the endothelial problems. In either case antiplatelet therapy might have a beneficial action in preventing or retarding the progression of pre-eclampsia. This underpins the use of fish oil supplements and also of low dose aspirin.

Anecdotal reports of the effectiveness of aspirin in preventing pre-eclampsia [131] were followed by controlled trials [22,376] of differing designs, using aspirin with or without another antiplatelet agent, dipyridamole. The results were promising and appear to have been confirmed by the meta-analyses of further small trials [77,159]. However, of three recent larger trials two [161,335] have failed to confirm the benefits promised. Both differed from the earlier studies in recruiting lower risk women; for example in the National Institutes of Health (NIH) trial [335] primigravidity was the entry criterion. The third [144] confirmed the promise of earlier studies.

The results of the Collaborative Low-dose Aspirin Study in Pregnancy (CLASP) organized by the Medical Research Council to which nearly 9500 women have been recruited worldwide became available in 1994 [72a]. Overall, the use of aspirin, 60 mg per day, was associated with a 12% reduction in the incidence of pre-eclampsia which was not significant though meta-analysis of all trials of antiplatelet therapy indicate a 25% reduction which is significant [72a]. There was suggestive evidence that low-dose aspirin may be more effective in reducing the risk of early-onset pre-eclampsia, i.e., that requiring delivery before 32 weeks' gestation [72a]. These results do not support routine prophylactic administration of aspirin to all women at increased risk of pre-eclampsia, though low-dose aspirin may be justified in women judged to be especially liable to pre-term delivery. Low-dose aspirin was generally safe for the fetus and newborn infant [72a].

Management of labour and delivery

If premature delivery is necessary then the question arises as to whether corticosteroids should be given to accelerate fetal pulmonary maturation. Although the original trial of their use suggested that in the context of pre-eclampsia there was a significantly worse perinatal outcome no further data on this subject have been presented and the current consensus is that they should be given as they would for any other pre-term delivery. They do not cause exacerbation of hypertension when given acutely.

The mode of delivery is determined amongst other variables by the speed with which it must be expedited, the ability of the fetus to withstand labour and the chances of successful induction of labour at early gestational ages. As in other circumstances, vaginal delivery is always to be preferred if it is safe.

Oxytocin (2–5 mu/min intravenously) is antidiuretic within 10–15 min [3]; if given with large volumes of 5 per cent dextrose and water, it can cause hyponatraemia and convulsions [228]. The drug causes peripheral vasodilatation with a reflex tachycardia which may stimulate significant increases in cardiac output. If cardiac function is already compromised, which happens in rare cases of severe pre-eclampsia, myocardial failure may occur [357].

When given ergometrine the pre-eclamptic patient is particularly prone to hypertension [15]; it can cause headaches, convulsions or even death [357]. For this reason Syntocinon, not ergometrine, should be used in the management of the third stage [108].

A woman with a shrunken intravascular compartment is less tolerant of blood loss than is the normal pregnant woman. Blood replacement must therefore be initiated sooner, at the same time very carefully, to guard against the dangers of underfilling or overfilling.

Analgesia and anaesthesia for labour and delivery

Epidural analgesia has [147,232] and has not [197,267] been recommended for the management of pre-eclamptic women in labour. Maternal cardiac output is unaffected [243], placental intervillous blood flow appears to be enhanced [168] and control of maternal blood pressure is improved [135,243, 395], although there is no effect on the maximum recorded pressures [136]. No controlled trials have been reported, but if it is done with care, the procedure seems to be safe for the baby [135,232]. Vasodilatation and pooling of the blood in the veins of the lower extremities may cause hypovolaemia. This problem can be anticipated and avoided by appropriate fluid loading so that the benefits seem to outweigh the disadvantages. However, epidural analgesia is contraindicated if there is evidence of actual or incipient DIC. A knowledge of at least the platelet count is essential and, if $<50 \times 10^9$/l, the procedure should be avoided. At counts between 50 and 100×10^9/l particular caution is necessary.

A caesarean section may have to be performed too quickly to consider using epidural anaesthesia. Although general anaesthesia allows more precise control of the speed and timing of surgery there are particular risks for pre-eclamptic women. Intubation may be difficult [169] or impossible [145] because of laryngeal oedema which may also cause post-operative respiratory obstruction and cardiac arrest [361]. Laryngoscopy is a well-known cause of extreme transient reflex hypertension in all individuals. The problem is aggravated in pre-eclamptic women [149] and may be so extreme as to cause acute pulmonary oedema [109]. The blood pressure swings at laryngoscopy are ameliorated if adequate control has been gained before the anaesthetic is given. Pretreatment with either nitroglycerine [204] or labetalol [275] has been given acutely to attenuate this problem. Laryngeal oedema is one of the few indications for the use of diuretics in pre-eclampsia; if it is anticipated, an experienced and well-briefed anaesthetist should perform the intubation.

Post-partum hypertension

The arterial pressure progressively rises during the first 5 days after normal delivery [380]. This trend may be exaggerated in hypertensive women, so that the highest readings of all can be recorded during this period. Concurrently, the signs and symptoms of severe pre-eclampsia can appear for the first time, with the onset of epigastric pain [226] or eclampsia. A maternal death with an eclamptic convulsion on the 6th day after delivery has been reported [56]. It is relatively unusual for these potential problems to be anticipated after delivery, so that inappropriately early post-partum discharge has been identified as one preventable factor associated with maternal death from pre-eclampsia or eclampsia [148].

Post-partum hypertension needs to be managed, as is ante-partum hypertension, with treatment titrated to prevent severe hypertension. It is better not to use methyldopa because of the tiredness and depression that it causes. Of the β blocking agents, labetalol has the advantage of a quick onset of action but postural hypotension can be a problem. For this reason the author prefers oxprenolol starting at 80 mg four times per day. Women with a history of asthma should be excluded and offered nifedipine on its own. The patient usually can be discharged 6–8 days after delivery. Within 2–3 weeks of discharge antihypertensive treatment can usually be reduced or stopped — a decision which can be delegated to the general practitioner.

Summary of treatment of pre-eclampsia

The correct treatment for pre-eclampsia is delivery. Antihypertensive drugs should be used to ensure that the maternal blood pressure remains below 170/110. Anticonvulsant drugs will rarely be needed to prevent or treat eclamptic convulsions. No medical treatment has yet been conclusively shown to prevent or retard the development of pre-eclampsia although low dose aspirin may prove to be effective.

Chronic hypertension (CHT) in pregnancy

This group comprises women with essential and renal hypertension, and hypertension caused by miscellaneous but rare conditions. The first is most common. Women with essential hypertension tend to be older and therefore more likely to be parous, heavier and to have a family history of hypertension (Table 6.3).

As outlined above, the physiological decline in blood pressure in early pregnancy is exaggerated in women with CHT [60] so that the underlying situation may be masked. Conversely in later pregnancy the normal rise in blood pressure is exaggerated.

Table 6.3. Characteristics of women with and without hypertension: chronic and pre-eclamptic

	Normal	Chronic hypertension	Pre-eclampsia
Number	14 109	485	1617
Age (years)*	27.5 ± 5.0	28.5 ± 5.2	26.6 ± 4.9
Weight/height^2 (g/cm^2)*	24 ± 4	27 ± 6	24 ± 4
Primigravidae	40.6%	41.4%	60.7%
Proteinuria	0.5%	2.4%	5.5%
Birthweight (kg)*	3.34 ± 0.52	3.26 ± 0.63	3.17 ± 0.65
Maturity at delivery (days)*	279 ± 13	273 ± 17	274 ± 16
Perinatal deaths			
Primigravidae	51/5731 (0.89%)	6/201 (2.99%)	11/981 (1.12%)
Multigravidae	75/8378 (0.90%)	2/284 (0.70%)	8/636 (1.26%)

* Means ± SD.

All women presented for care in the John Radcliffe Hospital, Oxford, before 20 weeks of gestation in 1981–84. The definitions classifying the groups are those of [288].

Thus a woman with CHT may be normotensive when she starts antenatal care early in the second trimester but then develops hypertension in the third trimester; she thus presents as PIH and appears to be developing early pre-eclampsia.

This has led to considerable diagnostic confusion but explains why third trimester hypertension segregates into two groups: (a) non-recurrent, affecting primigravidae, associated with a raised perinatal mortality; and (b) recurrent, affecting multiparae, with a good perinatal outcome [6,215]. The former group would have pre-eclampsia as defined in this chapter, the latter probably have CHT. Thus the only sure way to detect CHT in pregnancy is to refer to pre-pregnancy readings, or, if as is usual, these are not available, to reassess the blood pressure at a remote time after delivery. However, if blood pressures are consistently at or above 140/90 in the first half of pregnancy then CHT can be inferred. Not uncommonly the presentation is of mild hypertension alone in the second half of pregnancy without any antecedent readings at all. It is not, in these circumstances, possible to distinguish CHT from pre-eclampsia with absolute certainty.

CHT is one of the major predisposing factors to pre-eclampsia so that the two conditions, which in their pure forms are easily separable, may commonly occur together. Pre-eclampsia superimposed on CHT tends to be recurrent in later pregnancies whereas in a normotensive individual, pre-eclampsia tends not to recur. If a blood pressure of 140/90 in the first half of pregnancy is evidence of CHT then the affected individuals are about five times more likely to get pre-eclampsia than normotensive individuals [46]. This close link between the two conditions led earlier clinicians to conclude that CHT is extremely dangerous when combined with pregnancy [43]. It is now clear that the particular risks of CHT in pregnancy are entirely attributable to the increased chance of developing superimposed pre-eclampsia, and that the majority of chronically hypertensive women who do not get pre-eclampsia can expect a normal and uncomplicated perinatal outcome [55].

The signs of pre-eclampsia in chronically hypertensive women are the same as in other women except that the blood pressure levels start from a higher baseline. Thus the demonstration of a rise in the blood pressure (for example +30/+15 mmHg from baseline), of a progressive hyperuricaemia, or abnormal activation of the clotting system is evidence of superimposed pre-eclampsia which will progress to proteinuria unless pre-empted by delivery. When proteinuria develops, intrauterine growth retardation is almost the rule. The easiest diagnostic guide is the maternal plasma urate level. Values below 0.30 mmol/l are not in favour of pre-eclampsia and in a hypertensive woman would suggest the diagnosis of a chronic problem. Overall the differential diagnosis of chronic from pre-eclamptic hypertension rests on the demonstration of the absence of pre-eclamptic features such as a change in the blood pressure from the baseline, a rise in maternal plasma urate levels, and absence of proteinuria and activation of the clotting system.

Another complication is that of abruptio placentae. Although it is said to be more common in women with CHT [394], some disagree [250]. The reported incidence has varied from 0.45 to 5.6 per cent (reviewed in [334]). These data include all the unmeasured biases that arise in studies of hospital-based populations, which would be expected to lead to an overestimate of the problem. All that can be said is that it is a relatively rare complication (about 1 per cent); so that none of the clinical trials have been large enough to determine if antihypertensive treatment modifies the risk. Nor is there an *a priori* reason why it should.

Treatment of CHT in pregnancy

If antihypertensive treatment has been started before conception, the patient may seek advice about the possible effects of her medication on the growth and development of her fetus. None of the commonly used antihypertensive drugs is known to be teratogenic. This does not exclude the possibility of subtle problems which are as yet unknown. For this reason it is appropriate that women with no more than moderate hypertension should stop treatment before conception; so that only those whose hypertension is an immediate health hazard need continue on medication throughout the first trimester. By the 12th week the normal fall in blood pressure is such that the need for treatment is either temporarily diminished or no longer present.

If CHT is diagnosed for the first time in pregnancy, it is necessary to treat those in whom it presents an immediate (as opposed to a long-term) hazard to the patient. The precise levels for treatment have not been agreed upon; we take a cut-off point at or above 170/110.

The problem of less severe CHT (i.e. 140–170/90–110 mmHg) needs to be considered. In general medical practice the purpose of treating this degree of hypertension is to prevent long-term complications which are not relevant for the brief period of gestation. For this reason the only indication for antihypertensive treatment in these women would be if it could prevent the superimposition of pre-eclampsia which is the major short-term problem. There is evidence from randomized controlled trials that the early control of moderate CHT does not lessen the eventual incidence of superimposed pre-eclampsia [277,336]. Thus, there is no worthwhile fetal indication for the control of moderate hypertension in pregnancy, and consequently the medical management hinges entirely around considerations of maternal welfare.

Antihypertensive agents that are used in CHT

The choice of drugs is dictated by fetal considerations. Methyldopa is preferred because its fetal effects have been defined much more clearly than those of any other drug. Its antihypertensive action and side-effects are the same as in non-pregnant individuals. Detailed developmental follow-ups of drug-exposed fetuses to the age of 7 years confirm the absence of any significant adverse drug reaction [74,237,238,249]. Fetuses exposed *in utero* to methyldopa for the first time between 16 and 20 weeks gestation may have slightly reduced head circumferences [231]. The effect is of minor clinical relevance. In the first place at 16–20 weeks, the blood pressure is at its gestational nadir so there is little need to start treatment at this time. Second, the effect on the babies is so small as to be of doubtful importance — and the long-term follow-up of the affected children shows totally normal development [289]. The usual treatment schedule is 1–4 g/day in divided doses. Methyldopa can be supplemented with nifedipine for the treatment of pre-eclamptic hypertension.

β adrenergic blocking agents (β blockers)

Labetalol is the drug most used by obstetricians in the UK for the management of pre-eclampsia [157]. But the possible fetal effects of β blockers have not been so completely evaluated as they have for methyldopa.

There has been a tendency for β blockers to be associated with smaller fetuses [47] or placentas [359]. One report suggests the contrary effect, of oxprenolol *promoting* fetal growth [115], not confirmed in a similar study [104]. The adverse effect on fetal growth was so striking in one study [47], that β blockers should not be used for the long-term treatment of hypertension in pregnancy. This does not preclude their short-term use in the third trimester, for the treatment of pre-eclampsia or PIH, which has not been associated with adverse effects on the fetus (e.g. [306]). Occasionally it may be necessary to use β blockers for other reasons, such as the treatment of dysrhythmias (see Chapter 5), hyperthyroidism (see Chapter 12) or migraine (see Chapter 15).

Other drugs

If diuretics are essential for good blood pressure control they can be continued throughout pregnancy, but their use carries certain disadvantages if pre-eclampsia should supervene, as already discussed. Clonidine [364] and prazosin [208] have both been used in pregnancy but their effect on the fetus has not been fully defined.

Angiotensin-converting enzyme (ACE) inhibitors are now used more widely for the treatment of various forms of long-term hypertension in non-pregnant patients. Although ACE inhibitors have been given to women who have had successful pregnancies [179] there are anxieties about their safety for the fetus, based on animal experiments and the high incidence of fetal death and neonatal renal failure in the offspring of treated women [304]. For this reason although they seem to be safe in the first trimester and the puerperium they should not be used during the second two trimesters. The selection of antihypertensive drugs for use in pregnancy is summarized in Table 6.4.

Table 6.4. Antihypertensive drugs in pregnancy

Trimester	Relatively contraindicated drugs	Absolutely contraindicated drugs	Possible agents
First	None known	None known	Avoid all if possible
Second	β blockers Diuretics	ACE inhibitors	Methyldopa Clonidine Nifedipine
Third	Diuretics	ACE inhibitors	Methyldopa Nifedipine β blockers
Puerperium	Methyldopa	None known	β blockers Nifedipine ACE inhibitors Diuretics

Unusual causes of hypertension in pregnancy

Phaeochromocytoma

This is a rare but dangerous complication of pregnancy. Maternal mortality has previously been as high as 50 per cent [83]. The presentation frequently simulates severe pre-eclampsia [183] with extreme but unstable hypertension, proteinuria and pre-eclamptic-like symptoms such as headaches [315]. For this reason all patients with proteinuric hypertension in pregnancy should be screened for phaeochromocytoma, although even then the diagnosis can be missed by false negative results [75]. Provided the condition can be identified and treated before delivery the maternal mortality is reduced, to zero in cases where α adrenergic blockade has been used [143]. Methods of diagnosis are the same as in non-pregnant individuals and include examination of the adrenals by ultrasound, MRI or computerized tomography. Treatment with α adrenergic blockade with or without addition of β adrenergic blockade is compatible with normal fetal survival. Given adequate medical treatment tumour resection can be successfully accomplished early in pregnancy [143], at delivery by caesarean section [45] or at a later elective date [315]. Both malignant and ectopic tumours have been reported in pregnancy [100,339].

Coarctation of the aorta (see also Chapter 5)

Previously this condition was associated with a high enough mortality in pregnancy for termination to be recommended [88]. Maternal death was primarily from dissection or rupture of the aorta. Contemporary experience is more favourable and decisions about the advisability of a pregnancy may depend more on related factors such as associated cardiac malformation. Surgical resection during pregnancy is not advisable [133]. A previous successful resection is not a contraindication to undertaking pregnancy.

Cushing's syndrome (see also Chapter 13)

Amenorrhoea and menstrual irregularities are common features of Cushing's syndrome so that the likelihood of conception is diminished. Many of the features of the syndrome — increased pigmentation, striae, weight gain, hyperglycaemia and hypertension — may occur during pregnancy in the absence of the disease. Difficulties of diagnosis are further compounded because normal pregnancy causes increased bound and unbound plasma cortisol with blunting of its diurnal variation, increased urinary free cortisol, and moderately increased 17-hydroxysteroids and 17-ketosteroids [276]. Suppression of cortisol production by dexamethasone is the appropriate diagnostic test although normally this is less complete than in non-pregnant subjects. There is a relatively high incidence of primary adrenal tumours including carcinoma in rare instances [180]. For these reasons surgical exploration and removal should be considered once the diagnosis is made. Adrenalectomy during pregnancy with a later successful outcome has been reported [32] as has trans-sphenoidal pituitary adenectomy [52]. Fetal loss is high in Cushing's syndrome and there may be neonatal adrenal insufficiency [180]. The subject is reviewed in more detail elsewhere [254].

Conn's syndrome

This is a rare cause of hypertension in pregnancy. It has usually been diagnosed either before or after pregnancy on the basis of hypokalaemia combined with hypertension [82,134]. During pregnancy both plasma concentrations and urinary excretion of aldosterone are increased which makes diagnosis difficult. Remission of the disorder may occur during pregnancy possibly caused by progesterone which antagonizes the renal action of aldosterone [8]. Successful pregnancies with and without medical treatment have been reported.

Long-term sequelae of hypertension in pregnancy

Severe pre-eclampsia and eclampsia can cause irreversible maternal damage, particularly acute renal cortical necrosis or cerebral haemorrhage. In the absence of these complications there is no evidence at the present time that long-term health is impaired by a pre-eclamptic illness. However, in terms of life expectancy, pre-eclamptic women fall into two groups. Those who have an episode in the first pregnancy only and become normotensive soon after delivery, have a normal life expectancy. The second group have recurrent pre-eclampsia in several pregnancies, or blood pressures which remain elevated in the puerperium. They have a higher incidence of later cardiovascular disorders and a reduced life expectancy compatible with the diagnosis that the initial episode of pre-eclampsia was superimposed on pre-existing hypertension [63]. In terms of long-term follow-up a remote postnatal reassessment is therefore desirable after a hypertensive pregnancy. This should include measurements of blood pressure and renal function. If there has been significant proteinuria an intravenous pyelogram is indicated. If the proteinuria persists, further investigation including a renal biopsy may be indicated.

Contraception

Since the first report [44], oral contraceptives have been implicated as a cause of hypertension which may be severe and very rarely malignant [398]. For this reason chronic hypertension is a relative contraindication to their use. It has been suggested [51] but not confirmed [268] that pre-eclampsia may be associated with hypertension induced by oral contraceptives. The advice given to post-partum women should therefore be guided by whether or not hypertension persists as a chronic problem. If a pre-eclamptic woman's blood pressure returns to normal, there seems little reason to deny her the benefits of oral contraceptives provided adequate and continuing medical supervision is available.

Conclusions

1 Hypertension is an artificial concept.

2 A raised blood pressure is one of many secondary effects of pre-eclampsia on the maternal system.

3 In pre-eclampsia the main differential diagnosis is from chronic hypertension which in its pure form does not share the renal, coagulation, hepatic and placental abnormalities of pre-eclampsia.

4 The perinatal risks of chronic hypertension in pregnancy result from superimposed pre-eclampsia.

5 Extreme hypertension in pregnancy is as dangerous as it is in any other medical situation and demands urgent treatment.

6 The early treatment of mild CHT does not prevent the later superimposition of pre-eclampsia.

7 Methyldopa is the most thoroughly tested antihypertensive agent in pregnancy. Apart from a possible effect on fetal head growth, if treatment is started between 16 and 20 weeks' gestation no significant adverse reaction has been observed.

8 β blocking agents are safe for short-term use but cause significant fetal growth retardation if administered over longer periods (from the second trimester). The clinical trial data are less complete than for methyldopa.

9 Diuretics should primarily be reserved for the treatment of heart failure complicating pre-eclampsia.

10 ACE inhibitors are contraindicated for use in pregnancy because of adverse effects on fetal renal function.

References

1 Aalkjaer C, Danielsen H, Johannesen P, Pedersen EB, Rasmussen A & Mulvany MJ. Abnormal vascular function and morphology in pre-eclampsia: a study of isolated resistance vessels. *Clinical Science* 1985; **69**: 477–82.

2 Aarnoudse JG, Houthoff HJ, Weits J, Vellenga E & Huisjes H. A syndrome of liver damage and intravascular coagulation in the last trimester of normotensive pregnancy. *British Journal of Obstetrics and Gynaecology* 1986; **93**: 145–5.

3 Abdul-Karim RW & Rizk PT. The effect of oxytocin on renal hemodynamics, water and electrolyte excretion. *Obstetrics and Gynecology Survey* 1970; **25**: 805–13.

4 Abitbol MM. Weight gain in pregnancy. *American Journal of Obstetrics and Gynecology* 1969; **104**: 140–56.

5 Abitbol MM. Hemodynamic studies in experimental toxemia of the dog. *Obstetrics and Gynecology* 1977; **50**: 293–8.

6 Adams EM & MacGillivray I. Long-term effect of pre-eclampsia on blood pressure. *Lancet* 1961; **ii**: 1373–5.

7 Ahmed Y, Sullivan MHF & Elder MG. Detection of platelet desensitization in pregnancy-induced hypertension is dependent on the agonist used. *Thrombosis and Haemostasis* 1991; **65**: 474–7.

8 Aoi W, Doi Y, Tasaki S, Mitsuoka J, Suzuki S & Hashiba K. Primary aldosteronism aggravated during peripartum period. *Japanese Heart Journal* 1978; **19**: 946–53.

9 Arias F & Mancilla-Jimenez R. Hepatic fibrinogen deposits in pre-eclampsia. *New England Journal of Medicine* 1976; **295**: 578–82.

10 Assali NS, Kaplan S, Oighenstein S & Suyemoto R. Hemodynamic effects of 1-hydrazinophthalazine in human pregnancy; results of intravenous administration. *Journal of Clinical Investigation* 1953; **32**: 922–30.

11 August P, Marcaccio B, Gertner JM, Druzin ML, Resnick LM & Laragh JH. Abnormal 1,25-dihydroxyvitamin D metabolism in preeclampsia. *American Journal of Obstetrics and Gynecology* 1992; **166**: 1295–9.

12 Ayhan A, Akkok E, Urman B, Yarali H, Dundar S & Kirazli S. Beta-thromboglobulin and platelet factor 4 levels in pregnancy and preeclampsia. *Gynecology and Obstetric Investigation* 1990; **30**: 12–14.

13 Aznar J, Gilabert J, Estelles A & Espana F. Fibrinolytic activity and protein C in preeclampsia. *Thrombosis and Haemostasis* 1986; **55**: 314–17.

14 Bader RA, Bader ME, Rose DJ & Braunwald E. Hemodynamics at rest and during exercise in normal pregnancy as studied by cardiac catheterisation. *Journal of Clinical Investigation* 1955; **34**: 1524–36.

15 Baillie TW. Vasopressor activity of ergometrine maleate in anaesthetised parturient women. *British Medical Journal* 1963; **1**: 585–8.

16 Baird D. Epidemiological aspects of hypertensive pregnancy. *Clinical Obstetrics and Gynecology* 1977; **4**: 531–48.

17 Baker PN, Broughton Pipkin F & Symonds EM. Platelet angiotensin II binding and plasma renin concentration, plasma renin substrate and plasma angiotensin II in human pregnancy. *Clinical Science* 1990; **79**: 403–8.

18 Baker PN, Broughton Pipkin F & Symonds EM. Platelet angiotensin II binding sites in normotensive and hypertensive women. *British Journal of Obstetrics and Gynaecology* 1991; **98**: 436–40.

19 Ballegeer VC, Spitz B, De Baene LA, Van Assche AF, Hidajat M & Criel AM. Platelet activation and vascular damage in gestational hypertension. *American Journal of Obstetrics and Gynecology* 1992; **166**: 629–33.

20 Barton JR, Hiett AK, O'Connor WN, Nissen SE & Greene JWJ. Endomyocardial ultrastructural findings in preeclampsia. *American Journal of Obstetrics and Gynecology* 1991; **165**: 389–91.

21 Barton JR, Prevost RR, Wilson DA, Whybrew WD & Sibai BM. Nifedipine pharmacokinetics and pharmacodynamics during the immediate postpartum period in patients with preeclampsia. *American Journal of Obstetrics and Gynecology* 1991; **165**: 951–4.

22 Beaufils M, Uzan S, Donsimoni R & Colau JC. Prevention of eclampsia by early antiplatelet therapy. *Lancet* 1985; **i**: 840–2.

23 Beck DW & Menezes AH. Intracerebral hemorrhage in a patient with eclampsia. *Journal of the American Medical Association* 1981; **246**: 1442–3.

24 Beeson JH & Duda EE. Computed axial tomography scan demonstration of cerebral edema in eclampsia preceded by blindness. *Obstetrics and Gynecology* 1982; **60**: 529–32.

25 Belfort MA & Moise KJJ. Effect of magnesium sulfate on maternal brain blood flow in preeclampsia: a randomized, placebo-controlled study. *American Journal of Obstetrics and Gynecology* 1992; **167**: 661–6.

26 Belfort MA, Uys P, Dommisse J & Davey DA. Haemodynamic changes in gestational proteinuric hypertension: the effects of rapid volume expansion and vasodilator therapy. *British Journal of Obstetrics Gynaecology* 1989; **96**: 634–41.

27 Belizan JM & Villar J. The relationship between calcium

intake and edema-, proteinuria-, and hypertension-gestosis: an hypothesis. *American Journal of Clinical Nutrition* 1980; **33**: 2202–10.

28 Belizan JM, Villar J, Gonzales L, Campodonico L & Bergel E. Calcium supplementation to prevent hypertensive disorders of pregnancy. *New England Journal of Medicine* 1991; **325**: 1399–405.

29 Beller FK, Ebert C & Dame WR. High molecular fibrin derivatives in pre-eclamptic and eclamptic patients. *European Journal of Obstetrics, Gynecology and Reproductive Biology* 1979; **9**: 105–10.

30 Benedetti TJ & Carlson RW. Studies of colloid osmotic pressure in pregnancy induced hypertension. *American Journal of Obstetrics and Gynecology* 1979; **135**: 308–11.

31 Benedetti TJ, Cotton DB, Read JC & Miller FC. Hemodynamic observations in severe pre-eclampsia with a flow-directed pulmonary artery catheter. *American Journal of Obstetrics and Gynecology* 1980; **136**: 465–70.

32 Bevan JS, Gough MH, Gillmer MDG & Burke CW. Cushing's syndrome in pregnancy: The timing of definitive treatment. *Clinical Endocrinology Oxford* 1987; **27**: 225–33.

33 Bhose L. Postpartum eclampsia. *American Journal of Obstetrics and Gynecology* 1964; **89**: 898–902.

34 Bienarz J, Crottogini JJ *et al*. Aortocaval compression by the uterus in late human pregnancy. *American Journal of Obstetrics and Gynecology* 1968; **100**: 203–17.

35 Bing RF & Smith AJ. Plasma and interstitial volumes in essential hypertension: relationship to blood pressure. *Clinical Science* 1981; **61**: 287–293.

36 Bis KA & Waxman B. Rupture of the liver associated with pregnancy: a review of the literature and report of 2 cases. *Obstetrics and Gynecology Survey* 1976; **31**: 763–73.

37 Blair RG. Phaeochromocytoma and pregnancy. *Journal of Obstetrics and Gynaecology of the British Commonwealth* 1963; **70**: 110–19.

38 Blake S & MacDonald D. The prevention of the maternal manifestations of pre-eclampsia by intensive antihypertensive treatment. *British Journal of Obstetrics and Gynaecology* 1991; **98**: 244–8.

39 Blumenthal I. Diet and diuretics in pregnancy and subsequent growth of offspring. *British Medical Journal* 1976; **ii**: 733.

40 Boneu B, Fournie A, Sie P, Grandjean H, Bierme R & Pontonnier G. Platelet production time, uricemia and some hemostasis tests in pre-eclampsia. *European Journal of Obstetrics, Gynaecology and Reproductive Biology* 1980; **11**: 85–94.

41 Boyd PA, Lindenbaum RH & Redman CWG. Pre-eclampsia and trisomy 13: a possible association. *Lancet* 1987; **ii**: 425–7.

42 Brosens I & Renaer M. On the pathogenesis of placental infarcts in pre-eclampsia. *Journal of Obstetrics and Gynaecology of the British Commonwealth* 1972; **79**: 794–9.

43 Browne FJ & Dodds GH. Pregnancy in the patient with chronic hypertension. *Journal of Obstetrics and Gynaecology of the British Empire* 1942; **49**: 1–17.

44 Brownrigg GM. Toxemia in hormone-induced pseudopregnancy. *Canadian Medical Association Journal* 1962; **87**: 408–9.

45 Burgess GE. Alpha blockade and surgical intervention of pheochromocytoma in pregnancy. *Obstetrics and Gynecology* 1979; **53**: 266–70.

46 Butler NR & Bonham DG. *Perinatal Mortality*. Edinburgh, E & S Livingstone, 1963: 87–100.

47 Butters L, Kennedy S & Rubin PC. Atenolol in essential hypertension during pregnancy. *British Medical Journal* 1990; **301**: 587–9.

48 Byrom FB. The pathogenesis of hypertensive encephalopathy and its relation to the malignant phase of hypertension. Experimental evidence from the hypertensive rat. *Lancet* 1954; **ii**: 201–11.

49 Campbell DM & MacGillivray I. The effect of a low calorie diet or a thiazide diuretic on the incidence of pre-eclampsia and on birthweight. *British Journal of Obstetrics and Gynaecology* 1975; **82**: 572–7.

50 Campbell DM & MacGillivray I. Pre-eclampsia in second pregnancy. *British Journal of Obstetrics and Gynaecology* 1985; **82**: 131–40.

51 Carmichael SM, Taylor MM & Ayers CR. Oral contraceptives, hypertension and toxemia. *Obstetrics and Gynecology* 1970; **35**: 371–6.

52 Casson IF, Davis JC, Jeffreys RV, Silas JH, Williams J & Belchetz PE. Successful management of Cushing's disease during pregnancy by transsphenoidal adenectomy. *Clinical Endocrinology Oxford* 1987; **27**: 423–8.

53 Cavanagh D, Rao PS, Tsai CC & O'Connor TC. Experimental toxemia in the pregnant primate. *American Journal of Obstetrics and Gynecology* 1977; **128**: 75–85.

54 Chamberlain GVP, Lewis PJ, de Swiet M & Bulpitt JJ. How obstetricians manage hypertension in pregnancy. *British Medical Journal* 1978; **i**: 626–9.

55 Chamberlain G, Philipp E, Howlett B & Masters K. *British Births 1970*, Volume 2. *Obstetric Care*. London, Heinemann, 1978: 39–53.

56 Chapman K & Karimi R. A case of post partum eclampsia of late onset confirmed by autopsy. *American Journal of Obstetrics and Gynecology* 1973; **117**: 858–61.

57 Chesley LC. *Hypertensive Disorders in Pregnancy*. New York, Appleton-Century-Crofts, 1978: 9–11.

58 Chesley LC. *Hypertensive Disorders of Pregnancy*. New York, Appleton-Century-Crofts, 1978: 124–6.

59 Chesley LC. *Hypertensive Disorders in Pregnancy*. New York, Appleton-Century-Crofts, 1978: 210.

60 Chesley LC. *Hypertensive Disorders in Pregnancy*. New York, Appleton-Century-Crofts, 1978: 478.

61 Chesley LC. Habitus and eclampsia. *Obstetrics and Gynecology* 1984; **64**: 315–18.

62 Chesley LC, Annitto JE & Cosgrove RA. The familial factor in toxemia of pregnancy. *Obstetrics and Gynecology* 1968; **32**: 303–11.

63 Chesley LC, Annitto JE & Cosgrove RA. The remote prognosis of eclamptic women. Sixth periodic report. *American Journal of Obstetrics and Gynecology* 1978; **124**: 446–59.
64 Chesley LC, Annitto JE & Jarvis DG. A study of the interaction of pregnancy and hypertensive disease. *American Journal of Obstetrics and Gynecology* 1947; **53**: 851–63.
65 Chesley LC & Cooper DW. Genetics of hypertension in pregnancy: possible single gene control of pre-eclampsia and eclampsia in the descendants of eclamptic women. *British Journal of Obstetrics and Gynaecology* 1986; **93**: 898–908.
66 Chesley LC, Valenti C & Rein H. Excretion of sodium loads by non-pregnant and pregnant normal, hypertensive and pre-eclamptic women. *Metabolism* 1958; **7**: 575–88.
67 Chesley LC & Williams LO. Renal glomerular and tubular functions in relation to the hyperuricemia of pre-eclampsia and eclampsia. *American Journal of Obstetrics and Gynecology* 1945; **50**: 367–75.
68 Chesrow EJ, Bernstein M, Weiss D & Marquardt GH. Comparison of mebutamate, phenobarbital and placebo in the treatment of mild essential hypertension. *American Journal of Medical Science* 1966; **251**: 166–74.
69 Chester EM, Agamanolis DP, Banker BQ & Victor M. Hypertensive encephalopathy: a clinicopathologic study of 20 cases. *Neurology* 1978; **28**: 928–39.
70 Chua S & Redman CWG. Are prophylactic anticonvulsants required in severe pre-eclampsia? *Lancet* 1991; **337**: 250–1.
71 Chun D, Braga C, Chow C & Lok L. Clinical observations on some aspects of hydatidiform moles. *Journal of Obstetrics and Gynaecology of the British Commonwealth* 1964; **71**: 180–4.
72 Clarke E & Murphy EA. Neurological manifestations of malignant hypertension. *British Medical Journal* 1956; **ii**: 1319–26.
72a CLASP (Collaborative Low-dose Aspirin Study in Pregnancy) Collaborative Group. CLASP: a randomized trial of low-dose aspirin for the prevention and treatment of pre-eclampsia among 9364 pregnant women. *Lancet* 1994; **343**: 619–29.
73 Cloeren SE & Lippert TH. Effect of plasma expanders in toxemia of pregnancy. *New England Journal of Medicine* 1972; **278**: 1356–7.
74 Cockburn J, Moar VA, Ounsted M & Redman CWG. Final report of study on hypertension during pregnancy: the effects of specific treatment on the growth and development of the children. *Lancet* 1982; **i**: 647–9.
75 Coden J. Phaeochromocytoma in pregnancy. *Journal of the Royal Society of Medicine* 1972; **65**: 863.
76 Cohn JN. Blood pressure measurement in shock. *Journal of the American Medical Association* 1967; **199**: 972–6.
77 Collins R. Antiplatelet agents for IUGR and pre-eclampsia. In: Chambers I (ed), *Oxford Database of Perinatal Trials*, Version 1.2, Disk Issue 5, 1991. Oxford Electronic Publishing, Oxford.
78 Collins R, Yusuf S & Peto R. Overview of randomised trials of diuretics in pregnancy. *British Medical Journal* 1985; **290**: 17–23.
79 Connon AF & Wadsworth RJ. An evaluation of serum uric acid estimations in toxaemia of pregnancy. *Australia and New Zealand Journal of Obstetrics and Gynaecology* 1968; **8**: 197–201.
80 Cooper EH & Cranston W. A comparison of the effects of phenobarbitone and reserpine in hypertension. *Lancet* 1957; **i**: 396–7.
81 Cotton DB, Longmire S, Jones MM, Dorman KF, Tessem J & Joyce TH. Cardiovascular alterations in severe pregnancy-induced hypertension: effects of intravenous nitroglycerin coupled with blood volume expansion. *American Journal of Obstetrics and Gynecology* 1986; **154**: 1053–9.
82 Crane MG, Andes JP, Harris JJ & Slate WG. Primary aldosteronism in pregnancy. *Obstetrics and Gynecology* 1964; **23**: 200–8.
83 Cree JE, Meyer J & Hailey DM. Diazepam in labour: its metabolism and effect on the clinical condition and thermogenesis of the newborn. *British Medical Journal* 1973; **iv**: 251–5.
84 D'Angelo EK, Singer HA & Rembold CM. Magnesium relaxes arterial smooth muscle by decreasing intracellular Ca^{2+} without changing intracellular Mg^{2+}. *Journal of Clinical Investigation* 1992; **89**: 1988–94.
85 Davey DA & MacGillivray I. The classification and definition of the hypertensive disorders of pregnancy. *American Journal of Obstetrics and Gynecology* 1988; **158**: 892–8.
86 Davies MH, Wilkinson SP *et al.* Acute liver disease with encephalopathy and renal failure in late pregnancy and the early puerperium: a study of fourteen patients. *British Journal of Obstetrics and Gynaecology* 1980; **87**: 1005–14.
87 de Boer K, ten Cate JW, Sturk A, Borm JJ & Treffers PE. Enhanced thrombin generation in normal and hypertensive pregnancy. *American Journal of Obstetrics and Gynecology* 1989; **160**: 95–100.
88 Deal K & Wooley CF. Coarctation of the aorta and pregnancy. *Annals of Internal Medicine* 1973; **78**: 706–10.
89 Dennis EJ, Smythe CM, McIver FA & Howe HG. Percutaneous renal biopsy in eclampsia. *American Journal of Obstetrics and Gynecology* 1963; **87**: 364–71.
90 Dommisse J. Phenytoin sodium and magnesium sulphate in the management of eclampsia. *British Journal of Obstetrics and Gynaecology* 1990; **97**: 104–9.
91 Douglas BH & Langford HG. Post-term blood pressure elevation produced by uterine wrapping. *American Journal of Obstetrics and Gynecology* 1969; **97**: 231–4.
92 Douglas JT, Shah M, Lowe GDO, Belch JJF, Forbes CD & Prentice CRM. Plasma fibrinopeptide A and beta-

thromboglobulin in pre-eclampsia and pregnancy hypertension. *Thrombosis and Haemostasis* 1982; **47**: 54–5.

93 Duffus G & MacGillivray I. The incidence of pre-eclamptic toxaemia in smokers and non-smokers. *Lancet* 1968; **i**: 994–5.

94 Duffus GM, MacGillivray I & Dennis KJ. The relationship between baby weight and changes in maternal weight, total body water, plasma volume, electrolytes and proteins and urinary oestriol excretion. *Journal of Obstetrics and Gynaecology of the British Commonwealth* 1971; **78**: 97–104.

95 Dunlop W, Hill LM, Landon MJ, Oxley A & Jones P. Clinical relevance of coagulation and renal changes in pre-eclampsia. *Lancet* 1978; **ii**: 346–50.

96 Easterling TR, Benedetti TJ, Schmucker BC & Millard SP. Maternal hemodynamics in normal and pre-eclamptic pregnancies: a longitudinal study. *Obstetrics and Gynecology* 1990; **76**: 1061–9.

97 Eden TW. Eclampsia: a commentary on the reports presented to the British Congress of Obstetrics and Gynaecology. *Journal of Obstetrics and Gynaecology of the British Empire* 1922; **29**: 386–401.

98 Eisenbud E & Lobue CC. Hypocalcemia after therapeutic use of magnesium sulfate. *Archives of Internal Medicine* 1976; **136**: 688–91.

99 Eskenazi B, Fenster L & Sidney S. A multivariate analysis of risk factors for preeclampsia. *Journal of the American Medical Association* 1991; **266**: 237–41.

100 Fawcett FJ & Kimbell NKB. Phaeochromocytoma of the ovary. *British Journal of Obstetrics and Gynaecology* 1971; **78**: 458–9.

101 Felding CF. Obstetric aspects in women with histories of renal disease. *Acta Obstetricia Gynaecologica Scandinavica* 1969; **48** (suppl. 2): 1–43.

102 Fenakel K, Fenakel G, Appelman Z, Lurie S, Katz Z & Shoham Z. Nifedipine in the treatment of severe preeclampsia. *Obstetrics and Gynecology* 1991; **77**: 331–7.

103 Fidler J, Bennett MJ, de Swiet M, Ellis C & Lewis PJ. Treatment of pregnancy hypertension with prostacyclin. *Lancet* 1980; **ii**: 31–2.

104 Fidler J, Smith V & de Swiet M. Randomised controlled comparative study of methyl dopa and oxprenolol for the treatment of hypertension in pregnancy. *British Medical Journal* 1983; **286**: 1927–30.

105 Fish SA, Morrison JC, Bucovaz ET, Wiser WL & Whybrew WD. Cerebral spinal fluid studies in eclampsia. *American Journal of Obstetrics and Gynecology* 1972; **112**: 502–12.

106 Fisher ER, Pardo V, Paul R & Hayashi TT. Ultrastructural studies in hypertension. IV. Toxemia of pregnancy. *American Journal of Pathology* 1969; **55**: 109–31.

107 Fisher KA, Ahuja S, Luger A, Spargo B & Lindheimer M. Nephrotic proteinuria with pre-eclampsia. *American Journal of Obstetrics and Gynecology* 1977; **129**: 643–6.

108 Forman JB & Sullivan RL. The effects of intravenous injections of erogonovine and methergine on the post partum patient. *American Journal of Obstetrics and Gynecology* 1952; **63**: 640–4.

109 Fox EJ, Sklar GJ, Hill CH, Villanueva R & King BD. Complications related to the pressor response. *Anesthesiology* 1977; **47**: 524–5.

110 Freis ED & Kenny JF. Plasma volume, total circulating protein and available fluid abnormalities in pre-eclampsia and eclampsia. *Journal of Clinical Investigation* 1948; **27**: 283–9.

111 Freis ED, Rose JA, Higgins TF, Finnerty FA, Kelly RT & Partenope EA. The hemodynamic effects of hypotensive drugs in man IV. 1 — Hydrazinophthalazine. *Circulation* 1953; **8**: 199–204.

112 Fullerton WT, Hytten FE, Klopper AI & McKay E. A case of quadruplet pregnancy. *Journal of Obstetrics and Gynaecology of the British Commonwealth* 1965; **72**: 791–6.

113 Gaitz JP & Bamford CR. Unusual computed tomographic scan in eclampsia. *Archives of Neurology* 1982; **39**: 66.

114 Gallery EDM, Mitchell MDM & Redman CWG. Fall in blood pressure in response to volume expansion associated with hypertension (pre-eclampsia): why does it occur? *Journal of Hypertension* 1984; **2**: 177–82.

115 Gallery EDM, Ross ME & Gyory AZ. Antihypertensive treatment in pregnancy: analysis of different responses to oxprenolol and methyldopa. *British Medical Journal* 1985; **291**: 563–6.

116 Gallery EDM, Ross M, Hunyor SN & Gyory AZ. Predicting the development of pregnancy-associated hypertension. *Lancet* 1977; **i**: 1273–5.

117 Gallery EDM, Saunders DM, Hunyor SN & Gyory AZ. Randomised comparison of methyldopa and oxprenolol for treatment of hypertension in pregnancy. *British Medical Journal* 1979; **i**: 1591–4.

118 Gant NF, Daley GL, Chand S, Whalley PJ & MacDonald PC. A study of angiotensin II pressure response throughout primigravid pregnancy. *Journal of Clinical Investigation* 1973; **52**: 2682–9.

119 Gant NF, Madden JD, Chand S, Worley RJ, Siiteri PK & MacDonald PC. Metabolic clearance rate of dehydroisoandrosterone sulfate. VI. Studies of eclampsia. *Obstetrics and Gynecology* 1976; **47**: 327–30.

120 Garden A, Davey DA & Dommisse J. Intravenous labetalol and intravenous dihydralazine in severe hypertension in pregnancy. *Clinical and Experimental Hypertension [B]* 1982; **1**: 371–83.

121 Gedekoh RH, Hayashi TT & MacDonald HM. Eclampsia at Magee Womens Hospital 1970–1980. *American Journal of Obstetrics and Gynecology* 1981; **140**: 860–6.

122 Gertner JM, Coustan DR, Kliger AS, Mallette LE, Ravin N & Broadus AE. Pregnancy as state of physiologic absorptive hypercalciuria. *American Journal of Medicine* 1986; **81**: 451–6.

123 Giese J. Acute hypertensive vascular disease. 1. Relation between blood pressure changes and vascular lesions in different forms of acute hypertension. *Acta Pathologica Microbiologica Scandinavica* 1964; **62**: 481–96.

124 Gilabert J, Estelles A, Ridocci F, Espana F, Aznar J & Galbis M. Clinical and haemostatic parameters in the HELLP syndrome: relevance of plasminogen activator inhibitors. *Gynecology and Obstetrics Investigations* 1990; **30**: 81–6.

125 Giles C & Inglis TCM. Thrombocytopenia and macrothrombocytosis in gestational hypertension. *British Journal of Obstetrics and Gynaecology* 1981; **88**: 1115–19.

126 Ginsberg J & Duncan SB. Direct and indirect blood pressure measurement in pregnancy. *Journal of Obstetrics and Gynaecology of the British Commonwealth* 1969; **76**: 705–10.

127 Girard H, Brun J-L & Muffat-Joy M. An angiographic study of the sensitivity to epinephrine of the uterine arteries of the guinea pig: a comparison with angiotensin. *American Journal of Obstetrics and Gynecology* 1971; **111**: 687–91.

128 Glawanakowa W & Popowa G. Untersuchungen uber die desquamation des gefassendothels bei EPH-gestosen. *Cor Vasa* 1988; **30**: 140–5.

129 Goldby FS & Beilin LJ. Relationship between arterial pressure and the permeability of arterioles to carbon particles in acute hypertension in the rat. *Cardiovascular Research* 1972; **6**: 384–90.

130 Goodlin RC. Safety of sodium nitroprusside. *Obstetrics and Gynecology* 1983; **62**: 270.

131 Goodlin RC, Cotton DB & Haesslein HC. Severe edema-proteinuria-hypertension gestosis. *American Journal of Obstetrics and Gynecology* 1978; **132**: 595–8.

132 Goodlin RC, Haesslein HO & Fleming J. Aspirin for the treatment of recurrent toxaemia. *Lancet* 1978; **ii**: 51.

133 Goodwin JF. Pregnancy and coarctation of the aorta. *Clinical Obstetrics and Gynaecology* 1961; **4**: 645–64.

134 Gordon RD, Fishman LM & Liddle GW. Plasma renin activity and aldosterone secretion in a pregnant woman with primary aldosteronism. *Journal of Clinical Endocrinology and Metabolism* 1967; **27**: 385–8.

135 Graham C & Goldstein A. Epidural analgesia and cardiac output in severe pre-eclampsia. *Anaesthesia* 1980; **35**: 709–12.

136 Greenwood PA & Lilford RJ. Effect of epidural analgesia on maximum and minimum blood pressures during the first stage of labour in primigravidae with mild/moderate gestational hypertension. *British Journal of Obstetrics and Gynaecology* 1986; **93**: 260–3.

137 Grimes DA, Ekbladh LE & McCartney WH. Cortical blindness in pre-eclampsia. *International Journal of Gynaecology and Obstetrics* 1980; **17**: 601–3.

138 Groenendijk R, Trimbos JBMJ & Wallenburg HCS. Hemodynamic measurements in pre-eclampsia: preliminary observations. *American Journal of Obstetrics and Gynecology* 1984; **150**: 232–6.

139 Halligan A *et al*. Twenty-four-hour ambulatory blood pressure measurement in a primigravid population. *Journal of Hypertension* 1993; **11**: 869–73.

140 Hamlin RHJ. The prevention of eclampsia and pre-eclampsia. *Lancet* 1952; **i**: 64–8.

141 Hanretty KP, Whittle MJ, Howie CA & Rubin PC. Effect of nifedipine on Doppler flow velocity waveforms in severe pre-eclampsia. *British Medical Journal* 1989; **299**: 1205–6.

142 Harley JMG. Pregnancy in the chronic hypertensive woman. *Proceedings of the Royal Society of Medicine* 1966; **39**: 835–8.

143 Harper MA, Murnaghan GA, Kennedy L, Hadden DR & Atkinson AB. Phaeochromocytoma in pregnancy. Five cases and a review of the literature. *British Journal of Obstetrics and Gynaecology* 1989; **96**: 594–606.

144 Hauth JC, Goldenberg RL *et al*. Low-dose aspirin therapy to prevent preeclampsia. *American Journal of Obstetrics and Gynecology* 1993; **168**: 1083–93.

145 Heller PJ, Scheider EP & Marx GF. Pharolaryngeal edema as a presenting symptom in pre-eclampsia. *Obstetrics and Gynecology* 1983; **62**: 523–4.

146 Henrich WL, Cronin R, Miller PD & Anderson RJ. Hypertensive sequelae of diazoxide and hydralazine therapy. *Journal of the American Medical Association* 1977; **237**: 264–5.

147 Hibbard BM & Rosen M. The management of severe pre-eclampsia and eclampsia. *British Journal of Anaesthesia* 1977; **49**: 3–9.

148 Hibbard LT. Maternal mortality due to acute toxemia. *Obstetrics and Gynecology* 1973; **42**: 263–70.

149 Hodgkinson R, Husain PJ & Hayashi RH. Systemic and pulmonary blood pressure during cesarean section in parturients with gestational hypertension. *Canadian Anaesthesia Society Journal* 1980; **27**: 385–94.

150 Holmes F. Incidence of the supine hypotensive syndrome in late pregnancy. *Journal of Obstetrics and Gynaecology of the British Empire* 1960; **67**: 254–8.

151 Horn EH, Filshie M, Kerslake RW, Jaspan T, Worthington BS & Rubin PC. Widespread cerebral ischaemia treated with nimodipine in a patient with eclampsia. *British Medical Journal* 1990; **301**: 794.

152 Horne CHW, Howie PW & Goudie RB. Serum alpha2-macroglobulin, transferrin, albumin and IgG levels in preeclampsia. *Journal of Clinical Pathology* 1970; **23**: 514–16.

153 Howard W, Hunter C & Huber CP. Intervillous blood oxygen studies. *Surgical Gynecology and Obstetrics* 1961; **112**: 435–8.

154 Howie PW, Begg CB, Purdie DW & Prentice CRM. Use of coagulation tests to predict the clinical progress of preeclampsia. *Lancet* 1976; **ii**: 323–5.

155 Howie PW, Prentice CRM & Forbes CD. Failure of heparin therapy to affect the clinical course of severe pre-eclampsia. *British Journal of Obstetrics and Gynaecology* 1975; **82**: 711–17.

156 Hubel CA, Roberts JM, Taylor RN, Musci TJ, Rogers GM & McLaughlin MK. Lipid peroxidation in pregnancy: new perspectives on preeclampsia. *American Journal of Obstetrics and Gynecology* 1989; **161**: 1025–34.

157 Hutton JD, James DK, Stirrat GM, Douglas KA & Redman CWG. Management of severe pre-eclampsia and eclampsia by UK consultants. *British Journal of Obstetrics and Gynaecology* 1992; **99**: 554–6.

158 Hytten FE & Paintin DB. Increase in plasma volume during normal pregnancy. *Journal of Obstetrics and Gynaecology of the British Commonwealth* 1963; **70**: 402–7.

159 Imperiale TF & Petrulis AS. A meta-analysis of low-dose aspirin for the prevention of pregnancy-induced hypertensive disease. *Journal of the American Medical Association* 1991; **266**: 260–4.

160 Iseri LT & French JH. Magnesium: nature's physiologic calcium blocker. *American Heart Journal* 1984; **108**: 188–94.

161 Italian Study of Aspirin in Pregnancy. Low dose aspirin in prevention and treatment of intrauterine growth retardation and pregnancy-induced hypertension. *Lancet* 1993; **341**: 396–400.

162 Jacobs M. Mechanism of action of hydralazine on vascular smooth muscle. *Biochemistry and Pharmacology* 1984; **33**: 2915–19.

163 Jeffcoate TNA & Scott JS. Some observations on the placental factor in pregnancy toxemia. *American Journal of Obstetrics and Gynecology* 1959; **77**: 475–89.

164 Jellinek EH, Painter M, Prineas J & Russell RR. Hypertensive encephalopathy with cortical disorders of vision. *Quarterly Journal of Medicine* 1964; **33**: 239–56.

165 Johansson B, Strandgaard S & Lassen NA. On the pathogenesis of hypertensive encephalopathy. *Circulation Research* 1974; **34** (suppl. 1): 167–71.

166 Johnson T & Clayton CG. Diffusion of radioactive sodium in normotensive and pre-eclamptic pregnancies. *British Medical Journal* 1957; **i**: 312–14.

167 Jones HMR & Cummings AJ. A study of the transfer of α-methyldopa to the human fetus and newborn infant. *British Journal of Clinical Pharmacology* 1978; **6**: 432–4.

168 Jouppila P, Jouppila R, Hollmen A & Koivula A. Lumbar epidural analgesia to pre-eclampsia. *Obstetrics and Gynecology* 1982; **59**: 158–61.

169 Jouppila R, Jouppila P & Hollmen A. Laryngeal oedema as an obstetric anaesthesia complication: case reports. *Acta Anaesthesiologica Scandinavica* 1980; **24**: 97–8.

170 Jouppila P, Jouppila R & Koivula A. Albumin infusion does not alter the intervillous blood flow in severe pre-eclampsia. *Acta Obstetricia Gynaecologica Scandinavica* 1983; **62**: 345–8.

171 Jouppila P, Kirkinen P, Koivula A & Ylikorkala O. Effects of dihydralazine infusion on the fetoplacental blood flow and maternal prostanoids. *Obstetrics and Gynecology* 1985; **65**: 115–18.

172 Joyce DN & Kenyon VG. The use of diazepam and hydralazine in the treatment of severe pre-eclampsia. *Journal of Obstetrics and Gynaecology of the British Commonwealth* 1972; **79**: 250–4.

173 Katz VL & Cefalo RC. Maternal death from carotid artery thrombosis associated with the syndrome of hemolysis, elevated liver function, and low platelets. *American Journal of Perinatology* 1989; **6**: 360–2.

174 Katz VL, Thorp JMJ, Rozas L & Bowes WAJ. The natural history of thrombocytopenia associated with preeclampsia. *American Journal of Obstetrics and Gynecology* 1990; **163**: 1142–3.

175 Kawasaki N, Matsui K, Ito M, Ushijima H, Yoshimura T & Okamura H. Effect of increased calcium intake during the third trimester on the vascular sensitivity of angiotensin II. *Clinical and Experimental Hypertension in Pregnancy* 1990; **B9**: 19–26.

176 Killam A, Dillard S, Patton R & Pederson P. Pregnancy-induced hypertension complicated by acute liver disease and disseminated intravascular coagulation. *American Journal of Obstetrics and Gynecology* 1975; **123**: 823–8.

177 Kirby JC & Jaindl JJ. Cerebral CT findings in toxemia of pregnancy. *Radiology* 1984; **151**: 114.

178 Kirkendall WM, Feinleib M, Freis ED & Mark AL. Recommendations for human blood pressure determination by sphygmomanometers. Sub-committee of the AHA postgraduate education committee. *Hypertension* 1981; **3**: 510A–19.

179 Kreft-Jais C, Plouin PF, Tchobroutsky C & Boutry M. Angiotensin converting enzyme inhibitors during pregnancy: a survey of 22 patients given captopril and nine given enalapril. *British Journal of Obstetrics and Gynaecology* 1988; **95**: 420–2.

180 Kreines K & Devaux WD. Neonatal adrenal insufficiency associated with maternal Cushing's syndrome. *Pediatrics* 1971; **47**: 516–19.

181 Kuzniar J, Piela A, Skret A, Szmigiel ZB & Zaczek T. Echocardiographic estimation of hemodynamics in hypertensive pregnancy. *American Journal of Obstetrics and Gynecology* 1982; **144**: 430–7.

182 Ladner C, Brinkman CR, Weston P & Assali NS. Dynamics of uterine circulation in pregnant and non-pregnant sheep. *American Journal of Physiology* 1970; **218**: 257–63.

183 Lamming GD, Symonds EM & Rubin PC. Phaeochromocytoma in pregnancy: Still a cause of maternal death. *Clinical and Experimental Hypertension Part B. Hypertension in Pregnancy* 1990; **9**: 57–68.

184 *Lancet* Editorial. Acute fatty liver of pregnancy. *Lancet* 1983; **i**: 339.

185 *Lancet* Editorial. Bed rest and non-proteinuric hypertension in pregnancy. *Lancet* 1992; **339**: 1023–4.

186 Lancet M & Fisher IL. The value of blood uric acid levels in toxaemia of pregnancy. *Journal of Obstetrics and Gynaecology of the British Commonwealth* 1956; **63**: 116–19.

187 Lang RM, Pridjian G, Feldman T, Neumann A,

Lindheimer MD & Borow KM. Left ventricular mechanics in preeclampsia. *American Heart Journal* 1991; **121**: 1768–75.

188 Larkin JG, Butler E & Brodie MJ. Nifedipine for epilepsy? A pilot study. *British Medical Journal* 1988; **296**: 530–1.

189 Lean TH, Ratnam SS & Sivasamboo R. The use of chlordiazepoxide in patients with severe pregnancy toxaemia. *Journal of Obstetrics and Gynaecology of the British Commonwealth* 1968; **75**: 853–5.

190 Leather HM, Humphreys DM, Baker P & Chadd MA. A controlled trial of hypotensive agents in hypertension in pregnancy. *Lancet* 1968; **ii**: 488–90.

191 Ledingham JGG & Rajagopalan B. Cerebral complications in the treatment of accelerated hypertension. *Quarterly Journal of Medicine* 1979; **48**: 25–41.

192 Lees MM, Scott DB, Kerr MG & Taylor SH. The circulatory effects of recumbent postural change in late pregnancy. *Clinical Science* 1967; **32**: 453–65.

193 Lees MM, Taylor SH, Scott DB & Kerr MG. A study of cardiac output at rest throughout pregnancy. *Journal of Obstetrics and Gynaecology of the British Commonwealth* 1967; **74**: 319–27.

194 Liebowitz HA. Cortical blindness as a complication of eclampsia. *Annals of Emergency Medicine* 1984; **13**: 365–7.

195 Lin M-S, McNay JL, Shepherd AMM, Musgrave GE & Keeton TK. Increased plasma norepinephrine accompanies persistent tachycardia after hydralazine. *Hypertension* 1983; **5**: 257–63.

196 Lindberg BS & Sandstrom B. How Swedish obstetricians manage hypertension in pregnancy. A questionnaire study. *Acta Obstetricia Gynaecologica Scandinavica* 1981; **60**: 327–31.

197 Lindheimer MD & Katz AI. Hypertension in pregnancy. *New England Journal of Medicine* 1985; **313**: 675–80.

198 Lindheimer MD, Spargo BH & Katz AI. Eclampsia during the 16th week of gestation. *Journal of the American Medical Association* 1974; **230**: 1006–8.

199 Linton AL, Gavras H & Gleadle RI. Microangiopathic haemolytic anaemia and the pathogenesis of malignant hypertension. *Lancet* 1969; **i**: 1277–82.

200 Lipsitz PJ. The clinical and biochemical effects of excess magnesium in the newborn. *Pediatrics* 1971; **47**: 501–9.

201 Liston WA & Kilpatrick DC. Is genetic susceptibility to pre-eclampsia conferred by homozygosity for the same single recessive gene in mother and fetus? *British Journal of Obstetrics and Gynaecology* 1991; **98**: 1079–86.

202 Little WA. Placental infarction. *Obstetrics and Gynecology* 1960; **15**: 109–30.

203 Long RG, Scheuer PJ & Sherlock S. Pre-eclampsia presenting with deep jaundice. *Journal of Clinical Pathology* 1977; **30**: 212–15.

204 Longmire S, Leduc L, Jones MM, Hawkins JL, Joyce TH & Cotton DB. The hemodynamic effects of intubation during nitroglycerin infusion in severe preeclampsia. *American Journal of Obstetrics and Gynecology* 1991; **164**: 551–6.

205 Lopez-Llera M, Linares GR & Horta JLH. Maternal mortality rates in eclampsia. *American Journal of Obstetrics and Gynecology* 1976; **124**: 149–55.

206 Lorentzen B, Endresen MJ, Hovig T, Haug E & Henriksen T. Sera from preeclamptic women increase the content of triglycerides and reduce the release of prostacyclin in cultured endothelial cells. *Thrombosis Research* 1991; **63**: 363–72.

207 Lowe CR. Toxaemia and pre-pregnancy weight. *Journal of Obstetrics and Gynaecology of the British Commonwealth* 1961; **68**: 622–7.

208 Lubbe WF & Hodge JV. Combined α- and β-adrenoceptor-antagonism with prazosin and oxprenolol in control of severe hypertension in pregnancy. *New Zealand Medical Journal* 1981; **94**: 169–72.

209 Lunell NO, Lewander R, Nylund L, Sarby B & Thornstrom S. Acute effect of dihydralazine on uteroplacental blood flow in hypertension during pregnancy. *Gynecological and Obstetric Investigation* 1983; **16**: 274–82.

210 Lunell NO, Nylund L, Lewander R & Sarby B. Acute effect of an anti-hypertensive drug, labetalol, on uteroplacental blood flow. *British Journal of Obstetrics and Gynaecology* 1982; **89**: 640–4.

211 Mabie WC, Ratts TE & Sibai BM. The central hemodynamics of severe pre-eclampsia. *American Journal of Obstetrics and Gynecology* 1989; **161**: 1443–8.

212 MacGillivray I. Some observations on the incidence of pre-eclampsia. *Journal of Obstetrics and Gynaecology of the British Commonwealth* 1959; **65**: 536–9.

213 MacGillivray I. Hypertension in pregnancy and its consequences. *Journal of Obstetrics and Gynaecology of the British Commonwealth* 1961; **68**: 557–69.

214 MacGillivray I. The significance of blood pressure and body water changes in pregnancy. *Scottish Medical Journal* 1967; **12**: 237–45.

215 MacGillivray I. Pregnancy hypertension — is it a disease? In: Sammour MB, Symonds EM, Zuspan FP & El-Tomi N (eds), *Pregnancy Hypertension*. Cairo, Ain Shams University Press 1982: 1–15.

216 MacGillivray I, Rose GA & Rowe B. Blood pressure survey in pregnancy. *Clinical Science* 1969; **37**: 395–407.

217 Martin JNJ, Blake PG, Lowry SL, Perry KGJ, Files JC & Morrison JC. Pregnancy complicated by preeclampsia-eclampsia with the syndrome of hemolysis, elevated liver enzymes, and low platelet count: how rapid is postpartum recovery? *Obstetrics and Gynecology* 1990; **76**: 737–41.

218 Mathews DD. A randomised controlled trial of bed rest and sedation or normal activity and non-sedation in the management of non-albuminuric hypertension in late pregnancy. *British Journal of Obstetrics and Gynaecology* 1977; **84**: 108–14.

219 Mathews DD, Agarwal V & Shuttleworth TP. A

randomised controlled trial of complete bed rest versus ambulation in the management of proteinuric hypertension during pregnancy. *British Journal of Obstetrics and Gynaecology* 1982; **89**: 128–31.

220 Maxwell MH, Waks AU, Schroth PC, Karam M & Dornfeld LP. Error in blood-pressure measurement due to incorrect cuff size in obese patients. *Lancet* 1982; **i**: 33–5.

221 McCall ML. Cerebral circulation and metabolism in toxemia of pregnancy. Observations on the effects of veratvum viride and Apresoline (1-hydrazinophthalazine). *American Journal of Obstetrics and Gynecology* 1953; **66**: 1015–30.

222 McCarron DA & Morris CD. Blood pressure response to oral calcium in persons with mild to moderate hypertension. A randomized, double-blind, placebo-controlled, crossover trial. *Annals of Internal Medicine* 1985; **103**: 825–31.

223 McClure Browne JC & Veall N. The maternal placental blood flow in normotensive and hypertensive women. *Journal of Obstetrics and Gynaecology of the British Empire* 1953; **60**: 141–7.

224 McCubbin JH, Sibai BM, Abdella TN & Anderson GD. Cardiopulmonary arrest due to acute maternal hypermagnesaemia. *Lancet* 1981; **i**: 1058.

225 McFarlane CN. An evaluation of the serum uric acid level in pregnancy. *Journal of Obstetrics and Gynaecology of the British Commonwealth* 1963; **70**: 63–8.

226 McKay DG. Hematologic evidence of disseminated intravascular coagulation in eclampsia. *Obstetrical and Gynecological Survey* 1972; **27**: 399–417.

227 McKay DG, Merrill SJ, Weiner AE, Hertig AT & Reid DE. The pathologic anatomy of eclampsia, bilateral renal cortical necrosis, pituitary necrosis, and other acute fatal complications of pregnancy, and its possible relationship to the generalised Shwartzman phenomenon. *American Journal of Obstetrics and Gynecology* 1953; **66**: 507–39.

228 McKenna P & Shaw RW. Hyponatremic fits in oxytocin-augmented labours. *International Journal of Gynaecology and Obstetrics* 1979; **17**: 250–2.

229 Maclean PR, Paterson WG, Smart GE, Petrie JJB, Robson JS & Thomson P. Proteinuria in toxaemia and abruptio placentae. *Journal of Obstetrics and Gynaecology of the British Commonwealth* 1972; **79**: 321–6.

230 Milliez J, Dahoun A & Boudraa M. Computed tomography of the brain in eclampsia. *Obstetrics and Gynecology* 1990; **75**: 975–80.

231 Moar VA, Jefferies MA, Mutch LMM, Ounsted MK & Redman CWG. Neonatal head circumference and the treatment of maternal hypertension. *British Journal of Obstetrics and Gynaecology* 1978; **85**: 933–7.

232 Moore TR, Key TC, Reisner LS & Resnik R. Evaluation of the use of continuous lumbar epidural anesthesia for hypertensive pregnant women in labour. *American Journal of Obstetrics and Gynecology* 1985; **152**: 404–12.

233 Mordes JP, Swartz R & Arky RA. Extreme hypermagnesemia as a cause of refractory hypotension. *Annals of Internal Medicine* 1975; **83**: 657–8.

234 Mordes JP & Wacker WE. Excess magnesium. *Pharmacology Review* 1978; **29**: 253–300.

235 Morris JA & O'Grady JP. Volume expansion in severe edema-proteinuria-hypertension gestosis. *American Journal of Obstetrics and Gynecology* 1979; **135**: 276.

236 Mule JG, Tatum HJ & Sawyer RE. Nitrogenous retention in patients with toxemia of pregnancy — an unusual complication of salt restriction. *American Journal of Obstetrics and Gynecology* 1957; **74**: 526–37.

237 Mutch LMM, Moar VA, Ounsted MK & Redman CWG. Hypertension during pregnancy, with and without specific hypotensive treatment. *Early Human Development* 1977; **1**: 47–57.

238 Mutch LMM, Moar VA, Ounsted MK & Redman CWG. Hypertension during pregnancy, with and without specific hypotensive treatment. II The growth and development of the infant in the first year of life. *Early Human Development* 1977; **1**: 59–67.

239 Naeye RL & Friedman EA. Causes of perinatal death associated with gestational hypertension and proteinuria. *American Journal of Obstetrics and Gynecology* 1979; **133**: 8–10.

240 National Health and Medical Research Council. *Report on Maternal Deaths in Australia 1976–1978*. Australian Government Publishing Service, Canberra, 1981.

241 National High Blood Pressure Education Program. National High Blood Pressure Education Program Working Group Report on High Blood Pressure in Pregnancy. *American Journal of Obstetrics and Gynecology* 1990; **163**: 1691–712.

242 Nelson TR. A clinical study of pre-eclampsia. *Journal of Obstetrics and Gynaecology of the British Empire* 1955; **62**: 48–57.

243 Newsome LR, Bramwell RS & Curling PE. Severe pre-eclampsia: hemodynamic effects of lumbar epidural anesthesia. *Anesthesia and Analgesia* 1986; **65**: 31–6.

244 Odendaal HJ, Pattinson RC, Bam R, Grove D & Kotze TJ. Aggressive or expectant management for patients with severe preeclampsia between 28–34 weeks' gestation: a randomized controlled trial. *Obstetrics and Gynecology* 1990; **76**: 1070–5.

245 Olsen KS & Beier Holgersen R. Fetal death following labetalol administration in pre-eclampsia. *Acta Obstetricia Gynaecologica Scandinavica* 1992; **71**: 145–7.

246 Olsen KS & Beier Holgersen R. Hemodynamic collapse following labetalol administration in preeclampsia. *Acta Obstetricia Gynaecologica Scandinavica* 1992; **71**: 151–2.

247 Olsen SF & Secher NJ. A possible preventive effect of low-dose fish oil on early delivery and pre-eclampsia: indications from a 50-year-old controlled trial. *British Journal of Nutrition* 1990; **64**: 599–609.

248 Overgaard J & Skinhoj E. A paradoxical cerebral hemodynamic effect of hydralazine. *Stroke* 1975; **6**: 402–4.

249 Ounsted MK, Moar VA, Good FJ & Redman CWG.

Hypertension during pregnancy with and without specific treatment; the children at the age of 4 years. *British Journal of Obstetrics and Gynaecology* 1980; **87**: 19–24.

250 Paterson ME. The aetiology and outcome of abruptio placentae. *Acta Obstetricia Gynaecologica Scandinavica* 1979; **58**: 31–5.

251 Paterson WG, Hobson BM, Smart GE & Bain AD. Two cases of hydatidiform degeneration of the placenta with fetal abnormality and triploid chromosomic constitution. *Journal of Obstetrics and Gynaecology of the British Commonwealth* 1971; **78**: 136–42.

252 People's League of Health. The nutrition of expectant and nursing mothers in relation to maternal and infant mortality and morbidity. *Journal of Obstetrics and Gynaecology of the British Empire* 1946; **53**: 498–509.

253 Perry IJ, Stewart BA *et al*. Recording diastolic blood pressure in pregnancy. *British Medical Journal* 1990; **301**: 1198.

254 Pickard J, Jochen AL, Sadur CN & Hofeldt FD. Cushing's syndrome in pregnancy. *Obstetric and Gynecological Survey* 1990; **45**: 87–93.

255 Pickering G. *High Blood Pressure*. London, J & A Churchill, 1968: 1–5.

256 Pickering G. *High Blood Pressure*. London, J & A Churchill, 1968: 9–12.

257 Pickering G. *High Blood Pressure*. London, J & A Churchill, 1968: 215–16.

258 Pickering G. *High Blood Pressure*. London, J & A Churchill, 1968: 412.

259 Pickering G. *High Blood Pressure*. London, J & A Churchill, 1968: 414–25.

260 Pirani BBK, Campbell DM & MacGillivray I. Plasma volume in normal first pregnancy. *Journal of Obstetrics and Gynaecology of the British Commonwealth* 1973; **80**: 884–7.

261 Plouin PF, Breart G *et al*. A randomized comparison of early with conservative use of antihypertensive drugs in the management of pregnancy-induced hypertension. *British Journal of Obstetrics and Gynaecology* 1990; **97**: 134–41.

262 Pollak VE & Nettles JB. The kidney in toxemia of pregnancy: a clinical and pathologic study based on renal biopsies. *Medicine* 1960; **39**: 469–526.

263 Porapakkham S. An epidemiologic study of eclampsia. *Obstetrics and Gynecology* 1979; **54**: 26–30.

264 Pritchard JA. The use of the magnesium ion in the management of eclamptogenic toxemias. *Surgical Gynecology and Obstetrics* 1955; **100**: 131–40.

265 Pritchard JA, Cunningham FG & Mason RA. Coagulation changes in eclampsia: their frequency and pathogenesis. *American Journal of Obstetrics and Gynecology* 1976; **124**: 855–64.

266 Pritchard JA, Cunningham FG & Pritchard SA. The Parkland Memorial Hospital protocol for treatment of eclampsia: evaluation of 245 cases. *American Journal of Obstetrics and Gynecology* 1984; **148**: 951–63.

267 Pritchard JA & Pritchard SA. Standardised treatment of 154 consecutive cases of eclampsia. *American Journal of Obstetrics and Gynecology* 1975; **123**: 543–9.

268 Pritchard JA & Pritchard SA. Blood pressure response to estrogen-progestin oral contraceptive after pregnancy-induced hypertension. *American Journal of Obstetrics and Gynecology* 1977; **129**: 733–9.

269 Pritchard JA & Stone SR. Clinical and laboratory observations on eclampsia. *American Journal of Obstetrics and Gynecology* 1967; **99**: 754–65.

270 Pritchard JA, Weisman R, Ratnoff OD & Vosburgh GJ. Intravascular hemolysis, thrombocytopenia and other hematologic abnormalities associated with severe toxemia of pregnancy. *New England Journal of Medicine* 1954; **250**: 89–98.

271 Raab W, Schroeder G, Wagner R & Gigee W. Vascular reactivity and electrolytes in normal and toxemic pregnancy. *Journal of Clinical Endocrinology* 1956; **16**: 1196–216.

272 Raftery EB & Ward AP. The indirect method of recording blood pressure. *Cardiovascular Research* 1968; **2**: 210–18.

273 Rail DL & Perkin GD. Computerised tomographic appearance of hypertensive encephalopathy. *Archives of Neurology* 1981; **37**: 310–11.

274 Rakoczi I, Tallian F, Bagdany S & Gati I. Platelet lifespan in normal pregnancy and pre-eclampsia as determined by a non-radioisotope technique. *Thrombosis Research* 1979; **15**: 553–6.

275 Ramanathan J, Sibai BM, Mabie WC, Chauhan D & Ruiz AG. The use of labetalol for attenuation of the hypertensive response to endotracheal intubation in preeclampsia. *American Journal of Obstetrics and Gynecology* 1988; **159**: 650–4.

276 Ramsay ID. The adrenal gland. In: Hytten F & Chamberlain G (eds) *Clinical Physiology in Obstetrics*. Oxford, Blackwell Scientific Publications, 1980: 415–16.

277 Redman CWG. Treatment of hypertension in pregnancy. *Kidney International* 1980; **18**: 267–78.

278 Redman CWG. The definition of pre-eclampsia. In: Sharp F & Symonds EM (eds) *Hypertension in Pregnancy*. Perinatology Press, 1987: 317.

279 Redman CWG. Current topic: pre-eclampsia and the placenta. *Placenta* 1991; **12**: 301–8.

280 Redman CWG, Allington MJ, Bolton FG & Stirrat GM. Plasma β-thromboglobulin in pre-eclampsia. *Lancet* 1977; **ii**: 248.

281 Redman CWG, Beilin LJ & Bonnar J. Renal function in pre-eclampsia. *Journal of Clinical Pathology* 1976; **10** (Supplement Royal College of Pathologists): 91–4.

282 Redman CWG, Beilin LJ & Bonnar J. Variability of blood pressure in normal and abnormal pregnancy. In: Lindheimer MD, Katz AI & Zuspan FP (eds) *Hypertension in Pregnancy*. New York, John Wiley, 1976: 53–60.

283 Redman CWG, Beilin LJ & Bonnar J. Treatment of hypertension in pregnancy with methyldopa: blood

pressure control and side effects. *British Journal of Obstetrics and Gynaecology* 1977; **84**: 419–26.

284 Redman CWG, Beilin LJ, Bonnar J & Ounsted MK. Fetal outcome in trial of antihypertensive treatment in pregnancy. *Lancet* 1976; **ii**: 753–6.

285 Redman CWG, Beilin LJ, Bonnar J & Wilkinson RH. Plasma-urate measurements in predicting fetal death in hypertensive pregnancy. *Lancet* 1976; **i**: 1370–3.

286 Redman CWG, Bonnar J & Beilin LJ. Early platelet consumption in pre-eclampsia. *British Medical Journal* 1978; **i**: 467–9.

287 Redman CWG, Denson KWE, Beilin LJ, Bolton FG & Stirrat GM. Factor VII consumption in pre-eclampsia. *Lancet* 1977; **ii**: 1249–52.

288 Redman CWG & Jefferies M. Revised definition of pre-eclampsia. *Lancet* 1988; **i**: 809–12.

289 Redman CWG & Ounsted MK. Safety for the child of drug treatment for hypertension in pregnancy. *Lancet* 1982; **i**: 1237.

290 Reinthaller A, Mursch-Edlmayr G & Tatra G. Thrombin-antithrombin III complex levels in normal pregnancy and hypertensive disorders and after delivery. *British Journal of Obstetrics and Gynaecology* 1990; **97**: 506–10.

291 *Report on Confidential Enquiries into Maternal Deaths in England and Wales 1973–1975*. London, HMSO, 1979: 21–9.

292 *Report on Confidential Enquiries into Maternal Deaths in England and Wales 1976–1978*. London, HMSO, 1982: 19–25.

293 *Report on Confidential Enquiries into Maternal Deaths in England and Wales 1979–1981*. London, HMSO, 1986: 13–21.

294 *Report on Confidential Enquiries into Maternal Deaths in England and Wales 1982–1984*. London, HMSO, 1989: 10–19.

295 *Report on Confidential Enquiries into Maternal Deaths in the United Kingdom 1985–1987*. London, HMSO, 1991: 17–27.

296 *Report on Confidential Enquiries into Maternal Deaths in the United Kingdom 1988–1990*. London, HMSO, 1994: 22–33.

297 Rippmann ET. Gestosis of late pregnancy. *Gynaecologia* 1968; **165**: 12–20.

298 Roberts JM, Taylor RN, Musci TJ, Rodgers GM, Hubel CA & McLaughlin MK. Preeclampsia: an endothelial cell disorder. *American Journal of Obstetrics and Gynecology* 1989; **161**: 1200–4.

299 Robertson EG. The natural history of oedema during pregnancy. *Journal of Obstetrics and Gynaecology of the British Commonwealth* 1971; **78**: 520–9.

300 Robertson WB, Brosens I & Dixon HG. The pathological response of the vessels of the placental bed to hypertensive pregnancy. *Journal of Pathology and Bacteriology* 1967; **93**: 581–92.

301 Robertson WB, Brosens I & Dixon G. Uteroplacental vascular pathology. *European Journal of Obstetrics Gynecology and Reproductive Biology* 1975; **5**: 47–65.

302 Robinson M. Salt in pregnancy. *Lancet* 1958; **i**: 178–81.

303 Rodgers GM, Taylor RN & Roberts JM. Preeclampsia is associated with a serum factor cytotoxic to human endothelial cells. *American Journal of Obstetrics and Gynecology* 1988; **159**: 908–14.

304 Rosa FW, Bosco LA, Graham CF, Milstein JB, Dreis M & Creamer J. Neonatal anuria with maternal angiotensin-converting enzyme inhibition. *Obstetrics and Gynecology* 1989; **74**: 371–4.

305 Rovinsky JJ & Jaffin H. Cardiovascular hemodynamics in pregnancy I. Blood and plasma volumes in multiple pregnancy. *American Journal of Obstetrics and Gynecology* 1965; **193**: 1–15.

306 Rubin PC, Butters L *et al*. Placebo-controlled trial of antenolol treatment of pregnancy-associated hypertension. *Lancet* 1983; **i**: 431–4.

307 Rubin PC, Butters L & McCabe R. Nifedipine and platelets in preeclampsia. *American Journal of Hypertension* 1988; **1**: 175–7.

308 Ryan G, Lange IR & Naugler MA. Clinical experience with phenytoin prophylaxis in severe preeclampsia. *American Journal of Obstetrics and Gynecology* 1989; **161**: 1297–304.

309 Saftlas AF, Olson DR, Franks AL, Atrash HK & Pokras R. Epidemiology of preeclampsia and eclampsia in the United States, 1979–1986. *American Journal of Obstetrics and Gynecology* 1990; **163**: 460–5.

310 Samuels B. Postpartum eclampsia. *Obstetrics and Gynecology* 1960; **15**: 748–52.

311 Sanchez Ramos L, Jones DC & Cullen MT. Urinary calcium as an early marker for preeclampsia. *Obstetrics and Gynecology* 1991; **77**: 685–8.

312 Sanders TG, Clayman DA, Sanchez Ramos L, Vines FS & Russo L. Brain in eclampsia: MR imaging with clinical correlation. *Radiology* 1991; **180**: 475–8.

313 Sbabarti R, de Boer M, Marzilli M, Scarlattini M, Rossi G & van Mourik JA. Immunologic detection of endothelial cells in human whole blood. *Blood* 1991; **77**: 764–9.

314 Scanlon MF. Hypertension in pregnancy. *Journal of Obstetrics and Gynaecology of the British Commonwealth* 1974; **81**: 539–44.

315 Schenker JG & Chowers I. Pheochromocytoma and pregnancy. *Obstetrical and Gynecological Survey* 1971; **26**: 739–47.

316 Scher J, Hailey DM & Beard RW. The effects of diazepam on the fetus. *Journal of Obstetrics and Gynaecology of the British Commonwealth* 1972; **79**: 635–8.

317 Schramm M. Prophylactic anticoagulation in the management of recurrent pre-eclampsia and fetal death. *Australia and New Zealand Journal of Obstetrics and Gynaecology* 1979; **19**: 230–2.

318 Schwaighofer BW, Hesselink JR & Healy ME. MR demonstration of reversible brain abnormalities in

eclampsia. *Journal of Computer Assisted Tomography* 1989; **13**: 310–12.

319 Schwartz ML & Brenner W. Toxemia in a patient with none of the standard signs and symptoms of pre-eclampsia. *Obstetrics and Gynecology* 1985; **66**: 19S–21S.

320 Scott JS. Pregnancy toxaemia associated with hydrops foetalis, hydatidiform mole and hydramnios. *Journal of Obstetrics and Gynaecology of the British Empire* 1958; **65**: 689–701.

321 Seely EW, Wood RJ, Brown EM & Graves SW. Lower serum ionized calcium and abnormal calciotropic hormone levels in preeclampsia. *Journal of Clinical Endocrinology and Metabolism* 1992; **74**: 1436–40.

322 Seligman SA. Diurnal blood-pressure variation in pregnancy. *British Journal of Obstetrics and Gynaecology* 1971; **78**: 417–22.

323 Shanklin DR & Sibai BM. Ultrastructural aspects of preeclampsia. I. Placental bed and uterine boundary vessels. *American Journal of Obstetrics and Gynecology* 1989; **161**: 735–41.

324 Sheehan HL & Lynch JB. *Pathology of Toxaemia in Pregnancy*. London, Churchill-Livingstone, 1973: 328–30.

325 Sheehan HL & Lynch JP. *Pathology of Toxaemia of Pregnancy*. London, Churchill-Livingstone, 1973: 340–83.

326 Sheehan HL & Lynch JP. *Pathology of Toxaemia in Pregnancy*. London, Churchill-Livingstone, 1973: 384–97.

327 Sheehan HL & Lynch JB. *Pathology of Toxaemia in Pregnancy*. London, Churchill-Livingstone, 1973: 413–53.

328 Sheehan HL & Lynch JP. *Pathology of Toxaemia in Pregnancy*. London, Churchill-Livingstone, 1973: 524–53.

329 Shennan AH, Kissane J, de Swiet M. Validation of the Spacelabs 902207. *British Journal of Obstetrics and Gynaecology* 1993; **100**: 904–8.

330 Sheppard BL & Bonnar J. The ultrastructure of the arterial supply of the human placenta in pregnancy complicated by fetal growth retardation. *British Journal of Obstetrics and Gynaecology* 1976; **83**: 948–59.

331 Shoemaker CT & Meyers M. Sodium nitroprusside for control of severe hypertensive disease of pregnancy: a case report and discussion of potential toxicity. *American Journal of Obstetrics and Gynecology* 1984; **149**: 171–3.

332 Shukla PK, Sharma D & Mandal RK. Serum lactate dehydrogenase in detecting liver damage associated with pre-eclampsia. *British Journal of Obstetrics and Gynaecology* 1978; **85**: 40–2.

333 Sibai BM. The HELLP syndrome (hemolysis, elevated liver enzymes, and low platelets): much ado about nothing? *American Journal of Obstetrics and Gynecology* 1990; **162**: 311–16.

334 Sibai BM. Diagnosis and management of chronic hypertension in pregnancy. *Obstetrics and Gynecology* 1991; **78**: 451–61.

335 Sibai BM, Caritis SN *et al*. Prevention of pre-eclampsia with low-dose aspirin in health nulliparous pregnant women. *New England Journal of Medicine* 1993; **329**: 1213–18.

336 Sibai BM, Mabie WC, Shamsa F, Villar MA & Anderson GD. A comparison of no medication versus methyldopa or labetalol in chronic hypertension during pregnancy. *American Journal of Obstetrics and Gynecology* 1990; **162**: 960–6.

337 Sibai BM, McCubbin JH, Anderson GD, Lipshitz J & Dilts PV. Eclampsia. I Observations from 67 recent cases. *Obstetrics and Gynecology* 1981; **58**: 609–13.

338 Sibai BM, Taslimi M, Abdella TN, Brooks TF, Spinnato JA & Anderson GD. Maternal and perinatal outcome of conservative management of severe preeclampsia in midtrimester. *American Journal of Obstetrics and Gynecology* 1985; **152**: 32–7.

339 Simanis J, Amerson JR, Hendee AE & Anton AH. Unresectable pheochromocytoma in pregnancy. *American Journal of Medicine* 1972; **53**: 381–5.

340 Simanowitz MD, MacGregor WG & Hobbs JR. Proteinuria in pre-eclampsia. *Journal of Obstetrics and Gynaecology of the British Commonwealth* 1973; **80**: 103–8.

341 Slater RM, Wilcox FL *et al*. Phenytoin infusion in severe pre-eclampsia. *Lancet* 1987; **i**: 1417–21.

342 Smith K, Browne JCMc, Shackman R & Wrong OM. Renal failure of obstetric origin. *British Medical Bulletin* 1968; **24**: 49–58.

343 Spargo B, McCartney CP & Winemiller R. Glomerular capillary endotheliosis in toxemia of pregnancy. *Archives of Pathology* 1959; **68**: 593–9.

344 Stewart A & Hewitt D. Toxaemia of pregnancy and obesity. *Journal of Obstetrics and Gynaecology of the British Empire* 1960; **67**: 812–18.

345 Strandgaard S, Olesen J, Skinhoj E & Lassen NA. Autoregulation of brain circulation in severe arterial hypertension. *British Medical Journal* 1973; **i**: 507–10.

346 Strauss RG, Keefer JR, Burke T & Civetta JM. Hemodynamic monitoring of cardiogenic pulmonary edema complicating toxemia of pregnancy. *Obstetrics and Gynecology* 1980; **55**: 170–4.

347 Stubbs TM, Lazarchik J, Van Dorsten JP, Cox J & Loadholt CB. Evidence of accelerated platelet production and consumption in nonthrombocytopenic pre-eclampsia. *American Journal of Obstetrics and Gynecology* 1986; **155**: 263–5.

348 Studd JWW, Blainey JD & Bailey DE. Serum protein changes in the pre-eclampsia–eclampsia syndrome. *Journal of Obstetrics and Gynaecology of the British Commonwealth* 1970; **77**: 796–801.

349 Suonio S, Saarikoski S, Tahvanainen K, Paakkonen A & Olkkonen H. Acute effects of dihydralazine mesylate, furosemide, and metoprolol on maternal hemodynamics in pregnancy-induced hypertension.

American Journal of Obstetrics and Gynecology 1986; **155**: 122–5.

350 Szekely P & Snaith L. The heart in toxaemia of pregnancy. *British Heart Journal* 1947; **9**: 128–37.

351 Talledo OE, Chesley LC & Zuspan FP. Renin-angiotensin system in normal and toxemic pregnancies III. Differential sensitivity to angiotensin II and nor-epinephrine in toxemia of pregnancy. *American Journal of Obstetrics and Gynecology* 1968; **100**: 218–21.

352 Tatum HJ & Mule JG. Puerperal vasomotor collapse in patients with toxemia of pregnancy — A new concept of the etiology and a rational plan of treatment. *American Journal of Obstetrics and Gynecology* 1956; **71**: 492–501.

353 Taufield PA, Ales KL, Resnick LM, Druzin ML, Gertner JM & Laragh JH. Hypocalciuria in preeclampsia. *New England Journal of Medicine* 1987; **316**: 715–18.

354 Taylor HC, Tillman AJ & Blanchard J. Fetal losses in hypertension and pre-eclampsia. *Obstetrics and Gynecology* 1954; **3**: 225–39.

355 Taylor RN, Crombleholme WR, Friedman SA, Jones LA, Casal DC & Roberts JM. High plasma cellular fibronectin levels correlate with biochemical and clinical features of preeclampsia but cannot be attributed to hypertension alone. *American Journal of Obstetrics and Gynecology* 1991; **165**: 895–901.

356 Templeton A & Campbell D. A retrospective study of eclampsia in the Grampian Region 1965–1977. *Health Bulletin* 1979; **37**: 55–9.

357 Tepperman HM, Beydoun SN & Abdul-Karim RW. Drugs affecting myometrial contractility in pregnancy. *Clinical Obstetrics and Gynecology* 1977; **20**: 423–45.

358 Thomson AM, Hytten RE & Billewicz WZ. The epidemiology of edema during pregnancy. *Journal of Obstetrics and Gynaecology of the British Commonwealth* 1967; **74**: 1–10.

359 Thorley KJ. Randomised trial of atenolol and methyl dopa in pregnancy related hypertension. *Clinical and Experimental Hypertension* 1984; **B3**: 168.

360 Thornton JG & Onwude JL. Pre-eclampsia: discordance among identical twins. *British Medical Journal* 1991; **303**: 1241–2.

361 Tillmann Hein HA. Cardiorespiratory arrest with laryngeal oedema in pregnancy-induced hypertension. *Canadian Anesthesia Society Journal* 1984; **31**: 210–12.

362 Trofatter KFJ, Howell ML, Greenberg CS & Hage ML. Use of the fibrin D-dimer in screening for coagulation abormalities in preeclampsia. *Obstetrics and Gynecology* 1989; **73**: 435–40.

363 Tsukimori K, Maeda H, Shingu M, Koyanagi T, Nobunaga M & Nakano H. The possible role of endothelial cells in hypertensive disorders during pregnancy. *Obstetrics and Gynecology* 1992; **80**: 229–33.

364 Turnbull AC & Ahmed S. Catapres in the treatment of hypertension in pregnancy. In: Conolly ME (ed.) *Catapres in Hypertension*. London, Butterworths, 1969: 237–45.

365 Tzoumaka Bakoula C, Lekea Karanika V, Golding J & Thomas P. Hypertensive disorders of pregnancy in Greece. *European Journal of Obstetrics, Gynecology and Reproductive Biology* 1989; **31**: 127–31.

366 Ueland K, Novy MJ, Peterson EN & Metcalfe J. Maternal cardiovascular dynamics. IV The influence of gestational age on the maternal cardiovascular response to posture and exercise. *American Journal of Obstetrics and Gynecology* 1969; **104**: 856–64.

367 Ulmsten U. Treatment of normotensive and hypertensive patients with preterm labor using oral nifedipine, a calcium antagonist. *Archives of Gynecology* 1984; **236**: 69–72.

368 Underwood P, Hester LL, Lafitte T & Gregg KV. The relationship of smoking to the outcome of pregnancy. *American Journal of Obstetrics and Gynecology* 1965; **91**: 270–6.

369 Valentine BH & Baker JL. Treatment of recurrent pregnancy hypertension by prophylactic anticoagulation. *British Journal of Obstetrics and Gynaecology* 1977; **84**: 309–11.

370 Vardi J & Fields GA. Microangiopathic hemolytic anemia in severe pre-eclampsia. *American Journal of Obstetrics and Gynecology* 1974; **119**: 617–22.

371 Vink GJ & Moodley J. The effect of low-dose dihydralazine on the fetus in the emergency treatment of hypertension in pregnancy. *South African Medical Journal* 1982; **62**: 475–7.

372 Vink GJ, Moodley J & Philpott RH. Effect of dihydralazine on the fetus in the treatment of maternal hypertension. *Obstetrics and Gynecology* 1980; **55**: 519–22.

373 Visser W & Wallenburg HCS. Central hemodynamic observations in untreated preeclamptic patients. *Hypertension* 1991; **17**: 1072–7.

374 Vosburgh GJ. Blood pressure, edema and proteinuria in pregnancy-edema relationships. *Progress in Clinical and Biological Research* 1976; **7**: 155–68.

375 Waisman GD, Mayorga LM, Camera MI, Vignolo CA & Martinotti A. Magnesium plus nifedipine: potentiation of hypotensive effect in preeclampsia? *American Journal of Obstetrics and Gynecology* 1988; **159**: 308–9.

376 Wallenburg HCS, Dekker GA, Makovitz JW & Rotmans P. Low-dose aspirin prevents pregnancy-induced hypertension and pre-eclampsia in angiotensin-sensitive primigravidae. *Lancet* 1986; **i**: 1–3.

377 Wallenburg HCS & Hutchinson DL. A radioangiographic study of the effects of catecholamines on uteroplacental blood flow in the rhesus monkey. *Journal of Medical Primatology* 1979; **8**: 57–65.

378 Wallenburg HCS, Stolte LAM & Janssens J. The pathogenesis of placental infarction I. A morphologic study in the human placenta. *American Journal of Obstetrics and Gynecology* 1973; **116**: 835–40.

379 Walters BNJ & Redman CWG. Treatment of severe pregnancy-associated hypertension with the calcium antagonist nifedipine. *British Journal of Obstetrics and Gynaecology* 1984; **91**: 330–6.

380 Walters BNJ, Thompson ME, Lee A & de Swiet M. Blood pressure in the puerperium. *Clinical Science* 1986; **71**: 589–94.

381 Walters WAW. Effects of sustained maternal hypertension on fetal growth and survival. *Lancet* 1966; **ii**: 1214–17.

382 Walters WAW, MacGregor WG & Hills M. Cardiac output at rest during pregnancy and the puerperium. *Clinical Science* 1966; **30**: 1–11.

383 Wang YP, Walsh SW, Guo JD & Zhang JY. The imbalance between thromboxane and prostacyclin in preeclampsia is associated with an imbalance between lipid peroxides and vitamin E in maternal blood. *American Journal of Obstetrics and Gynecology* 1991; **165**: 1695–700.

384 Wardle EN & Wright NA. Role of fibrin in a model of pregnancy toxemia in the rabbit. *American Journal of Obstetrics and Gynecology* 1973; **115**: 17–26.

385 Wasserstrum N, Kirshon B, Rossavik IK, Willis RS. Moise JJ & Cotton DB. Implications of sino-aortic baroreceptor reflex dysfunction in severe preeclampsia. *Obstetrics and Gynecology* 1989; **74**: 34–9.

386 Wasserstrum N, Kirshon B, Willis RS, Moise KJJ & Cotton DB. Quantitative hemodynamic effects of acute volume expansion in severe preeclampsia. *Obstetrics and Gynecology* 1989; **73**: 546–50.

387 Watson DL, Sibai BM, Shaver DC, Dacus JV & Anderson GD. Late postpartum eclampsia: an update. *Southern Medical Journal* 1983; **76**: 1487–9.

388 Weiner CP, Kwaan HC, Chu XUC, Paul M, Burmeister L & Hauck W. Antithrombin III activity in women with hypertension during pregnancy. *Obstetrics and Gynecology* 1985; **65**: 301–6.

389 Weinstein L. Syndrome of hemolysis, elevated liver enzymes, low platelet count: a severe consequence of hypertension on pregnancy. *American Journal of Obstetrics and Gynecology* 1982; **142**: 159–67.

390 Weisman Y, Harell A, Edelstein S, David M, Spirer Z & Golander A. 1 alpha, 25-dihydroxyvitamin D3 and 24,25-dihydroxyvitamin D3 *in vitro* synthesis by human decidua and placenta. *Nature* 1979; **281**: 317–19.

391 Whigham KAE, Howie PW, Drummond AH & Prentice CRM. Abnormal platelet function in pre-eclampsia. *British Journal of Obstetrics and Gynaecology* 1978; **85**: 28–32.

392 Whitelaw A. Maternal methyldopa treatment and neonatal blood pressure. *British Medical Journal* 1981; **283**: 471.

393 Wiggers CJ. Dynamic patterns induced by compression of an artery. *Circulation Research* 1956; **4**: 4–7.

394 Williams MA, Lieberman E, Mittendorf R, Monson RR & Schoenbaum SC. Risk factors for abruptio placentae. *American Journal of Epidemiology* 1991; **134**: 965–72.

395 Willocks J & Moir D. Epidural analgesia in the management of hypertension in labour. *Journal of Obstetrics and Gynaecology of the British Commonwealth* 1968; **75**: 225–8.

396 Woods LL. Importance of prostaglandins in hypertension during reduced uteroplacental perfusion pressure. *American Journal of Physiology* 1989; **257**: R1558–61.

397 Zabriskie JR. Effect of cigarette smoking during pregnancy. Study of 2000 cases. *Obstetrics and Gynecology* 1963; **21**: 405–11.

398 Zech P, Rifle G, Lindner A, Sassard J, Blanc-Brunat N & Traeger J. Malignant hypertension with irreversible renal failure due to oral contraceptives. *British Medical Journal* 1975; **iv**: 326–7.

399 Zeek PM & Assali NS. Vascular changes with eclamptogenic toxemia of pregnancy. *American Journal of Clinical Pathology* 1950; **20**: 1099–109.

400 Zinaman M, Rubin J & Lindheimer MD. Serial plasma oncotic pressure levels and echoencephalography during and after delivery in severe pre-eclampsia. *Lancet* 1985; **i**: 1245–7.

Further reading

Chesley LC. Vascular reactivity in normal and toxemic pregnancy. *Clinical Obstetrics and Gynecology* 1966; **9**: 871–81.

Chesley LC & Annitto JE. Pregnancy in the patient with hypertensive disease. *American Journal of Obstetrics and Gynecology* 1947; **53**: 372–81.

Clarke HGM, Freeman T & Pryse-Phillips W. Serum proteins in normal pregnancy and mild pre-eclampsia. *Journal of Obstetrics and Gynaecology of the British Commonwealth* 1971; **78**: 105–9.

Page EW & Christianson R. The impact of mean arterial pressure in the middle trimester upon the outcome of pregnancy. *American Journal of Obstetrics and Gynecology* 1976; **125**: 740–6.

Sibai BM, Gonzalez AR, Mabie WC & Moretti M. A comparison of labetalol plus hospitalization versus hospitalization alone in the management of pre-eclampsia remote from term. *Obstetrics and Gynecology* 1987; **70**: 323–7.

7

Renal Disease

John Davison & Christine Baylis

The kidney in normal pregnancy, 227
- Anatomical changes
- Functional changes
- Physiological consequences of altered renal haemodynamics

Chronic renal disease and pregnancy, 233
- Pathophysiology of renal dysfunction
- Pre-pregnancy counselling
- Renal function and the impact of pregnancy
- Management of chronic renal disease in pregnancy
- Diagnosis during pregnancy
- Decisions regarding treatment of hypertension
- Fetal surveillance
- Decisions regarding delivery
- Specific problems in relation to certain types of renal disease

Asymptomatic bacteriuria, 254
- Diagnostic pitfalls
- Clinical implications

Acute symptomatic urinary tract infection, 258
- Acute cystitis
- Acute pyelonephritis

Haematuria during pregnancy, 259

Acute hydronephrosis and hydroureter, 260
- Non-traumatic rupture of the urinary tract

Pregnancy in renal transplant patients, 261
- Pregnancy counselling
- Management of renal transplant recipient in pregnancy
- Immunosuppressive therapy during pregnancy
- Decisions regarding delivery
- Paediatric management
- Postnatal assessment and long-term maternal follow-up
- Potential long-term paediatric problems

Pregnancy in haemodialysis patients, 274
- Pregnancy counselling
- General management plan

Pregnancy in patients on peritoneal dialysis, 276

Acute renal failure, 277
- Perspective
- Pathology
- Phases of acute renal failure
- Diagnosis and investigation
- Diagnostic pitfalls
- General management plan

Acute renal failure and septic shock, 281
- Pathology
- Diagnosis and investigation
- Diagnostic pitfalls
- General management plan

Acute renal failure in pre-eclampsia/eclampsia, 284

Acute renal failure and pyelonephritis, 285

Haemolytic uraemia syndrome, 285
- Pathophysiology and diagnosis
- Treatment and outcome

Bilateral renal cortical necrosis in pregnancy, 286

Miscellaneous causes of renal failure, 286

Obstetric renal failure: some conclusions, 286

Women with renal problems often consult the clinician on the advisability of becoming pregnant or continuing a pregnancy already in progress. When counselling such women, emotions must not be allowed to override objectivity and this requires knowledge of the physiological changes which occur during normal pregnancy and of the various pitfalls in the detection and diagnosis of obstetric renal problems. In some areas accurate information is lacking from clinical practice and animal models have therefore been carefully developed in order to examine rigorously the mechanisms controlling the altered renal function of normal pregnancy as well as the long-term consequences of pregnancy in health and disease. Therefore, this chapter first summarizes the changes that occur in the urinary tract in pregnancy, including data derived from animal models, and then discusses the management of problems associated with chronic renal disease.

The kidney in normal pregnancy

Anatomical changes

The kidney increases approximately 1 cm in length during normal pregnancy. More striking, however, are the anatomical changes in the calyces, renal pelvis and ureter, which dilate markedly, often giving the erroneous impression of obstructive uropathy [18,366,402].

By the third trimester some 80 per cent of women show evidence of stasis or hydronephrosis [87, 189], with fetal pyelectasis more likely to occur in such women. Dilatation is more pronounced in the right than in the left urinary tract at all stages of pregnancy perhaps related to the customary dextro-rotation of the uterus. Ultrasound studies suggest that renal parenchymal volumes also increase during pregnancy [39] probably the result of increases in intrarenal fluid [84,144]. It appears that an increment of some 70 per cent has occurred by the beginning of the third trimester with a slight reduction during the last weeks of pregnancy [88].

These anatomical changes have important clinical implications.

1 Dilatation of the urinary tract may lead to collection errors in tests based on timed urine volume (e.g. 24-hour creatinine or protein excretion).

2 Urinary stasis within the ureters may predispose pregnant women with asymptomatic bacteriuria to develop acute symptomatic pyelonephritis.

3 Acceptable norms of kidney size should be increased by 1 cm if estimated during pregnancy or immediately after delivery. Since dilatation of the ureters persists into the puerperium elective radiological examination of the urinary tract should be deferred until at least 16 weeks after delivery.

4 Rarely the changes may be extreme and precipitate the 'overdistension syndrome' (see below) and/or hypertension [413].

Functional changes

Renal haemodynamic changes in normal pregnancy

When a woman becomes pregnant her glomerular filtration rate (GFR) increases by about 50 per cent (Fig. 7.1), reaching the maximum at the end of the

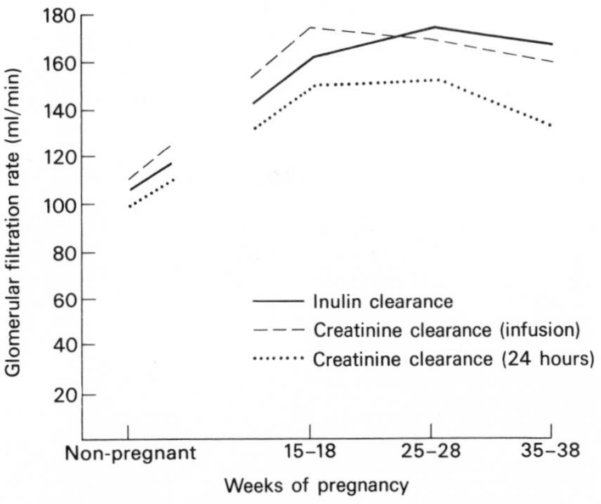

Fig. 7.1. Mean GFR in 10 healthy women during pregnancy and 8–12 weeks after delivery (non-pregnant). (Modified from [122].)

first trimester and is maintained at this augmented level until at least the 36th gestational week [121, 122]. Since GFR increases less than renal plasma flow (RPF) during early pregnancy, the ratio of GFR : RPF, the filtration fraction (FF) decreases. Late pregnancy is associated with an increase in FF to values similar to the non-pregnant norm [164].

Endogenous 24-hour creatinine clearance is a convenient, non-invasive method which measures GFR when inulin infusion studies are impracticable. Studies performed at weekly intervals after conception have shown that 24-hour creatinine clearance increases by 25 per cent 4 weeks after the last menstrual period and by 45 per cent at 9 weeks [127] (see Fig. 7.2). During the third trimester a consistent and significant decrease towards non-pregnant values occurs preceding delivery [129] and daily measurements post-partum have suggested a small transient increase during the first few days of the puerperium [121].

In the rat, pregnancy lasts 22 days and GFR increases early to a maximum (+30–40 per cent) which is maintained throughout pregnancy, until near term when a return towards non-pregnant values is evident [198]. The rise in GFR is paralleled by an increase in RPF due to a fall in renal vascular resistance (RVR) which reaches a nadir by mid-pregnancy. The pressures and flows at the glom-

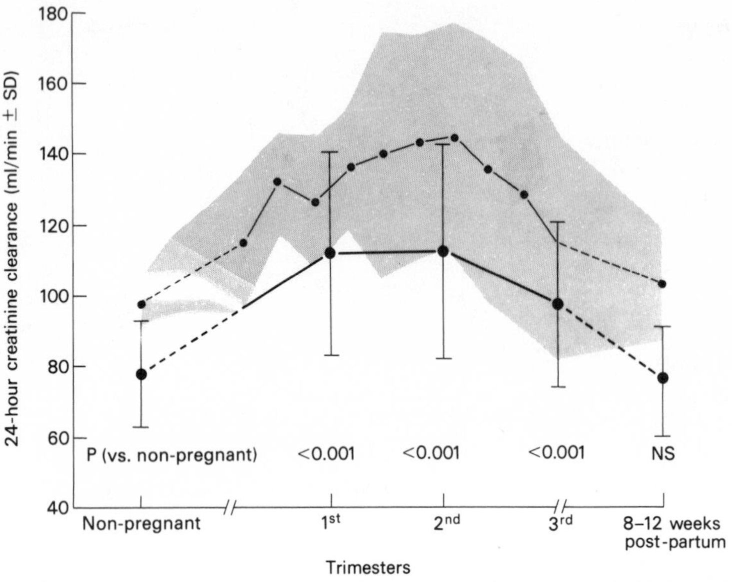

Fig. 7.2. ● Serial 24-hour creatinine clearances (mean ± 1 SD) during pregnancy complicated by chronic renal disease. Thirty-three pregnancies of 26 women studied preconception, each trimester and 8–12 weeks after delivery. Measurements from 10 healthy women (mean ± 1 SD) shown by shaded area (•). (From [246].)

erulus that determine GFR of a single nephron (SNGFR) are controlled by the tone of the pre-glomerular (afferent) and post-glomerular (efferent) resistance vessels. The ratio of the tone of these resistances determines the glomerular blood pressure, P_{GC}, which is directly related to SNGFR. The overall level of tone controls glomerular plasma flow, which is also directly related to SNGFR. Micropuncture studies allow measurement of SNGFR and all its determinants and in the pregnant rat show 30 per cent increases in superficial cortical SNGFR by mid-pregnancy. This is the result exclusively of a proportional increase in glomerular plasma flow, since the oncotic pressure of systemic blood, (π_A), the intraglomerular hydrostatic pressure, P_{GC}, the glomerular hydrostatic pressure gradient (dP) and the glomerular capillary ultrafiltration coefficient, K_f (the product of filtration surface area and water permeability), are unchanged by mid-pregnancy and therefore do not contribute to the gestational rise in SNGFR. Micropuncture studies show no sustained rise in P_{GC} in pregnant Munich–Wistar rats [26,27,28,30], despite the renal vasodilatation of pregnancy, due to close proportionality in the declines in pre-glomerular and efferent arteriolar resistances.

In normal human pregnancy computer simulation of the glomerulus using theoretical models of hindered solute transport that represent the capillary wall as a heteroporous membrane suggests that P_{GC} is unchanged [132,135]. Thus all the evidence points to the increased GFR being due entirely to the increment in RPF.

Renal ultrasound assessment in the human, with colour flow mapping displays a real-time map of the mean Doppler shift within blood vessels on a colour overlay on the B-mode image. Analysis of waveforms from interlobar and interlobular arteries have failed to reveal any change in pregnancy, which is surprising as the large increments in renal blood flow are thought to be due to reduced renal vascular resistances [450]. It is likely, however, that waveform pulsatility reflects an interaction of several haemodynamic factors many of which are altered during pregnancy. As yet it is not yet possible to access the individual effect on renal waveform variation of changes in maternal heart rate, stroke volume, blood pressure and blood flow because alterations in one variable affects the others. Haemodynamic modelling suggests that pulsatility (as indexed by pulsatility index and A:B ratio) correlates closely with vascular resistance [280], an effect that is independent of flow and pressure, but the relationship has not been specifically tested for the unique conditions of the renal circulation in pregnancy.

INITIATION OF GESTATIONAL RENAL CHANGES

The causes of the renal and peripheral vasodilatation and of the plasma volume expansion of pregnancy remain unknown although it has been suggested that the primary change is a fall in total peripheral resistance which creates an underfill signal, thus stimulating sodium retention and plasma volume expansion [420]. However, this view is not universally accepted because animal evidence indicates that plasma volume expansion in early pregnancy occurs in the absence of renal sodium retention and must be due to redistribution of fluids between body fluid compartments [40] with renal sodium retention only evident later on in pregnancy [86, 289]. Also, increased RPF and GFR occur early in both human and rodent pregnancy so renal vasodilatation may precede peripheral vasodilatation [31] and the increases can be dissociated from the plasma volume expansion [386]. Maternal influence must initiate the renal vasodilatation and plasma volume expansion of pregnancy, since the pseudopregnant rat, in whom the fetoplacental unit is absent, also undergoes a renal vasodilatation and plasma volume expansion [28].

Functional characteristics of the renal vasculature in pregnancy

RENAL AUTOREGULATION DURING PREGNANCY

The kidney is able to maintain blood flow and GFR over a range of blood pressure (i.e. autoregulation) mainly by variations in pre-glomerular arteriolar tone [352]. In rats and rabbits, with renal blood flow and GFR elevated, renal autoregulatory ability is similar in pregnant and virgin [387,497], thus gestational renal vasodilation does not alter this intrinsic renal characteristic. The fall in blood pressure in late pregnancy in rats does not impair autoregulation of renal blood flow and there may be a downward re-setting in the 'threshold' [387] which could protect the kidney at this time from periods of renal hypoperfusion.

RESPONSIVENESS OF THE RENAL VASCULATURE IN PREGNANCY

In normal non-pregnant humans and animals, a protein meal or an amino acid infusion elicit substantial increases in GFR due to a selective renal vasodilatation with increased RPF [57,77,215,332]. The mid-pregnant rat, which exhibits the maximal gestational renal vasodilatation, responds to an acute amino acid infusion with further substantial rises in both GFR and SNGFR, due solely to further increases in plasma flow [32].

In the human, observations have been conflicting. One group observed a substantial rise in creatinine clearance following a meat meal [60] and others demonstrated marginal increments in inulin and *para*-aminohippuric acid (PAH) clearances [24]. Healthy pregnant women, in response to intravenous amino acids, however, do show a marked renal vasodilatory response [451]. Overall, therefore the kidneys in pregnancy do possess a significant reserve of vasodilatory capacity despite a state of chronic renal vasodilatation.

RESPONSES TO VASOACTIVE HORMONES

Various hormone systems may play roles in mediating these gestational changes. Increased urinary prostaglandin and prostacyclin levels have been reported in pregnant women and rats [99,166] but there is also evidence against prostaglandins mediating the gestational rise in GFR [30,99]. The renin/angiotensin II (AII) system is greatly modified with increases in plasma renin activity and plasma AII and decreased responsivity to administered AII [25,179,361]. Whether this loss of sensitivity to the vasoconstrictor actions of AII extends to the renal resistance vessels and the glomerulus is not certain but there are animal studies which indicate that renal resistance vessels and glomerular AII receptors are as responsive as in the non-pregnant state [326]. Of importance, however, renal haemodynamics in normal unstressed pregnant and non-pregnant rats are not dependent on AII [37,45], thus loss of renal responsivity to AII cannot be the mechanism of the renal vasodilatation of pregnancy and furthermore, the close to term fall in GFR and RPF is not mediated by AII [37]. Although peripheral responsivity to administered norepinephrine (NE) and arginine vasopressin (AVP) is also reduced during pregnancy [25,99,361] these systems have not been extensively studied with regard to control of renal haemodynamics. Acute α_1 adrenoceptor blockade has similar depressor and renal vasoconstrictor effects in non-pregnant and pregnant rats [34] and blockade of the vascular AVP (V_1) receptor has no renal haemodynamic or blood pressure effects in pregnancy [35].

Vascular responsiveness to atrial natriuretic peptide (ANP) is unchanged during pregnancy [269,347] but normal women show moderate increases in plasma ANP during the second and third trimesters [73]. ANP is, however, unlikely to be involved in the renal vasodilatation of pregnancy since although pharmacological doses of ANP increase GFR, this is by a complex mechanism which includes *increases* in efferent resistance and P_{GC} [145] a pattern which differs from the glomerular haemodynamic alterations of normal pregnancy [31]. Also, non-pregnant and pregnant rats, have similar renal haemodynamic responses to administered ANP but the pregnant animal is refractory to its natriuretic effects [326].

RENAL VASODILATORY CAPACITY

The mechanism(s) causing renal vasodilatation, decreased total peripheral resistance, refractoriness to pressor agents and plasma volume expansion of normal pregnancy remain elusive. A recently discovered endothelial control system has major impacts on the physiological regulation of blood pressure and renal function: vascular endothelium makes an endothelial derived relaxing factor (EDRF), nitric oxide (NO), which acts via cyclic guanosine monophosphate (cGMP) [339]. Vascular endothelial cells contain a constitutive NO synthase that continually produces a basal release of NO [339] which controls peripheral resistance and blood pressure, both by direct vasodilatory actions and by blunting the responsiveness to vasoconstrictor factors [339]. A number of studies have investigated whether enhanced production of and/or sensitivity to NO occurs in normal pregnancy, causing the decrease peripheral resistance and/or blunted responsiveness to pressor agents. It is known that plasma and urinary levels of cGMP (NO second messenger) increase during pregnancy in women and rats and urinary cGMP increases in pseudopregnant rats [100], which probably reflects increased tissue production of cGMP since metabolic clearance rate is unaffected [100]. In guinea pigs, *in vitro* studies suggest enhancement of agonist-stimulated NO in pregnancy [487] and *in vitro* and *in vivo* studies suggest that NO is responsible for the pregnancy-associated refractoriness to administered vasoconstrictors [338,488]. In contrast, acute systemic NO blockade in late pregnant rats produces similar increases in blood pressure and bradycardia as in non-pregnancy [474]; however, these rats did not show the normal late fall in BP. Also, NO activity is similar in isolated thoracic aortic segments from pregnant and non-pregnant rats [444].

In non-pregnant animals, NO plays a major physiological role in control of renal function [38,405]. Acute systemic NO blockade in the conscious male rat produces profound renal vasoconstriction, a fall in RPF and a smaller fall in GFR [38]. Micropuncture studies [136] have shown complex glomerular haemodynamic changes with an increase in P_{GC} and fall in K_f suggesting that segmental arteriolar resistances and mesangial cell tone are tonically controlled by NO in the normal kidney. There are regional differences in NO control of vascular beds and the kidney is particularly sensitive, since falls in renal cortical blood flow occur with low doses of NO inhibitors which fail to influence blood pressure [371,482]. In pregnancy the chronic NO blockade model of hypertension shows no plasma volume expansion, no mid-term renal vasodilatation and no late fall in blood pressure. Also, proteinuria develops and there are poor maternal and fetal outcomes compared to normal animals [39]. These observations suggest that an intact NO system is necessary for expression of the antihypertensive effect of pregnancy.

Physiological consequences of altered renal haemodynamics

Since GFR increases without substantial alterations in the production of creatinine and urea, plasma levels of these solutes decrease. Creatinine levels change from a non-pregnant value of 73 μmol/l to 60, 54 and 64 μmol/l in successive trimesters (Table 7.1).

Average plasma urea levels are 3.5, 3.3 and 3.1 mmol/l in successive trimesters, rising to 4.3 mmol/l 6 weeks post-partum. Urea levels can be reported in a number of different ways; results may be given as either plasma (or serum) or whole blood levels, the latter being 10 per cent below plasma levels. Some of the fall in plasma urea may be due to reduced protein degradation as well as increased clearance of this solute.

Normal pregnancy induces relative hypouricaemia. Plasma urate concentrations decrease by over 25 per cent as early as week 8 of pregnancy, but increase again during the third trimester to attain levels close to the non-pregnant mean. The main reason for this is alteration in the renal handling of urate which, although freely filtered, is subsequently so actively re-absorbed that only about 10 per cent of the original filtered load appears in the urine. Later in pregnancy the kidney appears to excrete an even smaller proportion of the filtered urate load and it is this increase in net reabsorption that is associated with an increase in plasma urate concentration [76].

A number of other changes in normal pregnancy, [452] including increased excretion of nutrients, calcium (along with an inhibitor of crystalluria) and protein, are due to alterations in tubular function as well as augmented renal haemodynamics [114, 115]. Recently, it has been suggested that urinary protein excretion changes little if at all during pregnancy [27].

Plasma osmolality is markedly reduced (by 8–10 mosmol/l) from the early weeks of pregnancy [133] but this is not associated with the water diuresis which would occur in the non-pregnant individual. Whilst the process of osmoregulation is effective during pregnancy, it is now clear that there are important changes in the osmotic thresholds which trigger control mechanisms such as the sensation of thirst and the release of the antidiuretic hormone, arginine vasopressin (AVP) [133,134]. Other changes include a substantial increase in the metabolic clearance rate (MCR) of AVP, which rises fourfold after the first trimester, paralleling the appearance of, and marked increases in, circulating levels of a placental enzyme vasopressinase (also called oxytocinase), which is a cystine aminopeptidase capable of inactivating large quantities of AVP *in vitro*. The MCR of 1-deamino-8-D-AVP (desmopressin acetate, dDAVP), an analogue of vasopressin that is resistant to degradation by vasopressinase, is unaltered during pregnancy, suggesting that the aminopeptidase enzymes are also active *in vivo* [132,305].

Clinical consequences of functional changes

It is important to realize the extent to which the

Table 7.1. Changes in common indices of renal function during pregnancy (mean ± SD)

	Non-pregnant	First trimester	Second trimester	Third trimester
Effective renal plasma flow (ml/min)	480 ± 72	841 ± 144	891 ± 279	771 ± 175
Glomerular filtration rate (ml/min)				
Inulin clearance	105 ± 24	162 ± 19	174 ± 24	165 ± 22
24-h creatinine clearance	98 ± 8	151 ± 11	154 ± 15	129 ± 10
Plasma				
Creatinine (μmol/l)	73 ± 10	60 ± 8	54 ± 10	64 ± 9
Urea (mmol/l)	4.3 ± 0.8	3.5 ± 0.7	3.3 ± 0.8	3.1 ± 0.7
Urate (μmol/l)	246 ± 59	189 ± 48	214 ± 71	269 ± 56
Osmolality (mosmol/kg)	290 ± 2.2	280 ± 3.4	279 ± 2.9	279 ± 5.0

(From [121,122,127,129,133,143,144,294,452].)

dramatic alterations in physiological norms may affect clinical interpretation in pregnancy (see Figs 7.1, 7.2 and 7.3 and Table 7.1).

1 Values considered normal in non-pregnant women may reflect decreased renal function during pregnancy. Plasma levels of creatinine and urea exceeding 75 μmol/l and 4.5 mmol/l, respectively, should alert the clinician to investigate renal function further.

2 Urate concentration is significantly higher in pregnancies complicated by pre-eclampsia. Above a critical blood level of 350 μmol/l there is significant excess perinatal mortality in hypertensive patients and serial measurements can be used to monitor progress in pre-eclampsia (see Chapter 6). It must be remembered, however, that physiological variability can be such that some healthy women have high blood levels without problems and that single random measurements are of no use clinically [294].

3 Glycosuria in pregnancy reflects an alteration in renal physiology and does not necessarily signify hyperglycaemia [121].

4 Increased urinary protein excretion should not be considered abnormal until it exceeds 500 mg in 24 hours [115] and increasing proteinuria in women with chronic renal disease does not necessarily signify deterioration.

5 The osmoregulatory changes must be taken into account when managing women with known central diabetes insipidus (DI) (see Chapter 13) and when diagnosing the rare syndrome of 'transient diabetes insipidus of pregnancy', which usually presents during the second half of pregnancy and remits post-partum [23] (see Chapter 13).

Long-term significance of augmented renal haemodynamics

In animal models and in humans sustained increments in GFR — whether induced by excessive protein intake, hyperglycaemia, partial renal ablation or compensatory changes in the remaining glomeruli of kidneys with renal disease — can cause progressive glomerular injury [61]. The so-called hyper-filtration can be due to an increase in renal plasma flow or in glomerular capillary hydraulic pressure, or in both. It has been suggested that it is sustained glomerular hypertension that actually initiates the structural damage or sclerosis. There is, however, no agreement on what constitutes a reliable clinical marker of such glomerular damage. In diabetes mellitus for example, GFR can be considerably augmented [440] and long-term renal impairment is known to occur [216], but neither microalbuminuria which fluctuates considerably, nor albumin to creatinine ratios necessarily change significantly, and long-term improvement in metabolic control may have no effect.

Could the glomerular hyperfusion of pregnancy lead to similar progressive nephropathy? The augmented GFR of pregnancy is probably due exclusively to an increase in glomerular plasma flow, without coexistent glomerular hypertension and the evidence so far, albeit limited, argues against hyperfiltration sclerosis in normal pregnancy. A study of glomerular function and morphology in rats revealed no sustained increase in P_{GC}, no loss of nephrons, no persistent proteinuria and no morphological change in animals which had completed five consecutive cycles of pregnancy and lactation (a long period in the lifespan of this species), when compared with age-matched virgin controls [42].

Data are limited for human pregnancy [118,123]. There is certainly an increase in total protein excretion [111] and a small increase in albumin excretion particularly during the third trimester and early puerperium [311], changes related to altered tubular and probably not glomerular function. Recently, Wright *et al.* [498,499], although unable to detect an overall increase in albumin excretion during normal pregnancy, reported that ratios between clearances and urinary concentrations of albumin and creatinine increased progressively throughout pregnancy. The same group of workers have also suggested that these changes may indicate altered glomerular function and are more marked in women of high than of low parity, approximately matched for age. These results, however, were based upon urine collections during the afternoon, a protocol which must give rise to reservations about the validity of creatinine clearance estimations [144].

With the exception of the aforementioned report the consensus is that there is no irreversible deterioration in renal function during normal pregnancy or as a result of successive pregnancies, whether assessed by 24-hour creatinine clearance, by inulin clearance or by total protein excretion [115,117]. Furthermore women studied in consecutive pregnancies show similar GFR increments in the later compared with the first pregnancy and it is known that women do not show any tendency for GFR to decline during the reproductive years; overall they show far less of an age-dependent decline than men [68].

This important area has been reviewed elsewhere [31] and further investigation is needed. The clinical implications of the effect of pregnancy on glomerular physiology in the presence of chronic renal pathology are discussed later.

Volume homeostasis

Healthy women eating an unrestricted diet gain an average of 12.5 kg during their first pregnancy and 11.5 kg in subsequent pregnancies. Until fairly recently, clinicians regarded published averages as the upper limits of permissible weight gain, forgetting that there is a plus as well as a minus to deviations about a mean. Consequently many pregnant women were admonished for excessive weight gain and their intakes of calories, sodium or both were needlessly restricted.

The increase in weight is largely fluid, total body water increasing by 6–8 l, 4–6 l of which are extracellular [81,300]. There is also cumulative retention of approximately 900 mmol of sodium distributed between the products of conception and the maternal extracellular space. This accumulation occurs gradually and even in late pregnancy, the period of most rapid maternal weight gain, the amount retained is only 3–4 mmol/day, which is too small to be detected by conventional balance techniques.

Most of the maternally sequestered sodium is located in the extracellular space. Plasma volume increases by 40–50 per cent, starting in the first trimester, accelerating to a peak in the second and remaining elevated until near term (see Chapter 2). However, increases in maternal interstitial volume (as well as fetal storage of sodium) are greatest in the third trimester. The increase in maternal plasma volume and interstitial space constitute a physiological hypervolaemia (Fig. 7.3). However, the mother's volume receptors sense these changes as normal; when salt restriction or diuretic therapy limits the expansion, the maternal response resembles that of salt-depleted non-pregnant subjects. Whether or not the increases in the fluid spaces are 'necessary' remains to be elucidated, but this seems to be likely, since failure of plasma volume to increase appropriately has been correlated with poor reproductive performance [300].

Chronic renal disease and pregnancy

Pregnancy will usually end successfully if there is no significant hypertension or overt renal insufficiency prior to conception. If hypertension is present and it requires more than one drug for control than obstetric success is substantially reduced. There is no evidence that pregnancy accelerates the progress of renal disease.

Pathophysiology of renal dysfunction

To assess pregnancy and its altered renal physiology

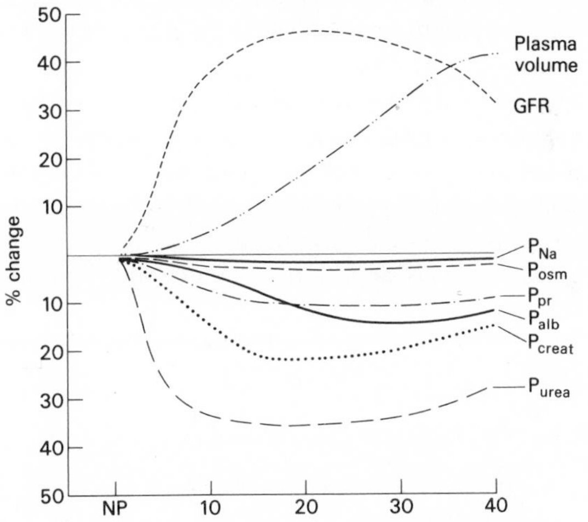

Fig. 7.3. Physiological changes induced by pregnancy. Increments and decrements in various parameters are shown in percentage terms with reference to the non-pregnant baseline. GFR, glomerular filtration rate; P_{Na}, plasma sodium; P_{osm}, plasma osmolality; P_{pr}, plasma proteins; P_{alb}, plasma albumin; P_{creat}, plasma creatinine; P_{urea}, plasma urea; NP, non-pregnant; 10–40, weeks of pregnancy.

in the presence of chronic renal disease it is necessary to understand what happens when nephron mass has been lost. The relationship between plasma creatinine concentration, creatinine clearance (GFR) and nephron population shown in Fig. 7.4 reveals that an individual may lose about 50 per cent of renal function and still have a plasma creatinine <130 μmol/l. However, if renal function is more severely compromised then a small decrease in GFR causes a marked increase in plasma creatinine. Nevertheless, a patient who has lost 75 per cent of her nephrons may have only lost 50 per cent of function and may have a deceptively normal plasma creatinine. Thus evaluation of renal function should be based on the clearance of creatinine rather than on its plasma concentration.

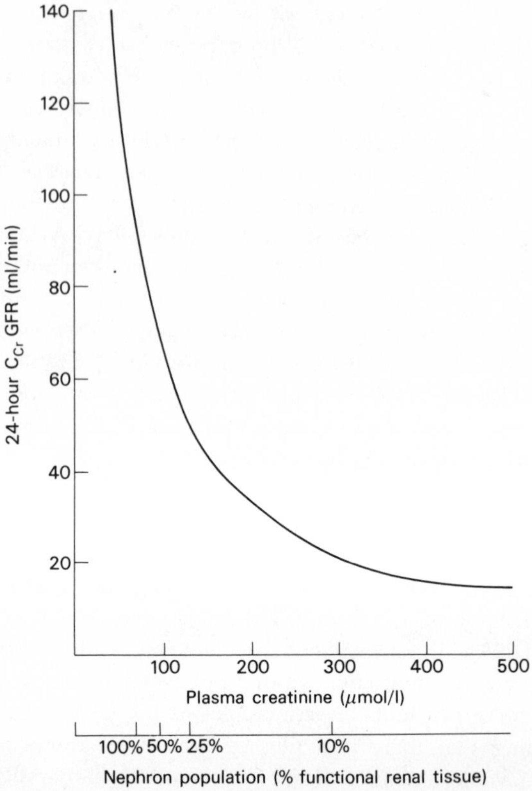

Fig. 7.4. Relationship of clearance of creatinine (GFR) in ml/min to plasma creatinine concentration (μmol/l) and nephron population (per cent) assuming a constant 24-hour creatinine excretion of about 11.5 mmol. (Non-pregnant data: J. Davison, unpublished observations.)

Pre-pregnancy counselling (see Box 7.1)

In patients with renal disease, pathology may be both clinically and biochemically silent. Most individuals remain symptom-free until their GFR falls to <25 per cent of its original level. Many plasma constituents are frequently normal until a late stage of the disease.

As renal function declines so does the ability to conceive and to sustain a viable pregnancy. Degrees of impairment that do not cause symptoms or appear to disrupt homeostasis in non-pregnant individuals, can jeopardize pregnancy. Normal pregnancy is rare when non-pregnant plasma creatinine and urea levels exceed 275 μmol/l and 10 mmol/l, respectively. These increments above normal non-pregnant levels appear trivial, but they represent decrements in function of more than 50 per cent (Fig. 7.4).

Assessment of a patient with chronic renal disease presents two basic and often conflicting issues: fetal prognosis and the maternal prognosis, both during pregnancy and in the long term. These issues must be carefully weighed and this delicate 'balance' is illustrated in Fig. 7.5.

Box 7.1. Pre-pregnancy counselling

- Type of chronic renal disease under consideration
- General health considerations
- Diastolic BP <80 mmHg
- Renal function:
  - Plasma creatinine <250 μmol/l
  - Plasma urea <10 mmol/l
  - Presence or absence of proteinuria
- Need to review pre-pregnancy drug therapy

Renal function and the impact of pregnancy

Because of the different obstetric and remote prognoses in women with different degrees of renal insufficiency, the impact of pregnancy should be considered by categories of functional renal status prior to conception (Table 7.2).

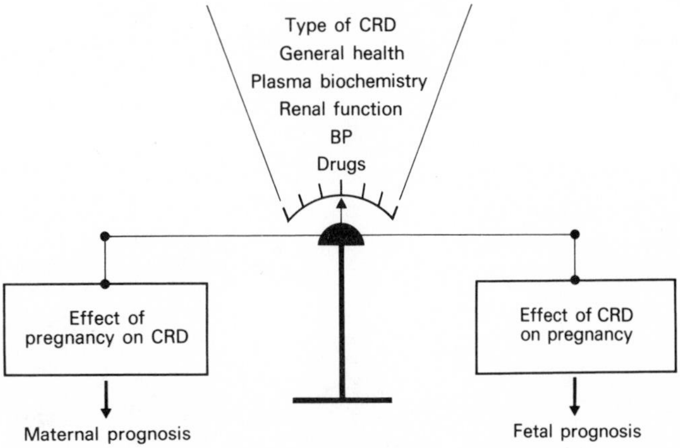

Fig. 7.5. Pregnancy and chronic renal disease (CRD) depicting the balance between maternal and fetal prognosis and the role of factors such as the type of CRD, the degree of renal insufficiency, the presence or absence of hypertension and the type of drug therapy that is needed.

Table 7.2. Pre-pregnancy renal functional status

Classification	Plasma creatinine (μmol/l)
Preserved/mildly impaired renal function	≤125
Moderate renal insufficiency	≥125
Severe renal insufficiency	≥250

Preserved/mildly impaired renal function

Women with chronic renal disease, but normal or mildly decreased pre-pregnancy renal function (plasma creatinine <125 μmol/l), usually have a successful obstetric outcome and pregnancy does not adversely affect the course of their disease [1, 2, 3, 4, 19, 48, 110, 165, 169, 204, 229, 238, 242, 246, 248, 262, 283, 446, 454, 489] (Table 7.3 and Fig. 7.6).

Although true for most patients, some authors suggest that this statement be tempered somewhat in lupus nephropathy, membranoproliferative glomerulonephritis, focal glomerular sclerosis and perhaps IgA and reflux nephropathies, which appear more sensitive to intercurrent pregnancy [301].

Most show increments in GFR, but less than those of normal pregnant women. Increased proteinuria is common, occurring in 50 per cent of pregnancies (although rarely in women with chronic pyelonephritis), and it can be massive (often exceeding 3 g in 24 hours), with nephrotic oedema. Two recent retrospective studies emphasize several important issues: Abe [1] analysed 240 pregnancies in 166 women and Jungers *et al.* [238] 254 pregnancies in 148 women, all with biopsy-proven disease. Perinatal outcome was poor in the presence of poorly controlled hypertension, nephrotic range proteinuria in early pregnancy and/or GFR ≤70 ml/min prior to pregnancy, or in the first trimester, whatever the type of renal disease.

The prevalence of hypertension, renal functional

Table 7.3. Pregnancy prospects for women with chronic renal disease

Renal status	Plasma creatinine (μmol/l)	Problems in pregnancy (%)	Successful obstetric outcome (%)	Problems in long term (%)
Mild	≤125	26	96 (85)	<3 (9)
Moderate	≥125	47	89 (59)	25 (71)
Severe	≥250	86	46 (8)	53 (92)

Estimates based on 1902 women/2813 pregnancies (1973–1993) which attained at least 28 weeks gestation (J. Davison and C. Baylis, unpublished data). Figures in brackets refer to prospects when complications developed prior to 28 weeks gestation.

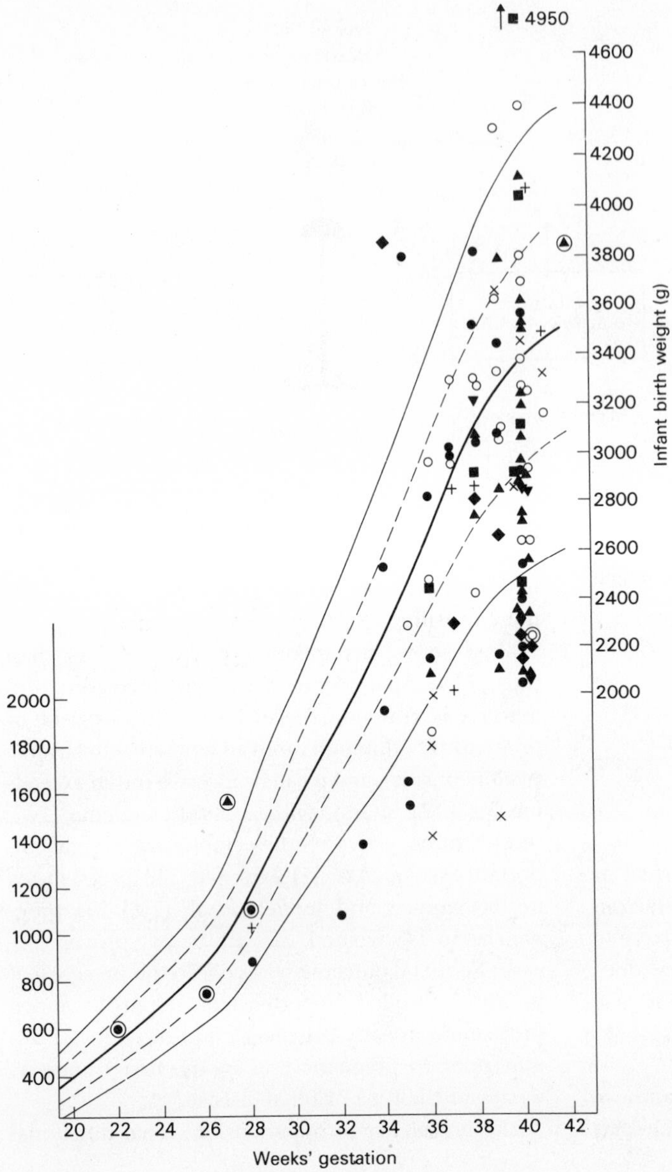

Fig. 7.6. Birthweight in relation to gestational age for 111 live births in women with chronic renal disease [246]. Lines represent mean weight ± 1 and 2 SD of 608 live births at University Hospital of Cleveland, Ohio, USA (1958–68) compiled by Dr H. Hendricks. ● Diffuse glomerulonephritis; ⦿ Diffuse glomerulonephritis + neonatal death; ▲ focal glomerulonephritis; Ⓐ focal glomerulonephritis + neonatal death; ▼ membrano-proliferative glomerulonephritis; ■ membranous nephropathy; ◆ lipoid nephrosis and focal glomerulosclerosis; ○ interstitial nephritis; ◎ interstitial nephritis + neonatal death: × arteriolar nephrosclerosis; + miscellaneous kidney disease; ◯ neonatal death. There is a high incidence of growth retardation.

abnormalities and proteinuria, as well as their severity, are considerably lower between pregnancies and during long-term follow-up. When renal failure does supervene, it usually reflects the inexorable course of a particular renal disease.

Moderate renal insufficiency

Prognosis is more guarded where renal function is moderately impaired before pregnancy (plasma creatinine 125–250 μmol/l). It is difficult to draw firm conclusions about pregnancy in these women, chiefly because the number of cases reported is still small. In one series, a high incidence of renal morbidity occurred early in pregnancy; nearly half (five of 11) developed serious deterioration of renal function culminating in terminal renal failure several months post-partum [256]. Due to this experience and the fact that apparent deterioration also was seen in an occasional patient with stable renal function, we have adopted a rather cautious approach to pregnancy in women with both mild and moderate renal disease.

Another study of the influence of pregnancy [48] revealed no immediate loss of renal function in 29 patients whose creatinine levels were <135 μmol/l. In contrast, four to eight patients with initial creatinine levels >145 μmol/l experienced significant further increases during pregnancy, which was complicated in virtually every case. Four patients in this group progressed to end stage renal failure within 18 months of delivery. It is now recognized that uncontrolled hypertension is a very important factor in the overall deterioration [147,217,218,230, 231,239,240] (Tables 7.4 and 7.5).

The customary recommendation has been that pregnancy is best avoided in women who have lost 50 per cent of their kidney function. Recent studies, however, have reopened the question [59,224]. Hou *et al.* [224] recorded a successful obstetrical outcome in 92 per cent of the pregnancies in 22 women with creatinine levels of 150–240 μmol/l, whose pregnancies were allowed to go beyond the second trimester. Many of these patients had escalating hypertension and in 25 per cent there was an accelerated decline in renal function. Cunningham *et al.* [110] had succesful obstetric outcome in 85 per cent of pregnancies in 26 women.

Severe renal insufficiency

Most women in this category (plasma creatinine >250 μmol/l) are amenorrhoeic and/or anovulatory [292]. The likelihood of conception, let alone having a normal pregnancy and delivery, is low but not, as some have been misled to believe, impossible. The risk of severe maternal complications is greater than the probability of a successful obstetric outcome [231] (see Table 7.3). Realistically, these patients should not take additional health risks. The aim should be to preserve what little renal function remains and/or to achieve renal rehabilitation via a dialysis and transplant programme, after which the question of pregnancy can be considered if appropriate.

Management of chronic renal disease in pregnancy

(see Box 7.2)

Antenatal care

There is good evidence from the studies of Katz

Table 7.4. Effect of blood pressure on pregnancy complications in 123 pregnancies in 86 women with chronic renal disease [454]

	Intrauterine growth retardation (%)	Pre-term delivery (%)	Renal deterioration (%)
Normotension	2.3	11.4	3.0
Hypertension	15.6	20.0	15.0

Table 7.5. Effect of blood pressure and/or renal deterioration on fetal mortality in 240 pregnancies in 122 women with chronic renal disease [239]

	Fetal mortality (%)		
	Hypertension	Renal deterioration	Both
Absent throughout pregnancy	18	12	10
Present at some time during pregnancy	34	27	40
Present from first trimester and controlled	20	—	—
Present from first trimester and uncontrolled	100	—	—
Present only during third trimester	12	—	—

Box 7.2. Management during pregnancy

- Type of chronic renal disease, if known
- General health considerations
- Effect of pregnancy on blood pressure
- Effect of pregnancy on renal function and plasma biochemistry
- Past obstetric history
- Use of drug therapy

et al. [246,247] and Klockars *et al.* [262] that one of the main factors in reducing maternal and perinatal morbidity and mortality is good antenatal care. The value of such care is greatly enhanced by early and regular attendance so that trends may be detected and the significance of an abnormal observation assessed when taken in context with previous observations. Where patients have chronic renal disease the following factors are important:
1 careful monitoring of blood pressure; detection of hypertension and assessment of its severity and long-term effects;
2 assessment of renal function (by 24-hour creatinine clearance and protein excretion) and also nutritional status in heavily proteinuric patients;
3 assessment of the size, development and well-being of the fetus;
4 early detection of asymptomatic bacteriuria or confirmation of urinary tract infection.

Criteria for hospital admission

As long as the antenatal course is uncomplicated the patient should be seen at 2-weekly intervals until 32 weeks gestation and then weekly thereafter. Immediate hospital admission is indicated in the following circumstances:
1 deterioration of renal function as evidenced by decrements in creatinine clearance to 20 per cent and/or the onset of proteinuria or marked increases in proteinuria which persist;
2 development of even moderate hypertension, i.e. blood pressure >140/90 on two or more occasions separated by an interval of at least 6 hours;
3 signs of intrauterine growth retardation and/or deterioration of placental function;
4 change in rate of weight gain, either cessation or excess;
5 symptomas of impending eclampsia.

Diagnosis during pregnancy

When the question of renal disease is raised for the first time during a pregnancy it is essential to try to establish a diagnosis and a course of management that will be helpful to both mother and fetus. When a patient presents with hypertension, proteinuria and/or abnormal renal function it is difficult to distinguish parenchymal renal disease from pre-eclampsia. A previous history of renal disorders, abnormal urine analysis, a family history of renal disease or a history of systemic illness known to involve the kidneys is obviously helpful, but even so parenchymal renal disease and pre-eclampsia may coexist. Also, think about the diagnosis of renal artery stenosis [210] (see Table 7.7).

The assessment of the patient and subsequent blood and urine testing are similar to those of non-pregnant patients but the definitive diagnosis usually has to wait until after delivery. Such patients should be hospitalized and their pregnancies allowed to continue if renal function and blood pressure remain stable. However, since pre-eclampsia is so serious, the pregnancy should be terminated if deterioration occurs. The use of interim haemodialysis to 'buy time' has been advocated but this is not established practice [185,335,351,358,467].

The role of renal biopsy in obstetric practice

Experience with renal biopsy in pregnancy is sparse, mainly because clinical circumstances rarely justify the minimal risks of biopsy at this time and the procedure is usually deferred to the post-partum period [298]. Reports of excessive bleeding and other complications in pregnant women have led some to consider pregnancy a relative contraindication to renal biopsy [417], although others have not observed any increased morbidity [306]. When the biopsy is performed in the immediate puerperium in subjects with well-controlled blood pressure and normal coagulation indices, the morbidity is certainly similar to that reported in non-pregnant patients [307].

Packham and Fairley [360] have recently reported on 111 biopsies in pregnant women, all pre-term, confirming and extending the impression that risks of the procedure resemble those in the non-pregnant population. In fact, their incidence of transient gross haematuria, 0.9 per cent (all patients undergoing biopsy have microscopic haematuria unless the kidney has been missed), was considerably lower than in non-pregnant patients, where it is 3–5 per cent. Such excellent statistics no doubt reflect the experience and technical skills of the unit and statistics have also been improved by refinement of the pre-biopsy evaluation, which includes verifying that the patient is not significantly hypertensive and has not ingested drugs that interfere with clotting (i.e. aspirin) for at least 7–10 days prior to the procedure, as well as the usual tests to exclude bleeding diatheses.

There can be no doubt that given these recent data, it is in order to re-state that pregnancy adds little or no risk to the procedure. However, because complications do occur, it is still important to have specific indications for renal biopsy in pregnancy. Packham and Fairley [360] suggest that closed (percutaneous) needle biopsy should be undertaken quite often, because they believe certain glomerular disorders to be adversely influenced by pregnancy, and that this effect might be blunted by specific therapy, such as antiplatelet agents. The consensus goes against such broad indications and reiterates that renal biopsy should be performed infrequently *during* gestation [296,303]. (Even in non-pregnant populations the reasons for renal biopsy are not clearly defined, and experts categorize indications as 'most useful', 'possibly useful' and of 'little or no use' [111].) The few widely agreed indications for ante-partum biopsy are as follows.

1 When there is a sudden deterioration of renal function prior to 32 weeks gestation and with no obvious cause. This is because certain forms of rapidly progressive glomerulonephritis may respond to aggressive treatment with steroid 'pulses', chemotherapy and perhaps plasma exchange, when diagnosed early.

2 When there is symptomatic nephrotic syndrome occurring before the 32nd week of gestation. While some might consider a therapeutic trial of steroids in such cases, it is best to determine beforehand whether the lesion is likely to respond to steroids, because pregnancy is itself a hypercoagulable state prone to worsening by such treatment. On the other hand, proteinuria alone in a normotensive woman with well-preserved renal function, and who has neither marked hypoalbuminaemia nor intolerable oedema, would mean that the patient should be examined at more frequent intervals and biopsy deferred to the post-partum period. This is because the consensus amongst most investigators [4,19,239,246,301,454] is that prognosis is determined primarily by the level of renal function and the presence or absence of hypertension. A similar approach applies in the management of pregnancies with asymptomatic microscopic haematuria alone when neither stone nor tumour is suggested by ultrasonography.

3 Where there is a presentation characterized by 'active urinary sediment' (red and white blood cells and casts) with proteinuria and 'borderline' renal function, in a patient who has not been evaluated in the past. This is a controversial area and it could be argued that diagnosis of a collagen disorder such as scleroderma or periarteritis would be grounds for termination of the pregnancy, or that classification of the type of lesion in a woman with systemic lupus erythematosus (SLE) would determine the type and intensity of therapy. The first two diseases are only infrequently diagnosed by renal biopsy, and a normotensive woman with stable renal function and neither systemic involvement nor laboratory evidence of these collagen disorders is watched closely without intervening. Biopsy may be indicated, however, in the latter condition, i.e. in selected patients with SLE and lupus nephropathy of uncertain histopathology.

Assessment of renal function in pregnancy

Serial data on renal function are needed to supplement routine antenatal observations. Tests that are available for use in routine clinical practice include the estimation of plasma creatinine, urea and electrolytes and determination of the clearances of creatinine and urea. A few words of caution are needed. Although plasma creatinine, its reciprocal or its logarithm are often used to estimate or even calculate GFR (in relation to age, height and weight), this approach should *not* be used in pregnancy, because bodyweight or size does not reflect kidney size. Ideally, evaluation of renal function in pregnancy should be based on the serial surveillance of clearance and not plasma concentration of creatinine, even though this is not the ideal measure of GFR. As creatinine levels may increase shortly after ingesting cooked meat (because cooking converts pre-formed creatine into creatinine), the timing of the blood sample during a clearance period must take meals and their content into account [233].

When reporting renal function values it must be remembered that correcting data to a standard body surface area of 1.73 m^2 (and thus, by implication, to a standard kidney size) is *not* applicable in pregnancy [82]. Serial renal function tests should be performed and where possible compared to pre-pregnancy values.

If renal function deteriorates during any stage of pregnancy, reversible causes should be sought such as urinary tract infection or obstruction and dehydration or electrolyte imbalance, which may be subtle, perhaps secondary to diuretic therapy. (Near term, a 15 per cent decrement in function which affects plasma creatinine minimally is normal [129].) Failure to detect a reversible cause for the decrease is an indication for ending the pregnancy by elective delivery. The use of dialysis to 'buy time', without really knowing the cause of the renal deterioration, is not generally accepted. If hypertension accompanies any observed decrease in renal function the outlook is usually more serious and the fetus should be delivered.

Decisions regarding treatment of hypertension

This is perhaps the most controversial area in the management of renal disease during pregnancy and is also discussed in Chapter 6. Most current practices have not been validated by controlled trials in pregnant patients so that many clinicians, not cognisant of pregnancy pathophysiology, prescribe therapy that has been determined to be appropriate by careful studies in non-pregnant populations but which may be unwise in pregnant women. Caution is certainly needed in treating pregnant women and, more important, there is a need for more concentrated and collaborative efforts in evaluating therapy in pregnancy.

Most of the specific risks of hypertension appear to be mediated through superimposed pre-eclampsia. There is still controversy about the incidence of pre-eclampsia in women with pre-existing renal disease [81,169,170]. The diagnosis cannot be made with certainty on clinical grounds alone, because hypertension and proteinuria may be manifestations of the underlying renal disease. Incidentally, a report [228] states that 90 per cent of women developing pre-eclampsia prior to 37 weeks gestation will have chronic renal disease superimposed on essential hypertension. This is a remarkable finding, but it has been contested [295].

In deciding what, if any, treatment is appropriate for hypertension several factors should be considered. These are thoroughly discussed in Chapter 6 and include the level of hypertension under consideration, the underlying cause of the hypertension, the effects on maternal complication rate and on perinatal morbidity and mortality, the detrimental effects of any treatment and lastly, the effect on long-term maternal prognosis.

Control of blood pressure in severe chronic hypertension

This is invariably as a continuation of treatment started before conception. If a woman is stabilized effectively with drugs not specifically contraindicated in pregnancy, these drugs (with the exception of diuretics) should be continued during pregnancy. The most obvious contraindicated drugs are angiotensin-converting enzyme inhibitors. Hospitalization is necessary for initiation or alteration of therapy.

Prevention or amelioration of superimposed pre-eclampsia in severe chronic hypertension

The earlier the presentation the more justified it is to attempt conservative management in order to allow fetal maturation, provided there are no other features necessitating delivery. If *de novo* treatment is indicated in pregnancy it must take place in hospital where the responses can be monitored. If the hypertension is not severe enough to require this, then it does not require treatment. If treatment is indicated for maternal reasons then hospital admission is mandatory. Antihypertensive therapy merely controls only one of the potentially dangerous problems but it allows further maturation before delivery becomes necessary for maternal and fetal reasons.

Control of acute severe hypertension

This is usually due to pre-eclampsia and includes hypertensive emergencies. Where such acute episodes occur early in the third trimester without marked deterioration in renal function, then some attempt might be made to control the blood pressure in the short term to enhance neonatal survival. Despite lowering the blood pressure to protect the mother against dangerous consequences, the other changes of pre-eclampsia will progress. Blood pressure may prove increasingly difficult to control and, if blood pressure 'escapes', this is then an indication to end the pregnancy by elective delivery.

Diuretics

The claim that diuretics reduce the incidence of pre-eclampsia and reduce perinatal mortality has not been confirmed in carefully controlled studies [94]. Diuretics may successfully mobilize fluid and oedema in overt pre-eclampsia, but this is controlling a sign without modifying whatever causes the pre-eclampsia.

Any approach to diuretic therapy must be based on the current concepts of volume homeostasis in pregnancy, described earlier (see above). Many pregnant women can have asymptomatic oedema at some time during pregnancy, and in the absence of pre-eclampsia, the offspring of women with oedema of hands and face weigh more at birth than do infants of women without oedema [226].

As diuretics do not prevent pre-eclampsia and do not have a favourable effect on the cause of the disorder they should not be used, particularly as administration of these agents is not without risk (see Chapter 6). This does not ignore the fact that oedema does occur in pre-eclampsia and therefore, in this context, is significant; it merely emphasizes that in the mild case, the differentiation between physiological and early pre-eclamptic oedema may not be possible. The only patients for whom diuretics should be prescribed unhesitatingly are pregnant women with heart failure and possibly for the treatment of pharyngolaryngeal oedema [209].

The use of volume expansion therapy, prostaglandin infusion and antiplatelet agents such as aspirin (which may also prevent pre-eclampsia) is discussed in Chapter 6.

Fetal surveillance

Serial assessment of fetal well-being is essential because renal disease can be associated with intrauterine growth retardation and, when complications do arise, the judicious moment for intervention is influenced by fetal status [461,481]. Current technology should minimize intrauterine fetal death as well as neonatal morbidity and mortality. Regardless of gestational age, most babies weighing 1500 g or more survive better in a special care nursery than in a hostile intrauterine environment. More and more, there is reliance on deliberate pre-term delivery if there are signs of impending intrauterine fetal death, if renal function deteriorates substantially, if uncontrollable hypertension supervenes or if eclampsia occurs (Table 7.6). It must be realized, however, that 'buying time' for the immature fetus, for example by attempting to control escalating hypertension, is really only controlling a sign without necessarily modifying the underlying disorder.

Decisions regarding delivery

If pregnancy proceeds satisfactorily it is probably advisable to induce labour at 38 weeks because prolonging the pregnancy beyond this time can be associated with a greater risk of placental failure and intrauterine death. Moreover, at this gestation, the fetus should be relatively free of risks if the expected date of delivery is correct.

Delivery before 38 weeks may be necessary if renal function deteriorates markedly, if there are signs of impending intrauterine death, if uncontrollable hypertension supervenes or if eclampsia occurs. Patients should be delivered where full facilities and personnel are available for fetal monitoring, operative delivery and neonatal resuscitation. The use of epidural block in labour is discussed in Chapter 6.

Table 7.6. Changing prospects and pre-term delivery in women with chronic renal disease (J. Davison & C. Baylis, unpublished data)

		Decade				
Renal status		1950s	1960s	1970s	1980s	1990s
Mild	Pre-term delivery	9	10	19	25	28
	Perinatal mortality	18	15	7	<5	<3
Moderate	Pre-term delivery	15	21	40	52	57
	Perinatal mortality	58	45	23	10	10
Severe	Pre-term delivery	100	100	100	100	100
	Perinatal mortality	99	91	59	52	51

Estimates based on 2570 women and 4280 pregnancies (1954–93). All results expressed as a percentage.

Blood transfusion policy in hypertensive emergencies

A woman with a shrunken intravascular compartment is less tolerant of blood loss than is the normal pregnant woman [458]. Blood replacement must therefore be initiated sooner, though managed very carefully, to guard against the dangers of underfilling and overfilling. Close monitoring of the central venous pressure (CVP) is helpful, especially where there is oliguria.

Specific problems in relation to certain types of renal disease

Table 7.7 summarizes the course of pregnancy in a number of specific diseases. Tables 7.8–7.10, from an in-depth review by Imsasciati and Ponticelli [229] describe outcomes in over 1000 women with a variety of specific renal lesions, usually documented by kidney biopsy. Therapeutic abortions were excluded when pregnancy success rates were calculated.

Table 7.7. Pregnancy and specific renal diseases

Renal disease	Effects
Chronic glomerulonephritis	Usually no adverse effect in the absence of hypertension. One view is that glomerulonephritis is adversely affected by the coagulation changes of pregnancy. Urinary tract infections may occur more frequently
Focal glomerulosclerosis	Risks of escalating hypertension and renal deterioration often not reversed post-partum. Increased fetal losses are likely
IgA nephropathy	Risks of uncontrolled and/or sudden escalating hypertension and worsening of renal function
Pyelonephritis	Bacteriuria in pregnancy can lead to exacerbation. Multiple organ system derangements may ensue including adult respiratory distress syndrome
Reflux nephropathy	Risks of sudden escalating hypertension and worsening of renal function

Continued

Table 7.7. (*Continued*)

Renal disease	Effects
Urolithiasis	Infections can be more frequent, but ureteral dilatation and stasis do not seem to affect natural history. Data on lithotripsy in pregnancy are limited.
Polycystic disease	Functional impairment and hypertension usually minimal in childbearing years
Diabetic nephropathy	Usually no adverse effect on the renal lesion, but there is increased frequency of infection, oedema, and/or pre-eclampsia
Systemic lupus erythematosus	Controversial; prognosis most favourable if disease in remission >6 months prior to conception. Steroid dosage should be increased post-partum
Periarteritis nodosa	Fetal prognosis is dismal and maternal death often occurs
Scleroderma	If onset during pregnancy then can be rapid overall deterioration. Reactivation of quiescent scleroderma may occur post-partum.
Previous urinary tract surgery	Might be associated with other malformations of the urogenital tract. Urinary tract infection common during pregnancy. Renal function may undergo reversible decrease. No significant obstructive problem but caesarean section often needed for abnormal presentation and/or to avoid disruption of the continence mechanism if artificial sphincter present
After nephrectomy, solitary kidney and pelvic kidney	Might be associated with other malformations of urogenital tract. Pregnancy well tolerated; dystocia rarely occurs with a pelvic kidney
Wegener's granulomatosis	Limited information. Proteinuria (±hypertension) is common from early in pregnancy. Immunosuppressives are safe but cytotoxic drugs are best avoided
Renal artery stenosis	May present as chronic hypertension or as recurrent isolated pre-eclampsia. If diagnosed then transluminal angioplasty can be undertaken in pregnancy if appropriate

Acute glomerulonephritis

Acute post-streptococcal glomerulonephritis complicating pregnancy is very rare but does occur [175, 348,431], and has been mistaken for pre-eclampsia.

Chronic glomerulonephritis [4,74,224,239,240,454]

The prognosis of chronic glomerulonephritis during pregnancy is hard to evaluate primarily because most reports are poorly documented, often failing to list the degree of functional impairment, the blood pressure prior to conception and the histology of 'glomerulonephritis'.

Table 7.8. Fetal and maternal outcome of pregnancies in women with primary glomerulonephritis. Data are the proportion (%) of all pregnancies. From Imbasciati and Ponticelli [229]. See [229] for details of the six reports surveyed in this table

					Renal function decrease		Blood pressure increase	
Histology	Pregnancies/ patients	Spontaneous abortion (%)	Perinatal loss (%)	Pre-term delivery (%)	Reversible (%)	Progressive (%)	Reversible (%)	Permanent (%)
Focal glomerulosclerosis	85/61	3	23	32	13	5	32	10
Membranous nephropathy	110/70	12	4	35	3	2	22	3
Membranoproliferative	165/98	17	8	19	6	3	20	12
IgA nephritis	268/166	5	15	21	12	2	25	12
Mesangial proliferative	278/163	5	12	9	2	3	36	7
All types	906/558	8	13	19	8	3	27	9

Table 7.9. Systemic lupus erythematosus and pregnancy. From Imbasciati and Ponticelli [229]. See [229] for details of literature surveyed in this table

	Pregnancies	Spontaneous abortions (%)	Perinatal loss (%)	Fetal loss (%)
1952–70	587	20	9	29
1971–80	184	20	5	25
1981–88	224	13	13	26

Table 7.10. Outcome of pregnancy in women with diabetic nephropathy, polycystic kidney disease and reflux nephropathy. Data are the proportion (%) of all pregnancies. From Imbasciati and Ponticelli [229]. See [229] for details of five reports surveyed in this table

Nephropathy	Pregnancies/ patients	Perinatal loss (%)	Pre-term delivery (%)	Renal function decrease (%)	Blood pressure increase (%)	Progressive course after delivery
Diabetic nephropathy	97/94	6	36	32	58	13
Polycystic disease	464/242	3	10	3	14	0.3
Reflux nephropathy	137/53	7	15	0.7	11	3

The Melbourne group [161,254,255,256] have stated that pregnancy tends to aggravate most glomerular diseases due to the hypercoagulable state that accompanies pregnancy; in particular they claim that crescentric glomerular lesions occur more readily. They also indicate that such patients are more prone to superimposed pre-eclampsia or hypertensive crises early in pregnancy. Other experience is that kidney function decreases most often in patients where hypertension is severe; nonetheless, most pregnancies are successful [246,247]. The subtypes of primary glomerulonephritis are all now regarded as distinct and separable disease entities and with few exceptions can be specifically distinguished only by renal biopsy. Those subtypes present in women of childbearing age are given in Table 7.11.

Table 7.11. Subtypes of primary glomerulonephritis (GN) in women of childbearing age

Name (abbreviation)	Synonyms
Focal glomerulosclerosis (FGS)	Focal and segmental glomerulosclerosis Focal and segmental hyalinosis Focal sclerosing GN
Membranous glomerulonephritis (MGN)	Membranous nephropathy
Diffuse proliferative GN (DPGN)	(Mesangial proliferative GN) (Endocapillary proliferative GN)
Membranoproliferative GN (MPGN)	Mesangiocapillary GN (Type II = dense deposit disease)
Mesangial IgA nephropathy (IgA-GN)	Berger's nephritis Focal proliferative GN
Minimal change nephrotic syndrome (MCNS)	Lipoid nephrosis Idiopathic nephrotic syndrome Minimal change glomerulonephritis

Focal glomerulosclerosis (FGS)

Increased proteinuria and hypertension during pregnancy are frequent but usually reversible. The renal lesion may be accelerated by pregnancy but this is rare if pre-pregnancy renal function is normal. Overall fetal loss rates are about 25 per cent.

Membranous glomerulonephritis

If renal function is satisfactory and stable and hypertension absent or under control then the outlook is good. Pregnancy does not damage the renal lesion.

Diffuse proliferative glomerulonephritis (DPGN)

This label covers a heterogeneous group of patients with prolonged proteinuria. Hypertension and proteinuria invariably worsen during pregnancy but the rate of subsequent progression into renal failure is not hastened. Fetal loss rates average 15 per cent.

Membranoproliferative glomerulonephritis (MPGN)

It is difficult to assess whether the course of MPGN, which is usually not good, is worsened by pregnancy. Certainly hypertension arising in pregnancy invariably persists afterwards and even when pre-pregnancy status is 'mild' (plasma creatinine <125 μmol/l) pregnancy can have an overall deleterious effect and fetal loss rates may be as high as 50 per cent. Some women with persistent hypocomplementaemia have a circulating antibody 'C3 nephritic factor' and placental transmission and transient neonatal hypocomplementaemia (without long-term sequelae) have been described [253] (see Table 7.8).

Mesangial IgA nephropathy (IgA-GN)

The risk of hypertension during pregnancy is probably higher than for other subtypes and its persistence after delivery can be problematical. If pre-pregnancy status is 'moderate' (plasma creatinine 125–250 μmol/l) then progressive renal failure after delivery is highly likely, but of course this may have happened anyway. Fetal loss rates are around 15 per cent except in the Melbourne series [254] where the figure is 30 per cent, perhaps related to a selected referral pattern. IgA-GN is associated with HLA-BW35 and in some cases may be an inheritable disease but as yet the genetic counselling implications are unclear. Abe [1,2,3] has examined the impact of IgA nephropathy and pregnancy on each other. Consistent findings were that (a) pregnancy is well tolerated without effect on the course of the disease if blood pressure is normal and GFR is >70 ml/min before conception; (b) the live birth rate is extremely low if hypertension exists before pregnancy and/or is not well controlled during pregnancy.

Minimal change nephrotic syndrome (MCNS)

Most women of childbearing age are in stable remission with 'mild' status and pregnancy is well tolerated without risk of relapse. For women who are 'frequent relapsers' prednisone can be restarted or continued throughout pregnancy [476] but some decide to stop therapy and take a calculated risk of further relapse during pregnancy.

Hereditary nephritis

Most cases (85 per cent) of this disorder are in males who have inherited the disease as an X-linked dominant disorder [191]. The majority of female carriers manifest mild abnormalities of renal function and urinary microscopy as dictated by the Lyon hypothesis. The remaining patients are examples of autosomal dominant or recessive inheritance. These diseases, therefore, may not become clinically manifest until pregnancy. Pregnancy in these women is usually successful from a renal viewpoint but can be complicated by bleeding problems usually due to disordered platelet morphology and function [192,194]. There is an interesting report of two sisters with this disorder who developed rapidly progressive crescentric glomerulonephritis associated with pregnancy [201].

This heterogeneous group, sometimes called familial glomerulonephritis, raises the question of renal disease transmission to the next generation, a problem not seen in any of the primary glomerulonephritis group, except possibly IgA-GN. The inheritance of Alport's syndrome (familial glomerulonephritis with deafness) is usually through less affected females and typically has greater expression in males. Benign familial haematuria syndrome is inheritable sometimes as an autosomal dominant disease [404].

Collagen diseases or diffuse connective tissue diseases (DCTD) (see also Chapter 8)

SLE

This relatively common disease with or without other DCTDs (overlap syndrome) has a predilection for the childbearing age group and coincidence with pregnancy poses complex clinical problems due to the profound disturbance of the immunological system and multiple organ involvement in SLE and the complicated immunology of pregnancy itself [271,341]. The majority of pregnancies succeed, especially when the maternal disease is in complete clinical remission for 6 months prior to conception, even if there were severe pathological changes in the original renal biopsy and heavy proteinuria in the early stages of the disease [206,237]. Continued signs of disease activity or increasing renal dysfunction certainly reduce the likelihood of an uncomplicated pregnancy and the clinical course [205] (see Table 7.9).

SLE nephropathy may sometimes become manifest during pregnancy and when accompanied by hypertension and renal dysfunction may be mistaken for pre-eclampsia. From recent reviews of the literature it appears that as many as 19 per cent (progressive in 8 per cent) and 42 per cent experience decrements in GFR and hypertension, respectively. The figures are worse if renal insufficiency (plasma creatinine >125 μmol/l) antedates the pregnancy [229,354].

Some patients have a definite tendency to relapse, occasionally severely in the puerperium, and therefore it is prudent to prescribe or increase steroids at this time [285,374]. Rarely a particularly severe postpartum syndrome may develop consisting of pleural effusion, pulmonary infiltration, fever, ECG abnormalities and even cardiomyopathy, with extensive IgG, IgM, Ig and C3 deposition in the myocardium [170]. The concept of the 'stormy puerperium' has been disputed [309]. Many now observe postpartum patients and do not institute or increase steroid therapy unless signs of increased disease activity are noted.

The fetal and thrombotic implications of the presence of maternal lupus anticoagulant, anticardiolipin antibodies and extractable nuclear antigen (ENA) antibodies (e.g. anti-Ro) are discussed in Chapter 8.

SYSTEMIC SCLEROSIS

Scleroderma is a term which includes a heterogeneous group of limited and systemic conditions causing hardening of the skin. Systemic sclerosis implies involvement of both skin and other sites, particularly certain internal organs. Renal involvement is thought to occur in about 60 per cent of patients with systemic sclerosis, usually within 3–4 years of diagnosis. The presentation may be the sudden onset of malignant hypertension, rapidly progressive renal failure or slowly worsening proteinuria and/or azotemia.

The combination of systemic sclerosis and pregnancy is unusual because systemic sclerosis occurs most often in the fourth and fifth decades and patients with systemic sclerosis are usually infertile. When systemic sclerosis has its onset in pregnancy, there is a much greater tendency for deterioration. Patients with scleroderma and no evidence of renal involvement prior to conception can develop severe kidney disease in pregnancy. There are also instances when pregnancy has been uneventful and successful but many required the use of converting enzyme inhibitors. Most maternal deaths involve rapidly progressive scleroderma with severe pulmonary complications, multiple infections, hypertension and/or renal failure [320].

The extent of systemic involvement is probably more important than the duration of the disease and limited mild disease carries a better prognosis. Sclerosis usually spares the abdominal wall skin but there is one report of hydronephrosis, presumed secondary to thickened skin and decreased abdominal wall compliance, in a twin pregnancy complicated by polyhydramnios [340].

WEGENER'S GRANULOMATOSIS

There is a paucity of information on pregnancy course and outcome in women with granulomatosis. Proteinuria is common from early in pregnancy [167] and reports to date have described both complicated and uneventful pregnancies [52,343], including women taking either azathioprine or cyclophosphamide (see also Chapter 1).

Periarteritis nodosa

The outcome of pregnancy in women with renal involvement due to periarteritis nodosa is very poor, largely because of the associated hypertension which is frequently malignant. Although a few successful pregnancies have been reported, in most cases fetal prognosis is dismal and many have ended with maternal death. This may merely reflect the nature of the disease itself, but it is an important consideration when making decisions about pregnancy. Early therapeutic termination has less maternal risk [350].

Diabetic nephropathy (see Chapter 11)

Because many patients have been diabetic since childhood, they probably already have microscopic changes in their kidneys [104,207]. Maternal hazards and perinatal loss are twice as common in diabetics with clinically overt renal disease as in those without (see Table 7.10).

During pregnancy, diabetic women have an increased prevalence and incidence of covert bacteriuria (and may be more susceptible to urinary tract infection), pre-eclampsia, peripheral oedema and occasionally severe, but transient, nephrotic syndrome [363]. Most women with diabetic nephropathy demonstrate the normal GFR increment and pregnancy does not accelerate renal deterioration [101,259,390].

There is a report of diabetic women with moderate renal dysfunction (plasma creatinine >125 μmol/l) whose renal function permanently deteriorated in pregnancy in comparison to the changes before and afterwards — GFR decrements of 1.8 ml/min/month in pregnancy and 1.4 ml/min/month post-partum until the start of dialysis [53]. Such changes occurred despite good metabolic control and might have been related to hypertension which often accelerates in late pregnancy, regardless of intensified treatment. It should be remembered, however, that these observations are uncontrolled. The condition of non-pregnant diabetics with plasma creatinines >125 μmol/l too often progresses rapidly to renal failure.

Whether or not hypertension should be treated more aggressively, especially before conception, is open to question [365]. Diabetes already causes glomerular hyperfiltration which theoretically may be further exacerbated by pregnancy if renal autoregulation fails to prevent excessive transmission of arterial pressure to the glomerular capillaries. Normalizing pressures may help to prevent (further) glomerular damage. Of course, some of the antihypertensive agents used pre-pregnancy, in particular angiotensin-converting enzyme inhibitors, may be contraindicated during pregnancy [191,376] (see Chapter 6). The use of microalbuminuria as a monitor for diabetic nephropathy is controversial.

Pyelonephritis (tubulo-interstitial disease)

Acute pyelonephritis will be dealt with separately (see later). In chronic pyelonephritis (tubulo-interstitial disease) the prognosis in pregnancy is similar to that of patients with glomerular disease, in that outcome is best in patients with adequate renal function and normal blood pressure. Compared to the non-pregnant state, there is an increased frequency of symptomatic infection in pregnant women, but overall, they have a more benign antenatal course than do women with glomerular disease [301].

Of interest is a report suggesting that women who develop frank pyelonephritis manifest greater degrees of pelvicalyceal dilatation in pregnancy, that may not regress after delivery, and which underscores the need for post-partum investigation of this population [472].

Reflux nephropathy

This term is used to describe renal morphological and functional changes which are the urodynamic consequence of vesicoureteric and intrarenal reflux, often complicated by recurrent infection. There are glomerular lesions (focal and segmental hyalinosis and sclerosis) and parenchymal atrophy and scarring. It is one of the most frequent renal diseases in women of childbearing age; a third of cases are clinically unmasked by pregnancy; up to 30 per cent of women developing end-stage renal failure have reflux nephropathy and this is usually present before 40 years.

It is frequently associated with hypertension and moderate to severe renal dysfunction features which, as discussed earlier (see above), adversely affect pregnancy outcome [50,241]. Specific obstetric worries in these patients include severe fetal intra-uterine growth retardation and the risk of sudden rapid worsening of hypertension and renal function with accelerated progression to renal failure.

As the disease may be inherited, children born to parents with vesicoureteric reflux or reflux nephropathy, or who have affected siblings, should be screened in infancy [17].

Urolithiasis

The prevalence of urolithiasis in pregnancy is 0.03–0.35 per cent [41,205]. Most stones contain calcium salts and some are infectious in origin. Occasionally the more malicious struvite stones (e.g. staghorn) are seen. Uric acid and cystine stones are much more infrequent [11]. Renal and ureteric calculi are one of the most common causes of non-uterine abdominal pain severe enough to necessitate hospital admission during pregnancy [260]. Despite these dramatic complications, pregnancy in fact has little influence on the course of stone disease, although there may be an increased incidence of both urinary tract infection and perhaps spontaneous abortion, as well as premature labour. The relatively benign prognosis is surprising, because pregnant women are normally hypercalciuric and their urinary supersaturation ratios for calcium oxalate and phosphate are substantially increased. This, in the face of urethral dilatation, stasis and perhaps obstruction, raises the question of why stone disease is not more prevalent in pregnancy. The answer to this, however, may be that there is concomitant increase in the excretion of magnesium and citrate as well as several glycoproteins which inhibit stone formation (i.e. nephrocalcin) [132,321].

Management should be conservative initially, with adequate hydration, appropriate antibiotic therapy and pain relief with systemic analgesics [447]. The use of continous segmental [T11–L2) epidural block has been advocated, as in non-pregnant patients with ureteric colic and may even favourably influence spontaneous passage of stone(s) [386]. With good pain relief, the patient micturates without difficulty, moves without assistance and is less at risk from thromboembolic problems than if drowsy, nauseated and bedridden with pain.

When there are complications that might need surgical intervention, then pregnancy should not be a deterrent to intravenous urography (IVU), even though there is an understandable reluctance to consider radiological investigation. Specific clinical criteria should be met before undertaking an IVU: (a) microscopic haematuria; (b) recurrent urinary tract symptoms; and (c) sterile urine culture: the presence of two of these indicates a diagnosis of calculi in 60 per cent of women [333].

Alternative management, avoiding X-rays during pregnancy, has recently been proposed which involves the placement of an internal ureteral tube, or stent, between bladder and kidney, under local anaesthesia using cystoscopy or endoluminal ultrasound [312,496]. The stent retains its position because it has a pigtail or J-like curve at each end (double-J) and to prevent encrustation it can be changed every 8 weeks. Early empirical use for presumed stone obstruction in pregnant women with flank pain could be helpful especially when hydration, analgesia and antibiotics do not resolve pain or fever. When the pregnancy is over the usual X-ray films should be obtained and standard management resumed.

Sonographically guided percutaneous nephrostomy is another effective and safe method of treating pregnant women with ureteric colic or symptomatic obstructive hydronephrosis [477]. The procedure is rapid, requires minimal anaesthesia and is perhaps a preferable alternative to retrograde stenting or more invasive approaches. Information on lithotripsy during pregnancy is limited and the procedure is best avoided.

In patients with cystinuria, assiduous maintenance of high fluid intake is the mainstay of management. Although D-penicillamine appears relatively safe it should only be used for severe cases, where urinary cystine excretion is known to be very high [190].

Polycystic kidney disease (PKD)

This is an autosomal dominant disorder, spontaneous mutations occurring in less than 10 per cent of cases [176]. It is the most common single-gene genetic disease of humans with an incidence of perhaps about one in 400–1000 [112,176]. Most cases do not have clinical manifestations until the fourth and fifth decade — only 17 per cent are diagnosed by the age of 25 [47]. It may therefore remain undetected during pregnancy, but careful questioning for a history of familial problems and the use of ultrasonography may lead to earlier detection. Patients do well when functional impairment is minimal and hypertension absent, as is often the case in childbearing years. Compared to the pregnancies of sisters unaffected by this autosomal dominant disease, they do have an increased incidence of hypertension late in pregnancy (20 versus 2 per cent) and a slightly higher perinatal mortality [334].

Women with advanced renal failure are best advised against pregnancy, although use of prophylactic dialysis has been advocated, despite lack of controlled studies, for just this type of patient [9].

Liver cysts are larger and more prevalent in women, especially those who have been pregnant and enlargement of cysts, but not rupture, may occur during pregnancy [176].

It has been suggested that multiparity (three or more pregnancies) leads to an earlier onset of renal insufficiency [176], which might reflect the effects of pregnancy once moderate renal insufficiency was present. The consensus view, however, is that pregnancy has no long-term effect on renal prognosis [334].

If one or other parent has PKD they may seek genetic counselling. Patients from families where there is evidence of clustering of intracranial aneurysms or subarachnoid haemorrhage should be screened before considering pregnancy [493]. There will be a 50 per cent chance of transmitting the disease to their offspring. DNA probe techniques are now being developed so that antenatal diagnosis is possible by chronic villus sampling allowing women to undergo selective termination of pregnancy [391].

Permanent urinary diversion

Permanent urinary diversion is still used in the management of patients with congenital lower urinary tract defects but its use has declined for neurogenic bladders since the introduction of self-catheterization. The most common complication of pregnancy is urinary infection. Pre-term labour occurs in 20 per cent and the use of prophylactic antibiotics throughout pregnancy may reduce its incidence. Decline in renal function may occur, invariably related to infection and/or intermittent obstruction. With an ileal conduit, or augmentation cystoplasty, elevation and compression by the expanding uterus can cause outflow obstruction whereas with a ureterosigmoid anastomosis, actual ureteral obstruction may occur [20,211]. The changes usually reverse after delivery.

The mode of delivery is dictated by obstetric factors. Abnormal presentation accounts for a caesarean section rate of 25 per cent, related no doubt to minor genital tract abnormalities. Vaginal delivery is safe but as the continence of a ureterosigmoid anastomosis depends on an intact anal sphincter, this must be protected with a mediolateral episiotomy.

Inherited renal disease

Inherited renal disorders are not rare, autosomal dominant PKD affecting one in 400–1000 individuals [176] (see below). Some of the rarer hereditary diseases manifest during childhood and then progress to end-stage renal failure before or by adolescence (i.e. cystinosis and nephronophthisis. Here pregnancy has occurred when on dialysis or after transplantation [390]. In contrast, the most prevalent disorders, hereditary nephritis (see above) and polycystic disease (see below) have a later onset. Table 7.12 gives examples of inherited kidney disorders in which antenatal diagnosis is technically possible [263]. All such women contemplating pregnancy or in early pregnancy should be referred for genetic counselling.

Tuberous sclerosis is an autosomal dominant disease, comprising skin lesions, involvement of the central nervous system and visceral lesions, including renal angiomyolipoma [446].

Table 7.12. Examples of inherited kidney diseases in which antenatal diagnosis may be technically possible

	Mode of inheritance	Biochemical diagnosis	DNA study: Linkage analysis	DNA study: Gene defect*
Polycystic kidney disease	AD		+	
Alport's syndrome	XD		+	+
	AR		+	+
Primary hyperoxaluria	AR	+		
Fabry's disease	XR	+	+	+
Finnish congenital nephrotic syndrome	AR	+ (raised amniotic fluid α-fetoprotein concentration)		
Congenital diabetes insipidus	XR		+	+
Oculocerebrorenal syndrome of Lowe	XR		+	+
von Hippel–Lindau disease	AD		+	

AD, autosomal dominant; AR, autosomal recessive; XD, X-linked dominant; XR, X-linked recessive.
* In certain families in which the gene defect has been identified.

Renal involvement in the von Hippel–Landau disease includes cysts and bilateral multifocal renal cell carcinoma and 25 per cent of these women have phaeochromocytomata, often bilateral (which may cluster in families, and be the only manifestation of the disorder [353]). Therefore there is substantial risk of fatal outcome especially in pregnancy and women with this condition should be screened to rule out phaeochromocytoma as well as for the haemangioblastomas involving retina or central nervous system.

The solitary kidney

Some patients have either a congenital absence of one kidney or marked unilateral hypoplasia. Most, however, have had a previous nephrectomy because of pyelonephritis (with abscess of hydronephrosis), unilateral tuberculosis, congenital abnormalities, trauma or a tumour. Occasionally the woman may have been a living-related kidney donor [71]. It is important to know the indication for and the time since the nephrectomy [260]. In patients with an infectious and/or structural renal problem sequential pre-pregnancy investigation is needed for detection of any persistent infection.

There is no difference whether the right or left kidney remains as long as it is located in the normal anatomical position. If function is normal and stable, all women with this problem seem to tolerate pregnancy well despite the superimposition of GFR increments on already hyperfiltering nephrons.

Ectopic kidneys (usually pelvic) are more vulnerable to infection and are associated with impaired fetal outcome, probably because of associated malformations of the urogenital tract [260]. If infection occurs in a solitary kidney during pregnancy and does not quickly respond to antibiotics, then termination may have to be considered for preservation of renal function. Pregnancy in women who have survived childhood treatment for a nephroblastoma (Wilms' tumour) has a 30 per cent perinatal loss, perhaps because of the late effects of radiotherapy on the uterus [288].

Nephrotic syndrome and pregnancy

The most common cause of nephrotic syndrome in late pregnancy is pre-eclampsia [168,169]. This form of pre-eclampsia has a poorer fetal prognosis than pre-eclampsia with less heavy proteinuria, but the maternal prognosis is similar.

Other causes of nephrotic syndrome in pregnancy include membranous nephropathy, proliferative or membranoproliferative glomerulonephritis, lipid nephrosis, lupus nephropathy, hereditary nephritis, diabetic nephropathy, renal vein thrombosis, amyloidosis, sarcoidosis and secondary syphilis [270, 298]. Some of these possibilities emphasize the importance of establishing a tissue diagnosis before initiating steroid therapy [476].

If renal function is adequate and hypertension is absent, there should be few complications during pregnancy: however, several of the physiological changes occurring during pregnancy may simulate aggravation or exacerbation of the disease. For example, increments in renal blood flow as well as increase in renal vein pressure may enhance protein excretion. Levels of serum albumin usually decrease by 5–10 g/l in normal pregnancy, and the further decreases that can occur in the nephrotic syndrome may enhance the tendency toward fluid retention. Despite oedema, diuretics should not be given as these patients have a decreased intravascular volume and this therapy could further compromise uteroplacental perfusion or aggravate the increased tendency to thrombotic episodes.

While the majority of these pregnancies succeed and are maintained near to term, there is evidence that the hypoalbuminaemia and the associated decreased intravascular volume may cause small-for-dates infants [337]. Furthermore, there is a report that infants of normotensive mothers who had heavy proteinuria during pregnancy manifested impaired neurological and mental development [406].

Long-term effects of pregnancy in renal disease

CLINICAL STUDIES

Pregnancy does not cause any deterioration or otherwise affect the rate of progression of the disease beyond what might be expected in the non-pregnant state, provided kidney dysfunction was minimal and hypertension was absent before pregnancy [229,303]. An important factor in remote prognosis could be the sclerotic effects that hyperfiltration might already have had in the residual (intact) glomeruli of kidneys of these patients. The situation may be worse in a single diseased kidney where presumably more sclerosis has occurred within the fewer (intact) glomeruli. Theoretically further progressive loss of renal function could ensue in pregnancy. Nevertheless, in some women with renal disease there can be unpredicted, accelerated and irreversible renal decline in pregnancy or immediately afterwards. The mechanisms which are unknown, will be slow to emerge from human data, if they are ever available from this source, and therefore animal research must be considered [29,31,301].

STUDIES IN ANIMALS

Animal models have been developed to elucidate the mechanisms involved in renal dysfunction when pregnancy and disease interact as well as to assess longer term renal prognosis [37]. In particular the role of P_{GC} is examined because of its importance in the development of glomerular injury.

Unilateral nephrectomy

The long-term effects of superimposition of repetitive pregnancies on a state of chronic underlying renal vasodilation induced by uninephrectomy plus high dietary protein feeding have been examined [43]. GFR and SNGFR were lower in repetitively pregnant compared to non-pregnant rats but of interest, the functional renal vasodilatory response to intravenous amino-acid infusion was intact in repetitively pregnant rats whereas this renal reserve was absent in the non-pregnant. Neither morphological evidence of damage nor proteinuria were worse in repetitively pregnant versus non-pregnant controls. P_{GC} was elevated by long-term uninephrectomy plus high dietary protein feeding but not worsened by pregnancy, which may explain the lack of exacerbation of the underlying glomerular impairment due to sequential pregnancies.

Spontaneously hypertensive rat (SHR)

Glomerular injury develops with advancing age although its evolution is much slower in females than males [163,164]. Repetitive pregnancies have no long-term effect on glomerular function and structure or protein excretion in 1-year-old SHRs nor is the already high P_{GC} further elevated [33]. It had been anticipated that in the presence of severe systemic hypertension (as occurs in the SHR) superimposed pregnancy would expose the kidney to additional increases in P_{GC} and injury, but the normal gestational renal vasodilatation was not seen in the pregnant SHR; this is quite unexpected as pregnancy is almost always associated with increases in GFR and RPF, providing renal function is not already seriously impaired. This lack of a renal vasodilatory response in the pregnant SHR, despite peripheral vasodilatation (blood pressure falls markedly in pregnancy) [15,456] may reflect a protective mechanism, guarding the maternal kidney.

Infarction and reduction of renal mass

With 5/6 reduction of renal mass alone, systemic hypertension was evident together with high P_{GC} in controls and despite the marked chronic compensatory renal vasodilatation, the remnant kidney was still capable of an additional renal vasodilatation during pregnancy with pre-glomerular and efferent arteriolar resistances decreasing in parallel. Since blood pressure also fell, there was no change in P_{GC} and no worsening of proteinuria, thus no haemodynamic basis for pregnancy to exacerbate the glomerular injury. Studies by others have shown no long-term damage by pregnancy in this model [279].

Experimentally produced hypertension

Attempts to produce a model of 'pre-eclampsia' by superimposition of pregnancy on a range of experimentally induced or genetic hypertensive states in the rats have been unsuccessful and pregnancy in hypertensive rodents is uniformly and powerfully antihypertensive [15,137]. In the model of systemic hypertension with renal disease produced by chronic NO blockade (see above) renal and peripheral vasodilatation as well as plasma volume expansion were absent, blood pressure remained elevated and proteinuria developed at term [39]. Thus, an intact NO system appears to be essential for expression of the antihypertensive response to pregnancy. Indeed, in the SHR the marked antihypertensive response to pregnancy is due to enhanced NO production [8].

Antibasement membrane nephritis

The effect of superimposition of pregnancy on the glomerular functional alterations in a rat model of anti-glomerular basement membrane glomerulonephritis [44] produced significant proteinuria, high P_{GC}, low K_f and mild impairment in function such that SNGFR and GFR were maintained at near normal values. Despite the underlying glomerulonephritis, moderate renal vasodilatation occurred in mid-pregnancy with increases in RPF but without worsening the already increased P_{GC} [44]. There was no difference in proteinuria and glomerular damage in non-pregnant and pregnant rats.

Heymann nephritis

The Fx1A antibody produces Heymann nephritis, a model of membraneous glomerulonephritis, with sustained and heavy proteinuria, mild impairment in glomerular function and high P_{GC} [45]. Superimposition of pregnancy normalizes P_{GC} due predominantly to increased pre-glomerular tone and although proteinuria remains unchanged there are substantial decrements in GFR and SNGFR, with marked functional impairment by late pregnancy. However, since P_{GC} is not increased, there is no haemodynamic basis to anticipate long-term exacerbation of this disease by pregnancy.

In summary, none of the models of normotensive renal disease thus far studied (where underlying glomerular damage is due to ablation of renal mass or immune stimuli or in the SHR) is associated with a pregnancy-induced increment in P_{GC} or any acute or chronic worsening of the underlying renal injury. Therefore, the chronic renal vasodilatation of pregnancy does not appear to be a damaging entity. When pregnancy is superimposed on chronic blockade of EDRF, however, hypertension occurs and renal function declines, indicative of further endothelial damage or dysfunction.

Renal disease and pregnancy: some conclusions

1 A balance must be struck between pregnancy outcome and the impact pregnancy has in the long term [50,248]. Crucial determinants are pre-pregnancy renal functional status, the absence or presence of hypertension (and its management) and the kidney lesion itself, as well as better fetal surveillance, more timely delivery and improvements in neonatal care (see Tables 7.3 and 7.6).
2 Once a renal disease patient always a renal disease patient. If a woman with chronic renal disease wishes to have children, the sooner she sets about it the better, because renal function will in any case diminish with age.
3 Absence of severe hypertension or renal insufficiency before pregnancy is favourable. If dysfunction is moderate, there is still a fair chance that pregnancy will succeed, but the risks are much greater (see Table 7.3).
4 Type of renal disease will influence outcome. Pregnancy outcome in the presence of FGS, membranoproliferative glomerulonephritis, the collagen disorders and IgA and reflux nephropathies is controversial.
5 Review of medication is essential.
6 Proteinuria is common during pregnancy (up to 3 g/24 hours).
7 Severe hypertension is a much greater adverse feature than low but stable renal function. Beware of controlling a sign without modifying the basic disorder.
8 Pre-eclampsia cannot be diagnosed clinically with certainty.
9 Deteriorating renal function, even without hypertension, is ominous.

Asymptomatic bacteriuria

In this condition, also labelled covert bacteriuria, true bacteriuria exists but there are no symptoms or signs of acute urinary tract infection (see also Chapter 16).

Diagnostic pitfalls

Pregnant women often complain of or will admit to symptoms of urgency, frequency, dysuria and nocturia, occurring singly or in combination. These symptoms are not in themselves diagnostic of urinary tract infection and can be elicited from women with sterile urine.

Urine collection and examination

The growth of bacteria on qualitative culture of a urine specimen may represent either true bacteriuria (the multiplication of bacteria within the urinary tract) or contamination of the urine with urethral or perineal organisms at the time of collection. True bacteriuria can be separated from contamination on the basis of colony counts from a freshly obtained midstream urine specimen (MSU), with 100 000 colonies/ml of urine as the dividing line [245]. Two consecutive clean-voided specimens containing the same organism in numbers greater than 100 000 colonies/ml of urine represents true bacteriuria, as does a single suprapubic aspiration with any bacterial growth [317,356].

The use of the clean-catch or clean-void technique is satisfactory provided each clinic determines the number of cultures needed to achieve a 95 per cent or greater level of confidence that bacteriuria exists [75,93]. The use of antiseptic solutions for vulval cleansing should be avoided as contamination of the urine may result in a false negative culture [403]. A plain soap solution or distilled water is satisfactory.

A number of presumptive tests based on changes in chemical indicators are available but the dependability of these varies greatly [327].

Recent studies raise the possibility that women with more than usual glycosuria in pregnancy may have sustained renal tubular damage from earlier untreated urinary tract infections, even though the women may be no longer bacteriuric when pregnant

[149]. Why infection might cause an alteration in the renal handling of glucose is not known. Certainly infection can impair distal tubular function, as evidenced by reduced urine concentrating ability, a manifestation of tubular dysfunction that is reversed once infection is eradicated. However, with regard to the renal handling of glucose, full recovery may not occur.

Site of infection

Asymptomatic bacteriuria is a heterogenous condition and several different approaches have attempted to differentiate between upper and lower urinary tract bacteriuria [108,300]. Ureteric catheterization, bladder washout techniques, renal biopsy, urinary concentration tests, determination of serum antibody titres and identification of antibody-coated bacteria in the urine have all been tried [89,148,161,208,344,468]. No single test is sufficiently precise, however, to give complete confidence in localizing the site of infection.

Source of infection

It is probable that bacteria originate from the large bowel and colonize the urinary tract transperineally. By far the most common infecting organism is *Escherichia coli*, which is responsible for 75–90 per cent of bacteriuria during pregnancy. The pathogenic virulence of this organism, which is not the most plentiful in faeces, appears to derive from a number of factors including resistance to vaginal acidity, rapid multiplication in urine, possession of adhesions (characterized as fimbriae) allowing adherence to uroepithelial cells and production of chemicals which decrease ureteric peristalsis and inhibit phagocytosis [316]. Other organisms frequently responsible for urinary tract infection include *Klebsiella*, *Proteus*, coagulase-negative staphylococci and *Pseudomonas*.

The stasis associated with ureteropelvic dilation and/or partial ureteric obstruction, increased nutrient content of the urine and the presence of potential pathogens are present in most gravidas [310]; yet only a small minority develop bacteriuria. Susceptible women may differ immunologically from those who resist infection: they are less likely to express antibody to the O antigen of *E. coli* on the vaginal epithelium and may display less effective leucocyte activity against the organism.

Clinical implications

Incidence

The reservoir of young women with asymptomatic bacteriuria acquired during childhood has been estimated at 5 per cent but only 1.2 per cent are infected at any one time. The incidence increases after puberty coincident with sexual activity and varies from 2 to 10 per cent depending on the techniques employed for testing and the socio-economic status of the patients [356,414]. There is some evidence to suggest that prophylactic antibiotics given to schoolgirls with asymptomatic bacteriuria prevent subclinical renal damage [131], which would in any case only be unmasked by the physiological demands of pregnancy.

In pregnancy, true asymptomatic bacteriuria is invariably diagnosed at the first antenatal visit if tested for at that time and <1.5 per cent subsequently acquire bacteriuria in late pregnancy. A recent antenatal study [443], in which 99 per cent of women took part in at least one screening, indicated that the risk of onset of bacteriuria was highest between the ninth and 17th weeks of gestation. The 16th week was the optimal time for a single screen for bacteriuria, calculated on the numbers of bacteria-free gestational weeks gained by treatment.

Importance of diagnosis

It is important to identify and treat the infected group because up to 40 per cent develop acute symptomatic urinary tract infection [490]. Treating this group should prevent approximately 70 per cent of all cases of acute urinary tract infection (Fig. 7.7).

The need for and cost-effectiveness of routine screening for bacteriuria in pregnancy, however, have been seriously questioned [75,276,277]. It is known that 2 per cent of those with negative cultures will also develop acute infections. Thus of the 90–98 per cent that do not have asymptomatic bacteriuria at the booking visit (and therefore will not be treated) the number actually at risk of developing an acute urinary tract infection is quite

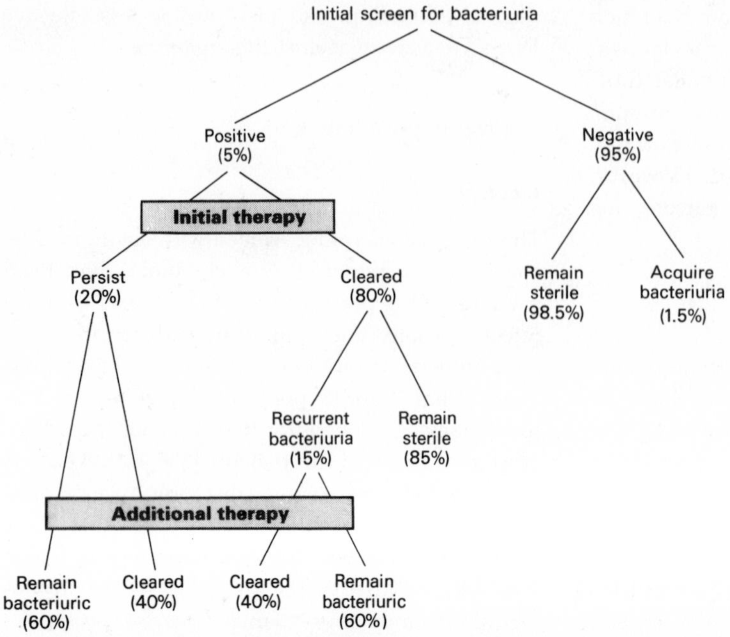

Fig. 7.7. Natural history of asymptomatic bacteriuria and effects of treatment in pregnancy. Approximate percentages are given in parentheses.

significant and accounts for about 30 per cent of all cases of acute urinary tract infection in pregnancy.

A positive history of previous urinary tract infection may be almost as effective as screening in predicting urinary tract infection in pregnancy [83]. Furthermore, the combination of bacteriuria with a history of urinary tract infection gives the most accurate prediction. Such women are at 10 times greater risk than those with neither feature, and four times greater risk than those with asymptomatic bacteriuria alone.

Any other postulated benefits of eradication of asymptomatic bacteriuria are unsubstantiated. The available data suggest that the association of asymptomatic bacteriuria and increased fetal loss, prematurity, pre-eclampsia, and anaemia are unproven [69,95,300,327]. Several of these apparent correlations may have resulted from inaccuracies in matching cases and controls and none appears to be supported by recent studies [134,324]. However, when evidence of previous parenchymal damage is present there may be a great propensity to hypertension [314]. Also there is good evidence of an association between any type of urinary tract infection in pregnancy and sudden unexpected infant death [180].

Some 30–40 per cent of pregnant women with asymptomatic bacteriuria may have upper (renal) urinary tract infection and these women may be a special population at greatest risk of pregnancy problems as well as of acute urinary tract infection. This assumption has been questioned by a study specifically designed to determine what adverse effects asymptomatic renal bacteriuria had on maternal and fetal well-being [184]. In a prospective study pregnancy outcomes in women with treated asymptomatic bacteriuria of renal origin (diagnosed by the antibody-coated bacteria technique, with a 20 per cent false positive rate), were compared to outcomes in those with treated bladder bacteriuria as well as non-infected control subjects. Women with asymptomatic renal bacteriuria appeared to be at no greater risk than abacteriuric women of developing pregnancy problems, nor were their progeny at greater risk. Nevertheless, even though the impact of asymptomatic renal infection on ultimate pregnancy outcome is minimal, the need for screening for and eradication of asymptomatic bacteriuria in order to prevent pyelonephritis is still important. This study [184] also reconfirmed the fact that symptomatic infections may be implicated in delivery of low birthweight infants when acute pyelonephritis complicates pre-term labour, suggesting a causal role in its initiation.

Where underlying undiagnosed chronic pyelonephritis is present this could be responsible for the reported obstetric complications and increased perinatal losses (see Fig. 7.6).

Choice of drug

The choice of drug must be based on the sensitivity of the isolated organim(s). Short-acting sulphonamides or nitrofurantoin derivatives are often the initial therapy [13,327]. Other drugs are reserved for treatment of failures and for symptomatic infection. Ampicillin and the cephalosporins can be safely used in pregnancy. Tetracyclines are contraindicated because of staining of the teeth of infants by binding with orthophosphates, as well as the rare maternal complication of acute fatty liver of pregnancy if they are given parenterally (see Chapter 9). If sulphonamides are prescribed in late pregnancy they should be withheld during the last 2–3 weeks since they compete with bilirubin for albumin binding sites, increasing the risk of fetal hyperbilirubinaemia and kernicterus. Nitrofurantoin used during the last few weeks may precipitate haemolytic anaemia due to glucose-6-phosphate dehydrogenase deficiency in the newborn. Trimethoprim, a constituent of Bactrim and Septrin, is not recommended for use in pregnancy since it is a folic acid antagonist. Nevertheless, it is extensively used and probably safe, though not a drug of first choice.

Duration of therapy

Opinions on optimal duration of therapy differ. Continuous antibiotic therapy from the time of diagnosis until after delivery has been recommended because of the belief that renal parenchymal involvement causes a high relapse rate. However, at least 60 per cent of patients have bladder involvement alone and the administration of short-term therapy (2 weeks) should be satisfactory. Furthermore, if patient follow-up is meticulous, there is no advantage in using continuous long-term administration of antibiotics and the possible hazards of such therapy to the fetus are avoided. Urine cultures should be obtained 1 week after therapy is discontinued and then at regular intervals throughout the pregnancy.

Relapses and re-infections

Relapse is the recurrence of bacteriuria caused by the same organism, usually within 6 weeks of the initial infection. *Re-infection* is the recurrence of bacteriuria involving a different strain of bacteria, after successful eradication of the initial infection [469]. Most patients with re-infections have infections limited to the bladder, usually occurring at least 6 weeks after therapy.

Approximately 15 per cent of patients will have a recurrence during pregnancy and a second course of treatment should be given, based on a repeat culture with sensitivity testing. In the group of patients who relapse or who are resistant to the first course of therapy, only about 40 per cent will have the asymptomatic bacteriuria cleared with subsequent therapy [284]. Since *E. coli* causes the majority of initial infections as well as recurrences, it may be necessary to employ an *E. coli* serotyping system to precisely distinguish different stains, although this does not help in clinical management.

Long-term considerations

As the interval between treatment of bacteriuria in pregnancy and post-partum follow-up becomes longer, the influence of the initial course of treatment on the incidence of bacteriuria becomes less noticeable [327]. Ten or more years after an initial episode of bacteriuria of pregnancy, the prevalence of bacteriuria in women not treated during pregnancy (25 per cent) is virtually the same as in those women who were treated (29 per cent). In contrast, women who have never been bacteriuric during pregnancy have rates of bacteriuria of about 5 per cent. Thus a single course of treatment during the index pregnancy does not appear to protect against persistent or recurrent bacteriuria years later. There are few prospective studies available, but there is no evidence that persistent asymptomatic bacteriuria in women with normal urinary tracts causes long-term renal damage or that treatment reduces the incidence of chronic renal disease [69].

Post-partum IVU

There is no consensus of opinion regarding the need for post-partum IVU in patients who have had bacteriuria [14]. It is known that 20 per cent of all patients with asymptomatic bacteriuria have IVU abnormalities [379] and this percentage is increased amongst patients with acute infections during pregnancy or with infections that have been difficult to eradicate [188].

The significance of an IVU abnormality is not so certain [65]. It may signify a predisposition to infection; it may result from infection or it may be unrelated to infection. Most abnormalities are minor and probably do not result from or cause renal infection. Furthermore, the role of infection in childhood, as indicated by scars on the IVU, is controversial [188].

In order to detect about 90 per cent of the women with major urinary tract abnormalities or to document a non-obstructed urinary tract, an IVU should be performed in women who have asymptomatic bacteriuria during pregnancy who fulfil the following additional criteria:

1 difficulty in eradicating the bacteriuria during the pregnancy;

2 episode(s) of acute symptomatic urinary tract infection during the pregnancy;

3 history of acute infection(s) prior to the index pregnancy;

4 persistence/recurrence of asymptomatic bacteriuria or acute infection post-partum.

Those patients who do have major abnormalities demonstrated post-partum are more likely to require careful long-term follow-up for eradication of bacteriuria rather than surgery. However, a non-functioning kidney may be removed and major drainage anomalies may be corrected.

Acute symptomatic urinary tract infection (UTI)

Where there is symptomatic UTI, two clinical syndromes are recognized: lower UTI or cystitis and upper UTI or acute pyelonephritis. The latter is the most common renal complication of pregnancy occurring in 1–2 per cent of all pregnancies. It has been blamed as a cause of intrauterine growth retardation, congenital abnormalities, fetal death and can certainly cause premature labour [69,95,108,183,184].

Acute cystitis

This occurs in about 1 per cent of pregnant women of whom 60 per cent have a negative initial screen. The symptoms are often difficult to distinguish from those due to pregnancy itself. Features indicating a true infection include haematuria, dysuria and suprapubic discomfort, as well as a positive urine culture. The spectrum of organisms found is the same as in women with asymptomatic bacteriuria (see above). Similar treatment is recommended with the aims of abolishing symptoms and preventing occurrence of acute pyelonephritis.

Acute pyelonephritis

The differential diagnosis includes other urinary tract pathology, other causes of pyrexia such as respiratory tract infection, viraemia, listeriosis (see Chapter 16) or toxoplasmosis (appropriate serological screening should be performed) and other causes of acute abdominal pain such as acute appendicitis, biliary colic, gastroenteritis, necrobiosis of a uterine fibroid or placental abruption.

Pneumonia on the affected side should present no difficulties if attention is paid to the type of respiration, the respiratory rate and the physical signs in the chest. It should be noted, however, that so-called adult respiratory distress syndrome (ARDS), with accompanying liver and haematopoietic dysfunction, can be a significant complication of pyelonephritis [20,382]. These problems are all probably due to lipopolysaccharide-induced red cell membrane damage [105].

Acute appendicitis can be a difficult diagnosis to make, especially in the third trimester. Usually at the onset of appendicitis the pain is referred to the centre of the abdomen, vomiting is not a marked feature, the pyrexia is not as high as in acute pyelonephritis and rigors rarely occur.

Once the diagnosis of pyelonephritis is considered, an MSU sample should be sent for culture and sensitivities. Antibiotic treatment should be aggressive and must be undertaken in a hospital setting. It should be started once the diagnosis has been made and before the sensitivities are available. If the patient is dehydrated, due to vomiting and sweating, then intravenous fluids should be given. Regular assessment of renal function should be undertaken: although the infective attack is said to have little effect on renal function in non-pregnant patients, such attacks during pregnancy have been observed to cause transient but marked decrements in GFR [491]. Ultrasonographic examination of the renal tract of pregnant women with pyelonephritis has revealed significantly increased pelvicalyceal dilatation compared to normal physiological dilatation of pregnancy, but as treatment does not produce a consistent decrease, the anomaly may antedate the acute infection [472]. The use of tepid sponging and antipyretic drugs such as paracetamol may reduce the incidence of premature labour.

Choice and duration of therapy

Dogmatic statements cannot be justified regarding the type of antimicrobial therapy for acute UTI and the appropriate duration of regimens is also debatable [327]. Treatment should aim at giving the most effective drug to eradicate a particular infection without exposing the fetus to an unnecessarily harmful agent.

Antibiotics producing high blood levels and resultant high renal parenchymal concentrations are favoured, although the importance of these factors is still undetermined [331]. Two suitable groups of antibiotics are the broad spectrum penicillins, e.g. ampicillin, and the cephalosporins; *E. coli* is the most common organism isolated in urinary infections and is usually sensitive to either of them. Trimethoprim/sulphonamide combinations, such as Septrin, are also used (see above). Aminoglycosides, such as kanamycin and gentamicin, can be given if there are problems with microbial resistance. Treatment should be monitored by blood levels. Whilst the patient is febrile, it is preferable to give intravenous antibiotics which can be continued orally when the pyrexia has settled. Antibiotic sensitivities should be reviewed within 48 hours.

The duration of treatment should be 2–3 weeks. In patients showing clinical deterioration or whose urine cultures reveal bacteria resistant to the selected antibiotic, repeat urine cultures are mandatory and alternative antibiotic therapy should be considered. In ill patients blood culture specimens should be taken. After the completion of the course of treatment urine cultures should be taken at every antenatal visit for the rest of the pregnancy.

Gram-negative sepsis

This can occur in severely ill patients with acute pyelonephritis but the situation is commonly associated with instrumentation of an infected urinary tract. An aminoglycoside antibiotic is best because it is effective against nearly all of the Gram-negative urinary bacteria. Enterococci less commonly cause bacteraemia but because of resistance to aminoglycosides ampicillin can be used combined with an aminoglycoside until culture results are available. Patients who are sensitive to penicillin should receive a cephalosporin. Haematological aspects of the management of Gram-negative sepsis are considered in Chapter 3.

Acute renal failure and pyelonephritis

This is discussed later.

Haematuria during pregnancy

The excretion of red blood cells increases (and one to two red cells per high power field may be acceptable in the urine of pregnant women) but whether leucocyturia occurs is unclear [178]. Spontaneous gross or microscopic haematuria can be due to a variety of causes [464]. UTIs, particularly those associated with congenital anomalies are difficult to eradicate and predispose to haematuria, especially if pyelonephritis is present. Rupture of small veins about the dilated renal pelvis may also cause bleeding. Spontaneous or traumatic rupture of the kidney can occur, usually where there are underlying anatomical abnormalities [323]. Spontaneous non-traumatic renal rupture, however, is very rare. Acute glomerulonephritis has been discussed earlier.

Haematuria may be secondary to any type of primary neoplasm, metastatic neoplasms, haemangiomata, calculi or fungal diseases involving the urinary system. Endometriosis, inflammatory bowel lesions, leucoplakia, amyloidosis and granulomata may involve the urinary tract and produce haematuria. The ureteral stump after a nephrectomy (for either benign or malignant disease) may be involved by any of the aforementioned conditions and should be investigated.

An aggressive approach to evaluation is needed. This may be deferred until after delivery but the clinician should assess all the circumstances to decide whether or not it takes absolute priority. In the absence of any demonstrable cause, haematuria can be classified as idiopathic and recurrences are unlikely in the current or subsequent pregnancy [113,393].

Acute hydronephrosis and hydroureter

Very occasionally pregnancy can precipitate acute hydronephrosis or hydroureter. There is a broad spectrum of the so-called 'overdistension syndrome' [149,331]. Obstruction may occur at varying levels at or above the pelvic brim (Table 7.13). This condition is not to be confused with the massive ureteral and renal pelvic dilatations (as well as slight reduction in cortical width) that can occasionally occur in normal pregnancy without ill-effect [67].

The condition should be suspected when there are recurrent episodes of loin or low abdominal pain radiating to the groin and repeat MSU specimens are sterile. There may be small increments in plasma creatinine levels but urinalysis contains few or no red cells and repeat MSU specimens are negative. Diagnosis can be confirmed using excretory urography or ultrasound (no evidence of stone) and ureteral catheterization. If positioning the patient on the unaffected side (with antibiotic therapy if appropriate) fails to relieve the situation, then ureteral catheterization or nephrostomy may be required. Typically, the pain is immediately relieved by ureteric catheterization or sonographically guided percutaneous nephrotomy so that corrective surgery can be delayed until the postpartum period [328,418,477].

Non-traumatic rupture of the urinary tract

The intrusion of unremitting pain and haematuria upon the course of pyelonephritis or the 'overdistension syndrome' suggests rupture of the urinary tract (Table 7.14). Furthermore, this complication can masquerade as other obstetric and surgical abdominal catastrophes, including appendicitis, pelvic abscess, cholecystitis, urolithiasis (see later) or abruptio placentae. Prompt recognition may prevent a small tear and urine leak, treatable by postural or tube drainage, from extending and/

Table 7.13. Clinical entities associated with pregnancy-induced urinary tract dilatation

Clinical entity	Clinical features
Overdistension syndrome	Flank pain, renal colic
Pyelonephritis	Flank pain, fever, bacteriuria
Urinary tract rupture	
Retroperitoneal	
parenchymal	Flank pain Mass: abscess, haematoma Anaemia/hypotension due to blood loss Haematuria
collecting system	Flank pain Mass: perinephric or subcapsular urinoma Haematuria (microscopic)
Intraperitoneal	
parenchymal	Peritonitis
collecting system	Flank pain Anaemia/hypotension due to blood loss Haematuria

Table 7.14. Factors contributing to rupture of the urinary tract

Traumatic	Precipitating factor: trauma
Non-traumatic	
parenchymal	Congenital: tuberose sclerosis Tumour, especially hamartoma Pyelonephritis or abscess Vasculitis (polyarteritis nodosa) Cystic disease
non-parenchymal (obstructive)	Urolithiasis Reflux, stricture Infection

or expanding. Rupture of the renal parenchyma, with haemorrhagic shock, formation of a flank mass or dissection of urinary tract contents intraperitoneally compels prompt surgical intervention, usually with nephrectomy [331].

Pregnancy in renal transplant patients

The abnormal reproductive function and sexual disorders of haemodialysed women are usually reversed after renal transplantation. (The option of sterilization should not have been offered at this time.) The resumption of regular menstruation and ovulation correlate closely with the level of function achieved by the graft [64,292,330]. With the increase in the number of transplanted women of childbearing age and more recently those with pancreatic grafts [342] clinicians must now both counsel such patients as to whether or not they should conceive and also manage the pregnancies of those who do. It has been estimated that one of every 50 women of childbearing age who have a functional renal transplant will become pregnant [63].

Recent reviews of such pregnancies have emphasized the difficulty in assessing the exact incidence of the various management problems because some of the data in the literature are incomplete and many more pregnancies than those reported have occurred [116, 117, 119, 120, 124, 125, 126, 197, 258, 329, 358,367,392,398,400,401]. Excluding the large Denver series [369,370] where 75 per cent of patients had received kidneys from living donors, only 20 per cent of births occurred in recipients of living donor grafts. Transplants have been performed with surgeons unaware that the allograft recipient was in fact pregnant, and obstetric success in such cases does not negate the importance of contraception counselling for all renal failure patients including the exclusion of pregnancy prior to transplantation.

Despite publication of numerous case reports, several series and registry data from the USA and Europe, little has been done to establish guidelines on the management of the transplant recipient who conceives. In some instances pregnancy is not diagnosed until the second or even the third trimester and many patients are under the impression that they could not conceive. Medical concern seems to be concerned with the management of the pregnancy rather than the advisability of the initial conception.

Pregnancy counselling

Management should start by counselling all couples who want a child, with a discussion of the implications of pregnancy as well as long-term prospects.

Pre-pregnancy assessment

Individual centres have their own specific guidelines. Most advise a wait of about 2 years post-transplant. This has turned out to be good advice because the patient will have recovered from the major surgical sequelae by then and renal function will have stabilized with a very high probability of allograft survival at 5 years. Immunosuppression will also be at maintenance levels which may account for higher birthweight babies in mothers becoming pregnant 2 years post-transplant as opposed to in those conceiving earlier. In one series the mean birth weight was 2.9 kg in 18 pregnancies conceived on average 60 months after transplantation, compared to 1.7 kg in seven similar pregnancies conceived 16 months after transplantation [110].

A suitable set of guidelines is given here [130], the absence of some of which is only a relative contraindication to pregnancy:

1 good general health for 2 years after transplantation;
2 stature compatible with good obstetric outcome;
3 no proteinuria;
4 no significant hypertension;
5 no evidence of graft rejection;
6 no evidence of pelvicalyceal distension on a recent excretory urogram;
7 plasma creatinine of 180 μmol/l or less;
8 drug therapy: prednisone, 15 mg/day or less and azathioprine 2 mg/kg/day or less. A safe dose of cyclosporin A has not yet been established because of limited experience, but quoted anecdotally is 5 mg/kg/day or less or even changing from cyclosporin A to azathioprine before or in early pregnancy.

After full pre-pregnancy assessment, advice can be given, but it can only be advice, since patients must ultimately decide for themselves what degree of risk is acceptable. If the situation is tackled prospectively the final decision is more of an agreement than a judgement.

Long-term considerations and allograft survival

The ultimate measure of transplant success is the long-term survival of the patient and the graft. As it is only just over 30 years since this procedure became widely employed in the management of end-stage renal failure, there are few long-term data from sufficiently large series from which to draw conclusions. Furthermore, it must be emphasized that the long-term results for renal transplants relate to a period when several aspects of management would be unacceptable by present day standards. Average survival figures of large numbers of patients worldwide indicate that 70–80 per cent of recipients of kidneys from related living donors are alive 5 years after transplantation and with cadaver kidneys the figure is 40–50 per cent [62,117,396,473]. Five-year survival is increased to about 80 per cent if renal function is normal 2 years post-transplant, and this is probably the optimal time to contemplate pregnancy.

Even after transplantation and the joy of new-found health, everyday life still has a baseline of uncertainty. Nevertheless, many patients will choose parenthood in an effort to renew a normal life and possibly in defiance of the sometimes negative attitudes of the medical and nursing establishments. Couples should be aware of all implications including the harsh realities of maternal survival prospects. A major concern is that even in the medium term the mother may not survive or remain well enough to rear the child she bears.

Pregnancy does not necessarily cause irreversible decline in renal function or affect the natural history of the allograft [302,304]. The first proper study (in 1983), albeit on a very small scale, concluded that pregnancy had no effect on graft survival or function [492]. Data from the Registry of the European Dialysis and Transplant Association (EDTA), limited to approximately 3 years post-pregnancy follow-up did not reveal any adverse influence of pregnancy on graft function [401]. Of interest is a survey which contained a considerable number of women in the 'poorer prognosis' category (hypertension, moderate renal insufficiency and long-standing diabetes mellitus): 18 women who underwent 34 pregnancies post-transplant were compared in case-control analysis with 18 allograft recipients who had never conceived. In a post-transplant follow-up in each group averaging 12 years (with a mean time from initial pregnancy of 5 years) there was no significant difference in GFR (inulin clearance or prevalence of hypertension) [449] (Fig. 7.8). These data are now contested by another study [410] based on plasma creatinine levels which suggests that pregnancy could significantly jeopardize allo-

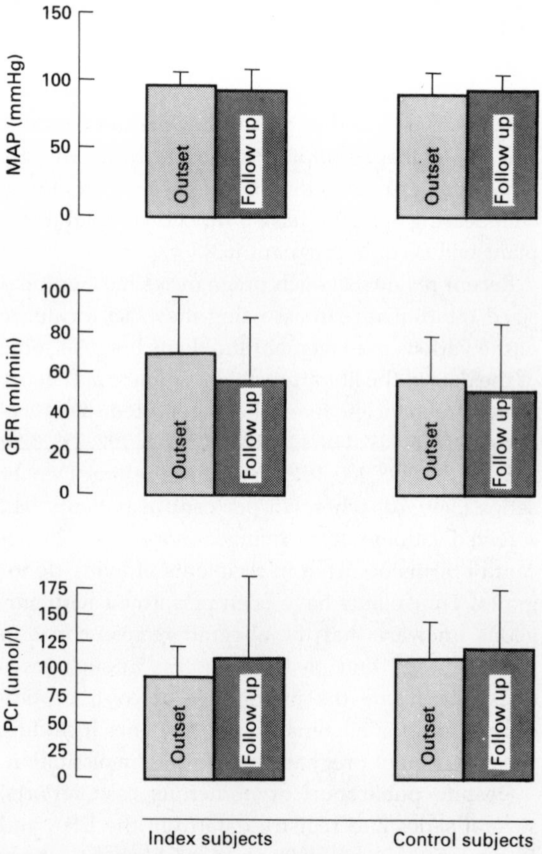

Fig. 7.8. Mean arterial pressure (MAP), GFR (inulin clearance) and PCr (plasma creatinine) in renal transplant recipients ($n = 18$) who underwent pregnancy (index subjects) compared to control subjects ($n = 18$) who never conceived. Open bars (±SEM) at onset just after transplantation and closed bars at end of follow up, averaging 12 years (modified from [449]).

grafts. However, the significance of this study is derived from the very unusual feature that the control group suffered no graft failures in 10 years [304].

Reviews of the literature indicate that about 12 per cent of women will have new long-term medical problems after pregnancy, although it is difficult to know whether such problems are merely time related or actually precipitated by pregnancy (Table 7.15) [117,120]. Interestingly, the incidence of later problems is doubled (25 per cent) if pregnancy complications occur prior to the 28th week. Registry data indicate that 10 per cent of mothers die within 1–7 years following childbirth. More long-term studies are needed to assess this (especially with the advent of the new immunosuppressive drugs), so that counselling is thorough and based on recorded experience and not clinical anecdote.

Table 7.15. Pregnancy prospects for renal allograft recipients

Problems in pregnancy (%)	Successful obstetric outcome (%)	Problems in long term (%)
49	93 (70)	12 (25)

Estimates based on 2409 women in 3382 pregnancies which attained at least 28 weeks gestation (1961–94). Figures in brackets refer to prospects when complications developed prior to 28 weeks gestation (from [120]).

Management of renal transplant recipient in pregnancy (see Box 7.3)

At the outset certain facts emerge from the literature [120]. About 35 per cent of all conceptions do not go beyond the first trimester mainly because of therapeutic and spontaneous abortions. The overall complication rate in pregnancies going beyond the first trimester is 49 per cent (Table 7.15). If complications (usually uncontrolled hypertension, renal deterioration or rejection) occur prior to the 28th gestational week then successful obstetric outcome occurs in 70 per cent compared to 93 per cent when pregnancy is trouble-free prior to 28 weeks. Remote problems occur in 12 per cent of women after delivery but where the pregnancy is complicated prior to 28 weeks remote problems occur in 25 per cent, although it is difficult to know whether such problems are precipitated by pregnancy or are time dependent and would have occurred any way. This sets the scene.

Box 7.3. Pregnancy management

- Hospital-based antenatal care in conjunction with nephrologists
- Surveillance of renal function
- Graft rejection
- Hypertension/pre-eclampsia
- Maternal infection
- Intrauterine growth retardation
- Pre-term labour
- Effects of drug therapy on fetus and neonate
- Decision on timing and route of delivery

Antenatal care

Patients must be monitored as high risk cases. Management requires attention to serial assessment of renal function, diagnosis and treatment of rejection, blood pressure control, prevention or early diagnosis of anaemia, treatment of any infection as well as the meticulous assessment of fetal well-being.

Antenatal visits should be 2-weekly up to 32 weeks and weekly thereafter. At each visit routine antenatal care should be supplemented with the following:

1 full blood count, including platelets (Coulter counter analysis);

2 blood urea, creatinine, electrolyte and urate levels;

3 24-hour creatinine clearance and protein excretion;

4 MSU specimen for microscopy and culture;

5 plasma protein, calcium and phosphate levels [265] and liver function tests should be checked at 6-weekly intervals;

6 cytomegalovirus (CMV) and herpes homini virus (HHV) titres should be checked in each trimester if the initial screen is negative.

If the patient has diabetes mellitus then a very strict management protocol is needed. It is evident that the complication rate is at least double that in other pregnant renal allograft recipients [359,479]. This may relate to the cardiovascular changes that accompany diabetes. The outlook may be considerably better when women have received a pancreas as well as a kidney allograft and successful pregnancies are increasing [73,156,359,471,479]. In one patient, however, the pancreatic graft was unexpectedly lost in acute rejection immediately after delivery, having functioned normally for 3 years prior to the pregnancy. For the future, the consensus generally is that simultaneous kidney/pancreas transplants are considered to be a treatment of choice for patients with diabetic nephropathy: inevitably such women will be potential mothers [290].

Screening all rhesus (Rh) negative recipients for Rh antibodies is mandatory. In selecting donors for renal transplantation Rh antigens are usually disregarded because they are found only on red cells and not on leucocytes or other tissue cells. Nevertheless, several cases of Rh antibody response have occurred as a result of sensitization to the transplant and it is possible for these antibodies to contribute to transplant failures since they bind to the allograft. Rhesus isoimmunization and a rising antibody titre in a pregnant transplant patient could theoretically have serious renal as well as the better known fetal consequences.

Immunosuppressive therapy is usually maintained at pre-pregnancy levels but adjustments may be needed if there are decreases in the maternal leucocyte and platelet counts, so as to at least ensure that the neonate is born with a normal blood count [128]. Azathioprine liver toxicity and the rarer interstitial pneumonitis usually respond to dose reduction or changing to cyclosporin A therapy, if necessary. Other controversies concerning immunosuppressives in pregnancy will be discussed later (see below).

Dietary counselling

Haematinics, vitamin D and calcium supplements should be prescribed if indicated [362,383]. (Metabolic bone disease in renal failure is mentioned in Chapter 14.) The role of dietary protein in augmenting glomerular function in pregnancy is controversial [31] but it is important in these patients because their kidney is already hypertrophied. It has been suggested that graft failure may be hastened by hyperfiltration [162]. For safe dietary recommendations, more information is urgently needed about the intrarenal effects and the long-term renal sequelae of dietary protein manipulation as well as the effect restriction might have on fetal outcome, particularly central nervous system development.

Early pregnancy problems

Spontaneous abortion occurs in about 14 per cent, the same as for the normal pregnant population. Between 0.2 and 0.5 per cent of all conceptions are ectopic pregnancies. Hydatidiform mole has been reported in a transplant recipient and the potential for malignant transformation is possibly enhanced by immunosuppressive drugs [322]. Ovarian tumours in early pregnancy must be distinguished from pelvic blood vessel anomalies [364].

THERAPEUTIC TERMINATION

This procedure is an obvious option. In fact, 20 per cent of pregnancies are terminated for various indications: psychosocial problems associated with an unplanned pregnancy, uncertainty about long-term maternal prognosis, renal dysfunction before pregnancy and deteriorating renal function and/or severe hypertension during pregnancy [116].

ECTOPIC PREGNANCY

These patients may be at higher risk of ectopic pregnancy because of pelvic adhesions due to previous urological surgery, peritoneal dialysis or pelvic inflammatory disease. The diagnosis can be difficult because irregular bleeding and amenorrhoea accompany deteriorating renal function or even an intrauterine pregnancy [424]. The main clinical problem is that symptoms secondary to genuine pelvic pathology are erroneously attributed to the transplant.

Allograft function (Fig. 7.9)

Serial surveillance of creatinine clearance is essential. The following points are important.

1 The increase in GFR characteristic of early preg-

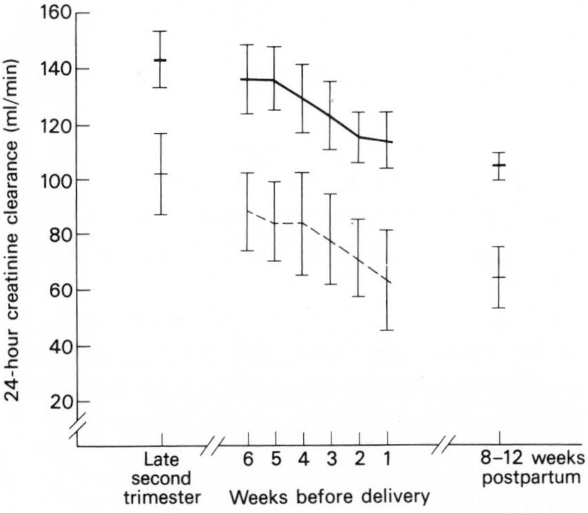

Fig. 7.9. Changes in 24-hour creatinine clearance in late pregnancy in 10 healthy women (upper) compared to 10 renal allograft recipients (lower) mean ± SEM. (Compiled from data of [124,125,129]).

nancy and maintained thereafter, is surprisingly also evident in transplant recipients even though the allograft is ectopic, denervated, possibly from an old donor, potentially damaged by previous ischaemia and immunologically different from both recipient and her fetus [102,103,130].

2 The better the renal function before pregnancy, the greater is the increment in GFR during pregnancy.

3 There can be a transient reduction in GFR during the third trimester [330,484] just as occurs in normal pregnancy [129] and such a change does not necessarily represent a deteriorating situation with permanent impairment.

4 In 15 per cent of patients significant impairment of renal function develops during pregnancy and may persist following delivery [330]. As a gradual decline in allograft function is a common occurrence in non-pregnant patients, it is difficult to delineate the specific role of pregnancy. Subclinical chronic rejection, with declining renal function, may occur as a late result of tissue damage after acute rejection or when immunosuppression has not been adequate.

5 There may be a non-immune contribution to chronic graft failure due to the damaging effect of hyperfiltration through remnant nephrons [162], perhaps even exacerbated during pregnancy (see above).

6 Proteinuria occurs near term in about 40 per cent of patients but disappears post-partum and in the absence of hypertension is not significant [115].

7 If renal function deteriorates by >15 per cent at any stage of pregnancy, reversible causes should be sought such as UTI, subtle dehydration or electrolyte imbalance (occasionally precipitated by inadvertent diuretic therapy); allograft rejection must of course be considered. Inability to detect a treatable cause of a significant functional decrement is a reason to end the pregnancy by elective delivery. When proteinuria occurs and persists, but renal function is preserved and blood pressure is normal, the pregnancy can be allowed to continue.

Allograft rejection

It has been reported that serious rejection episodes occur in 9 per cent of women with pregnancies lasting into the third trimester [408]. Whilst the incidence of rejection is no greater than expected for non-pregnant transplant patients it might be considered unusual because it had always been assumed that the privileged immunological state of pregnancy would benefit the transplant. Furthermore, there are reports of reduction or cessation of immunosuppressive therapy during pregnancy without rejection episodes [249,398].

Chronic rejection may be a problem in all recipients and probably has a progressive subclinical course. If this is somehow influenced by pregnancy there do not appear to be any consistent factors serving to predict which patients will develop rejection episodes, as there is no relationship to prior rejection episodes, HLA types, the transplant-pregnancy time interval or problems in previous pregnancies [196]. The following points are important:

1 rejection at any time is difficult to diagnose;

2 if any of the clinical hallmarks such as fever, oliguria, or deteriorating renal function associated with renal enlargement and tenderness are present, then the diagnosis must be considered;

3 ultrasonography can be helpful because alterations in the echogenicity of the renal parenchyma and the presence of an indistinct corticomedullary junction are indicative of rejection [273];

4 without renal biopsy, rejection cannot be distinguished from acute pyelonephritis, recurrent glomerulopathy, possible severe pre-eclampsia and even cyclosporin A nephrotoxicity;

5 the diagnosis must be beyond doubt before embarking upon anti-rejection therapy;

6 rejection occasionally occurs in the puerperium [362,398]; and this may be the result of the return to a normal immune state (despite immunosuppression) or possibly a rebound effect from the altered immunoresponsiveness associated with pregnancy.

Hypertension and pre-eclampsia

The appearance of hypertension and proteinuria in the third trimester and their relationship to deteriorating renal function, to the possibility of chronic underlying pathology and to pre-eclampsia are difficult diagnostic problems. Hypertension, particularly before 28 weeks gestation, is associated with adverse perinatal outcome [448], which may be due to covert cardiovascular changes that accompany or are aggravated by chronic hypertension.

Pre-eclampsia is diagnosed clinically in about 30 per cent of pregnancies and, interestingly, is not related to the chronological age of the donor organ [102]. Although many of the hypertensive syndromes are quite severe, there is only one report of a woman (a primigravida) where there was rapid progress to eclampsia and interestingly, she subsequently had an uncomplicated successful pregnancy [494,498].

Unlike the situation in normal pregnant women, changes in urinary protein excretion, plasma urate levels, platelet count or liver function tests do not appear to be useful markers for either the onset or the severity of pre-eclampsia, as all of these parameters can be substantially changed in otherwise uncomplicated pregnancies. The following points are important:

1 many of the specific risks of hypertension are mediated through superimposed pre-eclampsia, a diagnosis which cannot be made with certainty on clinical grounds alone, because proteinuria, hypertension and renal deterioration may be manifestations of underlying transplant dysfunction or even rejection;

2 it is not known whether systemic hypertension has any significant intrarenal effect in pregnancy although in the single kidney situation, with or without pregnancy, it could theoretically contribute further to glomerular hyperfiltration and possibly glomerular hypertension and injury (reviewed by [31,43]);

3 treatment of mild hypertension is not necessary during normal pregnancy but many would treat transplant patients more aggressively, believing this preserves renal function.

Infections

Although some reports describe an increased incidence of all types of infection, this is controversial [214,422]. Nevertheless, there can be no doubt that immunosuppression, anaemia and debility make all recipients susceptible to infection. Infection with uncommon organisms is common and cultures should always be obtained when infection is suspected. Fungal and related infections occur less frequently now that transplant teams have learnt more about the limits of the various immunosuppressive regimens. *Aspergillus*, *Mycobacterium tuberculosis*, *Listeria monocytogenes* and *Pneumocystis* have all been reported. The incidence of urinary tract infection may be as high as 40 per cent and is said to occur in all women in whom chronic pyelonephritis was a primary cause of the renal failure. Viral infections, mainly CMV, herpes simplex (HSV) and hepatitis B, are always a potential hazard to mother and fetus [158,318,441].

Gastrointestinal disorders

Dyspepsia can cause considerable distress in any allograft recipient particularly in pregnancy. Although there is no correlation between dyspepsia and total steroid dosage, it does appear that problems are less common with low dose immunosuppressive regimens.

Parathyroid dysfunction (see also Chapter 14)

Up to 20 per cent of women with successful renal

transplants develop tertiary hyperparathyroidism. If maternal hyperparathyroidism is untreated (or undiagnosed) there is the risk of maternal hypercalcaemia followed by neonatal hypocalcaemia [419]. If parathyroidectomy is undertaken there is then the risk of hypoparathyroidism [383] with maternal hypocalcaemic seizures as well as congenital hypo- and hyperparathyroidism. Calcium and phosphate levels therefore need careful monitoring during pregnancy.

Immunosuppressive therapy during pregnancy

As mentioned above routine clinical practice is to maintain therapy at pre-pregnancy levels. Changes in therapy must not jeopardize overall suppression even though there are some reports where therapy was reduced or stopped during pregnancy without invoking rejection [249,398]. At no point after transplantation, barring serious drug toxicity, is it prudent to stop all immunosuppressive therapy [196].

The commonly used maintenance regimen is a combination of prednisone and azathioprine. Cyclosporin A is a relatively new immunosuppressive agent and preliminary evidence suggests that it may be more effective than the conventional drugs [72,157] but experience in pregnancy is still limited [7,171,202,252,287].

Prednisone

This steroid decreases cell-mediated responses to the allograft with the disadvantages of increased risks of infection and/or malignancy and poor healing. Additional maternal side-effects include glucose intolerance, peptic ulcer development, osteoporosis and weakening of connective tissues, which may have predisposed to uterine rupture in one patient [398].

Prednisone crosses the placenta to a limited extent (see Chapter 1) and is converted to prednisolone which, although not suppressing fetal adrenocorticotrophic hormone (ACTH), may have other adverse fetal effects (see later). Augmenting steroids post-partum to cover so-called 'rebound immunoresponsiveness' is controversial [275,367] and the consensus is that it is neither necessary nor beneficial.

Azathioprine

This purine analogue decreases delayed hypersensitivity and cellular cytoxicity while leaving antibody-mediated responses relatively intact. In the mother the primary hazards are increased risk of infection and/or neoplasia. Azathioprine crosses the placenta and the fetal and paediatric implications will be discussed later (see below). In theory, the fetus should be protected from the effects of azathioprine in early pregnancy, as it then lacks the enzyme inosinate pyrophosphorylase which converts azathioprine to thioinosinic acid, the metabolite active on dividing cells [408,495].

The most sensitive method of monitoring azathioprine dosage and bioavailability is the measurement of red cell 6-thioguanine nucleotides (6-TGN), which are metabolites of both azathioprine and 6-mercaptopurine and whose formation is catalysed by red cell thiopurine methyltransferase (TPMT). Low TPMT activity may be a risk factor for the development of thiopurine toxicity and there certainly are large individual variations in red cell 6-TGN amongst patients receiving identical azathioprine dosage [281,286]. One in 300 patients inherits a lack of TPMT activity and identification of such patients could be important, especially in pregnancy, if side-effects are to be avoided. A less sensitive, but nevertheless safe, approach involves adjustments in azathioprine dosage to maintain maternal leucocyte count within normal limits for pregnancy thus ensuring that the neonate is born with a normal blood count [128].

Cyclosporin A

This fungal metabolite's major inhibitory effect is on the T lymphocyte and other cells mediating allograft rejection. There is wide individual sensitivity and it is plasma rather than whole blood drug levels that correlate best with toxicity. The widely differing accumulation seen in various human tissues is related to variations in cyclophilin, the major intracellular cyclosporin A binding protein.

Although renal allograft survival data are better with cyclosporin A [72,157], it actually reduces compensatory hyperfunction at the time of the transplant and has long-term nephrotoxic effects.

Consequently most patients have plasma creatinine levels of 100–260 μmol/l compared to 70–180 μmol/l in those on routine immunosuppression [462]. Whether the usual relationship between higher plasma creatinine values and worse gestational outcome applies in cyclosporin A treated patients has not yet been established [116]. As well as nephrotoxicity other adverse effects include neoplasia, hepatic dysfunction, tremor, convulsions, glucose intolerance, hypertension, haemolytic uraemic syndrome (HUS) and predisposition to thromboembolic phenomena. The latter four are particularly significant and worrying in relation to pregnancy.

Little is known about either the maternal or fetal effects of this drug in pregnancy. Theoretically some of the maternal physiological adaptations could be blunted by cyclosporin A, for example its depressive effects on extracellular volume and renal haemodynamics [140,244,381,462]. In the few cases in the literature, however, renal function was not adequately documented and whether the kidney in pregnancy is more vulnerable to cyclosporin A is not known [10,171,252,287]. Interestingly, the presence of *E. coli* kidney infection can increase susceptibility to nephrotoxicity and yet absence of renal innervation, as in a transplant, possibly affords some protection.

More pregnancy information is emerging [16,138, 171,202,375] but there are still theoretical worries that cyclosporin A reduces a women's ability to cope with the challenge of pregnancy on renal function and the placental circulation. Overall, the pregnancy success rate with cyclosporin A seems comparable to that with azathioprine [90]. Reports from the recently established US National Transplantation Pregnancy Registry are particularly enlightening [7,16] with over 300 patients enrolled by 1993. In 154 pregnancies in 115 women on cyclosporin A (54 per cent of whom had required antihypertensive therapy prior to pregnancy) birthweights were overall reduced and specifically, intrauterine growth retardation was greater, but this may relate more to hypertension and decreased renal function than to cyclosporin A. We suggest that if possible, dosage be maintained between 2–4 mg/kg day.

Decisions regarding delivery

Pre-term delivery is common (45–60 per cent) because of intervention for obstetric reasons and the common occurrences of pre-term rupture of membranes and pre-term labour. Pre-term labour is commonly associated with poor renal function and this may be a contributory factor in transplant patients [165]. In some, however, there is no obvious explanation and it has been postulated that long-term steroid therapy may weaken connective tissue and contribute to the increased incidence of pre-term rupture of membranes [408].

Management during labour

Vaginal delivery should be the aim and there is no evidence that there is any extra risk of mechanical injury to the transplanted kidney. Unless there are problems or unusual circumstances [319,409], the onset of labour should be spontaneous but of course induction should be undertaken if there are specific indications.

Careful monitoring of maternal fluid balance, cardiovascular status and temperature is essential. Aseptic technique is mandatory at all times [345]: any surgical procedure, however trivial, such as an episiotomy, should be covered with prophylactic antibiotics (ampicillin and metronidazole). Indeed, surgical induction of labour by amniotomy might be considered to warrant antibiotic cover.

Augmentation of steroids is necessary to cover the stress of delivery. A reasonable dose would be intramuscular hydrocortisone, 100 mg every 6 hours during labour. Pain relief is conducted as for healthy women. If there are problems with acute hypertension then management should be as discussed in Chapter 6.

Fetal electronic monitoring should be undertaken. If fetal scalp blood samples are taken then a fetal platelet count would help to exclude fetal thrombocytopenia, which increases the risk of fetal intracerebral haemorrhage and is an indication for caesarean section [425] (but see also Chapter 3).

Role of caesarean section

Although obstructed labour due to the position of

the graft has been reported [355], the kidney does not usually obstruct the birth canal. Caesarean section is only necessary for purely obstetrical reasons [319,409]. However, from the literature, the 25 per cent caesarean section rate is certainly much higher than might be expected, presumably reflecting fear of the unknown, rather than certainty that vaginal delivery would be hazardous for mother and/or child.

The following are important when making a final decision on the route of delivery.

1 Transplant patients may have pelvic osteodystrophy related to their previous renal failure (and dialysis) or prolonged steroid therapy, particularly if it occurred before puberty [225]. For instance, avascular necrosis, particularly of the femoral head, is a common problem, occurring in 20 per cent of all transplant patients [153,227]. Patients with pelvic problems should be recognized antenatally and delivered by caesarean section if there is cephalopelvic disproportion.

2 Some authors have recommended that if there is any question of disproportion or kidney compression, then simultaneous intravenous urogram and X-ray pelvimetry should be performed at 36 weeks gestation [398].

3 When a caesarean section is performed, a lower segment approach is usually feasible but previous urological surgery may make this difficult [106,159]. Care must be taken that the ureter and/or the graft blood supply are not damaged or compromised.

Box 7.4. Factors causing neonatal problems in offspring of renal allograft patients

- Pre-term delivery/small for gestational age
- Respiratory distress syndrome
- Depressed haemopoiesis
- Lymphoid/thymic hypoplasia
- Adrenocortical insufficiency
- Septicaemia
- CMV infection
- Hepatitis B surface antigen carrier state
- Congenital abnormalities
- Immunological problems
  - Reduced lymphocyte PHA reactivity
  - Reduced T lymphocytes
  - Reduced immunoglobulin levels
- Chromosome aberrations in leucocytes

Paediatric management (see Box 7.4)

Pre-term delivery

Pre-term delivery (<37 weeks' gestation) is common (45–60 per cent) because of intervention for obstetric reasons and the tendency to pre-term labour, which although commonly associated with renal impairment, is not always the obvious explanation. It has been suggested that long-term steroid therapy weakens connective tissue and contributes to the increased incidence of pre-term rupture of membranes.

Average birthweights are low since most deliveries are pre-term (Fig. 7.10). Additionally, the incidence of intrauterine growth retardation is 20 per

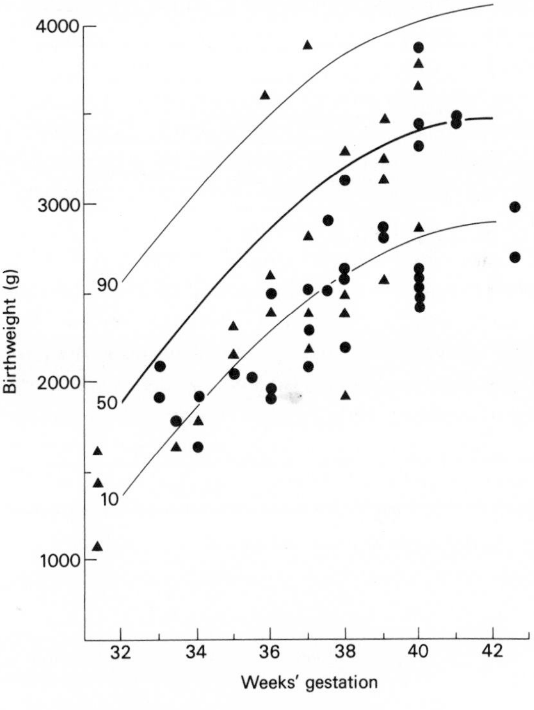

7.10. Birthweight and gestational age of infants born to renal allograft recipients, who all received azathioprine prior to and throughout pregnancy (modified from [423]). 10th, 50th and 90th centiles are shown. Twenty-five cases managed in Newcastle upon Tyne (1976–92) are shown as ▲.

cent (range 8–40 per cent in the literature) and is not necessarily related to the severity of renal impairment, vascular disease or hypertension [377] (Table 7.16). Certainly, immunogenetic disparity between conceptus and mother is advantageous, and placentae and fetuses are bigger when there is smaller maternofetal histocompatibility. Thus, in the renal transplant mother non-specific depression of the maternal immune system by immunosuppressives may contribute to fetal growth retardation. Congenital CMV infection may also be a contributory factor [158].

Immediate problems

Over 50 per cent of live-borns have no neonatal problems. As pre-term delivery is common (45–60 per cent) small-for-dates infants are delivered in at least 20 per cent of cases and as occasionally the two problems occur together neonatal paediatric management must be available. There are also some special problems in these babies such as thymic atrophy, transient leucopenia, CMV and hepatitis B infection, bone marrow hypoplasia, reduced blood levels of IgG and IgM, septicaemia, chromosome aberrations and polymorphism in lymphocytes, hypoglycaemia, hypocalcaemia and adrenocortical insufficiency [182,385,408,486].

Cord blood samples should be taken at delivery with the aim of excluding these problems. Adrenocortical insufficiency due to maternal steroid therapy increases the risk of overwhelming neonatal infection. Occasionally the neonate collapses shortly after delivery with overwhelming infection, and adrenocortical insufficiency should be suspected [369]. Once the diagnosis has been considered, the proper therapy consists of steroids, antibiotics, γ globulin and appropriate electrolyte solutions.

Congenital abnormalities

No frequent or predominant development abnormalities have been reported. Azathioprine is teratogenic in animals but only with large doses, equivalent to >6 mg/kg bodyweight/day, much more than the modest ones (2 mg/kg/day or less) required by women with stable renal function [412, 495]. In one series, however, where birth anomalies were present in seven out of 103 offspring, the mothers of abnormal babies had been taking a significantly higher daily dose of azathioprine than those who had normal babies: 2.64 mg/kg versus 2.02 mg/kg [392]. (There was no significant difference in the daily dose of prednisone between the two groups.) This was based on a relatively small number of abnormal babies and could still be due to chance.

Very large doses of steroids in experimental animals can produce congenital abnormalities but the risk to the fetus from doses used after transplantation is small. Cyclosporin A is embryo- and fetotoxic in animals when given in doses 2–5 times greater than the human dose.

Viral infections

INFECTIOUS HEPATITIS

It is likely that children born to renal transplant mothers who are carriers of HBsAg (during and after pregnancy) become antigen carriers themselves [385,434]. Of interest is the fact that any woman with acute hepatitis in late pregnancy or within 2 months after delivery transmits HBsAg to her offspring in at least 75 per cent of cases, whereas in asymptomatic carriers the risk of the children becoming antigen positive is much less

Table 7.16. Possible effects (%) of immunosuppression during pregnancy (from [377])

Women	Pregnancies	Oligo-hydramnios	Intrauterine growth retardation	In labour: Meconium	In labour: Fetal distress
Renal transplants (18)	20	20	40	45	25
Controls (3410)	5012	2	8	12	2

(see Chapter 9). Even if there is little effect on general health, however, serum aminotransferases may be elevated perhaps signifying chronic persistent hepatitis, which in some cases has been verified by biopsy [181].

The use of hyperimmunoglobulin against HBsAg given prophylactically to neonates has been investigated and it is known that the carrier state can be prevented in 75 per cent if newborns are given hepatitis B immunoglobulin immediately after birth [172,342,388,503] (see also Chapter 9). Recently it has been shown that if hyperimmunoglobulin is given with hepatitis B virus vaccine within a few hours of birth this regimen is 90 per cent effective in reducing the HBsAg carrier state in infants, but not if administration is delayed beyond 48 hours or if either is given alone [49].

CMV

CMV infection, a major cause of morbidity in transplant recipients, can present in a variety of ways in the mother including fever, leucopenia, thrombocytopenia and pneumonia as well as liver and renal dysfunction. CMV immunoglobulin can provide effective prophylaxis in women at risk for primary infection [455] and perhaps all potential mothers should be treated if appropriate.

Of most importance to the pregnant transplant recipient and her fetus are the implications of congenital CMV infection [235]. Therapeutic termination is not a practical approach because maternal infections are mostly symptomless, detectable only by serological monitoring and many infants born to women with CMV infection are not seriously damaged but can be growth retarded. If primary maternal CMV infection is responsible for the majority of damaged CMV-infected infants, there may be a case for pre-pregnancy testing followed by CMV immunoglobulin or even CMV vaccination [51]. Live CMV vaccines are available but it is not known whether they can prevent congenital CMV infection.

HSV

Primary maternal infection prior to 20 weeks is associated with an increased rate of abortion. Caesarean section should be undertaken if a cervical culture is positive for HSV at term, since the risk of neonatal infection resulting from vaginal delivery is at least 50 per cent (see Chapter 16).

Postnatal assessment and long-term maternal follow-up

A major concern is that the mother may or may not survive or remain well enough to rear the child she bears. It has been calculated that 10 per cent will be dead within 7 years of pregnancy and 50 per cent dead within 15 years [107], data that perhaps should be presented cautiously when undertaking pre-pregnancy assessment and long-term counselling (see above). Many women, however, will choose parenthood in an effort to re-establish a normal life and possibly in defiance of the sometimes negative attitudes of the medical establishment.

Contraception

All women should be routinely counselled about contraception. The choice depends on balancing the desirability of pregnancy prevention against the potential risks of the contraceptive method. Contraceptive steroids can produce subtle changes in the immune system [250], but this is not necessarily a contraindication to their use. Low dose oestrogen–progesterone preparations can be prescribed although some have avoided them because of the possibility of causing or aggravating hypertension or further increasing the incidence of thromboembolism [384,459]. If the oral contraceptive is prescribed, careful and frequent surveillance is needed.

An intrauterine contraceptive device (IUCD) can aggravate any tendency towards menstrual problems and these in turn may confuse the signs and symptoms of abnormalities in early pregnancy, such as threatened abortion or ectopic pregnancy [424]. The risks of pelvic infection are increased and this could be disastrous in an immunosuppressed patient [457]. Insertion or replacement of an IUCD is normally associated with bacteraemia in at least one in every 10 women so in transplant patients antibiotic cover is essential at this time [342a]. Furthermore, there is a higher incidence of fungal infections with a plastic IUCD (42 per cent) compared to a copper-containing device (2 per cent). The efficacy of the IUCD may be reduced by immunosuppressive and anti-inflammatory agents, possibly due to modification of the leucocyte response [460,502]. Nevertheless, many request this method. Careful counselling and follow-up are essential.

Gynaecological problems

These patients have the same problems that afflict the normal female population. There is a danger, however, that symptoms secondary to genuine gynaecological pathology may be erroneously attributed to the transplant due to its location near the pelvis. Transplant patients might be at slightly higher risk of ectopic pregnancy because of pelvic adhesions due to previous urological surgery, peritoneal dialysis, pelvic inflammatory disease or the use of an IUCD [502]. Diagnosis can be overlooked because irregular bleeding and amenorrhoea may be associated with deteriorating renal function as well as intrauterine pregnancy.

Transplant recipients receiving immunosuppressive therapy have a *de novo* malignancy rate estimated to be 100 times greater than normal and the female genital tract is no exception [78,198,213, 429]. For instance, there are reports of cervical changes ranging from cellular atypia through carcinoma *in situ* to invasive squamous cell carcinoma [378]. The malignancy association is probably related to factors such as loss of immune surveillance, chronic immunosuppression allowing tumour proliferation and/or prolonged antigenic stimulation of the reticuloendothelial system [368]. Regular gynaecological assessment is essential and any treatment should be conventional, with outcome unlikely to be influenced by stopping or reducing immunosuppression.

Breast feeding

Steroids are secreted in breast milk but not in sufficient quantity to affect the infant at therapeutic doses. In theory, if the baby has been exposed to azathioprine and its metabolites throughout pregnancy, it should be well accustomed to them and if their concentrations in breast milk are minimal then breast feeding would not be contraindicated. Despite the beneficial effects of breast feeding, more specific information is needed about whether the amounts of azathioprine and its metabolites are trivial or substantial from a biological point of view [102,160] and only then can sound advice be given. Cyclosporin A is excreted in breast milk in amounts <2 per cent of the maternal dose, but little is known about the potential effects of this drug in children [171]; therefore breast feeding should be discouraged until more definitive data are forthcoming.

Potential long-term paediatric problems

If azathioprine causes chromosome aberrations in fetal lymphocytes (see Table 7.17) [380] — however transient — the fear is that these anomalies may not be temporary in other somatic cells not studied and in the germ cells. The sequelae could be future development of malignancies or impairment of reproduction in the affected offspring. There is some evidence concerning this from animal studies [394]. The ovaries of female offspring of mice treated with 6-mercaptopurine (the principal metabolite of azathioprine): equivalent to 3 mg/kg contained fewer oöcytes and ovarian follicles compared to offspring of mothers that had not received the drug. Furthermore, these mice had fertility problems when they were bred. Despite normal bodyweight and general appearance, many proved to be sterile or if they became pregnant, had smaller litters and more dead fetuses (Table 7.18).

This effect was probably initiated while the offspring were developing in the uteri of their mothers during treatment. It is unlikely that such damage would be eliminated or repaired, as seems to happen in somatic cells, because synthesis of DNA stops when the germ cells are arrested in the prophase of the first meiotic division *in utero*, and no new DNA is synthesized until after fertilization.

Thus exposure of the fetus to low doses of potential mutagens may not cause immediate, obvious effects such as morbidity or birth defects, but may have severe consequences when otherwise normal female offspring reach puberty. As yet, there are no animal data on the reproductive performance of the male offspring.

Table 7.17. Chromosome aberrations* (per cent) in cultured lymphocytes of two renal transplant mothers and their offspring compared to non-pregnant transplant patients and the normal population (modified from [380])

		Infant		
	Adult	Birth	6 months	>6 months
Mother 1	25	16	8	10
Mother 2	12	18	14	0
Renal transplant patients (non-pregnant)	26			
Normal	2.5	0.5–1	0.5–1	0.5–1

* Gaps, fragments, deletions, rings, etc. studied in metaphase.

Table 7.18. Effect of 6-mercaptopurine (6-MP) in pregnancy in the mouse on subsequent reproduction of offspring. Mean ± SEM (from [394])

6-MP dose to mother (mg/kg/day)	Weight of ovaries of offspring (mg)	Number of offspring bred	Number of offspring achieving pregnancy	Number of fetuses per pregnancy	Percentage of dead fetuses
0	8.6 ± 0.4	33	33	13.0 ± 0.4	13
0.5	8.7 ± 0.3	46	44	12.8 ± 0.3	18
1.5	7.3 ± 0.6	33	26	10.6 ± 0.5	25
3.0	2.2 ± 0.6	9	2	6.5 ± 3.5	46

It is reassuring that, to date, information about general progress in infancy and early childhood of the offspring of renal transplant mothers has been good but there have been no studies of possible impairment of fertility [267,367,408,486]. Of course, with the introduction of cyclosporin A new evaluations are urgently required and need to be balanced against its other worrying maternal side-effects. Above all it is imperative that any child exposed to immunosuppressive therapy *in utero* has a careful evaluation of the immune system and long-term follow-up.

Renal transplants and pregnancy: some conclusions

1 The reproductive endocrinology of uraemia is complex and has been reviewed elsewhere [292]; renal transplantation is usually quickly followed by improvements in reproductive function.

2 The possibility of conception in women of child-bearing age emphasizes the need for compassionate and comprehensive counselling. Couples who want a child should be encouraged to discuss all the implications, including long-term maternal survival prospects.

3 Therapeutic abortion is an option taken up by one in every five women.

4 The spontaneous abortion rate is about 14 per cent (the same as for the normal population) and of the conceptions that go beyond first trimester, 93 per cent end successfully.

5 In most women, renal function is augmented during pregnancy, but permanent impairment occurs in 15 per cent of pregnancies. In others there may be transient deterioration in late pregnancy (with or without proteinuria).

6 There is a 30 per cent chance of developing hypertension, pre-eclampsia or both.

7 Pre-term delivery occurs in 45–60 per cent and intrauterine growth retardation in at least 20 per cent of pregnancies. The incidence is 30–40 per cent in women taking cyclosporin A.

8 Despite its pelvic location, the transplanted kidney rarely obstructs labour and is not injured during vaginal delivery. Caesarean section should be reserved for obstetric reasons only.

9 Neonatal complications include respiratory distress syndrome, leucopenia, thrombocytopenia, adrenocortical insufficiency and infection. No predominant or frequent developmental abnormalities have been described and data on progress in infancy and childhood are encouraging.
10 There is no room for complacency and further data are needed to improve understanding and management in the following areas: pre-pregnancy assessment criteria, the mechanisms of gestational renal dysfunction and proteinuria, the side-effects and implications of immunosuppression in pregnancy and the remote effects of pregnancy on both maternal renal prognosis and the offspring.

Pregnancy in haemodialysis patients

It has been several decades since the first documentation of conception and successful delivery in a patient undergoing chronic haemodialysis [96] and since then further case reports and registry data have been published [6,12,22,80,141,151,218,219, 221,265,249,389,392,401,415,432,465,467,475]. In one of the cases reported [475] the renal function was so good that success might have been achieved without dialysis.

Any optimism must be tempered by remembering that clinicians are reluctant to publish their failures and consequently the true incidence of unsuccessful pregnancies and their sequelae in women on haemodialysis cannot be determined. There is no doubt that the high surgical abortion rate (albeit decreasing in recent years) in these patients indicates that those who become pregnant do so accidentally, probably because they are unaware that pregnancy is a possibility.

Pregnancy counselling

In spite of irregular or absent menstruation [293], decreased libido and potency, and impaired fertility, women undergoing haemodialysis should always use contraception if they wish to avoid pregnancy [64,292,439]. The introduction of recombinant human erythropoietin (rHuEpo) to the treatment of women with renal failure appears to be associated in some cases with return of normal menses (and ovulation), probably because of correction of hyperprolactinaemia and/or improved overall health [416].

There are substantial arguments against pregnancy and these should be pointed out, not least the risks to the patient and the greatly reduced likelihood of succesful outcome [304]. Even when therapeutic terminations are excluded, there is generally about a 20–30 per cent likelihood of success (Table 7.19) [119,218,220,265,349]. A recent report [222] indicates that 52 per cent are 'successful' even though several were extremely premature and several had disturbing maternal problems.

General management plan

Early pregnancy assessment

Early diagnosis of pregnancy can be a problem.

Table 7.19. Dialysis and pregnancy

Number of pregnancies (year)	*182 (1989)	*287 (1992)	†56 (1992)
Pregnancy rate (%)	0.5	1.0	1.2
Therapeutic abortion (%)	40	22	9
Spontaneous abortion (%)	47	50	48
Perinatal loss (%)	3	10	13
Successful outcome (%)	10	18	30
(excluding therapeutic abortion) (%)	19	23	33

* Cumulative literature surveys (J. Davison and C. Baylis, unpublished data).
† Questionnaire survey of 206 dialysis units in 10 States in the USA [220].

Irregular menstruation is common and a missed period will usually be ignored [155,292]. The big mistake the clinician may make is not even to consider the possibility of pregnancy. As urine pregnancy tests are unreliable [212], even if there is any urine available, early diagnosis and estimation of gestational age are best accomplished by ultrasound.

Management objectives

For a successful outcome, scrupulous attention must be paid to blood pressure control, fluid balance, increased dialysis requirements and provision of good nutrition [22,92,146,152,221,389,501]. It should be emphasized that this will place many demands on the hospital team as well as the patient's family. It might even be considered to be a misuse of scarce resources and manpower.

Strategy during pregnancy

Women with residual renal function and satisfactory daily urine volumes, in whom biochemical control is easier, are more likely to become pregnant. Some patients show increments in GFR even if the level of renal function is too poor to sustain life without haemodialysis. The dialysis strategy should have the following aims.

1 Maintain plasma urea at <20 mmol/l. It has been suggested that intrauterine death is likely if levels are much in excess of 20 mmol/l [463] but in one case report [6] success was achieved despite levels of 25 mmol/l for many weeks.

2 Maintain pH and electrolyte levels near pregnancy norms. For instance, daily haemodialysis with dialysate bicarbonate reduced to 18–20 mmol/l may be needed in women who have no renal function.

3 Ensure good control of blood pressure.

4 Avoid hypotension during dialysis. In late pregnancy the gravid uterus and the supine posture may aggravate this by decreasing venous return.

5 Be on guard for dialysis-induced uterine contractions.

6 Ensure minimal fluctuations in fluid balance and limit volume changes.

7 Avoid maternal hypercalcaemia: the placenta produces 1,25-hydroxy vitamin D and oral supplementation may have to be reduced.

8 Attempt to minimize heparin use, although this may be difficult as pregnancy is a hypercoaguable state.

9 Limit interdialysis weight gain to 0.5 kg until late pregnancy.

Inevitably this strategy means increased length and frequency of dialysis — in some instances by as much as 50 per cent [265]. There is no doubt that frequent dialysis renders dietary management and control of weight gain much easier but the domestic problems caused might require that a combination of home and hospital dialysis is used.

In a recent report from Saudi Arabia of 27 pregnancies in 22 women, only 10 went beyond 28 weeks gestation and eight of these were successful. Comparing the pregnancies that ended before 28 weeks with those that went beyond, the authors found no significant differences in blood pressure, haemoglobin, creatinine levels, type of dialysate, post-obstetric history or years on dialysis. Dialysis hours were, however, significantly longer in the successful group.

Anaemia

Increasing anaemia causes concern for maternal and fetal welfare. Patients are usually anaemic and blood transfusion may be needed, especially before delivery, for safe obstetric management [265,399]. Caution is needed because transfusion may exacerbate hypertension and might also impair the ability to control circulatory overload, even with extra dialysis. Fluctuations in blood volume can be minimized, however, if nitrogen-frozen packed red cells are transfused during dialysis.

rHuEpo has been used in pregnancy without ill-effect [22,315]. Specifically, the theoretical risks of hypertension and thrombotic complications have not been encountered so far [500]. No adverse effects have been noted in neonates in whom haematological indices and erythropoietin concentrations for gestational age suggest that rHuEpo does not have significant transplacental effects [223].

Unnecessary blood sampling should be avoided and, in any case, lack of venepuncture sites can be a problem. The protocol for the various routine tests performed in a particular unit should be followed meticulously, removing no more blood per venepuncture than is absolutely necessary. Screening for Australia antigen is mandatory.

Hypertension

Blood pressure can fluctuate wildly. These patients have such abnormal lipid profiles and accelerated atherogenesis that it is difficult to predict the ability of the cardiovascular system to tolerate the stresses of pregnancy. Diabetic women on dialysis who have become pregnant are those in whom cardiovascular problems are most evident. Normal blood pressure is reassuring. Unfortunately, hypertension is a common problem, though it may be possible to control this by ultrafiltration to reduce circulating blood volume, provided exacerbation does not occur between dialysis. Any other measures must be carefully assessed in the light of possible side-effects.

Dietary counselling

Despite more frequent dialysis, free dietary intake should be discouraged. An oral intake of at least 70 g protein, 1500 mg calcium, 50 mmol potassium and 80 mmol sodium per day is advised and oral supplements of dialysable vitamins should be given. Vitamin D supplements can be difficult to judge in patients who have had a parathyroidectomy. It is not clear to what extent these dietary factors and maternal uraemia affect the fetus and its nutrition. The use of parenteral nutrition supplementation in pregnancy has been advocated [66].

Delivery

Caesarean section should only be necessary for obstetric reasons, although it could be argued that an elective caesarean section would always minimize potential problems of volume and blood pressure control during labour. In fact, pre-term labour is generally the rule and the role of caesarean section under these circumstances needs to be carefully considered [291].

Pregnancy in patients on peritoneal dialysis

Since 1976 chronic ambulatory peritoneal dialysis (CAPD) and chronic cycling peritoneal dialysis (CCPD) have been utilized more frequently in the management of patients with all forms of renal insufficiency. Several features of peritoneal dialysis make it an attractive approach for the management of renal failure in pregnancy.

1 Maintenance of a more stable environment for the fetus in terms of fluid and electrolyte concentrations.
2 Avoidance of episodes of abrupt hypotension — a frequent occurrence during haemodialysis, which can cause fetal distress.
3 Continuous allowance for extracellular fluid volume control so that blood pressure control is augmented.
4 Lack of systemic heparinization.
5 Achievement of better maternal nutrition by allowing semi-restricted diet.
6 Better blood sugar control in women with diabetes mellitus via intraperitoneal insulin.
7 Theoretically permitting safe use of intraperitoneal magnesium facilitating prevention and treatment of premature labour and possibly pre-eclampsia.

Young women can be managed with this approach and a few successful pregnancies have been reported [152,177,223,232,257,389,501]. Although anticoagulation and some of the fluid balance and volume problems of haemodialysis are avoided in these women, they nevertheless face the same problems — placental abruption, pre-term labour, sudden intrauterine death and hypertension. Furthermore, it should be remembered that peritonitis can be a severe complication of CAPD and accounts for the majority of therapy failures [186,187]. This, superimposed on a pregnancy, can present a confusing diagnostic picture with the potential for a whole series of treatment problems.

There are reports of gynaecological sequelae in these patients. Reflux of menstrual blood can occur through the intraperitoneal catheter under normal circumstances as well as due to possible endometriosis [54]. Severe pelvic peritonitis is always a possibility [407]. Psychosocial problems are common and can influence libido (and potency in males) [55].

Lastly, it has been argued that if dialysis is to be used in pregnancy then peritoneal dialysis is the method of choice and if a woman is already on haemodialysis then a change should be considered [389]. We, however, prefer that women continue on the mode of dialysis of the time of conception.

Acute renal failure

Acute renal failure is a clinical syndrome characterized by a sudden and marked decrease in glomerular filtration, rising plasma urea and creatinine levels, and usually by a decrease in urine output to <400 ml in 24 hours. As a clinical diagnosis the term only describes *the functional state of the kidneys* without distinguishing between the different forms of underlying pathology [266] (Table 7.20). For the most part, acute renal failure occurs in persons with previously healthy kidneys but it may also complicate the course of patients with pre-existing renal disease [266,470].

Before anuria or oliguria are ascribed to acute renal failure, obstruction to the renal outflow must be excluded, usually by infusion urography, if investigation is needed. This is particularly pertinent in obstetric practice, since it is all too easy to unwittingly damage the urinary tract when performing emergency surgery for obstetric disasters, such as post-partum haemorrhage, which are themselves causes of acute renal failure.

Rarely hydronephrosis leading to acute renal failure in late pregnancy can be due to obstruction from an enlarging uterus with or without polyhydramnios [286,480] a situation which resolves immediately after amniotomy [57], or if delivery is not appropriate then ultrasound-guided percutaneous nephrostomy is safe and reliable [477]. The effects of polyhydramnios are very occasionally added to by a fetal abdominal mass [426].

Perspective

Twenty years ago the incidence of acute renal failure in pregnancy was 0.02–0.05 per cent [251] and

Table 7.20. Some causes of obstetric acute renal failure

Volume contraction/hypotension	Ante-partum haemorrhage due to placenta praevia Post-partum haemorrhage: from uterus or extensive soft tissue trauma Abortion Hyperemesis gravidarum Adrenocortical failure; usually failure to augment steroids to cover delivery in patient on long-term therapy
Volume contraction/hypotension and coagulopathy	Ante-partum haemorrhage due to abruptio placentae Pre-eclampsia/eclampsia Amniotic fluid embolism Incompatible blood transfusion Drug reaction(s) Acute fatty liver Haemolytic uraemic syndrome
Volume contraction/hypotension, coagulopathy and infection	Septic abortion Chorioamnionitis Pyelonephritis Puerperal sepsis
Urinary tract obstruction	Damage to ureters: during caesarean section and repair of cervical/vaginal lacerations Pelvic haematoma Broad ligament haematoma

represented about 2 per cent of cases reported of renal failure of all causes. At that time acute renal failure was a substantial cause of maternal mortality, as at least 20 per cent of women with this complication died [437].

Recently there has been a marked decline in cases of acute renal failure related to obstetrics, largely attributable to liberalization of abortion laws and improvements in perinatal care which had reduced complications, such as sepsis, eclampsia, hypovolaemia and severe haemorrhage [46,203,445,470]. The current incidence is <0.005 per cent, but complications with transient decrements in GFR of a mild to moderate degree probably occur in one in 8000 deliveries [268]. Acute renal failure still has a bimodal distribution corresponding to septic abortion in early pregnancy and pre-eclampsia and bleeding problems in the third trimester [204,308, 372,373]. There are still parts of the world where the incidence of acute obstetric renal failure remains high (0.06 per cent) and in one unit in Northern India 10 per cent of all renal failure cases are related to pregnancy [85].

Pathology

There are three common patterns of altered renal function and anatomy, which are probably part of a spectrum of increasing severity of the same pathological process: pre-glomerular vasoconstriction causing renal hypoperfusion with preferential cortical ischaemia [333,346] (see Table 7.21).

Pre-renal failure or vasomotor nephropathy

This is a relatively mild form of acute renal failure and is caused by moderate degrees of renal ischaemia. It is partly a functional disorder, there are no changes in renal morphology and it is reversible if renal perfusion is improved.

Acute tubular necrosis

This occurs if renal ischaemia is more severe or persistent. Damage is limited to the most metabolically active tubular cells. Blood vessels and glomeruli do not show significant alteration. It

Table 7.21. Differential diagnosis of oliguria

	Pre-renal failure (vasomotor nephropathy)	Acute tubular necrosis
History/background	Vomiting, diarrhoea, dyhydration	Dehydration, ischaemic insult, ingestion of nephrotoxin (no specific history in 50%)
Physical examination	Decreased blood pressure, increased pulse, poor skin turgour	May have signs of dehydration, but physical examination often normal
Urinalysis	Concentrated urine; few formed elements on sediment, many hyaline casts	Isosthenuria; sediment contains renal tubular cells and pigmented casts, but may be normal
Urinary sodium	<20 mmol/l; most <10 mmol/l	≥25, usually >60 mmol/l
U : P ratios	High	Low
Osmolality	Often ≥1.5	<1.1
Urea	≥20	≤3
Creatinine	>40	<15
Fractional sodium excretion ($U:P_{Na}/U:P_{creatinine}$)	<1%	>1%
Renal failure index	<1	>1
($U:P_{Na}/U:P_{creatinine}$)	<1	>1

Modified from Lindheimer MD, Davison JM: *In* Medical Disorders during Pregnancy. Barron WM, Lindheimer MD (eds), Mosby-Yearbook, 1991.
U : P, urine/plasma ratio.

is also reversible after a variable period of renal shutdown.

Acute cortical necrosis

This occurs if renal ischaemia is very severe or protracted or when there is intense intravascular coagulation. There is complete disintegration of glomeruli and tubules throughout the entire cortex of both kidneys, usually with an irreversible clinical course. In pregnancy, however, renal involvement may be patchy.

Phases of acute renal failure

Traditionally there are three consecutive phases and these have important management implications.

Oliguria

Urine volumes are <400 ml in 24 hours. This phase may last from a few days to several weeks. Complete anuria is uncommon in acute tubular necrosis and is usually a manifestation of massive acute cortical necrosis or complete obstruction. Non-oliguric forms of acute cortical necrosis may be occasionally encountered in which urine volumes seem adequate but renal function is severely impaired [478] (see Table 7.21).

Polyuria

Urine volumes increase markedly and can be up to 10 l in 24 hours. The polyuria may last from several days to 2 weeks. The urine is dilute and, despite the large volumes excreted, metabolic waste products are not efficiently eliminated. Consequently plasma urea and creatinine levels will continue to rise for several days in parallel with increased urine output. Profound fluid and electrolyte losses can endanger survival if not adequately replaced.

Recovery

Urine volumes decrease towards normal. Renal function gradually improves, nearing the level before the acute renal failure developed.

Diagnosis and investigation

A carefully taken history may reveal a background of abortion, severe hyperemesis gravidarum, haemorrhage, sensitization to drugs, incompatible blood transfusion, pre-eclampsia and/or neglect of recent steroid intake (see Table 7.20). Once the diagnosis has been entertained, the possible causes must be pursued and, in conjunction with a nephrologist, a full initial assessment should be undertaken. The assessment should include the following.

1 Blood specimens: full blood count (Coulter counter analysis), urea, electrolytes and osmolality, glucose, liver function tests, amylase, plasma proteins, in particular albumin, coagulation indices, acid–base status (arterial blood sample).

2 Urine specimens: specific gravity and osmolality, electrolyte concentrations, protein excretion.

3 Bacteriological assessment: blood cultures (aerobic and anaerobic), vaginal swabs, MSU.

4 Electrocardiogram (ECG): abnormalities do not necessarily correlate with the degree of hyper- or hypokalaemia. Initially, in hyperkalaemia, there are peaked T waves with QRS prolongation and then disappearance of P waves with deformation of the QRS complex.

5 Assessment of fluid balance: the bladder should be catheterized and continuous drainage allowed so that hourly volumes can be recorded. A CVP line should be established, preferably via the antecubital vein. Where the patient is deeply shocked the subclavian vein may be used, but this route should be avoided when artificial ventilation is likely, because of the danger of pneumothorax. This complication is unlikely to arise using the right internal jugular vein, a route that has the added advantage that the catheter tip invariably enters the right atrium. The right atrial pressure (RAP) serves as an indicator of volume of blood returning to the right side of the heart and the response of the right ventricle to a volume load.

A separate intravenous therapy line, preferably also in a central vein, should be established. Exact therapy will depend on the biochemical disturbance(s) and CVP or RAP readings.

Administration of large amounts of fluid in acute tubular necrosis is both useless and fraught with danger. Blood loss must be taken into account; it is frequently underestimated especially if there has been an ante-partum haemorrhage, which is often concealed.

6 Fetal salvage: if this has to be taken into consideration then a decision will have to be made regarding the timing and route of delivery.

Diagnostic pitfalls

It is difficult and often impossible to decide which of the three types of acute renal failure (acute tubular necrosis, acute cortical necrosis, pre-renal failure) is present. Total anuria or alternating periods of anuria and polyuria strongly suggests obstruction, but normal urine volumes do not exclude obstruction. Complete anuria and/or evidence of disseminated intravascular coagulation (DIC) are suggestive of acute cortical necrosis but this diagnosis can only be firmly established by renal biopsy [372].

The differential diagnosis between functional renal insufficiency caused by dehydration or hypotension (pre-renal failure or vasomotor nephropathy) and acute tubular or cortical necrosis is of practical importance as their therapy is diametrically different (see Table 7.21).

Urine/plasma (U : P) osmolality ratio. This ratio is the single most valuable indicator of early acute renal failure [313]. Pre-renal failure is suggested when the ratio is >1.5, whereas in acute tubular or cortical necrosis it is closer to unity.

Urine specific gravity. This is inadequate because misleadingly high values may be caused by sugar or protein admixture and comparison with plasma is not possible.

Urinary sodium concentration. This index is only useful when oliguria is present because a low sodium concentration can be found in non-oliguric acute renal failure [317]. In pre-renal failure the urine is concentrated with low sodium concentration (<20 mmol/l) and in acute tubular necrosis the urine is isotonic to plasma with a relatively high sodium concentration (>60 mmol/l) [313].

Trial intravenous infusion of 100 ml 25 per cent mannitol. Mannitol infusion is a relatively safe therapeutic test and may be helpful in distinguishing between reversible pre-renal failure and established acute tubular necrosis provided the period of oliguria does not exceed 48 hours and the U : P osmolality ratio is >1.05 [313].

If a diuresis is established within 3 hours (>50 ml/hour or double the previous urine volume) then urine output should be replaced exactly with intravenous isotonic saline in an attempt to sustain adequate urine flow for at least 24–36 hours, after which the danger of acute tubular necrosis has probably passed. By determining urinary electrolytes the losses can be replaced accordingly. If urine flow subsequently decreases to <30 ml then the mannitol infusion can be repeated 6–8 hourly.

If attempts to increase urine flow are unsuccessful, the objective is to support the functionally anephric patient until the kidneys recover.

Use of diuretics. Increments in urine flow produced by 'loop diuretics' such as frusemide may represent conversion of oliguric renal failure to a polyuric form, rather than reversal of pre-renal failure. Furthermore, there is no evidence of any beneficial effect of frusemide on the period of oliguria, immediate prognosis or mortality [236].

Role of renal biopsy. Since acute cortical necrosis is usually irreversible, biopsy is indicated in patients with protracted oliguria or anuria who fail to improve, in order to allow an assessment of prognosis [296]. Diagnosing acute cortical necrosis early, however, is not mandatory, since the management of the acute stage is no different from that of acute tubular necrosis.

General management plan

Pre-renal failure or vasomotor nephropathy

The basic principle is to adequately replace blood and fluid losses and maintain blood pressure at levels that will permit adequate renal perfusion. Evidence of continuing blood loss calls for localization and control of the bleeding. Volume correction should always precede the use of diuretics, with the exception of mannitol (both a volume expander and an osmotic diuretic) which may usefully reduce endothelial cell swelling and thereby help to restore renal blood flow.

Volume and metabolic control

Fluid intake and output must be determined daily. Insensible fluid losses cannot be measured directly, but weighing the patient every day is helpful in assessing the state of hydration, and haematocrit and total protein determinations are additional evaluators.

Volume balance is achieved by allowing the adult, non-febrile patient an intake of 500 ml of fluid plus the total output of the preceding 24 hours. If the patient is febrile 200 ml of additional intake is needed for each 1°C increment. If fluid volume is in balance then bodyweight should decrease approximately 0.3–0.5 kg per 24 hours because of tissue catabolism. Overhydration must be avoided and if present must be promptly corrected, if necessary by dialysis. Continuous careful supervision and replacement of urinary fluid electrolyte losses is even more important in the polyuric phase, as 50 per cent of deaths occur at this time.

There is a need for oral or parenteral administration of at least 1500 calories of a protein-free fat/carbohydrate combination which is low in potassium and sodium. Carbohydrate calories are important for decreasing gluconeogenesis from protein (protein-sparing effect), thus retarding the development of azotaemia/acidosis. Volume limitations dictate that glucose should be administered as a hypertonic (up to 50 per cent) solution via a central vein.

Administration of essential L-amino acids improve wound healing, result in reductions of plasma potassium, magnesium and phosphate levels, and generally improve survival and hasten recovery [5].

In such circumstances dialysis should be started regardless of plasma biochemistry, but when creatinine and urea levels rise rapidly because of a hypercatabolic state, dialysis is indicated even if clinical symptoms have not yet appeared. Early 'prophylactic' dialysis, before the onset of uraemic symptoms, allows more liberal intake of protein, salt and water as well as preventing hyperkalaemic emergencies [308]. Furthermore, it decreases the incidence of infectious complications, improves wound healing, increases patient comfort and appears to improve patient survival.

Peritoneal dialysis

Peritoneal dialysis has many advantages and can be used in pregnant or recently delivered women [218, 323]. It is easily available, simple, inexpensive and has a relatively low complication rate. There are no absolute contraindications and it can be used even in the presence of pelvic peritonitis. Relative contraindications are intraperitoneal adhesions, open wounds or drains in the abdomen and recent retroperitoneal operations [261]. Occasionally peritoneal dialysis may be complicated by peritonitis or trauma to the intra-abdominal viscera.

Haemodialysis

Haemodialysis depends on an adequate shunt blood flow and has limited usefulness in the presence of hypotension. It is contraindicated in the actively bleeding patient, since even well controlled regional heparinization does not ensure the safety of the procedure.

Acute renal failure and septic shock

(see also above)

Septicaemia associated with pregnancy is commonly due to septic abortion whereas pyelonephritis, chorioamnionitis and puerperal sepsis occur less frequently [85,203,373]. Only occasionally is the abortion spontaneous, although detailed questioning may be required to elicit evidence that abortifacients have been used. Although this life-threatening condition is now very rare the clinician should not be lulled into a false sense of security given the ever present potential of antibiotic-resistant bacterial strains.

Pathology

There are many reasons why acute renal failure should be associated with septic abortion. The patient is both dehydrated and hypotensive — a combination which leads to considerable renal ischaemia. Haemoglobinuria (due to haemolysis) and DIC are often present and soap and lysol (common abortifacients) have specific nephrotoxic effects [21]. The severity of the renal dysfunction associated with clostridial infections suggest that clostridia produce a specific nephrotoxin [397]. However, most pregnancy sepsis is due to Gram-negative bacteria (clostridia is responsible for only 0.5 per cent), so that marked haemolysis due to bacteria and/or abortifacients is sufficient by itself to provoke renal shutdown, although it is now apparent that antilipopolysaccharide antibodies may have a role [264].

Diagnosis and investigation

The presentation can be quite dramatic, especially in cases of *E. coli* and clostridia infection. There is an abrupt rise in temperature (to 40°C) often associated with myalgias, vomiting and diarrhoea, the latter occasionally bloody.

Once symptoms commence, hypotension, tachypnoea and progression to acute shock occur rapidly. The patients are usually jaundiced, with a particular bronze-like colour ascribed to the association of jaundice with cutaneous vasodilation, cyanosis and pallor. Despite the presence of fever, the extremities are often cold, with purplish areas which may be precursors of small patches of necrosis on the toes, fingers or nose.

There is laboratory evidence of severe anaemia due to haemolysis with hyperbilirubinaemia of the direct type. There are also alterations in clotting factors which suggest DIC (see Chapter 3). Leucocytosis (25×10^9/l) with marked shifts to the left are the rule and thrombocytopenia of $<50 \times 10^9$/l is often observed. Hypocalcaemia, severe enough to provoke tetany, can occur [203].

Abdominal X-ray may demonstrate air in the uterus or abdomen — the result of gas-forming organisms and/or perforation. Despite this toxic and septicaemic picture bacterial identification may be difficult and the situation is further confused because clostridia are normally present in the female genital tract [438].

Full initial assessment should be conducted with an intensive care physician and a nephrologist [150] along the lines discussed for acute renal failure with the following additional important points:

Skin and core temperature differential. The relationship of skin temperature to central body temperature serves as an indicator of adequacy of peripheral perfusion. Peripheral temperature can be measured from the medial aspect of the big toe and central body temperature by a probe placed in the rectum, in the lumen of the oesophagus or over the sternum. A large difference between the two (>2°C) implies poor peripheral perfusion. This is commonly associated with lactic acidosis and occasionally with DIC.

Serum albumin. This should always be assessed in any patient with severe sepsis. Levels <25 g/l are commonly found, predisposing the patient to pulmonary oedema. Albumin replacement should be considered.

Blood sugar. Diabetes must be excluded. Blood from a finger prick should not be used if there is poor skin perfusion.

Acid–base status. The patient may be hypoxic, through ventilation–perfusion inequality. The P_{aCO_2} is usually low in order to compensate for the increasing metabolic acidosis. An elevated P_{aCO_2} is unusual: it may imply deterioration in the level of consciousness with loss of respiratory drive or, occasionally, may precede respiratory failure or depression due to sedative drugs.

Metabolic acidosis is generally related to inadequate peripheral oxygenation, anaerobic metabolism and the onset of lactic acid acidosis. An increasing and irreversible metabolic acidosis following initial resuscitation is a bad prognostic sign.

Coagulation indices (see Chapter 3). Hypercoagulability may be seen early and can alternate with hypocoagulability. Haematological evidence of DIC correlates with the severity of the shock and poor peripheral oxygenation. The potential for blood loss in septic abortion increases the susceptibility to DIC. Thrombocytopenia alone can occur in the presence of significant sepsis.

Cardiovascular investigation. Routine cardiovascular assessment may be insufficient for haemodynamic evaluation [150]. More elaborate investigations may be needed such as right ventricular output assessment or pulmonary capillary wedge pressure (PCWP), and these require skilled personnel as well as specialized equipment. Therefore, should a patient fail to respond to volume replacement, metabolic correction and antibiotics or be severely shocked, treatment must be conducted in an appropriately equipped intensive therapy unit.

Diagnostic pitfalls

The clinician may be misled by an asymptomatic patient admitted with an incomplete abortion who rapidly becomes shocked within hours. The generalized muscular pains, often most intense in the thorax and abdomen, may lead to confusion with intra-abdominal inflammatory processes; this is especially true when a history of provoked abortion is denied or not sought, since heavy vaginal bleeding is often not a prominent feature.

Recent treatment with antibiotics or other drugs must be pursued as it will give pointers to bacterial resistance, suppressed infection and drug-modified physiology.

General management plan

The initial steps include vigorous supportive therapy and the use of antibiotics in high doses. The use of clostridia antitoxin, steroids and the role of surgical intervention are controversial.

The role of surgery

Three or four decades ago women with septicaemia due to septic abortion were usually considered too ill to undergo surgery. It was later suggested that in such patients the placenta served as a huge culture site for bacterial growth, from which bacteria and toxins could easily pass into the maternal circulation [453]. This led to the hypothesis that if this nidus could be contained by securing the ovarian and uterine vessels, the patient's blood pressure would respond favourably and rapidly. In a series of 77 women with soap-provoked septic abortion, 60 per cent of patients who underwent surgery survived compared to 30 per cent of those treated by supportive therapy alone [234]. Bartlett and Yahia [21] described five successive gravely ill women whose abortion had been induced by soap and/or phenol: each of them survived, and this success rate was attributed to the rapid performance of abdominal hysterectomy.

Such results led many to advocate a radical approach, where abdominal hysterectomy is performed in patients who are responding poorly to volume replacement and vasoactive agents [79,154]. However, this approach was questioned by Hawkins *et al.* [203] who described 20 patients managed with intensive antibiotic therapy, dialysis as required, and an absolute minimum of surgical intervention: 17 out of 19 of these patients survived while a 20th patient who had undergone hysterectomy died. These authors state that modern antibiotic therapy alone is usually capable of confining the infection to the pelvis and eventually eradicating it from the uterus. They further noted that many young women with septic abortion may want a pregnancy in the future, and in their series of 11 women who subsequently attempted to conceive, seven achieved normal pregnancies.

The debate concerning radical versus conservative treatment continues [308]. Data supporting the surgical approach have not always been as favourable as the small series of Bartlett and Yahia [21], and none of the reported studies was controlled. On the other hand, the picture of a necrotic and grossly infected uterus that often accompanies these chemically produced abortions is sufficient to convince many that hysterectomy is necessary. Whilst the results of Hawkins *et al.* [203] are impressive, it should be noted that most of their patients were transferred from other hospitals, and constituted a group that had already survived for several days with a conservative approach.

Volume and metabolic control

It is essential to restore an adequate circulating volume as soon as possible, and the volume infused must be regulated according to CVP or RAP readings. When both the blood pressure and the CVP are low, fluid should be infused until the systolic pressure rises to 100 mmHg or higher and/or the CVP is up to 8 cmH_2O. An increase in urinary output to >40 ml/hour is an excellent prognostic sign.

The fluid selected for volume replacement will depend upon whether there is an obvious electrolyte deficit, possible albumin depletion, or fluid is merely required to increase the circulating volume. Plasma protein fraction (PPF) is the solution of choice for volume replacement. Should the urinary output improve, potassium supplementation is generally necessary.

Sodium chloride (as normal saline) should only be given when there has been obvious sodium loss. A low serum sodium is common in the septic patient but does not necessarily reflect a fall in total body sodium. Blood should not be used for volume replacement, unless the haematocrit is 30 per cent or less, because it increases viscosity and hence may encourage capillary sludging. Dextran 70 should not be used if there is evidence of a bleeding diathesis or a history of skin allergy or bronchospasm.

In an appreciable number of cases anuria may persist for up to 3 or more weeks [199]. Often it is just when the patient is thought to have cortical rather than tubular necrosis that the diuretic phase commences. Some women with septic abortion do develop cortical necrosis, however, perhaps due to a severe ischaemic insult or massive DIC.

Digoxin should be used (provided the plasma potassium is normal) when there is evidence of myocardial failure or the patient develops atrial flutter or fibrillation. Other drugs which may improve the haemodynamic state include dopamine, isoprenaline and phentolamine; their use must be based on expert assessment of the haemodynamic situation [200].

Bacteriological control

Appropriate antibiotic therapy is essential but in the shocked patient it is of secondary importance to restoration of adequate perfusion. Before antibiotics are given the appropriate specimens for aerobic and anaerobic cultures must be taken. A bactericidal antibiotic may produce temporary clinical deterioration because of breakdown of bacteria and endotoxin release. This is an additional reason for performing basic resuscitation procedures before starting antibiotic therapy.

In patients without previous antibiotic therapy, it is reasonable to commence with a combination of a cephalosporin and metronidazole. Should the shock be severe and a *Pseudomonas* or *Proteus* infection be diagnosed or a resistant *Klebsiella* or coliform be suspected, then gentamicin should be included. The dosage of gentamicin must be regulated according to daily blood levels. Once the sensitivities are available, the antibiotic therapy may need to be modified. Antibiotics should be given intravenously at first, changing to the oral route once the shock phase is over.

Haematological control

Sequential assessment of the coagulation indices is essential. A steady deterioration may be seen consistent with a diagnosis of DIC, and is commonly associated with overall clinical deterioration. Active treatment is not required where there are minor changes in the coagulation indices without clinical evidence of bleeding and where shock is rapidly corrected.

Should the clotting factors continue to deteriorate, in spite of the preceding resuscitative measures, fresh frozen plasma (FFP) should be given. Heparin may be considered if there is a further fall in the fibrinogen titre, in spite of FFP. A persistent thrombocytopenia (platelet count $<40 \times 10^9$/l) and capillary oozing in spite of replacement of clotting factors is an indication for an infusion of platelets or platelet-enriched plasma.

Other measures

Hyperbaric oxygen and exchange transfusion have both been used to treat clostridial sepsis, but results are too fragmentary to recommend specific protocols [148].

Acute renal failure in pre-eclampsia/eclampsia (see also Chapter 6)

The cause of renal failure in pre-eclampsia/eclampsia is considered in Chapter 6, but the situation may be aggravated by haemorrhage or even inappropriate drug therapy [67]. If the renal failure is related solely to pre-eclampsia without chronic hypertension, renal disease or both (before pregnancy) then normal renal function resumes in about 80 per cent of cases in the long-term. Underlying renal problems reduce this to 20 per cent, with the remainder needing permanent renal replacement therapy.

Treatment should follow the standard approach, although recently more specific therapies have been tested such as prostacyclin infusion [174].

Acute renal failure and pyelonephritis

Acute pyelonephritis is the most common renal complication during pregnancy [108]. In the absence of complicating features such as obstruction, calculi, papillary necrosis and analgesic nephropathy, acute pyelonephritis is an extremely rare cause of acute renal failure in non-pregnant subjects, but this association appears to be more frequent in pregnant women [357]. The reason is obscure. It is known that, in pregnant women, acute pyelonephritis is accompanied by marked decrements in GFR as well as significant increments in plasma creatinine levels [491] and this contrasts with the situation in non-pregnant patients. The vasculature in pregnancy may be more sensitive to the vasoactive effect of bacterial endotoxins [109].

Haemolytic uraemia syndrome (HUS)

This rare and often lethal syndrome was first described 20 years ago [71] and named 'irreversible post-partum renal failure'. Several other labels have been used since then including 'idiopathic post-partum renal failure', 'post-partum malignant nephrosclerosis', 'idiopathic post-partum renal failure' and most commonly 'post-partum HUS'. The haematological manifestations of HUS are considered in Chapter 3.

Pathophysiology and diagnosis

HUS is characterized by the onset of renal failure 3–10 weeks into the puerperium [204,272,278] after the patient has had an uneventful pregnancy and delivery. She develops marked azotemia and severe hypertension frequently associated with microangiopathic haemolytic anaemia and platelet aggregation with formation of microthrombi in the terminal portions of the renal vasculature. It should be remembered that renal failure, microangiopathic haemolytic anaemia and thrombocytopenia may be associated in pregnant women with severe pre-eclampsia, the so-called HELLP syndrome (haemolysis, elevated liver enzymes, low platelets [589]), acute fatty liver of pregnancy and thrombotic thrombocytopenic purpura. Distinction between HUS and some of these disorders may be difficult since they may persist in the post-partum period. Although there is clinically a broad overlap between these conditions, correct identification is necessary since specific investigations or therapy are needed in some [139,411].

The pathophysiology is unknown and the controversies about management reflect this uncertainty [142,427,453]. HUS has a poor prognosis: in a review of 49 patients with HUS by Segonds *et al.* [427], death occurred in 61 per cent, complete recovery of renal function in only 9.5 per cent and 12 per cent of the patients had terminal renal failure requiring maintenance dialysis.

It has been suggested that endothelial damage is the key lesion in HUS. This may involve the Sanarelli–Schwartzman reaction [97], the action of an *E. coli* produced vero-cell toxin (verotoxin) [243] and/or platelet aggregation and deposition. It has recently been demonstrated that endothelial production of NO (see p. 230) may be critical to prevent endotoxin-induced glomerular thrombosis [421]. Genetic and environmental factors have been implicated as they have in post-pill HUS, idiopathic HUS and thrombocytopenic purpura. Of interest are recent reports of two HLA-identical sisters, one of whom developed post-partum HUS and the other post-pill HUS [337] and familial occurrence of thrombotic thrombocytopenic purpura during pregnancy. A pathogenic role for immunological factors has also been proposed as transient hypocomplementaemia can occur.

Treatment and outcome

Treatment has been with dialysis or plasma phoresis, immunosuppression, heparin, streptokinase, dipyridamole, acetylsalicylic acid and corticosteroids in various combinations. Other forms of management have evolved in recent years and have been used with some success. A supposed lack of plasma prostacyclin (PGI_2) — a powerful vasodilator and potent endogenous inhibitor of platelet aggregation — can be counteracted by exchange transfusion or even plasma infusion alone [395] on the basis of its successful use in thrombotic thrombocytopenic purpura or in adult HUS [336]. Prolonged PGI_2 infusions have been tried with the aim of restoring the deficiency, thus controlling hypertension and reversing platelet consumption [485].

Because DIC may be of pathogenic significance, with placental thromboplastin release during labour, antithrombin III (ATIII) may have a protective effect. ATIII can be given as a concentrate and there have been reports of low plasma ATIII concentrations at the onset of the syndrome [58]. Interestingly, heparin increases the turnover rate of ATIII, and giving heparin to patients with potentially decreased plasma ATIII levels may therefore paradoxically increase an existing risk of thrombosis. Lastly, renal transplantation may be successful but there is a chance of recurrence of the HUS lesion in the allograft.

Bilateral renal cortical necrosis (BRCN) in pregnancy

Renal cortical necrosis is an extremely rare complication which at one time seemed to be more common in pregnant compared to non-pregnant populations [373] but most recently its incidence during pregnancy has decreased to below one in 80 000. It is characterized by tissue death throughout the cortex with sparing of the medullary portions [193,194,195]. Although it may develop in patients with DIC or overwhelming septicaemia most cases present in the third trimester or the puerperium when septic complications occur less often and when it is associated with specific obstetric complications such as placental abruption, unrecognized long-standing intrauterine death and occasionally pre-eclampsia [372]. Multigravidas beyond the age of 30 are more likely to develop this condition. It has been considered the clinical counter-part of the experimental Sanarelli–Schwartzman reaction [97].

While cortical necrosis may involve the entire renal cortex resulting in irreversible renal failure, it is the 'patchy' variety that occurs more often in pregnancy. This is characterized by an initial episode of severe oliguria, which lasts much longer than in uncomplicated acute tubular necrosis, followed by a variable return of function and stable period of moderate renal insufficiency. Years later, for reasons still obscure, renal function may decrease again, often leading to end-stage renal failure.

Miscellaneous causes of renal failure

Acute renal failure can occur during pregnancy in a variety of situations similar to those causing renal dysfunction in non-pregnant patients. These situations include primary renal diseases (acute nephritis, sarcoidosis, lymphoma, Goodpasture's syndrome), those related to systemic illnesses (endocarditis, ingestion of nephrotoxins, incompatible blood transfusions) and structural infiltrations of the kidneys secondary to extrarenal disease [430]. Acute renal failure in acute fatty liver of pregnancy is considered in Chapter 9.

Obstetric renal failure: some conclusions

1 Acute renal failure can occur during pregnancy in a variety of situations similar to those causing sudden renal dysfunction in non-pregnant patients [373]. Pathology peculiar to pregnancy, however, must always be considered. Acute fatty liver can be complicated by renal failure and its early recognition with prompt treatment could reduce fetal and maternal mortality rate. HUS is also associated with a high morbidity and mortality.

2 The need to actively treat acute renal failure cannot be questioned but, the importance of reaching an early (histological) diagnosis of its cause must not be forgotten [483].

3 Treatment of sudden renal failure resembles that used in non-pregnant populations and aims at retarding the appearance of uraemic symptomatology, acid–base and electrolyte disturbances and volume problems. There must be constant awareness of the propensity of patients with acute renal failure to become infected, a complication which can be serious in pregnant women.

4 Some of the problems can be dealt with by judicious conservative management, but if such an approach is unsuccessful dialysis will be necessary.

5 Dialysis in patients with acute renal failure is prescribed 'prophylactically'; that is prior to the appearance of electrolyte, acid–base disturbances imbalance or uraemic symptoms. Furthermore, as urea, creatinine and a presumed variety of metabolic waste products cross the placenta 'prophylactic' dialysis could be more compelling in pre-partum patients with immature fetuses and in whom temporization is desired. The policy of 'buying time' without modifying the underlying pathology should be continually reviewed.

6 The method of dialysis (peritoneal or haemodialysis) should be dictated by facilities available and by clinical circumstances. Peritoneal dialysis is effective and safe as long as the catheter is inserted high in the abdomen under direct vision through a small incision. It probably minimizes rapid metabolic pertubations.

7 Controlled anticoagulation with heparin (preferably including monitoring of activated clotting time to maintain it between 150 and 180 seconds) is desirable during haemodialysis. Volume shifts during haemodialysis must be minimized to avoid impairment of uteroplacental blood flow.

8 Increments in uterine activity or the onset of labour frequently occur during or immediately after dialysis. Therefore, when possible, early delivery (as dictated by fetal maturity) should be undertaken.

9 At or after delivery blood loss should be replaced quickly to the point of slight overtransfusion, because any haemorrhage may be underestimated.

10 The neonate can be subject to rapid dehydration because increased levels of urea and other solutes within the fetal circulation precipitate an osmotic diuresis in the neonate shortly after birth.

References

1 Abe S. An overview of pregnancy in women with underlying renal disease. *American Journal of Kidney Diseases* 1991; **17**: 112–15.

2 Abe S. Pregnancy in IgA nephropathy. *Kidney International* 1991; **40**: 1098–102.

3 Abe S. The influence of pregnancy on the long-term renal prognosis of IgA nephropathy. *Clinical Nephrology* 1994; **41**: 61–4.

4 Abe S, Amagasaki Y, Konishi K, Kato E, Sakaguchi H & Iyori S. The influence of antecedent renal disease on pregnancy. *American Journal of Obstetrics and Gynecology* 1985; **153**: 508–14.

5 Abel RM, Abbott WM & Fischer JE. Intravenous essential L-amino acids and hypertonic dextrose in patients with acute renal failure. *American Journal of Surgery* 1973; **123**: 695–9.

6 Ackrill P, Goodwin FJ, Marsh FP, Stratton D & Wagman H. Successful pregnancy in patient on regular dialysis. *British Medical Journal* 1975; **ii**: 172–4.

7 Ahlswede KM, Armenti VT & Mokritz MJ. Premature births in female transplant recipients: degree and effect of immunosuppressive regimen. *Surgical Forum* 1992; **43**: 524–5.

8 Ahokas RA, Mercer BM & Sibai BM. Enhanced endothelium-derived relaxing factor activity in pregnant, spontaneously hypertensive rats. *American Journal of Obstetrics and Gynecology* 1991; **165**: 801–7.

9 Alcaly M, Blau A & Barkai G. Successful pregnancy in a patient with polycystic disease and advanced renal failure: the use of prophylactic dialysis. *American Journal of Kidney Diseases* 1992; **19**: 382–4.

10 Al-Khader A, Absy M, Al-Hasani MK, Joyce B & Sabbagh T. Successful pregnancy in renal transplant recipients treated with cylosporine. *Transplantation* 1988; **45**: 987–8.

11 Alexopoulos E, Tampakoudis P, Bili H & Mantalenakis S. Acute uric acid nephropathy in pregnancy. *Obstetrics and Gynecology* 1992; **80**: 488–9.

12 Amoah E & Arab H. Pregnancy in a hemodialysis patient with no residual renal function. *American Journal of Kidney Diseases* 1991; **17**: 585–7.

13 Andriole VT. Bacterial infections. In: Burrow GN & Ferris TF (eds), *Medical Complications During Pregnancy*. WB Saunders & Company, Philadelphia, 1975: 382–95.

14 Andriole VT & Patterson TF. Epidemiology, natural history and management of urinary tract infection in pregnancy. *Medical Clinics of North America* 1991; **75**: 359–73.

15 Aol W, Gable D, Cleary RE, Young PCM & Weinberger MH. The antihypertensive effect of pregnancy in spontaneously hypertensive rats. *Proceedings of Society of Experimental Biology and Medicine* 1976; **153**: 13–15.

16 Armenti VT, Ahlswede BA, Moritz MJ & Jarrell BE. National Transplantation Registry: Analysis of pregnancy outcomes of female kidney recipients with relation to time interval from transplantation to conception. *Transplantation Proceedings* 1993; **25**: 1036–7.

17 Bailey RR. Vesicoureteric reflux and reflux nephropathy. In: Cameron JS, Davison AM, Grunfeld JP, Kerr D & Ritz E (eds) *Oxford Textbook of Clinical Nephrology*. Oxford, Oxford University Press, 1992: 1983–2001.

18 Bailey RR & Rolleston GL. Kidney length and ureteric dilation in the puerperium. *Journal of Obstetrics and Gynaecology of the British Commonwealth* 1971; **78**: 55–61.

19 Barcelo P, Lopez-Lillo J, Caberto L & Del Rio G. Successful pregnancy in primary glomerular disease. *Kidney International* 1986; **30**: 914–19.

20 Barrett RJ & Peters WA. Pregnancy following urinary diversion. *Obstetrics and Gynecology* 1983; **62**: 582–56.

21 Bartlett RH & Yahia C. Management of septic abortion with renal failure: Report of five consecutive cases with five survivors. *New England Journal of Medicine* 1969; **281**: 747–50.

22 Barri YM, Al-Furayh O, Qunibi WY & Rahman F. Pregnancy in women on regular hemodialysis. *Dialysis and Transplantation* 1991; **20**: 652–7.

23 Barron WM. Water metabolism and vasopressin secretion during pregnancy. *Clinical Obstetrics and Gynaecology* 1987; **1**: 853–871.

24 Barron WM, Bailin J & Lindheimer MD. Effect of oral protein loading in pregnant and postpartum women: How well does it predict renal reserve? *B. Clinical Experimental Hypertension* 1989; **B8**: 208A.

25 Bay WH & Ferris TF. Factors controlling plasma renin and aldosterone during pregnancy. *Hypertension* 1979; **1**: 410–15.

26 Baylis C. The mechanism of the increase in glomerular filtration rate in the 12 day pregnant rat. *Journal of Physiology* 1980; **305**: 405–14.

27 Baylis C. Effect of early pregnancy on glomerular filtration rate and plasma volume in the rat. *Renal Physiology* 1980; **2**: 333–9.

28 Baylis C. Glomerular ultrafiltration in the pseudopregnant rat. *American Journal of Physiology* 1982; **243**: F300–5.

29 Baylis C. Renal disease in gravid animal models. *American Journal of Kidney Diseases* 1987; **9**: 350–3.

30 Baylis C. Renal effects of cyclooxygenase inhibition in the pregnant rat. *American Journal of Physiology* 1987; **253**: F158–63.

31 Baylis C. Glomerular filtration and volume regulation in gravid animal models. *Clinical Obstetrics and Gynaecology* 1987; **1**: 789–814.

32 Baylis C. Effect of amino acid infusion as an index of renal vasodilatory capacity in pregnant rats. *American Journal of Physiology* 1988; **254**: F650–6.

33 Baylis C. Immediate and long term effects of pregnancy on glomerular function in the SHR. *American Journal of Physiology* 1989; **257**: F1140–5.

34 Baylis C. Effects of acute blockade of α-1 adrenoceptors in virgin, midterm pregnant and late pregnant conscious rats. *Clinical and Experimental Hypertension. B Hypertension in Pregnancy* 1991; **10**: 212A.

35 Baylis C. Blood pressure and renal hemodynamic effects of acute blockade of the vascular actions of arginine vasopressin in normal pregnancy in the rat. *Hypertension in Pregnancy* 1993; **12**: 93–102.

36 Baylis C. Glomerular filtrators and volume regulation in gravid animal models. *Clinical Obstetrics and Gynaecology* 1994; **8**: 235–64.

37 Baylis C & Collins RC. Angiotensin II inhibition on blood pressure and renal hemodynamics in pregnant rats. *American Journal of Physiology* 1986; **250**: F308–14.

38 Baylis C & Davison J. The urinary system. In: Hytten F & Chamberlain G (eds) *Clinical Physiology in Obstetrics*. Blackwell Scientific Publications, Oxford, 1990: 245–302.

39 Baylis C & Engels K. Adverse interactions between pregnancy and a new model of systemic hypertension produced by chronic blockade of endothelial derived relaxing factor (EDRF) in the rat. *Clinical and Experimental Hypertension* 1992; **B11**: 117–29.

40 Baylis C & Munger K. Persistence of maternal plasma volume expansion in midterm pregnant rats maintained on a zero sodium intake: evidence that early gestational volume expansion does not require renal sodium retention. *Clinical and Experimental Hypertension* 1990; **B9**: 237–47.

41 Baylis C & Reckelhoff JF. Renal haemodynamics in normal and hypertensive pregnancy; lessons from micropuncture. *American Journal of Kidney Diseases* 1991; **17**: 98–104.

42 Baylis C & Rennke HG. Renal hemodynamics and glomerular morphology in repetitively pregnant aging rats. *Kidney International* 1985; **28**: 140–5.

43 Baylis C & Wilson CB. Sex and the single kidney. *American Journal of Kidney Diseases* 1989; **13**: 290–8.

44 Baylis C, Reese K & Wilson CB. Glomerular effects of pregnancy in a model of glomerulonephritis in the rat. *American Journal of Kidney Diseases* 1989; **14**: 452–60.

45 Baylis C, Deng A, Samsell L, Boles J & Couser WG. Superimposition of pregnancy in the Fx1A model of membranous glomerulonephritis is antihypertensive and lowers glomerular blood pressure. *Journal of American Society of Nephrology* 1992; **3**: 558A.

46 Beaman M, Turney JH, Rodger RSC, McGonigle RSJ, Adu D & Michael J. Changing pattern of acute renal failure. *Quarterly Journal of Medicine* 1987; **62**: 15–23.

47 Bear JC, McManamon P & Morgan P. Age at clinical onset and at ultrasonographic detection of adult polycystic kidney disease: data for genetic counselling. *American Journal of Medical Genetics* 1984; **18**: 45–9.

48 Bear RA. Pregnancy in patients with renal disease: A study of 44 cases. *Obstetrics and Gynecology* 1976; **48**: 13–18.

49 Beasley RP, Hwang L-U & Lee GY. Prevention of perinatally transmitted hepatitis B virus infections with hepatitis B immune globulin and hepatitis B vaccine. *Lancet* 1983; **ii**: 1099–102.

50 Becker GJ, Ihle BO, Fairley KF, Bastos M & Kincaid-Smith P. Effect of pregnancy on moderate renal failure in reflux nephropathy. *British Medical Journal* 1986; **292**: 796–8.

51 Best JM. Congenital cytomegalovirus infection. *British Medical Journal* 1987; **294**: 1440–1.

52 Biesenbach G, Stöger H & Zazgornik J. Successful

pregnancy of twins in a renal transplant patient with Wegener's granulomatosis. *Nephrology Dialysis Transplantation* 1991; **6**: 139–40.

53 Biesenbach G, Stöger H & Zaztgornik J. Influence of pregnancy on progression of diabetic nephropathy and subsequent requirements of renal replacement therapy in type 1 diabetic patients with impaired renal function. *Nephrology Dialysis and Transplantation* 1992; **7**: 105–9.

54 Blumenkrantz MJ, Gallagher N, Bashore RA & Teuckhoff MD. Retrogade menstruation in women undergoing chronic peritoneal dialysis. *Obstetrics and Gynecology* 1981; **57**: 667–70.

55 Borgeson BD. Continuous ambulatory peritoneal dialysis (CAPD): some psychosocial observations. *Dialysis and Transplantation* 1982; **11**: 54–6.

56 Bosch JP, Saccaggi A, Lauer A, Ronco A, Belledonne M & Glabman S. Renal functional reserve in humans: effect of protein intake on glomerular filtration rate. *American Journal of Medicine* 1983; **75**: 943–50.

57 Brandes JC & Fritsche C. Obstructive acute renal failure by a gravid uterus: a case report and review. *American Journal of Kidney Diseases* 1991; **18**: 398–401.

58 Brandt P, Jesperson J & Gregerson G. Post-partum haemolytic-uraemic syndrome successfully treated with antithrombin III. *British Medical Journal* 1980; **i**: 449.

59 Brem AS, Singer D, Anderson L, Lester B & Abuelo JG. Infants of azotemic mothers: a report of three live births. *American Journal of Kidney Diseases* 1988; **12**: 299–303.

60 Brendolan A, Bragantini L *et al*. Renal functional reserve in pregnancy. *Kidney International* 1985; **28**: 232A.

61 Brenner BM, Meyer TW & Hostetter TH. Dietary protein intake and the progressive nature of the kidney disease: The role of hemodynamically mediated glomerular injury in the pathogenesis of progressive glomerular sclerosis in ageing, renal ablation and intrinsic renal disease. *New England Journal of Medicine* 1982; **307**: 652–9.

62 Briggs JD & Junor BJR. Longterm complications and results in the transplant patient. In: Cameron JS, Davison AM, Grunfeld JP, Kerr DNS & Ritz E (eds) *Oxford Textbook of Nephrology*. Oxford, Oxford University Press, 1992: 1570–94.

63 *British Medical Journal* editorial. Pregnancy after renal transplantation. *British Medical Journal* 1976; **i**: 733–4.

64 *British Medical Journal* editorial. Effect of transplantation on non-renal effects of renal failure. *British Medical Journal* 1981; **284**: 221–2.

65 Briedahl P, Hurst PE, Martin JD & Vivian AB. The post-partum investigation of pregnancy bacteriuria. *Medical Journal of Australia* 1972; **2**: 1174–7.

66 Brookhyser J. The use of percutanel nutrition supplementation in pregnancy complicated end-stage renal disease. *Journal of American Dietetics Association* 1989; **89**: 93–4.

67 Brown MA. Urinary tract dilatation in pregnancy. *American Journal of Obstetrics and Gynecology* 1990; **164**: 641–3.

68 Brown WW, Davis BB, Spray LA, Wongsurawat N, Malone JD & Domoto DT. Aging and the kidney. *Archives of Internal Medicine* 1986; **146**: 1790–6.

69 Brumfitt W. The significance of symptomatic and asymptomatic infection in pregnancy. *Contributions to Nephrology* 1981; **25**: 23–9.

70 Burke JF. The National Transplant Registry: An analysis of 325 pregnancies in female kidney recipients. *Journal of American Society of Nephrology* 1992; **3**: 851P.

71 Buszta C, Steinmuller DR *et al*. Pregnancy after donor nephrectomy. *Transplantation* 1985; **40**: 651–5.

72 Calne RY. Cyclosporin in cadaveric renal transplantation: 5-year follow-up of a multi-centre trial. *Lancet* 1987; **ii**: 506–7.

73 Calne RY, Brons EGM, Williams PF, Evans EB, Robinson RE & Dossa M. Successful pregnancy after paratopic segmental pancreas and kidney transplantation. *British Medical Journal* 1988; **296**: 1709.

74 Cameron JS & Hicks J. Pregnancy in patients with pre-existing glomerular disease. *Contributions to Nephrology* 1984; **37**: 1459–55.

75 Campbell-Brown M, McFadyen IR, Seal DV & Stephenson ML. Is screening for bacteriuria in pregnancy worthwhile? *British Medical Journal* 1987; **294**: 1579–82.

76 Cano RI, Delman MR, Pitchumoni CS, Lev R & Fosenberg WS. Acute fatty liver of pregnancy. Complication of disseminated intravascular coagulation. *Journal of the American Medical Association* 1975; **231**: 159–61.

77 Castellino P, Coda B & Defronzo RA. Effect of amino acid infusion on renal hemodynamics in humans. *American Journal of Physiology* 1986; **251**: F132–40.

78 Caterson RJ, Furber J, Murray J, McCarthy W, Mahony JF & Shiels AGR. Carcinoma of the vulva in two young renal allograft recipients. *Transplant Proceedings* 1984; **16**: 559–61.

79 Cavanaugh D & Singh KB. Endotoxin shock in abortion. In: Schurmer W & Nyhus LM (eds), *Corticosteroids in the Treatment of Shock*. University of Illinois Press, Illinois, 1970: 86.

80 Challah S, Wing AW, Broyer M & Rizzoni G. Successful pregnancy in women or regular dialysis treatment and women with a functioning transplant. In: Andreucci VF (ed.), *The Kidney in Pregnancy*. Martinus Nijhoff, Boston, 1986; 185–94.

81 Chesley LC. *Hypertension in Pregnancy*. Appleton-Century-Crofts, New York, 1978.

82 Chesley LC & Williams LO. Renal glomerular and tubular function in relation to the hyperuricaemia of pre-eclampsia and eclampsia. *American Journal of Obstetrics and Gynecology* 1945; **50**: 367–75.

83 Chng PK & Hall MH. Antenatal prediction of urinary tract infection in pregnancy. *British Journal of Obstetrics and Gynaecology* 1982; **89**: 8–11.
84 Christensen T, Klebe JG *et al*. Changes in renal volume during normal pregnancy. *Acta Obstetrica et Gynaecologica Scandinavica* 1989; **68**: 541–3.
85 Chugh KS, Singhal PC *et al*. Acute renal failure of obstetric origin. *Obstetrics and Gynecology* 1976; **48**: 642–6.
86 Churchill SE, Bengele HH & Alexander EA. Sodium balance during pregnancy in the rat. *American Journal of Physiology* 1980; **239**: R143–8.
87 Cietak KA & Newton JR. Serial qualitative maternal nephrosonography in pregnancy. *British Journal of Radiology* 1985; **58**: 399–404.
88 Cietak KA & Newton JR. Serial quantitative nephrosonography in pregnancy. *British Journal of Radiology* 1985; **58**: 405–13.
89 Clark H, Ronald AR, Cutler RE & Turck M. The correlation between site of infection and maximal concentrating ability in bacteriuria. *Journal of Infectious Diseases* 1969; **120**: 47–53.
90 Cockburn I, Krupp P & Monka C. Present experience of Sandimmun® in pregnancy. *Transplantation Proceeding* 1989; **21**: 3730–2.
91 Coe FC, Parks JH & Lindheimer MD. Nephrolithiasis during pregnancy. *New England Journal of Medicine* 1978; **298**: 324–6.
92 Cohen D, Frenkley Y, Maschiach S & Eliahou HE. Dialysis during pregnancy in advanced chronic renal failure patients: outcome and progression. *Clinical Nephrology* 1988; **29**: 144–8.
93 Cohen SN & Kass EH. A simple method for quantitative urine culture. *New England Journal of Medicine* 1967; **277**: 176–80.
94 Collins R, Yusuf & Peto R. Overview of randomised trials of diuretics in pregnancy. *British Medical Journal* 1985; **290**: 17–23.
95 Condie AP, Brumfitt W, Reeves DS & Williams JD. The effects of bacteriuria in pregnancy on fetal health. In: Brumfitt W & Asscher AW (eds), *Urinary Tract Infection*. Oxford University Press, London, 1973: 108–16.
96 Confortini P, Galanti G, Ancona G, Giongo A, Bruschi E & Lorenzini E. Full term pregnancy and successful delivery in a patient on chronic haemodialysis. In: Cameron JS (ed.), *Proceedings of the European Dialysis and Transplant Association*. Pitman Medical Limited, London, 1971: 74–8.
97 Conger JD, Falk SA & Guggenhheim SJ. Glomerular dynamics and morphologic changes in the generalised Schwartzman reaction in postpartum rats. *Journal of Clinical Investigation* 1981; **67**: 1334–46.
98 Conrad K. Possible mechanisms for changes in renal hemodynamics during pregnancy: studies from animal models. *American Journal of Kidney Diseases* 1987; **9**: 253–9.
99 Conrad KP & Colpoys MC. Evidence against the hypothesis that prostaglandins are the vasodepressor agents of pregnancy. *Journal of Clinical Investigation* 1986; **77**: 236–45.
100 Conrad KP & Vernier KA. Plasma levels, urinary excretion and metabolic production of cGMP during gestation in rats. *American Journal of Physiology* 1989; **257**: R847–53.
101 Coombs GA & Kitzmiller JL. Diabetic nephropathy and pregnancy. *Clinical Obstetrics and Gynecology* 1991; **5**: 505–15.
102 Coulam CB, Moyer TP, Jiang MS & Zincke H. Breastfeeding after renal transplantation. *Transplantation Proceedings* 1985; **14**: 605–9.
103 Coulam CB & Zincke H. Successful pregnancy in a renal transplant patient with a 75-year-old kidney. *Surgical Forum* 1981; **32**: 457–9.
104 Cousins L. Pregnancy complications among diabetic women: Review 1965–1985. *Obstetrical and Gynecological Survey* 1987; **42**: 140–9.
105 Cox SM, Shelburne P, Mason RA, Guss S & Cunningham FG. Mechanisms of hemolysis and anemia associated with acute antepartum pyelonephritis. *American Journal of Obstetrics and Gynecology* 1991; **164**: 587–90.
106 Coyne SS, Walsh JW *et al*. Surgically correctable renal transplant complications: An integrated clinical and radiologic approach. *American Journal of Radiology* 1981; **136**: 113–19.
107 Crespigny PCD & d'Apice AJF. Parenthood after renal transplantation. *Australian and New Zealand Journal of Medicine* 1986; **16**: 245–9.
108 Cunningham FG & Lucas MJ. Urinary tract infections complicating pregnancy. *Clinical Obstetrics and Gynaecology* 1994; **8**: 353–74.
109 Cunningham FG, Lucas MJ & Hankins GDV. Pulmonary injury complicating ante-partum pyelonephritis. *American Journal of Obstetrics and Gynecology* 1987; **156**: 797–807.
110 Cunningham FG, Cox SM, Harstad TW, Mason RA & Pritchard JA. Chronic renal disease and pregnancy outcome. *American Journal of Obstetrics and Gynecology* 1990; **163**: 453–9.
111 Cutler RD & Striker GE. Renal biopsy. In: Massry SG & Glassock RJ (eds), *Textbook of Nephrology*. Williams & Wilkins Co, Baltimore, 1983.
112 Dalgaard OZ. Bilateral polycystic disease of the kidneys: a follow-up of 284 patients and their families. *Acta Medica Scandinavica* 1957; **328** (suppl): 1–10.
113 Danielli L, Korchazak D, Beyar H & Lotan M. Recurrent hematuria during multiple pregnancies. *Obstetrics and Gynecology* 1987; **69**: 446–8.
114 Davison JM. Renal nutrient excretion. *Clinics in Obstetrics and Gynaecology* 1987; **2**: 365–80.
115 Davison JM. The effect of pregnancy on kidney function in renal allograft recipients. *Kidney International* 1985; **27**: 74–9.
116 Davison JM. Renal transplantation and pregnancy.

American Journal of Kidney Diseases 1987; **9**: 374–80.
117 Davison JM. Pregnancy in renal allograft recipients: prognosis and management. *Clinical Obstetrics and Gynaecology* 1987; **1**: 1027–45.
118 Davison JM. The effect of pregnancy on long term renal function in women with chronic renal disease and single kidneys. *Clinical and Experimental Hypertension* 1988; **B8**: 222A.
119 Davison JM. Dialysis, transplantation and pregnancy. *American Journal of Kidney Diseases* 1991; **27**: 127–32.
120 Davison JM. Pregnancy in renal allograft recipients: prognosis and management. *Clinical Obstetrics and Gynaecology* 1994; **8**: 501–25.
121 Davison JM & Dunlop W. Changes in renal haemodynamics and tubular function induced by normal human pregnancy. *Seminars in Nephrology* 1984; **4**: 198–207.
122 Davison JM & Hytten FE. Glomerular filtration during and after pregnancy. *Journal of Obstetrics and Gynaecology of the British Commonwealth* 1974; **81**: 588–95.
123 Davison JM & Hytten FE. Can normal pregnancy damage your health? *British Journal of Obstetrics and Gynaecology* 1987; **94**: 385–6.
124 Davison JM & Lindheimer MD. Gynaecological and obstetrical problems after renal transplantation. *Nieren und Hochdruckkrankheiten* 1982; **11**: 258–65.
125 Davison JM & Lindheimer MD. Pregnancy in renal transplant recipients. *Journal of Reproductive Medicine* 1982; **27**: 240–7.
126 Davison JM & Lindheimer MD. Pregnancy in women with renal allografts. *Seminars in Nephrology* 1984; **4**: 240–7.
127 Davison JM & Noble MCB. Serial changes in 24-hour creatinine clearance during normal menstrual cycles and the first trimester of pregnancy. *British Journal of Obstetrics and Gynaecology* 1981; **88**: 10–17.
128 Davison JM, Dellagrammatikas H & Parkin JM. Maternal azathioprine therapy and depressed haemopoiesis in the babies of renal allograft recipients. *British Journal of Obstetrics and Gynaecology* 1985; **92**: 233–9.
129 Davison JM, Dunlop W & Ezimokhai M. Twenty-four hour creatinine clearance during the third trimester of normal pregnancy. *British Journal of Obstetrics and Gynaecology* 1980; **87**: 106–9.
130 Davison JM, Lind T & Uldall PR. Planned pregnancy in a renal transplant recipient. *British Journal of Obstetrics and Gynaecology* 1976; **83**: 518–27.
131 Davison JM, Sprott MS & Selkon JB. The effect of covert bacteriuria in schoolgirls on renal function at 18 years and during pregnancy. *Lancet* 1984; **ii**: 651–5.
132 Davison JM, Nakagawa Y, Coe FL & Lindheimer MD. Increases in urinary inhibiter activity and excretion of an inhibitor of crystalluria in pregnancy: a defense against the hypercalciuria of normal gestation. *Hypertension in Pregnancy* 1993; **12**: 25–35.
133 Davison JM, Shiells EA, Philips PR & Lindheimer MD. Serial evaluation of vasopressin release and thirst in human pregnancy: the role of human chorionic gonadotrophin in the osmoregulatory changes of gestation. *Journal of Clinical Investigation* 1988; **81**: 798–806.
134 Davison JM, Gilmore EA, Durr J, Robertson GL & Lindheimer MD. Altered osmotic thresholds for vasopressin secretion and thirst in human pregnancy. *American Journal of Physiology* 1984; **246**: F105–9.
135 Davison JM, Shiells EA, Kirkley M, Sturgiss SN & Lindheimer MD. Use of glomerular sieving of neutral dextrans and a heteroporous membrane model to study renal function in human pregnancy. *Journal of the American Society of Nephrology* 1992; **3**: 560.
136 Deng A & Baylis C. Locally produced EDRF controls preglomerular resistance and the ultrafiltration coefficient. *American Journal of Physiology* 1993; **264**: F212–15.
137 Deng A, Samsell L & Baylis C. Rats with 5/6th reduction of renal mass exhibit renal vasodilation at midterm pregnancy. *Journal of the American Society of Nephrology* 1983; **3**: 560.
138 Derfler K, Schaller A *et al*. Successful outcome of a complicated pregnancy in a renal transplant recipient taking cyclosporine-A. *Clinical Nephrology* 1988; **29**: 96–102.
139 de Swiet M. Some rare medical complications of pregnancy. *British Medical Journal* 1985; **290**: 2–3.
140 Devarajan P, Kaskel FJ, Arbeit LA & Moore LC. Cyclosporine nephrotoxicity: blood volume, sodium conservation and renal haemodynamics. *American Journal of Physiology* 1989; **256**: F71–8.
141 Dominguez N, Cruz N, Ramos-Barroso A & Ramos-Umpierre E. Pregnancy in chronic hemodialysis. *Transplantation Proceedings* 1991; **23**: 1836–7.
142 Drummond KN. Hemolytic uremic syndrome — then and now. *New England Journal of Medicine* 1985; **312**: 116–18.
143 Dunlop W. Serial changes in renal haemodynamics during normal human pregnancy. *British Journal of Obstetrics and Gynaecology* 1981; **88**: 1–9.
144 Dunlop W & Davison JM. Renal haemodynamics and tubular function in human pregnancy. *Clinical Obstetrics and Gynaecology* 1987; **1**: 769–88.
145 Dunn BR, Ichikawa I, Pfeffer JM, Troy JL & Brenner BM. Renal and systemic hemodynamic effects of synthetic atrial natriuretic peptide in the anesthetized rat. *Circulation Research* 1986; **59**: 237–46.
146 Durant AQ. Treatment guidelines in a pregnant hemodialysis patient. *Dialysis and Transplantation* 1989; **18**: 86–90.
147 Easterling TR, Brateng D, Goldman ML, Strandness DE & Zaccardi MJ. Renal vascular hypertension during pregnancy. *Obstetrics and Gynecology* 1991; **78**: 921–5.
148 Eaton CJ & Peterson EP. Diagnosis and acute management of patients with advanced clostridial sepsis

complicating abortion. *American Journal of Obstetrics and Gynecology* 1971; **109**: 1162–5.
149 Eckford SD & Gingell JC. Ureteric obstruction in pregnancy-diagnosis and management. *British Journal of Gynaecology* 1991; **98**: 1337–40.
150 Edwards JD. Management of septic shock. *British Medical Journal* 1993; **306**: 1661–4.
151 Ehrich JHH, Rizzoni G *et al*. Combined report on regular dialysis and transplantation of children in Europe 1989. *Nephrology, Dialysis and Transplantation* 1991; **6**: 37–47.
152 Elliott JP, O'Keefe DF, Schon DA & Cherem LB. Dialysis in pregnancy: a critical review. *Obstetrical and Gynecological Survey* 1991; **46**: 319–24.
153 Elmstedt E. Avascular bone necrosis in the renal transplant patient. *Clinical Orthopaedics and Related Research* 1981; **158**: 149–57.
154 Emmanouel DS & Katz AI. Acute renal failure in obstetric shock. Current views on pathogenesis and management. *American Journal of Obstetrics and Gynecology* 1973; **117**: 145–9.
155 Emmanouel DS, Lindheimer MD & Katz AI. Pathogenesis of endocrine abnormalities in uremia. *Endocrine Reviews* 1980; **1**: 28–44.
156 Endler M, Derfler K, Schaller A & Nowotny C. Schwangerschaft und Geburt nach Nierentransplantation unter Cyclosporin A. *Fallbericht und Literaturubersicht Geburtshilfe Frauenheilkd* 1987; **47**: 660–3.
157 European Multicentre Trial. Cyclosporin A as sole immunosuppressive agent in recipients of kidney allografts from cadaver donors. Preliminary results of a European multicentre trial. *Lancet* 1982; **ii**: 57–60.
158 Evans TJ, McCollum JPK & Valdimasson H. Congenital cytomegalovirus infection after maternal renal transplantation. *Lancet* 1975; **i**: 1359–60.
159 Faber M, Kennison RD, Jackson HT, Sbarra AJ & Widnere B. Successful pregnancy after renal transplantation. *Obstetrics and Gynecology* 1976; **48**: 2–4.
160 Fagerholm MI, Coulam CB & Moyer TP. Breast feeding after renal transplantation: 6-mercaptopurine content of human breast milk. *Surgical Forum* 1980; **31**: 447–9.
161 Fairley KF, Whitworth JS & Kincaid-Smith P. Glomerulonephritis and pregnancy. In: Kincaid-Smith P, Mathew TH & Becker EL (eds), *Glomerulonephritis* Part II Wiley, New York, 1973: 997–1011.
162 Feehally J, Bennett SE, Harris KPG & Walls J. Is chronic renal transplant rejection a non-immunological phenomenon? *Lancet* 1986; **ii**: 486–8.
163 Feld LG, Brentjens JR & Van Liew JB. Renal injury and proteinuria in female spontaneously hypertensive rats. *Renal Physiology* 1981; **4**: 46–56.
164 Feld LG, Van Liew JB, Galaske RG & Boylan JW. Selectivity of renal injury and proteinuria in the spontaneously hypertensive rat. *Kidney International* 1977; **12**: 332–43.
165 Felding CF. Obstetric aspects in women with histories of renal disease. *Acta Obstetrica et Gynecology Scandinavica* 1969; **48**: 2–43.
166 Ferris TF. Prostanoids in normal and hypertensive pregnancy. In: Rubin PC (ed.) *Handbook of Hypertension. Volume 10: Hypertension in Pregnancy*. London, Elsevier Science Publishers, 1988: 102–17.
167 Fields CL, Ossorio MA, Roy TM & Bunke CM. Wegener's granulomatosis complicated by pregnancy: A case report. *Journal of Reproductive Medicine* 1991; **36**: 463–6.
168 First MR, Ooi BS, Wellington J & Pollak VE. Preeclampsia with the nephrotic syndrome. *Kidney International* 1978; **13**: 166–77.
169 Fisher KA, Luger A, Spargo BH & Lindheimer MD. A biopsy study of hypertension in pregnancy. In: Bonnar J, MacGillivray I & Symonds EM (eds), *Pregnancy Hypertension*. MTP Press, Lancaster, 1980: 333–8.
170 Fisher K, Luger A, Spargo BH & Lindheimer MD. Hypertension in pregnancy: Clinical-pathological correlations and remote prognosis. *Medicine* 1981; **60**: 267–74.
171 Flechner SM, Katz AR, Rogers AJ, van Buren C & Kahan BD. The presence of cyclosporine in body tissues and fluids during pregnancy. *American Journal of Kidney Diseases* 1985; **5**: 6–63.
172 Flewett TH. Can we eradicate hepatitis B? *British Medical Journal* 1986; **293**: 404–5.
173 Fournier A, El Esper GN *et al*. Atrial natriuretic factor in pregnancy and pregnancy-induced hypertension. *Canadian Journal of Physiology and Pharmacology* 1991; **69**: 1601–8.
174 Fox JG, Sutcliffe NP, Walker JJ & Allison M. Postpartum eclampsia and acute renal failure: treatment with prostacyclin. Case report. *British Journal of Obstetrics and Gynaecology* 1991; **98**: 400–2.
175 Gabert HA & Miller JM. Renal disease in pregnancy. *Obstetrical and Gynecological Survey* 1985; **40**: 449–61.
176 Gabow PA. Autosomal dominant polycystic kidney disease. *New England Journal of Medicine* 1993; **329**: 332–42.
177 Gadallah MF, Bashir A & Karubian F. Pregnancy in patients on chronic ambulatory peritoneal dialysis. *American Journal of Obstetrics and Gynecology* 1992; **20**: 407–10.
178 Gallery EDM, Ross M & Gyory AZ. Urinary red blood cell and cast excretion in normal and hypertensive human pregnancy. *American Journal of Obstetrics and Gynecology* 1993; **168**: 67–70.
179 Gant NF, Whalley PJ, Everett RB, Worley RJ & Macdonald PC. Control of vascular reactivity in pregnancy. *American Journal of Kidney Diseases* 1987; **9**: 303–7.
180 Gardner A. Urinary tract infection during pregnancy and sudden unexpected infant death. *Lancet* 1985; **ii**: 495.
181 Gerety RJ & Schweitzer IL. Viral hepatitis B during pregnancy, the neonatal period and infancy. *Journal of Paediatrics* 1977; **90**: 368–74.
182 Ghahranmains N, Attaipour Y & Ghods AJ.

Chromosomal aberrations among offspring of female renal transplant recipients. *Transplantation Proceedings* 1993; **25**: 2190.
183 Gilstrap LC, Cunningham FG & Whalley PJ. Acute pyelonephritis in pregnancy: an anterospective study. *Obstetrics and Gynecology* 1981; **57**: 408–13.
184 Gilstrap LC, Leveno KJ, Cunningham FG, Whalley PJ & Roark ML. Renal infection and pregnancy outcome. *American Journal of Obstetrics and Gynecology* 1981; **141**: 709–16.
185 Goldsmith JH, Menzies DN, De Boer CH & Caplan W. Delivery of healthy infants after five week's dialysis treatment for fulminating toxaemia of pregnancy. *Lancet* 1971; **ii**: 738–40.
186 Goodship THJ, Heaton A, Rodger RSC, Ward MK, Wilkinson R & Kerr DNS. Factors affecting development of peritonitis in continuous ambulatory peritoneal dialysis. *British Medical Journal* 1984; **289**: 1485–6.
187 Gotloib L, Shustak A, Varka I, Haas R, Mines M & Weiss Z. What is the acute incidence of peritonitis in maintenance peritoneal dialysis? A prospective study. *Artificial Organs* 1985; **9**: 160–3.
188 Gower PE, Haswell B, Sidaway ME & de Wardener HE. Follow-up of 164 patients with bacteriuria of pregnancy. *Lancet* 1968; **i**: 990–4.
189 Graif M, Kessler A *et al*. Renal pyelectasis in pregnancy. Correlative evaluation of fetal and maternal collecting systems. *American Journal of Obstetrics and Gynecology* 1992; **167**: 1304–6.
190 Gregory MC & Mansell MA. Pregnancy and cystinuria. *Lancet* 1983; **ii**: 1158–60.
191 Grünfeld J-P. Alport's syndrome. In: Cameron JS, Davison AM, Grünfeld JP, Kerr D & Ritz E (eds), Oxford, Oxford University Press, 1992: 2197–205.
192 Grünfeld J-P, Boise EP & Hinglais N. Progressive and non-progressive hereditary chronic nephritis. *Kidney International* 1973; **4**: 216–20.
193 Grünfeld J-P, Ganeval D & Bournerias F. Acute renal failure in pregnancy. *Kidney International* 1980; **18**: 179–91.
194 Grünfeld J-P, Noel LH, Hafez S & Droz D. Renal prognosis in women with hereditary nephritis. *Clinical Nephrology* 1985; **23**: 267–70.
195 Grünfeld J-P & Pertuiset N. Acute renal failure in pregnancy. *American Journal of Kidney Diseases* 1987; **9**: 359–62.
196 Guttman RD. Renal transplantation (I and II). *New England Journal of Medicine* 1979; **301**: 975–81 and 1038–48.
197 Hadi HA. Pregnancy in renal transplant recipients: A review. *Obstetrical and Gynecological Survey* 1986; **41**: 264–71.
198 Halpert R, Fruchter RG, Sedlisi A, Butt K, Boyce JG & Sillman FH. Human papillomavirus and lower genital neoplasia in renal transplant patients. *Obstetrics and Gynecology* 1986; **68**: 251–8.
199 Hamburger J, Richet G, Crosnier J, Funck-Brentano JL, Mery JP & Moutera HD. Acute tubular and interstitial nephritis ('acute tubular necrosis'). *Nephrology*, Volume 1. WB Saunders Co., Philadelphia, 1968: 501.
200 Hanson GC. Shock and infection. In: Hanson GC & Weight PL (eds), *The Medical Management of the Critically Ill*. Academic Press, London, 1978; 367–73.
201 Harris JP, Rakowski JA & Argy WP. Alport's syndrome presenting as crescentric glomerulonephritis. A report of two siblings. *Clinical Nephrology* 1978; **10**: 245–9.
202 Haugen G, Fauchald P, Sodal G, Halvorsen S, Oldereid N & Moe N. Pregnancy outcome in renal allograft recipients: influence of cyclosporin A. *European Journal of Obstetrics Gynaecology and Reproductive Biology* 1991; **29**: 25–9.
203 Hawkins DF, Sevitt IH, Fairbrother PF & Tothil AU. Management of chemical septic abortion with renal failure: use of a conservative regimen. *New England Journal of Medicine* 1975; **292**: 722–5.
204 Hayslett JP. Postpartum renal failure. *New England Journal of Medicine* 1985; **312**: 1556–9.
205 Hayslett JP. The effect of systemic lupus erythematosus on pregnancy and pregnancy outcome. *American Journal of Reproductive Immunology* 1992; **28**: 199–204.
206 Hayslett JP & Lynn RI. Effect of pregnancy in patients with lupus nephropathy. *Kidney International* 1980; **18**: 207–20.
207 Hayslett JP & Reece EA. Managing diabetic patients with nephropathy and other vascular complications. *Clinical Obstetrics and Gynaecology* 1994; **8**: 405–24.
208 Heineman HS & Lee JH. Bacteriuria in pregnancy. *Obstetrics and Gynecology* 1973; **41**: 22–6.
209 Heller PJ, Schneider EP & Marx GF. Pharyngolaryngeal edema as a presenting symptom in preeclampsia. *Obstetrics and Gynecology* 1983; **62**: 523–4.
210 Heybourne KD, Schultz MF, Goodlin RC & Durham JD. Renal artery stenosis during pregnancy: a review. *Obstetrical and Gynecological Survey* 1991; **46**: 509–14.
211 Hill DE, Chantigan PM & Kramer SA. Pregnancy after augmentation cystoplasty. *Surgery, Gynecology and Obstetrics* 1990; **170**; 485–7.
212 Hogan WJ & Price JW. Proteinuria as a cause of false positive results in pregnancy tests. *Obstetrics and Gynecology* 1967; **29**: 585–9.
213 Hoover R & Fraumeni JR. Risk of cancer in renal transplant recipients. *Lancet* 1973; **ii**: 55–7.
214 Horbach J, van Liebergen F, Mastboom J & Wijdeveld P. Pregnancy in a patient after cadaveric renal transplantation. *Acta Medica Scandinavica* 1973; **194**: 237–40.
215 Hostetter TH. Human renal response to a meat meal. *American Journal of Physiology* 1984; **250**: F613–18.
216 Hostetter TH. Diabetic nephropathy. *New England Journal of Medicine* 1985; **312**: 642–3.
217 Hou S. Pregnancy in women with chronic renal disease. *New England Journal of Medicine* 1985; **312**: 836–9.
218 Hou S. Peritoneal and hemodialysis in pregnancy.

Clinical Obstetrics and Gynaecology 1987; **1**: 1009–26.
219 Hou S. Pregnancy in organ transplant recipients. *Medical Clinics of North American* 1989; **73**: 667–83.
220 Hou S. Incidence and outcome of pregnancy in end-stage renal disease (ESRD). *Journal of American Society of Nephrology* 1992; **3**: 77P.
221 Hou S. Peritoneal and haemodialysis in pregnancy. *Clinical Obstetrics and Gynaecology* 1994; **8**: 481–500.
222 Hou S. Frequency and outcome of pregnancy in women on dialysis. *American Journal of Kidney Disease.* 1994; **23**: 60–3.
223 Hou S, Orlowski J, Pahl M, Ambrose S, Hussey M & Wong D. Pregnancy in women with end-stage disease: treatment of anaemia and premature labor. *American Journal of Kidney Diseases* 1993; **21**: 16–22.
224 Hou SH, Grossman SD & Madias NE. Pregnancy in women with renal disease and moderate renal insufficiency. *American Journal of Medicine* 1985; **78**: 185–94.
225 Huffer WF, Kuzela D & Popovtzer MM. Metabolic bone disease in chronic renal failure. II. Renal transplant patients. *American Journal of Pathology* 1975; **78**: 385–98.
226 Hytten FE & Thomson AM. Weight gain in pregnancy. In: Lindheimer MD, Katz AI & Zuspan FP (eds), *Hypertension in Pregnancy*. John Wiley & Sons, New York, 1976: 179–87.
227 Ibels LS, Alfrey AC & Huffer WE. Aseptic necrosis of bone following renal transplantation: experience in 194 transplant recipients and review of the literature. *Medicine (Baltimore)* 1978; **57**: 25–45.
228 Ihle BU, Long P & Oats J. Early onset pre-eclampsia: recognition of underlying renal disease. *British Medical Journal* 1987; **294**: 79–81.
229 Imbasciati E & Ponticelli C. Pregnancy and renal disease: predictors for fetal and maternal outcome. *American Journal of Nephrology* 1991; **11**: 353–62.
230 Imbasciati E, Pardi G *et al*. Pregnancy in women with chronic renal failure. *Proceedings IVth World Congress of International Society Study of Hypertension in Pregnancy* 1984; **78A**.
231 Imbasciati E, Pardi G *et al*. Pregnancy in women with chronic renal failure. *American Journal of Nephrology* 1986; **6**: 193–8.
232 Jacobi P, Ohel G, Szylman P, Levit A, Lewin M & Paldi E. Continuous ambulatory peritoneal dialysis as the primary approach in the management of severe renal insufficiency in pregnancy. *Obstetrics and Gynecology* 1992; **79**: 808–10.
233 Jacobsen FK, Christensen CK, Mogensen CE & Heilskow HCS. Evaluation of kidney function after meals. *Lancet* 1980; **i**: 319.
234 Janovski NS, Weimer LE & Ober WB. Soap intoxication following criminal abortion. *New York Medical Journal* 1963; **63**: 1463–5.
235 Jeffries DU. Cytomegalovirus infections in pregnancy. *British Journal of Obstetrics and Gynaecology* 1984; **91**: 305–96.
236 Jorgensen KA. Acute renal failure: diuretic treatment. *Scandinavian Journal of Urology* 1981; (suppl 57): 31–5.
237 Jungers P, Dougados M & Pelissies C. Lupus nephropathy and pregnancy. *Archives of Internal Medicine* 1982; **142**: 771.
238 Jungers P, Houillier P, Forget D & Henry-Amar M. Specific controversies concerning the natural history of renal disease in pregnancy. *American Journal of Kidney Diseases* 1991; **17**: 166–71.
239 Jungers P, Forget D, Henry-Amar M & Grünfeld J-P. Chronic kidney disease and pregnancy. *Advances in Nephrology* 1986; **15**: 103–41.
240 Jungers P, Forget D, Houillier P, Henry-Amar M & Grünfeld J-P. Pregnancy in IgA nephropathy, reflux nephropathy and focal glomerular sclerosis. *American Journal of Kidney Diseases* 1987; **9**: 334–8.
241 Jungers P, Joillier P & Forget D. Reflux nephropathy and pregnancy. *Clinical Obstetrics and Gynaecology* 1987; **1**: 955–70.
242 Kaplan AI, Smith JP & Tillman AJB. Healed acute and chronic nephritis in pregnancy. *American Journal of Obstetrics and Gynecology* 1962; **83**: 1519–25.
243 Karmali MA, Petric M, Steele BT & Lim C. Sporadic cases of haemolytic uraemic syndrome associated with faecal cytotoxin and cytotoxin-producing *Escherichia coli* in stools. *Lancet* 1983; **i**: 619–29.
244 Kaskel TM, Devarajan P, Arbeit LA, Partin JS & Moore LC. Cyclosporine nephrotoxicity: sodium excretion, autoregulation and angiotensin II. *American Journal of Physiology* 1987; **252**: F733–42.
245 Kass EH. Asymptomatic infections of the urinary tract. *Transactions of the Association of American Physicians* 1956; **60**: 56–63.
246 Katz AI, Davison JM, Hayslett JP, Singson E & Lindheimer MD. Pregnancy in women with kidney disease. *Kidney International* 1980; **18**: 192–206.
247 Katz AI, Davison JM, Hayslett JP & Lindheimer MD. Effect of pregnancy on the natural history of kidney disease. *Contributions to Nephrology* 1981; **25**: 53–60.
248 Katz AI & Lindheimer MD. Does pregnancy aggravate primary glomerular disease? *American Journal of Kidney Diseases* 1985; **6**: 261–5.
249 Kaufmann JJ, Dignam W, Goodwin WE, Martin DC, Goldman R & Maxwell MH. Successful normal childbirth after kidney homotransplantation. *Journal of the American Medical Association* 1967; **200**: 162–5.
250 Keller AJ, Irvine WJ, Jordan JJ & London NB. Phytohemagglutin-induced lymphocyte transformation in oral contraceptive users. *Obstetrics and Gynecology* 1976; **49**: 83–91.
251 Kerr DNS & Elliott RW. Renal disease in pregnancy. *Practitioner* 1963; **190**: 459–64.
252 Khawar M, Pomrantz & Tejani A. Two successful pregnancies in a cadaveric renal allograft recipient on cyclosporine (CsA) as the sole maintenance immunosuppressive. *Proceedings Xth International Congress of Nephrology* 1987; **620A**.

253 Kim Y, Shvil Y & Michael AF. Hypocomplementuria in a newborn infant caused by placental transfer of C3 nephritic factor *Journal of Pediatrics* 1978; **92**: 88–90.

254 Kincaid-Smith P & Fairley KF. Renal disease in pregnancy. Three controversial areas: Mesangial IgA nephropathy, focal glomerular sclerosis (focal and segmental hyalinosis and sclerosis) and reflux nephropathy. *American Journal of Kidney Diseases* 1987; **9**: 328–33.

255 Kincaid-Smith P, Fairley KF & Bullen M. Kidney disease and pregnancy. *Medical Journal of Australia* 1967; **2**: 1155–9.

256 Kincaid-Smith P, Whitworth JA & Fairley KF. Mesangial IgA nephropathy in pregnancy. *Clinical and Experimental Hypertension* 1980; **2**: 821–38.

257 Kioko EM, Shaw KM, Clark AD & Warren DJ. Successful pregnancy in a diabetic patient treated with continuous ambulatory peritoneal dialysis. *Diabetes Care* 1983; **6**: 298–300.

258 Kirk EP. Organ transplantation and pregnancy. *American Journal of Obstetrics and Gynecology* 1991; **164**: 1629–34.

259 Kitzmiller JI, Brown ER *et al*. Diabetic nephropathy and perinatal outcome. *American Journal of Obstetrics and Gynecology* 1981; **141**: 741–51.

260 Klein EA. Urologic problems of pregnancy. *Obstetrical and Gynecological Survey* 1983; **39**: 605–15.

261 Kleinknecht D, Grünfeld JP, Gomez PC, Moreau JF & Garcia-Torres R. Diagnostic procedures and long-term prognosis in bilateral renal necrosis. *Kidney International* 1973; **4**: 390–400.

262 Klockars M, Saarikoski S, Ikonen E & Kuhlback P. Pregnancy in patients with renal disease. *Acta Medica Scandinavica* 1980; **207**: 207–14.

263 Knebelmann B, Antiganac C, Gubler MC & Grünfeld JP. A molecular approach to inherited kidney disorders. *Kidney International* 1994 (in press).

264 Kniaz D, Eisenberg G & Elrad H. Postpartum hemolytic uremic syndrome associated with antiphospholipid antibodies. A case report and review of the literature. *American Journal of Nephrology* 1992; **12**: 126–33.

265 Kobayashi H, Matsumoto Y, Otsubo O, Otsubo K & Naito T. Successful pregnancy in a patient undergoing chronic hemodialysis. *Obstetrics and Gynecology* 1981; **57**: 382–6.

266 Kon V & Ichikawa I. Physiology of acute renal failure. *Journal of Pediatrics* 1984; **105**: 351–7.

267 Korsh BM, Klein JD, Negrete VF, Henderson DJ & Fine RN. Physician and psychological follow-up on offspring of renal allograft recipients. *Pediatrics* 1980; **65**: 275–83.

268 Krane NK. Acute renal failure in pregnancy. *Archives of Internal Medicine* 1988; **148**: 2347–57.

269 Kristensen CG, Nakagawa Y, Coe FL & Lindheimer MD. Effect of atrial natriuretic factor in rat pregnancy. *American Journal of Physiology* 1986; **250**: R589–94.

270 Kublickas M, Bergström I, Randmaa I, Lunell N-O, Westgren M. Sarcoidosis in pregnancy: a review with reference to kidney involvement. *Current Obstetrics and Gynaecology* 1994; **4**: 32–6.

271 Kuo VS, Koumantakis G & Gallery EDM. Proteinuria and its assessment in normal and hypertensive pregnancy. *American Journal of Obstetrics and Gynecology* 1992; **167**: 723–38.

272 *Lancet* editorial. Haemolytic uraemic syndrome. *Lancet* 1984; **ii**: 1078–9.

273 *Lancet* editorial. Imaging the transplanted kidney. *Lancet* 1986; **i**: 781–3.

274 *Lancet* editorial. Pregnancy and glomerulonephritis. *Lancet* 1989; **333**: 253–4.

275 Lau RJ & Scott JR. Pregnancy following renal transplantation. *Clinical Obstetrics and Gynecology* 1985; **28**: 339–50.

276 Lawson DH & Miller AWF. Screening for bacteriuria in pregnancy. *Lancet* 1971; **i**: 9–11.

277 Lawson DH & Miller AWF. Screening for bacteriuria in pregnancy: a critical reappraisal. *Archives of Internal Medicine* 1973; **132**: 925–8.

278 Lazebnik N, Jaffa J & Peyeser MR. Hemolytic-uremic syndrome in pregnancy: Review of the literature and report of a case. *Obstetrical and Gynecological Survey* 1985; **40**: 618–21.

279 Leaker B, Becker GJ, El-Khatib M, Hewitson TD & Kincaid-Smith PS. Repeated pregnancy does not accelerate glomerulosclerosis in rats with subtotal renal ablation. *Hypertension in Pregnancy* 1992; **B11**: 1–23.

280 Legarth J & Thorup E. Characteristics of Doppler blood velocity waveforms in a cardiovascular *in-vitro* model. II. The influence of peripheral resistance, perfusion pressure and blood flow. *Scandinavian Journal of Clinical and Laboratory Investigation* 1989; **49**: 459–64.

281 Lennard L, Brown CB, Fox M & Maddocks JL. Azathioprine metabolism in kidney transplant patients. *British Journal of Clinical Pharmacology* 1984; **18**: 693–700.

282 Lennard L, van Loon JA, Lilleyman JL & Weinshilboum MD. Thiopurine pharmacogenetics in leukemia: Correlation of erythrocyte thiopurine methyltransferase activity and 6-thioguanine nucleotide concentrations. *Clinical Pharmacology and Therapeutics* 1987; **41**: 18–22.

283 Leppert P, Tisher CC, Shu-Chung SC & Harlan WR. Antecedent renal disease and the outcome of pregnancy. *Annals of Internal Medicine* 1979; **90**: 747–51.

284 Leveno KJ, Harris RE, Gilstrap LC, Whalley PJ & Cunningham FG. Bladder versus renal bacteriuria during pregnancy: recurrence after treatment. *American Journal of Obstetrics and Gynecology* 1981; **139**: 403–6.

285 Levy G. Pharmacokinetics in renal disease. *American Journal of Medicine* 1977; **62**: 461–5.

286 Lewis GJ, Chatterjee SP & Rowse AD. Acute renal failure presenting in pregnancy secondary to idio-

pathic hydronephrosis. *British Medical Journal* 1985; **290**: 1250–1.

287 Lewis GJ, Lamont CAR, Lee HA & Slapak M. Successful pregnancy in a renal transplant recipient taking cyclosporin A. *British Medical Journal* 1983; **286**: 603.

288 Li FP, Gimbrere K & Gelber RD. Outcome of pregnancy in survivors of Wilm's tumor. *Journal of the American Medical Association* 1987; **257**: 216–19.

289 Lichton IJ. Salt saving in the pregnant rat. *American Journal of Physiology* 1961; **201**: 765–8.

290 Light JA. Experience with 50 kidney/pancreas transplants at the Washington Hospital Center. *Dialysis and Transplantation* 1993; **22**: 522–32.

291 Lim DTY & Fairweather DVI. The management of preterm labour. In: Elder MG & Hendricks CH (eds) *Preterm Labour*. Butterworths, London, 1981: 231–58.

292 Lim VS. Reproductive endocrinology in uremia. *Clinical Obstetrics and Gynaecology* 1994; **8**: 469–80.

293 Lim VS, Henriquez C, Sievertsen G & Frohman LA. Ovarian function in chronic renal failure: Evidence suggesting hypothalamic anovulation. *Annals of Internal Medicine* 1980; **57**: 7–12.

294 Lind T, Godfrey KA, Otun H & Philips PR. Changes in serum uric acid concentrations during normal pregnancy. *British Journal of Obstetrics and Gynaecology* 1984; **91**: 128–32.

295 Lindheimer MD & Chesley LC. Early onset preeclampsia: recognition of underlying renal disease. *British Medical Journal* 1987; **294**: 1547–8.

296 Lindheimer MD & Davison JM. Renal biopsy during pregnancy: 'To b...or not to b... ' *British Journal of Obstetrics and Gynaecology* 1987; **94**: 932–4.

297 Lindheimer MD & Davison JM. Renal disorders. In: Barron WM & Lindheimer MD (eds) *Medical Disorders during Pregnancy*. CV Mosby, 1991.

298 Lindheimer MD & Katz AI. *Kidney Function and Disease in Pregnancy*. New York, Lea and Febiger, 1977.

299 Lindheimer MD & Katz AI. Pathophysiology of preeclampsia. *Annual Review of Medicine* 1981; **32**: 273–89.

300 Lindheimer MD & Katz AI. The renal response to pregnancy. In: Brenner BM & Rector FC Jr (eds), *The Kidney*. WB Saunders, Philadelphia, 1981: 1762–815.

301 Lindheimer MD & Katz AI. Gestation in women with kidney disease: prognosis and management. *Clinical Obstetrics and Gynaecology* 1987; **1**: 921–38.

302 Lindheimer MD & Katz AI. Pregnancy in the renal transplant patient. *American Journal of Kidney Diseases* 1992; **19**: 173–6.

303 Lindheimer MD & Katz AI. Gestation in women with kidney disease: prognosis and management. *Baillière's Clinical Obstetrics and Gynaecology* 1994; **8**: 387–404.

304 Lindheimer MD, Katz AI. Pregnancy in women receiving renal replacement therapy. *Kidney: A Current Survey of World Literature* 1994; **3**: 135–7.

305 Lindheimer MD, Barron WM & Davison JM. Osmoregulation and vasopressin release in pregnancy. *American Journal of Physiology* 1989; **257**: F159–69.

306 Lindheimer MD, Spargo BH & Katz AI. Renal biopsy in pregnancy-induced hypertension. *Journal of Reproductive Medicine* 1975; **15**: 189–94.

307 Lindheimer MD, Fisher KA, Spargo BH & Katz AI. Hypertension in pregnancy: a biopsy study with long term follow-up. *Contributions to Nephrology* 1981; **25**: 71–7.

308 Lindheimer MD, Katz AI, Ganeval D & Grünfeld JP. Renal failure in pregnancy. In: Brenner BM, Lazarus JH & Myers BD (eds), *Acute Renal Failure*. WB Saunders, Philadelphia, 1982.

309 Lockshin MD, Reinitz E & Druzin NL. Case control prospective study demonstrating absence of lupus exacerbation during and after pregnancy. *American Journal of Medicine* 1984; **77**: 893–8.

310 Lomberg H, Jodal U, Lefler H, DeMan P, Svanborg C. Blood group non-secretors have an increased inflammatory response to urinary tract infection. *Scandinavian Journal of Infectious Diseases* 1992; **24**: 7.

311 Lopez-Espinoza I, Dhar H, Humphreys S & Redman CWG. Urinary albumin excretion in pregnancy. *British Journal of Obstetrics and Gynaecology* 1986; **93**: 176–81.

312 Loughlin KR & Bailey RB. Internal ureteral stents for conservative management of ureteral calculi during pregnancy. *New England Journal of Medicine* 1986; **315**: 1647–9.

313 Luke RG, Linton AI, Briggs JD & Kennedy AC. Mannitol therapy in acute renal failure. *Lancet* 1965; **i**: 980–32.

314 McGladdery SL, Aparicio S & Verrier-Jones K. Outcome of pregnancy in an Oxford–Cardiff cohort of women with previous bacteriuria. *Quarterly Journal of Medicine* 1992; **303**: 533–9.

315 McGregor E, Stewart G, Junor BJR & Rodger RSC. Successful use of recombinant human erythropoietin in pregnancy. *Nephrology Dialysis and Transplantation* 1991; **6**: 292–3.

316 McFadyean IR. Urinary tract infection in pregnancy. In: Andreucci VE (ed.), *The Kidney*. Martinus Nijhoff, Boston, 1986: 195–229.

317 McFadyen IR, Eykryn SJ *et al*. Bacteriuria of pregnancy. *Journal of Obstetrics and Gynaecology of the British Commonwealth* 1973; **80**: 385–405.

318 MacLean AB, Abbott GD, Aickin DR, Bailey RR, Bashford DH & Little PJ. Successful pregnancy after renal transplantation. *Australian and New Zealand Journal of Obstetrics and Gynaecology* 1977; **17**: 224–8.

319 MacLean AB, Sharp F, Briggs JD & MacPherson SG. Successful triplet pregnancy following renal transplantation. *Scottish Medical Journal* 1980; **25**: 320–2.

320 Magmon R & Fejgin M. Scleroderma in pregnancy. *Obstetrical and Gynecological Survey* 1989; **44**: 530–4.

321 Maikrantz P, Holley JL & Parks JH. Gestational hypercalciuria causes pathological urine calcium oxalate supersaturation. *Kidney International* 1989; **36**: 108–13.

322 Manifold IH, Champsion AE, Goepel JR, Ramsewak S

& Mayor PE. Pregnancy complicated by gestational trophoblastic disease in a renal transplant recipient. *British Medical Journal* 1983; **287**: 1025–6.

323 Maresca L & Koucky CJ. Spontaneous rupture of the renal pelvis during pregnancy presenting as acute abdomen. *Obstetrics and Gynecology* 1981; **58**: 745–7.

324 Martinell J, Jodall U & Lipiu-Janson G. Pregnancies in women with and without renal seaming after urinary infections in childhood. *British Medical Journal* 1990; **300**: 840–4.

325 Masilamani S & Baylis C. Pregnant rats are refractory to the natriuretic action of administered atrial natriuretic peptide. *Clinical Research* 1993; **41**: 327A.

326 Masilamani S & Baylis C. The renal vasculature does not participate in the peripheral refractoriness to administered angiotensin II in the late pregnancy rat. *Journal of American Society of Nephrology* 1992; **3**: 566.

327 Mead PB & Gump DW. Asymptomatic bacteriuria in pregnancy. In: de Alvarez RR (ed.) *The Kidney*. John Wiley & Sons, New York, 1976: 45–67.

328 Meares EM. Urologic surgery during pregnancy. *Clinics in Obstetrics and Gynecology* 1978; **21**: 907–15.

329 Meier PR & Makowski EL. Pregnancy in the patient with a renal transplant. *Clinics in Obstetrics and Gynecology* 1984; **27**: 903–13.

330 Merkatz IR, Schwartz GH, David DS, Stenzel KH, Riggio RR & Whitsell JC. Resumption of female reproductive function following renal transplantation. *Journal of the American Medical Association* 1971; **216**: 1749–54.

331 Meyers SJ, Lee RV & Munschauer RW. Dilatation and nontraumatic rupture of the urinary tract during pregnancy: a review. *Obstetrics and Gynecology* 1983; **66**: 809–15.

332 Meyer TM, Ichikawa I, Zatz R & Brenner BM. The renal hemodynamic response to amino acid infusion in the rat. *Transactions of the Association of American Physicians* 1983; **96**: 76–83.

333 Miller DR & Kakkis J. Prognosis, management and outcome of obstructive renal disease in pregnancy. *Journal of Reproductive Medicine* 1982; **27**: 199–201.

334 Milutinovic J, Fialkow PJ & Agodoa LY. Fertility and pregnancy complications in women with autosomal dominant polycystic kidney disease. *Obstetrics and Gynecology* 1983; **61**: 566–70.

335 Mitra S, Vertes V, Roza O & Berman LB. Periodic haemodialysis in pregnancy. *American Journal of Medical Science* 1970; **259**: 333–9.

336 Moake JL. An update on the therapy of the thrombotic thrombocytopenic purpura. In: Kaplan BS, Trompeter RS & Moake JL (eds) *Hemolytic Uremic Syndrome and Thrombotic Thrombocytopenic Purpura*. Marcel Dekker, New York: 541–6.

337 Modesto A, Durand D, Orfila C & Suc JM. Syndrome hemolytique uremique chez deux germanius HLA identiques. *Nephrologie* 1984; **5**: 47.

338 Molnar M & Hertelendy F. Nω-nitro-L-arginine, an inhibitor of nitric oxide synthesis, increases blood pressure in rats and reverses the pregnancy-induced refractoriness to vasopressor agents. *American Journal of Obstetrics and Gynecology* 1992; **166**: 1560–7.

339 Moncada S, Palmer RMJ & Higgs EA. Biosynthesis and endogenous roles of nitric oxide. *Pharmacological Reviews* 1991; **43**: 109–42.

340 Moore M, Saffon JE & Barof HSB. Systemic sclerosis and pregnancy complicated by obstructive uropathy. *American Journal of Obstetrics and Gynecology* 1985; **153**: 893–5.

341 Mor-Josef S, Navot D, Rabinowitz R & Sehenker JG. Collagen disease in pregnancy. *Obstetrical and Gynecological Survey* 1984; **39**: 67–83.

342 Mulley AG, Silverstein MD & Dienstag JL. Indications for use of hepatitis B vaccine, based on cost-effectiveness analysis. *New England Journal of Medicine* 1982; **307**: 644–52.

343 Murty GE, Davison JM & Cameron DS. Wegener's granulomatosis complicating pregnancy: first report of a case with a traceostomy. *Journal of Obstetrics and Gynecology* 1991; **10**: 399–403.

344 Mundt KA & Polk BF. Identification of urinary tract infections by antibody-coated bacteria assay. *Lancet* 1979; **ii**: 1172–5.

345 Myerowitz RL, Medeiros AA & O'Brien TF. Bacterial infection in renal homotransplant recipients: a study of fifty-three bacteremic episodes. *American Journal of Medicine* 1972; **53**: 308–14.

346 Myers BD & Moran SM. Hemodynamically mediated acute renal failure. *New England Journal of Medicine* 1972; **314**: 97–105.

347 Nadel AS, Ballerman BJ, Anderson S & Brenner BM. Interrelationships among atrial peptides, renin and blood volume in pregnant rats. *American Journal of Physiology* 1988; **254**: R793–800.

348 Nadler N, Salinas-Madrigal L, Charles AG & Pollak VE. Acute glomerulonephritis during late pregnancy. *Obstetrics and Gynecology* 1969; **34**: 277–80.

349 Nageotte MP & Grundy HO. Pregnancy outcome in women requiring chronic hemodialysis. *Obstetrics and Gynecology* 1988; **72**: 456–9.

350 Nagey DA, Fortier KJ & Linden J. Pregnancy complicated by periarteritis nodosa: Induced abortion as an alternative. *American Journal of Obstetrics and Gynecology* 1983; **147**: 103–95.

351 Nalk RB, Clark AD & Warren DJ. Acute proliferative glomerulonephritis with crescents and renal failure in pregnancy successfully managed by intermittent haemodialysis. *British Journal of Obstetrics and Gynaecology* 1979; **86**: 819–22.

352 Navar LG. Renal autoregulation: perspectives from whole kidney and single nephron studies. *American Journal of Physiology* 1978; **234**: F357–70.

353 Neumann HPH. von Hippel–Lindau syndrome. In: Morgan S & Grunfeld JP (eds) *The Investigation*

and Management of Inherited Disorders of the Kidney. Oxford, Oxford University Press, 1994.

354 Nicklin JL. Systemic lupus erythematosus and pregnancy at the Royal Women's Hospital, Brisbane 1979–1989. *Australian and New Zealand Journal of Obstetrics and Gynaecology* 1991; **31**: 128–33.

355 Nolan GH, Sweet RL, Laros RK & Roure CA. Renal cadaver transplantation followed by successful pregnancies. *Obstetrics and Gynecology* 1974; **43**: 732–9.

356 Norden CW & Kass EH. Bacteriuria of pregnancy — a critical reappraisal. *Annual Review of Medicine* 1968; **19**: 431–70.

357 Ober WE, Reid DE, Romney SL & Merrill JP. Renal lesions and acute renal failure in pregnancy. *American Journal of Medicine* 1956; **21**: 781–810.

358 O'Donnell D, Sevitz H, Seggie JL, Meyers AM, Botha JR & Myburgh JA. Pregnancy after renal transplantation. *Australian and New Zealand Journal of Medicine* 1985; **15**: 320–32.

359 Ogburn PL, Kitzmiller JL *et al*. Pregnancy following renal transplantation in Class T diabetes mellitus. *Journal of American Medical Association* 1986; **310**: 146–50.

360 Packham D & Fairley KF. Renal biopsy; indications and complications in pregnancy. *British Journal of Obstetrics and Gynaecology* 1987; **94**: 935–9.

361 Paller MS. Mechanism of decreased pressor responsiveness to ANG II, NE and vasopressin in pregnant rats. *American Journal of Physiology* 1984; **247**: H100–8.

362 Parsons V, Bewick M, Elias J, Snowden SA, Weston MJ & Rodeck CH. Pregnancy following transplantation. *Journal of the Royal Society of Medicine* 1979; **72**: 815–17.

363 Patterson KR, Lunan CB & MacCuish AC. Severe transient nephrotic syndrome in diabetic pregnancy. *British Medical Journal* 1985; **291**: 1612.

364 Parer JT, Lichtenberg ES, Callen PW & Feduska N. Iliac venous aneurysm in a pregnant patient with a renal transplant. *Journal of Reproductive Medicine* 1987; **29**: 869–71.

365 Parving H-H, Andersen AR, Smidt UM, Hommonel E, Mathiesen ER & Svendsen PA. Effect of antihypertensive treatment on kidney function in diabetic nephropathy. *British Medical Journal* 1987; **294**: 1443–7.

366 Peake SL, Roxburgh HB & Langlois S. Ultrasonic assessment of hydronephrosis of pregnancy. *Radiology* 1983; **128**: 167–70.

367 Penn I. Pregnancy following renal transplantation. In: Andreucci VE (ed.) *The Kidney in Pregnancy*. Martinus Nijhoff, Boston, 1985: 195–204.

368 Penn I. Cancers complicating organ transplantation. *New England Journal of Medicine* 1990; **323**: 1767–8

369 Penn I & Makowski EL. Parenthood following renal and hepatic transplantation. *Transplantation* 1980; **30**: 297–9.

370 Penn I, Makowski EL & Harris P. Parenthood following renal transplantation. *Kidney Internationał* 1980; **18**: 221–33.

371 Perrella MA, Hildebrand FL Jr, Margulies KB & Burnett JC Jr. EDRF in regulation of basal cardiopulmonary and renal function. *American Journal of Physiology* 1991; **261**: R323–8.

372 Pertuiset N & Grünfeld J-P. Acute renal failure in pregnancy. *Clinical Obstetrics and Gynaecology* 1987; **1**: 873–90.

373 Pertiset N & Grünfeld JP. Acute renal failure in pregnancy. *Baillière's Clinical Obstetrics and Gynaecology* 1994; **8**: 333–54.

374 Petri M, Howard D & Repke J. Frequency of lupus flare in pregnancy: The Hopkins Lupus Pregnancy Center experience. *Arthritis and Rheumatism* 1991; **34**: 1538–45.

375 Pickrell MD, Sawers R & Michael J. Pregnancy after renal transplantation: severe intrauterine growth retardation during treatment with cyclosporin A. *British Medical Journal* 1988; **296**: 825.

376 Piper JM, Ray WA & Rosa FW. Pregnancy outcome following exposure to angiotensin converting enzyme inhibitors. *Obstetrics and Gynecology* 1992; **80**: 429–32.

377 Pirson Y, Van Lierde M, Ghysen J, Squifflet JP, Alexandre GPJ & Van Ypersele de Strihou C. Retardation of fetal growth in patients receiving immunosuppressive therapy. *New England Journal of Medicine* 1985; **313**: 328.

378 Porreco R, Penn I, Droegemneller W, Greer B & Makowski EL. Gynecologic malignancies in immunosuppressed organ homograft recipients. *Obstetrics and Gynecology* 1975; **45**: 359–64.

379 Powers RD. New directions in the diagnosis and therapy of urinary tract infections. *American Journal of Obstetrics and Gynecology* 1991; **164**: 1387–9.

380 Price HV, Salaman JR, Laurence KM & Langmaid H. Immunosuppressive drugs and the fetus. *Transplantation* 1976; **21**: 294–8.

381 Provoost AP. Cyclosporine nephrotoxicity in rats with an acute reduction of renal function. *American Journal of Kidney Diseases* 1986; **8**: 314–18.

382 Pruett K & Faro S. Pyelonephritis associated with respiratory distress. *Obstetrics and Gynecology* 1987; **69**: 444–6.

383 Rabau-Friedman E, Maschiach S, Cantor E & Jacob ET. Association of hypoparathyroidism and successful pregnancy in kidney transplant recipient. *Obstetrics and Gynecology* 1982; **59**: 126–8.

384 Rao VK, Smith EJ & Alexander JW. Thromboembolic disease in renal allograft recipients, *Archives of Surgery* 1976; **111**: 1086–92.

385 Rasmussen P, Fasth A, Ahlmen J, Brynger H, Iwarson S & Kjellmer I. Children of female renal transplant recipients. *Acta Paediatrica Scandinavica* 1981; **70**: 869–75.

386 Reckelhoff JF, Samsell L & Baylis C. Failure to duplicate the glomerular haemodynamic changes of pregnancy by an acute moderate PVE. *Clinical and Experimental Hypertension* 1989; **B8**: 533–49.

387 Reckelhoff JF, Yokota S & Baylis C. Autoregulation of renal blood flow in the mid and late pregnant rat. *American Journal of Obstetrics and Gynecology* 1992; **166**: 1546–50.

388 Recommendations of the Immunization Practices Advisory Committee. Immune globulins for protection agains viral hepatitis. *Annals of Internal Medicine* 1982; **96**: 193–7.

389 Redrow M, Cherem L *et al*. Dialysis in the management of pregnant patients with renal insufficiency. *Medicine* 1988; **67**: 199–208.

390 Reece EA, Coustan DR & Hayslett JP. Diabetic nephropathy. Pregnancy performance and fetal maternal outcome. *American Journal of Obstetrics and Gynecology* 1988; **159**: 56–66.

391 Reeders ST, Zerres K *et al*. Prenatal diagnosis of autosomal dominant polycystic kidney disease with a DNA probe. *Lancet* 1986; **ii**: 6–7.

392 Registration Committee of the European Dialysis and Transplant Association. Successful pregnancies in women treated by dialysis and kidney transplantation. *British Journal of Obstetrics and Gynaecology* 1980; **87**: 839–45.

393 Reid DE, Ryan KJ & Benirschke K. Medical and surgical diseases in pregnancy. In: *Principles and Management of Human Reproduction*. WB Saunders Co., Philadelphia, 1972: 734.

394 Reimers TJ & Sluss PM. 6-Mercaptopurine treatment of pregnant mice. Effects on second and third generations. *Science* 1978; **201**: 65–7.

395 Remuzzi G, Misiani R *et al*. Treatment of hemolytic uremic syndrome with plasma. *Clinical Nephrology* 1979; **12**: 279–84.

396 Renal Transplant Registry Advisory Committee. The 13th report of the human renal transplant registry. *Transplant Proceedings* 1977; **9**: 9–26.

397 Richet G & Alagille D. La proteolyse precose au course des anuries hemolytiques du postabortum. *Revue Française d'Etudes Cliniques et Biologiques* 1975; **2**: 475–9.

398 Rifle G & Traeger J. Pregnancy after renal transplantation? An international review. *Transplant Proceedings* 1975; **7** (Suppl. 1): 723–8.

399 Rigenbach M, Renger B, Beavais P, Imbs JF, Eschbach J & Frey G. Grosesse et accouchment d'un enfant vivant chez une patiente traitée par haemodialyse interative. *Journal d'urologie et de nephrologie* 1978; **84**: 360–6.

400 Rizzoni G, Ehrich JHH *et al*. Combined report on regular dialysis and transplantation of children in Europe 1988. *Nephrology, Dialysis and Transplantation* 1989; **4**: 31–40.

401 Rizzoni G, Ehrich JHH *et al*. Successful pregnancies in women on renal replacement therapy: Report from the EDTA Registry. *Nephrology, Dialysis and Transplantation* 1992; **7**: 1–9.

402 Roberts J. Hydronephrosis of pregnancy. *Urology* 1976; **8**: 1–5.

403 Roberts AP, Robinson RE & Beard RW. Some factors affecting bacterial colony counts in urinary infection. *British Medical Journal* 1967; **i**: 400–3.

404 Rogers PW, Kurtzman NA & Bunn SM. Familial benign essential hematuria. *Archives of Internal Medicine* 1973; **131**: 257–9.

405 Romero JC, Lahera V, Salom MG & Biondi ML. Role of endothelium dependent relaxing factor nitric oxide on renal function. *Journal of American Society Nephrology* 1992; **2**: 1371–87.

406 Rosenbaum AL, Churchill JA, Shakhasashiri ZA & Moody RL. Neuropsychologic outcome of children whose mothers had proteinuria during pregnancy. *Obstetrics and Gynecology* 1969; **33**: 118–23.

407 Rubin J, Rogers WA *et al*. Peritonitis during continuous ambulatory peritoneal dialysis. *Annals of Internal Medicine* 1980; **92**: 7–13.

408 Rudolph JE, Shwihizir RT & Barius SA. Pregnancy in renal transplant patients: A review. *Transplantation* 1979; **27**: 26–9.

409 Salant DJ, Marcus RG & Milne FJ. Pregnancy in renal transplant recipients. *South African Medical Journal* 1976; **50**: 1288–92.

410 Salmela KT, Kyllonen LEJ, Homberg C, Grönhagen-Riska C. Impaired renal function after pregnancy in renal transplant recipients. *Transplantation* 1993; **56**: 1372–5.

411 Saltiel C, Legendre C, Descamps JP, Hecht M & Grünfeld J-P. Hemolytic and uremic syndrome in association with pregnancy. In: Kaplan BS, Thrompeter RS & Moake JL (eds), *Hemolytic Uremic Syndrome and Thrombocytopenic Purpura*. Marcell Dekker, New York, 1992: 241–54.

412 Sarramon JP, Lhez JM *et al*. Grossesse chez les transplantes renales. *Annals of Urology* 1985; **19**: 57–9.

413 Satin AJ, Seikin GL & Cunningham FG. Reversible hypertension in pregnancy caused by obstructive uropathy. *Obstetric Gynecology* 1993; **81**: 823–5.

414 Savage WE, Hajj SN & Kass EH. Demographic and prognostic characteristics of bacteriuria in pregnancy. *Medicine (Baltimore)* 1967; **46**: 385–407.

415 Savdie E, Caterson RJ, Mahoney JF, Clifton-Bligh I, Birrell W & John E. Successful pregnancies in women treated by hemodialysis. *Medical Journal of Australia* 1982; **2**: 9.

416 Schaefer RM, Kokot F & Wernze H. Improved sexual function in hemodialysis patients on recombinant erythropoietin: a possible role for prolactin. *Clinical Nephrology* 1989; **31**: 1–5.

417 Schewitz LJ, Friedman EA & Pollak VE. Bleeding after renal biopsy in pregnancy. *Obstetrics and Gynecology* 1965; **26**: 295–304.

418 Schloss WA & Solomkin M. Acute hydronephrosis of pregnancy. *Journal of Urology* 1952; **68**: 885–8.
419 Schoenike SL, Kaldenburgh HH & Kaplan AM. Transient hypoparathyroidism in an infant of a mother with a renal transplant. *American Journal of Diseases of Childhood* 1978; **132**: 530–2.
420 Schrier RTW. Body fluid volume regulation in health and disease: a unifying hypothesis. *Annals of Internal Medicine* 1990; **113**: 155.
421 Schultz PJ & Raij L. Endogenously synthesized nitric oxide prevents indotoxin-induced glomerular thrombosis. *Journal of Clinical Investigation* 1992; **90**: 1718–25.
422 Sciarra JJ, Toledo-Pereyra LH, Bendel RP & Simmons RI. Pregnancy following renal transplantation. *American Journal of Obstetrics and Gynecology* 1975; **123**: 411–25.
423 Scott JR. Fetal growth retardation associated with maternal administration of immunosuppressive drugs. *American Journal of Obstetrics and Gynecology* 1977; **128**: 668–76.
424 Scott JR, Cruikshank DP & Corry. Ectopic pregnancy in kidney transplant patients. *Obstetrics and Gynecology* 1978; **51**: 565–85.
425 Scott JR, Cruikshank DP, Kochenour NK, Pitkin RM & Warenski JC. Fetal platelet counts in the obstetric management of immunologic thrombocytopenic purpura. *American Journal of Obstetrics and Gynecology* 1980; **136**: 459–9.
426 Seeds JW, Cefalo RC, Herbert WNP & Bowes WA. Hydramnios and maternal renal failure: Relief with fetal therapy. *Obstetrics and Gynecology* 1984; **64**: 268–95.
427 Segonds A, Louradour N, Suc JM & Orfila C. Postpartum hemolytic uremic syndrome: A study of three cases with a review of the literature. *Clinical Nephrology* 1979; **12**: 229–42.
428 Sheehan HL. The pathology of acute yellow atrophy and delayed chloroform poisoning. *Journal of Obstetrics and Gynaecology of the British Empire* 1940; **47**: 49–56.
429 Sheil AGR. Cancer in organ transplant recipients: part of an induced immune deficiency syndrome: *British Medical Journal* 1984; **288**: 659–61.
430 Sheil O, Redman CWG & Pugh C. Renal failure in pregnancy due to primary lymphoma. Case Report. *British Journal of Obstetrics and Gynaecology* 1991; **98**: 216–17.
431 Shepherd J & Shepard C. Poststreptococcal glomerulonephritis: a rare complication of pregnancy. *Journal of Family Practice* 1992; **34**: 630–2.
432 Sheriff MHR, Hardman M, Lamont CAR, Shepherd R & Warrent DJ. Successful pregnancy in a 44-year-old haemodialysis patient. *British Journal of Obstetrics and Gynaecology* 1978; **85**: 386–9.
433 Sibai BM, Villar M, Mabic BC. Acute renal failure in the hypertensive disorders of pregnancy. *American Journal of Obstetrics and Gynecology* 1990; **162**: 777–83.
434 Skinhöj P, Cohn J & Bradburne AF. Transmission of hepatitis type B from healthy HBsAg-positive mothers. *British Medical Journal* 1976; **i**: 10–11.
435 Smith CA. Progressive systemic sclerosis and postpartum renal failure complicated by peripheral gangrene. *Journal of Rheumatology* 1982; **9**: 455–60.
436 Smith K, Browne JCM, Shackman R & Wrong OM. Acute renal failure of obstetric origin. An analysis of 70 patients. *Lancet* 1965; **ii**: 351–4.
437 Smith K, Browne JCM, Schackman R & Wrong OM. Renal failure of obstetric origin. *British Medical Bulletin* 1968; **24**: 49–64.
438 Smith LP, MacLean APH & Maughan GB. *Clostridium welchii* septicaemia: a review and report of three cases. *American Journal of Obstetrics and Gynecology* 1971; **110**: 135–40.
439 Soffer O. Sexual dysfunction in chronic renal failure. *Southern Medical Journal* 1980; **73**: 1599–601.
440 Solling K, Christensen CK, Solling J, Sandahl-Christiansen J & Mogense CE. Effect on renal haemodynamics, glomerular filtration rate and albumin excretion of high oral protein load. *Scandinavian Journal of Clinical and Laboratory Investigation* 1986; **46**: 351–7.
441 Spencer ES & Anderson HK. Viral infections in renal allograft recipients treated with long-term immunosuppression. *British Medical Journal* 1979; **ii**: 829–30.
442 Souqiyyeh MZ, Huraib SO, Mohd Salem AC & Aswad S. Pregnancy in chronic hemodialysis patients in the Kingdom of Saudia Arabia. *American Journal of Kidney Diseases* 1991; **19**: 235–8.
443 Stenquist K, Dahlin-Nilsson I & Lidin-Janson G. Bacteriuria in pregnancy. Frequency and risk of acquisition. *American Journal of Epidemiology* 1989; **129**: 372–9.
444 St-Louis J & Sicotte B. Prostaglandin- or endothelium-mediated vasodilation is not involved in the blunted responses of blood vessels to vasoconstrictors in pregnant rats. *American Journal of Obstetrics and Gynecology* 1992; **166**: 684–92.
445 Stratta P, Canavese C & Dolgiani M. Pregnancy-related acute and renal failure. *Clinical Nephrology* 1988; **32**: 14–20.
446 Strauch BS & Hayslett JP. Kidney disease and pregnancy. *British Medical Journal* 1974; **iv**: 378–82.
447 Strong DW, Murchison RJ & Lynch DF. The management of ureteral calculi during pregnancy. *Surgery, Gynecology and Obstetrics* 1978; **146**: 604–8.
448 Sturgiss SN & Davison JM. Perinatal outcome in renal allograft recipients: prognostic significance of hypertension and renal function before and during pregnancy. *Obstetrics and Gynecology* 1991; **78**: 573–7.
449 Sturgiss SN & Davison JM. Effect of pregnancy on longterm function of renal allografts. *American Journal of Kidney Diseases* 1992; **19**: 167–72.
450 Sturgiss SN, Martin K, Whittingham TA & Davison JM. Assessment of the renal circulation during preg-

nancy with colour Doppler ultrasonography. *American Journal of Obstetrics and Gynecology* 1992; **167**: 1250–4.
451 Sturgiss SN, Wilkinson R & Davison JM. Renal haemodynamic reserve (RHR) during normal human pregnancy. *Journal of Physiology (London)* 1992; **452**: 317P.
452 Sturgiss SN, Dunlop W & Davison JM. Renal haemodynamics and tubular function in human pregnancy. *Baillière's Clinical Obstetrics and Gynaecology* 1994.
453 Sun NCJ, Johnson WJ, Sung DTW & Woods JE. Idiopathic postpartum renal failure: Review and case report of a successful renal transplantation. *Mayo Clinic Proceedings* 1975; **50**: 395–401.
454 Surian M, Imbasciati E *et al*. Glomerular disease and pregnancy: A study of 123 pregnancies in patients with primary and secondary glomerular disease. *Nephrology* 1984; **36**: 101–5.
455 Syndman DR, Werner BG *et al*. Use of cytomegalovirus immune globulin to prevent cytomegalovirus disease in renal transplant recipients. *New England Journal of Medicine* 1987; **317**: 1049–54.
456 Takeda T. Experimental study on the blood pressure of pregnant hypertensive rats. I. Effect of pregnancy on the course of experimentally and spontaneously hypertensive rats. *Japanese Circulation Journal* 1964; **28**: 49–54.
457 Tatum HJ. Clinical aspects of intrauterine contraception: circumspection. *Fertility and Sterility* 1976; **28**: 3–27.
458 Tatum HJ & Mulé JG. Puerperal vasomotor tone in patients with toxemia of pregnancy: a new concept of the etiology and a rational plan of treatment. *American Journal of Obstetrics and Gynecology* 1956; **71**: 492–8.
459 Taylor ES. Editorial comments. *Obstetrical and Gynaecological Survey* 1975; **30**: 739.
460 Taylor ES, McMillan JH, Greer BE, Droegemueller W & Thompson HE. The intrauterine device and tubo-ovarian abscess. *American Journal of Obstetrics and Gynecology* 1975; **123**: 338–48.
461 Thacker SB & Berkelman RL. Assessing the diagnostic accuracy and efficacy of selected antepartum fetal surveillance techniques. *Obstetrics and Gynecology Survey* 1986; **41**: 121–41.
462 Thiel G. Experimental cyclosporine A nephrotoxicity: a summary of International Workshop. *Clinics in Nephrology* 1986; **25**: S205–10.
463 Tenney B & Dandrow BV. Clinical study of hypertensive disease in pregnancy. *American Journal of Obstetrics and Gynecology* 1961; **81**: 8–15.
464 Texter JH, Bellinger M, Kawamoto E & Koontz WE. Persistent haematuria during pregnancy. *Journal of Urology* 1980; **123**: 84–7.
465 Thomson NM, Rigby RJ, Atkins RC & Walters WAW. Successful pregnancy in a patient on recurrent haemodialysis. *Australian Society of Nephrology* 1978; **8**: 243.
466 Torres VE, King BF *et al*. The kidney in the tuberous sclerosis complex. *Advances in Nephrology* 1994 (in press).
467 Trebbin WM. Hemodialysis and pregnancy. *Journal of the American Medical Association* 1979; **241**: 1811–12.
468 Turck M. Localisation of the site of recurrent urinary tract infection in women. *Urology Clinics of North America* 1975; **2**: 433–4.
469 Turck M, Ronald AR & Petersdorf RG. Relapse and reinfection in chronic bacteriuria. II. The correlation between site of infection and pattern of recurrence in chronic bacteriuria. *New England Journal of Medicine* 1968; **278**: 422–7.
470 Turney JH, Ellis CM & Parson FM. Obstetric acute renal failure: 1956–1987. *British Journal of Obstetrics and Gynaecology* 1989; **96**: 679–87.
471 Tyden G, Brattstrom C *et al*. Pregnancy after combined pancreas–kidney transplantation. *Diabetes* 1989; **38** (Suppl 1): 43–5.
472 Twickler D, Little BB, Satin AJ & Brown CE. Renal pelvicalyceal dilation in antepartum pyelonephritis: ultrasonographic findings. *American Journal of Obstetrics and Gynecology* 1991; **165**: 1115–19.
473 *UK Transplant Service Report* 1986; 4–30.
474 Umans JG, Lindheimer MD & Barron WM. Pressor effect of endothelium derived relaxing factor inhibition in conscious virgin and gravid rats. *American Journal of Physiology* 1990; **259**: F 293–6.
475 Unzelman RF, Alderfer GR & Chojnacki RE. Pregnancy and chronic hemodialysis. *Transactions of the American Society of Artificial Internal Organs* 1973; **19**: 422–7.
476 Uribe LG, Thakur VD & Krane NK. Steroid-responsive nephrotic syndrome with renal insufficiency in the first trimester of pregnancy. *American Journal of Obstetrics and Gynecology* 1991; **164**: 568–9.
477 Van Sonnenberg E, Casola G, Talner LB, Wittich GR, Varney RR & D'Agostino HB. Symptomatic renal obstruction or urosepsis during pregnancy: treatment by sonographically guided percutaneous nephrostomy. *American Journal of Roentgenology* 1992; **158**: 91–4.
478 Vertel RM & Knochel JP. Non-oliguric acute renal failure. *Journal of the American Medical Association* 1967; **200**: 598–604.
479 Vinicor F, Golichowski A, Filo R, Smith EJ & Maxwell D. Pregnancy following renal transplantation in a patient with insulin-dependent diabetes mellitus. *Diabetes Care* 1984; **7**: 280–4.
480 Vintzileos AM, Turner GW, Campbell WA, Weinbaum PJ, Ward SM & Nochimson DJ. Polyhydramnios and obstructive renal failure: A case report and review of the literature. *American Journal of Obstetrics and Gynecology* 1985; **152**: 883–5.
481 Vintzileos AM, Campbell WA, Nochimson DJ & Weinbaum PJ. The use and misuse of the biophysical profile. *American Journal of Obstetrics and Gynecology* 1987; **156**: 527–33.
482 Walder CE, Thiemermann C & Vane JR. The involvement of EDRF in the regulation of renal cortical blood

flow in the rat. *British Journal of Pharmacology* 1991; **102**: 967–73.

483 Warren DJ. Acute renal failure: diagnosis of cause needed within hours. *British Medical Journal* 1987; **294**: 1569.

484 Warren SF, Mitas JA & Evertson LR. Pregnancy after renal transplantation: Reversible acidosis and renal dysfunction. *Southern Medical Journal* 1981; **74**: 1139–41.

485 Webster J, Rees AJ, Lewis PJ & Hensby CN. Prostacylin deficiency in haemolytic uraemic syndrome. *British Medical Journal* 1980; **281**: 271.

486 Weil R, Barfield N, Schröter GPJ & Bauling PC. Children of mothers with kidney transplants. *Transplant Proceedings* 1985; **17**: 1569–72.

487 Weiner C, Liu KZ, Thompson L, Herrig J & Chestnut D. Effect of pregnancy on endothelium and smooth muscle: their role in reduced adrenergic sensitivity. *American Journal of Physiology* 1991; **261**: H1275–83.

488 Weiner CP, Thompson LP, Kang-Zhu L & Herrig JE. Endothelium-derived relaxing factor and indomethacin-sensitive contracting factor alter arterial contractile responses to thromboxane during pregnancy. *American Journal of Obstetrics and Gynecology* 1992; **166**: 1171–81.

489 Werkö L & Bucht H. Glomerular filtration rate and renal blood flow in patients with chronic diffuse glomerulonephritis during pregnancy. *Acta Medica Scandinavica* 1956; **153**: 177–86.

490 Whalley PJ. Bacteriuria of pregnancy. *American Journal of Obstetrics and Gynecology* 1967; **97**: 723–38.

491 Whalley PJ, Cunningham FG & Martin FG. Transient renal dysfunction associated with acute pyelonephritis of pregnancy. *Obstetrics and Gynecology* 1975; **46**: 174–9.

492 Whetam JCG, Cardelle C & Harding M. Effect of pregnancy on graft function and graft survival in renal cadaver transplant recipients. *American Journal of Obstetrics and Gynecology* 1983; **145**: 193–7.

493 Wiebers DO & Torres VE. Screening for unruptured intracranial aneurysms in automsomal dominant polycystic kidney disease. *North of England Journal of Medicine* 1992; **327**: 953–5.

494 Williams PF & Jelen J. Eclampsia in a patient who had had a renal transplant. *British Medical Journal* 1979; **ii**: 972.

495 Williamson RA & Karp LE. Azathioprine toxicity: review of the literature and case report. *Obstetrics and Gynecology* 1981; **58**: 247–50.

496 Wolf MC, Hollander JB & Salisz JA. A new technique of ureteral stent placement during pregnancy using endoluminal ultrasound. *Surgical Gynecology and Obstetrics* 1992; **175**: 575–6.

497 Woods LL, Mizelle HL & Hall JE. Autoregulation of renal blood flow and glomerular filtration rate in the pregnant rabbit. *American Journal of Physiology* 1987; **252**: R69–72.

498 Wright A, McIntoch C, Steele P, Bennet J & Polat A. Urinary albumin excretion during normal pregnancy in women of low and high parity: evidence of albumin leakage after prolonged hyperfiltration. *Proceedings of Xth International Congress of Nephrology* 1987; 513A.

499 Wright A, Steele P, Bennett JR, Watts G & Polak A. The urinary excretion of albumin in normal pregnancy. *British Journal of Obstetrics and Gynaecology* 1987; **94**: 408–12.

500 Yankowitz J, Piraino B & Laifer SA. Erythropoietin in pregnancies complicated by severe anaemia of renal failure. *Obstetrics and Gynecology* 1992; **80**: 485–8.

501 Yasin SY & Bey Doun SN. Hemodialysis in pregnancy. *Obstetrical and Gynecological Survey* 1988; **43**: 655–68.

502 Zerner D, Doil KL & Drewry J. Intrauterine contraceptive device failures in renal transplant patients. *Journal of Reproductive Medicine* 1981; **26**: 99–101.

503 Zuckerman AJ. New hepatitis B vaccines. *British Medical Journal* 1985; **290**: 492–6.

Further reading

Aarnoudse JG, Houthoff HJ, Weits J, Vellenga E & Huisjes HJ. A syndrome of liver damage and intravascular coagulation in the last trimester of normotensive pregnancy. A clinical and histopathological study. *British Journal of Obstetrics and Gynaecology* 1986; **94**: 145–55.

Baethge BA & Wolf RE. Successful pregnancy with scleroderma renal disease and pulmonary hypertension in a patient using converting enzyme inhibitors. *Annals of Rheumatic Disease* 1989; **48**: 776–8.

Barclay CS, French MAH, Rose LD & Sokol RJ. Successful pregnancy following steroid therapy and plasma exchange in a woman with anti-Ro (SS-A) antibodies. Case report. *British Journal of Obstetrics and Gynaecology* 1987; **94**: 369–71.

Baylis C. Glomerular filtration dynamics. In: Lote CJ (ed.) *Advances in Renal Physiology*. Croom Helm, London, 1986: 33–83.

Baylis C. The determinants of renal hemodynamics in pregnancy. *American Journal of Kidney Diseases* 1987; **9**: 260–4.

Baylis C. Gentamicin-induced glomerulotocixity in the pregnant rat. *American Journal of Kidney Diseases* 1989; **13**: 108–13.

Baylis C, Harton P & Engels K. Endothelial derived relaxing factor (EDRF) controls renal hemodynamics in the normal rat kidney. *Journal of the American Society of Nephrology* 1990; **1**: 875–81.

Baylis C, Mitruka B & Deng A. Chronic blockade of nitric oxide synthesis in the rat produces systemic hypertension and glomerular damage. *Journal of Clinical Investigation* 1992; **90**: 278–81.

Baylis C, Engels K, Harton P & Samsell L. The acute effects of endothelial derived relaxing factor (EDRF) blockade in the normal conscious rat are not due to angiotensin II. *American Journal of Physiology* 1993; **264**: F74–8.

Beaufils M, Uzan S, Donsimoni R & Colan JC. Prevention of preeclampsia by early antiplatelet therapy. *Lancet* 1985; **i**: 840–42.

Calne RY, White DJJG *et al.* Cyclosporin A initially as the only immunosuppressant in 34 recipients of cadaveric organs: 32 kidneys, 2 pancreas, and 2 livers. *Lancet* 1979; **ii**: 1033–6.

Cammu H, Velkeniers B, Charels K & Amy JJ. Idiopathic acute fatty liver of pregnancy associated with transient diabetes insipidus. Case report. *British Journal of Obstetrics and Gynaecology* 1987; **94**: 173–8.

Chamberlain GVP, Lewis PJ, de Swiet M & Bulpitt CJ. How obstetricians manage hypertension in pregnancy. *British Medical Journal* 1978; **i**: 626–9.

Cotton DB, Gonik B & Spillman T. Intrapartum to postpartum changes in colloid osmotic pressure. *American Journal of Obstetrics and Gynecology* 1984; **149**: 174–8.

Coulam CB, Zincke H & Sterioff S. Relationship between donor age and outcome of pregnancy in a renal allograft population. *Transplantation* 1982; **33**: 97–9.

Crawford JS. Epidural analgesia in pregnancy hypertension. *Clinical Obstetrics and Gynecology* 1977; **4**: 735–49.

Cunningham RJ, Buszta C, Braun WE, Steinmuller D, Novick AC & Popowniak K. Pregnancy in renal allograft recipients and longterm follow-up of their offspring. *Transplantation Proceedings* 1983; **15**: 1067–70.

Davison JM. Changes in renal function in early pregnancy in women with one kidney. *Yale Journal of Biological Medicine* 1978; **51**: 347–9.

Davison JM, Shiells EA, Philips PR & Lindheimer MD. Metabolic clearance of vasopressin and an analogue resistant to vasopressinase in human pregnancy. *American Journal of Physiology* 1993; **264**: F348–53.

Davison JM, Shiells EA, Kirkley M, Sturgiss SN & Lindheimer MD. Application of glomerular sieving of neutral dextrans and heteroporous membrane modelling to the study of kidney function in pregnant women. *Hypertension in Pregnancy* 1993; **12**: 275.

Dunlop W & Davison JM. The effect of pregnancy upon the renal handling of uric acid. *British Journal of Obstetrics and Gynaecology* 1977; **84**: 13–21.

Fairley KF, Bond AG & Adey F. The site of infection in pregnancy bacteriuria. *Lancet* 1966; **i**: 939–41.

Fairley KF, Bond AG, Brown RB & Habasberger P. Simple test to determine the site of urinary-tract infection. *Lancet* 1967; **ii**: 427–9.

Folger GK. Pain and pregnancy: Treatment of painful states complicating pregnancy with particular emphasis on urinary calculi. *Obstetrics and Gynecology* 1955; **5**: 513–15.

Gallery EDM, Delprado W & Györy AZ. Antihypertensive effect of plasma volume expansion in pregnancy-associated hypertension. *Australian and New Zealand Journal of Medicine* 1981; **2**: 20–4.

Gallery EDM, Hunyor SM & Györy AZ. Plasma volume contraction: A significant factor in both pregnancy-associated hypertension (pre-eclampsia) and chronic hypertension in pregnancy. *Quarterly Journal of Medicine* 1979; **192**: 573–602.

Gant NF, Worley RJ, Everett RB & MacDonald PC. Control of vascular responsiveness during human pregnancy. *Kidney International* 1980; **18**: 253–8.

Graber LW, Spargo BH & Lindheimer MD. Renal pathology in preeclampsia. *Clinical Obstetrics and Gynaecology* 1987; **1**: 971–95.

Greiss Jr FC. Pressure-flow relationship in the gravid uterine vascular bed. *American Journal of Obstetrics and Gynecology* 1966; **96**: 41–8.

Gross A, Fein A, Serr DM & Nebel L. The effect of imuran on implantation and early embryonic development in rats. *Obstetrics and Gynecology* 1976; **50**: 713–18.

Hague WM & de Swiet M. A syndrome of liver damage and intravascular coagulation in the last trimester of normotensive pregnancy. A clinical and histopathological study. *British Journal of Obstetrics and Gynaecology* 1986; **93**: 1113–14.

Hall BM. Immunosuppression in renal transplantation. *Medical Journal of Australia* 1982; **2**: 415–18.

Hankins GP, Wendel GD, Cunningham FG & Leveno KG. Longitudinal evaluation of hemodynamic changes in eclampsia. *American Journal of Obstetrics and Gynecology* 1984; **150**: 506–9.

Harris RE & Dunnihoo DR. The incidence and significance of urinary calculi in pregnancy. *American Journal of Obstetrics and Gynecology* 1967; **99**: 237–43.

Hatfield AK, Stein H, Greenberger NJ, Abernathy RW & Ferris TF. Idiopathic acute fatty liver of pregnancy. *American Journal of Digestive Diseases* 1976; **17**: 167–71.

Hayslett JP. Maternal and fetal complications in pregnant women with systemic lupus erythematosus. *American Journal of Kidney Diseases* 1991; **17**: 123–6.

Hou S. Pregnancy in women with chronic renal disease. *New England Journal of Medicine* 1983; **312**: 830–9.

Houser MT, Fish AJ, Tegatz GE, Williams PP & Michael AF. Pregnancy and systemic lupus erythematosus. *American Journal of Obstetrics and Gynecology* 1980; **138**: 409–13.

Howie PW, Prentice CRM & Forbes CD. Failure of heparin therapy to affect the clinical course of severe pre-eclampsia. *British Journal of Obstetrics and Gynaecology* 1975; **82**: 711–17.

Joyce III TH, Debnath KS & Baker EA. Pre-eclampsia — relationship of CVP and epidural analgesia. *Anesthesiology* 1979; **51**: S297.

Karlan JR & Cook WA. Renal scleroderma and pregnancy. *Obstetrics and Gynecology* 1970; **44**: 349–52.

Kasinath BS & Katz AI. Delayed maternal lupus after delivery of offspring with congenital heart block. *Archives of Internal Medicine* 1983; **142**: 1217–18.

Kochenour NK, Branch WD, Rote NS & Scott JR. A new postpartum syndrome associated with antilipid antibodies. *Obstetrics and Gynecology* 1987; **69**: 460–8.

Kopp L, Paradiz G & Tucci JR. Urinary excretion of cyclic 3′,5′-adenosine monophosphate and cyclic 3′,5′-guanosine monophosphate during and after pregnancy.

Journal of Clinical Endocrinology and Metabolism 1977; **44**: 590–4.

Kraus GW & Marchese JR. Prophylactic use of hydrochlorothiazide in pregnancy. *Journal of the American Medical Association* 1966; **198**: 1150–4.

Lancet editorial. Aspirin and pre-eclampsia. *Lancet* 1986; **i**: 18–20.

Lancet editorial. Hydronephrosis, renal obstruction and renography. *Lancet* 1986; **i**: 1301–2.

Lancet editorial. Are ACE inhibitors safe in pregnancy? *Lancet* 1991; **338**: 482–3.

Lancet editorial. Systemic lupus erythematosus in pregnancy. *Lancet* 1991; **338**: 87–8.

Lattanzy DR & Cook WA. Urinary calculi in pregnancy. *Obstetrics and Gynecology* 1980; **56**: 462–70.

Leikin JB, Arof HM & Pearlman LM. Acute lupus pneumonitis in the postpartum period. A case history and review of the literature. *Obstetrics and Gynecology* 1986; **68**: 293–315.

Lewis PJ, Bulpit CJ & Zuspan FP. A comparison of current British and American practice in the management of hypertension in pregnancy. *American Journal of Obstetrics and Gynecology* 1982; **1**: 78–82.

Lindheimer MD & Katz AI. Hypertension and pregnancy. In: Genest J *et al.* (eds), *Hypertension: Physiopathology Treatment*. McGraw-Hill, New York, 1984.

Long RG, Scheur PJ & Sherlock S. Pre-eclampsia presenting with deep jaundice. *Journal of Clinical Pathology* 1977; **30**: 212–16.

Love PE & Santoro SA. Antiphospholipid antibodies: Anticardiolipin and the lupus anticoagulant in systemic lupus erythematosus (SLE) and in non-SLE disorders. *Annals of Internal Medicine* 1990; **112**: 682–98.

Lubbe WF, Butler WS, Palmer SJ & Liggins GC. Lupus anticoagulant in pregnancy. *British Journal of Obstetrics and Gynaecology* 1984; **91**: 357–63.

MacGillivray L, Rose GA & Rowe B. Blood pressure survey in pregnancy. *Clinical Science* 1969; **37**: 395–401.

McKee CM, Foser JH, Callender MD, Weir PE & Murnaghan GA. Acute fatty liver of pregnancy and diagnosis by computed tomography. *British Medical Journal* 1986; **292**: 291–4.

Maikranz P, Coe FL, Parks J & Lindheimer MD. Nephrolithiasis in pregnancy. *Clinical Obstetrics and Gynaecology* 1994; **8**: 375–86.

Moise KJ & Shah DM. Acute fatty liver of pregnancy etiology of fetal distress and fetal wastage. *Obstetrics and Gynecology* 1987; **69**: 482–5.

Molnar M & Hertelendy F. Pressor responsiveness to endothelin is not attenuated in gravid rats. *Life Sciences* 1990; **47**: 1463–8.

Murray S, Hickey J & Houang E. Significant bacteremia associated with replacement of intrauterine contraceptive device. *American Journal of Obstetrics and Gynecology* 1987; **156**: 698–9.

Nolten WE & Ehrlich EN. Sodium and mineralocorticoids in normal pregnancy. *Kidney International* 1980; **18**: 162–72.

Ockner SA, Brunt EM & Cohn SM. Fulminant hepatic failure caused by acute fatty liver of pregnancy treated by orthotopic liver transplantation. *Hepatology* 1990; **11**: 59–64.

Olah KS & Redman CWG. Overlap syndrome and its implications in pregnancy. Case report. *British Journal of Obstetrics and Gynaecology* 1991; **98**: 728–30.

Olah KS, & Gee H. Fetal heart block associated with maternal anti-Ro(SS-A) antibody current management. A review. *British Journal of Obstetrics and Gynaecology* 1991; **98**: 751–5.

Pinto A, Sorrentino R *et al.* Endothelial derived relaxing factor released by endothelial cells of human umbilical vessels and its impairment in pregnancy-induced hypertension. *American Journal of Obstetrics and Gynecology* 1991; **164**: 507–13.

Pockros PJ, Peters RL & Reynolds TB. Idiopathic fatty liver of pregnancy: findings in ten cases. *Medicine* 1984; **63**: 1–8.

Pritchard JA. Management of pre-eclampsia and eclampsia. *Kidney International* 1980; **18**: 259–66.

Quigley MM. Acute obstetric yellow atrophy presenting as idiopathic hyperuricemia. *Southern Medical Journal* 1974; **67**: 142–6.

Ready BL & Johnson ES. Epidural block for treatment of renal colic during pregnancy. *Canadian Anaesthetists Society Journal* 1981; **28**: 77–9.

Reece EA, Winn HN & Hayslett JP. Does pregnancy alter the rate of progression of diabetic nephropathy? *American Journal of Perinatology* 1990; **7**: 193–7.

Reiss RE, Kuwabara T & Smith M. Successful pregnancy despite placental cystine crystals in a woman with nephrotic cystinosis. *New England Journal of Medicine* 1988; **319**: 223–6.

Reye RDK, Morgan G & Banal J. Encephalopathy and fatty degeneration of the viscera. A disease entity in childhood. *Lancet* 1963; **ii**: 749–52.

Robertson EG & Cheyne GA. Plasma biochemistry in relation to oedema of pregnancy. *Journal of Obstetrics and Gynaecology of the British Commonwealth* 1972; **79**: 769–76.

Romagnoli A & Batra MS. Continuous epidural block in the treatment of impacted ureteric stones. *Canadian Medical Association Journal* 1973; **109**: 968.

Rosenkrantz JG, Githens JH, Cox SM & Kellum DL. Azathioprine (Imuran) and pregnancy. *American Journal of Obstetrics and Gynecology* 1967; **97**: 387–94.

Saarikoski S & Seppala M. Immunosuppression during pregnancy: transmission of azathioprine and its metabolites from mother to the fetus. *American Journal of Obstetrics and Gynecology* 1973; **115**: 1100–6.

Sacks SH, Verrier Jones K, Roberts R, Asscher AW & Ledingham JGG. Effect of symptomless bacteriuria in childhood on subsequent pregnancy. *Lancet* 1987; **ii**: 991–4.

Schiffer M. Fatty liver associated with administration of tetracycline in pregnant and non-pregnant women. *American Journal of Obstetrics and Gynecology* 1966; **96**: 326–32.

Scott JS, Maddison PJ, Taylor PV, Esscher E, Scott O &

Skinner RP. Connective-tissue disease, antibodies to ribonucleoprotein and congenital heart block. *New England Journal of Medicine* 1983; **309**: 209–12.

Seigler AM & Spain DM. Polyarteritis nodosa and pregnancy. *Clinical Obstetrics and Gynecology* 1965; **8**: 322–9.

Sheehan HL. Jaundice in pregnancy. *American Journal of Obstetrics and Gynecology* 1961; **81**: 427–33.

Sibai BM. Diagnosis and management of chronic hypertension in pregnancy. *Obstetrics and Gynecology* 1991; **78**: 451–61.

Singsen BH, Akhter JE, Weinstein MM & Sharp GC. Congenital complete heart block and SSA antibodies: obstetric implications. *American Journal of Obstetrics and Gynecology* 1985; **152**: 655–9.

Slavin MJ. Renal function and hypertension associated with pregnancy. *Journal of the American Obstetrics Association* 1980; **80**: 258–63.

Stamey TA, Goven DE & Palmer JM. The localisation and treatment of urinary tract infections: The role of bactericidal levels as opposed to serum levels. *Medicine (Baltimore)* 1965; **44**: 1–36.

Steen VD, Conte C & Day N. Pregnancy in women with systemic sclerosis. *Arthritis and Rheumatology* 1989; **32**: 151–7.

Steinhausen M, Dallenbach FD, Dussel R & Nelinski D. Pathophysiological mechanisms of acute renal failure. *Contributions to Nephrology* 1981; **25**: 151–6.

Studd JWW & Blainey JD. Pregnancy and the nephrotic syndrome. *British Medical Journal* 1969; **i**: 276–8.

Studdiford WF & Douglas GW. Placental bacteriuria: a significant finding in septic abortion accompanied by vascular collapse. *American Journal of Obstetrics and Gynecology* 1956; **71**: 842–7.

Swapp GH. Asymptomatic bacteriuria, birthweight and length of gestation in a defined population. In: Brumfitt W & Asscher AW (eds), *Urinary Tract Infection*. Oxford University Press, London, 1973: 92–102.

Taylor PV, Scott JS, Gerlis LM, Esscher E & Scott O. Maternal antibodies against fetal cardiac antigens in congenital complete heart block. *New England Journal of Medicine* 1986; **315**: 667–72.

Thomson AM, Billewicz WZ & Hytten FE. The assessment of fetal growth. *Journal of Obstetrics and Gynaecology of the British Commonwealth* 1968; **75**: 903–16.

Van Asche FA, Spitz B, Vermylen J & Deckmijn H. Preliminary observations on treatment of pregnancy-induced hypertension with a thromboxane synthetase inhibitor. *American Journal of Obstetrics and Gynecology* 1984; **148**: 216–18.

Wallenburg HCS, Dekker GA, Makovitz JW & Rotmans P. Low-dose aspirin prevents pregnancy-induced hypertension and pre-eclampsia in angiotensin-sensitive primigravidae. *Lancet* 1986; **i**: 1–3.

Waltzer WC. The urinary tract in pregnancy. *Journal of Urology* 1981; **125**: 271–6.

Waltzer WC, Coulam CB, Zincke H, Sterioff S & Frohnert PP. Pregnancy in renal transplantation. *Transplant Proceedings* 1980; **12**: 221–8.

Weber FL, Snodgrass PJ, Powell DE, Rao P, Hoffman SL & Brady PG. Abnormalities of hepatic mitochondrial urea-cycle enzyme activities and hepatic ultra-structure in acute fatty liver of pregnancy. *Journal of Laboratory and Clinical Medicine* 1979; **94**: 27–41.

Weinstein L. Preeclampsia/eclampsia with hemolysis, elevated liver enzymes and thrombocytopenia. *Obstetrics and Gynecology* 1985; **66**: 657–60.

Whalley PJ, Martin FG & Peters PC. Significance of asymptomatic bacteriuria detected during pregnancy. *Journal of the American Medical Association* 1965; **193**: 879–81.

Williams PF & Johnstone M. Normal pregnancy in renal transplant recipient with history of eclampsia and intrauterine death. *British Medical Journal* 1982; **285**: 1535.

Zinaman M, Rubin J & Lindheimer MD. Serial plasma oncotic pressure levels and echoencephalography during and after delivery in severe pre-eclampsia. *Lancet* 1985; **i**: 1245–57.

8

Systemic Lupus Erythematosus and Other Connective Tissue Diseases

Michael de Swiet

Systemic lupus erythematosus, 306
Effect of pregnancy on SLE
Effect of SLE on pregnancy
Management of SLE in pregnancy
Rheumatoid arthritis, 313
Sclerodema and other connective tissue diseases, 314

Systemic lupus erythematosus (SLE)

SLE is a multisystem disease which most frequently presents in young women. It is therefore relatively common in pregnancy, and it is certainly the connective tissue disease that has been studied most intensively. It is quite possible that SLE was the reason why Queen Anne lost 17 pregnancies and failed to produce an heir to the throne of England [41]. The apparent prevalence has increased as more mild forms of the disease are recognized. In 1974 Fessel [51] found the prevalence of SLE to be one in 700 women aged 15–64 years. In black women the prevalence was one in 245. Women in 'minority' races have a fivefold excess risk compared to white women [63]. The diagnosis may be based on the patient having at least four of the features noted by the American Rheumatism Association, either simultaneously or following each other (Box 8.1). However, the necessity to have four rather than three criteria has been challenged [113].

Since the publication of the American Rheumatism Association Criteria, the measurement of antinuclear factor and of anti-DNA antibodies has replaced the LE cell test in the diagnosis of SLE. In pregnancy, proteinuria and thrombocytopenia can lead to confusion with pre-eclampsia. The clinical features of pre-eclampsia, which usually run a much more acute course, remit after delivery, and are not associated with other features summarized in Box 8.1, normally distinguish the two conditions. However, proteinuria may occasionally appear early

Box 8.1. Criteria for the diagnosis of SLE as suggested by the American Rheumatism Association [150]. To substantiate the diagnosis, the patient should have at least four features, either simultaneously, or following each other

- Facial butterfly rash
- Discoid lupus
- Photosensitivity — skin rash as a result of unusual reaction to sunlight
- Oral or nasopharyngeal ulceration
- Non-erosive arthritis involving two or more peripheral joints
- Pleurisy or pericarditis
- Proteinuria >0.5 g/day or cellular casts
- Psychosis or convulsions
- One of:
  - haemolytic anaemia
  - leucopenia, wbc <4000/mm^3 on two or more occasions
  - lymphopenia <1500/mm^3 on two or more occasions
  - thrombocytopenia <100 000/mm^3
- Immunological disorder:
  - positive LE cell preparation
  - antibody to native DNA in abnormal titre
  - antibody to SM nuclear antigen
  - chronic false positive syphilis serology for 6 months
- Antinuclear antibody in abnormal titre

in pregnancy, the process may not be so acute, and in this situation, measurement of antinuclear factor and anti-DNA antibodies helps to distinguish SLE from other renal conditions and pre-eclampsia.

The disease runs a fluctuating course. In advanced forms, with severe nephritis or nervous system involvement, the overall prognosis is bad, but as less severe forms are recognized, the prognosis has improved so that many centres now report a >95 per cent survival at 5 years. If treatment is required, the drugs most commonly used are aspirin, prednisone and antimalarials such as hydroxychloroquine and azathioprine. (For other reviews of connective tissue disease [75] and SLE in pregnancy see [12,35,138,149].)

Overlap syndrome relates to diffuse connective tissue diseases overlapping in their clinical and immunological features. Olah and Redman [123] have described a single case where the fetus developed congenital heart block in association with anti-Ro antibodies (see below).

Effect of pregnancy on SLE

As is the case with most illnesses which run a fluctuating course, such as asthma or disseminated sclerosis, it is difficult to document any special effect of pregnancy on SLE. The general consensus is that pregnancy does not affect the long-term prognosis of SLE [58], but that pregnancy itself may be associated with more 'flare ups', particularly in the puerperium [55,107]. Since patients are usually observed more closely in pregnancy this is not surprising. Also, patients with SLE are normally advised against conceiving during an active phase of the disease and therefore conceive when they are well [44]. If the effect of pregnancy is judged by a comparison of the state of pregnancy with that before conception (see for example [170]), their condition can only either stay unchanged if they were well before pregnancy or deteriorate; this is a further cause of bias. However, in a comparison with the pre-pregnancy period, Garsenstein *et al.* [58] found that the exacerbation rate was three times greater in the first half of pregnancy, one and a half times greater in the second half, and at least six times greater in the puerperium — the time when maternal deaths have occurred [170]. These deaths have been due to pulmonary haemorrhage [145] or lupus pneumonitis [2] to which these women appear to be particularly susceptible [94].

Kincaid-Smith *et al.* [87] in Melbourne found specific renal biopsy changes in patients with renal 'flares' in pregnancy. These were similar to those found in haemolytic uraemic syndrome (HUS) and were also associated with microhaemangiopathic haemolytic anaemia. Treatment directed toward HUS (aspirin, fresh frozen plasma, plasmapheresis) may be helpful for renal 'flares' in pregnancy which may be an endothelial disease.

It is interesting that successive pregnancies do not necessarily affect an individual in the same way [44]. Chorea gravidarum is a rare complication of SLE in pregnancy [37,105].

The relationships of pregnancy to renal and skin diseases caused by SLE are also considered in Chapters 7 and 19 respectively.

Effect of SLE on pregnancy

There are three main ways in which SLE affects pregnancy and its outcome. First, SLE increases the risks of late pregnancy losses due to hypertension and renal failure; secondly, it is an important cause of heart block and other cardiac defects in the newborn. This effect may be part of a more general neonatal lupus syndrome. Thirdly, SLE increases the risk of abortion. Although technically most of the latter cases, being pregnancy losses before 28 weeks, should be classified as abortions, it is clear that they are quite different from most abortions which occur at about 12 weeks. The losses in association with SLE may occur at gestations up to and even after 28 weeks with a bias towards the later part of pregnancy. Even if the fetus does not die, it is at risk of developing fetal distress as judged by abnormal fetal heart rate traces [99].

Hypertension and renal failure

As indicated above, patients with trivial SLE, or even no clinical evidence of SLE, have a much higher risk of abortion. The other group of patients at risk of fetal morbidity are those with renal involvement who may also have hypertension. For example, Houser *et al.* [76] studied 18 pregnancies in patients with SLE. Ten occurred in patients with no evidence of renal disease and were uncomplicated. The remaining eight occurred in patients with renal disease. There were four abortions (one elective), three premature deliveries, and only one normal term delivery. It is difficult to be precise as to what level of renal impairment is significant, but a creatinine clearance of <65 ml/min/m^3 or proteinuria >2.4 g/24 hours would be ominous (see Chapter 7). Hayslett and Lynn [71] noted a 50 per cent fetal loss rate in mothers with a serum creatinine in excess of 132 mmol/l (1.5 mg/dl).

The neonatal lupus syndrome

This syndrome [92] includes haematological complications, cardiac abnormalities, babies in whom skin lesions are present [98] as the only abnormalities, and neonates who develop SLE in the absence of any involvement in the mother [64]. Maternal antibodies have been shown to cross the placenta [64] and it is likely that SLE is one of the conditions — such as rhesus disease, Graves' disease or myasthenia gravis — where transplacental passage of antibodies harms the fetus. However, in SLE, the precise antibody which affects the fetus has not been identified, and the fetal outcome cannot be correlated with fetal (or maternal) antibody levels apart from the relationship between congenital heart block and certain maternal antibodies (see below).

The haemotological abnormalities are haemolytic anaemia, leucopenia and thrombocytopenia. They are usually transient and not a major problem [118].

The cardiac abnormalities have been best defined by McCue *et al.* [110] and Esscher and Scott [43]. By far the most common abnormality is complete heart block which may be present and detected antenatally [3]. However, a variety of abnormalities have been described including endomyocardial fibrosis [43], pericarditis [38,53,132] and persistent sinus bardycardia [54]. Although the majority of infants born to mothers with SLE are normal, about one in three mothers (38 per cent) who deliver babies with congenital heart block have, or will have, a connective tissue disease [43]. Most frequently, the disease is SLE, but in 16 per cent of cases the mother had rheumatoid arthritis, and 25 per cent have a less well-defined form of connective tissue disease.

About 60 per cent of mothers who deliver a child with congenital heart block have antibodies to soluble tissue ribonucleoprotein antigen (anti-Ro or SS-A and anti-La or SS-B antibodies). Since the production of anti-Ro and anti-La antibodies is correlated with the presence of HLA antigen DR3 and is more common in patients with Sjögren's syndrome [79] such patients are at particular risk of having an infant with congenital heart block [126, 161]. The risk of congenital heart block is far greater with anti-Ro than with anti-La but must not be over-estimated. Anti-Ro antibodies are quite common so that the risk of congenital heart block in the presence of anti-Ro is at most one in 20 though this increases to one in three if the mother already has a child with congenital heart block [122]. In one prospective study there were no cases of heart block in 91 infants born to mothers with SLE despite 23 per cent of the mothers being Ro positive [102]. In one series, these autoantibodies were invariably present in the mothers with SLE that delivered an affected child but they were also present in some of those asymptomatic women who had a child with congenital heart block [109]. Antibody has been found in the site of the conducting tissue in the heart of a fetus that died with complete heart block. However, since it was both IgG and IgA antibody [97], some, the IgA antibody which does not cross the placenta, was presumably derived from the fetus. This is rather puzzling. In addition it is quite unclear why maternal cardiac conductive tissue is not affected by the anti-Ro antibody.

It has also been shown that the mothers and their offspring may also have an IgG antibody which reacts with fetal cardiac tissue [152]. This antibody may also be involved in the pathogenesis of congenital heart block and the presence of this and other autoantibodies may explain why the fetal prognosis is not invariably good even in the absence of well-established markers for fetal death such as anticardiolipin antibodies (see below). Thus although the baby usually survives the perinatal period, and often does not require pacing, in a few cases with congenital heart block and without cardiolipin antibodies the fetus dies antenatally or in labour [140]. Perhaps the antibodies directed against cardiac muscle are causing a fatal cardiomyopathy [73]. This would certainly be in keeping with findings of diffuse IgG antibody in all cardiac tissue of a fetus which died in association with high maternal titres of anti-Ro in early pregnancy [162] and with the clinical presentation before delivery as non-immune hydrops. In addition fatal cases may be associated with the other abnormalities noted above.

Of course fetuses may have congenital heart block because of a primary structural abnormality, frequently an A-V canal defect [139]. Under these circumstances there is usually no association with maternal connective tissue disease.

McCuiston and Shock [114] first described discoid skin lesions in a neonate whose mother subsequently developed SLE. The lesions are usually on the face or the scalp and are present at birth or develop after birth possibly because fetal skin does not contain the anti-Ro antigen [91]. They have normally disappeared by 1 year of life, and only rarely are associated with other organ involvement [164]. Some skin lesions have been associated with maternal and fetal antibodies to U1RNP (nRNP) a protein found in normal human skin cells [128].

Abortion and the cardiolipin syndrome [81]

The incidence of abortion in patients with SLE may be as high as 40 per cent [55]. On reviewing previous pregnancies, even those occurring before the onset of SLE, Fraga *et al.* [55] found that the incidence of abortion was 23 per cent — about twice as high as in a group of control patients. Chesley [25] also analysed the outcome of 630 pregnancies in mothers with SLE and found that there was a 36 per cent failure rate.

The risk of abortion is not clearly related to the severity of the condition. In SLE, abortion often occurs later than the usual 12–14 weeks gestation and, indeed, may occur at any gestation up to 28 weeks. The risk of abortion is not shared by other connective tissue diseases such as rheumatoid arthritis [83] or scleroderma [82]. Baesnihan *et al.* [6] showed a high titre of lymphocytotoxic antibodies in three or four patients with SLE, whose pregnancies ended in abortion. These antibodies can be absorbed by trophoblast which indicates a number of possible mechanisms for the cause of abortion in SLE [6]. For example, Abramowsky *et al.* [1] have described necrotizing decidual vascular lesions with immunoglobulin deposition in placentas of women whose pregnancies were complicated by SLE.

However, it is now realized that the presence of lupus anticoagulant and cardiolipin antibodies may be very closely related to the risk of abortion and later fetal loss [14,34,99,105–7,134]. It is probable that those women with clinical lupus who do not have significant cardiolipin antibodies or lupus anticoagulant do not have excess fetal risk apart from the slight excess that may be present in association with anti-Ro or anti-La antibodies (see above) or because of hypertension or renal disease. For example Lockshin *et al.* [99] studied 21 patients with lupus. Twelve had normal pregnancies; their mean cardiolipin titre was only marginally raised to 27 units. Nine had abnormal pregnancies with fetal death or fetal distress. Their mean cardiolipin titre was 212 units. In the larger series of Loizou [104] there were 129 pregnancies in women without cardiolipin antibodies; the abortion rate was 27 per cent, whereas in 37 pregnancies with high levels of cardiolipin antibodies the abortion rate was 89 per cent. The lupus anticoagulant is an inhibitor of the coagulation pathway found in 5–10 per cent of patients with SLE [137] which causes prolongation of the kaolin clotting time. In contrast to the situation in coagulopathies, this prolongation is not corrected by mixing the patient's plasma with control plasma. There are increasingly complicated haematological tests to detect lupus anticoagulant [13,45,130] with little standardization between laboratories. Paradoxically the lupus anticoagulant is associated with an increased risk of thromboembolism, both arterial and venous [90] (Chapter 4) and excessive bleeding is very rare [13,124]. Anticardiolipin antibodies are antibodies active against certain phospholipid components of cell walls. They are responsible for the 'false positive Wasserman reaction' which has been known to occur in SLE. The higher the titre of anticardiolipin antibodies, the greater the risk to the fetus [67]. Even in the absence of known lupus and without knowledge of cardiolipin antibody status, a retrospective study of patients with biologically false positive tests for syphilis showed an increased fetal loss rate [155].

The above and other clinical features of the 'cardiolipin syndrome' are summarized in Box 8.2 [80].

In patients with SLE who have a bad obstetric history, both antibodies are often present in high titre. Patients who have cardiolipin antibodies in high titre usually have high levels of lupus anticoagulant [65,66]. If they do not, the level of cardiolipin antibodies is usually considered to be a better predictor of fetal outcome [99,103] probably because it is subject to less variability [34]. Cardiolipin antibodies may belong to both IgG and IgM subtypes. The IgG antibodies seem to be better predictors of fetal outcome although the presence of IgM antibodies is not without risk to the fetus [103]. The levels of these antibodies may be elevated quite disproportionately to the clinical severity of lupus. Indeed some patients have a bad obstetric history with high titres of cardiolipin antibodies or lupus anticoagulant and almost no clinical evidence of lupus [52,57,99]. Careful questioning, however, will often elicit a history of mild joint pains, 'growing pains' as a child, or vitiligo or livedo reticularis. The risk to the fetus if the mother has lupus anticoagulant has been put at 85 [14] to 92 per cent [107] mortality. However, the series of Lubbé and Liggins [107] was culled from the literature and represents patients where the lupus anticoagulant was often measured because of the patient's bad obstetric history. In a group of women attending a rheumatology clinic for SLE who have the lupus anticoagulant, or cardiolipin antibodies, the risk to the fetus may be much less, although Lockshin's retrospective study [99] of cardiolipin antibodies in patients with SLE does not support this concept. The problem is compounded by considerable methodological variation in assay procedures [65, 68,101]. So what was thought to be a simple association between the presence of cardiolipin antibodies or lupus anticoagulant and high fetal risk has become rather blurred [165]. Furthermore although the presence of these antibodies in the normal obstetric population is low, between 2 and 5 per cent depending on the cut-off point used, they may be present in low titre in up to 30 per cent of patients with severe hypertension in pregnancy [15,151] or even in 10 per cent of non-pregnant patients with endometriosis [151].

Box 8.2. Clinical features of the cardiolipin syndrome [80]

- Thrombosis
  - Venous
    - recurrent DVT (also axillary, IVC, and retinal vein thromboses)
  - Arterial
    - cerebrovascular accidents
    - peripheral arterial gangrene
    - coronary thrombosis
    - retinal artery thrombosis
  - Other
    - pulmonary hypertension
    - ? avascular necrosis
- Abortion
  - recurrent IUD, placental thrombosis and infarction
- Thrombocytopenia
  - Intermittent, often acute
- Other occasional features
  - Coombs' positivity
  - Livedo reticularis
  - Migraine
  - Chorea
  - Epilepsy
  - Chronic leg ulcers
  - ? Endocardial disease
  - ? Progressive dementia due to repeated cerebrovascular thromboses

The problem is further confounded by studying patients with early fetal loss. In patients presenting with unexplained recurrent abortion the incidence of subclinical autoimmune disease varies between 1 and 29 per cent [29]. The clearest association between cardiolipin antibodies and fetal loss is with second and third trimester losses. There may well be an increased risk of first trimester loss, but first trimester loss is so common that it is much more difficult to know whether the presence of cardiolipin antibodies relates to first trimester loss in an individual patient. Since the prevalence of cardiolipin antibodies is higher in patients with recurrent early abortion than with single early abortions, these antibodies are more likely to be relevant with patients who have had many miscarriages.

It is, therefore, clear that the fetus of the woman

who has lupus anticoagulant or cardiolipin antibodies is at risk, but it is difficult to quantify that risk [134] and difficult to state what its excess risk is over that of the normal population [85,127,138]. This is of particular relevance to treatment options, some of which are not without maternal risk (see below). In addition lupus anticoagulant levels show spontaneous variation between non-pregnancy and pregnancy [85] and even within the same pregnancy. Measurement of anticardiolipin antibody has been proposed for screening the normal population [86] but in general it does not select a high risk group [10] nor does it distinguish between normal pregnancy and all cases of fetal death including abortion [81]. Maternal thrombocytopenia in association with platelet antibodies appears to be an additional risk factor for fetal death in patients with the cardiolipin syndrome [111].

The mechanism(s) by which these agents might affect the fetus is unknown. The placenta is usually severely infarcted and the fetus is often growth retarded. Even in the pregnancies of those fetuses that survive, severe pre-eclampsia is very common. Current theories centre round the damage to placental vascular endothelium caused by cardiolipin antibodies, platelet desposition and imbalance in thromboxane/prostacyclin production tilted towards too much thromboxane and too little prostacyclin [22,33]. If the primary problem is maternal placental vasculopathy [37], measurement of maternal placental vascular resistance by Doppler ultrasound might be the way to monitor these pregnancies.

Inhibition of protein C [21,27] and of tissue plasminogen activator [163] have been postulated as the mechanisms whereby lupus anticoagulant may cause thrombosis.

Management of SLE in pregnancy

Maternal considerations

The drugs most frequently used for the treatment of SLE [19] are simple analgesics such as paracetamol and non-steroidal anti-inflammatory drugs including aspirin. In more severe cases antimalarial drugs, corticosteroids, other immunosuppressives and cytotoxic agents are used.

Paracetamol has been used widely in pregnancy with no adverse effects in normal therapeutic doses. Aspirin has been extensively studied. Three large prospective studies [16,142,157], including the Perinatal Collaborative Project of over 14000 women exposed to aspirin in the USA, have shown no teratogenic risk [142]. However, salicylate and other non-steroidal anti-inflammatory agents have been associated with neonatal haemorrhage because of their action in inhibiting platelet function [148,157]. In addition there is the risk that prostaglandin synthetase inhibitors will cause premature closure of the ductus arteriosus and pulmonary hypertension [89]. This appears to be more of a theoretical than a practical risk [74]. So far, only occasional cases have been reported following maternal indomethacin treatment [61]. There were no such complications in over 200 infants exposed to indomethacin in studies of its effect in pre-term labour [40,120]. Chloroquine causes choroidoretinitis [131] though not usually in the doses employed for malaria prophylaxis or treatment [168]. However, withdrawal of chloroquine is associated with a high risk of SLE flare [20]. Therefore it would seem sensible not to withdraw chloroquine in pregnancy but to treat exacerbations of SLE in pregnancy by an increase in steroid therapy rather than the *de novo* introduction of chloroquine.

The safety of steroids is considered in Chapter 1. Azathioprine is the cytotoxic agent that is most commonly used in rheumatic conditions and the only cytotoxic agent that can be considered for use in pregnancy. The possibility of induction of chromosome breaks and their long-term consequences for female fetuses is discussed in Chapter 7.

In summary, paracetamol is the best agent to use as an analgesic and an antirheumatic in pregnancy. Non-steroidal anti-inflammatory agents are best avoided in normal therapeutic doses in the last trimester and if a patient requires extra therapy for this relatively short time, corticosteroids should be used. Since the ESR is elevated in normal pregnancy, reduction of C_3 complement can be used as an objective index of disease activity [171]. In patients taking long-term corticosteroids, parenteral steroid cover should be given in labour. Our practice is to use intramuscular hydrocortisone 100 mg

6-hourly, until the patient is taking oral medication. Because of the risk of dangerous exacerbation of SLE in the puerperium, steroid dosage should only be reduced with great care after delivery. Some authors [169] have even arbitrarily increased steroid therapy in all patients from the 30th week of pregnancy until 4 weeks after delivery. The use of azathioprine should be reserved for cases where steroid therapy has failed or is contraindicated.

Plasmapheresis has been successfully used in pregnancy for maternal reasons in a patient with SLE and severe proximal myopathy induced by steroids. The fetus was already growth retarded but did not appear to suffer further from the procedure [154]. A single successful case raises the possibility that plasmapheresis and steroid therapy may decrease the risk of the development of complete heart block in a patient who is anti-Ro positive [8] but there have also been failures.

In breast-feeding women, the non-steroidal anti-inflammatory drugs with short half-lives and rapidly elevated or inactive metabolites are best, i.e. ibuprofen, flurbiprofen and diclofenac [19]. Salicylates and antimalarial drugs should be avoided for the reasons given above. Minute quantities of prednisolone are secreted in breast milk and this drug should therefore be considered safe.

Fetal considerations

It was originally hoped that the use of corticosteroids would decrease the high abortion rate associated with SLE. In general, this has not been the case [55]. However, it has been reported that aggressive treatment with aspirin 75–300 mg/day and prednisone in doses increasing to 60 mg/day can suppress lupus anticoagulant and anticardiolipin antibodies and consequently improve fetal outcome. Lubbé *et al.* [106] and Branch *et al.* [14] have reported two series of 10 and eight patients in which the outcome (50 and 62 per cent survival) was much superior to that expected in untreated patients (see above). In addition there have been several case reports of similar successes [50,146]. However, the dose of prednisone often makes the patients Cushingoid [106] and induces diabetes which requires further treatment. There is an increased risk of infection with *Listeria monocytogenes* [129] amongst other organisms. One patient has died of miliary tuberculosis [42]. Even with such treatment the pregnancies are usually complicated by hypertension and/or growth retardation and require very carefully monitoring [14].

Removal of anticardiolipin antibodies and lupus anticoagulant is not a guarantee of success [14,100], nor is failure to remove the antibodies a guarantee of fetal death [85,127,130]. Furthermore we still do not know the significance in fetal terms of these antibodies in an unselected population (see above). Therefore controlled clinical trials of this aggressive form of therapy are urgently required [50,146]. For example a preliminary trial suggests that heparin and aspirin may be preferable to prednisone and aspirin in high risk patients [30]. In another study, high dose subcutaneous heparin (24 000 ± 7000 units/day) was associated with success in 14 of 15 high risk lupus pregnancies [135]. Because of the Cowchock study referred to above [30], I now prefer to use aspirin and heparin rather than aspirin and steroids. At present I reserve steroid or heparin therapy for patients who have antibodies and a bad obstetric history. Patients who have antibodies but a good obstetric history or no obstetric history (primigravidae) are treated with aspirin 75 mg/day only. In patients where heparin, steroid and aspirin therapy has been unsuccessful, a variety of additional therapies have been tried including azathioprine [24,62], plasmapheresis, immunoglobulin and plasma exchange. Nevertheless the place of these therapies is even less clear than the place of aspirin and steroid therapy.

Similarly it is not clear how to manage patients with recurrent early pregnancy loss who have lupus anticoagulant or cardiolipin antibodies. Low dose aspirin has been used from before conception but this too should be subjected to clinical trial.

Patients who also have a past history of thromboembolism, arterial or venous, should be treated with subcutaneous heparin throughout pregnancy in addition to any aspirin and prednisone therapy that might be considered necessary. The heparin is given as described for patients with thromboembolism in pregnancy (Chapter 4). Although this treatment will exacerbate any bone loss associated with steroid therapy, I believe it to be necessary in view of the dire consequences, particularly of cerebral arterial thrombosis [49]. Patients with lupus anticoagulant and/or cardiolipin antibodies and no history of thromboembolism are treated with low dose aspirin alone (75 mg/day) unless it is judged that they also require steroids for fetal reasons.

The timing of delivery in patients with SLE or the cardiolipin syndrome depends on the severity of the condition and whether the patients have renal involvement or hypertension. If there are none of these complications, the patient should be delivered at term. Increasing degrees of renal failure or hypertension will necessitate early delivery, either for these reasons alone or because of evidence of fetal compromise, as judged by poor growth, or cardiotocography or Doppler ultrasound measurement of fetal and maternal placental blood flow. With the advent of cardiotocography and widespread use of ultrasound to measure fetal growth, there is little need for measurement of oestriol levels. These can also be depressed purely by corticosteroid therapy, although usually only in dosages >75 mg cortisol per day [121].

Congenital heart block should be diagnosed before delivery from routine auscultation of the fetal heart and subsequent cardiotocography when bradycardia is discovered. If possible a detailed ultrasound examination of the fetal heart should then be performed. This will show atrioventricular dissociation confirming complete heart block and also demonstrate any structural heart disease which is present in 15–20 per cent of cases [147]. If the fetus has complete heart block, it is difficult to assess its general condition *in utero* since accurate assessment usually depends on measurement of fetal heart rate and its variability. However, it is possible to measure the atrial rate and its variability by detailed ultrasound. Measurement of umbilical blood flow by Doppler ultrasound can be of value [88] and antenatal fetal blood sampling to measure fetal blood gases [119,144] is of real value in this situation. Labour can be monitored by repeated fetal blood gas estimation [126] but many such fetuses are understandably delivered by elective caesarean section.

The greatest problems occur in fetuses with heart block who are hydropic. They have low output intrauterine heart failure either due to the slow heart rate alone or to an additional cardiomyopathic process. The use of plasmapheresis and/or immunosuppressive or steroid therapy to prevent heart block occurring in high risk cases (anti-Ro positive, previously affected fetus) has been mentioned above but there is no evidence that this form of treatment is of benefit once heart block has developed [18]. Nevertheless glucocorticoids which cross the placenta such as dexamethasone are frequently used [17,18,53] with the aim of achieving viability at which time the fetus should be delivered by caesarean section.

Rheumatoid arthritis

The finding by Hench [72] that rheumatoid arthritis improved in 24 of 30 pregnancies, coupled with a belief that cortisol levels were markedly elevated in pregnancy, was so important that it led to the successful use of steroids in patients with rheumatoid arthritis who were not pregnant. These observations have been confirmed by Kaplan and Diamond [83], and difficulties in the management of rheumatoid arthritis are rare in pregnancy, although exacerbations may occur in the puerperium. The subject has been extensively reviewed by Thurnau [156]. Unger *et al.* [160] have correlated the improvement in rheumatoid arthritis with the level of pregnancy-associated α_2-glycoprotein which has immunosuppressive action. However, pregnancy induces many other changes in the immune system and therefore there may be other reasons why rheumatoid arthritis improves.

In contrast to SLE there is no increased risk of abortion in patients with rheumatoid arthritis [83]. As indicated above, there is a small risk of congenital heart block in the newborn. Other potential problems are in abduction of the hip during vaginal delivery, or extension of the neck and opening of the mouth for intubation in general anaesthesia.

The most common difficulty concerns drug administration. As indicated above, the dangers of steroid therapy have been exaggerated, and paracetamol is a better analgesic for use in pregnancy than aspirin. However, if paracetamol is inadequate it seems reasonable to use aspirin and other prostaglandin antagonists at least in the first two trimesters. However, there are case reports of convulsions in a breast-fed infant, after the mother had taken indomethacin for analgesia [40,47], and therefore indomethacin should not be used in women who are breast feeding.

There is little experience with the use of phenylbutazone in pregnancy. In non-pregnant patients, phenylbutazone can cause sodium retention and bone marrow dyscrasias. It is not known whether these and other abnormalities occur in the fetus exposed to phenylbutazone before delivery but in any case phenylbutazone should now be reserved for the inpatient treatment of (non-pregnant) patients with ankylosing spondylitis. The situation is similar concerning gold therapy. In the adult, gold causes blood dyscrasias, drug rashes and nephropathy. However, gold is very strongly protein-bound and little appears to cross the placenta [133].

Antimalarial drugs such as chloroquine are also used in the treatment of rheumatoid arthritis. Chloroquine has been reported to cause chromosome damage, but there is no evidence that this results in stable chromosome abnormalities which might be of genetic or neoplastic significance [59]. A greater worry is that chloroquine may cause retinopathy in the neonate because it is concentrated in the fetal uveal tract [158]. Congenital deafness has also been reported [69]. Antimalarial drugs should therefore not be used in the treatment of rheumatoid arthritis in pregnancy, particularly since alternative treatments exist. Nevertheless, the risks of their use have probably been exaggerated. Because there is no alternative, women must, and do, take antimalarial drugs for the treatment or prophylaxis of malaria in pregnancy [95] (see Chapter 16); a high incidence of fetal damage associated with malaria has not been reported.

Sulphasalazine is increasingly used as second line treatment for rheumatoid arthritis. Its safety in pregnancy is documented in Chapter 10.

Immunosuppressive drugs are occasionally used in the treatment of rheumatoid arthritis. Azathioprine is the drug that has been used most frequently and it appears to be relatively safe, although it has still not been extensively tried (Chapter 7). Penicillamine is also used in the treatment of rheumatoid arthritis. There are occasional reports of suspected teratogenesis [143] and neonatal abnormalities of connective tissue [115], which may be irreversible or reversible [96]. However, there are two series (totalling 56 pregnancies) in which the only abnormality (which could have occurred by chance) was one child with a small ventricular septal defect [108,136]. It would therefore seem that penicillamine is reasonably safe in pregnancy (see Chapter 9).

In summary, if a patient with rheumatoid arthritis requires treatment in pregnancy, she should be given paracetamol. If this does not give adequate relief in the first two trimesters, aspirin or other non-steroidal anti-inflammatory drugs may be used. If these are inadequate and in the last trimester corticosteroids should be used. Penicillamine treatment also appears to be safe.

Scleroderma and other connective tissue diseases

Scleroderma is a connective tissue disease affecting the skin, gastrointestinal tract (oesophagus), kidneys (see Chapter 7) and lungs. The cause is unknown and there is no known cure or disease modifying therapy. There have been five series of 87 patients [70,82,93,141] and several case reports [84], describing the interaction of scleroderma and pregnancy (see also review in [11]). Scleroderma has been divided into localized cutaneous and diffuse cutaneous forms. In the localized cutaneous form the scleroderma process is localized usually to the hands and arms distal to the elbow; it is associated with Raynaud's phenomenon and without organ involvement. The prognosis is good in general and in particular in pregnancy although occasionally Raynaud's phenomenon may first appear as an aggressive manifestation of scleroderma in pregnancy [5]. Diffuse cutaneous scleroderma has more widespread cutaneous manifestations and is a much more aggressive illness. Raynaud's phenomenon is less common and the patient may have SCL-70 antibodies. Organ involvement is frequent affecting heart, lungs and kidneys and is the cause of death. Not surprisingly the prognosis in general and in pregnancy in particular is far worse; since many patients deteriorate, they have been advised against pregnancy [84] particularly since they may not be able to look after their children even if they survive pregnancy; but we still do not know whether pregnancy itself accelerates the deterioration that is inevitable in these patients.

The fetal outcome is also impaired. In a review of 17 pregnancies reported in the literature, Karlen and Cook [84] documented five perinatal deaths, and five instances of premature delivery. Involvement of the cervix has been implicated as a cause of dystocia [9]. These patients often have sclerotic skin and blood vessels making venepuncture, venous access and blood pressure measurement difficult. Both regional and general anaesthesia are associated with technical problems particularly the difficulty of endotracheal intubation [153]. Such patients should see an anaesthetist early in their pregnancy so that anaesthetic management can be planned rather than guessed at in an emergency. The one patient that we have managed at Queen Charlotte's Maternity Hospital with scleroderma had a growth-retarded infant in each of two pregnancies. She did not have renal involvement but did have a severe reduction of pulmonary transfer factor. Captopril has been advocated as treatment for crises in patients with scleroderma [112]. It is usually used as an antihypertensive drug but should be avoided in pregnancy because of concern about the fetus (see Chapter 6).

Other connective tissue diseases which rarely complicate pregnancy are polyarteritis nodosa [125, 32], dermatomyositis [145] relapsing polychondritis [77] and Wegener's granulomatosis. Wegener's granulomatosis has already been considered in Chapter 1. In all these conditions there is insufficient experience to be confident of the effect of pregnancy. Since some patients have deteriorated in pregnancy, termination has been suggested for cases of polyarteritis nodosa [125] but this may not be justified [32].

Relapsing polychondritis is a condition where cartilage is inflamed and loses its structural integrity. Four cases have been described in pregnancy [77]. The most recent patient deteriorated in pregnancy and required a tracheotomy [77]. In one case the neonate was also affected [4] suggesting transplacental passage of autoantibodies.

Finally, it has recently been suggested that patients are particularly at risk from developing polymyositis, an autoimmune disease of muscle, in the puerperium.

References

1 Abramowsky CR, Vegas ME, Swinehart G & Gyves MT. Decidual vasculopathy of the placenta in lupus erythematosus. *New England Journal of Medicine* 1980; **303**: 668–72.

2 Ainslie WH, Britt K & Moshipur JA. Maternal death due to lupus pneumonitis in pregnancy. *Mount Sinai Journal of Medicine* 1979; **46**: 494–9.

3 Altenburger KM, Jedziniak M, Roper WL & Hernandez J. Congenital complete heart block with hydrops fetalis. *Journal of Pediatrics* 1977; **91**: 618–20.

4 Arundell FD & Haserick JR. Familial chronic atrophic polychondritis. *Archives of Dermatology* 1960; **82**: 439.

5 Avrech OM. Raynaud's phenomenon and peripheral gangrene complicating scleroderma in pregnancy. *British Journal of Obstetrics and Gynaecology* 1992; **99**: 850–1.

6 Baesnihan B, Grigor RR *et al*. Immunological mechanism for spontaneous abortion in systemic lupus erythematosus. *Lancet* 1977; **ii**: 1205–7.

7 Ballou SP, Morley JJ & Kushner I. Pregnancy and systemic sclerosis. *Arthritis and Rheumatism* 1984; **27**: 295–8.

8 Barclay CS, French MAH, Ross LD & Sokol RJ. Successful pregnancy following steroid therapy and plasma exchange in a woman with anti-Ro (SS-A) antibodies. Case report. *British Journal of Obstetrics and Gynaecology* 1987; **94**: 369–71.

9 Bellucci MJ, Coustan DR & Plotz RD. Cervical scleroderma: a case of soft tissue dystocia. *American Journal of Obstetrics and Gynecology* 1984; **150**: 891–2.

10 Bendon RW, Hayden LE *et al*. Perinatal screening for anticardiolipin antibody. *American Journal of Perinatology* 1990; **7**: 245–50.

11 Black CM & Stevens WM. Scleroderma. *Rheumatoid Disease Clinics of North America* 1989; **15**: 193–212.

12 Boelaert J, Ryckaert R, Tser Kezoglou A & Daneels R. Systemic lupus erythematosus and pregnancy. *Acta Clinica Belgica* 1980; **35**: 183–92.

13 Boxer M, Ellman L & Carvalho A. The lupus anticoagulant. *Arthritis and Rheumatism* 1976; **19**: 1244–8.

14 Branch WD, Scott JR, Kochenour NK & Hershgold E. Obstetric complications associated with the lupus anticoagulant. *New England Journal of Medicine* 1985; **313**: 1322–6.

15 Branch WD Rote NS, Scott RJ & Edwin S. The association of antiphospholipid antibodies with severe preeclampsia. *Clinical Experiments in Rheumatology* 1988; **6**: 198.

16 Buckfield P. Major congenital faults in newborn infants: a pilot study in New Zealand. *New Zealand Medical Journal* 1973; **78**: 159–204.

17 Bunyon JP, Roubey R *et al*. Complete congenital heart block: Risk of occurrence and therapeutic approach to prevention. *Journal of Rheumatology* 1988; **15**: 1104–8.

18 Bunyon JP, Swersey SH, Fox HE, Bierman F &

Winchester RJ. Intrauterine therapy for presumptive fetal myocarditis with acquired heart block due to systemic lupus erythematism. *Arthritis and Rheumatism* 1987; **30**: 44–9.

19 Byron MA. Treatment of rheumatic diseases. *British Medical Journal* 1987; **294**: 236–8.

20 Canadian Hydroxychloroquine Study Group. A randomized study of the effect of withdrawing hydroxychloroquine sulfate in systemic lupus erythematosus. *New England Journal of Medicine* 1991; **324**: 150–4.

21 Cariou T, Tobelem G, Soria C & Caen J. Inhibition of Protein C activation by endothelial cells in the presence of lupus anticoagulant. *New England Journal of Medicine* 1986; **314**: 1193–4.

22 Carreras LO, Defreyn G *et al*. Arterial thrombosis, intrauterine death and 'lupus' anticoagulant: detection of immunoglobulin interfering with prostacyclin formation. *Lancet* 1981; **i**: 244–6.

23 Carreras LO, Perez GN, Vega HR & Gasavilla F. Lupus anticoagulant and recurrent fetal loss: Successful treatment with gammaglobulin. *Lancet* 1988; **ii**: 393–4.

24 Chan JKM, Marris EN & Hughes GRV. Successful pregnancy following suppression of cardiolipin antibodies and lupus anticoagulant with azathioprine in systemic lupus erythematosus. *Journal of Obstetrics and Gynaecology* 1986; **7**: 16–17.

25 Chesley LC. *Hypertensive Disorders in Pregnancy*. Appleton-Century-Crofts, New York, 1978: 504.

26 Collins E & Turner G. Maternal effects of regular salicylate ingestion in pregnancy. *Lancet* 1975; **ii**: 335–8.

27 Comp PC, De Bault LE, Esmon NL & Esmon CT. Human thrombomodulin is inhibited by IgG from two patients with non-specific anticoagulants. *Blood* 1983; **1** (suppl): 1099.

28 Copelrud CP. Scleroderma. *Clinical Obstetrics and Gynecology* 1983; **26**: 587–91.

29 Cowchock S, Dehoratius RD, Wapner RJ & Jackson LG. Subclinical autoimmune disease and unexplained abortion. *American Journal of Obstetrics and Gynecology* 1984; **150**: 367–71.

30 Cowchock FS, Reece EA, Balaban D, Ware Banch D & Plouffe L. Repeated fetal losses associated with antiphospholipid antibodies: A collaborative randomized trial comparing prednisone with low-dose heparin treatment. *American Journal of Obstetrics and Gynecology* 1992; **166**: 1318–23.

31 Creagh MD, Malia RG, Cooper SM, Smith AR, Duncan SLB & Greaves M. Screening for lupus anticoagulant and anticardiolipin antibodies in women with fetal loss. *Journal of Clinical Pathology* 1991; **44**: 45–47.

32 Debeukelaer MM, Travis LB & Roberts DK. Polyarteritis and pregnancy: report of a successful outcome. *Southern Medican Journal* 1973; **66**: 613–15.

33 de Castellarnau C, Vila L. Sancho MJ, Borrell M, Fontcuberta J & Rutllant ML. Lupus anticoagulant, recurrent abortion, and prostacyclin production by cultured smooth muscle cells *Lancet* 1988; **ii**: 1137–8.

34 Derue GJ, Englert MJ *et al*. Fetal loss in systemic lupus: association with anticardiolipin antibodies. *Journal of Obstetrics and Gynaecology* 1985; **5**: 207–9.

35 Devoe LD & Taylor RL. Systemic lupus erythematosus in pregnancy. *American Journal of Obstetrics and Gynecology* 1979; **135**: 473–9.

36 De Wolf F, Carreras LO, Moerman P, Vermylen J, Van Assche A & Renaer M. Decidual vasculopathy and extensive placental infraction in a patient with repeated thromboembolic accidents, recurrent fetal loss, and lupus anticoagulant. *American Journal of Obstetrics and Gynecology* 1982; **142**: 829.

37 Donaldson LM & Espiner EA. Disseminated lupus erythematosus presenting as chorea gravidarum. *Archives of Neurology* 1971; **25**: 240–4.

38 Doshi N, Smith B & Klionsky B. Congenital pericarditis due to maternal lupus erythematosus. *Journal of Pediatrics* 1980; **96**: 699–701.

39 Dudley DKL & Mardie MJ. Fetal and neonatal effects of indomethacin used as a tocolytic agent. *American Journal of Obstetrics and Gynecology* 1985; **151**: 181–4.

40 Eeg-Olofsson O, Malmros I, Elwin C & Steen B. Convulsions in a breast-fed infant after maternal indomethacin. *Lancet* 1978; **ii**: 215.

41 Emson HE. For the want of an heir: the obstetrical history of Queen Anne. *British Medical Journal* 1992; **304**: 1365–6.

42 Englert MG, Derue GM, Loizous S, Hawkins DF, Elder MG & de Swiet M. Pregnancy and lupus: Prognostic indications and response to treatment. *Quarterly Journal of Medicine* 1988; **66**: 125–36.

43 Esscher E & Scott JS. Congenital heart block and maternal systemic lupus erythematosus. *British Medical Journal* 1979; **i**: 1235–8.

44 Estes D & Larson DL. Systemic lupus erythematosus and pregnancy. *Clinical Obstetrics and Gynecology* 1965; **8**: 307–21.

45 Exner T, Rickard KA & Kronenberg H. A sensitive test demonstrating lupus anticoagulant and its behavioural patterns. *British Journal of Haematology* 1978; **40**: 143–51.

46 Exner T, Triplett DA, Taberner DA & Harris EN. Comparison of test methods for the lupus anticoagulant: International survey on lupus anticoagulants-1 (ISLA-1). *Thrombosis and Haemostasis* 1990; **64**: 478–84.

47 Fairhead FW. Convulsions in a breast-fed infant after maternal indomethacin. *Lancet* 1978; **ii**: 576.

48 Farquharson RG, Pearson JF & John L. Lupus anticoagulant and pregnancy management. *Lancet* 1984; **ii**: 228–9.

49 Farquharson RG, Compston A & Bloom AL. Lupus anticoagulant: a place for pre-pregnancy treatment? *Lancet* 1985; **ii**: 842–3.

50 Freinstein DI. Lupus anticoagulant, thrombosis and fetal loss. *New England Journal of Medicine* 1985; **313**: 1348–50.
51 Fessel WJ. Systemic lupus erythematosus in the community. Incidence, prevalence, outcome and first symptoms; the high prevalence in black women. *Archives of Internal Medicine* 1974; **134**: 1027–35.
52 Firkin BG, Howard MA & Radford N. Possible relationship between lupus inhibitor and recurrent abortion in young women. *Lancet* 1980; **ii**: 366.
53 Fox R & Hawkins DF. Fetal-pericardial effusion in association with congenital heart block and maternal systemic lupus erythematosus. Case report. *British Journal of Obstetrics and Gynaecology* 1990; **97**: 638–40.
54 Fox R, Lumb MR & Hawkins DF. Persistent fetal sinus bradycardia associated with maternal anti-Ro antibodies. Case report. *British Journal of Obstetrics and Gynaecology* 1990; **97**: 1151–3.
55 Fraga A, Mintz G, Orozco J & Orozco JH. Sterility and fertility rates, fetal wastage and maternal morbidity in systemic lupus erythematosus. *Journal of Rheumatology* 1974; **1**: 1293–8.
56 Fulcher D, Stewart G, Exner T, Trudinger B & Jeremy R. Plasma exchange and the anticardiolipin syndrome in pregnancy. *Lancet* 1989; **ii**: 171.
57 Gardlund B. The lupus inhibitor in thromboembolic disease and intrauterine death in the absence of systemic lupus. *Acta Medica Scandinavica* 1984; **215**: 293–8.
58 Garsenstein M, Pollak VE & Karik RM. Systemic lupus erythematosus and pregnancy. *New England Journal of Medicine* 1962; **267**: 165–9.
59 Gifford RH. Rheumatic diseases. In Burrow GN & Ferris TF. (eds), *Medical Complications during Pregnancy*. WB Saunders, Philadelphia, 1975.
60 Gopelrud CP. Scleroderma. *Clinical Obstetrics and Gynecology* 1983; **26**: 587–91.
61 Goudie BM & Dossetor JFB. Effect on the fetus of indomethacin given to suppress labour. *Lancet* 1979; **ii**: 1187–5.
62 Gregorini G, Setti G & Remuzzi G. Recurrent abortion with lupus anticoagulant and preeclampsia: a common final pathway for two different diseases? Case report *British Journal of Obstetrics and Gynaecology* 1986; **93**: 194–6.
63 Grimes DA, Le Bolt SA, Grimes RR & Wingo PA. Systemic lupus erythematosus and reproductive function: a case-control study. *American Journal of Obstetrics and Gynecology* 1985; **153**: 179–86.
64 Hardy JD, Solomon S, Banwell GS, Beach R, Wright V & Howard FM. Congenital complete heart block in the newborn associated with maternal systemic lupus erythematosus and other connective tissue disease. *Archives of Disease in Childhood* 1979; **54**: 7–13.
65 Harris ENH, Gharavi AE *et al.* Anticardiolipin antibodies: detection by radioimmunoassay and association with thrombosis in systemic lupus erythematosus. *Lancet* 1983; **ii**: 1211–14.
66 Harris EN, Louizou S *et al.* Anticardiolipin antibodies and lupus anticoagulant. *Lancet* 1984; **ii**: 1099.
67 Harris EN, Chan J, Asherson R, Charavi A & Hughes GRV. Predictive value of the anticardiolipin antibody for thrombosis, fetal loss and thrombocytopoenia. *Clinical Science* 1986; **70**: 56P.
68 Harris EN & Hughes GRV. Standardising the anticardiolipin antibody test. *Lancet* 1987; **i**: 277.
69 Hart CW & Nauton RF. The ototoxicity of chloroquine phosphate. *Archives of Otolaryngology* 1964; **80**: 407.
70 Haynes DM. Collagen diseases in pregnancy. In: Haynes DM (ed), *Medical Complications during Pregnancy*. McGraw Hill, New York, 1969.
71 Hayslett JP & Lynn RI. Effect of pregnancy in patients with lupus nephropathy. *Kidney International* 1980; **18**: 207.
72 Hench AB. The ameliorating effect of pregnancy on chronic atrophic (infectious rheumatoid) arthritis; fibrositis and intermittent hydrothosis. *Proceedings of the Mayo Clinic* 1938; **13**: 161.
73 Herreman G & Galelowski N. Maternal connective tissue disease and congenital heart block. *New England Journal of Medicine* 1985; **312**: 1329.
74 Heymann MA. Non steroidal anti-inflammatory agents. In: Eskes TKAB & Finster M (eds), *Drug Therapy during Pregnancy*. Butterworths, London, 1985: 85–99.
75 Horowitz GM & Hankins GDV. Cutaneous manifestations of collagen vascular disease in pregnancy. *Clinical Obstetrics and Gynecology* 1990; **33**: 759–76.
76 Houser MT, Fish AJ, Tagatz GE, Williams PP & Michael AF. Pregnancy and systemic lupus erythematosus. *American Journal of Obstetrics and Gynecology* 1980; **138**: 409–13.
77 Howard RJ & Tuck SM. Caesarean section in a pregnancy complicated by relapsing polychondritis. *Journal of Obstetrics and Gynaecology* 1992; **12**: 120.
78 Hughes GRV. Thrombosis, abortion, cerebral disease and the lupus anticoagulant. *British Medical Journal* 1983; **287**: 1088–9.
79 Hughes GRV. Autoantibodies in lupus and its variants: experience in 1000 patients. *British Medical Journal* 1984; **289**: 339–42.
80 Hughes GRV, Harris EN & Gharavi AE. The anticardiolipin syndrome. *Journal of Rheumatology* 1986; **13**: 486–9.
81 Infante-Rivard C, David M, Gauthier R & Rivard GE. Lupus anticoagulants, anticardiolipin antibodies, and fetal loss. A case-control study. *New England Journal of Medicine* 1991; **325**: 1063–6.
82 Johnson TR, Banner EA & Winkelmann RK. Scleroderma and pregnancy. *Obstetrics and Gynecology* 1964; **23**: 467–9.
83 Kaplan D & Diamond H. Rheumatoid arthritis and pregnancy. *Clinical Obstetrics and Gynecology* 1965; **8**: 286–303.

84 Karlen JG & Cook WA. Renal scleroderma and pregnancy. *Obstetrics and Gynecology* 1974; **44**: 349–54.

85 Kilpatrick DC. Anti-phospholipid antibodies and pregnancy wastage. *Lancet* 1986; **ii**: 185–6.

86 Kilpatrick DC & Liston WA. Obstetric significance of cardiolipin antibodies in subjects without systemic lupus erythematosus. *Journal of Obstetrics and Gynaecology* 1992; **12**: 82–6.

87 Kincaid-Smith P, Fairley KF & Kloss M. Lupus anticoagulant associated with renal thrombotic microangiopathy and pregnancy related renal failure. *Quarterly Journal of Medicine* 1988; **69**: 795–815.

88 Kleinman CS, Copel JA & Hobbuns JL. Combined echocardiographic and Doppler assessment of fetal congenital atrioventricular block. *British Journal of Obstetrics and Gynaecology* 1987; **94**: 967–74.

89 *Lancet* editorial. PG-synthetase inhibition in obstetrics and after. *Lancet* 1980; **ii**: 185–6.

90 *Lancet* editorial. Anticardiolipin antibodies a risk factor for venous and arterial thrombosis. *Lancet* 1985; **i**: 912–13.

91 *Lancet* editorial. Neonatal lupus syndrome. *Lancet* 1987; **ii**: 489–90.

92 Lee LA, Bias WB *et al*. Immunogenetics of the neonatal lupus syndrome. *Annals of Internal Medicine* 1983; **99**: 592–6.

93 Leinwald I & Durgee AW. Scleroderma. *Annals of Internal Medicine* 1954; **41**: 1033–41.

94 Leung ACT & Bolton Jones M. Why do patients with lupus nephritis die? *British Medical Journal* 1985; **290**: 937.

95 Lewis R, Lauersen NH & Birn Baum S. Malaria associated with pregnancy. *Obstetrics and Gynecology* 1973; **42**: 696–700.

96 Linares A, Zarranz JJ, Rodriguez-Alarcon J & Diaz-Perez JL. Reversible cutis laxa due to maternal D-penicillamine treatment. *Lancet* 1979; **ii**: 43.

97 Litsey SE, Noonan JA, O'Connor WM, Cottrill CM & Mitchell B. Maternal connective tissue disease and congenital heart block. Demonstration of immunoglobulin in cardiac tissue. *New England Journal of Medicine* 1985; **312**: 98–100.

98 Lockshin MD. Anticardiolipin antibodies in pregnant patients with systemic lupus erythematosus. *New England Journal of Medicine* 1986; **314**: 1392–3.

99 Lockshin MD, Gibofsky A, Peebles CL, Gigli I, Fotino M & Hurwitz S. Neonatal lupus erythematosus with heart block: family study of a patient with anti-SS-A and SS-B antibodies *Arthritis and Rheumatism* 1983; **26**: 210–13.

100 Lockshin MD, Druzin ML *et al*. Antibody to cardiolipin as a predictor of fetal distress or death in pregnant patients with systemic lupus erythematosus. *New England Journal of Medicine* 1985; **313**: 152–6.

101 Lockshin MD & Druzin ML. Antiphospholipid antibodies and pregnancy. *New England Journal of Medicine* 1985; **313**: 1351.

102 Lockshin MD, Bonfa E, Elkon K & Druzin ML. Neonatal lupus risk to newborns of mothers with systemic lupus erythematosus. *Arthritis and Rheumatism* 1988; **31**: 697–701.

103 Lockwood CJ, Reece EA, Romero R & Hobbins JC. Antiphospholipid antibody and pregnancy wastage. *Lancet* 1986; **ii**: 742–3.

104 Loizou S, Byron MA, Englert HJ, David J, Hughes GR & Walport MJ. Association of quantitative anticardiolipin antibody levels with fetal loss and time of loss in systemic lupus erythematosus. *Quarterly Journal of Medicine* 1988; **68**: 525–31.

105 Lubbé WF & Walker EB. Chorea gravidarum associated with lupus anticoagulant: successful outcome of pregnancy with prednisone therapy. *British Journal of Obstetrics and Gynaecology* 1983; **90**: 487–90.

106 Lubbé WF & Liggins GC. Lupus anticoagulant and pregnancy. *American Journal of Obstetrics and Gynecology* 1985; **153**: 322–7.

107 Lubbé WF, Butler WS, Palmer SJ & Liggins GC. Lupus anticoagulant in pregnancy. *British Journal of Obstetrics and Gynaecology* 1984; **91**: 357–63.

108 Lyle WH. Penicillamine in pregnancy. *Lancet* 1978; **i**: 606–7.

109 Maddison PJ, Skinner RP, Esscher E, Taylor PV, Scott O & Scott JS. Serological studies in congenital heart block. *Annals of the Rheumatic Diseases* 1983; **42**: 218–19.

110 McCue CM, Matakas ME, Tinglesrad JB & Ruddy S. Congenital heart block in newborns of mothers with connective tissue disease. *Circulation* 1977; **56**: 82–90.

111 McCormack MJ, Adu D, Weaver J, Michael J & Kelley J. Anti-platelet antibodies: A prognostic marker in pregnancies associated with lupus nephritis. Case reports. *British Journal of Obstetrics and Gynaecology* 1991; **98**: 324–5.

112 McKenna F, Martin MFR, Bird HA & Wright V. Captopril. *British Medical Journal* 1983; **287**: 1299.

113 Manu P. Serial probability analysis of the 1982 revised criteria for the classification of systemic lupus erythematosus. *New England Journal of Medicine* 1983; **309**: 1460.

114 McCuiston CH & Shock EP. Possible discoid lupus erythematosus in a newborn infant, report of a case with subsequent development of acute systemic lupus erythematosus in the mother. *Archives of Dermatology and Syphilology* 1954; **70**: 782–5.

115 Mjolnerod JK, Rasmussen K, Dommerud SA & Gjeruldsen ST. Congenital connective tissue defect probably due to D-penicillamine treatment in pregnancy. *Lancet* 1971; **i**: 673–5.

116 Mund A, Simson J & Rothfield N. Effect of pregnancy on course of systemic lupus erythematosus. *Journal of the American Medical Association* 1963; **183**: 917–20.

117 Nagey DA, Fortier KI & Linder J. Pregnancy complicated by periarteritis nodosa. Induced abortion as an alternative. *American Journal of Obstetrics and Gynecology* 1983; **147**: 103–5.

118 Nathan DJ & Snapper I. Simultaneous placental trans-

fer of factors responsible for LE cell formation and thrombocytopenia. *American Journal of Medicine* 1958; **25**: 647.

119 Nicolaides KH, Soothill PW, Rodeck CH & Campbell S. Ultrasound-guided sampling of umbilical cord and placental blood to assess fetal wellbeing. *Lancet* 1986; **i**: 1065–7.

120 Niebyl JR & Witter FR. Neonatal outcome after indomethacin treatment for preterm labour. *American Journal of Obstetrics and Gynecology* 1986; **155**: 747–9.

121 Oakey RE. The interpretation of urinary oestrogen and pregnanediol excretion in women receiving corticosteroids. *Journal of Obstetrics and Gynaecology of the British Commonwealth* 1970; **77**: 922–7.

122 Olah KS & Gee H. Fetal heart block associated with maternal anti-Ro (SS-A) antibody — current management. A review. *British Journal of Obstetrics and Gynaecology* 1991; **98**: 751–5.

123 Olah KS & Redman CWG. Overlap syndrome and its implications in pregnancy. Case report. *British Journal of Obstetrics and Gynaecology* 1991; **98**: 728–30.

124 Ordi J, Vilardel M *et al*. Bleeding in patients with lupus anticoagulant. *Lancet* 1984; **ii**: 868–9.

125 Owen J & Hauth JC. Polyarteritis nodosa in pregnancy: A case report and brief literature review. *American Journal of Obstetrics and Gynecology* 1989; **160**: 606–7.

126 Paredes RA, Morgan H & Lachelin GCL. Congenital heart block associated with maternal Sjörgren's syndrome. Case report. *British Journal of Obstetrics and Gynaecology* 1983; **90**: 870–1.

127 Prentice RL, Gatenby PA, Loblay RM, Shearman RP, Kronenberg M & Basten A. Lupus anticoagulant in pregnancy. *Lancet* 1984; **ii**: 464.

128 Provost TT, Watson R, Gammon WR, Radowsky M, Harley JB & Riechlin M. The neonatal lupus syndrome associated with U 1 RNP (nRNP) antibodies. *New England Journal of Medicine* 1987; **316**: 1135–8.

129 Ramsden GH, Johnson PM, Hart CA & Farquharson RG. Listeriosis in immunocompromised pregnancy. *Lancet* 1989; **i**: 794.

130 Reece EA, Romero R, Clyne LP, Kriz NS & Hobbins JC. Lupus like anticoagulant in pregnancy. *Lancet* 1984; **i**: 344–5.

131 Rees RB & Maubach MM. Chloroquine: a review of reactions and dermatologic indications. *Archives of Dermatology* 1963; **88**: 96–105.

132 Richards DS, Wagman AJ & Cabaniss ML. Ascites not due to congestive heart failure in a fetus with lupus-induced heart block. *Obstetrics and Gynecology* 1990; **76**: 957–9.

133 Rocker I & Henderson WJ. Transfer of gold from mother to fetus. *Lancet* 1976; **ii**: 1246.

134 Ros JO, Tarres MV, Baucells MV, Maired JJ & Solano J. Prednisone and maternal lupus anticoagulant. *Lancet* 1983; **ii**: 576.

135 Rosove MH, Tabsh K, Wasserstrum N, Howard P, Hahn BH & Kalunian KC. Heparin therapy for pregnant women with lupus anticoagulant or anticardiolipin antibodies. *Obstetrics and Gynecology* 1990; **75**: 630–4.

136 Scheinberg IH & Sternlieb I. Pregnancy in penicillamine-treated patients with Wilson's disease. *New England Journal of Medicine* 1975; **293**: 1300–2.

137 Schlieder MA, Nachman RL, Jaffe EA & Coleman MA. Clinical study of the lupus anticoagulant. *Blood* 1976; **48**: 499–509.

138 Scott JS. Systemic lupus erythematosus and allied disorders in pregnancy. *Clinics in Obstetrics and Gynaecology* 1979; **6**: 461–71.

139 Shenker L, Reed KL, Anderson CF, Marx GR, Sobonya LE & Graham AR. Congenital heart block and cardiac anomolies in the absence of maternal connective tissue disease. *American Journal of Obstetrics and Gynecology* 1987; **157**: 248–53.

140 Singsen BM, Akhter JE, Weinstein MW & Sharp GC. Congenital complete heart block and SSA antibodies: obstetric implications. *American Journal of Obstetrics and Gynecology* 1985; **152**: 655–8.

141 Slate WG & Graham AR. Scleroderma and pregnancy. *American Journal of Obstetrics and Gynecology* 1968; **101**: 335–41.

142 Slone D, Sisilind V, Heinonen OP, Monson RR, Kaufman DW & Shapiro S. Aspirin and congenital malformations. *Lancet* 1976; **i**: 1373–5.

143 Solomon L, Abrams G, Dinner M & Berman L. Neonatal abnormalities associated with D-Penicillamine, treatment during pregnancy. *New England Journal of Medicine* 1977; **296**: 54–5.

144 Soothill PW, Nicolaides KH, Rodeck CH & Campbell S. The effect of gestational age on blood gas and acid–base values in human pregnancy. *Fetal Therapy* 1986; **7**: 166–73.

145 Speira IE. Connective tissue disease in pregnancy. *Mount Sinai Journal of Medicine* 1980; **47**: 438–41.

146 Spitz B, Van Assche FA & Vermylen J. Lupus anticoagulant and pregnancy. *American Journal of Obstetrics and Gynecology* 1986; **154**: 1169.

147 Stephensen O. Cleland WP & Hallidie-Smith K. Congenital heart block and persistent ductus arteriosus associated with maternal systemic lupus erythematosus. *British Heart Journal f48 1981;* **46**: 101.

148 Stuart MJ, Gross SJ, Ellad H & Graeber JE. Effects of acetylsalicylic-acid ingestion on maternal and neonatal hemostasis. *New England Journal of Medicine* 1982; **307**: 909–12.

149 Syrop CH & Varner MW. Systemic lupus erythematosus. *Clinical Obstetrics and Gynecology* 1983; **26**: 547–57.

150 Tan EM, Cohan AS *et al*. The 1982 revised criteria for the classification of systemic lupus erythematosus. *Arthritis and Rheumatism* 1982; **25**: 1271–7.

151 Taylor PV & Skerrow SM. Pre-eclampsia and antiphospholipid antibody. *British Journal of Obstetrics and Gynaecology* 1991; **98**: 604–6.

152 Taylor PV, Scott JS, Gerlis LM, Esscher E & Scott O.

Maternal autoantibodies against fetal cardiac antigens in congenital complete heart block. *New England Journal of Medicine* 1986; **315**: 667–72.
153 Thompson J & Conklin KA. Anesthetic management of a pregnant patient with scleroderma. *Anesthesiology* 1983; **59**: 69–71.
154 Thomson BJ, Watson ML, Liston WA & Lambie AT. Plasmaphaeresis in a pregnancy complicated by acute systemic lupus erythematosus. Case report. *British Journal of Obstetrics and Gynaecology* 1985; **92**: 532–4.
155 Thornton JR, Scott JS & Tovey LAD. Anticardiolipin antibodies in pregnancy. *British Medical Journal* 1984; **289**: 697.
156 Thurnau GR. Rheumatoid arthritis. *Clinical Obstetrics and Gynecology* 1983; **26**: 558–78.
157 Turner G & Collins E. Fetal effects of regular salicylate ingestion in pregnancy. *Lancet* 1975; **ii**: 338–9.
158 Ullberg S, Lindquist NG & Sjostrand SE. Accumulation of retinotoxic drugs in the foetal eye. *Nature* 1970; **227**: 1257.
159 Unander AM, Norberg R, Hahn L & Arfors L. Anticardiolipin antibodies and complement in ninety-nine women with habitual abortion. *American Journal of Obstetrics and Gynecology* 1987; **156**: 114–19.
160 Unger A, Kay A, Griffin AJ & Panayi GS. Disease activity and pregnancy associated α_2-glycoprotein in rheumatoid arthritis during pregnancy. *British Medical Journal* 1983; **286**: 750–2.
161 Veille JC, Sunderland C & Bennett RM. Complete heart block in a fetus associated with maternal Sjögren's syndrome. *American Journal of Obstetrics and Gynecology* 1985; **151**: 660–1.
162 Venning MC, Burn DJ, Ward RM, Henry JA & Davison JM. Neonatal lupus syndrome: Optimism justified? *Lancet* 1988; **i**: 640.
163 Violi F, Ferro D *et al*. Tissue plasminogen activator inhibitor in patients with systemic lupus erythematosus and thrombosis. *British Medical Journal* 1990; **300**: 1099–102.
164 Vonderheid EC, Koblenzer PJ, Ming P, Ming L & Burgoon CF. Neonatal lupus erythematosus, report of four cases with a review of the literature. *Archives of Dermatology* 1976; **112**: 698–705.
165 Walport MJ. Pregnancy and antibodies to phospholipids. *Annals of Rheumatological Disease* 1989; **48**: 795–7.
166 Wapner RJ, Cowchock FS & Shapiro SS. Successful treatment in two women with antiphospholipid antibodies and refactory pregnancy losses with intravenous immunoglobulin infusions. *American Journal of Obstetrics and Gynecology* 1989; **161**: 1271–2.
167 Watson KV & Schorer AE. Lupus anticoagulant inhibition of in vitro prostacyclin release is associated with a thrombosis-prone subset of patients. *American Journal of Medicine* 1991; **90**: 47–53.
168 Wolfe MS & Cordero JF. Safety of chloroquine in chemosuppression of malaria during pregnancy. *British Medical Journal* 1985; **290**: 1466–7.
169 Wong KL, Chan FY & Lee CP. Outcome of pregnancy in patients with systemic lupus erythematosus: A prospective study. *Archives of Internal Medicine* 1991; **151**: 269–73.
170 Zulman JI, Talal N, Hoffman GS & Epstein WV. Problems associated with the management of pregnancies in patients with systemic lupus erythematosus. *Journal of Rheumatology* 1980; **7**: 37–49.
171 Zurier RB, Argyros TG, Urman JD, Warren J & Rothfield NF. Systemic lupus erythematosus. Management during pregnancy. *Obstetrics and Gynecology* 1978; **51**: 178–80.

9

Disorders of the Liver, Biliary System and Pancreas

Elizabeth A. Fagan

Physiology, biochemistry and anatomy, 321
Hyperbilirubinaemia and the fetus, 322
Liver diseases peculiar to pregnancy, 323
- Hyperemesis gravidarum
- Hepatic disorders associated with hypertension
- Intrahepatic cholestasis of pregnancy

Liver diseases incidental to pregnancy, 333
- Viral hepatitis A to E
- Herpes viruses
- AIDS and the liver
- Acute liver failure
- Liver transplantation
- Chronic hepatitis
- Budd–Chiari syndrome
- Congenital disorders of metabolism of bilirubin and lipids
- Inflammatory bowel disease and the liver
- Acute porphyria
- Hepatic abscess
- Polycystic liver disease
- Hepatic tumours

Gallbladder and biliary tract, 361
- Anatomy and physiology
- Cholesterol cholelithiasis
- Cholelithiasis in pregnancy

Pancreas, 363
- Acute pancreatitis
- Malignancies

Diseases of the liver remain rare in pregnancy. Only 50 cases from 56 000 pregnancies were recorded in one non-specialized centre [204]. The majority are conditions unique to pregnancy. Most often these do not adversely affect maternal and fetal outcome. Early diagnosis of the exceptions is important because multidisciplinary management in a referral centre can improve outcome. Liver disease is now a major cause of maternal mortality in the UK (see below).

Physiology, biochemistry and anatomy

In a normal pregnancy with adequate nutrition, the metabolic changes seem to be without significant effect on liver metabolism and function. Table 9.1 summarizes the physiological changes observed in standard liver function tests. Abnormalities on liver function testing suggest liver disease or an hepatic complication. In the non-pregnant individual, hepatic blood flow represents 25–35 per cent of the cardiac output [310]. In pregnancy, absolute hepatic blood flow is not increased significantly. Therefore a smaller proportion of the increased cardiac output (approximately 25 per cent) passes through the liver. The total blood volume in pregnancy increases by up to 50 per cent and is partly redistributed into the splanchnic circulation and great veins. Portal vein pressure is increased in late pregnancy. The additional pressure of the gravid uterus on the vena cava results in divertion of a portion of the venous return through the azygous system [195]. Venous pressure increases in the oesophagus leading to transient engorgement of oesophageal veins (varices) in up to 60 per cent of healthy pregnant women [195] (see below).

The liver in pregnancy shows no undue susceptibility to drugs and toxins. Clearance of drugs with high hepatic extraction ratios is unlikely to be altered significantly [310]. However, hepatic clearance may be reduced for those drugs which rely on blood flow due to the larger volume of distribution [382].

Serum levels of alkaline phosphatase, aspartate aminotransferase (AST – serum glutamic oxaloacetic transaminase, SGOT) and lactic acid dehydro-

Table 9.1. Liver function tests and pregnancy

Serum tests	Non-pregnant	Change in pregnancy	
General			
Bilirubin	2–17 μmol/l	No change	Alteration signifies hepatic dysfunction
Transaminase	7–40 IU/l	No change	
γGT	<30 IU/l	No change	
5-nucleotidase	2–17 IU/l	No change	
Prothrombin time	12–14 seconds	No change	
Proteins			
Total protein	65–80 g/l	Fall	By 10 g/l by 16th–20th week
Albumin	35–55 g/l	Fall	By 10 g/l mostly in first trimester
Globulin	30–50 g/l	Rise	Progressive increase to term
Fibrinogen	2–4 g/l	Rise	Progressive increase to term
Lipids			
Cholesterol	4–6.5 mmol/l	Rise	Progressive increase to term
Triglyceride	<1.5 mmol/l	Rise	Progressive increase to term
Enzymes			
Alkaline phosphatase	30–130 IU/l	Rise	Progressive increase after 5th week to term (1.5 × normal) — placental component — skeletal component

genase (LDH) rise during labour and delivery. The alkaline phosphatase may remain elevated for up to 6 weeks post-partum but levels rarely exceed two times upper normal limits [114]. Levels of serum albumin fall through haemodilution in pregnancy by up to 25 per cent. Serum α_1, α_2 and β globulins show a progressive rise by up to 50 per cent but levels of γ globulin remain essentially unchanged [382].

Hypercholesterolaemia in pregnancy is well documented [114]. Plasma cholesterol rises by approximately 50 per cent by the third trimester and triglycerides may rise two to three times upper normal limits. Serum levels of the bile acids chenodeoxycholic and cholic acids rise but remain within normal limits in most women.

In the third trimester, the liver occupies a more posterosuperior position with displacement to the right and subsequent reduction in dullness to percussion. A palpable liver suggests underlying liver disease. Histopathological studies show no specific changes apart from mild steatosis. Percutaneous liver biopsy is safe in expert hands within the limitations of normal coagulation and ultrasonographic imaging.

Palmar erythema and spider naevae are common in normal pregnancy. These stigmata are not specific for chronic liver disease and can be seen in acute liver failure.

Hyperbilirubinaemia and the fetus

Placental transfer of unconjugated bilirubin from the fetus into the maternal system provides the major pathway for conjugation and subsequent elimination of bilirubin and its degradation products. Only minor amounts are handled directly by the fetus or excreted into amniotic fluid [33]. Fetal exposure to high maternal levels of unconjugated and conjugated bilirubins may result in high circulating fetal levels since the unconjugated form can cross the placenta in both directions [33,388]. No simple relation has been found between maternal and fetal levels of the bilirubins [17,388]. Prolonged exposure to elevated levels of unconjugated bilirubin and toxic metabolites, such as in maternal liver failure, does not result in neurological and developmental abnormalities [17,388]. Disruption of the fetal blood–brain barrier is as important as the level of unconjugated bilirubin for the development of kernicterus [229].

Certain maternal disorders are peculiar to pregnancy; others occurring coincidentally will be considered separately.

Liver diseases peculiar to pregnancy

Hyperemesis gravidarum (see Chapter 10)

Hepatic dysfunction from vomiting sufficient to require hospitalization is more common than previously thought [143,334]. Elevations in serum levels of AST to four times upper normal limits have been found in 15–25 per cent of women with hyperemesis gravidarum. The biochemical abnormalities reverse rapidly with restoration of fluid balance, improved nutrition and cessation of vomiting [221,261]. Hepatic synthetic function, as measured by the prothrombin ratio, remains normal except with marked cholestasis and vitamin K deficiency.

Pathogenetic mechanisms are unclear. Earlier reports included cases of viral hepatitis, drug-related hepatotoxicity and coincidental thyrotoxicosis. Current hypotheses favour a multifactorial origin for the liver injury including adverse effects of starvation and dehydration, high levels of oestrogens and a genetic predisposition. Abnormal liver function tests occur but do not correlate with severe ketonuria levels [261]. Serum levels of AST up to 22 times upper normal limits have been recorded [221] but synthetic function remains normal. Reduced flow of bile and bile salts, as measured by impaired excretion of bromosulphthalein, has been demonstrated in Kwashiorkor and in late pregnancy in women who experienced emesis in the first trimester [178]. Liver dysfunction responds promptly to control of vomiting and correction of dehydration and malnutrition [221]. The main differential diagnoses are viral hepatitis and thyrotoxicosis. Liver biopsy usually is not required. The histopathology shows only non-specific changes.

Hepatic disorders associated with hypertension (see Chapter 6)

The most common liver diseases in late pregnancy are associated with hypertension. Acute fatty liver, HELLP syndrome (haemolysis, elevated liver enzymes and low platelet count) and hepatic rupture and infarction [114,212,322] form a spectrum but their related aetiologies remain obscure. Improvements in non-invasive imaging techniques, specialized haematological tests and liver histology have led to re-appraisal of the hepatic abnormalities.

Early clinical features can be vague, overlap and make diagnosis difficult [131]. Epigastric pain from hepatic tenderness, nausea and vomiting are common in pre-eclampsia. Jaundice is uncommon but abnormal liver function occurs frequently. Elevated levels of serum AST (SGOT) are common to many conditions, including those unrelated to pregnancy (Box 9.1).

Abdominal pain can occur in many conditions (Box 9.1) [95]. The prothrombin ratio and fibrinogen levels typically are normal [200,393].

The liver is not involved primarily in pre-eclampsia but becomes the target organ in severe

Box 9.1. Differential diagnosis of hepatic disorders and hypertension

- HELLP
- Acute fatty liver
- Alcoholic hepatitis
- Biliary colic
- Budd–Chiari syndrome
- Cholecystitis
- Cocaine abuse
- Dissecting aortic aneurysm
- Disseminated intravascular coagulation
- Hepatic necrosis
- Hiatus hernia
- Pancreatitis
- Peptic ulcer
- Pyelonephritis
- Septicaemias
- SLE
- Thrombocytopenias
- Viral hepatitis

cases. Liver disease most often occurs in fulminating pre-eclampsia but may also occur in milder forms of pre-eclampsia due to inadequate antenatal care. The associated constellation of signs and symptoms typically include marked hypertension (diastolic blood pressure >110 mmHg) and proteinuria with renal impairment (oliguria and raised serum creatinine), cerebral and visual disturbances and intrauterine growth retardation.

Macroscopically, the liver in pre-eclampsia shows diffuse petechial haemorrhages over Glisson's capsule and the cut surface. Histopathological features are seen in over three-quarters of cases at post-mortem [249]. Prominent features are hepatocellular necrosis with haemorrhage in the periportal regions and deposits of fibrin without any inflammatory infiltrate. Thrombi can be detected in capillaries in the portal tract and occasionally in branches of hepatic arteries and portal vein [312]. These features have been attributed to disseminated intravascular coagulation (DIC) [160] and resemble those of thrombotic thrombocytopenic purpura [80]. However, they are unlikely to be primary events because coagulation abnormalities are seen only in the minority of causes of pre-eclampsia complicated by liver disease [14,143]. Hormonal factors may play a role because the clinical features can be imitated with administration of massive doses of oestrogen [128].

A vascular theory is now favoured for many of the features of pre-eclampsia [312]. Segmental vasospasm results in injury to endothelial cells and exposure of subendothelial collagen leading to platelet adherence and aggregation and precipitation of fibrin [312]. In dilated segments there is separation of endothelial cells and increased intraluminal pressure. The mechanisms whereby these abnormalities can lead to hepatic rupture and infarction are discussed below.

The HELLP syndrome

Some patients with hypertension in the third trimester may present principally with hepatic dysfunction and laboratory evidence of the HELLP syndrome [393]. Occasionally presentation may precede the 20th week or occur post-partum. Hepatic dysfunction in patients with hypertension is more common than previously thought. In two North American referral centres, HELLP syndrome was diagnosed in around 15 per cent of patients with hypertension [70].

Elevations in levels of many tests occur including unconjugated bilirubin, creatinine, LDH, fibrin degradation products, fibrin D-dimer, plasminogen activator inhibitor, protein C, anaphylatoxins (C3a, C5a) and creatinine. There is a microangiopathic haemolytic anaemia with DIC. Unfortunately, many of these values show too much variation for clinical use. Levels of antithrombin III often are reduced. Synthetic function of the liver, as measured by the prothrombin ratio, is usually normal or near normal as are the partial thromboplastin time and level of fibrinogen. Elevation in levels of serum AST and unconjugated bilirubin reflects the severity of the haematological disturbances but does not correlate with trimester of presentation, clinical severity or propensity for complications and recovery. Typically, the serum level of AST will recover within days after delivery whereas the thrombocytopenia may be protracted.

There are no universally accepted criteria for the diagnosis of HELLP syndrome. Some authorities do not separate this from other conditions associated with hypertension — most will accept raised levels of AST (SGOT) above 50 IU/l ($n < 40$) and lactate dehydrogenase above 180 IU/l with a platelet count $<100 \times 10^9$/l and haemolysis. The AST level usually is below 10 times upper normal limits but occasionally can exceed 1000 IU/l.

The spectrum has widened to include milder cases with epigastric pain, elevated serum levels of AST and DIC but with normal or mild elevations in blood pressure and no significant proteinuria [1,133]. This is probably only another example of the well-recognized temporal dissociation of the various clinical features of pre-eclampsia (see Chapter 6). Deposition of fibrin in the periportal regions and, especially, the sinusoids is found early in the HELLP syndrome, including the milder cases. Fibrin is best demonstrated using immunofluorescence techniques [1,133]. Similar changes are found in pregnancy-associated hypertension with abnormal serum liver biochemistry but without evidence of HELLP, some cases of viral hepatitis and drug-related hepatotoxicity [1].

Some patients with mild HELLP syndrome may improve with conservative management and proceed to spontaneous vaginal delivery but intrauterine growth retardation is common [1]. Correction of hypertension followed by immediate delivery by caesarean section is the treatment of choice for severe cases. Prompt delivery may allow therapeutic manoeuvres for the mother that had previously been considered unsafe for the fetus.

Provision should be made for all patients with HELLP to be delivered with intensive care facilities for mother and child. As with acute fatty liver of pregnancy, post-partum recovery is rapid. Medical expertise may be necessary for the management of liver failure for the mother, including provision for liver transplantation [140].

Hepatic rupture and infarction

Spontaneous rupture of the liver was reported by Abercrombie in 1844 [2]. A recent survey gives its occurrence as about one in 45 000 live births [343]. The majority are associated with severe hypertension including the HELLP syndrome. Rupture is most common in the third trimester but can occur at any time, including early in the puerperium [2,38, 240,342]. As in the non-pregnant patient, liver rupture can be precipitated by trauma, vomiting and convulsions. Vascular malformations, polyarteritis nodosa, mycotic aneurysms, fibromuscular dysplasia, amoebic abscess and tumours account for a minority of cases in pregnancy [350].

The pathogenetic mechanisms of spontaneous rupture remain obscure. Subcapsular haemorrhages in the liver are found in 80 per cent of cases of pre-eclampsia and eclampsia [242] in association with DIC. The altered haematological state may favour pathological deposition of fibrin thrombi in vessels and sinusoids leading to focal, and later confluent, subcapsular haemorrhagic necrosis [16,54,129] prior to rupture. This hypothesis has been challenged by the finding of a coagulopathy which developed after onset of rupture and following surgical repair [154]. The elevation in serum AST (SGOT) is accompanied usually by a rise in serum LDH and probably reflects red cell destruction [157]. Extensive necrosis of hepatocytes and a coagulopathy will result in high levels of AST (>1000 IU/l) [235,240] and impaired synthetic function reflected in the elevated prothrombin ratio [154].

Occlusion of the hepatic artery does not lead to widespread infarction because additional blood is supplied from the portal vein. Hepatic infarction more likely results from several factors including gross ischaemia and obstruction to sinusoidal blood flow by deposited fibrin and relative hypovolaemia. Differential diagnosis and management are similar to that of acute liver failure (see below).

Rupture and infarction can occur at any time including in the puerperium. Onset is sudden with upper abdominal pain, nausea and vomiting. Usually the lower abdomen is soft and uterus not tender [175]. Severe cases may be heralded by shock, hypotension, fever, vomiting, absent fetal heart sounds and vaginal bleeding with a haemorrhagic diathesis. Hepatic encephalopathy is compounded by severe hypoglycaemia. Levels of serum transaminases typically are grossly elevated (>10 times upper normal limits) and the prothrombin ratio is prolonged. Haemoperitoneum may be discovered at laparotomy for suspected perforated viscus, abruptio placenta and ruptured uterus. A subcapsular tear and haematoma may be seen with liver rupture. In over 90 per cent these involve the anterosuperior aspect of the right lobe. Until recently, diagnosis was delayed until late and maternal mortality was as high as 75 per cent [38,155].

Hepatic rupture should be suspected with the triad of pre-eclampsia, right upper quadrant pain typically referred to the shoulder tip and shock. Urgent provision should be made for a general surgeon and obstetrician to proceed to theatre. In 10 per cent of cases the left lobe of the liver is involved and a subcapsular haematoma may be overlooked at surgery [97]. Bleeding also may occur at intracerebral, intrathoracic and retroperitoneal sites [97].

The prognosis of liver rupture has improved with increased awareness of the complications of hypertension and advances in imaging techniques. Serial scanning for suspected haematoma, hepatic rupture and infarction is essential. Computed tomography (CT) scanning and magnetic resonance imaging (MRI) may be necessary if results of ultrasonography are negative. CT imaging typically reveals a crescentic or oval lesion of low attenuation without distortion of the hepatic vasculature (absence of mass effect). In hepatic infarction, enhancement after intravenous contrast medium is not seen, though it is seen with haemorrhage, infection and malignancy. Diagnostic hepatic arteriography offers the option of transcatheter embolization early in the process when the patient is haemodynamically stable and without intraperitoneal haemorrhage. Percutaneous diagnostic peritoneal lavage under aseptic technique should be carried out for suspected liver rupture. The presence of blood and haemodynamic instability should prompt urgent combined surgical and obstetrical intervention. Packing with drainage is preferred to radical hepatic resection [112]. Transcatheter embolotherapy also can be considered especially with haemodynamic instability and when the risk of surgery is high. In expert hands, selective catheterization and embolization of the offending vessels can arrest bleeding abruptly but cessation may be temporary. Non-selective embolization may result in complications such as hepatic abscess, sepsis and ischaemia of the gallbladder [390]. Laparotomy is essential if arteriography fails. Hepatic resection is carried out only if the more conservative packing procedures fail.

Several authors favour immediate caesarean section although still-birth and perinatal mortality remain high [97,137,316,400]. Earlier diagnosis may improve fetal and maternal outcome and obviate the need for surgery. Between 1984 and 1985, in a total of 10 patients reported by three separate groups [100,136,245] diagnosis was made of intrahepatic haematoma with subcapsular haematoma in six before delivery, who then proceeded to caesarean section for fetal distress, and in four post-partum. All recovered without surgery and serial scans showed regression of the haematoma over weeks to 6 months. Later, uneventful pregnancies have been recorded in survivors of previous hepatic rupture [293,316,400]. One [20] non-pregnant patient presented in shock and survived a 50 per cent hepatic resection for rupture of a hepatic adenoma in the left lobe and excision of an unruptured adenoma in the right lobe. This patient conceived 5 months later and proceeded with an uneventful pregnancy to an elective caesarean section at term. Serial scans showed no recurrence (see hepatic tumours below).

Acute fatty liver of pregnancy (AFLP)

The separate recognition of AFLP is usually attributed to Stander and Cadden [347], although similar features were described by Rokitansky in 1843 and Tarnier in 1856 [368]. Differentiation from fulminant viral hepatitis is attributed to Sheehan [334].

Estimates of occurrence rate are one in 9000–13 300 deliveries [291,299]. The greater awareness of this condition and improvements in imaging have led to the recognition of milder cases and the reporting of survivors [189,292]. Collected data from four series (Table 9.2) of biopsy-proven AFLP published from 1980 show a reduction in mortalities: the maternal to as low as 18 per cent and fetal to 23 per cent [34,49,75,291].

These advances have not been matched in general obstetric practice. The number of maternal deaths from AFLP seems to be increasing and accounted for six of the 20 direct other deaths in the UK between 1985 and 1987 [87]. This is as many as for each category of death attributed to sepsis, ruptured uterus, abortion and anaesthesia. The diagnosis of AFLP was considered difficult in all cases and in

Table 9.2. Survival in biopsy-proven acute fatty liver of pregnancy

			Mothers		Infants	
Author	Reference		Number	Survival	Number	Survival
Davies *et al.*	[75]	1980	6	5	7*	4
Burroughs *et al.*	[49]	1982	12	8	15***	6**
Bernuau *et al.*	[34]	1983	5	4	6*	5*
Pockros *et al.*	[292]	1984	10	9	12**	10**

Sets of twins: * 1 set, ** 2 sets, *** 3 sets.

only one of the six was this made pre-mortem. In three, jaundice was not obvious, two had additional hepatitis B and hypoparathyroidism, and one presentation was in the second week post-partum after an uneventful pregnancy and delivery. The typical pre-mortem diagnoses were adult respiratory distress syndrome, DIC and cholecystitis requiring surgery.

AFLP typically occurs in the obese woman in the third trimester. The predeliction for primaparae is not emphasized in more recent series [291,311]. Multiparous women have presented as late as the 11th gestation [144,311]. Common independent associations are pre-eclampsia in approximately 30–60 per cent [49,144], twin pregnancy in 9–25 per cent [49,144] and a male rather than female fetus (ratio 3 : 1) [144,189]. Distributions in age, parity and race do not differ significantly from normal obstetric practice [144,311]. The frequency of presentation rises after the 13th week but onset has been reported in the 20th week [143] and post-partum [49,144,384].

Symptoms develop acutely but are non-specific such as abdominal pain (40–58 per cent), nausea and vomiting (35–88 per cent), headache (1–17 per cent) and jaundice (50–90 per cent) [44,87,144,291]. Signs associated with pre-eclampsia such as hypertension, oedema and proteinuria occur in over 50 per cent. More variable features are pruritus in 5–30 per cent [144,291], fever in 40–53 per cent [144,291], ascites (40 per cent) [291], necrotizing enterocolitis [384] and clinical or post-mortem evidence of pancreatitis in 16–100 per cent [144, 150,166,311]. The more severe cases may progress rapidly with impairment of conscious level, often related to profound hypoglycaemia, and development of acute liver failure, renal failure, bleeding diatheses, coma and death [49,144,189,291,311].

Laboratory findings include a marked neutrophil leucocytosis often $>15\,000/\text{mm}^3$ and occasionally $>30\,000/\text{mm}^3$ with left shift. Other findings may be DIC and microangiopathic haemolytic anaemia with thrombocytopenia, abnormal red cell forms (burr cells, schistocytes, nucleated forms), elevated levels of fibrin degradation products and reduced levels of antithrombin III [49,130,144,222,231,291]. Oliguria with elevated serum levels of creatinine and severe metabolic acidosis are common in severe cases [144,291,311]. The serum level of uric acid often is elevated out of proportion to the impairment of renal function but this is considered a variable and not distinguishing finding [291]. Serum levels of bilirubin may be normal on presentation but rise with delayed delivery [189]. Serum AST is elevated between three and 10 times upper normal limits [144,291,311]. The association of a modest rise in serum AST and disproportionate elevations in serum alkaline phosphatase and uric acid are no longer considered discriminative for AFLP. Markedly elevated levels of serum AST (>1000 IU/l) are found with shock, hepatic ischaemia and profound hypoglycaemia [311]. Some milder cases exhibited only minor elevations in serum alkaline phosphatase [291]. Profound hypoglycaemia is common and, if unrecognized, contributes significantly to mortality [291,311].

Morphological changes at post-mortem in severe cases are widespread. Fatty infiltration and haemorrhages occur in many organs especially the gastrointestinal tract, pancreas, kidney, brain and bone marrow [311,312,341]. The liver is small and grossly yellow from steatosis [312]. The distribution of fat and necrosis characteristically is panlobular with sparing of periportal areas (Figs 9.1 & 9.2). Microvesicular steatosis commonly is accompanied by intrahepatic cholestasis with canalicular plugs of bile and an acute cholangiolitis. There may be extramedullary haemopoiesis and hyperplastic collections of Kupffer cells [312]. The differential diagnosis from other causes of jaundice and encephalopathy, especially in the third trimester (see viral hepatitis, acute liver failure below), is wide (see Box 9.1). Diagnosis has become more difficult with inclusion of more mild cases of AFLP with overlapping features. The main differential diagnosis is between other causes of acute liver failure such as viral hepatitis and drug hepatotoxicity, severe pre-eclamptic toxaemia and alcoholic hepatitis [80,312]. Serological markers will distinguish viral causes such as hepatitis A, B (not C necessarily: see viral hepatitis below), D, E and the herpes group. Distinction from hepatitis due to viruses and alcohol may be impossible, especially in mild AFLP. Several histological features overlap and cytoplasmic ballooning can mask the characteristic microvesicular steatosis [312]. Other con-

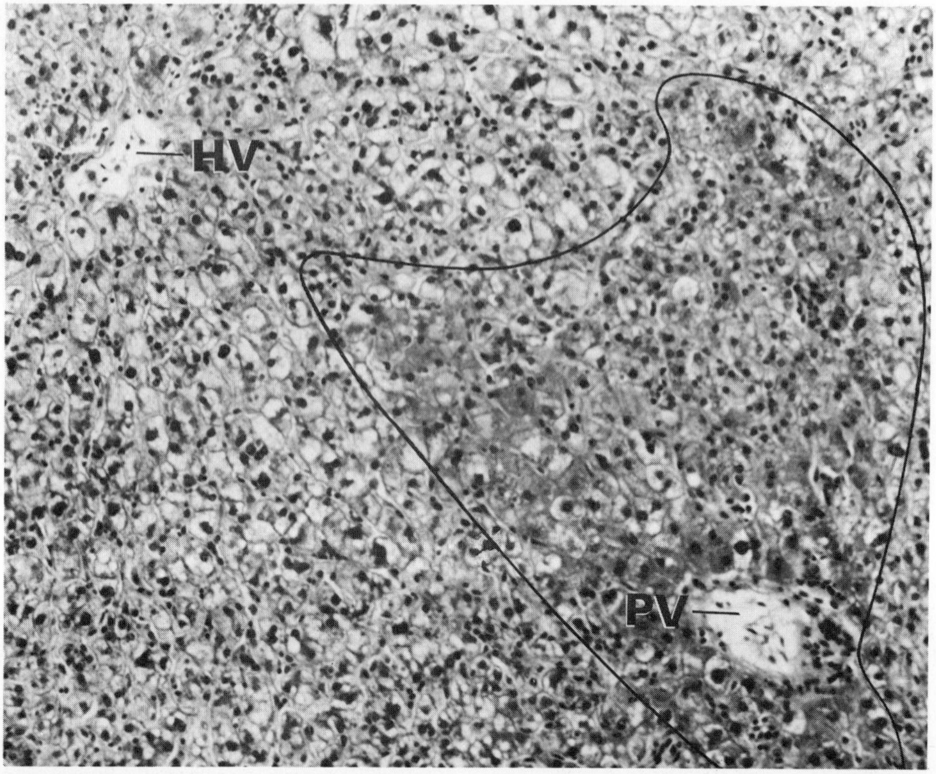

Fig. 9.1. Acute fatty liver of pregnancy (H&E, × 150) showing typical sparing of periportal area (ringed). HV hepatic vein; PV, portal vein.

fusing clinical conditions include a constellation of disorders such as haemolytic uraemic syndrome (HUS), thrombocytopenic purpura and the HELLP syndromes. Thrombotic thrombocytopenic purpura and HUS are considered a spectrum of overlapping disorders with microhaemangiopathic haemolytic anaemia, thrombocytopenia, renal failure and neurological disturbance [80]. Common associations are with DIC and sepsis [44,80,222]. The degree of liver dysfunction is minor in these predominantly haematological conditions and elevations in levels of serum biochemistry such as the AST and bilirubin reflect haemolysis rather than abnormal liver function. Differential diagnosis of AFLP from the HELLP syndromes and toxaemia may only be possible using immunofluorescent techniques on liver histology [312].

No specific diagnostic features are found on clinical examination. AFLP should be considered in any pregnant woman presenting with one or more of the following: epigastric pain, symptoms suggestive of reflux oesophagitis, nausea, vomiting, jaundice and a bleeding diathesis even in the absence of hepatic encephalopathy [49]. Backache may indicate underlying pancreatitis. The differential diagnosis of DIC in emergency obstetric practice is wide. In abruptio placentae, intrauterine death, amniotic fluid embolism, toxaemia and sepsis the haematological disorder usually is manifest before the onset of liver failure [222].

Microvesicular steatosis has been described in other conditions which usually do not occur in pregnancy such as alcoholic hepatitis and hepatotoxicity due to tetracycline, sodium valproate and salicylates, vomiting disease of Jamaica, yellow fever, Reye's syndrome in children, Wolman's disease and deficiencies of congenital urea cycle enzymes with fatty acid oxidation. Abnormalities

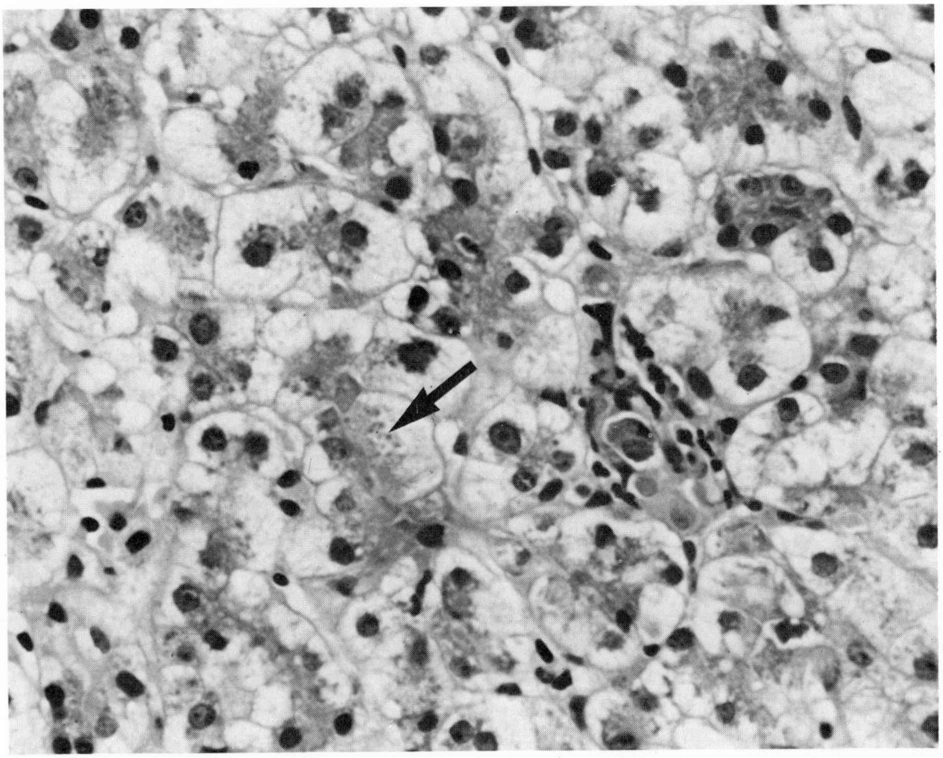

Fig. 9.2. Acute fatty liver of pregnancy (H&E, × 600) showing perinuclear microvesicular steatosis (arrowed).

in neutral triglycerides and fatty acid oxidation have been implicated in AFLP [321] as well as some of these other disorders [312].

The aetiology of AFLP and related disorders remains obscure. Possible predisposing factors have included toxins, viruses and pre-eclampsia [189]. Pyelonephritis and urinary tract infection have been found in up to 25 per cent of reports [144,214] and respiratory tract infection is common [144]. Histopathological similarities are seen with jejuno-ileal bypass and protein malnutrition [148] but most cases recently have been well nourished [144]. Depression of protein synthesis by tetracyclines may have accounted for some of the early reports especially those presenting before the 28th week [144]. Discrimination from idiopathic AFLP is usually possible on histological criteria [312]. The chemical syndrome and liver histology of AFLP is very similar to that of Reye's syndrome in children [312]. Transient deficiency of ornithine transcarbamylase and carbamyl synthetase has been described in both conditions [385] but their significance remains obscure and the findings on electron microscopy are different [189,312]. Abnormal predisposition to development of AFLP has been suggested by the finding of an elevated serum cholinesterase activity in a subsequent pregnancy in one case report of a survivor of AFLP 18 months previously [338]. Serum cholinesterase levels show a progressive fall in normal pregnancy suggesting altered metabolism of lipid in AFLP [317].

No consistent abnormalities have been found on examination of a limited number of fetal livers and placentae [49].

OVERLAP WITH PREGNANCY-INDUCED HYPERTENSION AND HELLP

Pre-eclampsia is present in 30–100 per cent of AFLP [49,317]. HELLP and AFLP present typically in the third trimester with non-specific symptoms and the haematological and histological features overlap [49,153,291]. In a detailed study from Japan using oil red O on frozen liver sections, microvesicular fat was detected in all 41 women presenting with pre-eclampsia, including those with normal liver function tests [256]. Importantly, fat may be overlooked with conventional histopathological stains. Electron microscopic examination is sensitive for detecting non-membrane-bound fat in the hepatocytes and the abnormally large needle-shaped mitochondria containing large crystalline inclusions. The risk of perinatal mortality rises with the quantity of fat, elevation in serum level of uric acid and reduction in platelet count.

Neonatal abnormalities are less common with severe AFLP than HELLP. Widespread fatty infiltration in the offspring has been reported after several months of age in isolated cases [321]. Whether these families represent distinct recessive genetic errors of fatty metabolism, requires further study (see below).

Ultrasonographic findings of increased reflectivity are consistent with fat — CT and MRI may show low attenuation. These tests are safe in pregnancy. A single 'slice' over the liver using modern CT equipment exposes the fetus to less irradiation than a conventional plain abdominal radiograph [250]. Overall, these tests are insensitive. A negative result does not exclude AFLP and related conditions. Liver histology may help occasionally to time delivery for mild disease and an immature fetus. Percutaneous sampling often is precluded by abnormal coagulation. The transjugular route can be successful in expert hands. Maternal and fetal outcome depend on clinical assessment of disease severity (see below) and not the AST levels.

Management principles

Optimal management for hypertension and liver dysfunction involves early discussion and transferral to a tertiary referral centre with intensive care facilities for managing hepatological, haematological and obstetric emergencies. Emphasis is on early diagnosis aided by improvements in radiological imaging techniques and intensive treatment of complications such as profound hypoglycaemia, gastrointestinal haemorrhage, pancreatitis and sepsis [291,384]. The paediatric department needs facilities for dealing with small-for-dates, pre-term babies, fetal hypoxia and profound hypoglycaemia [169]. Impaired hepatic synthetic function, neonatal thrombocytopenia, neutropenia and hypoprothrombinaemia unrelated to vitamin K and hypoalbuminaemia, have been reported in newborns when there was maternal hypertension. Calcium supplements may be necessary following maternal pancreatitis and additional vitamin K_1 to prevent excess bleeding.

General measures include bed rest, strict control and frequent monitoring of arterial blood pressure, blood sugar, coagulation status and acid–base balance. The hypoglycaemia may be profound and protracted for many days following delivery, accounting for the continued deterioration in conscious level [75]. A large centrally placed venous catheter is essential for delivery of large amounts of glucose and monitoring of glucose levels. Fluid balance should be controlled with a Swan–Ganz catheter. Low levels of glucose and calcium may be aggravated by pancreatitis. Some authors have recommended reduction in intake of dietary cholesterol as prophylaxis against development of AFLP which is commonly associated with hyperlipidaemia [255] but this remains unproven. Correction of bleeding tendencies with fresh frozen plasma, clotting factor concentrates, vitamin K_1 therapy or fresh whole blood has improved the prognosis in severe cases [169,291]. Some authorities have advocated correction of the deficiency of antithrombin III using fresh plasma and/or antithrombin III concentrate [231]. Others have stressed correction of hypovolaemia and oligohydramnios with plasma [130]. The consumption coagulopathy may continue and be exacerbated following delivery [291] so life-threatening post-partum haemorrhage is not uncommon [49].

Replacement of clotting factors with fresh frozen plasma and factor concentrates and platelets may be necessary. For caesarean section and vaginal delivery, platelet transfusions should be given for counts $<30 \times 10^9$/l. Plasma exchange [244] and antithrombotic agents [338], including infusions of prostaglandin derivatives and inhibitors of thromboxane synthetase, have shown benefit in isolated severe cases of HELLP syndrome [244] but these treatments have not yet been fully evaluated.

Correction of hypertension should be followed by delivery by caesarean section for presentations beyond the 34th week. Spontaneous vaginal delivery is possible in exceptional mild cases but close monitoring is essential to anticipate further impairment of liver function.

General and epidural anaesthesia should be carried out by an experienced anaesthetist. Epidural anaesthesia should be avoided with coagulopathy. The catheter should be removed as soon as possible after delivery. The nadir in the platelet count occurs typically 24–72 hours post-partum and may precipitate haemorrhage.

It is argued whether early delivery really does lead to improved prognosis for mother and child [291,292]. In one series of 12 patients with AFLP, the eight survivors had proceeded to immediate delivery via induced labour or caesarean section [49]. However, two of the four maternal deaths occurred in the induced pregnancies [49]. In addition several survivors, albeit more recently, have proceeded to term with spontaneous vaginal delivery of a live fetus in up to 70 per cent of cases [291]. Many of the cases reported after 1980 have been mild and based on clinical but not haematological criteria [34,291,292]. Nevertheless, the striking improvement in liver function and conscious status achieved with rapid delivery and the absence of spontaneous recovery of a proven case of AFLP prior to delivery argue strongly for induction of labour and delivery by caesarean section in the severe case (Table 9.2).

Maternal recovery is rapid following delivery but intensive care facilities should be available. The risk of liver rupture and infarction, hypoglycaemia, pancreatitis and pseudocyst formation, and neurological complications continues post-partum. Liver transplantation for severe AFLP has been successful, including post-partum [11].

Subsequent normal pregnancies have been reported for survivors of HELLP, AFLP and liver rupture. There are isolated reports of histologically proven recurrent AFLP and of HELLP in a successive pregnancy. A maternal defect in oxidation of long chain fatty acids was demonstrated in one woman with AFLP occurring in successive pregnancies. Both infants died within the first year and autopsy revealed widespread fatty infiltration of their livers [321].

Advice given to survivors of AFLP who desire a further pregnancy must be optimistic but recurrences may be more common than realized. Some multiparous patients presenting with AFLP have documented hypertension in a preceding pregnancy.

Intrahepatic cholestasis of pregnancy (IHCP)

IHCP is second only to viral hepatitis as a cause of jaundice in pregnancy and accounts for up to 20 per cent of cases [312] in some countries. IHCP is the most common condition perculiar to pregnancy. Geographical variation in incidence is wide. IHCP has been reported in up to 2 per cent of deliveries [31,302,333] in Scandinavia [31,217], Mediterranean countries [29], Poland [314], Chile, [305,306], Canada [333], Australia [349] and China [302]. The suggestion that the incidence of IHCP is falling [31,305] is offset by the recent publications of mild cases [31,199].

The original description of generalized pruritus, mild jaundice and intrahepatic cholestasis occurring predominantly in the third trimester was attributed to Thorling [370], but was described 100 years before [6]. Svanborg [358] described seven women with similar features. He noted fatigue, mild abdominal pain and subsidence after delivery with recurrence in some in subsequent pregnancies. Today, the classical and dominant feature is generalized pruritus. Itching develops characteristically after the 30th week and becomes progressively severe but typically is relieved within 48 hours following delivery [31,143,302,333]. In some, no further symptoms will develop — 'pruritus gravidarum' (see Chapter 19). More typically, jaundice develops 2–4 weeks after the debut of pruritus and resolves rapidly post-partum. Nocturnal itching of trunk, palms and soles can be severe with insomnia and fatigue. Anorexia, malaise, epigastric discomfort, steatorrhoea and dark urine are common. Cases have been reported with pruritus commencing as early as the sixth week [31,302,333]. The frequency with which pruritus develops increases rapidly after the third month through to term [31]. For reasons which remain unclear, the onset of pruritus is distinctly uncommon in the seventh month [31,370]. Occasionally, clearance of jaundice has been delayed for up to 2 months post-partum [258,302]. The predominantly conjugated hyperbilirubinaemia (total serum bilirubin <100 μmol/l) is mild and serum levels of AST, alanine aminotransferase (ALT) and alkaline phosphatase [31,143,302,333] rarely exceed two times upper limits of normal [258]. Elevation in prothrombin ratio relates usually to vitamin K deficiency and is rapidly corrected by replacement therapy. Mild right upper quadrant pain is present in a minority. Any marked pain, hepatomegaly, splenomegaly or other findings should prompt exclusion of other causes of pruritus and jaundice, especially the cholestatic phase of viral hepatitis and gallstones. The increased risk of gallstones in IHCP probably relates to the combined presence of lithogenic factors such as the increased gallbladder volume, reduced ejection fraction of bile and rise in serum bile acids [202].

IHCP probably arises from a genetic predisposition and increased sensitivity to sex steroids with altered membrane composition of bile ducts and hepatocytes. Seasonal variation, with more cases reported in the winter in some Scandinavian countries [31], points to an additional environmental factor. A positive family history is found in up to half of the patients [31,302,305,333] in association with the histocompatibility antigen haplotypes HLA-B8 and HLA-BW16. This genetic predisposition favours transmission as an autosomal dominant trait and fathers transmit the susceptibility to daughters [167].

A central theory is suggested for the pruritus and increased availability of brain opiate receptors for binding their agonist ligands in cholestasis [183]. Intrahepatic cholestasis has recurred with menstruation [209], with oral contraceptive therapy and at the menopause [93,180,209,283,286,380] and severe cases may be associated with multiple pregnancies [217]. Measurement of oestrogenic components show conflicting results [5,31,152a,217,371, 372]. Progestogens may play a synergistic role [290].

Numerous biochemical abnormalities have been reported in maternal serum including elevated levels of copper [293,294].

Reversal of the cholestasis and abolition of pruritus has been described after high dose S-adenosyl-L-methionine pointing to an underlying metabolic defect and susceptibility [115,382]. Serum levels of cholic acid, chenodeoxycholic acid and total 3α-hydroxy bile acids are elevated from 10- to 100-fold in patients with IHCP compared to healthy matched pregnant contols [31,217,294,333,371]. In general, serum levels of bile acids correlate with severity of maternal pruritus and increased risk of fetal distress [31,217,333] which is a feature of IHCP.

Management principles

All women with suspected IHCP should be screened for viral markers of hepatitis (see below) since presentation in the cholestatic phase of hepatitis is common. Autoimmune diseases should be sought by screening for autoantibodies, especially for antimitochondrial antibodies (see below). Hepatic ultrasonography should be carried out and repeated to exclude extrahepatic cholestasis including gallstones and cholangiocarcinoma (see below). Percutaneous liver biopsy, always under ultrasonographic guidance, may be indicated in atypical cases to exclude other causes of intrahepatic cholestasis such as drug hepatotoxicity and the Dubin–Johnson syndrome (see below). Clinical anatomical relationships may have altered, especially in the third trimester and there is a risk of puncturing the exceptionally large gallbladder in IHCP [202]. Histological confirmation of an acinar cholestasis with bile plugs in the canaliculi may be useful when jaundice occurs without pruritus, symptoms commence before the 20th week and serum levels of bilirubin remain high 8 weeks or more after delivery [258]. Hepatocellular necrosis and an inflammatory cell infiltrate, typical of hepatitis, are absent in IHCP [312].

Premature labour has been reported in up to 59 per cent of cases. Fetal distress and meconium staining are common [302,304,333,399] especially with severe cholestasis [302,304,399]. Intrauterine death and still-birth have been reported even in clinically mild IHCP [217,333]. Some studies have reported more optimistic findings with no increase in number of pre-term deliveries [31] or an increase in pre-term labour but with less fetal loss [182]. These discordant findings relate probably to inclusion of mild cases in reported series [31].

Close monitoring of fetal well-being is essential in all cases of IHCP although it is not clear which parameter predicts accurately the risk of intrauterine death. As the risks of intrauterine death and fetal distress seem to increase near to term, provision should be made for early delivery and for changes on fetal cardiotocography indicating fetal distress [217]. Vitamin K therapy should be administered immediately post-partum to the baby to prevent intracranial bleeding, especially if the mother has been receiving cholestyramine for pruritus [230]. Rising maternal serum bile acids may indicate cases at increased risk of fetal complications [31,202,217,333,371].

The mother with IHCP should be reassured of the generally good outlook. Itching and jaundice will usually resolve immediately following delivery but may recur in subsequent pregnancies. In one study of 27 multiparous women with IHCP, 15 experienced pruritus or jaundice in one subsequent pregnancy and three in more than one pregnancy. The remaining nine were not affected in later pregnancies [117]. The recurrence rate was 40 and 45.4 per cent in subsequent pregnancies in China [302] and Canada [333] and included two successive fetal losses for one patient [302]. Women with a history of IHCP should be warned that symptoms can recur on oral contraceptive therapy.

Treatment for pruritus with cholestyramine up to 20 g/day and phenobarbitone has been disappointing [333]. Cholestyramine, overall seems to be safe in pregnancy [230]. This non-absorbable anion-exchange resin binds bile acids, anionic drugs and fat soluble vitamins. Binding of vitamin K may result in elevations in prothrombin ratio. Post-partum haemorrhage has been reported in 8–22 per cent of cases following delivery [302,333] and may be exacerbated by vitamin K deficiency. Vitamin K_1 should be administered regularly to women with IHCP throughout pregnancy, especially those receiving cholestyramine. Results from controlled trials of intravenous *S*-adenosyl-L-methionine (800 mg daily) have shown variable relief of pruritus with lessening of jaundice. This agent seems non-toxic to the fetus.

Liver diseases incidental to pregnancy

Viral hepatitis A to E

Viral hepatitis remains the most common cause of jaundice in pregnancy. General reviews have been published concerning the non-pregnant patient [164,415]. The main hepatotropic agents likely to be seen in pregnancy are listed in Table 9.3.

Clinical and epidemiological features overlap. Diagnosis relies on detection of specific serological markers of acute and chronic infection. Presentation typically is delayed until the cholestatic phase with pruritus, jaundice and steatorrhoea. The main differential diagnosis is from other causes of cholestasis such as alcoholic hepatitis, biliary obstruction, intrahepatic cholestasis of pregnancy (see above), drugs and autoimmune liver diseases (see below). In addition viral infections may be detected during pregnancy as a result of screening, such as for hepatitis B, or because of reactivation, such as in the herpes viruses.

Areas of concern in obstetric practice are the adverse effects on the pregnant woman and her fetus including the risks of transmission to the newborn infant.

Despite numerous studies spanning more than 30 years, there is still uncertainty concerning the effects of viral hepatitis in pregnancy and conclusions must be drawn with caution. Many reports suggesting viral hepatitis pursued a more severe course in pregnancy [40,124] pre-dated discriminative testing. Most later reports [8,378,379] from developing countries have highlighted severe cases. Acute viral hepatitis in an adult in a high prevalence country such as India is more likely to be due to hepatitis type E or B than A. There is widespread exposure to hepatitis A in childhood and subsequent long-term immunity. In contrast, studies from Europe [370], the USA [161] and Zagreb [288] suggest no overall increase in severity but detail is lacking.

In developing countries malnutrition, poor socio-economic conditions and suboptimal obstetric care may combine significantly to contribute to the unusually severe outcome of hepatitis but information is conflicting. Data from Israel [331] support these conclusions. Studies before 1960 [289],

Table 9.3. Serological diagnosis of acute viral hepatitis

Name	Antibodies	Other markers
Hepatitis A	IgM antihepatitis A virus (HAV)	Nil
Hepatitis B	IgM antihepatitis B core antigen (HBc)	Hepatitis B virus DNA clearance
Hepatitis C	Core region*	Hepatitis C virus RNA clearance*
Hepatitis D	IgM anti-HDV	Hepatitis B virus DNA clearance (hepatitis D virus can interfere with B) Hepatitis D virus RNA clearance
Hepatitis E	IgM-anti-hepatitis E virus*	Hepatitis E virus RNA clearance IgG antibodies*
Herpes viruses (simplex, zoster, cytomegalovirus Epstein–Barr)	IgM antibodies	Paired sera, cultures, liver inclusions and *in situ* hybridization
Exotic viruses	Panels	Cytopathic effects in cell culture

* Under evaluation.

coinciding with poor socioeconomic conditions, reported an increased severity of hepatitis in pregnant, compared with non-pregnant, women. In contrast, between 1967 and 1977, which marked rising socioeconomic progress, severity was similar [331]. A comparable study from Saudi Arabia [124] spanned more than 20 years and included a prospective period (1963–75) of rising socioeconomic growth. This showed a fall in mortality from 70.8 per cent (1953–62) to 14.3 per cent (1963–75) amongst pregnant women with viral hepatitis. The mortality amongst non-pregnant women fell similarly; 26.7 per cent to 5.6 per cent for the two respective time periods [124] indicating a high relative risk of death (approximately 4 : 1) for pregnancy. Maternal and fetal outcome may depend more on improvements in medical care than a reduction in severity of hepatitis in pregnancy. Whether malnutrition affects outcome also remains controversial. Prospective studies from India for non-A, non-B hepatitis [198] and Libya for unspecified varieties of predominantly non-B viral hepatitis [59] have shown either a persistence of high attack rate and mortality in pregnancy despite adequate nutrition or a similar outcome for non-A, non-B hepatitis despite malnutrition [340]. Other factors suggested as contributary to the adverse outcome of acute viral hepatitis in pregnancy have included hormonal changes [40] which may impair cellular immunity [378] but proof is lacking. Furthermore, evidence has accumulated that enhanced, rather than impaired, cellular immunity may play a role in the development of severe, including fulminant, viral hepatitis B. The suggestion that an enhanced coagulopathy may contribute to the excess mortality in pregnant women [124], does not take into account the common observation of the severely deranged coagulation status seen in all varieties of acute liver failure regardless of pregnancy [239,285]. Evidence from one large surveillance programme in Boston [270] indicated that viral hepatitis occurred more frequently in women using oral contraceptive therapy. Therefore some authorities recommend discontinuation of combined therapy until normalization of liver serum biochemistry [294]. Others concluded that oral contraceptive therapy has no adverse effect on acute viral hepatitis [325] and chronic liver disease [179] but modern data relating to the individual viral agents are lacking.

Avoidance of sexual contact as a major route of transmission of many of the hepatotropic agents, is important in limiting spread. Age and parity have no overriding effect on maternal and fetal outcome [161,331]. Most, although not all [370], studies have shown an increase in rate of intrauterine death and still-births [8,124,251,340] and prematurity [8,161, 251,331,340]. No excess in incidence of congenital abnormalities has been reported in retrospective [161,246] and prospective [90,330] studies.

The majority of studies relating severity of hepatitis to maternal and fetal outcome have come from regions such as India and North Africa where there are severe epidemics of hepatitis E reported among pregnant women. More research is needed to assess maternal and fetal outcome in relation to influence of individual virus type. Variables to be considered are geographical region, socioeconomic status, nutrition, duration of immunity and temporal changes in prevalence of viral hepatitis within a given community.

Hepatitis A

Hepatitis A virus is an enteric RNA-containing virus spread predominantly by ingesting water contaminated with sewage (faeco-oral route) [227]. The prevalence of previous infection, determined by detecting IgG-antihepatitis A antibodies, relates inversely to standards of sanitation. Almost universal exposure occurs in infancy and childhood in the developing countries especially in Asia and the East, Africa, India, certain Mediterranean countries and South America. In contrast, infections among children and young adults in northern Europe, including the UK and the USA have fallen in response to improved standards of hygiene [116]. In low prevalence countries, the infection typically shows seasonal variation. The peak in autumn and early winter usually indicates virus imported from a higher prevalence area. Hepatitis A virus has a short incubation of approximately 4 weeks (range 14–50 days). Discrimination from other viruses based on incubation periods and clinical features can be misleading. Presenting symptoms often are abrupt but non-specific with a flu-like illness, headache, fatigue, nausea, anorexia, vomiting and diarrhoea. Cholestatic jaundice with pale stools, dark urine and pruritus usually follows within days of the prodrome and is a common mode of presentation. Differentiation from other causes of jaundice may be difficult. Alcoholic hepatitis, biliary obstruction and intrahepatic cholestasis and chronic liver diseases such as primary biliary cirrhosis may present in pregnancy. Diagnosis of acute infection relies on the detection of IgM antihepatitis A antibodies in serum (see Table 9.3). In pregnancy, testing is mandatory to make a diagnosis and exclude other causes. Testing for IgG antihepatitis A is useful to demonstrate immunity in patients exposed to an index case and prior to travel abroad.

Management of hepatitis A is similar regardless of pregnancy. Hepatitis A and other causes of viral hepatitis occur more frequently as pregnancy progresses with a peak onset in the third trimester [161,288]. Whether symptoms and jaundice are more likely than in anicteric cases, remains uncertain and may reflect the bias of reporting severe cases. In one prospective study [288] only 28.5 per cent of cases were anicteric compared to 77.7 per cent for non-A, non-B and 4.5 per cent for hepatitis B.

Hepatitis A is a self-limiting illness noted for its complete recovery. A chronic carrier state is not recognized in humans. Occasionally, recovery may be delayed with protracted cholestasis and a biphasic course. Acute liver failure is rare [285] and not especially common in pregnancy (in contrast to herpes hepatitis, see below).

Little information exists regarding risks of transmission to the newborn. Only one of six infants born to women who developed hepatitis A (one in the second and five in the third trimester) showed a minor and transient elevation in serum aminotransferase [375]. Two further developed detectable antihepatitis A antibodies. Pre-term delivery has been documented in several early studies of acute viral hepatitis in late pregnancy [161,370]. These predated discriminative diagnosis on serological testing but undoubtedly included hepatitis A. In a prospective study from Zagreb [288], of 43 pregnant women with serologically defined acute uncomplicated viral hepatitis (A: 18.4 per cent; B: 57.9 per cent; non-A, non-B: 23.7 per cent), pre-term delivery occurred in 27 per cent but there was no direct information for the eight with hepatitis A. There is no increased risk of spontaneous abortion, still-birth, intrauterine growth retardation or congenital abnormalities following hepatitis A in pregnancy [161,288] although large specific surveys are lacking.

PROTECTION AND IMMUNOPROPHYLAXIS

Hepatitis A is most infectious in the pre-symptomatic phase prior to jaundice and early symptomatic phase when the virus is excreted in the stool. Poor personal hygiene and sanitation favour epidemics. Exposure to the virus is almost universal in promiscuous subjects, especially with oro-anal intercourse [105]. The risk of transmission rapidly wanes with development of symptoms and jaundice. Hepatitis A virus is resistant to several chlorinated disinfectants which ordinarily destroy bacteria and survives heating to 60°C for 30 min. The virus is destroyed by boiling (100°C) for 1 min and autoclaving [298].

Immunoglobulin contains antibodies to hepatitis A (and also hepatitis B; see below) and has been used as effective passive immunoprophylaxis for more than 40 years [262,264]. Intramuscular immunoglobulin is safe if prepared to standards agreed by the World Health Organization and when given intramuscularly [262,264]. A single dose of 0.02 ml/kg given by deep intramuscular injection immediately following an exposure, gives a protective efficacy rate of around 80 per cent in the short term. Immunoglobulin can protect or attenuate the illness if given up to 2 weeks following exposure (in contrast to hepatitis B). This is surprising for a virus with an average incubation of 4 weeks. Immunoglobulin is recommended following close and sexual contacts with an index case and during an epidemic. Day-care centres for infants and institutions for custodial care are important settings for transmission. Immediate contacts of an index case should receive immunoprophylaxis [262,264].

Post-exposure immunoprophylaxis may not prevent virus shedding in the stool. Isolation of potentially infectious subjects is important in limiting spread in epidemics. No specific recommendations have been drawn for immunoglobulin during pregnancy. The outcome of hepatitis A to mother and child seems to be similar to that of the non-pregnant population [288,375] but large-scale documentation is lacking. Immunoglobulin should be given to symptomless women in contact with an index case during the third trimester in view of the increased rate of pre-term deliveries [288]. Pregnant women about to travel to high prevalence areas should be considered for prophylaxis with immunoglobulin. Travellers should be prescreened for IgG antihepatitis A antibodies to prevent unnecessary immunization of at least one-third who will be found to be immune [63].

Faecal contamination during delivery is a potential source for transmission to the newborn. In practice, transmission is rare owing to the limited interval for faecal excretion. Neonatal hepatitis A should be considered if the mother develops features of infection in the puerperium or has been given immunoglobulin which may prolong the period of faecal excretion. Neonatal immunoprophylaxis is rarely necessary. Most neonatal infections are mild and life-long immunity follows recovery.

In 1992 in Europe at least one inactivated, whole-virus hepatitis A vaccine was licensed for parenteral administration. No information is available for pregnancy but early data are encouraging on safety and immunogenicity in the non-pregnant population.

Hepatitis E

A distinct variety of epidemic, predominantly water-borne, non-A, non B hepatitis was described in several cities in India between 1955 and 1982 [9,108]. Similar epidemics were reported in South East Asia including Nepal and Burma (1973–77), in Rangoon (1982–85), north Africa [27,281] and the central Asian area of the Commonwealth of Independent States. All outbreaks resembled hepatitis A with a short incubation period, faeco-oral mode of spread and lack of chronic sequelae. Unlike hepatitis A, the incubation period was longer (about 40 days) and the attack rate was highest in young adults in countries known to be endemic for hepatitis A in childhood, suggesting limited immunity. Furthermore, secondary (horizontal) spread was uncommon and there was an excess severity and mortality in pregnancy [9,108,198]. Subsequently, hepatitis E virus has been identified by electron microscopy in stools derived from these epidemics. Cloning of the RNA genome has shown some homology to caliciviruses.

In the study from Kashmir [198] acute liver failure was reported in 22.2 per cent of pregnant, compared with <3 per cent of non-pregnant women. The hepatitis was more frequent and severe in late pregnancy; 8.8 per cent developed hepatitis in the first trimester. This rose to approximately 19 per cent in the second and third trimesters. Maternal deaths (44.4 per cent) only occurred in late pregnancy [198]. In Rangoon, of 399 cases of hepatitis, the case/fatality rate amongst pregnant women was up to 12 times that for non-pregnant females and males for non-A, non-B but not hepatitis B [272]. In the Rangoon study [272] there was a sixfold excess risk of household contacts developing non-A, non-B hepatitis suggesting person-to-person contact via faeco-oral spread.

Whether the severe outcome in pregnancy in developing countries reflects virus virulence, variants or host factors, especially malnutrition, remains inconclusive. Epidemic forms of non-A, non-B hepatitis from Japan [408] showed no special adverse outcome in pregnancy. Further atypical features included the longer than usual incubation period (up to 5 months), general lack of severe symptoms and failure to implicate contaminated water supplies. These features are prominent in the majority of epidemics with an adverse outcome amongst pregnant women [188,198,272,281].

Hepatitis E has not been reported within the UK except in travellers returning from areas of high prevalence such as the Indian subcontinent, the Commonwealth of Independent States, Nepal, Burma, Africa and Mexico. Antibody immunoassays are available in some reference centres and can discriminate acute infection (IgM isotype) from previous exposure (IgG isotype) (see Table 9.3).

Management of a pregnant woman with suspected hepatitis E does not differ from her non-pregnant counterpart. This is optimal in a centre with expertise in maternal and fetal intensive care, hepatology and infectious diseases. Secondary spread to contacts is uncommon but handling of faeces and bile should be minimized by washing hands thoroughly and the disposal of contaminated clothes and fomites by autoclaving and incineration. There are no forms of immunoprophylaxis. Pregnant personnel are best advised to avoid contact with cases of suspected hepatitis E.

Hepatitis C

Hepatitis C virus, an RNA-containing virus related to the pestiviruses and flaviviruses, is a major cause of parenterally transmitted (post-transfusion non-A, non-B) hepatitis. Cloning of part of the virus genome was published in 1989 alongside development of an antibody test [58,215]. Since 1990, all blood donors in Europe and the USA have been tested routinely for antibodies. Diagnosis depends first on detection of antibodies to a panel of recombinant (cDNA) antigens, synthetic peptides (sp) and glycoproteins (gp) representing the more conserved regions of the virus genome [102,103]. Second generation antibody tests (recombinant immunoblot and enzyme linked immunosorbent assays) show improved sensitivity and specificity over first generation tests. Diagnosis of acute infection can be overlooked; seroconversion can be delayed many weeks and discrimination from chronic infection is difficult. Results correlate well with detection of hepatitis C virus RNA using the polymerase chain reaction (PCR) technique. This detects viraemia by amplifying as little as one of virus particle. Unfortunately, the PCR is labour intensive, expensive and difficult to adapt for routine testing [102].

Hepatitis C is common amongst intravenous drug users, multiply transfused individuals and human immunodeficiency virus (HIV) seropositive subjects. Hepatitis C virus is a major cause of sporadic (community acquired) hepatitis. In the USA the estimated annual incidence of new infections is between 150 000 and 170 000 [265]. Chronic hepatitis and cirrhosis commonly follow acute infection. Primary liver cancer associated with cirrhosis is common especially in Japan. Vertical and sexual transmission are less frequent than for hepatitis B [237]. The risk of transmission to the neonate depends on the trimester at exposure. No perinatal transmission has been shown after acute maternal infection in the second trimester. Based on the few reported cases, chronic maternal infection or acute infection in the third trimester may result in neonatal infection in 45–87 per cent [237]. Selective screening of high risk patients is recommended. There are no specific recommendations against pregnancy for seropositive individuals and no special precautions for the pregnant woman or her fetus [265].

Trials of antiviral therapies, especially interferons, are underway. Normalization of serum AST levels is easier to achieve with lower doses and more rapid than for chronic hepatitis B. Interferons are contraindicated in pregnancy.

Hepatitis B

Hepatitis B is a global public health problem. Worldwide, at least 280 million individuals are chronically infected with the hepatitis B virus. This is a major cause of liver disease, including chronic hepatitis, cirrhosis and primary liver cancer. Hepatitis B is second only to tobacco as a global cause of cancer. Worldwide, primary liver cancer (hepatoma, hepatocellular carcinoma) is probably the most common cancer, at least in males. Hepatitis B has been implicated in over 80 per cent of cases [23]. The 750 000 deaths per annum from primary liver cancer are expected to continue rising with the increase in the population and a reduction in infant mortality.

In the West, the chronic carrier rate is between 0.5 and 5 per cent of the general population. In prospective studies from Sydney [47] and Montreal [83] the prevalence of HBsAg seropositivity amongst blood donors and pregnant women was 0.07 per cent [47] and 1.9 per cent [83]. HBsAg positivity amongst native Australian antenatal patients correlated with previous intravenous drug use, hepatitis, occupational exposure, blood transfusion, living in an institution, and birth in Indo-China [47] and Africa [83]. The Montreal questionnaire was completed by 30 315 pregnant women from nine hospitals between 1982 and 1984 [83]. Only about half of the seropositive Canadians declared a risk factor. Exposure to intravenous recreational drugs was sought only in the Australian study and found to be common.

In the USA, the reservoir of infectious carriers may be as high as 1 000 000 [265]. More than 300 000 Americans become infected annually. Up to 30 000 of these can be expected to become HBsAg seropositive chronic carriers. Each year, more than 4000 Americans die from related cirrhosis and 800 from primary liver cancer [168,265].

Transmission is mostly horizontal from person to person especially via intravenous drug use in young males and heterosexual contact in young females. Consecutive surveys from the Centers of Disease Control (CDC) [10] between 1981 and 1988 showed that the number of reports of acute hepatitis B attributed to parenteral drug use rose by 80 per cent and to heterosexual contact by 38 per cent. The peak prevalence was in individuals aged 15–29 years, compared with <1 per cent below 15 years and 26 per cent for those of 30–44 years.

The impact of hepatitis B in obstetric practice is greatly underestimated. Transmission typically goes unnoticed. Symptoms are uncommon and non-specific and disease becomes manifest only after many years. Three major, interrelated areas are of concern: (a) vertical transmission in neonates and horizontal transmission in early childhood; (b) the propensity of the newborn of an infected mother to become a chronic carrier and its consequences; and (c) the potential to eradicate hepatitis B via immunoprophylaxis.

ACUTE HEPATITIS B

Infection may remain symptomless and anicteric. Any symptoms are non-specific such as a 'flu-like' illness, malaise, anorexia, nausea and vomiting and occasionally arthralgia and a skin rash. Clinically, hepatitis B cannot be distinguished easily from hepatitis due to other viruses, drugs, alcohol and autoimmune diseases. Clinical recovery from uncomplicated infection may take several months. A biphasic illness with resurgence of serum levels of transaminase and bilirubin is seen more commonly than with hepatitis A. At the other end of the spectrum is progression to acute liver failure with a mortality of >50 per cent. Fortunately this is rare, especially in pregnancy [17,239], and accounts for <1 per cent of hospitalized cases of acute viral hepatitis [109].

There is no evidence that a pregnant woman with acute hepatitis B pursues a more severe course than her non-pregnant counterpart. As with other types of acute viral hepatitis, the frequency of pre-term delivery is increased when acute hepatitis B is contracted in the third trimester [161].

SEROLOGICAL RESPONSES

Hepatitis B virus is not cytopathic and clearance of virus depends on the host's immune attack (reviewed in [415]). Serological responses remain the cornerstone of diagnosis of acute (see Table 9.3) and chronic infection. Acute infection typically leads to the detection of HBsAg in blood 2–8 weeks before development of abnormal serum liver biochemistry and onset of symptoms. Serum HBsAg usually remains detectable until the convalescent phase. Hepatitis B 'e' antigen (HBeAg) becomes detectable soon after HBsAg. HBeAg is a marker of high infectivity and is closely associated with the inner core (HBcAg) and hepatitis B virus DNA. IgG antihepatitis B core antigen (IgG anti-HBc) is present in the serum of HBsAg positive chronic carrier mothers and may play an important role in immunomodulation of fetal serological responses to hepatitis B virus infection. In uncomplicated acute hepatitis B, recovery is associated with rapid clearance of serum hepatitis B virus DNA and detection of anticore antibodies (IgM and, soon after, IgG), shortly followed by antihepatitis B e antigen, with decline and disappearance of HBeAg and HBsAg antigenaemia within 3 months. The subsequent 'window' phase, defined by the serological presence of antihepatitis B core antigen in the absence of HBeAg and antihepatitis B surface antigen persists for 2–16 weeks. This phase terminates with detection of antihepatitis B surface antigen signalling recovery, viral clearance and immunity from future hepatitis B infection. The window phase probably is an artefact. HBsAg can be detected using monoclonal antibodies and hepatitis B virus DNA by PCR. Importantly, a pregnant woman who presents with acute hepatitis B, especially acute liver failure, may be misdiagnosed as having a non-B hepatitis if only HBsAg is sought using conventional polyclonal reagents. Serological testing for high titre IgM antihepatitis B core antigen (IgM anti-HBc) is mandatory for the diagnosis of acute infection. Additional infection with hepatitis delta virus can lead to an inhibition of the serological markers of hepatitis B (see Table 9.3 and below).

ROUTES OF TRANSMISSION

The predominant route in any given community has important implications for developing strategies for immunoprophylaxis.

Vertical transmission

Acute hepatitis B infection occurring in late pregnancy and around delivery [64,161,253,324] favours vertical transmission from mother to child before or peri-partum. In one study from California [375] the risk of vertical transmission for mothers with acute hepatitis B manifest during the first (0 per cent) and second trimesters (6 per cent) respectively was significantly less than that for the third trimester (67 per cent) and within 5 weeks post-partum (100 per cent).

Up to 40 per cent of all chronic carriers of hepatitis B virus arise following vertical transmission. Babies born of HBsAg positive mothers with serological evidence of virus replication — HBeAg and hepatitis B virus DNA [81] — have between a 20 and 95 per cent chance of becoming infected, depending on the maternal ethnic origin [104,138,174,176,352,405]. Ethnic origin, especially the Far East, is important even for mothers residing in low prevalence countries [43,47,89,352,405]. As part of a large scale controlled prospective study on the efficacy of the hepatitis B vaccine amongst babies born of HBeAg positive mothers in Taiwan, 95 per cent who received no immunoprophylaxis became infected acutely and 93 per cent became infected chronically by the sixth month of follow-up [25]. Studies from Hong Kong [404] showed a similar attack rate in unprotected infants.

Why vertical transmission from high risk carrier mothers is much less frequent in certain regions, particularly in Senegal and Kenya (approximately 20 per cent), than in the Far East, is not completely understood [243]. Ethnic differences may reflect maternal levels of hepatitis B virus DNA [138,152, 225] but this has been disputed [44]. Vertical transmission can occur in up to 25 per cent of cases where the HBsAg positive mother is HBeAg negative and in up to 12 per cent of cases where the mother is antihepatitis B e antigen positive [264, 267]. There was no correlation with maternal seropositivity for IgM antihepatitis B core antigen, an indirect measure of virus replication, in chronic carrier mothers and subsequent vertical transmission in Taiwan [174].

Until recently transmission was assumed to occur at or around the time of birth. Suggested mechanisms during delivery and post-partum have included mixing of maternal and fetal blood [224], contact with cervicovaginal epithelial cells shown to be positive for hepatitis B virus DNA and ingestion of amniotic fluid [224] and breast milk which are known to contain detectable HBsAg [42,233].

Up to recently it was believed that hepatitis B virus does not traverse the placenta. There is little serological evidence of infection in the newborn for acute hepatitis B before the third trimester [64,161,165,253,324]. In the infected neonate, serum HBsAg becomes detectable typically around 3 months implicating transmission around delivery. Specific high titre IgM antihepatitis B core antigen, an accurate predictor of recent infection, is absent in neonatal sera [135]. HBsAg, if present in cord blood, often is in low titre and reflects contamination with maternal blood during delivery. The most pursuasive argument against infection occurring *in utero* is the success of perinatal immunoprophylaxis [24,25,352,404] (see immunoprophylaxis below).

But evidence has accumulated in favour of infection *in utero* in some cases. Avoidance of breast feeding, delivery by caesarean section and immediate separation from the infectious mother do not prevent subsequent infection within the first 6 months. Transplacental transmission seems to be common at least in the Far East. Hepatitis B virus DNA was detected in 44 per cent of fetal livers from HBsAg seropositive Chinese mothers following abortion [366]. This route may explain failure to protect up to 15 per cent of neonates born of HBsAg positive mothers despite optimum administration of immunoprophylaxis post-partum [352,366]. Also, after administration at birth of hepatitis B immunoglobulin (HBIG) containing high titre antibodies against hepatitis B surface and core antigens, after their predicted falls in titre within 3 months (see below), levels of antihepatitis B surface antigen rise again in the majority of babies [25]. This pattern suggests passive–active immunity from exposure pre-dating immunoprophylaxis. In the HBsAg seropositive mother, maternal antihepatitis B core antibody traverses the placenta leading to immunomodulation of fetal responses to the virus. Maternal antihepatitis B core antibody can suppress expression of viral antigens (HBsAg, HBcAg) and replication in the fetus which only responds to hepatitis B virus associated antigens when levels of maternal antibodies fall, typically around 3–6 months of age. HBIG may prevent neonatal infection by protracting the time period of effective inhibitory antibody on virus replication until maturation of the fetal immune system occurs after the first 2 months of life. Thereafter, the baby can mount an effective immune response, clear hepatitis B virus and develop immunity (antihepatitis B surface and core antibodies) to future infection. In acute infection, HBcAg and HBsAg are expressed on the surface of infected hepatocytes. Maternal IgG antihepatitis B core antibodies may block recognition of virus-infected cells by cytotoxic T cells. Early exposure to soluble virus protein may induce a state of immune tolerance to virus antigen via induction of specific T suppressor cells which also serve to inhibit the host's cytotoxic attack. Also, maturation of the hepatocyte may be a pre-requisite before virus replication can occur.

Horizontal transmission

Person-to-person contact [280], especially in communal living conditions [41], is important in the West, the Mediterranean littoral [39], the Middle East, Saudi Arabia and parts of Africa including Kenya [138], Senegal [243], Namibia [41], Nigeria [361], Zambia [262], Liberia [296] and New Zealand and Pacific Islands [271]. Up to 60 per cent of neonates born of HBsAg seropositive mothers who seem to escape vertical transmission become infected within 5 years [242]. Other routes postulated but unproven include ritual scarification and blood-sucking vectors.

OUTCOME OF NEONATAL INFECTION

Factors other than maternal antihepatitis B core antigen influence the development of the chronic carrier state following neonatal infection. Development of a chronic carrier state correlates with the finding of high titre [24,25,405] HBsAg found in cord blood which probably relates to the presence of maternal hepatitis B virus DNA. Chronic carriage is uncommon in babies born following acute hepatitis B in the third trimester [125], and of carrier mothers with serological evidence of low levels of virus replication [113,337]. In the California study of acute hepatitis B in late pregnancy [375], HBsAg was detected in 12 of 18 (67 per cent) babies at 1–3 months of age but none became chronic carriers. In contrast, over 90 per cent of babies born to HBeAg positive chronically infected mothers eventually showed serological evidence of infection [23–25]. Furthermore, the vast majority will become chronic carriers — i.e. HBsAg positive for more than 6 months — into adult life [23–25]. This compares with only 1–10 per cent of otherwise healthy adults becoming chronic carriers (Fig. 9.3) [12] following transmission in adulthood.

Chronic carriage is common amongst children born of HBsAg positive carrier (HBeAg negative/antihepatitis B e antigen negative) mothers if exposure to infection is delayed beyond the first year [243]. In Senegal where horizontal transmission predominates, acquisition of hepatitis B infection is typically delayed beyond the first 5 months of life [243]. Out of 34 such babies who showed no serological evidence of infection until the second year, four of six eventually became chronic carriers; none developed acute liver failure [243].

Chronic infection is uncommon in babies born to HBsAg positive mothers with antihepatitis B e antigen [337] and mothers also seronegative for HBeAg. Instead, these babies are at risk of severe acute neonatal hepatitis, including progression to acute liver failure [26,84,101,339,374]. Survivors show serological evidence of clearance of virus and subsequent immunity (antihepatitis B surface antigen) to future infection [374].

All neonates born to HBsAg positive, HBeAg positive mothers who have HBeAg detected in uncontaminated cord blood are infected. Persistence of HBeAg beyond the second month also is predictive of chronic carriage. Conversely, a rapid reduction in titre of HBeAg after birth may predict subsequent clearance of virus and seroconversion to antihepatitis B surface antigen [176].

In adults as well as babies, chronicity tends to follow a mild anicteric illness [374]. The risk of developing the chronic carrier state in neonatal life and infancy is related to gender of the child and inversely to age at exposure (Fig. 9.3) [67]. Risk of chronicity does not depend on gestational age, birthweight and subtype of the virus [125]. In Senegal where horizontal transmission is important, 155 infants with serological evidence of infection (100 HBsAg, 55 antihepatitis B core antigen) were serially studied during a 7-year period [67]. Chronic carriage was observed in 68 per cent of those infected within the first year compared with 25 per cent between the first and second years and 6 per cent for years 3–7 respectively [67]. A gradation of risk of chronic carriage also was demonstrated within the first year; 82 per cent of those infected before 6 months compared with 54 per cent for infections between 6 and 12 months [67]. Males were more likely (87.5 per cent) to become carriers than females (55.2 per cent). This sex difference holds for infections acquired in adult life suggesting an inherent susceptibility to hepatitis B of the male or protective factors in the female.

For Senegal, there is no correlation between maternal HBsAg status and epidemiological factors

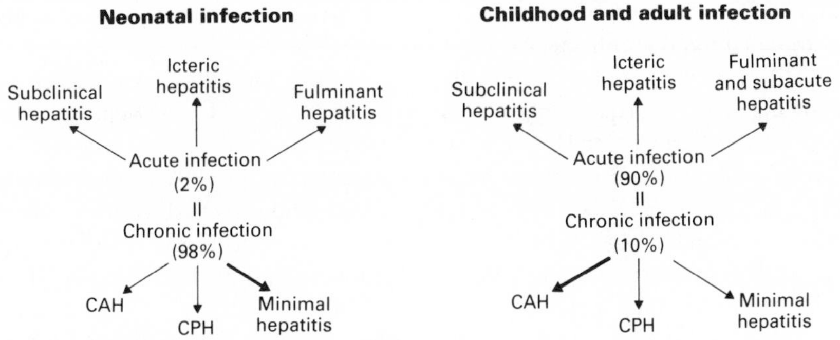

Fig. 9.3. Contrasting presentations and outcomes between neonatal and adult hepatitis B virus infection. CAH, chronic active hepatitis; CPH, chronic persistent hepatitis.

such as parity, age, tribal origin, previous blood transfusion and caesarean section [138]. Other horizontally acting factors must explain the vast excess over anticipated numbers of chronic carriers. Direct evidence is lacking but scarification rituals, blood-sucking vectors and close person-to-person contact may account for some of the spread. The risk of spread from an infected neonate to susceptible members of an adopted, new household can be significant [39] even after early cessation of contact with the original mother [280].

Evidence has been cited for [364] and against [166] perinatal transmission of virus, HBsAg antigenaemia and the subsequent development of immune complex-associated glomerulonephritis with membranous nephropathy reported in Japanese HBsAg positive children.

Also, at least one retrospective [161] and one prospective study [90] have failed to demonstrate any increase in congenital abnormalities, in particular Down's syndrome [213,353], following maternal acute and chronic hepatitis B virus infection.

THE CHRONIC CARRIER

At least half of long-term chronic carriers will die eventually from virus-related liver disease including chronic active hepatitis, cirrhosis and its complications (see above). The lifetime risk of a chronic carrier from neonatal infection developing primary liver cancer may be as high as 40 per cent, at least in high prevalence areas [23]. These risks may be less in the West but hepatitis B virus remains an important cause of chronic liver disease, cirrhosis and primary liver cancer. Spontaneous seroconversion from HBeAg to antihepatitis B e antigen and from HBsAg to antihepatitis B surface antigen with clearance of virus following neonatal acquisition of virus is uncommon [67,236]. Furthermore, an HBsAg seropositive carrier with antihepatitis B e antigen may have detectable hepatitis B virus DNA. Virus replication may continue despite HBeAg negativity due to the presence of variants unable to produce HBeAg [51]. In long-standing infection, persistence of circulating HBsAg may result from integration of the gene for surface antigen (S gene) into the hepatocyte genome with production of non-infectious subunit (22 nm) HBsAg particles. Hepatitis B virus DNA has been detected in all body fluids of chronic carriers including seminal fluid. Testing of potential donors to sperm banks should be extended to seminal fluid. Contamination with hepatitis B of culture medium used for *in vitro* fertilization procedures has been reported [381].

Long-standing virus persistence, impaired cell-mediated host defences and tolerance to the virus may explain the disappointing results of antiviral therapies for neonatally acquired infection. The long-term success of eradicating neonatally acquired hepatitis B virus infection will depend on clearance of infected hepatocytes before integration of viral sequences and development of cirrhosis has occurred. Both seem to be important determinants in the future development of primary liver cancer.

ANTENATAL SCREENING

All pregnant women should be screened for HBsAg. Seropositive mothers must be identified before delivery. Neonatal immunoprophylaxis is most efficient if given at birth. Universal prenatal screening in the USA is estimated to identify 22 000 HBsAg seropositive women per year. This strategy should prevent annually 3000 chronic infections and is cost-effective [267]. Previous strategies from the National Center of Health Statistics in the USA until 1988 selected only high risk women for screening. One half or less of seropositive women are identified from demographic and epidemiological characteristics [39,267]. High risk mothers include first and second generation residents from high prevalence countries. Apart from Asian descent, no other risk factor was identified easily from histories [10].

Testing for HBsAg should be repeated in late pregnancy and post-partum in seronegative mothers with suspected acute infection or continued exposure to an HBsAg positive subject via sexual, ocular and mucosal contact, needle-stick injury, intravenous drug use, blood transfusion and other parenteral exposures [262,263].

Mothers with suspected *acute* infection should be tested also for IgM antihepatitis B core antigen as a reliable marker of recent infection (see Table 9.3). The finding of an HBsAg positive mother should trigger serological screening for all household and other close, especially sexual, contacts. Sero-negativity for HBsAg, antihepatitis B core and surface antigens identifies susceptible individuals who require immunization. A mother belonging to high risk groups (Box 9.2) who presents in labour without pre-screening, should be managed as high risk until results become available. Her newborn must be considered high risk and immunoprophylaxis commenced immediately, if necessary, before serological tests are confirmed. The decision to complete the immunization schedule should be assessed on the basis of risk of future exposure via horizontal transmission (see above) [41,138,243,271,296,361,362], serological results in the mother and cost of completion and follow-up. Babies born to mothers only identified as HBsAg positive more than 1 month after birth, such as at the postnatal visit, should be screened for HBsAg as evidence of recent infection and for antihepatitis B core and surface antigens as markers of previous exposure with immunity. Sero-negative babies should commence an immunization course without delay (see below).

Box 9.2. High risk women for hepatitis B presenting in pregnancy (after [262]).

- Women from high prevalence areas, whether immigrant or UK born:
  - The Far East, SE Asia, Mediterranean, Middle East, United Arab Emirates, Sub-Saharan Africa, Haiti, Asian, Pacific Island or Alaskan Eskimo.
- Women with histories of:
  - Acute or chronic liver disease
  - Frequent occupational exposure to blood in medical or dental care:
    - e.g. work or treat high-risk patients, e.g. in haemodialysis
    - e.g. work or residing in institutions for the mentally handicapped
  - Rejection as a blood donor
  - Multiple transfusions
  - Tattoos from a high risk area of the world or suspected contaminated needles
  - Intravenous drug use
  - Impaired immune responses
  - Episodes of venereal disease
  - Household and/or sexual contact with suspected HBV carrier:
    - e.g. from high risk groups: with a bisexual partner, high risk immigrant

ANTIVIRAL THERAPIES

Following delivery, HBsAg seropositive carriers with serological evidence of virus replication (hepatitis B virus DNA) should be considered for treatment with interferons. Interferon-induced clearance of HBsAg with seroconversion eventually to anti-hepatitis B surface antigen status can be achieved in around half of adult females with recent infection and chronic active hepatitis. The disappointing results for neonatally acquired infection reflects long-term virus persistence with integration of hepatitis B virus DNA into the hepatocyte genome and impaired cell-mediated host defences favouring tolerance to hepatitis B virus.

PREVENTION OF TRANSMISSION TO THE NEONATE

Caesarean section does not prevent transmission from an HBsAg positive mother to her newborn. Provided immunization has commenced, the neonate need not be isolated from its mother and breast feeding is not contraindicated [267]. Care should be taken to prevent the infant from coming into direct contact with blood-soaked dressings and pads. Lactation is not a contraindication to receiving the hepatitis B vaccine.

PASSIVE IMMUNOPROPHYLAXIS

HBIG contains high titre antihepatitis B surface and core antigens and offers good passive protection if given (0.06 ml/kg, intramuscularly) within 36 hours of exposure to an HBsAg positive subject or material [266]. Exposure includes babies born of infectious mothers and following needle-stick injury, sexual, ocular and mucosal contact [262,263,401]. Immunoglobulin, previously denoted as γ globulin, is used primarily as passive immunoprophylaxis against hepatitis A. Immunoglobulin contains moderate titres of antihepatitis B surface antigen (as well as antihepatitis B viral antibodies) and should be used if HBIG is not available. The immunoglobulins offer only temporary protection. They are expensive, limited in supply and effective only if given immediately following a definite exposure. Many subjects requiring immediate protection remain at future risk from repeated exposure and should be assessed for vaccine. Examples include babies born of infectious mothers with acute [374] and chronic hepatitis B, the sexual partner of an HBsAg positive carrier, an intravenous drug user and health-care personnel.

Passive immunoprophylaxis has been administered effectively and safely for more than 20 years. No specific adverse effects have been reported among many women later discovered to be pregnant. There is no evidence that preparations made to the specifications of the World Health Organization and administered intramuscularly transmit any blood-borne infections including HIV implicated in acquired immune deficiency syndrome (AIDS) [262,263].

ACTIVE IMMUNOPROPHYLAXIS

Hepatitis B immunization has been reviewed elsewhere [10,164,242]. Safe and efficacious vaccines have been licensed for clinical practice in the UK and USA since 1982. Several recombinant vaccines have been manufactured and licensed for clinical use since the late 1980s in the USA and Europe. In the West in clinical practice, these have superseded the plasma-derived vaccines. The HBsAg subunits (approximately 20 nm) are synthesized by molecular biological techniques rather than harvested from plasma of chronic carriers prior to rigorous inactivation. The recombinant and plasma vaccines share similar immunogenic properties including immunization schedules and numbers of suboptimal responses. Their safety has been endorsed by the World Health Organization [82] and the Immunization Practices Advisory Committee [267]. Serious adverse reactions are rare. Soreness at the site of injection and a low grade fever occur in <5 per cent of vaccinees.

MATERNAL IMMUNIZATION

Prudent practice dictates that no immunization be offered routinely in pregnancy and for known allergy to the individual vaccine components such as alum adsorbent and preservative. Manufacturers do not recommend immunization in pregnancy. However, in obstetric practice, there are no specific contraindications to administering HBIG and a licensed hepatitis B vaccine. No specific adverse consequences have been reported amongst many women who received intramuscular immunoglobulins and vaccine and later were found to be pregnant. There is no possibility of transmission of viruses. The licensed vaccines are not made from whole virus and inactivation procedures are exhaustive.

Immunization should not be withheld during pregnancy and lactation if a woman is perceived to be at risk from hepatitis B infection and provided each is assessed carefully and counselled. She should be pre-screened to avoid unnecessary immunization. Immunization with vaccine and HBIG should be offered only to susceptible women defined as seronegative for HBsAg, antihepatitis B core and surface antigens and who remain at risk from repeated exposure from a regular HBsAg seropositive sexual partner, occupation and intravenous drug use [262, 263]. Immunization should be postponed if there is intercurrent infection to avoid exacerbation of fever.

All licensed vaccines require multiple, spaced doses administered as a deep intramuscular injection in the deltoid or anterior thigh. Antihepatitis B surface antigen levels are lower when administered into the fatty buttock or intradermally. Concern over the safety of multisite, automatic injectors for mass immunization and reduced efficacies of routes other than intramuscular have limited their appeal in mass immunization [414].

The spacing of doses at times 0, 1, 2, and 12 months is superior to original recommendations for 0, 1 and 6 months in terms of speed of development and duration of detectable antihepatitis B surface antigen levels. The immunogenicity and protective efficacy rates exceed 90 per cent in young adults. In adults, HBIG usually is given as a single dose (500 IU) by deep intramuscular injection at a contralateral site to the vaccine, and using a new disposable needle and syringe. There is no evidence of interaction when active and passive immunization are administered concurrently at separate sites [103].

Prior to the advent of effective vaccines, a second dose of HBIG was recommended 1 month later to complete post-exposure passive prophylaxis [262, 263]. This is unnecessary when a vaccine course has commenced unless there is uncertainty over the immune responsiveness of the vaccinee (see below). Proof of additional protective efficacy in the adult following a second dose of HBIG is lacking and doses should be conserved where supplies are limited. HBIG has limited protective efficacy if delayed 48 hours or more after an exposure. In contrast, the hepatitis B vaccine can offer protection even if administered up to 2 weeks following an exposure [263]. Hepatitis B infection may be detected serologically but symptoms are uncommon and minor; seroconversion to antihepatitis B surface antigen is rapid and chronic carriage uncommon [263]. No information is available regarding transmission to the fetus following maternal immunization for acute hepatitis B virus infection in pregnancy but an optimistic outcome is likely in view of the rapid seroconversion in the mother.

PROTECTION OF HEALTH-CARE PERSONNEL

Immunization is recommended for all clinical health-care personnel in direct and regular contact with patients [82,86]. In the USA, an Occupational Safety Health Administration (OSHA) directive in 1990 recommended all health-care personnel in the USA be immunized against hepatitis B [111]. Screening for immunity (antihepatitis B surface and core antigens) is not cost-effective in low prevalence areas of the world, including the UK [106]. Prescreening may prevent unnecessary immunization in health-care personnel belonging to high-risk groups, including high prevalence countries for hepatitis B [262,263]. Testing for antihepatitis B core and surface antigens identifies previous exposure and immunity. Antihepatitis B core antigen seropositivity alone does not discriminate between carriers and non-carriers but overcomes the dilemma of detecting an HBsAg positive subject.

Isolation and barrier nursing are unnecessary but direct contact with blood-soaked dressings and pads should be avoided. All attendants should wear protective clothing, cover exposed cuts and abrasions and handle body fluids with care. Goggles and masks should be worn for anticipated splashes onto ocular and mucosal surfaces [265]. Five of 12 clusters involving transmission of hepatitis B virus from health-care personnel to patients involved obstetricians and gynaecologists performing invasive procedures [266].

NEONATAL IMMUNIZATION

In 1992, the World Health Assembly endorsed the universal immunization targets for 1997 set by their Global Advisory Group to integrate hepatitis B vaccine into the Expanded Programme of Immunization (EPI). The strategy favouring universal immunization replaces selective targeting of high risk groups which has failed to make any epidemiological impact on hepatitis B infection. In the USA, the Immunization Practices Advisory Committee has recommended universal immunization of all babies regardless of maternal hepatitis B status and teenagers and young adults where intravenous drug use and sexually transmitted diseases are common [267]. In countries with limited resources immunoprophylaxis should be given as priority to all infants born of HBsAg positive mothers regardless of maternal ethnic origin and HBeAg and antihepatitis B e antigen status.

Concurrent active and passive immunization is the prophylaxis of choice for preventing hepatitis B infection. Results with recombinant and plasma-derived vaccines are similar. In two seminal randomized controlled trials from Taiwan [23] and Hong Kong [402] the overall protective efficacy rate for dual immunoprophylaxis exceeded 93 per cent. Confirmation of the superiority of combined immunoprophylaxis for interruption of vertical transmission has been demonstrated amply in many prospective trials with high risk infants in high and low prevalence countries for hepatitis B infection such as in China [234], the USA [352] and Europe [98,410]. HBIG must be given in adequate dose as soon as possible after delivery (Table 9.4). Ideally, vaccine should be administered at the same time but at a different site and using a different disposable needle and syringe. There is no contraindication to the concurrent administration of other vaccines against polio, diphtheria, tetanus or pertussis [267].

Table 9.4. Hepatitis B virus perinatal post-exposure recommendations of the Immunization Practices Advisory Committee (after [267])

HBIG		Vaccine*	
Dose	Timing	Dose†	Timing
0.5 ml (250 IU)	Within 12 hours	5–10 μg i.m.	Within 12 hours

* First dose given concurrently with HBIG at different intramuscular sites. Schedules for basic course: 0, 1, 2 and 12 months or 0, 1 and 6 months.
† Dose and schedule depends on recommendations of the manufacturer.

In the neonate, vaccine, but not HBIG, may be postponed up to 7 days after delivery with preservation of good (>90 per cent) protective efficacy [24,262,263,360]. Whether any longer delay is justified in a high risk neonate with an intercurrent bacterial infection is undecided.

Typical schedules are doses at 0, 1, 2 and 12 months and 0, 1 and 6 months. Doses vary according to the recommendations of the manufacturer. Protective efficacy has been proven in New Zealand following low dose (around 20 per cent of recommended) immunization of schoolchildren.

Testing for antihepatitis B surface antigen after completion of the basic schedule usually is considered unnecessary in neonates (but see below). Ideally, testing for HBsAg, antihepatitis B surface and core antigens is recommended at 1 year to assess outcome. Maternal antihepatitis B core antigen may persist beyond 1 year [390] but usually detection of IgM antihepatitis B core antigen indicates recent infection [262,263].

A good responder tested 1–3 months after completing a basic immunization schedule will have high levels of antihepatitis B surface antigen (>100 mIU/ml) [106]. Antibody levels fall exponentially in all vaccinees [66,106,181,220] and typically fall below 20 per cent of the test level within 2 years [106,181]. In the good responder, antihepatitis B surface antigen levels rise exponentially again on challenge with an additional dose indicating a responsive immune memory [106]. The duration of protection from hepatitis B infection is unknown but outlives detectable levels of antihepatitis B surface antigen in the good responder [142,359]. Immune responsiveness may dictate the duration of protection afforded long after antihepatitis B surface antigen levels have fallen.

The minimum level of antihepatitis B surface antigen antibody guaranteeing protection from hepatitis B infection is unknown but poor responders probably are not protected from future infection. Studies in male homosexuals with suboptimal responses have shown little reduction in annual attack rates for hepatitis B infection after additional doses of vaccine [142,359].

IMMUNIZATION FAILURES

The licensed hepatitis B vaccines are highly immunogenic and efficacious, especially in neonates. Approximately 5 per cent of neonates and children and 10–20 per cent of adults make a poor response (antihepatitis B surface antigen <100 m IU/ml). Failures are attributed to a genetically predetermined poor response, infection *in utero* (see above), immunosuppression from intercurrent infection, in particular HIV [53], drugs, other diseases and the emergence of antibody escape variants of the hepatitis B virus.

Normally, antihepatitis B surface antigen antibody neutralizes hepatitis B virus by binding to the dominant epitopes — the 'a' determinant — on HBsAg. There are reports of babies who tested positive for HBsAg beyond 6 months despite circulating antihepatitis B surface antigen. A point mutation (glycine substituted for arginine) found in the second loop of the 'a' determinant abrogated the neutralizing effects of antihepatitis B surface antigen antibody [52,149].

No decision has been reached regarding the need

to offer additional 'booster' doses to vaccinees on long-term follow-up [264]. The optimal policy for the poor responder groups has not been defined. The safest policy for poor responder adults continually exposed, such as health-care personnel, would be to ignore previous immunization. Instead, poor responders should be offered HBIG (and an additional dose of vaccine if some response is anticipated) following a definite exposure such as needle-stick injury and await arrival of more immunogenic vaccines. Whether additional doses are justified in paediatric practice in the hope of some protection in poor and non-responders has not been decided.

Hepatitis D

Patients with acute and chronic hepatitis B infection are at risk from the additional problem of hepatitis delta virus [275,309]. Importantly, prevention of hepatitis B via immunization will protect against hepatitis delta infection.

This highly pathogenic RNA-containing virus is very small and relies on hepatitis B for helper functions. Hepatitis D virus is found wherever hepatitis B virus is endemic. High prevalence areas of the world for hepatitis B and D virus include the Mediterranean littoral, especially southern Italy and Israel, South America and the Middle East. Here over half of the HBsAg positive individuals show serological evidence (anti-delta antibody, delta antigen) of additional infection with hepatitis D virus. In northern Europe and the USA, dual infection predominantly is confined to high risk groups specifically intravenous drug users, immigrants from high prevalence areas and the multiply transfused. Simultaneous co-infection of hepatitis D virus with B accounts for a significant number of cases of acute liver failure in intravenous drug users and their sexual contacts [332].

Evidence for horizontal transmission of hepatitis D virus comes from Italy. Clustering of cases is seen within HBsAg positive families without obvious risk factors [50]. The relative roles of intimate contact between sexual partners and spread between siblings are unclear. Why the spread of hepatitis D virus via sexual contact amongst heterosexuals and homosexuals who are not intravenous drug users is uncommon, is not clearly understood.

Vertical transmission of hepatitis D virus may require high levels of hepatitis B virus replication. In one study from Italy [412] where hepatitis B and D virus are common, out of 481 symptomless HBsAg positive carrier mothers, 36 (7.5 per cent) were found to have hepatitis D superinfection based on serological detection of total anti-delta antibodies (IgM and IgG). Serological and biochemical evidence of vertical transmission in the newborn was found in one neonate from each group. Incidentally, neither had received HBIG at birth [412]. In an earlier report [411], development of anti-HDV positivity as evidence of vertical transmission of hepatitis D infection was found in one of seven babies of HBsAg positive mothers who were also anti-HDV positive. Transmission of hepatitis D virus occurred in the sole mother who was HBeAg positive. More studies are required where the status of virus replication (hepatitis B virus DNA) in the mother is confirmed.

Hepatitis D virus can suppress replication of hepatitis B virus, measured by falling titres of serum HBsAg, hepatitis B virus DNA and IgM antihepatitis B core antigen, leading to misdiagnosis. Testing must include HDVAg, hepatitis D virus RNA and antihepatitis D virus antibodies and markers of hepatitis B viral infection and be repeated in suspected cases (see Table 9.3).

Successful immunoprophylaxis against hepatitis B viral infection should protect against hepatitis D regardless of route of transmission. Vertical transmission is unlikely to play as significant role as that for hepatitis B because the majority of subjects infected with hepatitis D virus have sufficient liver disease to impair fertility and preclude pregnancy (see above).

Herpes viruses

Herpes simplex is the only virus in the West which seems to have an especial predeliction for severe hepatitis in pregnancy. Early diagnosis and treatment with acyclovir can be successful. All members of the herpes group — herpes simplex, varicella zoster, cytomegalovirus and Epstein–Barr virus

(EBV) — can cause hepatitis. Hepatitis due to herpes simplex is very uncommon in adults but well recognized in neonates. Less than 100 cases due to herpes simplex have been reported in the literature [402]. More than half were associated with immunosuppression but some were women in the third trimester [136,156,177,315,394,402,409]. Presenting features are non-specific and lead to delays in diagnosis. Mucocutaneous stigmata may be absent and jaundice is not invariable [136,177,336]. Herpes simplex hepatitis carries a grave prognosis. Mortality exceeds 90 per cent even with treatment [402]. Types I and II are represented. Herpes simplex type II is most common in the third trimester and most patients have cervical and genital lesions [409]. Genital herpes infection has been found in the non-pregnant patient with fulminant hepatitis [315,396]. Mechanisms predisposing towards dissemination of the virus during pregnancy remain unclear. Impaired immune surveillance, as implicated in the predisposition to disseminated EBV infection, may play a role [301].

Herpes simplex II commonly reactivates in pregnancy. Symptoms are three times more common in the pregnant than in the non-pregnant patient [363]. Herpes simplex virus crosses the placenta but there seems to be no relation with congenital malformations [363] (in contrast to cytomegalovirus, see below). In recurrent infection, high maternal levels of antibody offer some protection to the newborn. The risks of congenital dissemination are more common if primary infection occurs during pregnancy and increase to term. Herpes simplex acquired at birth from cervical and vaginal contamination can lead to disseminated infection in over half of the babies with 90 per cent mortality from meningoencephalitis. Delivery by caesarean section has been considered in suspected cases of maternal primary infection [363]. Diagnosis depends on a battery of tests including serological markers and demonstration of inclusion bodies on histological examination of liver tissue (see Table 9.3). Viral DNA detected by *in situ* hybridization in liver tissue can provide a rapid diagnosis if sampling is feasible [402]. Antiviral therapy such as acyclovir can be successful if given early [206]. Hepatitis due to varicella zoster has been reported rarely in children [73]. Details for pregnancy are lacking.

EBV and cytomegalovirus

Both viruses are ubiquitous; more than 50 per cent of adults have detectable antibodies. Common transmission routes include sexual contact via body fluids such as saliva and blood, especially from leucocyte fractions [105].

EBV

Transmission via blood is uncommon but outbreaks of hepatitis have been noted in haemodialysis units. Most primary infections occur in otherwise healthy children and young adults as infectious mononucleosis ('glandular fever'). Less than 5 per cent of all cases develop an hepatitis. This typically is symptomless but represents a significant number of cases. Acute liver failure is rare [285] and there is no especial predeliction for pregnancy.

CYTOMEGALOVIRUS

This is probably the most common cause of post-transfusion hepatitis in seronegative neonates and children in the West [4] (compare with hepatitis C in adults). Over 30 per cent of the population acquire cytomegalovirus during the first few months of life. After primary infection, the virus probably persists for life. Reactivation of latent infection is common in pregnancy and 3–5 per cent of otherwise healthy women show a viruria [162,307]. Virus can be detected in 0.3–3 per cent of babies screened routinely in pregnancy [35,252,348]. Up to 2 per cent of neonates have signs of infection [226]. Following infection during pregnancy up to 10 per cent will be severely handicapped [35]. This assessment is more optimistic than in previous reports [245] but, for England and Wales alone, cytomegalovirus accounts for 180 children per annum with severe and permanent handicaps [35]. Various neonatal syndromes have been recorded following maternal reactivation including midbrain damage and cytomegalic inclusion disease [363]. Five per cent of congenital infections include a neonatal hepatitis with hepatosplenomegaly, pneumonitis, chorioretinitis and a myriad of central nervous system disorders. Primary maternal infection in the first and second trimesters is associated with brain damage to the fetus.

Diagnosis of maternal infection relies on serological tests; (IgM anticytomegalovirus), rising titres of antibody from paired sera and detection of viruria. The finding of cytomegalovirus in cervical swabs in up to 28 per cent of healthy women [282,385] does not always equate with congenital infection [363]. Instead, cultures of nasopharyngeal secretions and urine from the newborn provide a ready and more reliable diagnosis. Cytomegalovirus has been isolated from cultures of bile and body fluids. Virus can be detected in liver biopsy specimens by visualizing inclusions and using monoclonal antibodies and DNA probes.

Passive immunization using specific, high titre immunoglobulin can offer some protection against primary infection after accidental exposure. This is very expensive and no information is available for use against primary infection during pregnancy. No vaccines are available. Studies to develop recombinant vaccines are in progress in Europe, the USA and Japan but fears remain over establishing long-term latency for viruses with oncogenic potential.

AIDS and the liver (see also Chapter 17)

Concurrent liver disease is common in late HIV infection and AIDS. Liver disease accounted for 4 per cent of deaths in HIV seropositive American women aged 15–44 years up until 1987 [60]. Confounding factors include all the hepatotropic agents, side-effects of medicinal drugs such as antituberculosis therapies and recreational drugs such as cocaine.

The presenting features are protean with fever, hepatosplenomegaly and elevated serum levels of alkaline phosphatase and γ glutamyl transpeptidase. Histological changes are wide and commonly include viral hepatitis and granulomata from opportunistic infections and drugs. Opportunistic infections, especially cryptosporidium and cytomegalovirus, can cause biliary tract abnormalities resembling sclerosing cholangitis and extrahepatic duct obstruction. Cryptococcosis, histoplasmosis and, rarely, pneumocystis may cause granulomatous hepatitis. Differential diagnosis is correspondingly wide and includes all causes of cholestatic jaundice and biliary tract infections (see below).

Liver biopsy can provide a valuable source of fresh tissue for culture and fixed material to assist in the diagnosis of many opportunistic infections.

Acute liver failure

This rare and complex medical emergency requires early discussions and referral to a specialized centre with facilities for managing multi-organ failure and liver transplantation. Early transfer is essential. Grade III encephalopathy is associated with clinical onset of cerebral oedema and exacerbated by travel [284,285]. Early diagnosis is essential because prognosis without grafting depends on aetiology.

Fulminant hepatic failure (FHF) is defined as the development of hepatic encephalopathy caused by severe liver dysfunction within 8 weeks of onset of symptoms in a patient with a previously normal liver [377]. Late onset hepatic failure (LOHF; subacute hepatic necrosis) defines the development of encephalopathy between 8 and 26 weeks after onset of symptoms [126].

Clinical features of acute liver failure are non-specific and non-diagnostic (see above). The liver is usually small in severe cases regardless of aetiology; hepatomegaly suggests infiltration. Splenomegaly is uncommon but seen in Wilson's disease and other chronic liver diseases. Systolic hypertension may be marked with cerebral oedema. A polymorphonuclear leucocytosis can be found in any liver failure complicated by microbial infection. Haematological features of DIC occur regardless of the aetiology. A haemolytic anaemia should prompt exclusion of Wilson's disease. Levels of serum transaminase (AST or ALT), reported as relatively low in acute fatty liver and the HELLP syndrome amongst others (see above), can rise (>2000 IU/l) with hepatic necrosis from infarction and rupture. Relatively low serum levels of bilirubin and transaminase may indicate extensive hepatocellular necrosis with lack of regeneration of hepatocytes and, consequently, a poor prognosis.

The concern in obstetric practice is the differential diagnosis which may alter obstetric management, the benefits of early delivery and management prior to transfer to a referral centre.

DIFFERENTIAL DIAGNOSIS AND OBSTETRIC OUTCOME

The most common causes of acute liver failure likely to be encountered in pregnancy and anticipated outcome following delivery are given in Table 9.5. Paracetamol (acetaminophen) overdose is the most common cause of FHF in the UK and is prevalent in young women of childbearing age. Serum levels should be sought in all patients. Hepatotoxicity of the fetal liver from metabolites of paracetamol can lead to impaired coagulation and intraventricular haemorrhage [216]. *N*-acetyl-cysteine given up to 36 hours following the overdose can prevent the onset of hepatic encephalopathy [285]. The very limited information suggests that this antidote is safe in pregnancy [216].

In the West, sporadic non-A, non-B, non-C, non-E is the most common presumed viral cause of acute liver failure but data in pregnancy are lacking. Viral causes are rare in pregnancy but prevalent amongst series reported in Europe. Hepatitis E is prevalent in the developing countries and travellers returning from high prevalence countries (see above). Exotic agents such as Rift Valley fever, dengue and other arboviruses cause haemorrhagic fevers. These should be considered in travellers bitten by insects in endemic areas such as the African countries. Other, non-viral causes include paracetamol overdose, other drugs including anti-epileptics and non-steroidal anti-inflammatory agents, carbon tetrachloride, halothane and poisonous mushrooms (*Amanita phalloides*).

Rapid serological diagnosis is essential for the correct management of viral hepatitis. In expert hands, survival rates of 40–60 per cent with medical management alone can be achieved for non-pregnant patients with hepatitis A and B who are referred early but progress through grades III–IV encephalopathy [108,285]. In contrast, the uniformly poor prognosis of most other causes of acute liver failure requires early assessment of the suitability for liver transplantation which has revolutionized maternal outcome (see below).

Table 9.5. Acute liver failure in pregnancy

Aetiology	Maternal outcome following delivery
Viral hepatitis	No effect
Drugs	No effect
Acute fatty liver	Improved
HELLP	Improved

Serological markers remain the cornerstone for the diagnosis of viral hepatitis (see Table 9.3). Seronegativity for antibodies to hepatitis C does not exclude the diagnosis because seroconversion can be delayed. A negative test for HBsAg does not exclude hepatitis B since this antigen is abnormally rapidly cleared in acute liver failure [108]. Similarly, HBsAg if present and persisting in high titre, may indicate a chronic carrier with an additional aetiology for the liver failure. Multiple viral aetiologies should be sought using panels of tests and repeated (see Table 9.3) in doubtful cases.

In obstetric practice the major differential diagnoses include viral hepatitis, AFLP, severe pre-eclampsia and toxaemia of pregnancy, the HELLP syndrome and overlapping conditions such as thrombotic thrombocytopenic purpura and HUS (see above). Other confusing conditions include severe hyperemesis gravidarum, Budd–Chiari syndrome, alcoholic hepatitis, pancreatitis, septicaemias and other severe infections such as leptospirosis. In addition, chronic liver disease, especially Wilson's disease, and autoimmune chronic active hepatitis, and malignant infiltrations of the liver from lymphomas and metastases may present with a picture indistinguishable from acute liver failure.

MANAGEMENT

This is similar regardless of pregnancy. Any of the following features, namely hepatic encephalopathy (grade II, III or IV), elevated prothrombin ratio (e.g. > twice normal control), renal impairment, metabolic acidosis (blood pH <7.3), hypotension, hyponatraemia and thrombocytopenia should prompt discussion and referral to a specialized centre [284,285].

The prothrombin time is the most sensitive indicator of the severity of liver dysfunction, and hence prognosis (Table 9.6), and should be tested frequently. Administration of fresh frozen plasma is best avoided without overt bleeding because outcome is not affected and interpretation of the prothrombin time can be difficult. Fresh blood and blood products should be available to support any surgical intervention and following delivery to help minimize blood loss. Parenteral vitamin K_1 and folinic (folic) acid should be given routinely. Blood glucose levels should be monitored closely and immediate provision made to administer large quantities (10–50 per cent) via a central venous catheter to prevent hypoglycaemia which remains a common cause of fetal and maternal death. Early manifestations of cerebral oedema include peaks of systolic hypertension and tachycardia and should be treated by mannitol-induced diuresis (100 ml of 20 per cent as a bolus). Mannitol is nephrotoxic and ineffective in the presence of renal failure. Ultrafiltration and haemodialysis may be required to remove excess fluid. Levels of blood urea may be misleadingly low. Renal function is best monitored by serial levels of serum creatinine and its clearance. Gastrointestinal bleeding from erosions is decreased by the prophylactic administration of an H_2 antagonist. Elective endotracheal intubation and assisted ventilation may be required especially prior to travel and before the development of overt cerebral oedema. The intubation must be carried out by an experienced anaesthetist. All sedation and dietary protein should be withdrawn.

Corticosteroids are of no proven benefit in acute liver failure and may exacerbate complications such as infection. Microbial, including fungal, infection is very common in liver failure. Detailed microbiological cultures and analyses should be carried out routinely and serially on all body fluids including blood, urine, sputum and ascites.

The place for antiviral agents which inhibit virus replication seems limited from results of small uncontrolled trials mostly for hepatitis B. Interferons have been given to three pregnant women with fulminant viral hepatitis and two of these survived [228]. Data on controlled trials in fulminant viral hepatitis are lacking. In fulminant hepatitis B and D, virus replication is less than in uncomplicated acute infection and may have ceased before presentation. For continuing replication, the extent of liver damage may preclude regeneration.

Insulin–glucagon infusions promoted rapid liver cell regeneration in controlled studies in animal models but results in humans are conflicting. Prostaglandin E_1 by continuous infusion was associated with improvements and no mortality in acute liver failure from hepatitis B and presumed non-A, non-B hepatitis. Results from larger controlled studies are awaited. Prostaglandin E will of course induce labour.

Unlike AFLP and some cases of HELLP (see above), delivery for viral hepatitis does not necessarily improve maternal outcome (see Table 9.5) but controlled studies are lacking. Equally there are no data to indicate that delivery causes viral hepatitis to deteriorate.

Table 9.6. Poor prognostic indicators in acute liver failure (after [284])

Paracetamol	Other causes
All three of these	*Any* three of these
Grade III encephalopathy	Aetiology, e.g. non- A, B, C
Prothrombin time >100 seconds	Age <10 or >40 years
Creatinine >300 μmol/l	Prothrombin time >50 seconds
	Serum bilirubin >300 μmol/l
	Jaundice >7 days before encephalopathy
And/or:	Or
Arterial pH <7.3	Prothrombin time >100 seconds

These are for guidance only: other factors must be considered.

Survival of the fetus in severe liver failure is exceptional. Often the fetus is dead on presentation and this relates to profound fetal and maternal hypoglycaemia.

SCREENING CONTACTS

Close, especially sexual, contacts of the patient with viral hepatitis should be screened for virological markers and public health officials notified. Susceptible contacts should be offered HIBG for hepatitis B and immunoglobulin for hepatitis A (see above) and vaccines considered (see above). In practice, a patient with advanced acute liver failure due to hepatitis A or B probably is not very infectious to health-care personnel. Nevertheless, attendants should remain cautious in the handling of patients and body fluids. Protective clothing should be worn. Non-immunized pregnant attendants should not be allowed to nurse patients with viral hepatitis.

Liver transplantation

Comparable survival rates to those in the non-pregnant population can be achieved for acute liver failure with early referral to a transplantation centre. Assessment includes the potential for recovery and suitability for grafting based on prognostic indicators (see Table 9.6). Knowledge of the patient's blood group is important for matching potential donors. Microbial infections should be sought and treated aggressively. Tests should be commenced to exclude Wilson's disease (see below).

The uniformly poor survival for acute liver failure excluding hepatitis A and B has emphasized the place of early liver grafting. Successful maternal and fetal outcomes have been reported for pregnant women grafted for fulminant hepatitis B [15,110, 218,239], AFLP [11] HELLP syndrome [140] and Budd–Chiari syndrome [201,320]. Re-infection following transplantation in non-pregnant survivors has been documented for hepatitis B, D and C with variable clinical outcomes. Data on the efficacy of immunoprophylaxis and antiviral therapies are sparse. Re-infection seems less likely for fulminant hepatitis B and D if HBIG is used.

The menstrual cycle returns soon after successful grafting [48,72,78]. Amenhorrhoea continuing after grafting may signify early pregnancy. Patients should be offered early advice on contraception. Pregnancy does not increase the risk of graft rejection. Deferral of pregnancy until beyond the first year seems sensible because morbidity and mortality are greatest within this time. Oral contraceptive drugs can enhance the hepatotoxicity of cyclosporin [88] and are contraindicated in thrombogenic disorders such as Budd–Chiari syndrome.

Successful pregnancies have been reported in grafted women maintained on cyclosporin, azathioprine and corticosteroids. Graft function and survival seem unaffected by pregnancy [218]. Cyclosporin is nephrotoxic, crosses the placenta and can impair fetal growth [72] but long-term survivors seem unaffected. Blood levels of cyclosporin should be monitored very frequently. Divided daily doses may reduce maximum peaks. Pregnancy in recipients of hepatic allografts is associated with good perinatal outcome, but there is an increased risk of pre-eclampsia, worsening hypertension, anaemia and pre-term delivery. Shared management is essential between transplant specialists and perinatologists.

Chronic hepatitis

Chronic hepatitis is an histopathological diagnosis and does not discriminate the many causes of chronic liver disease. Reliance on detection of clinical stigmata and liver serum biochemistry to monitor underlying disease activity may be misleading. Liver biopsy performed during pregnancy is safe in expert hands when assisted by ultrasonographic imaging and when carried out within recommended limitations of normal parameters of coagulation. Attention must be given to anatomical displacement of the liver especially in the third trimester.

Chronic persistent hepatitis is characterized by the presence of a chronic inflammatory infiltrate confined to the portal tracts. It may follow acute viral hepatitis B and C and is common in symptomless HBsAg positive carriers with normal liver function tests. Chronic persistent hepatitis is generally considered a benign disease unless it progresses to chronic active hepatitis (see below). Women who are HBsAg positive and have additional evidence of virus replication (HBeAg, serum hepatitis B virus DNA) should be considered for antiviral therapy after delivery.

Chronic active hepatitis

In the West, the majority of cases in young women have autoimmune features with hypergammaglobulinaemia, autoantibodies to smooth muscle, specific proteins (anti-LSP) and nuclear factor (ANF). Some may be related to viral hepatitis, drugs including methyldopa and isoniazid or genetic causes such as Wilson's disease (see below). The histological features include a chronic inflammatory cell infiltrate in the portal tracts extending beyond the limiting plate to surround islands of hepatocytes ('piecemeal necrosis'). The inflammation and necrosis can extend towards the hepatic vein in the hepatic lobule ('bridging necrosis').

Untreated autoimmune chronic active hepatitis is associated with amenorrhoea and infertility. Progression to cirrhosis and decompensated liver disease is not uncommon. Introduction of corticosteroids and azathioprine has led to increased fertility [351] and a marked improvement in prognosis, including in pregnancy. Liver function during pregnancy is preserved with well-controlled disease activity but fetal prematurity and low birthweight have been recorded [351]. Obstetrical complications such as urinary infections and toxaemia are common. In some series [351,395] fetal loss reached 55 per cent but there was no increased incidence of congenital malformations. Prednisolone therapy for autoimmune hepatitis should be continued throughout pregnancy in conventional doses (10–20 mg/day) and increased for suspected relapse [395], although this is unusual (10–15 per cent) [351]. Uncontrolled disease and frequent relapses should prompt re-appraisal of the diagnosis and exclusion of other conditions especially Wilson's disease and viral hepatitis (see below). Regardless of pregnancy, azathioprine is considered an established therapy in the treatment of autoimmune chronic active hepatitis (50–100 mg/day) with prednisolone [351]. No specific adverse effects on the fetus have been reported when azathioprine was used in larger doses as an immunosuppressant in pregnant renal transplant recipients [223] (see Chapter 7). Maintenance of well-controlled disease may be possible with azathioprine alone, after cautious withdrawal of corticosteroids [190]. Whether monotherapy should be contemplated during pregnancy is debatable. The risks to the fetus are high should relapse occur and evidence is lacking for adverse effects of corticosteroids in this condition.

Hepatitis B and C can progress from chronic persistent to chronic active hepatitis and cirrhosis with continuing virus replication (hepatitis B virus DNA, hepatitis C virus RNA) and superinfection with other agents such as hepatitis D virus. Corticosteroids and other immunosuppressant drugs are contraindicated in viral hepatitis. Women with hepatitis B or C should be considered for antiviral therapy following delivery (see above).

Cirrhosis

Pregnancy remains uncommon in advanced cirrhosis although there have been over 100 reports [46,55,211,323,368] the first [318] in 1923. Information from two independent series [46,55] and a collective review of the literature [323] have identified the prognosis for mother and fetus, the effects of pregnancy on coexisting liver disease and the role of surgical portal decompression [323].

EFFECTS ON FERTILITY

Infertility reflects the degree of hepatic dysfunction [46]. Irregular menses are common [383] and result from disturbances of the hypothalamopituitary axis rather than directly from the liver disease [71]. Malnutrition and altered hepatic metabolism of sex steroids may play a role but data are lacking. Fertility is normal or near-normal with well-compensated cirrhosis due to autoimmune and Wilson's disease.

EFFECTS ON PREGNANCY

Fetal loss is high in advanced cirrhosis. In early pregnancy there is an increased risk of spontaneous abortion (10–11 per cent) [46,171,383] and this risk worsens without portosystemic shunt decompression [55,323]. In late pregnancy, only 45 babies from 69 pregnancies without surgical portal decompression [323] survived the neonatal period. Stillbirth was reported in 17 (24.5 per cent) and there were five (7.2 per cent) neonatal deaths. Prognosis for the fetus was better with previous portosystemic shunts (median 3 years) prior to delivery: 80 per cent of 30 pregnancies ended in live births [323].

EFFECTS OF PREGNANCY ON DISEASE

The once gloomy prognosis for mother and child has improved. Maternal prognosis depends more on the degree of hepatic dysfunction during pregnancy than aetiology although well-compensated biliary and post-necrotic cirrhosis carry the best prognosis. Some early studies reported improved liver function during pregnancy in primary biliary cirrhosis [6] and Wilson's disease [36,92,335]. In Cheng's literature survey [55], around half the women with documented severe cirrhosis had successful term pregnancies without maternal complications.

Bleeding from oesophageal varices remains the most significant complication in pregnancy [319], especially in the second and third trimester. The progressive increase in circulating blood volume, elevations in portal pressure and added pressure from the gravid uterus on the inferior vena cava coincide to divert a greater proportion of the venous return through the azygous system [195]. The resultant increase in oesophageal pressure leads to transient oesophageal varices in at least half of healthy pregnant women [195,323]. Two papers [46, 323] report divergent views on the outcomes of oesophageal varices in pregnancy. In the study by Britton [46], out of 160 pregnancies with documented coexisting oesophageal varices, bleeding occurred on 38 occasions. Associated maternal mortalities from variceal bleeds was 18 and 2 per cent in cirrhotic and non-cirrhotic groups respectively. In a literature review up until 1982 [323], gastrointestinal haemorrhage, from presumed oesophageal varices, occurred in eight of 60 (13.3 per cent) cases without previous surgical portal decompression. Maternal mortality was high. Seven of 10 deaths in the non-shunted group were due to gastrointestinal bleeding. These figures, when compared with a 38 per cent mortality in a non-pregnant cirrhotic control group [46], suggest that there is no increased risk of fatal haemorrhage from oesophageal varices during pregnancy [46]. The literature survey [323] did not include a non-pregnant control group. However, a comparison was made with the maternal outcome for pregnant women who had previously undergone portosystemic shunting prior to pregnancy [323]. Only one of 23 pregnancies (21 mothers) resulted in a maternal death. This was due to hepatic coma on the eighth day post-partum and not gastrointestinal bleeding. In a further seven cases, in which surgical portal decompression was performed during pregnancy (median 4 months prior to delivery), there were no maternal and fetal deaths [323].

The discordance between the two reports [46,323] can be partly explained. The literature review [323] highlighted the dangers of the post-partum period accounting for five of the seven deaths from gastrointestinal haemorrhage. This challenges the physiological explanation of haemodynamic alterations during pregnancy [195]. Other post-partum complications included early uterine haemorrhage (5.8 per cent versus 16.6 per cent), hepatic coma (3.3 per cent versus 4.3 per cent) and ascites (17.4 versus 0 per cent) in the shunted and non-shunted groups respectively [323].

MANAGEMENT

General advice to any pregnant women with cirrhosis and portal hypertension should include avoidance of situations which raise portal pressure such as straining, stooping and avoidance of alcohol. Re-bleeding and death are likely in those patients with oesophageal varices who do not maintain complete abstinence from alcohol [319]. No specific measures to protect the oesophagus are of proven benefit in the absence of oesophageal reflux [319]. A pregnancy with well-compensated cirrhosis without jaundice and previously impaired liver function should be allowed to proceed to term. Attention should be paid to rest, vitamin supplementation and diet high in carbohydrate, low in protein in advanced cirrhosis and following surgical portal decompression. A high fibre diet should be encouraged to avoid constipation. Lactulose seems safe but specific data for human pregnancy are lacking. Along with all drugs, laxatives should be used with caution in the first trimester. Vaginal delivery is safe in the majority of cases [46] but a protracted second stage should be avoided and interrupted by early forceps delivery to avoid excess straining with subsequent rise in portal pressure. The selection of forceps may explain the improved fetal outcome in shunted (26.6 per cent) over non-shunted (13 per cent) groups in the literature survey [323]. Excess blood loss, especially in the puerperium [323], should be anticipated. Delivery should take place in a centre with expertise in handling bleeding oesophageal varices. Vitamin K_1, fresh frozen plasma and additional coagulation factors and platelets may be required. Sedatives, anaesthetics and diuretics should be used with caution since these and other factors, including excess blood loss, hypotension, occult infection, hypoglycaemia and constipation can precipitate hepatic encephalopathy.

Ascites should be managed with restriction of dietary sodium and, if severe, fluids. In the non-pregnant patient with ascites, spironolactone remains the drug of choice. Unfortunately, spironolactone crosses the placenta and may affect the male fetus in particular since it is an anti-androgen. The thiazide diuretics can precipitate hepatic coma in pregnant patients with cirrhosis [13,230]. Metabolites of spironolactone cross into breast milk and breast feeding is not recommended [230]. An ascitic tap carried out under ultrasonographic imaging should be analysed for a leucocytosis (>250 cells/mm^3), microbial organisms and an acid pH (<7.35). Any one of these usually signifies peritonitis; fever and a peripheral blood leucocytosis may be absent. The prognosis with untreated spontaneous bacterial peritonitis or other sepsis is poor and frequently confounded by recurrent bleeding from the gastrointestinal tract, including from oesophageal varices. Appropriate antimicrobial therapy to cover gut-related organisms, such as *E. coli*, should be instigated without delay. Tetracyclines are contraindicated in pregnancy (see Chapter 1) and in patients with liver disease.

Caesarean section should be reserved for urgent situations to save the baby in the presence of rapidly deteriorating maternal liver function. The prognosis in these circumstances remains poor for mother and child [55]. Abdominal surgery may be technically difficult due to the large collateral circulation and adhesions from previous shunt surgery. Local anaesthesia with an epidural or pudendal block can be carried out safely [346] but advantages must be balanced against the increased risk of bleeding from the raised venous pressure and abnormal coagulation (compare with HELLP syndrome, see above). Elective termination of pregnancy should be considered only for decompensated cirrhosis in the first trimester. A woman presenting in pregnancy with suspected cirrhosis and portal hypertension requires full medical investigation.

If the patient has gastrointestinal haemorrhage upper oesophagogastroduodenoscopy should be carried out and, if necessary, liver biopsy. Both techniques are safe in expert hands with the usual reservations over normal coagulation and use of ultrasonography for liver biopsy. Survivors of a variceal bleed usually have end-stage irreversible disease. Even in the presence of large varices remission may be induced by additional medical therapy such as corticosteroids for autoimmune chronic active hepatitis, D-penacillamine for Wilson's disease and abstinence from alcohol in alcoholic cirrhosis [319]. Management of bleeding oesophageal varices has been simplified by the use of sclerosing agents to obliterate venous channels [28,207]. Several controlled trials, comparing the use of endoscopic sclerotherapy with surgical intervention (portosystemic shunting, oesophageal transection), have shown a significant reduction in re-bleeding from varices in non-pregnant patients who present at the time of bleeding and are treated by sclerotherapy, but not by surgery [28,319]. Portal pressure can be reduced by drugs such as β blockers and vasodilators. Venoconstriction and shunting of blood away from the oesophagus can be promoted using a combination of a vasoconstrictor and nitrate [28,319]. None of these measures has been shown to be superior to a course of sclerotherapy or to prevent bleeding which typically recurs within 8 weeks [319]. No data are available on trials of sclerotherapy for bleeding varices in pregnancy but this technique seems relatively safe and less traumatic than previously recommended surgical interventions [211,323,368]. Upper endoscopy should be repeated for each presentation of gastrointestinal bleeding. Interventional sclerotherapy is best carried out early in the course of bleeding and other non-variceal causes may be found.

Cirrhosis is the main cause of intrahepatic portal hypertension. Non-cirrhotic causes of portal hypertension which may require different medical management include sarcoidosis, tuberculosis, schistosomiasis [346], metastatic malignancy, Gaucher's disease [247] polycystic liver disease, congenital hepatic fibrosis [28] and AFLP [34].

Primary biliary cirrhosis (PBC)

PBC has a wide spectrum of disease and variable natural history [279] and is more common than previously thought. PBC may be diagnosed on routine testing of liver function. The pregnant woman may be symptomless with elevated levels of serum alkaline phosphatase (liver isoenzyme) and γ glutamyl transpeptidase. Diagnosis relies on detection of mitochondrial antibodies in almost all patients and characteristic liver histology in the absence of other biliary diseases.

Differential diagnosis includes intrahepatic cholestasis of pregnancy (see above) which resolves in the puerperium and sclerosing cholangitis which may be associated with covert inflammatory bowel disease and cholelithiasis.

Maternal and fetal outcomes are variable. Prognosis is good for well-compensated disease. Drug therapy is non-specific and aimed at relieving symptoms such as pruritus (see above). Cholestyramine resin binds fat soluble vitamins (A, D, E and K) and vitamin K_1 supplements should be given especially before delivery. There are no studies relating to the prognosis of PBC presenting in pregnancy.

Wilson's disease

Pregnancy is uncommon in untreated disease [35, 373,391], especially with advanced cirrhosis and portal hypertension. Subfertility and amenorrhoea are common, spontaneous abortions frequent, and there is high maternal morbidity and mortality in untreated disease. Treatment with D-penicillamine (35 cases) or triethylene tetramine dihydrochloride (trientine: nine cases) up until 1986 resulted in good maternal and fetal outcome [391,392]. Trientine is of equivalent cupriuretic value to D-penicillamine but possibly less toxic and was given for a mean of 5 years before conception. Seven of 11 pregnancies and their outcomes were normal up to 9 years of follow-up [392]. One further had a pre-term delivery at 36 weeks and two had miscarriages unrelated to the Wilson's disease. One patient delivered a baby with the isochromosome X abnormality at 31 weeks [392].

Oral zinc has been used but there are no data relating to trials in pregnancy. The use of chelating agents in pregnancy is generally considered safe for the mother. Therapy should not be discontinued because the relapse rate is high and a rapid deterioration in liver function can occur after many years of successful therapy. D-penicillamine can be toxic in doses >1.5 g/day but is well tolerated in Wilson's disease. The dose of chelating agent required for successful cupriuresis probably is less in pregnancy than otherwise and can be cautiously reduced [269] by 25–50 per cent should toxic symptoms occur. Toxicity is unusual and a full dose should be resumed immediately after delivery. In addition, note that chelating agents can reduce serum levels of iron and zinc and should not be administered simultaneously with oral iron supplements. Pyridoxine (vitamin B_6) should be supplemented by a minimum of 50 mg/week to counteract the anti-pyridine effects of D-penicillamine [391].

Reductions in maternal levels of serum copper also have been attributed to an oestrogen effect of elevating the serum level of caeruloplasmin [37] but these changes are not invariable in pregnancy [269, 392] or in patients taking oestrogen therapy [269].

A diagnosis of Wilson's disease should be considered in any young patient with undiagnosed liver disease, including acute liver failure, and especially with haemolysis. Specimens for analysis of urinary copper levels and diagnostic liver biopsy tissue must be handled in a copper-free environment to prevent contamination from skin, needles and containers. The demonstration of Kayser–Fleischer rings by slit lamp analysis assists the diagnosis. The rings may be absent especially when presenting with liver disease and can be found in

PBC. Family members should be investigated. Detection of symptomless but significant liver disease is common in siblings. The prognosis is favourable if therapy with chelating agents is commenced before onset of cirrhosis. Liver grafting has been successful with clinical resolution of hepatic and neurological dysfunction but no data are available for pregnancy.

FETAL ASPECTS

D-penicillamine crosses the placenta and the congenital abnormalities described are probably caused by the copper deficiency rather than direct effects of the chelating agent [191]. Three babies with abnormalities of skin and connective tissue were born of mothers taking between 0.9 and 2 g/day of D-penicillamine during pregnancy for cystinuria [260], rheumatoid arthritis [241,345] and Wilson's disease (two patients) [147,313,391]. One further baby with reversible cutis laxa followed maternal D-penicillamine therapy (1.5 g/day) for Wilson's disease [232]. Cerebral palsy with blindness and arthrogryposis multiplex have been reported with maternal exposure to D-penicillamine for Wilson's disease [313] but the pregnancies were complicated by other factors which could have influenced outcome.

Serum levels of copper and caeruloplasmin in cord blood and urinary levels of copper are normal in the heterozygote baby even if pre-term and with poor maternal compliance of drug therapy [37,269, 392]. Handling of copper by the fetus seems normal and there is no evidence of copper depletion [392]. Extraction of copper by the normal fetus may account for improvements in neurological status and liver function in some cases during pregnancy [36,92,335].

Budd–Chiari syndrome

The first description by Chiari in 1899 followed childbirth [57]. Over 30 cases have been described during pregnancy or, more commonly, post-partum [68,74,85,146,173,197,208].

This syndrome is defined as obstruction of the large hepatic veins which produces congestion and necrosis of the centrilobular areas of the liver [28]. Related disorders sharing clinical and haematological abnormalities include high inferior vena cava thrombosis, veno-occlusive disease with obstruction of centrilobular veins and peliosis hepatis with obstruction at the junction between hepatic sinusoids and centrilobular veins [28].

The aetiology of Budd–Chiari syndrome remains obscure. In the non-pregnant population in the West the most common associations are with polycythaemia rubra vera, paroxysmal nocturnal haemoglobinuria and altered coagulation. More than three-quarters arise without pregnancy, oral contraceptive therapy and overt haematological disease and occur in females. This predilection may be enhanced with further alterations in hormonal status such as pregnancy and oral contraceptive use [197,382] taken from 20 days up to 10 years before presentation [259]. In the past, affected females were dissuaded from pregnancy for fear of an increased risk of hepatic venous thrombosis [259]. Activities of clotting factors are altered in pregnancy but no specific abnormality has been found in Budd–Chiari syndrome following pregnancy [197]. Out of 105 patients with Budd–Chiari syndrome, 15 presented between 4 days and 4 weeks post-partum and one further presented during pregnancy [197].

Clinical features include rapid abdominal distension due to accumulation of ascites which may be painless or associated with a vague discomfort. The liver typically is enlarged and occasionally tender. Serum liver biochemistry shows an elevation in level of alkaline phosphatase above that considered to reflect normal placental function. The serum level of transaminase is usually modestly raised but can become markedly elevated causing diagnostic confusion with viral hepatitis. Rarely, the clinical presentation may be indistinguishable from acute liver failure (see above). The protein content of the ascitic fluid typically is an exudate (>40 g/l) but can be variable and not helpful. Diagnosis in pregnancy is best achieved by ultrasonographic Doppler flow studies and percutaneous liver biopsy. Percutaneous hepatic venous catheterization is diagnostic should these techniques fail. Liver histology is not specific but characteristically shows outflow block with centrizonal venous congestion, haemorrhage, hepatocellular necrosis, dilatation of the sinusoids and central veins [74,208,367]. A search for abnormal haematological features should include tests for detecting antithrombin III deficiency, lupus anticoagulant, paroxysmal nocturnal haemoglobinuria and other haemolytic anaemias. Analysis of bone marrow may detect abnormalities in erythroid precursors and polycythaemia rubra vera.

Management of Budd–Chiari syndrome in pregnancy has been disappointing. The fetus is not affected directly; outcome depends on maternal well-being. The ascites often is resistant to therapy with diuretics and salt restriction. Safety of spironolactone has not been established in human pregnancy [230]. Only two of 16 patients gained relief of symptoms despite a variety of treatments including anticoagulation, re-infusion of ascites and surgery involving portocaval, splenorenal or mesocaval shunts. Maternal mortality with surgical intervention was 50 per cent [197].

In general the prognosis for pregnancy is poor [350]. However, individual cases have been reported without maternal complications despite a mesocaval and cavo-atrial shunt and intrauterine death in the sixth month [173]. Five successful pregnancies following Budd–Chiari syndrome have been reported up to 1984 [173,295,386]. One occurred 2 years after developing Budd–Chiari syndrome attributed to oral contraceptive therapy. Two consecutive pregnancies followed 3 and 4 years after developing the syndrome in association with polycythaemia rubra vera [386]. Successful pregnancies have been reported following grafting (see above) but there is a moderately high chance of recurrent veno-occlusion even with anticoagulant therapy. Oral contraceptive drugs are contraindicated following grafting because the coagulation disorder remains.

Congenital disorders of metabolism of bilirubin and lipids

The hyperbilirubinaemias are relatively benign conditions characterized by persistent elevation in levels of serum bilirubin which is predominantly unconjugated (Gilbert's disease) or conjugated (Dubin–Johnson and Rotor's syndromes). The conjugated forms characteristically have bilirubinuria and deposition of dark, granular pigment in hepatocytes [94]. The patient typically is symptomless. Jaundice and dark urine may be noticed with excess alcohol, stress, fasting, exercise, oral contraceptive therapy and pregnancy [61,94,329].

The underlying mechanisms are not fully understood. The Dubin–Johnson syndrome is believed to relate to a functional inability to excrete organic ions including conjugated bilirubin, and certain dyes and porphyrins [15].

The only untoward effect in pregnancy is aggravation of jaundice [15] in up to half the women [329]. Fetal outcome is good. An unconjugated hyperbilirubinaemia has been described in the neonate of a mother with Dubin–Johnson syndrome [65] but there is no specific risk of kernicterus [229]. The syndrome has been implicated as a cause of fetal death in some [413], but not all [15] cases of Dubin–Johnson syndrome. The main concern in obstetric practice is the differential diagnosis from other causes of cholestasis and jaundice in pregnancy, especially IHCP, biliary disease and viral hepatitis which may have implications for the fetus and mother. Dubin–Johnson syndrome, unlike IHCP and many other causes of cholestasis, is not associated with pruritus and the serum alkaline phosphatase is within the normal range for pregnancy [61]. Haemolytic anaemias, including that in Wilson's disease, and gallstones should be excluded.

Hepatic steatosis has been described in many defects in fatty acid metabolism. Physiological alterations of fatty acid oxidation may precipitate carnitine deficiency in susceptible pregnant women. Some authorities suggest similar mechanisms may be involved in the pathogenesis of AFLP [321] but more studies are required.

Inflammatory bowel disease and the liver

Abnormal liver function tests, histological and radiological changes primarily affecting the biliary tract are common in ulcerative colitis and Crohn's disease. Surgical and post-mortem liver specimens show histological abnormalities in 50–95 per cent. The hepatic abnormalities do not seem to correlate with severity of inflammatory bowel disease. Symptomless patients may have significant sclerosing cholangitis and cholangiocarcinoma. Associations with the HLA system have been described but pathogenetic mechanisms remain obscure. There are no specific reports relating to outcome in pregnancy.

Acute porphyria (see also Chapter 15)

Single case reports have shown variable hepatic dysfunction and outcome, including uncomplicated consecutive pregnancies [187,254,365].

Hepatic abscess

Amoebic abscess presenting in pregnancy is rare [69,79,259a,274,389] but outcome can be poor because the diagnosis is easily overlooked until catastrophic rupture. Presentation typically is in the third trimester or puerperium [274,389]. Clinical features are non-specific with abdominal discomfort, occasional fever or pulmonary features such as pain, pleural effusion and an elevated right diaphragm [259a]. Rupture is common in late pregnancy and the puerperium [274]. Diagnosis is often late. Six of seven cases reviewed in one series [259a] were diagnosed only at laparotomy for suspected appendicitis. Survival has improved significantly with earlier diagnosis using ultrasonographic techniques and effective antimicrobial agents such as metronidazole.

A strongly positive complement fixation test is diagnostic. For reasons which remain unclear, pregnant patients with amoebiasis do not invariably have elevated serum levels of immunoglobulins [3]. Ultrasonographic analysis can also sometimes differentiate between a pyogenic abscess and a cyst due to *Echinococcus granulosus* (hydatid cyst).

Hydatid disease must be excluded prior to surgical manipulation. Aspiration of a hydatid cyst is contraindicated because dissemination of daughter scolices can prove fatal.

Polycystic liver disease

Polycystic liver disease shows an autosomal dominant inheritance and is found most often in multiparous women with concurrence of renal cysts [118]. Pregnant patients may present with abdominal pain due to enlargement of the cysts and infection and hepatomegaly. Several factors, including age, female sex, pregnancy and the degree of renal involvement and functional impairment may modify the expression of hepatic cystic disease [99]. Differential diagnosis of an enlarged liver includes polycystic liver disease and congenital hepatic fibrosis.

Hepatic tumours

ORAL CONTRACEPTIVE STEROIDS AND THE LIVER

A variety of benign and malignant hepatic lesions have been found more commonly in users than non-users of oral contraceptive steroids. Hepatic adenoma and follicular nodular hyperplasia are rare but recognized associations [326]. Development of hepatic adenomata was first linked to oral contraceptive use in 1973 [22]. This tumour has become more common since the dramatic rise in consumption of oral contraceptive steroids [76]. Overwhelming evidence for this association is available from controlled case studies. The relative risk after 5 years of oral contraceptive therapy has been estimated at between 100–500 times that of non-users [276]. Importantly, regression of the lesion follows cessation of therapy.

In pregnancy, the main concern is rupture of this very vascular tumour [192]. In the Confidential Enquiries Report on Maternal Deaths for England and Wales between 1979 and 1981 [86] one death occurred post-partum from haemoperitoneum due to a ruptured benign hepatic tumour. Successful pregnancy has been reported following partial hepatectomy for removal of multiple adenomata [20] (see hepatic rupture above).

PRIMARY LIVER CANCER (HEPATOCELLULAR CARCINOMA, HEPATOMA)

This is also linked with oral contraceptive use [276]. The number of cases in young women has risen since 1970 in line with rising use of oral contraceptive therapy [196]. One series from London reported that 18 to 26 white women aged under 50 years with tumour arising in a non-cirrhotic liver had used oral contraceptive steroids for a median of 8 years [276]. Short-term use below 8 years was not associated with an increased risk of tumour development. The risk increased 4.4-fold in users beyond 8 years and 7.2-fold when hepatitis B infection was excluded. These risks are significant but much less than for development of hepatic adenoma [276]. Other confounding factors include hepatitis B virus and smoking. High dose oestrogen (e.g. mestranol >50 μg) has been implicated in earlier studies but seven of the 17 women in the London survey had taken low dose oestrogen (<30 μg daily) [276]. Rarely, primary liver cancer may present in pregnancy and this can be associated with rapid growth of the tumour [328]. Some adenomata show histological features of focal nodular hyperplasia and malignant change. This interrelation between hepatic adenoma, focal nodular hyperplasia and carcinoma [76,203] casts doubt on their benign classification.

The prognosis for the mother with primary liver cancer is abysmal. No survivors have been reported following presentation in pregnancy and few pregnancies resulted in a live infant [328]. The clinical findings are similar to those without pregnancy. Most cases with cirrhosis show a marked elevation in serum level of α fetoprotein. The main differential diagnosis is from treatable causes of a rapidly expanding mass such as benign hepatic tumours requiring resection, hepatic abscess (see above) and metastatic malignancy. Serological tests should include screening for hepatitis B and C and an amoebic complement fixation test. Serum levels of carcino-embryonic antigen (CEA) and β human chorionic gonadotropin (bHCG) may be raised causing confusion with gestational trophoblastic disease (choriocarcinoma) [300] (see below).

Cholangiocarcinoma is very rare and the prognosis poor. Single case reports document presentation in pregnancy [96,273]. Clinically, the tumour presents with signs of extrahepatic cholestasis and pruritus. The main differential diagnosis is from the common causes of bile duct obstruction (see below), intrahepatic cholestasis, PBC and pancreatic abnormalities.

METASTATIC TROPHOBLASTIC DISEASE

Elevated or rising titres of serum and urinary bHCG after evacuation of a hydatidiform mole or antecedent pregnancy indicate residual functional trophoblastic tissue and, possibly, malignant transformation to gestational trophoblastic disease (choriocarcinoma) [139,172,277]. Patients with hepatic metastases from gestational trophoblastic disease are classified as high risk with a grave prognosis [19,145,403]. Overall survival in the poor prognosis category is 72 per cent but falls to 33 per cent with liver metastases [19]. In a study from North Carolina, USA, 15 of 126 women (12 per cent) followed with gestational trophoblastic disease between 1966 and 1980 had liver metastases from a previous hydatidiform mole (seven cases), a previous full-term delivery (six) and presumed aborted pregnancy (two) [19]. Similar findings were reported from Texas [134] and Hong Kong [403]. Survival in the American studies [19,134] was <40 per cent despite use of a modified Bagshawe regimen of multi-agent chemotherapy and sublethal hepatic irradiation [275]. The majority with hepatic metastases had other risk factors associated with a poor prognosis such as a previous term pregnancy [134], multiple sites and high titres (>40 000 IU/l) of bHCG in serum and urine [19]. More optimistic results were published from Hong Kong [403]. Complete remission was achieved in seven of 10 patients following vigourous multi-agent chemotherapy. Partial remission was achieved in a further two who were changed to etoposide following resistance to the modified Bagshawe regimen. Improved results were attributed to aggressive and flexible chemotherapy regimes. Interestingly, these patients also had additional risk factors but in only two did their metastases arise from a previous full-term pregnancy [403].

Previous reports have stressed that hepatic, gastrointestinal and splenic haemorrhage [387] are the most significant complications of liver metastases in gestational trophoblastic disease [210]. Haemorrhage was not common in the above studies [19,403], and seems amenable to embolization. Some authors recommended prophylactic irradiation to the liver [145]. The doses used were sublethal but not tumoricidal. No controlled trials have been carried out to prove the efficacy of sublethal irradiation in such patients [145]. Irradiation to the liver may result in enhanced hepatotoxicity in the presence of chemotherapeutic agents [19]. Other therapies tried for hepatic metastases have included embolization, surgical resection and regional perfusion with chemotherapeutic agents but with variable results [19]. Future approaches aim to improve delineation of hepatic metastases which place the patient into the high risk category and affect the choice of chemotherapy [19,406]. The superiority of individual radiographic techniques for visualization of hepatic metastases remains undecided. Ultrasonography for tissue characterization is very useful [406] although some lesions are very diffuse and only visualized by hepatic arteriography [403] and CT scanning.

Gestational trophoblastic disease believed to arise from abdominal pregnancy migrating to the liver (primary choriocarcinoma) has been reported [151]. Differentiation from primary hepatocellular carcinoma is difficult due to overlapping histological features and elevated levels of bHCG documented in up to 17 per cent of cases of primary liver cancer [300].

Gallbladder and biliary tract

Anatomy and physiology

Gallbladder size increases through pregnancy [21] and residual and fasting volumes are increased in late pregnancy [348]. Results of dynamic studies remain controversial. Rates of contraction and emptying measured by ultrasonographic imaging were similar to those of non-pregnant controls [303]. Gallbladder emptying was impaired in the luteal phase of the ovulatory cycle in one study [278] but was considered normal by others [100]. Oral contraceptive users may have normal gallbladder volumes and emptying [45] or increased fasting volumes on ultrasonographic imaging after a liquid meal [700]. The mean diameter of the common bile duct is increased through pregnancy compared to non-pregnant females [303] but this is not invariable [257]. The relaxant action of progestogens on smooth muscle does not correlate with early dysfunction because serum progestogens rise significantly only after the first trimester. Oestrogens may impair water absorption by the gallbladder by inhibiting the sodium–potassium adenosine triphosphatase (ATPase) pump [45,257]. In primates, oestriol can effect a dose-dependent reduction in volume of bile [257].

The United States Food and Drugs Safety Administration (FDA) require information on the increased risks of gallbladder disease be included with instructions to users of oral contraceptive steroids [111]. In Australia, a large case controlled study was conducted [327] on the interrelation between oral contraceptive steroids, pregnancy and gallbladder disease. Two hundred women with newly diagnosed gallstones based on ultrasonographic analysis were case matched with women with suspected, but unproven, cholelithiasis and healthy controls. The risk of developing gallstones rose with parity only in young women and declined with rising age at first pregnancy. There was a dose–response relation between the relative risk of developing gallstones and exposure to pregnancy in the young patient [327]. A subpopulation of women seem susceptible to early development of gallstones after exposure to oral contraceptive steroids and pregnancy. The mean duration of oral contraceptive exposure for women with gallstones (<1 year) was lower than for healthy controls indicating that the increase in relative risk was of short duration. The rate of development of cholelithiasis fell with increasing duration of contraceptive use. These findings may explain the significant risk found only in short-term follow-up of pregnant women and oral contraceptive users. The authors concluded that the degree, rather than period, of exposure to oestrogen increased significantly the risk of developing gallstones. The increased risk seen in subsequent pregnancies may be related to 'oestrogenic shift'. Links with oestrogens include the finding of elevated levels of urinary oestrone in women with gallstones [327] and the statistical correlation between vomiting in pregnancy, gallbladder disease and a known intolerance to oral contraceptive steroids. The hormonal load on the liver in early pregnancy may be similar to that with oral contraceptive steroids [178].

Cholesterol cholelithiasis

Cholesterol gallstones are common in the West and found in women more often than men [29] and in users of oral contraceptive steroids. The sex difference commences at the menarche and remains throughout reproductive life. Other established risk factors include obesity, gastrointestinal disorders with malabsorption of bile salts such as Crohn's disease and small bowel resection, liver diseases and diabetes mellitus. The impact of pregnancy and parity remains unresolved by the controversial results on biliary physiology.

A prerequisite for stone formation includes the hepatic secretion of lithogenic bile [100]. In the non-pregnant female when compared with the male there is a reduction in total bile acid pool, in particular for chenodeoxycholic acid (CDCA). In users of oral contraceptive steroids the ratio of cholate to CDCA falls rendering the bile more saturated — more lithogenic [194,382]. In the second and third trimesters there is a progressive decrease in the size of the CDCA, but not cholic acid, pool. As the overall rate of cholesterol secretion is unchanged, its concentration relative to the diminishing size of the bile acid pool is increased, rendering the bile more lithogenic [193,382]. Oestrogens and progestogens have marked, different effects on metabolism of bile salts, cholesterol and biliary lipids, at least in the rat [354]. Ethinyl oestradiol causes an increase in cholesterol content within the liver but decreases the secretion of bile salts [77]. Progesterone increases the rate of esterification, but not synthesis, of cholesterol and an increase in bile salt-independent bile secretion. The net effect is to increase saturation of the bile with cholesterol [354,382].

Cholelithiasis in pregnancy

Gallbladder disease in pregnancy is the most common non-obstetric condition requiring surgery after acute appendicitis [407]. Acute cholecystitis requiring surgery and cholecystectomy have been reported in around one in 1000 deliveries [163,186, 407]. Detection during pregnancy of symptomless gallstones by ultrasonography has varied between 2.5 (normal for non-pregnant young females) and 11.3 per cent [56,398] but was not influenced by gestation. Echogenic bile — 'biliary sludge' — was detected in 36 per cent of pregnant women serially examined using ultrasonography [21]. Gallstones were seen to develop at 37 weeks following echogenic bile at 31 weeks [21]. The variable literature reflects biased reporting, variation in equipment and user expertise, and the prevalence of obesity and parity of the population sampled [348,398].

The classical presentation is with pain in the right upper quadrant which may radiate through to the back [407]. Nausea and vomiting are frequent but weight loss, intolerance to fatty food and fever are uncommon. The gallbladder usually is not palpable [163,407]. A past medical history may suggest gallbladder disease. The differential diagnosis of acute cholecystitis is wide and includes other causes of cholestatic jaundice such as viral hepatitis, alcoholic hepatitis, acute pyelonephritis and other causes of infection, including AIDS.

Thickening of the gallbladder wall in severe pre-eclampsia probably reflects the marked hypoalbuminaemia and should not be mistaken for an attack of cholecystitis [119]. Cirrhosis and IHCP (see above) are associated with cholelithiasis.

MANAGEMENT

The role of routine screening for gallstones and management of the symptomless patient remains controversial [56,348]. Management of acute cholecystitis and biliary obstruction is the same as that in the non-pregnant patient. General measures are bed rest, withdrawal of oral feeding, rehydration with intravenous fluids and antibiotics which concentrate in bile. Detection of stones in the common bile duct is more difficult than those in the gallbladder [238]. Ultrasonography is not helpful for determining the state of the papilla of Vater and the presence of a biliary stricture. Coexisting pancreatitis may be overlooked by obscuring gas from a small bowel ileus [159]. The biliary tree can be outlined using a technetium^{99}-IDA (iododiethylacetic acid) scan with minimal irradiation to the fetus [159]. The use of endoscopic retrograde cholecystopancreatography and percutaneous transhepatic cholecystography are not justified if the fetus cannot be shielded from the significant doses of irradiation which are necessary [18]. A film-badge should be placed near the abdomen to monitor the exposure. Preference should be given to pre- and peri-operative ultrasonographic analysis. Fibre-optic endoscopic cannulation with retrieval of stones may be possible [18]. Laparoscopic cholecystectomy is contraindicated because of risks of bleeding and the enlarged uterus. Some authors [159] recommend delaying cholecystectomy until after delivery but recurrent attacks are common [163,407].

Medical management may be less successful post-partum and there is an increase in post-operative complications such as deep venous thrombosis [407]. Fetal outcome [159,407] is optimal for surgery carried out in the second trimester. This timing coincides with less risk from spontaneous abortion and before the uterus is sufficiently large to displace the liver significantly [159,407]. Clinical and biochemical evidence of pancreatitis is common especially with stones in the common bile duct [159]. The risk of maternal and fetal mortality rises significantly when cholelithiasis is associated with pancreatitis complicated by pseudocyst [297] (see below).

Stones in the common bile duct may be painless and jaundice in pregnancy is uncommon. The patient may develop a high fever, rigors and a polymorphonuclear leucocytosis due to cholangitis [407]. Surgical intervention is obligatory for large duct obstruction to avoid recurrent attacks and other complications including cholangitis, pancreatitis, and empyema of the gallbladder. Rarely, biliary obstruction may be due to cholangiocarcinoma (see above) or *Clonorchis sinensis* in patients from the Far East. Management is the same as for non-pregnant individuals. HIV infection is associated with acalculous cholangitis and large duct dilatation.

Bile acid therapy with chenodeoxycholic acid, ursocholic acid and their congeners which can dissolve cholesterol gallstones, is contraindicated in pregnancy [287]. Bile acids cross the placenta. Chenodeoxycholic acid has been linked to liver toxicity and teratogenicity in animals [287]. Lithotrypsy is contraindicated in pregnancy.

Pancreas

The normal range for serum amylase is wide and its behaviour in normal pregnancy remains controversial [122,185,356]. Amylase is secreted by the pancreas, salivary, sweat and lactating mammary glands [122]. Production by the fallopian tube accounts for the very elevated serum levels found in a ruptured ectopic pregnancy [122].

A markedly elevated level of serum amylase remains the cornerstone for diagnosing pancreatitis. In pregnancy this may be difficult because the values in serum of amylase, its ratio to creatinine and lipases may be misleadingly low, even normal, in the first trimester with severe pancreatitis. The high levels of serum triglycerides found in late pregnancy are associated with pancreatitis and can interfere with amylase levels. The renal clearances of amylase and creatinine are elevated in pregnancy. Whether the use of ratios is superior to a single elevated level of serum amylase, remains debatable. The level in serum lipase rises in parallel with amylase and may be of use in the diagnosis of acute pancreatitis in pregnancy but information is lacking.

Cystic fibrosis which can affect the pancreas in pregnancy is described in Chapter 1.

Acute pancreatitis

This is an uncommon cause of abdominal pain in pregnancy and has been reported in less than one in 1000 pregnancies [62,184,397]. Reported series are biased towards the severe end of the spectrum. Pregnancy and the post-partum period do not precipitate or protect against severe pancreatitis. Fewer cases occurred post-partum than at any time during pregnancy [205].

The morbidity and mortality from acute pancreatitis remains high regardless of pregnancy. In early surveys, maternal deaths were as high as 20 per cent [219,268] with neonatal losses in up to a half [268,397]. Series after 1980 suggest that maternal mortalities are similar to the non-pregnant and fetal losses are around 10 per cent [205].

The pathogenetic mechanisms causing acute pancreatitis are poorly understood except for a link with gallstones. There is no specific association between pancreatitis and pregnancy. Suggested but unproven mechanisms which predispose a pregnant patient to pancreatitis, excepting gallstones, include the relaxant effect of progestogens leading to atony of the biliary tract, bile stasis in the duodenum and reflux [184,382]. Extreme elevations in abdominal pressure from vomiting in toxaemia may promote a rise in intrapancreatic pressure, rupture of the ducts and release of enzymes [32]. These suggestions lack scientific data and ignore the confounding influence of diuretic therapies in the treatment of hypertension, which predisposes to pancreatitis [230]. Pancreatitis in the non-pregnant patient can be associated with an underlying hypertriglyceridaemia. Whether the elevation in triglycerides which occurs in normal pregnancy as an effect of oestrogens, predisposes women to pancreatitis remains an attractive possibility. Alternatively, pregnancy and oral contraceptive steroids may unmask an underlying lipid disorder associated with high levels of very low density lipoproteins (VLDL) and chylomicrons (type V hyperlipidaemia) or type I hyperlipidaemia [357].

Primary hyperparathyroidism remains a rare cause of pancreatitis during pregnancy, although over 50 cases have been reported [369]. Other uncommon associations are hyperfunctioning parathyroid carcinoma [158], alcoholism [62,248], thiazides and corticosteroids and infections such as mumps [32,376] and acute fatty liver [292] (see above).

CLINICAL PRESENTATION

Typically, this occurs in late pregnancy, possibly coinciding with the peak in serum levels of triglycerides. Acute pancreatitis can occur at any time and there seems to be no influence from maternal parity or age [205]. Abdominal pain is maximal in the epigastrum, often constant (not colicky) and may radiate through to the back. Pain is not invariable; up to one-quarter may present with only nausea and vomiting [62]. Physical examination may be unhelpful.

Severe, haemorrhagic pancreatitis presents with profound shock, hypotension and marked hypovolaemia. Other features include ecchymoses, pleural effusions, hypoxia due to adult respiratory distress syndrome and milky ascites. A paralytic ileus and enlarged uterus may obscure images on ultrasonographic analysis. The detection of gallstones may point to underlying pancreatitis. A markedly elevated level of amylase in various body fluids, including a pleural effusion may persist after serum levels return to normal.

Pancreatitis associated with gallstones in the common bile duct usually is associated with an elevation in serum alkaline phosphatase beyond that attributed to placental growth, and in elevated γ-glutamyl transpeptidase levels.

The differential diagnosis in pregnancy includes all other causes of abdominal pain, nausea and vomiting. This wide list includes acute appendicitis, peptic ulceration, hyperemesis gravidarum, pre-eclamptic toxaemia, renal infections and many liver disorders such as hepatitis, abscess and cholecystitis. The differential from a ruptured ectopic pregnancy and spleen may be difficult especially with bloody ascites. Severe, acute pancreatitis occurring in the puerperium may pose diagnostic problems leading to a delay in diagnosis and poor outcome for the mother [141].

MANAGEMENT

The aims are to induce a state of visceral rest and prevent complications. Nasogastric suction is traditional and comforting but lacks evidence for efficacy and may promote elevations in serum amylase and delay the return of bowel sounds. There are no specific therapies. Various agents have been used as inhibitors of pancreatic secretion including anticholinergic agents, glucagon, corticosteroids, prostaglandins, vasopressin, trypsin inhibitors and ε aminocaproic acid but results of trials are conflicting or absent. The H_2 antagonists inhibit the acid stimulus to pancreatic secretion but have no demonstrable effect on biliary and pancreatic secretion.

Total parenteral nutrition has been used successfully in a malnourished pregnant woman with alcoholism. Therapy was maintained for 83 days prior to elective caesarean section at 36 weeks of gestation with delivery of a 2.12 kg baby [127]. Total parenteral nutrition has been used in the third trimester for acute pancreatitis complicated by a pseudocyst and marked hypoalbuminaemia associated with intrauterine growth retardation [355].

A major consideration includes the prevention and management of complications. Hypovolaemia may be marked. Strict attention should be paid to central monitoring of fluid balance and replacement with colloid and crystalloid solutions. Other considerations include electrolyte imbalance with hypocalcaemia and hypomagnesaemia, carbohydrate intolerance, renal failure, fat necrosis, haemorrhage including DIC, venous thrombosis, ascites, peritonitis, intestinal damage, jaundice and hepatic and metabolic encephalopathies. Pulmonary oedema, pleural effusions and respiratory distress syndromes may produce profound hypoxia requiring assisted respiratory support and oxygen therapy.

In the majority of uncomplicated cases in pregnancy, the disease settles with conservative management. Pregnancy poses additional problems because the use of many of the therapeutic agents remains controversial. Termination of pregnancy is rarely indicated and does not seem to influence maternal outcome [397]. Elective induction of labour in the third trimester has been recommended [184, 397] but remains controversial and offers no guarantee of cessation of the pathological state after delivery.

The optimal timing for surgery for gallstones associated with pancreatitis is in the second trimester. Surgery is best performed during the same hospital admission but after the first attack has settled. Recurrent attacks of acute cholecystitis, biliary colic and pancreatitis are common.

Malignancies

In a 3-year survey from the CDC in the USA, 2.8 per cent of patients with malignancies in the reproductive age group had carcinoma of the pancreas [91]. There are reports in pregnancy and the puerperium of pancreatic adenocarcinoma [121], mucin-secreting cystadenoma and adenocarcinoma [344] and insulinoma [120]. The outcome of these malignant tumours is poor regardless of pregnancy. In insulinoma, early recognition of hypoglycaemia, neurological features and the finding of elevated levels of insulin, including C peptide, has led to early diagnosis, surgery and successful outcome in pregnancy [120].

Acknowledgement

This chapter is dedicated to Sir Francis Avery Jones. Dr Fagan is supported by fellowships from the Wellcome Trust and British Digestive Foundation, London, UK and Abbott Laboratories, Chicago, USA.

References

1 Aarnoudse JG, Houthoff HJ *et al*. A syndrome of liver damage and intravascular coagulation in the last trimester of normotensive pregnancy. A clinical and histopathological study. *British Journal of Obstetrics and Gynaecology* 1986; **93**: 145–55.

2 Abercrombie J. Case of haemorrhage of the liver. *London Medical Gazette* 1844; **34**: 792.

3 Abioye AA & Edington GM. Prevalence of amoebiasis at autopsy in Ibadan. *Transactions of the Royal Society of Tropical Medicine and Hygiene* 1972; **66**: 754–63.

4 Adler SP, Chandrika T *et al*. Cytomegalovirus infections in the neonate acquired by blood transfusion. *Paediatric Infectious Diseases* 1982; **2**: 114–18.

5 Adlercreutz H, Tikkanen MJ *et al*. Recurrent jaundice in pregnancy. IV. Quantitative determination of urinary and biliary estrogens, including studies in pruritus gravidarum. *Journal of Clinical Endocrinology and Metabolism* 1974; **38**: 51–7.

6 Ahlfeld F. *Berichte und arbeiten aus des gebutsflich-gynaekologischen Klinik 3er Giessen 1881–1882*. Grunow, Leipzig 1883, p. 148.

7 Ahrens EH & Payne MA. Primary biliary cirrhosis. *Medicine (Baltimore)* 1950; **29**: 299–364.

8 Akhtar KAK & Akhtar MA. Viral hepatitis in pregnancy. *Journal of the Pakistan Medical Association (Karachi)* 1979; **29**: 31–5.

9 Alter HJ & Dienstag JL. Non-A, non-B hepatitis: evolving epidemiologic and clinical perspectives. *Seminars in Liver Disease* 1986; **6**: 67–81.

10 Alter MJ, Hadler SC *et al*. The changing epidemiology of hepatitis B in the United States. Need for alternative vaccination strategies. *Journal of the American Medical Association* 1990; **263**: 1218–22.

11 Amon E, Allen SR *et al*. Acute fatty liver of pregnancy associated with preeclampsia: management of hepatic failure with postpartum liver transplantation. *American Journal of Perinatology* 1991; **8**: 278–9.

12 Anderson MG & Murray-Lyon IM. Natural history of

the chronic carrier. *Gut* 1985; **26**: 848–60.
13 Aneckstein AE & Weingold AD. Chlorthiazide-induced hepatic coma in pregnancy. *American Journal of Obstetrics and Gynecology* 1966; **95**: 136–7.
14 Antia FP, Bharadwaj TP *et al*. Liver in normal pregnancy, pre-eclampsia and eclampsia. *Lancet* 1958; **ii**: 776–8.
15 Arias IM. Inheritable and congenital hyperbilirubinemia. *New England Journal of Medicine* 1971; **285**: 1416–21.
16 Aziz S, Merrell RC *et al*. Spontaneous hepatic hemorrhage during pregnancy. *American Journal of Surgery* 1983; **146**: 680–2.
17 Baker VV & Cefalo RC. Fulminant hepatic failure in the third trimester of pregnancy. A case report. *Journal of Reproductive Medicine* 1985; **30**: 229–31.
18 Bar-Meir S & Rotmensch S. Investigation of obstructive jaundice by ultra-thin-caliber endoscope: a new technique for potential use in pregnancy. *American Journal of Obstetrics and Gynecology* 1984; **150**: 1003–4.
19 Barnard DE, Woodward KT *et al*. Hepatic metastases of choriocarcinoma: a report of 15 patients. *Gynecological Oncology* 1986; **25**: 73–83.
20 Barnes AD, Harder E *et al*. Successful pregnancy following partial hepatectomy for removal of hepatocellular adenomas. *American Journal of Obstetrics and Gynecology* 1984; **150**: 998.
21 Bartoli E, Calonaci N *et al*. Ultrasonography of the gallbladder in pregnancy. *Gastrointestinal Radiology* 1984; **9**: 35–8.
22 Baum JK, Holz F *et al*. Possible association between benign hepatomas and oral contraceptives. *Lancet* 1973; **ii**: 926–9.
23 Beasley RP. Hepatitis B virus as the etiologic agent in hepatocellular carcinoma-epidemiologic considerations. *Hepatology* 1982: **2** (suppl): 21S–6S.
24 Beasley RP, Hwang L-Y *et al*. Efficacy of hepatitis B immune globulin (HBIG) for prevention of perinatal transmission of the HBV carrier state: final report of a randomized, double-blind, placebo-controlled trial. *Hepatology* 1983; **3**: 135–41.
25 Beasley RP, Hwang L-Y *et al*. Prevention of perinatally transmitted hepatitis B virus infections with hepatitis B immune globulin and hepatitis B vaccine. *Lancet* 1983; **ii**: 1099–102.
26 Beath SV, Boxall EH *et al*. Fulminant hepatitis B in infants born to anti-HBe hepatitis B carrier mothers. *British Medical Journal* 1992; **304**: 1167–70.
27 Belabbes EH, Bouguermouh A *et al*. Epidemic non-A, non-B viral hepatitis in Algeria: strong evidence for its spreading by water. *Journal of Medical Virology* 1985; **16**: 257–63.
28 Benhamou JP & Lebrec D. Non-cirrhotic intrahepatic portal hypertension in adults. *Clinics in Gastroenterology* 1985; **14**: 21–31.
29 Bennett NMcK, Lehmann NI *et al*. Viral hepatitis and intrahepatic cholestasis of pregnancy. *Australian and New Zealand Journal of Medicine* 1979; **9**: 54–7.
30 Bennion LJ & Grundy SM. Risk factors for the development of cholelithiasis in man (second of two parts). *New England Journal of Medicine* 1978; **299**: 1221–7.
31 Berg B, Helm G *et al*. Cholestasis of pregnancy. Clinical and laboratory studies. *Acta Obstetrica Gynecologica Scandinavica* 1986; **65**: 107–3.
32 Berk JE, Smith BH *et al*. Pregnancy pancreatitis. *American Journal of Gastroenterology* 1971; **56**: 216–26.
33 Bernstein RB, Novy MJ *et al*. Bilirubin metabolism in the fetus. *Journal of Clinical Investigation* 1969; **48**: 1678–88.
34 Bernuau J, Degott C *et al*. Non-fatal acute fatty liver of pregnancy. *Gut* 1983; **24**: 340–4.
35 Best JM. Congenital cytomegalovirus infection. *British Medical Journal* 1987; **294**: 1440–1.
36 Bihl JH. Congenital cytomegalovirus infection. *British Medical Journal* 1959; **78**: 1182–8.
37 Biller J, Swiontoniowski M *et al*. Successful pregnancy in Wilson's disease: a case report and review of the literature. *European Neurology* 1985; **24**: 306–9.
38 Bis KA & Waxman B. Rupture of the liver associated with pregnancy: A review of the literature and report of two cases. *Obstetrical and Gynecological Survey* 1976; **31**: 763–73.
39 Bogomolski-Yahalom V, Granot E *et al*. Prevalence of HBsAg carriers in native and immigrant pregnant female populations in Israel and passive/active vaccination against HBV of newborns at risk. *Journal of Medical Virology* 1991; **34**: 217–22.
40 Borhanmanesh F, Haghighi P *et al*. Viral hepatitis during pregnancy: severity and effect on gestation. *Gastroenterology* 1973; **64**: 304–8.
41 Botha JF, Ritchie MJ *et al*. Hepatitis B virus carrier state in black children in Ovamboland: role of perinatal and horizontal transmission. *Lancet* 1984; **i**: 1210–12.
42 Boxall EH, Flewett TH *et al*. Hepatitis B surface antigen in breast milk. *Lancet* 1974; **ii**: 1007–8.
43 Boxall EH & Tarlow MJ. Hepatitis B vaccine in the prevention of perinatally transmitted hepatitis B virus infections: initial report of a study in the West Midlands of England. *Journal of Medical Virology* 1986; **18**: 255–60.
44 Brandt P, Jespersen J *et al*. Post-partum haemolytic uraemic syndrome treated with antithrombin III. *Nephron* 1981; **27**: 15–18.
45 Braverman DZ, Johnson ML *et al*. Effects of pregnancy and contraceptive steroids on gallbladder function. *New England Journal of Medicine* 1980; **302**: 362–4.
46 Britton RC. Pregnancy and esophageal varices. *American Journal of Surgery* 1982; **4**: 421–5.
47 Britton WJ, Parsons C *et al*. Risk factors associated with hepatitis B infection in antenatal patients. *Australian and New Zealand Journal of Medicine* 1985; **15**: 641–4.
48 Brown KA & Lucey MR. Liver transplantation restores

female reproductive endocrine function. *Hepatology* 1991; **13**: 1255–7.

49 Burroughs AK, Seong NH *et al*. Idiopathic acute fatty liver of pregnancy in 12 patients. *Quarterly Journal of Medicine* 1982; **204**: 481–97.

50 Caporaso N, Del Vecchio-Blano *et al*. Delta infection: intrafamily spreading. In: Verme G, Bonino F & Rizzetto M. (eds) *Viral Hepatitis and Delta Infection*. Alan R. Liss, New York, 1983: 139–43.

51 Carman WF, Jacyna MR *et al*. Mutation preventing formation of hepatitis B e antigen in patients with chronic hepatitis B infection. *Lancet* 1989; **ii**: 588–91.

52 Carman WF, Zanetti AR *et al*. Vaccine-induced escape mutant of hepatitis B virus. *Lancet* 1990; **336**: 325–9.

53 Carne CA, Weller IVD *et al*. Impaired responsiveness of homosexual men with HIV antibodies to plasma derived hepatitis B vaccine. *British Medical Journal* 1987; **294**: 866–8.

54 Castaneda H, Garcia-Romero H *et al*. Hepatic haemorrhage in toxaemia of pregnancy. *American Journal of Obstetrics and Gynecology* 1970; **107**: 578–84.

55 Cheng YS. Pregnancy in liver cirrhosis and/or portal hypertension. *American Journal of Obstetrics and Gynecology* 1977; **128**: 812–22.

56 Chesson RR, Gallup DG *et al*. Ultrasonographic diagnosis of asymptomatic cholelithiasis in pregnancy. *Journal of Reproductive Medicine* 1985; **30**: 920–2.

57 Chiari H. Uber die Selbstandige Endophlebitis Obiterans der Haupstamme der Venae Hepaticae als Todesurache. *Beitrage zur Pathologischen Anatomie* 1899; **26**: 1–18.

58 Choo Q-L, Kuo G *et al*. Isolation of a cDNA clone derived from a blood-borne non-A, non-B viral hepatitis genome. *Science* 1989; **244**: 359–61.

59 Christie AB, Allam AA *et al*. Pregnancy hepatitis in Libya. *Lancet* 1976; **ii**: 827–9.

60 Chu SY, Buehler JW *et al*. Impact of the human immunodeficiency virus epidemic on mortality in women of reproductive age, United States. *Journal of the American Medical Association* 1990; **264**: 225–9.

61 Cohen L, Lewis C *et al*. Pregnancy oral contraceptives and chronic familial jaundice with predominantly conjugated hyperbilirubinemia (Dubin–Johnson syndrome). *Gastroenterology* 1972; **62**: 1182–90.

62 Corlett RC & Mishell DR. Pancreatitis in pregnancy. *American Journal of Obstetrics and Gynecology* 1972; **113**: 281–90.

63 Cossar JH & Reid D. Not all travellers need immunoglobulin for hepatitis A. *British Medical Journal* 1987; **294**: 1503.

64 Cossart YE, Hargreaves FD *et al*. Australia antigen in the human fetus. *American Journal of Diseases of Children* 1972; **123**: 376–8.

65 Cotton DB. Infantile hepatic cholestasis with maternal Dubin–Johnson syndrome. *Southern Medical Journal* 1984; **77**: 1213–14.

66 Coursaget P, Yvonnet B *et al*. Seven year study of hepatitis B vaccine efficacy in infants from an endemic area (Senegal). *Lancet* 1986; **ii**: 1143–5.

67 Coursaget P, Yvonnet B *et al*. Age and sex-related study of hepatitis B virus chronic carrier state in infants from an endemic area (Senegal). *Journal of Medical Virology* 1987; **22**: 1–5.

68 Covillo FV, Nyong AO *et al*. Budd–Chiari syndrome following pregnancy. *Missouri Medicine* 1984; **81**: 356–8.

69 Cowan DB, Houlton MC. Rupture of an amoebic liver abscess in pregnancy. A case report. *South African Medical Journal* 1978; **53**: 460–1.

70 Crosby ET. Obstetrical anaesthesia for patients with the syndrome of haemolysis, elevated liver enzymes and low platelets. *Canadian Journal of Anaesthesiology* 1991; **38**: 227–33.

71 Cundy TF, Butler J *et al*. Amenorrhoea in women with non-alcoholic chronic liver disease. *Gut* 1991; **32**: 202–6.

72 Cundy TF, O'Grady JG *et al*. Recovery of menstruation and pregnancy after liver transplantation. *Gut* 1990; **31**: 337–8.

73 Da Silva O, Hammerberg O *et al*. Fetal varicella syndrome. *Pediatric Infectious Disease Journal* 1990; **9**: 854–5.

74 Datta DV, Chhuttani PN *et al*. Clinical spectrum of Budd–Chiari syndrome in Chandigarh with particular reference to obstruction of intrahepatic portion of the inferior vena cava. *Gut* 1972; **13**: 372–8.

75 Davies MH, Wilkinson SP *et al*. Acute liver disease with encephalopathy and renal failure in late pregnancy and early puerperium, a study of fourteen patients. *British Journal of Obstetrics and Gynaecology* 1980; **87**: 1005–14.

76 Davis M, Portmann B *et al*. Histological evidence of carcinoma in a hepatic tumour associated with oral contraceptives. *British Medical Journal* 1975; **iv**: 496–9.

77 Davis RA & Kern F. Effects of ethinyl estradiol and phenobarbital on bile acid synthesis and biliary bile acid and cholesterol excretion. *Gastroenterology* 1976; **70**: 1130–5.

78 De Koning ND & Haagsma EB. Normalization of menstrual pattern after liver transplantation: consequences for contraception. *Digestion* 1990; **46**: 239–41.

79 De Silva K. Intraperitoneal rupture of an amoebic liver abscess in a pregnant woman at term. *Ceylon Medical Journal* 1970; **15**: 51–3.

80 de Swiet M. Some rare medical complications of pregnancy (editorial). *British Medical Journal* 1985; **290**: 2–4.

81 De Virgiliis S, Frau F *et al*. Perinatal hepatitis B virus detection by hepatitis B virus-DNA analysis. *Archives of Disease in Childhood* 1985; **60**: 56–8.

82 Deinhardt F & Zuckerman AJ. Against hepatitis B: a report on a WHO meeting on viral hepatitis in Europe. *Journal of Medical Virology* 1985; **17**: 209–17.

83 Delage G, Montplaisir S *et al*. Prevalence of hepatitis

B virus infection in pregnant women in the Montreal area. *Canadian Medical Association Journal* 1986; **134**: 897–901.

84 Delaphane D & Shulman ST. Immunoprophylaxis for infants born to HBsAg positive mothers. *Lancet* 1983; **ii**: 170–1.

85 Dentsch V, Rosenthal T *et al*. Budd–Chiari syndrome. Study of angiographic findings and remarks on etiology. *American Journal of Roentgenology* 1972; **116**: 430–9.

86 Department of Health and Social Security. *Report on Confidential Enquiries into Maternal Deaths in England and Wales 1979–1981*. Report on health and social subjects. HMSO, London, 1986: 29.

87 Department of Health and Social Security. *Report on Confidential Enquiries into Maternal Deaths in the United Kingdom 1986–1987*. HMSO, London, 1991: 1–161.

88 Deray G, le Hoang P *et al*. Oral contraceptives interaction with cyclosporin (letter). *Lancet* 1987; **i**: 158–9.

89 Derso A, Boxall EH *et al*. Transmission of HBsAg from mother to infant in four ethnic groups. *British Medical Journal* 1978; **i**: 949–52.

90 Dietzman DE, Madden DL *et al*. Lack of relationship between Down's syndrome and maternal exposure to Australia antigen. *American Journal of Diseases of Children* 1972; **124**: 195–7.

91 Donegan WL. Cancer and pregnancy. *Cancer* 1983; **33**: 194–214.

92 Dreifuss FE & McKinney WM. Wilson's disease (hepatolenticular degeneration) and pregnancy. *Journal of the American Medical Association* 1966; **195**: 960–2.

93 Drill VA. Benign cholestatic jaundice of pregnancy and benign cholestatic jaundice from oral contraceptives. *American Journal of Obstetrics and Gynecology* 1974; **119**: 165–74.

94 Dubin IM & Johnson FB. Chronic idiopathic jaundice with unidentified pigment in liver cells: new clinicopathologic entity with report of 12 cases. *Medicine (Baltimore)* 1954; **33**: 155–97.

95 Egley CC, Gutliph J *et al*. Severe hypoglycaemia associated with HELLP syndrome. *American Journal of Obstetrics and Gynecology* 1985; **152**: 576–7.

96 Egwuatu VE. Primary hepatocarcinoma in pregnancy. *Transactions of the Royal Society of Tropical Medicine and Hygiene* 1980; **74**: 793–4.

97 Ekberg H, Leyon J *et al*. Hepatic rupture secondary to pre-eclampsia — A report of a case treated conservatively. *Annales Chirurgiae et Gynaecologiae* 1984; **73**: 350–3.

98 Esteban JI, Genesca J *et al*. Immunoprophylaxis of perinatal transmission of the hepatitis B virus: efficacy of hepatitis B immune globulin and hepatitis B vaccine in a low-prevalence area. *Journal of Medical Virology* 1986; **18**: 381–91.

99 Everson GT. Hepatic cysts in autosomal dominant polycystic kidney disease (comment). *Mayo Clinics Proceedings* 1990; **65**: 933–42.

100 Everson GT, McKinley C *et al*. Gallbladder function in the human female: effect of the ovulatory cycle, pregnancy and contraceptive steroids. *Gastroenterology* 1982; **82**: 11–19.

101 Ewing CI & Davidson DC. Fatal hepatitis B in infant born to an HBsAg carrier with HBeAb. *Archives of Disease in Childhood* 1985; **60**: 265–7.

102 Fagan EA. Testing for hepatitis C. *British Medical Journal* 1991; **303**: 535–6.

103 Fagan EA. Hepatitis A to G and beyond. *British Journal of Hospital Medicine* 1992; **47**: 127–31.

104 Fagan EA & Eddleston AWLF. Hepatitis vaccination. *Clinics in Immunology and Allergy* 1985; **5**: 43–85.

105 Fagan EA, Partridge M *et al*. Review of hepatitis non-A, non-B: the potential hazards in dental care. *Oral Surgery, Oral Medicine, Oral Pathology* 1988; **65**: 167–71.

106 Fagan EA, Tolley P *et al*. Hepatitis B vaccine: immunogenicity and follow-up including two year booster doses in high-risk health care personnel in a London teaching hospital. *Journal of Medical Virology* 1987; **21**: 49–56.

107 Fagan EA & Williams R. Non-A, non-B hepatitis. *Seminars in Liver Disease* 1984; **4**: 314–35.

108 Fagan EA & Williams R. Serological responses to HBV infection. *Gut* 1986; **27**: 858–67.

109 Fagan EA & Williams R. Fulminant viral hepatitis. *British Medical Bulletin* 1990; **46**: 462–80.

110 Fair J, Klein AS *et al*. Intrapartum orthotopic liver transplantation with successful outcome of pregnancy. *Transplantation* 1990; **50**: 534–5.

111 Federal Register. US Department of Labor, Occupational Safety Health Administration. Occupational exposure to bloodborne pathogens: proposed rule and notice of hearing. *Federal Register* 1989; **54**: 23042–139.

112 Feliciano DV, Mattox KL *et al*. Management of 1000 consecutive cases of hepatic trauma (1979–1984). *Annals of Surgery* 1986; **204**: 438–45.

113 Foschini M, De Toni A *et al*. Prevention of perinatally transmitted hepatitis B virus infection by hepatitis B immunoglobulin immunoprophylaxis: an account of 201 newborn babies of hepatitis Bs antigen carrier mothers. *Journal of Pediatric Gastroenterology and Nutrition* 1985; **4**: 523–7.

114 Freund G & Arvan DA. Clinical biochemistry of pre-eclampsia and related liver diseases of pregnancy: a review. *Clinica Chimica Acta* 1990; **191**: 123–51.

115 Frezza M, Pozzato G *et al*. Reversal of intrahepatic cholestasis of pregnancy in women after high dose *S*-adenosyl-L-methionine. *Hepatology* 1984; **4**: 274–8.

116 Frosner GG, Papaevangelou G *et al*. Antibody against hepatitis A in seven European countries. I. Comparison of prevalence data in different age groups. *American Journal of Epidemiology* 1979; **110**: 63–9.

117 Furhoff AK & Hellstrom K. Jaundice in pregnancy. A follow-up study of the sera of women originally reported by I.Thorling. I: The pregnancies. *Acta Medica Scandinavica* 1973; **193**: 259–66.
118 Gabow PA, Johnson AM *et al*. Risk factors for the development of hepatic cysts in autosomal dominant polycystic kidney disease. *Hepatology* 1990; **11**: 1033–7.
119 Gadwood KA, Reynes CJ *et al*. Gallbladder wall thickening in preeclampsia. *Journal of the American Medical Association* 1985; **253**: 71–3.
120 Galun E, Ben-Yehuda A *et al*. Insulinoma complicating pregnancy: a case report and review of the literature. *American Journal of Obstetrics and Gynecology* 1986; **155**: 64–5.
121 Gamberella FR. Pancreatic carcinoma in pregnancy: a case report. *American Journal of Obstetrics and Gynecology* 1984; **149**: 15–17.
122 Garrison R. Amylase. *Emergency Medical Clinics of North America* 1986; **4**: 315–27.
123 Gelpi AP. Fatal hepatitis in Saudi Arabian women. *American Journal of Gastroenterology* 1970; **53**: 41–61.
124 Gelpi AP. Viral hepatitis complicating pregnancy: mortality trends in Saudi Arabia. *International Journal of Gynaecology and Obstetrics* 1979; **17**: 73–7.
125 Gerety RJ & Schweitzer IL. Viral hepatitis, type B during pregnancy, the neonatal period and infancy. *Journal of Pediatrics* 1977; **90**: 368–74.
126 Gimson AES, O'Grady J *et al*. Late-onset hepatic failure: clinical, serological and histological features. *Hepatology* 1986; **6**: 288–94.
127 Gineston JL, Capron JP *et al*. Prolonged total parenteral nutrition in a pregnant woman with acute pancreatitis. *Journal of Clinical Gastroenterology* 1984; **6**: 249–52.
128 Glynn LE. Relation of nutrition of hepatic disease and toxaemias of pregnancy. In: *Toxemias of Pregnancy, Human and Vetinary*. Blaskiston Co., CIBA Foundation Symposium, Philadelphia, 1950: 19 et seq.
129 Gonzalez GD, Rubel HR *et al*. Spontaneous hepatic rupture in pregnancy: management with hepatic artery ligation. *Southern Medical Journal* 1984; **77**: 242–5.
130 Goodlin RC. Acute fatty liver of pregnancy (letter). *Acta Obstetricia et Gynecologica Scandinavica* 1984; **63**: 379.
131 Goodlin RC. Preeclampsia as the great impostor. *American Journal of Obstetrics and Gynecology* 1991; **164**: 1577–80.
132 Goodlin RC, Anderson JC *et al*. Conservative treatment of liver hematoma in the postpartum period: a report of two cases. *Journal of Reproductive Medicine* 1985; **30**: 368–70.
133 Goodlin RC & Holdt D. Impending gestosis. *Obstetrics and Gynecology* 1981; **58**: 743–5.
134 Gordon AN, Gershenson DM *et al*. High risk metastatic gestational trophoblastic disease. *Obstetrics and Gynecology* 1985; **65**: 550–6.
135 Goudeau A, Yvonnet B *et al*. Lack of anti-HBc IgM in neonates with HBsAg carrier mothers argues against transplacental transmission of hepatitis B virus infection. *Lancet* 1983; **ii**: 1103–4.
136 Goyert GL, Bottoms SF *et al*. Anicteric presentation of fatal herpetic hepatitis in pregnancy. *Obstetrics and Gynecology* 1985; **65**: 585–8.
137 Greca FH, Coelho JC *et al*. Ultrasonographic diagnosis of spontaneous rupture of the liver in pregnancy. *Journal of Clinical Ultrasound* 1984; **12**: 515–16.
138 Greenfield C, Osidiana V *et al*. Perinatal transmission of hepatitis B virus in Kenya: its relation to the presence of serum HBV DNA and anti-HBe in the mother. *Journal of Medical Virology* 1986; **19**: 135–42.
139 Grumbine FC, Rosenshein NB *et al*. Management of liver metastasis from gestational trophoblastic neoplasia. *American Journal of Obstetrics and Gynecology* 1980; **137**: 959–61.
140 Gubernatis G, Pichlmayr R *et al*. Auxilliary partial orthotopic liver transplantation (APOLT) for fulminant hepatic failure: first successful case report. *World Journal of Surgery* 1991; **15**: 660–5; discussion 665–6.
141 Guth A, Ekoundzola JR *et al*. Acute pancreatitis in the puerperium. Diagnostic problems following Caesarean section. *Journal de Gynecologie Obstetrique et Biologie de la Reproduction (Paris)* 1985; **14**: 753–6.
142 Hadler SC, Francis DP *et al*. Long-term immunogenicity and efficacy of hepatitis B vaccine in homosexual men. *New England Journal of Medicine* 1986; **315**: 209–14.
143 Haemmerli VP. Jaundice during pregnancy. In: Schiff L (ed), *Diseases of the Liver*. JB Lippincott, Philadelphia, 1975: 1336–8.
144 Hague WM, Fenton DW *et al*. Acute fatty liver of pregnancy. *Journal of the Royal Society of Medicine* 1983; **76**: 652–61.
145 Hammond CB, Berchert L *et al*. Treatment of metastatic trophoblastic disease. Good and poor prognosis. *American Journal of Obstetrics and Gynecology* 1973; **115**: 451–7.
146 Hancock KW. The Budd–Chiari syndrome in pregnancy. *Journal of Obstetrics and Gynaecology of the British Commonwealth* 1968; **75**: 746–8.
147 Harpey JP, Jaudon MC *et al*. Cutis laxa and low serum zinc antenatal exposure to penicillamine (letter). *Lancet* 1983; **ii**: 858.
148 Harrison RA & Araujo JG. Aetiology of acute fatty liver of pregnancy (letter). *Journal of the Royal Society of Medicine* 1983; **76**: 1079.
149 Harrison TJ & Zuckerman AJ. Variants of hepatitis B virus. *Vox Sanguinis* 1992; **63**: 161–7.
150 Hatfield AK, Stein JH *et al*. Idiopathic acute fatty liver of pregnancy. Death from extrahepatic manifestations. *American Journal of Digestive Diseases* 1972; **17**: 167–78.
151 Heaton GE, Matthews TH *et al*. Malignant tropho-

blastic tumors with massive hemorrhage presenting as liver primary. A report of two cases. *American Journal of Surgical Pathology* 1986; **10**: 342–7.

152 Heijtink RA, Boender PJ *et al*. Hepatitis B virus DNA in serum of pregnant women with HBsAg and HBeAg or antibodies to HBe (letter). *Journal of Infectious Diseases* 1984; **150**: 462.

152a Heikinheimo M, Aunnerus H *et al*. Pregnancy specific beta-1-glycoprotein levels in cholestasis of pregnancy. *Obstetrics and Gynecology* 1978; **52**: 276–8.

153 Heilmann L, Hojnacki B *et al*. Hemostasis and preeclampsia (German). *Gerburt Frauenheilkd* 1991; **51**: 223–7.

154 Heller TD & Goldfarb JP. Spontaneous rupture of the liver during pregnancy. A case report and review of the literature. *New York State Journal of Medicine* 1986; **86**: 314–16.

155 Henny CP, Lim AE *et al*. A review of the importance of acute multidisciplinary treatment following spontaneous rupture of the liver capsule during pregnancy. *Surgery, Gynecology and Obstetrics* 1983; **156**: 593–8.

156 Hensleigh PA, Glover BD *et al*. Systemic herpesvirus hominis in pregnancy. *Journal of Reproductive Medicine* 1979; **22**: 171–6.

157 Herbert WNP. Hepatic rupture and pregnancy. *New York State Journal of Medicine* 1986; **86**: 286–8.

158 Hess HM, Dickson J *et al*. Hyperfunctioning parathyroid carcinoma presenting as acute pancreatitis in pregnancy. *Journal of Reproductive Medicine* 1980; **25**: 83–7.

159 Hiatt JR, Hiatt JC *et al*. Biliary disease in pregnancy: strategy for surgical management. *American Journal of Surgery* 1986; **151**: 263–5.

160 Hibbard LT. Spontaneous rupture of the liver in pregnancy: a report of eight cases. *American Journal of Obstetrics and Gynecology* 1976; **126**: 334–8.

161 Hieber JP, Dalton D *et al*. Hepatitis and pregnancy. *Journal of Pediatrics* 1977; **91**: 545–9.

162 Hildebrandt RJ, Sever JL *et al*. Cytomegalovirus in the normal pregnant woman. *American Journal of Obstetrics and Gynecology* 1967; **98**: 1125–8.

163 Hill LM, Johnson CE *et al*. Cholecystectomy in pregnancy. *Obstetrics and Gynecology* 1975; **9**: 291–3.

164 Hollinger FB, Lemon SM & Margolis HS (eds) *Viral Hepatitis and Liver Disease. Proceedings of the 1990 International Symposium, Houston, Texas*. Williams & Wilkins, Baltimore, 1991: 1–916.

165 Holzbach RT. Australia antigen hepatitis in pregnancy: evidence against transplacental transmission of Australia antigen in early and late pregnancy. *Archives of Internal Medicine* 1972; **130**: 234–6.

166 Holzbach RT. Acute fatty liver of pregnancy with disseminated intravascular coagulation. *Obstetrics and Gynecology* 1974; **43**: 740–4.

167 Holzbach RT, Sivak DA *et al*. Familial recurrent intrahepatic cholestasis of pregnancy: a genetic study providing evidence for transmission of a sex-linked dominant trait. *Gastroenterology* 1983; **85**: 175–9.

168 Hoofnagle J, Shafritz DA *et al*. Chronic type B hepatitis and the 'healthy' HBsAg carrier state. *Hepatology* 1987; **7**: 758–63.

169 Hou SH, Levin S *et al*. Acute fatty liver of pregnancy. Survival with early Caesarian section. *Digestive Diseases and Sciences* 1984; **29**: 449–52.

170 Hsy H-C, Lin GH *et al*. Association of hepatitis B surface (HBs) antigenemia and membranous nephropathy in children in Taiwan. *Clinical Nephrology* 1983; **20**: 121–9.

171 Huchzermeyer H. Schwangershaft bei Leberzirrhose und chronischer Hepatitis (Pregnancy in patients with liver cirrhosis and chronic hepatitis). *Acta Hepatogastroenterologica (Stuttgart)* 1971; **18**: 294–305.

172 Huggins GR. Neoplasia and hormonal contraception. *Clinics in Obstetrics and Gynecology* 1981; **24**: 903–25.

173 Huguet C, Deliere T *et al*. Budd–Chiari syndrome with thrombosis of the inferior vena cava: long-term patency of mesocaval and cavoatrial prosthetic bypass. *Surgery* 1984; **95**: 108–11.

174 Hwang L-Y, Roggendorf M *et al*. Perinatal transmission of hepatitis B virus: role of maternal HBeAg and anti-HBc IgM. *Journal of Medical Virology* 1985; **15**: 265–9.

175 Ibrahim N, Payne E *et al*. Spontaneous rupture of the liver in association with pregnancy. Case report. *British Journal of Obstetrics and Gynaecology* 1985; **92**: 539–40.

176 Inaba N, Ijichi M *et al*. Placental transmission of hepatitis B e antigen and clinical significance of hepatitis B e antigen titers of children born to hepatitis B e antigen-positive carrier women. *American Journal of Obstetrics and Gynecology* 1984; **149**: 580–1.

177 Jacques SM, Qureshi F. Herpes simplex virus hepatitis in pregnancy: a clinicopathologic study of three cases. *Human Pathology* 1992; **23**: 183–7.

178 Jarnfelt-Samsioe A, Eriksson B *et al*. Serum bile acids, gamma glutamyltransferase and routine liver function tests in emetic and nonemetic pregnancies. *Gynecologic and Obstetric Investigation* 1986; **21**: 169–76.

179 Jenny S & Markoff N. Oral contraceptives in liver disease. *Schweizerische Medizinische Wochenschrift* 1967; **97**: 1502–5.

180 Jeppsson S & Rannevik G. Effect of oral 17-beta-oestradiol on the liver in women with intrahepatic cholestasis (hepatosis) during previous pregnancy. *British Journal of Obstetrics and Gynaecology* 1976; **83**: 567–71.

181 Jilg W, Schmidt M *et al*. Hepatitis B vaccination: how long does protection last? (letter) *Lancet* 1984; **ii**: 458.

182 Johnson WC & Baskett TF. Obstetric cholestasis. *American Journal of Obstetrics and Gynecology* 1979; **133**: 299–301.

183 Jones EA & Bergasa NU. The pruritus of cholestasis: from bile acids to opiate antagonists. *Hepatology* 1990; **11**: 884–7.

184 Jouppila P, Mokka R *et al*. Acute pancreatitis in pregnancy. *Surgery, Gynecology and Obstetrics* 1974; **139**: 879–82.
185 Kaiser R, Berk JE *et al*. Serum amylase changes during pregnancy. *American Journal of Obstetrics and Gynecology* 1975; **122**: 283–6.
186 Kammerer WS. Non-obstetric surgery during pregnancy. *Medical Clinics of North America* 1979; **6**: 1157–63.
187 Kanaan C, Veille JC *et al*. Pregnancy and acute intermittent porphyria. *Obstetrical and Gynecological Survey* 1989; **44**: 244–9.
188 Kane MA, Bradley DW *et al*. Epidemic non-A, non-B hepatitis in Nepal. Recovery of a possible etiologic agent and transmission studies in marmosets. *Journal of the American Medical Association* 1984; **252**: 3140–5.
189 Kaplan MM. Acute fatty liver of pregnancy. *New England Journal of Medicine* 1985; **313**: 367–70.
190 Keating JJ, O'Brien CJ *et al*. Influence of aetiology, clinical and histological features on survival in chronic active hepatitis: an analysis of 204 patients. *Quarterly Journal of Medicine* 1987; **62**: 59–66.
191 Keen CL, Cohen N *et al*. Low tissue copper and teratogenesis in trientine-treated rats. *Lancet* 1982; **i**: 1127.
192 Kent DR, Nissen ED *et al*. Effect of pregnancy on liver tumor associated with oral contraceptives. *Obstetrics and Gynecology* 1978; **51**: 148–51.
193 Kern F, Everson GT *et al*. Biliary lipids, bile acids and gallbladder function in the human female. Effects of pregnancy and the ovulatory cycle. *Journal of Clinical Investigation* 1981; **68**: 1229–42.
194 Kern F, Everson GT *et al*. Biliary lipids, bile acids and gallbladder function in the human female: effects of contraceptive steroids. *Journal of Clinical Investigation* 1982; **99**: 798–805.
195 Kerr MG, Scott DB *et al*. Studies of the inferior vena cava in late pregnancy. *British Medical Journal* 1964; **i**: 532–3.
196 Khoo SK. Cancer risks and the contraceptive pill. What is the evidence after nearly 25 years of use? *Medical Journal of Australia* 1986; **144**: 185–90.
197 Khuroo MS & Datta DV. Budd–Chiari syndrome following pregnancy. Report of 16 cases with roentgenologic, hemodynamic and histologic studies of the hepatic outflow tract. *American Journal of Medicine* 1980; **8**: 113–21.
198 Khuroo MS, Teli MR *et al*. Incidence and severity of viral hepatitis in pregnancy. *American Journal of Medicine* 1981; **70**: 252–5.
199 Kiilholma P. Serum copper and zinc concentrations in intrahepatic cholestasis of pregnancy: a controlled study. *European Journal of Obstetrics, Gynecology and Reproductive Biology* 1986; **21**: 207–12.
200 Killam AP, Dillard SH *et al*. Pregnancy-induced hypertension complicated by acute liver disease and disseminated intravascular coagulation. *American Journal of Obstetrics and Gynecology* 1975; **123**: 823–8.
201 Kirk EP. Organ transplantation and pregnancy. A case report and review. *American Journal of Obstetrics and Gynecology* 1991; **164**: 1629–34.
202 Kirkinen P, Ylostalo P *et al*. Gallbladder function and maternal bile acids in intrahepatic cholestasis of pregnancy. *European Journal of Obstetrics, Gynecology and Reproductive Biology* 1984; **18**: 29–34.
203 Klatskin G. Hepatic tumours: possible relationship to the use of oral contraceptives. *Gastroenterology* 1977; **73**: 386–94.
204 Klebanoff MA, Koslowe PA *et al*. Epidemiology of vomiting in early pregnancy. *Obstetrics and Gynecology* 1985; **66**: 612–16.
205 Klein KB. Pancreatitis in pregnancy. In Rustgi VK & Cooper JN (eds), *Gastrointestinal and Hepatic Complications in Pregnancy*. J. Wiley & Sons, New York, 1986: 138–61.
206 Klein NA, Mabie WC *et al*. Herpes simplex hepatitis in pregnancy. Two patients successfully treated with acyclovir. *Gastroenterology* 1991; **100**: 239–44.
207 Kochlar R, Goenka MK *et al*. Endoscopic sclerotherapy during pregnancy. *American Journal of Gastroenterology* 1990; **85**: 1132–5.
208 Krass IM. Chiari's syndrome: report of a case following pregnancy. *Journal of Obstetrics and Gynaecology of the British Empire* 1957; **64**: 715–19.
209 Kreek MJ, Sleisenger MH *et al*. Recurrent cholestatic jaundice of pregnancy with demonstrated estrogen sensitivity. *American Journal of Medicine* 1967; **43**: 795–803.
210 Kristoffersson A, Emdin S *et al*. Acute intestinal obstruction and splenic hemorrhage due to metastatic choriocarcinoma. A case report. *Acta Chirurgica Scandinavica* 1985; **151**: 381–4.
211 Krol Van Straaten J & De Maat CE. Successful pregnancies in cirrhosis of the liver before and after portacaval anastomosis. *Netherlands Medical Journal* 1984; **27**: 14–15.
212 Krueger KJ, Hoffman BJ *et al*. Hepatic infarction associated with eclampsia. *American Journal of Gastroenterology* 1990; **85**: 588–92.
213 Kucera J. Down's syndrome and infectious hepatitis. *Lancet* 1970; **i**: 569–70.
214 Kunelis CT, Peters JL *et al*. Fatty liver of pregnancy and its relationship to tetracycline therapy. *American Journal of Medicine* 1965; **38**: 359–77.
215 Kuo G, Choo Q-L *et al*. An assay for circulating antibodies to a major etiologic virus of human non-A, non-B hepatitis. *Science* 1989; **244**: 362–4.
216 Kurzel RB. Can acetaminophen excess result in maternal and fetal toxicity? *Southern Medical Journal* 1990; **83**: 953–5.
217 Laatikainen T & Tulenheiko A. Maternal serum bile acid levels and fetal distress in cholestasis of pregnancy. *International Journal of Gynaecology and Obstetrics* 1984; **22**: 91–4.

218 Laifer SA, Darby MJ *et al*. Pregnancy and liver transplantation. *Obstetrics and Gynecology* 1990; **76**: 1083–8.

219 Langmade CF & Edmondson HA. Acute pancreatitis during pregnancy and the postpartum period: report of 9 cases. *Surgery, Gynecology and Obstetrics* 1951; **92**: 43–52.

220 Laplanche A, Courouce A-M *et al*. Timing of hepatitis B revaccination in healthy adults (letter). *Lancet* 1987; **i**: 1206–7.

221 Larrey D, Rueff B *et al*. Recurrent jaundice caused by recurrent hyperemesis gravidarum. *Gut* 1984; **25**: 1414–15.

222 Laursen B, Frost L *et al*. Acute fatty liver of pregnancy with complicating disseminated intravascular coagulation. *Acta Obstetricia et Gynecologica Scandinavica* 1983; **62**: 403–7.

223 Lawson DH, Lovatt GE *et al*. Adverse effects of azathioprine. *Adverse Drug Reactions and Acute Poisoning Review* 1984; **3**: 161–71.

224 Lee AKY, Ip HMH *et al*. Mechanisms of maternal–fetal transmission of hepatitis B virus. *Journal of Infectious Diseases* 1978; **138**: 668–71.

225 Lee S-D, Lo J-K *et al*. Prevention of maternal–infant hepatitis B virus transmission by immunization: the role of serum hepatitis B virus DNA. *Hepatology* 1986; **6**: 369–73.

226 Leinikki P, Heinonen K *et al*. Incidence of cytomegalovirus infections in early childhood. *Scandinavian Journal of Infectious Diseases* 1972; **4**: 1–5.

227 Lemon SM. Type A viral hepatitis. New developments in an old disease. *New England Journal of Medicine* 1985; **313**: 1059–69.

228 Levin S, Leibowitz E *et al*. Interferon treatment in acute progressive and fulminant hepatitis. *Israeli Journal of Medical Science* 1989; **25**: 364–72.

229 Levine RL, Fredricks WR *et al*. Entry of bilirubin into the brain due to opening of the blood–brain barrier. *Pediatrics* 1982; **69**: 255–9.

230 Lewis JH & Weingold AB. The use of gastrointestinal drugs during pregnancy and lactation. *American Journal of Gastroenterology* 1985; **80**: 912–23.

231 Liebman HA, McGeehee WG *et al*. Severe depression of anti-thrombin III associated with disseminated intravascular coagulation in women with fatty liver of pregnancy. *Annals of Internal Medicine* 1983; **98**: 330–3.

232 Linares A, Zarranz JJ *et al*. Reversible cutis laxa due to maternal D-penicillamine treatment (letter). *Lancet* 1979; **ii**: 43.

233 Linneman CC & Goldberg S. HBsAg in breast milk (letter). *Lancet* 1974; **ii**: 1550.

234 Lo JK, Sai YTT *et al*. Immunoprophylaxis of infection with hepatitis B virus in infants born to hepatitis B surface antigen-positive carrier mothers. *Journal of Infectious Diseases* 1985; **152**: 817–22.

235 Loevinger EH, Vujic I *et al*. Hepatic rupture associated with pregnancy: treatment with transcatheter embolotherapy. *Obstetrics and Gynecology* 1985; **65**: 281–4.

236 Lok ASF, Lai C-L *et al*. Interferon therapy of chronic hepatitis B virus infection in Chinese. *Journal of Hepatology* 1986; **3** (suppl 2): S209–15.

237 Lynch-Salamon DI & Combs CA. Hepatitis C in obstetrics and gynecology. *Obstetrics and Gynecology* 1992; **79**: 621–9.

238 Machi J, Sigel B *et al*. Operative ultrasonography in the biliary tract during pregnancy. *Surgery, Gynecology and Obstetrics* 1985; **160**: 119–23.

239 Mallia CP & Nancekivell AF. Fulminant virus hepatitis in late pregnancy. *Annals of Tropical Medicine and Parasitology* 1982; **76**: 143–6.

240 Manas KJ, Welsh JD *et al*. Hepatic hemorrhage without rupture in preeclampsia. *New England Journal of Medicine* 1985; **312**: 424–6.

241 Marecek Z & Graf M. Pregnancy in penicillamine-treated patients with Wilson's disease. *New England Journal of Medicine* 1976; **295**: 841–2.

242 Margolis HS, Alter MJ *et al*. Hepatitis B: evolving epidemiology and implications for control. *Seminars in Liver Disease* 1992; **11**: 84–92.

243 Marinier E, Barrois V *et al*. Lack of perinatal transmission of hepatitis B virus infection in Senegal, West Africa. *Journal of Pediatrics* 1985; **106**: 843–9.

244 Martin JN, Files JC *et al*. Plasma exchange for preeclampsia-eclampsia with HELLP syndrome. *American Journal of Obstetrics and Gynecology* 1990; **162**: 126–37.

245 Marx JL. Cytomegalovirus: a major cause of birth defects. *Science* 1975; **190**: 1184–6.

246 Matsaniotis N, Kiossoglou K *et al*. Chromosomal aberrations in infectious hepatitis. *Journal of Clinical Pathology* 1970; **23**: 553–7.

247 Mazor M, Wiznitzer A *et al*. Gaucher's disease in pregnancy associated with portal hypertension. *American Journal of Obstetrics and Gynecology* 1986; **154**: 1119–20.

248 McKay AJ, O'Neill J *et al*. Pancreatitis, pregnancy and gallstones. *British Journal of Obstetrics and Gynaecology* 1980; **87**: 47–50.

249 McKay DG. Clinical significance of the pathology of toxemia of pregnancy. *Circulation* 1964; **30** (suppl 2): 66–75.

250 McKee CM, Weir PE *et al*. Acute fatty liver of pregnancy and diagnosis by computed tomography. *British Medical Journal* 1986; **292**: 291–2.

251 Mehrotra R. Histopathological and immunohistochemical changes in placenta due to acute viral hepatitis during pregnancy. *Indian Journal of Medical Research* 1986; **83**: 282–92.

252 Melish ME & Hanshaw JB. Congenital cytomegalovirus infection. Developmental progress of infants detected by routine screening. *American Journal of Diseases of Children* 1973; **126**: 190–4.

253 Merrill DA & Dubois RS. Neonatal onset of the

hepatitis-associated antigen carrier state. *New England Journal of Medicine* 1972; **287**: 1280–2.

254 Milo R, Neuman M *et al.* Acute intermittent porphyria in pregnancy. *Obstetrics and Gynecology* 1989; **73**: 450–2.

255 Minakami H, Kimura K *et al.* Acute fatty liver of pregnancy with hyperlipidemia, acute hemorrhagic pancreatitis and disseminated intravascular coagulation. *Asia-Oceania Journal of Obstetrics and Gynaecology* 1985; **11**: 371–6.

256 Minakami H, Oka N *et al.* Preeclampsia: a microvesicular fat disease of the liver. *American Journal of Obstetrics and Gynecology* 1988; **159**: 1043–7.

257 Mintz MC, Grumbach K *et al.* Sonographic evaluation of bile duct size during pregnancy. *American Journal of Roentgenology* 1985; **145**: 575–8.

258 Misra PS, Evanov FA *et al.* Idiopathic intrahepatic cholestasis of pregnancy. Report of an unusual case and review of the recent literature. *American Journal of Gastroenterology* 1980; **73**: 54–9.

259 Mitchell MC, Boitnott JM *et al.* Budd–Chiari syndrome: etiology, diagnosis and management. *Medicine (Baltimore)* 1982; **61**: 199–218.

259a Mitchell RW, Teare AJ. Amoebic liver abscess in pregnancy: Case report. *British Journal of Obstetrics and Gynaecology* 1984; **91**: 393–5.

260 Mjolnerod OK, Rasmunssen K *et al.* Congenital connective-tissue defect probably due to D-penicillamine in pregnancy. *Lancet* 1971; **i**: 673.

261 Morali GA & Braverman DZ. Abnormal liver enzymes and ketonuria in hyperemesis gravidarum. A retrospective review of 80 patients. *Journal of Clinical Gastroenterology* 1990; **12**: 303–5.

262 Morbidity Mortality Weekly Report (MMWR). Recommendations for protection against viral hepatitis. *Morbidity Mortality Weekly Report* 1985; **34**: 313–24.

263 Morbidity Mortality Weekly Report (MMWR). Leads from the MMWR. Recommendations for the protection against viral hepatitis. *Journal of the American Medical Association* 1985; **254**: 197–8.

264 Morbidity Mortality Weekly Report (MMWR). Centers for Disease Control: Protection against viral hepatitis. Recommendations of the Immunization Practices Advisory Committee (AICP). *Morbidity Mortality Weekly Report* 1990; **39**: 5–22.

265 Morbidity Mortality Weekly Report (MMWR). Public Health Service Interagency Guidelines for screening Donors of blood, plasma, organs, tissues, and semen for evidence of hepatitis B and hepatitis C. *Morbidity Mortality Weekly Report* 1991; RR4 **40**: 1–17.

266 Morbidity Mortality Weekly Report (MMWR). Recommendations for preventing transmission of human immunodeficiency virus and hepatitis B virus to patients during exposure-prone invasive procedures. *Morbidity Mortality Weekly Report* 1991; RR8 **40**: 1–9.

267 Morbidity Mortality Weekly Report. Update on adult immunization. Recommendations of the immunization Practices Advisory Committee. *Morbidity Mortality Weekly Report* 1991; RR 12 **40**: 33–89.

268 Montgomery WH & Miller FC. Views and reviews: pancreatitis and pregnancy. *Obstetrics and Gynecology* 1970; **35**: 658–65.

269 Morimoto I, Nonomiya H *et al.* Pregnancy and penicillamine treatment in a patient with Wilson's disease. *Japanese Journal of Medicine* 1986; **25**: 59–62.

270 Morrison AS, Jick H *et al.* Oral contraceptives and hepatitis: a report from the Boston Collaborative Drug Surveillance Program, Boston University Medical Center. *Lancet* 1977; **i**: 1142–3.

271 Moyes CD, Milne A *et al.* Very-low-dose hepatitis B vaccine in newborn infants: an economic option for control in endemic areas. *Lancet* 1987; **i**: 29–31.

272 Myint Hla, Soe MM *et al.* A clinical and epidemiological study of an epidemic of non-A, non-B hepatitis in Rangoon. *American Journal of Tropical Medicine and Hygiene* 1985; **34**: 1183–9.

273 Nakamoto SK & Van Sonnenberg E. Cholangiocarcinoma in pregnancy: the contribution of ultrasound guided interventional techniques. *Journal of Ultrasound Medicine* 1985; **4**: 557–9.

274 Navaratne RA. Postpartum intraperitoneal rupture of an amoebic liver abscess. *Ceylon Medical Journal* 1972; **17**: 160–3.

275 Negro F & Rizzetto M. Pathobiology of delta virus. In Hollinger FB, Lemon SM & Margolis HS (eds), *Viral Hepatitis and Liver Disease. Proceedings of the 1990 International Symposium, Houston, Texas.* Williams & Wilkins, Baltimore, 1991: 477–80.

276 Neuberger J, Forman D *et al.* Oral contraceptives and hepatocellular carcinoma. *British Medical Journal* 1986; **292**: 1355–7.

277 Newlands ES. Trophoblastic tumours. In: Studd J (ed), *Progress in Obstetrics and Gynaecology*, Churchill Livingstone, Edinburgh, 1983, p. 158.

278 Nilsson S & Stattin S. Gallbladder emptying during the normal menstrual cycle. *Acta Chirurgica Scandinavica* 1967; **133**: 648–52.

279 Nir A, Sorokin Y *et al.* Pregnancy and primary biliary cirrhosis. *International Journal of Obstetrics and Gynaecology* 1989; **28**: 279–82.

280 Nordenfelt E & Dahlquist E. HBsAg positive adopted children as a cause of intrafamilial spread of hepatitis B. *Scandinavian Journal of Infectious Diseases* 1978; **10**: 161–3.

281 Nouasria B, Larouze B *et al.* Epidemic non-A, non-B hepatitis in east Algeria. *Bulletin de la Societe de Pathologie Exotique et de ses Filiales* 1985; **78**: 903–6.

282 Numazaki Y, Yano N *et al.* Primary infection with human cytomegalovirus: virus isolation from healthy infants and pregnant women. *American Journal of Epidemiology* 1970; **9**: 410–17.

283 Ockner RK & Davidson CS. Hepatic effects of oral contraceptives. *New England Journal of Medicine* 1967; **276**: 331–4.

284 O'Grady J, Gimson ASE *et al*. Controlled trials of charcoal haemoperfusion and prognostic factors in fulminant hepatic failure. *Gastroenterology* 1988; **94**: 1186–92.
285 O'Grady J & Williams R. Acute liver failure. In: Gilmore I & Shields R (eds), *Gastrointestinal Emergencies*. Baillière Tindall, London, 1991: 104–22.
286 Orellana-Alcake JM & Dominguez JP. Jaundice and oral contraceptive drugs. *Lancet* 1966; **i**: 1278–80.
287 Palmer AK & Heywood R. Pathological changes in the rhesus fetus associated with oral administration of chenodeoxycholic acid. *Toxicology* 1974; **2**: 239–46.
288 Palmovic D. Acute viral hepatitis in pregnancy. Results of a prospective study of 99 pregnant women. *Lijecnicki Vjesnik* 1986; **108**: 296–300.
289 Peretz A, Paldi E *et al*. Infectious hepatitis in pregnancy. *Obstetrics and Gynecology* 1959; **14**: 435–41.
290 Perez V & Gorodisch S. Female sex hormones and the liver. In: Schaffner F, Sherlock S & Leevy CM (eds), *The Liver and its Diseases*. Georg Thieme, Stuttgart, 1974: 179.
291 Pockros PJ, Peters RI *et al*. Idiopathic fatty liver of pregnancy: findings in ten cases. *Medicine (Baltimore)* 1984; **63**: 1–11.
292 Pockros PJ & Reynolds TB. Acute fatty liver of pregnancy (letter). *Digestive Diseases and Sciences* 1985; **30**: 601–2.
293 Portnuff J & Ballon S. Hepatic rupture in pregnancy. *American Journal of Obstetrics and Gynecology* 1972; **114**: 1102–4.
294 Potts M & Diggory P (eds) *Textbook of Contraceptive Practice*. Cambridge University Press, Cambridge, 1983: 164.
295 Powell-Jackson PR, Melia W *et al*. Budd–Chiari syndrome: clinical patterns and therapy. *Quarterly Journal of Medicine* 1982; **201**: 29–88.
296 Prince AM, White T *et al*. Epidemiology of hepatitis B infection in Liberian infants. *Infection and Immunology* 1981; **32**: 675–80.
297 Printen KJ & Ott RA. Cholecystectomy during pregnancy. *American Journal of Surgery* 1978; **44**: 432–4.
298 Provost PJ, Wolanski BS *et al*. Physical, chemical and morphological dimensions of human hepatitis A virus strain. *Proceedings of the Society of Experimental Biology and Medicine* 1975; **148**: 532–9.
299 Purdie JM & Walters BN. Acute fatty liver of pregnancy: clinical features and diagnosis. *Australian and New Zealand Journal of Obstetrics and Gynaecology* 1988; **28**: 62–7.
300 Purtilo DJ, Clark JV *et al*. Hepatic malignancy in pregnant women. *American Journal of Obstetrics and Gynecology* 1975; **121**: 41–3.
301 Purtilo DT. Fulminant hepatic failure due to genital herpes in a healthy woman: was she healthy? (letter). *Journal of the American Medical Association* 1985; **254**: 3421–2.
302 Qui ZD, Wang QN *et al*. Intrahepatic cholestasis of pregnancy. Clinical analysis and follow-up study of 22 cases (English). *Chinese Medical Journal* 1983; **96**: 902–6.
303 Radberg G, Asztely M *et al*. Gastric and gallbladder emptying in relation to the secretion of cholecystokinin after a meal in late pregnancy. *Digestion* 1989; **42**: 174–80.
304 Reid R, Ivey KJ *et al*. Fetal complications of obstetric cholestasis. *British Medical Journal* 1976; **i**: 870–2.
305 Reyes H. The enigma of intrahepatic cholestasis of pregnancy: lessons from Chile. *Hepatology* 1982; **2**: 87–96.
306 Reyes H, Ribalda J *et al*. Idiopathic cholestasis in a large kindred. *Gut* 1976; **17**: 709–13.
307 Reynolds DW, Stagno S *et al*. Maternal cytomegalovirus excretion and perinatal infection. *New England Journal of Medicine* 1973; **289**: 1–5.
308 Riely CA, Latham PS *et al*. Acute fatty liver of pregnancy. A reassessment based on observations in nine patients. *Annals of Internal Medicine* 1987; **106**: 703–6.
309 Rizetto M, Ponzetto A *et al*. Hepatitis delta virus as a global health problem. *Vaccine* 1990; **8**: S10–14.
310 Robson SC, Mutch E *et al*. Apparent liver blood flow during pregnancy: a serial study using indocyanine green clearance. *British Journal of Obstetrics and Gynaecology* 1990; **97**: 720–4.
311 Rolfes DB & Ishak KG. Acute fatty liver of pregnancy: a clinicopathologic study of 35 cases. *Hepatology* 1985; **5**: 1149–58.
312 Rolfes DB & Ishak KG. Liver disease in pregnancy. *Histopathology* 1986; **10**: 555–70.
313 Rosa FW. Teratogen update: penicillamine. *Teratology* 1986; **33**: 127–31.
314 Roszkowski I & Wojcicka J. Jaundice in pregnancy. 1. Biochemical assays. *American Journal of Obstetrics and Gynecology* 1968; **102**: 839–46.
315 Rubin MH, Ward DM *et al*. Fulminant hepatic failure caused by genital herpes in a healthy person. *Journal of the American Medical Association* 1985; **253**: 1299–301.
316 Sakala EP & Moore WD. Successful term delivery after previous pregnancy with ruptured liver. *Obstetrics and Gynecology* 1986; **68**: 124–6.
317 Sakamoto S, Tsuji Y *et al*. Idiopathic fatty liver of pregnancy with a subsequent uncomplicated pregnancy and a progressive increase in serum cholesterase activity during the third trimester. A case report. *Hepatogastroenterology* 1986; **33**: 9–10.
318 Scaglione S. Cirrosi di Laennec in gravidanza. *Rivista Italiana di Ginecologia* 1923; **1**: 489.
319 Schalm SW & van Buuren HR. Prevention of recurrent variceal bleeding: non-surgical procedure. *Clinics in Gastroenterology* 1985; **14**: 209–32.
320 Schmid R & Newton JJ. Childbirth after liver transplantation (letter). *Transplantation* 1980; **29**: 432.
321 Schoeman MN, Batey RG *et al*. Recurrent acute fatty liver of pregnancy associated with a fatty-acid

oxidation defect in the offspring. *Gastroenterology* 1991; **100**: 544–8.

322 Schorr-Lesnick B, Lebovics E *et al*. Liver diseases unique to pregnancy. *American Journal of Gastroenterology* 1991; **86**: 659–70.

323 Schreyer P, Caspi E *et al*. Cirrhosis, pregnancy and delivery: a review. *Obstetrical and Gynecological Survey* 1982; **37**: 304–12.

324 Schweitzer IL & Spears RL. Hepatitis-associated antigen (Australia antigen) in mother and infant. *New England Journal of Medicine* 1970; **283**: 570–2.

325 Schweitzer IL, Weiner JM *et al*. Oral contraceptives in acute viral hepatitis. *Journal of the American Medical Association*. 1975; **233**: 979–80.

326 Scott LD, Katz AR *et al*. Oral contraceptives, pregnancy, and focal nodular hyperplasia of the liver. *Journal of the American Medical Association* 1984; **251**: 1461–3.

327 Scragg RK, McMichael AJ *et al*. Oral contraceptives, pregnancy and endogenous oestrogen in gall stone disease — a case control study. *British Medical Journal* 1984; **288**: 1795–9.

328 Seaward PG, Koch MA *et al*. Primary hepatocellular carcinoma in pregnancy. A case report. *South African Medical Journal* 1986; **69**: 700–1.

329 Seligsohn U & Shani M. The Dubin–Johnson syndrome and pregnancy. *Acta Hepatogastroenterologica* 1977; **24**: 167–9.

330 Sever JL, Kapikian AZ *et al*. Hepatitis A in Down's syndrome: lack of an association. *Journal of Infectious Diseases* 1976; **134**: 198–200.

331 Shalev E & Bassan HM. Viral hepatitis during pregnancy in Israel. *International Journal of Obstetrics and Gynaecology* 1982; **20**: 73–8.

332 Shattock AG, Irwin FM *et al*. Increased severity and morbidity of acute hepatitis in drug abusers with simultaneously acquired hepatitis B and hepatitis D virus infections. *British Medical Journal* 1985; **290**: 1377–80.

333 Shaw D, Frohlich J *et al*. A prospective study of 18 patients with cholestasis of pregnancy. *American Journal of Obstetrics and Gynecology* 1982; **142**: 621–5.

334 Sheehan HL. The pathology of hyperemesis and vomiting of late pregnancy. *Journal of Obstetrics and Gynaecology of the British Empire* 1939; **46**: 685–9.

335 Sherwin AL, Beck IT *et al*. The course of Wilson's diseases (hepatolenticular degeneration) during pregnancy and after delivery. *Canadian Medical Association Journal* 1960; **83**: 160–3.

336 Shlien RD, Meyers S *et al*. Fulminant herpes simplex hepatitis in a patient with ulcerative colitis. *Gut* 1988; **29**: 257–61.

337 Shiraki K, Yoshihara N *et al*. Acute hepatitis B in infants born to carrier mothers with the antibody to hepatitis B e antigen. *Journal of Pediatrics* 1980; **97**: 768–70.

338 Sibai BM. The HELLP syndrome (hemolysis, elevated liver enzymes, and low platelets): much ado about nothing? *American Journal of Obstetrics and Gynecology* 1990; **162**: 311–16.

339 Sinatra FR, Shah P *et al*. Perinatal transmitted acute icteric hepatitis B in infants born to hepatitis B surface antigen-positive and antihepatitis B c-positive carrier mothers. *Pediatrics* 1982; **70**: 557–9.

340 Singh DS, Balasubramaniam M *et al*. Viral hepatitis during pregnancy. *Journal of Indian Medical Research* 1979; **73**: 90–2.

341 Slater DN & Hague WM. Renal morphological changes in idiopathic acute fatty liver of pregnancy. *Histopathology* 1984; **8**: 567–81.

342 Sloan DA & Schlegel DM. Spontaneous hepatic rupture associated with pregnancy. *Contemporary Surgery* 1984; **24**: 39–42.

343 Smith LG, Moise KJ *et al*. Spontaneous rupture of the liver during pregnancy: current therapy. *Obstetrics and Gynecology* 1991; **77**: 171–5.

344 Smithers BM, Welch C *et al*. Cystadenocarcinoma of the pancreas presenting in pregnancy. *British Journal of Surgery* 1986; **73**: 591.

345 Solomon L, Abrams G *et al*. Neonatal abnormalities associated with D-penicillamine during pregnancy (letter). *New England Journal of Medicine* 1977; **296**: 54–5.

346 Soto-Albors CE, Rayburn WF *et al*. Portal hypertension and hypersplenism in pregnancy secondary to chronic schistosomiasis. A case report. *Journal of Reproductive Medicine* 1984; **29**: 345–8.

347 Stander HJ & Cadden JF. Acute yellow atrophy of the liver in pregnancy. *American Journal of Obstetrics and Gynecology* 1934; **28**: 61–9.

348 Stauffer RA, Adams A *et al*. Gallbladder disease in pregnancy. *American Journal of Obstetrics and Gynecology* 1982; **144**: 661–4.

349 Steel R & Parker ML. Jaundice in pregnancy. *Medical Journal of Australia* 1973; **1**: 461.

350 Steven MM. Pregnancy and liver disease. *Gut* 1981; **22**: 592–614.

351 Steven MM, Buckley JB *et al*. Pregnancy in chronic active hepatitis. *Quarterly Journal of Medicine* 1979; **48**: 519–33.

352 Stevens CE, Toy PT *et al*. Perinatal hepatitis B virus transmission in the United States. Prevention by passive-active immunization. *Journal of the American Medical Association* 1985; **253**: 1740–5.

353 Stoller A & Collmann RD. Incidence of infectious hepatitis followed by Down's syndrome nine months later. *Lancet* 1965; **ii**: 1221–3.

354 Stone B, Erickson SK *et al*. Regulation of rat biliary cholesterol secretion by agents which alter cholesterol metabolism. Evidence for a distinct biliary precursor pool. *Journal of Clinical Investigation* 1985; **76**: 1773–81.

355 Stowell JC, Bottsford JE *et al*. Pancreatitis with pseudocyst and cholelithiasis in third trimester of pregnancy:

management with total parenteral nutrition. *Southern Medical Journal* 1984; **77**: 502–4.

356 Strickland DM, Hauth JC *et al*. Amylase and isoamylase activities in serum of pregnant women. *Obstetrics and Gynecology* 1984; **63**: 389–91.

357 Stuvyt PMJ, Demaker PNM *et al*. Pancreatitis induced by oestrogen in a patient with type I hyperlipidaemia. *British Medical Journal* 1986; **293**: 734.

358 Svanborg A. A study of recurrent jaundice in pregnancy. *Acta Obstetrica et Gynecologica Scandinavica* 1954; **33**: 434–44.

359 Szmuness W, Stevens CE *et al*. A controlled clinical trial of the efficacy of the hepatitis B vaccine (heptavax B): a final report. *Hepatology* 1981; **1**: 377–85.

360 Tabor E. Hepatitis B vaccine: different regimens for different geographic regions (Editor's column). *Journal of Pediatrics* 1985; **106**: 777–8.

361 Tabor E & Gerety RJ. Hepatitis B virus infection in infants and toddlers in Nigeria: the need for early intervention. *Journal of Pediatrics* 1979; **95**: 647–50.

362 Tabor E, Bayley AC *et al*. Horizontal transmission of hepatitis B virus among children and adults in five rural villages in Zambia. *Journal of Medical Virology* 1985; **15**: 113–20.

363 Taina E, Hanninen P *et al*. Viral infections in pregnancy. *Acta Obstetricia et Gynecologica Scandinavica* 1985; **64**: 167–73.

364 Takekoshi Y, Tanaka M *et al*. Strong association between membranous nephropathy and hepatitis-B surface antigenaemia in Japanese children. *Lancet* 1978; **ii**: 1065–8.

365 Tanferna M, Panazzoloo A *et al*. Acute intermittent porphyria and pregnancy. *Minerva Ginecologica* 1986; **38**: 225–8.

366 Tang S. Study on the HBV intrauterine infection and its rate (Chinese). *Chung Hua Liu Hsing Ping Hsueh Tsa Chih* 1990; **11**: 328–30.

367 Tavill AS, Wood EJ *et al*. The Budd–Chiari syndrome. Correlation between hepatic scintigraphy and clinical, radiological and pathological findings in 19 cases of hepatic venous outflow obstruction. *Gastroenterology* 1975; **68**: 509–18.

368 Teisala K & Tuịmala R. Pregnancy and esophageal varices. *Annals of Chirurgiae et Gynaecologiae* 1985; **197** (suppl): 65–6.

369 Thomason JL, Sampson MB *et al*. Pregnancy complicated by concurrent primary hyperparathyroidism and pancreatitis. *Obstetrics and Gynecology* 1981; **57** (suppl 6): 34S–6.

370 Thorling L. Jaundice in pregnancy: clinical study. *Acta Medica Scandinavica* 1955; **302** (suppl): 1–123.

371 Tiitinen A, Laatikainen T *et al*. Placental protein 10 (PP10) in normal pregnancy and cholestasis of pregnancy. *British Journal of Obstetrics and Gynaecology* 1985; **92**: 1137–40.

372 Tikkanen MJ & Adlercreutz H. Recurrent jaundice in pregnancy. III. Quantitative determination of urinary estriol conjugates, including studies in pruritus gravidarum. *American Journal of Medicine* 1973; **54**: 600–4.

373 Toaff R, Toaff ME *et al*. Hepatolenticular degeneration (Wilson's disease) and pregnancy. A review and report of a case. *Obstetrical and Gynecological Survey* 1977; **32**: 497–507.

374 Tong MJ, Sinatra FR *et al*. Need for immunoprophylaxis in infants born to HBsAg-positive carrier mothers who are HBeAg negative. *Journal of Pediatrics* 1984; **105**: 945–7.

375 Tong MJ, Thursby M *et al*. Studies on the maternal–infant transmission of the viruses which cause acute hepatitis. *Gastroenterology* 1981; **80**: 999–1004.

376 Trapnell JE & Duncan EHL. Patterns and incidence of acute pancreatitis. *British Medical Journal* 1975; **ii**: 179–83.

377 Trey C & Davidson CS. The management of fulminant hepatic failure. *Progress in Liver Disease* 1970; **3**: 282–98.

378 Tripathi BM & Misra NP. Viral hepatitis with pregnancy. *Journal of the Association of Physicians of India* 1981; **29**: 463–9.

379 Tsega E. Viral hepatitis during pregnancy in Ethiopia. *East African Medical Journal* 1976; **53**: 270–7.

380 Urban E, Frank BW *et al*. Liver dysfunction with mestranol but not with norethynodrel in a patient with Enovid-induced jaundice. *Annals of Internal Medicine* 1968; **68**: 598–602.

381 Van Os HC, Drogendijk AC *et al*. The influence of contamination of culture medium with hepatitis B virus on the outcome of *in vitro* fertilization pregnancies. *American Journal of Obstetrics and Gynecology* 1991; **165**: 152–9.

382 Van Thiel D. Effects of pregnancy and sex hormones on the liver. *Seminars in Liver Disease* 1987; **7**: 1–66.

383 Varma RR, Michelsohn NH *et al*. Pregnancy in cirrhotic and non-cirrhotic portal hypertension. *Obstetrics and Gynecology* 1976; **50**: 217–22.

384 Varner M & Rinderknecht NK. Acute fatty metamorphosis of pregnancy. A maternal mortality and literature review. *Journal of Reproductive Medicine* 1980; **24**: 177–80.

385 Vesterinen E, Savolainen ER *et al*. Occurrence of herpes simplex and cytomegalovirus infections. *Acta Obstetrica et Gynecologica Scandinavica* 1977; **56**: 101–4.

386 Vons C, Smadja C *et al*. Successful pregnancy after Budd–Chiari syndrome (letter). *Lancet* 1984; **ii**: 975.

387 Vujic I, Stanley JH *et al*. Embolic management of rare hemorrhagic gynecologic and obstetrical conditions. *Cardiovascular and Interventional Radiology* 1986; **9**: 69–74.

388 Waffarn F, Carlisle S *et al*. Fetal exposure to maternal hyperbilirubinaemia. *Journal of Diseases of Children* 1982; **136**: 416–17.

389 Wagner VP, Smale LE *et al*. Amoebic abscess of the

liver and spleen in pregnancy and the puerperium. *Obstetrics and Gynecology* 1974; **45**: 562–5.

390 Wagner WH, Lundell CJ *et al*. Percutaneous angiographic embolization for hepatic arterial hemorrhage. *Archives of Surgery* 1985; **120**: 1241–9.

391 Walshe JM. Pregnancy in Wilson's disease. *Quarterly Journal of Medicine* 1977; **46**: 73–83.

392 Walshe JM. The management of pregnancy in Wilson's disease treated with trientine. *Quarterly Journal of Medicine* 1986; **58**: 81–7.

393 Weinstein L. Syndrome of hemolysis, elevated liver enzymes, and low platelet count; a consequence of hypertension in pregnancy. *American Journal of Obstetrics and Gynecology* 1982; **142**: 159–67.

394 Wertheim RA, Brooks BJ *et al*. Fatal herpetic hepatitis in pregnancy. *Obstetrics and Gynecology* 1983; **62**: 38–42.

395 Whelton MJ & Sherlock S. Pregnancy in patients with hepatic cirrhosis. Management and outcome. *Lancet* 1968; **ii**: 995–9.

396 Whorton CM, Thomas DM *et al*. Fatal herpes simplex virus type 2 infection in a healthy young woman. *Southern Medical Journal* 1983; **76**: 81–3.

397 Wilinson EJ. Acute pancreatitis in pregnancy: a review of 98 cases and a report of 8 new cases. *Obstetrics and Gynecological Survey* 1973; **28**: 281–303.

398 Williamson SL & Williamson MR. Cholecystosonography in pregnancy. *Journal of Ultrasound Medicine* 1984; **3**: 329–31.

399 Wilson BR & Haverkamp AD. Cholestatic jaundice of pregnancy; new perspectives. *Obstetrics and Gynecology* 1979; **54**: 650–2.

400 Winer Muram HT, Muram D *et al*. Hepatic rupture in preeclampsia: the role of diagnostic imaging. *Journal of the Canadian Association of Radiology* 1985; **36**: 34–6.

401 Winsnes R & Siebke JC. Efficacy of post-exposure prophylaxis with hepatitis B immunoglobulin in Norway. *Journal of Infection* 1986; **12**: 11–21.

402 Wolf H, Kuhler O *et al*. Leberdystrophie bei disseminierter Herpes-simplex-Infektion in der Schwangerschaft (Liver dystrophy in disseminated herpes simplex infection in pregnancy). *Geburtshilfe Frauenheilkd* 1992; **52**: 123–5.

403 Wong LC, Choo YC *et al*. Hepatic metastases in gestational trophoblastic disease. *Obstetrics and Gynecology* 1986; **67**: 107–11.

404 Wong VCV, Ip H *et al*. Prevention of the HBsAg carrier state in newborn infants of mothers who are chronic carriers of HBsAg and HBeAg by administration of hepatitis-B vaccine and hepatitis-B immunoglobulin. *Lancet* 1984; **i**: 921–6.

405 Woo D, Cummings M *et al*. Vertical transmission of hepatitis B surface antigen in carrier mothers in two west London hospitals. *Archives of Disease in Childhood*. 1979; **54**: 670–5.

406 Woo JS, Wong LC *et al*. Sonographic patterns of pelvic and hepatic lesions in persistent trophoblastic disease. *Journal of Ultrasound Medicine* 1985; **44**: 189–98.

407 Woodhouse DR & Haylen B. Gallbladder disease complicating pregnancy. *Australian and New Zealand Journal of Obstetrics and Gynaecology* 1985; **25**: 233–7.

408 Yamauchi M, Nakajima H *et al*. An epidemic of non-A/non-B hepatitis in Japan. *American Journal of Gastroenterology* 1983; **78**: 652–5.

409 Young EJ, Killam AP *et al*. Disseminated herpesvirus infection; association with primary genital herpes in pregnancy. *Journal of the American Medical Association* 1976; **235**: 2731–3.

410 Zanetti AR, Dentico P *et al*. Multicenter trial of the efficacy of HBIG and vaccine in preventing perinatal hepatitis B. Final report. *Journal of Medical Virology* 1986; **18**: 327–34.

411 Zanetti AR, Ferron P *et al*. Perinatal transmission of the hepatitis B virus and of the HBV associated delta agent from mothers to offspring in Northern Italy. *Journal of Medical Virology* 1982; **9**: 139–48.

412 Zanetti AR, Tanzi E *et al*. Vertical transmission of the HBV-associated delta agent. In: Verme G, Bonino F & Rizzetto M (eds), *Viral Hepatitis and Delta Infection*, Alan R. Liss, New York, 1983: 127–32.

413 Zoglio JDD & Cardillo E. The Dubin–Johnson syndrome and pregnancy. *Obstetrics and Gynecology* 1973; **42**: 560–3.

414 Zuckerman AJ. Preventative medicine. Appraisal of intradermal immunisation against hepatitis B. *Lancet* 1987; **1**: 435–6.

415 Zuckerman AJ. Viral hepatitis. *British Medical Bulletin* 1990; **46**: 1–564.

416 Zuckerman AJ & Thomas HC (ed.). *Viral hepatitis*. Churchill Livingstone, Edinburgh, 1994.

Further reading

Blumberg BS, Fredlander JS *et al*. Hepatitis and Australia antigen: autosomal recessive inheritance of susceptibility to infection in humans. *Proceedings of the National Academy of Science (USA)* 1969; **62**: 1108–15.

Bova JG & Schenker S. Acute fatty liver of pregnancy (letter). *New England Journal of Medicine* 1985; **313**: 1608.

Carman WF, Fagan EA *et al*. Association of a precore genomic variant of hepatitis B virus with fulminant hepatitis. *Hepatology* 1991; **14**: 219–23.

De Pagter AGF, Van Berge Henegouwen GP *et al*. Familial benign recurrent intrahepatic cholestasis. Interrelation with intrahepatic cholestasis of pregnancy and oral contraceptives? *Gastroenterology* 1976; **71**: 202–7.

Denney RC & Johnson R. Nutrition, alcohol and drug abuse. *Proceedings of the Nutrition Society* 1984; **43**: 265–70.

Eliakim M, Sadovsky E *et al*. Recurrent cholestatic jaundice of pregnancy. Report of five cases and electron microscopic observations. *Archives of Internal Medicine* 1966; **117**: 696–705.

Fagan EA, Partridge M *et al*. Review of the herpesviruses and hepatitis A: the potential hazards in dental care. *Oral Surgery, Oral Medicine, Oral Pathology* 1987; **64**: 693–7.

Food and Drug Administration (FDA), Department of Health, Education and Welfare. Oral contraceptive labelling. *Food and Drug Administration Drug Bulletin* 1978; **8**: 12–13.

Heyl PS. The fetal alcohol syndrome. In Rustgi VK & Cooper JN (eds), *Gastrointestinal and Hepatic Complications in Pregnancy*. J. Wiley & Sons, New York, 1986: 277–89.

Jarnfelt-Samsioe A, Eriksson B *et al*. Gallbladder disease related to use of oral contraceptives and nausea in pregnancy. *Southern Medical Journal* 1985; **78**: 1040–3.

Johnson P. Studies in cholestasis of pregnancy with special reference to lipids and lipoproteins. *Acta Obstetrica Gynecologica Scandinavica* 1973; **27** (suppl): 1–80.

Jones KL, Smith DW *et al*. Pattern of malformation in offspring of chronic alcoholic women. *Lancet* 1973; **i**: 1267–71.

Karayiannis P, Fowler MJF *et al*. Detection of serum HBV-DNA by molecular hybridization — correlation with HBeAg/anti-HBe status, racial origin, liver histology and hepatocellular carcinoma. *Journal of Hepatology* 1985; **1**: 99–106.

Kiilholma P, Erkkola R *et al*. Trace elements in postdate pregnancy. *Gynecological and Obstetrical Investigation* 1984; **18**: 45–8.

Machu JH, Duvaldestin P *et al*. Biliary transport of cholephilic dyes: evidence for two different pathways. *American Journal of Physiology* 1977; **232**: E445–50.

Margolis K & Naidoo BN. Spontaneous postpartum subcapsular haematoma of the liver. *South African Medical Journal* 1974; **48**: 1997–8.

Miles JF, Martin JN *et al*. Post-partum eclampsia: a recurring perinatal dilemma. *Obstetrics and Gynecology* 1990; **76**: 328–31.

Morbidity Mortality Weekly Report (MMWR). Hepatitis B virus: a comprehensive strategy for eliminating transmission in the United States through universal childhood vaccination. Report of the Immunization Proceedings Advisory Committee (ACIP). *Morbidity Mortality Weekly Report* 1991; **RR-13 40**: 1–25.

Radberg G, Friman S *et al*. The influence of pregnancy and contraceptive steroids on the biliary tract and its reference to cholesterol gallstone formation. *Scandinavian Journal of Gastroenterology* 1990; **25**: 97–102.

Ranta T, Vnnerus HA *et al*. Elevated plasma prolactin concentration in cholestasis of pregnancy. *American Journal of Obstetrics and Gynecology* 1979; **134**: 1–3.

Rosett HL, Weiner L *et al*. Patterns of alcohol consumption in fetal development. *Obstetrics and Gynecology* 1983; **61**: 539–46.

Scantlebury V, Gordon R *et al*. Childbearing after liver transplantation. *Transplantation* 1990; **49**: 317–21.

Sokol RJ. Alcohol and abnormal outcomes of pregnancy. *Canadian Medical Association Journal* 1981; **125**: 143–8.

Starr JG, Bart RD *et al*. Inapparent congenital cytomegalovirus infection. Clinical and epidemiologic characteristics in early infancy. *New England Journal of Medicine* 1970; **282**: 1075–8.

Stevens CE & Beasley RP. Lack of an autosomal recessive genetic influence in vertical transmission of hepatitis B antigen. *Nature* 1976; **260**: 715–16.

Streissguth AP. Fetal alcohol syndrome: epidemiologic perspective. *American Journal of Epidemiology* 1978; **107**: 467–78.

Summerskill WHJ & Walshe JM. Benign recurrent intrahepatic 'obstructive' jaundice. *Lancet* 1959; **ii**: 686–90.

Tada H, Yanagida M *et al*. Combined passive and active immunization for preventing perinatal transmission of hepatitis B virus carrier state. *Pediatrics* 1982; **70**: 613–19.

Tarnier M. Note sur l'état grassieux du foie dans la fièvre puerpérale. 1856. *Comptes Rendus Séances et Memoires Société De Biologie* 1856; **III**: 209–14.

Vyas GN. Evidence against a recessive inheritance of susceptibility to the chronic carrier state for hepatitis B antigen. *Nature* 1974; **248**: 159–60.

Walters RM. Alcohol and advice to the pregnant woman. *British Medical Journal* 1983; **286**: 640.

Wright JT, Waterson EJ *et al*. Alcohol consumption, pregnancy and low birthweight. *Lancet* 1983; **i**: 663–5.

10

Disorders of the Gastrointestinal Tract

Elizabeth A. Fagan

Management problems in pregnancy, 379
Dietary habits in pregnancy, 380
Disorders of the oral cavity, 380
- Aphthous stomatitis
- Hyperplastic gingivitis
- Dental caries

Gastro-oesophageal disorders, 381
- Gastro-oesophageal reflux
- Hiatus hernia
- Oesophagitis
- Nausea and vomiting

Gastrointestinal disorders, 387
- Gastric acid secretion
- Peptic ulceration
- Coeliac disease

Infections and infestations, 390
- Bacterial infections
- HIV, acquired immunodeficiency syndrome and the gastrointestinal tract
- Intestinal parasites and infestations
- Viral gastroenteritis

Inflammatory bowel disease, 397
- Management
- Ileostomy and colostomy

Appendicitis, 403
Intestinal obstruction, 404
Abdominal complications of tubal pregnancy, 405
Total parenteral nutrition (hyperalimentation), 405
Jejuno-ileal bypass, 405
Constipation, 406
Irritable bowel syndrome, 407
Anorectal and perineal disorders, 408
- Haemorrhoids
- Sphincter injuries
- Herpes simplex
- Papillomaviruses and warts

Gastrointestinal malignancies, 409

Management problems in pregnancy

Symptoms relating to the gastrointestinal tract, such as nausea, vomiting and constipation, are common in pregnancy. Alterations in the neuroendocrinological axis and gut motility have been implicated but the underlying physiological changes remain controversial. Delayed gastric emptying has been implicated in the impaired absorption of glucose in some [155] but not all [287] studies. Most recent data show no significant delay in gastric emptying and intestinal transit when compared with non-pregnant females. These gestational problems are self-limiting and most do not affect maternal and fetal outcome. Their importance in obstetric practice is to differentiate from the many diseases with similar presentations requiring specific diagnosis and management.

Advances in ultrasonographic techniques have revolutionized the diagnosis of many gastrointestinal disorders. These should be employed whenever possible, especially prior to surgery, to improve the specificity of diagnosis.

The fetal brain is especially sensitive to radiation damage between weeks 8 and 15 of gestation. There is some evidence that exposure of below 200 mGy is without apparent harmful effect on the developing fetal brain and well above that used for most diagnostic procedures today, using modern, well-maintained equipment [344]. A single film taken through the abdomen by a computerized tomography (CT) scan probably is safe. The effects of magnetic resonance imaging (MRI) have not been evaluated in pregnancy. The minimum number of films should be used and the fetus shielded. Flexible fibre-optic upper endoscopy is safe in expert hands and preferred to conventional barium studies for suspected gastro-oesophageal reflux, gastric lesions, peptic ulcer and coeliac disease. Flexible fibre-optic sigmoidoscopy is also safe if carried out with care and is essential for investigating persistent diarrhoea especially in the management of colonic inflammatory bowel disease.

Self-medication for gastrointestinal disorders is widespread. Proprietary antacids, anti-emetics, laxatives and antidiarrhoeal agents may be taken before awareness of pregnancy. Patients with pre-existing diseases, such as inflammatory bowel disease on regular medication, require close monitoring. The decision to alter treatment will depend on the relative risks to the fetus and mother, should she relapse.

Suggestions for therapy included in this chapter are given on the understanding that many drugs have not been subjected to extensive trials in pregnancy. A drug should always be prescribed with reluctance and only for disorders that are not self-limiting and of short duration. A decision to treat in the first trimester should be considered exceptional.

Dietary habits in pregnancy

Changes in dietary selection are common. Aversion to coffee, alcohol, cigarettes, fried food, poultry and herbs are common and exacerbated by nausea, vomiting and gastro-oesophageal reflux. Dietary cravings also are common but their mechanisms are poorly understood [155]. In a large study of 1772 women in the first trimester [383], dietary cravings were reported in 68 per cent of urban black, and 84 per cent of white, women. Typical tastes included sour, savoury and sweet and especially for fruit and milk. Aversions reported in 45 and 81 per cent respectively typically were against meat, fish, fatty foods and coffee [383].

Pica also is common [150]. Cravings admitted are for clay, chalk, starch, coal, soap, toothpaste and disinfectants [150,383]. Ethnic factors may play a role [150,383]. In the study by Walker *et al.* [383], pica, particularly for soil and ash, was reported in 38–44 per cent of black, compared with 5 per cent of Indian and white, women; the latter preferred chalk and ice. Underlying mechanisms are not understood. Pica is not related necessarily to gestational nausea and vomiting [383] or parity. The relation between geophagia (eating soil) and iron-deficiency anaemia [71,150], especially resulting from blood loss in the gastrointestinal tract [106], is debated. Geophagy is not exclusive to pregnancy but tends to be exacerbated. Geophagy usually resolves after delivery but typically recurs in later pregnancies. Pica usually is harmless but has been implicated in some cases of maternal and perinatal mortalities [150], chronic constipation, bowel obstruction and parasitosis such as toxoplasmosis [106] and congenital plumbism [283].

Disorders of the oral cavity

Aphthous stomatitis

Benign ulceration has been reported in up to 20 per cent of the general population [10]. Complaints amongst pregnant women are common but a literature review concluded there was no evidence for an association between aphthous stomatitis, the menstrual cycle, pregnancy or the menopause [230]. Large objective studies are lacking. Most cases are idiopathic and a family history is common. The importance is to recognize the exceptions which can herald many diseases such as coeliac disease, inflammatory bowel disease (IBD), Behçet's syndrome, Reiter's syndrome, nutritional deficiencies, immunodeficiencies, particularly human immunodeficiency virus (HIV) infection (see Chapter 16) and various haematological disorders.

The numerous and diverse medications testify to their limited success and understanding of the idiopathic form of ulceration. Management generally is palliative, aimed at relieving pain, reducing the number of ulcer days, extending the periods of remission and identifying and treating any underlying disorders, especially deficiency of vitamins such as folic acid and B_{12} and iron, and fungal infection. Treatment should focus on good dental hygiene, antifungal lozenges for superadded candidiasis and, if necessary, topical corticosteroids.

Hyperplastic gingivitis (see also Chapter 19)

Hyperplasia of gingival tissues can occur with puberty in association with elevated levels of gonadotrophins and sex hormones [127] as well as in pregnancy [211]. Loe and Silness [211] found gingivitis in all women between the second and eighth month, with regression at term and after delivery. Lobulated or nodulated gingival tissue (pregnancy tumour, pregnancy granuloma) has been reported in 2 per cent of pregnancies [405]. In extreme cases the gingival margin and interdental papillae may become a deep purple and red with excessive bleeding on contact [127]. Histological features may be similar to pyogenic granuloma and include nodular inflammatory hyperplasia with endothelial proliferation and vascular dilatation. Gingival oedema seems to be the primary feature; debris and other irritants are not considered to be the major cause [155]. Management is difficult as these conditions may recur. Some improvement can occur with attention to oral hygiene, removal of dental plaque and use of soft toothbrushes.

Dental caries

The increase in pregnancy by one to two times that of the non-pregnant population relates to the increase in incidence of acidophilic micro-organisms (*Streptococcus mutans, Lactobacillus acidophilus*) in plaque and subgingiva. Measurement of the pH of saliva has given conflicting results [155]. Predisposing factors include raised levels of sex hormones [192]. Deficiency of calcium plays only a secondary role.

Gastro-oesophageal disorders

Gastro-oesophageal reflux

Pathophysiology

Dyspepsia and heartburn due to gastro-oesophageal reflux are distressing symptoms that often commence in early pregnancy and occur in up to 80 per cent of pregnant women [105,369]. Reflux is most common in the third trimester [116] but can occur at any time during gestation. Various hypotheses have been postulated to explain the predisposition to reflux during pregnancy including mechanical factors such as changes in lower oesophageal sphincter pressure (LOSP) [20,53,87], increased intragastric pressure [50,67], reduced competence of the pyloric sphincter with backwash of alkaline bile [15], failure of acid clearance, diet and racial predisposition [30].

Gastro-oesophageal reflux is related to a reduced 'barrier' pressure — the difference between gastric and LOSP pressure — rather than an elevation in intragastric pressure alone [20,272,370]. LOSP is under control from a variety of humoral agents [370] including gut hormones, particularly motilin [128], acetylcholine, noradrenaline, histamine, 5-hydroxytryptamine (5-HT) and prostaglandins [128]. In the non-pregnant individual, there is an adaptive response to any rise in intragastric pressure with an increase in LOSP [67,370]. This response prevents reflux by maintaining the barrier pressure. In pregnancy, in women taking combined progesterone and oestrogen oral contraceptive therapy and in the luteal phase of the menstrual cycle [370] there is a failure of this adaptive response due to lowering of LOSP [20] under the combined influence of progesterone and oestrogen, rather than oestrogen alone [272]. Elevation in intragastric pressure commences from the first trimester but plays only a minor role [20] except, perhaps, in late pregnancy.

Factors which promote gastro-oesophageal reflux by lowering the LOSP include a variety of drugs, especially those used in anaesthesia such as atropine, halothane, enflurane, opiates and thiopentone, and tricyclic antidepressant agents [67]. Other factors in pregnancy include the impaired contractile response to exogenous stimuli such as a protein meal and pentagastrin [272,370] although plasma levels of gastrin, gastric pH and gastric acid output are unchanged by pregnancy [335].

Hiatus hernia

Hiatus hernia is common in the general population and can be demonstrated in about 10–20 per cent of women in late pregnancy [50]. Controversy continues over the relation between the 'barrier' pressure, symptoms of gastro-oesophageal reflux and the presence of a hiatus hernia [30,62].

Oesophagitis

Inflammation of the oesophageal mucosa results from contact with acid or alkaline gastric contents. The most common cause is gastro-oesophageal reflux of acid peptic juice with or without hiatus hernia [62] or vomiting [323]. Alkaline oesophagitis also may occur [175]. There is no direct correlation between severity of symptoms, the degree of gastro-oesophageal reflux [20], extent of oesophagitis seen at endoscopy and histopathology and the presence of an hiatus hernia.

Management

Gastro-oesophageal reflux and oesophagitis are distressing symptoms which often require treatment after exclusion of other disorders. Similar symptoms, especially dyspepsia, can herald many disorders ranging from infections and infestations, liver and biliary diseases, pancreatitis and myocardial infarction. Reflux can present as bronchospasm.

In early pregnancy, ingestion of small carbohydrate-rich meals with avoidance of excess fat and alcohol [145], and avoiding bending, stooping and lying supine, are sufficient to alleviate symptoms in over half of the patients. In late pregnancy and during labour and obstetrical anaesthesia there is additional concern regarding the increased risk of vomiting and regurgitation with tracheal aspiration of acid gastric contents leading to a chemical pneumonitis, hypoxia and pulmonary oedema (Mendelson's syndrome, see Chapter 1).

ANTACIDS

A retrospective study showed that up to one-third of women take antacids at some time during pregnancy [263]. Studies on the teratogenicity of conventional simple antacids containing aluminium, magnesium and calcium, suggest that they are safe [263], although prospective data from controlled trials are lacking [16]. Furthermore, aluminium and magnesium hydroxide do not cross into breast milk [208]. Magnesium trisilicate in high dose and over a protracted time should be avoided because respiratory distress, hypotonia, silica nephrolithiasis and cardiovascular complications have been reported [208]. First line therapy is with single preparations of magnesium trisilicate, magnesium hydroxide and non-absorbable alginates in doses of 10–15 ml two to three times daily, between meals and at night. Limited information on preparations containing alginates, such as alginic acid (Gaviscon), suggest these non-absorbed products probably are safe.

Proprietary antacids are best avoided. Many contain anticholinergic agents which are well absorbed, reduce LOSP [46,67,110] and are excreted into breast milk [397]. Sodium bicarbonate should be avoided; metabolic alkalosis and fluid overload can occur in the fetus and mother. Misoprostol, an analogue of prostaglandin E_1, increases uterine tone and contractions and is contraindicated in pregnancy because of the risks of abortion and congenital malformation. In patients with coeliac disease, milk and lactose intolerance, Nulacin, should be avoided because this contains gluten, milk fats and lactose. Cimetidine, ranitidine and other H_2 receptor antagonists have not been approved by the Food and Drugs Administration (FDA) for use during pregnancy and lactation. Sufficient data are lacking regarding their safety [208]. Cimetidine and ranitidine freely cross the placenta [118,243,298]. High levels have been achieved in breast milk compared to serum [5,298]. Anecdotal adverse effects have included hepatic dysfunction with severe jaundice in two newborn infants exposed to cimetidine 1 month prior to delivery [121]. Impaired masculinization has been demonstrated in rats after exposure to cimetidine, but not ranitidine, *in utero* or during the neonatal period [5,277]. Anti-androgenic effects of cimetidine, such as gynaecomastia and galactorrhoea, are recognized in humans. The significance of uterine H_2 receptors is unclear. In rabbits given H_1 and H_2 receptor blockers there was interference with the uterine vascular response at the time of implantation [149] but no adverse effects on fertility and gestation have been noted in humans. In conclusion, the H_2 receptor antagonists should be reserved for peptic ulceration in late pregnancy that has failed to show healing on effective antacid therapy and strict supervision of conservative measures.

Metoclopramide and domperidone raise LOSP [67] but experience in early pregnancy [83,138] is limited (see Anti-emetics below). Metoclopramide interacts with anticholinergic agents. Clinical trials in pregnancy have not been carried out for the long-acting H_2 blockers and omeprazole. Individual publications have reported safety and efficacy of omeprazole in the treatment of hyperemesis gravidarum and in prevention of gastric aspiration prior to anaesthesia. Their safety in human pregnancy and lactation remains to be established.

EMERGENCY ANAESTHESIA

Concern that commonly used antacid suspension gels may be pulmonary irritants if inhaled has led to the preferential use of non-particulate antacid solutions such as sodium citrate. These seem to mix more effectively with gastric juice than their particulate counterparts and probably are safer, at least in late pregnancy and prior to emergency anaesthesia [250]. Cimetidine and ranitidine continue to be used in preparation for obstetrical anaesthesia. Data concerning their efficacy in rapidly neutralizing gastric contents and so preventing pulmonary complications following gastric aspiration are limited. In a controlled trial in Italy of 75 women given ranitidine (50 mg intravenously) 30–60 min before caesarean section, this resulted in a significant reduction in gastric acidity (pH > 2.5) and gastric fluid volume (<25 ml) compared with no therapy [35]. Addition of metoclopramide was without extra benefit [35]. Gastric emptying can be delayed following extradural lumbar anaesthesia and fentanyl. The volume of gastric contents can be assessed using ultrasonography. Prior to anaesthesia, the pH of gastric contents should be raised with a non-particulate antacid such as sodium citrate and an H_2 antagonist. Parenteral anti-emetics commonly used are promethazine and promazine.

Nausea and vomiting

These occur so frequently [36,162,184,242,383] as to be considered by many as diagnostic of pregnancy and its normal physiological consequences. Risk factors implicated in some studies are active and passive smoking, intolerance to oral contraceptive therapy, gallbladder disease and twin pregnancy.

Hyperemesis gravidarum (see below)

This is defined as vomiting occurring before the 20th week and requiring admission to hospital [97]. Studies on hyperemesis have been hampered by variation in definition between centres [406] and a tendency for affected women to register early in pregnancy. Ptyalism (excessive salivation) can be a distressing accompaniment of severe vomiting and probably results from impaired ability of the nauseated woman to swallow normal quantities of saliva [155].

Epidemiology

Nausea and vomiting occur worldwide, crossing cultural, genetic and environmental boundaries [388,389]. Symptoms occur most commonly between the sixth and 16th week [184] but in 20 per cent of cases may continue into the second and third trimesters [242]. In a large prospective epidemiological study carried out between 1959 and 1966 by the National Institutes of Health (USA), 9098 healthy women without any predisposing factors were followed from the first trimester [184]. Vomiting (excluding hyperemesis gravidarum) was reported in 56 per cent and associated more commonly with being a white (but not black) primapara, young, of low education, non-smoker, obese and black as independent risk factors [184]. Several surprising factors considered not significant in the American study included the presence of a twin pregnancy (compared to singleton), black primagravida, smoking, degree of weight gain, known intolerance to oral contraceptive therapy and gallbladder disease [162], unplanned or planned pregnancy and a past obstetric history of fetal death, hypertension, diabetes and thyrotoxicosis [184]. A tendency to vomit in future pregnancies was significant even when adjusted for age and smoking history. In a prospective study in Sweden of 102 women followed through pregnancy, 61 per cent complained of vomiting in the first trimester [161,162]. In contrast to the American study [184], vomiting was more common in multiparae. Other significant risk factors included a short interpregnancy (<4 years) interval, and a higher diastolic blood pressure in late pregnancy in those who had emesis in the first trimester [161]. No correlation was found with previous intolerance to oral contraceptive therapy, motion sickness, alcohol intake and smoking and complications in late pregnancy such as oedema and eclampsia [161].

The risk for developing hyperemesis gravidarum was assessed between 1958 and 1965 amongst participants who enrolled in the Collaborative Perinatal Study [81]. The risk was increased by being white, reduced age (women aged <20 years had above twice the risk of those aged >35 years), nulliparous and of increased bodyweight. The increased risks for non-smokers [81], with passive smoking [406], parity and obesity, were not found significant in a retrospective study of 64 women with hyperemesis gravidarum [135]. These contradictions can be resolved only by large prospective studies which clearly define and separate hyperemesis gravidarum from uncomplicated gestational emesis and from nausea alone.

Factors associated with a reduced risk of gestational nausea and vomiting seem easier to identify than those associated with increased risk. In a multivariate analysis of 825 women in California surveyed between 1983 and 1984 a reduced risk of gestational nausea and vomiting was associated with being white, aged above 35 years, a history of infertility, of professional occupation, a history of drinking alcohol which pre-dated conception and no previous gestational nausea and vomiting if multiparous [388,389].

Mechanisms

These remain unclear. Altered gastric electrical rhythms documented in early pregnancy using manometric and neuroelectrical techniques [188] reverse 2 months after voluntary termination [297] but their relation to gestational nausea and vomiting remains unproven. Higher levels of β human chorionic gonadotrophin (bHCG) and a specific β_1 glycoprotein (schwangerschafts protein — SP1) have been found in vomiting pregnancies and in hyperemesis gravidarum in some [173,174,225], although not all [81,97,350] studies.

A central role for oestrogens is favoured but unproven. Neuroregulatory hormones such as the β lipotrophins (endorphins) are detectable in placenta and amniotic fluid. Their binding to opioid receptors in the vomiting centre in the hypothalamus which have been sensitized to (bHCG) may promote nausea and vomiting [343]. Other neurotransmitters implicated in vomiting are dopamine, 5-HT, acetylcholine and histamine but their role in gestational emesis remains unclear.

The mechanisms surrounding hyperemesis gravidarum (see below) and its association with uncomplicated gestational vomiting remain obscure. Whether there is an additional genetic predisposition for hyperemesis requires further study. Hyperemesis may represent the extreme end of the spectrum of gestational vomiting. Mean levels of total oestradiol were elevated above those seen in uncomplicated gestational vomiting in one study [81]. In hyperemesis, the elevated levels of serum cholesterol, triglycerides and phospholipids and alterations in low and high density lipoproteins (LDL, HDL) may reflect the effects of excess oestrogen on the liver.

The roles of progesterone, cortisol and thyroxine in gestational vomiting are controversial.

Elevated levels of free thyroxine (T_4) [38,42,48,163] and reverse tri-iodothyronine (rT_3) [38,168] have been found in several, although not all [94], studies in hyperemesis gravidarum and in uncomplicated vomiting [255]. The rise in levels of free T_4 and accompanying HCG were found to be proportional to the severity of nausea and vomiting [255]. These findings support the contention that activation of the thyroid gland in early pregnancy by HCG and/or related hormones is linked to gestational nausea and vomiting [255]. Vomiting may be the presenting symptom in thyrotoxicosis in the non-pregnant [307] and occult (biochemical) thyrotoxicosis is well recognized in trophoblastic tumours [34,48,268]. Assessment of the pituitary–thyroid–adrenal axis has been reported as normal [168,173] and abnormal [38,403]. The general consensus is that the thyrotoxicosis, if present in hyperemesis gravidarum, is occult and that biochemical parameters of thyroid function rapidly return to normal post-partum [38,48] (see also Chapter 12).

Management

Persistent vomiting requires full investigation to exclude pyelonephritis and other infections such as viral hepatitis, other liver disorders including acute liver failure, intestinal obstruction, appendicitis, raised intracranial pressure, thyrotoxicosis and Addison's disease [36,242,307] and ruptured tubal pregnancy and abdominal pregnancy [86] amongst many other disorders. In the third trimester vomiting may herald acute liver failure due to fatty liver, or HELLP syndrome (haemolysis, elevated liver enzymes and low platelet count); other causes are cholecystitis and pancreatitis.

GESTATIONAL VOMITING

Morning sickness does not influence health. Symptoms generally improve with re-assurance, small and dry carbohydrate-rich meals and avoidance of large volume drinks in the early morning [36]. Therapy with anti-emetics is rarely necessary (see below).

HYPEREMESIS GRAVIDARUM

Elevated levels of aspartate aminotransferases (AST; serum glutamic oxalo-acetic transaminase or SGOT) have been reported in 15–25 per cent independently of ketonuria but return to normal with cessation of vomiting and rehydration [253] (see Chapter 9).

Management involves removal from a stressful home environment, withdrawal of oral nutrition and fluids, rehydration with intravenous fluids, replacement of electrolytes and vitamins and treatment with antihistamine anti-emetics or metoclopramide [398]. Corticosteroids have been used in early studies with some reported success [391] but information from controlled trials is lacking.

Hyperemesis with protracted vomiting has been associated with various complications including the Mallory–Weiss oesophageal tear, neurological dysfunction specifically Wernicke's encephalopathy, Korsakoff's psychosis and central pontine myelinolysis [33], retinal haemorrhage and Mendelson's syndrome [97,335]. The neurological disturbances may result from deficiency of vitamin B_1 as assessed by low levels of red cell transketolase and elevated levels of thiamine pyrophosphate. These should respond to the urgent replacement of thiamine (vitamin B_1 complex) and expert, judicious attention to restoration of fluid, and acid–base balance. An elevated prothrombin ratio indicates marked cholestasis and vitamin K deficiency.

Total parenteral nutrition is recommended for severe cases, especially for suspected maternal protein–calorie malnutrition (see below) [124,222, 299,407]. Total parenteral nutrition, including with lipid preparations, is safe in expert hands with special care taken over insertion of the indwelling catheter, regular monitoring of maternal levels of nutrients and provision for delivery of preterm, small-for-dates infants.

Anti-emetic drug therapy. This continues to be widely used and prescribed by physicians in pregnancy [259]. None is approved specifically for use in early pregnancy. The majority of cases of 'morning sickness' can be managed without recourse to drug therapy. Prescription should be reserved for the exceptional case and only after exclusion of intercurrent disease. Pyridoxine hydrochloride (vitamin B_6) is safe and reduces gestational nausea and vomiting in randomized controlled trials although no relation was found between levels of pyridoxal 5′ phosphate and symptoms in 180 pregnant women with morning sickness in the first trimester [319]. Ginger significantly relieved symptoms in hyperemesis gravidarum compared with placebo in one study [110] and seems to be safe but detailed study is lacking. Drugs which block dopamine receptors such as metoclopramide, domperidone and phenothiazines seem safe but should be used with caution. Extrapyramidal side-effects can occur.

DRUG SAFETY

Concern over the teratogenic potential and consequent safety of many anti-emetics in humans following the thalidomide tragedy has led to the re-appraisal of the use of anti-emetic drugs for human pregnancy and the unreliability of some animal studies [205,228]. This concern remains despite encouraging data from large retrospective [263] and prospective [185,195] studies, suggesting that a variety of anti-emetics commonly used in early pregnancy including meclozine, cyclizine and dimenhydrinate probably do not cause a significant increase in congenital malformations [185].

The withdrawal of Bendectin/Debendox (doxylamine succinate, and pyridoxine hydrochloride) from the market in June 1983 for suspected [12,408], but unproved, teratogenicity is an example of public pressure forcing a manufacturer (Merrell Dow, USA) to discontinue a product despite several carefully controlled studies which failed to support an association with congenital abnormalities [104,263,329, 340]. Between 1956 and 1983, Bendectin (Debendox) had been used by over 30 million pregnant women [92] and was the only anti-emetic approved by the FDA for use in pregnancy. Withdrawal was forced after links with individual case reports of, predominantly, skeletal abnormalities [280,281]. Since then, one group [125] in Oxford reported a significant excess of cleft palate in infants born to mothers who had taken Debendox (Bendectin) compared to matched controls during pregnancy. The FDA, in association with the Boston Collaborative Drug Surveillance Program [93] and one other group [12], have found an increased risk of pyloric stenosis and, possibly, congenital heart disease [408]. These studies can be criticized for lack of experimental design allowing bias in data which rely on maternal recall [408], unstructured questioning and lack of matched case controls [93]. More carefully designed studies have failed to show a significant correlation with maternal Bendectin and pyloric stenosis. Future studies should take into account the fluctuation in incidence of congenital diseases such as pyloric stenosis [177].

The individual components of Bendectin (doxylamine, pyridoxine and, previously dicylomine) are available for use in pregnancy. They seem to be safe [247] but experience is small compared with that of Bendectin. Concern remains that these and other less well-tried drugs will be used instead [244,247]. In 1979, the FDA committee removed the restrictions on prescribing meclozine and cyclizine in pregnancy. Evidence to date fails to incriminate them as teratogenic in humans, although teratogenicity in rats is well documented [104]. There are isolated reports of cleft palate in babies born to mothers taking meclozine [204] and cyclizine [229]. Diphenhydramine has been linked to cleft palate [144] and trimethobenzamide, to other fetal anomalies [434]. Some phenothiazines are embryotoxic in animals and, in addition, jaundice and extrapyramidal effects have occurred in neonates of mothers receiving chlorpromazine during pregnancy [44]. Promethazine is probably safe in early pregnancy despite anecdotal reports of congenital hip dislocation [153,195]. Dimenhydrinate may be contraindicated because of anecdotal reports of premature labour [44].

Metoclopramide blocks central and peripheral dopamine D_2 receptors and, at high dose, 5-HT_3 receptors which are implicated in vomiting. Metoclopramide is a base which readily crosses the placenta and is excreted in breast milk [348]. Metoclopramide is generally considered to be safe, despite lack of data from controlled trials, and is finding increasing use in idiopathic vomiting of late pregnancy, labour [138,373] and during anaesthesia [83,342,381]. In the puerperium, metoclopramide causes hyperprolactinaemia and promotes lactation [318]. Other hormonal effects of unknown clinical significance include a reduction in levels of growth hormone, follicle-stimulating hormone and luteinizing hormone [342].

Droperidol, a major tranquillizer of the butyrophenone class, is being used increasingly to prevent vomiting in relation to spinal anaesthesia and caesarean section [314]. Whether it is more effective than metoclopramide when used as a post-operative anti-emetic is debatable [381] and information on its safety in early pregnancy is lacking. Prochlorperazine enjoyed popularity as a general anti-emetic in pregnancy until the 1960s, particularly for hyperemesis gravidarum, but has been superseded by metoclopramide which causes less systemic side-effects. Its use has also been limited because of possible links with cardiovascular and other abnormalities [44]. Ondansetron and granisetron are potent and highly selective 5-HT_3 receptor antagonists but their safety and efficacy have not been evaluated in trials in human pregnancy.

Fetal outcome

Birthweight is usually within the normal range. The incidence of miscarriage, still-birth and preterm delivery each is significantly less, even following hyperemesis gravidarum [81], compared with non-emetic pregnancies [184,237]. Meta-analyses confirm a small reduction in risk of spontaneous abortion before 20 weeks with gestational vomiting. No statistical association has been found between gestational nausea and vomiting, perinatal mortality and fetal anomalies [81]. Intrauterine growth retardation and small-for-dates babies can occur with severe hyperemesis gravidarum in association with maternal weight loss [135] and multiple hospital admissions [124]. In a retrospective study of 64 women, intrauterine growth retardation occurred in 32 per cent of babies where mothers lost more than 5 per cent of bodyweight through vomiting compared with 6 per cent born if mothers maintained their weight [135].

Vomiting *per se* is not considered to be teratogenic. The Collaborative Perinatal Project group at the National Institutes of Health (USA) conducted a prospective study on the epidemiology of vomiting in pregnancy in the 1960s which involved 16 398 women registered before the 20th week and, subsequently, 1046 (6.4 per cent) abnormalities and 1387 minor anomalies [184]. No single category of congenital defects was found to be significantly different between vomiting pregnancies on no therapy and non-vomiting pregnancies [184]. In addition, there were no significant differences for congenital defects between cases of 'morning sickness', those with hyperemesis gravidarum and non-vomiting pregnancies [124,135,184] except for macrosomia in severe hyperemesis reported in one study [135]. These findings support earlier studies in which a smaller number of mothers of infants born with major abnormalities required anti-emetics in the first trimester (7.4 per cent) than mothers of normal infants (13.1 per cent), suggesting an inverse relation between nausea and vomiting (anti-emetic therapy) and fetal abnormalities [263].

Gastrointestinal disorders

Gastric acid secretion

Studies on gastric physiology during pregnancy are limited. The consensus from early papers is that basal and maximal acid outputs are not altered significantly [335,369]. Variation between and within individuals is wide, yielding conflicting results [155]. Any reduction in outputs is limited to the second trimester [154,155]. Serum pepsinogen, an indirect marker of acid output, does not change significantly through pregnancy and the puerperium [382]. Serum levels of gastrin rise significantly only as term approaches and peak soon after birth [306].

Any reduction in acid output during pregnancy is insufficient to explain the reported reduction in peptic ulcer symptoms [276,382]. However, the rise in level of serum gastrin, which peaks post-partum, corresponds with the resurgence of ulcer symptoms. Oestrogens may play a role in cytoprotection, independent of effects on acid output, since clinical trials have shown improved healing in men taking stilboestrol [362]. The reduction in symptoms of peptic ulceration seen during pregnancy also have been attributed to a healthier diet, increased intake of foods such as milk, emotional tranquillity and medical supervision [68].

Peptic ulceration

Prevalence

Peptic ulceration arising *de novo* in pregnancy is remarkably uncommon. In nearly 23 000 deliveries, only six women had proven active ulceration [22]. In a study of 118 women with peptic ulceration documented prior to pregnancy, 89 per cent improved clinically or became symptomless [68]. Despite these encouraging reports peptic ulceration is probably underrecognized. Symptoms do not correlate with disease severity. There remains a reluctance to use diagnostic fibre-optic endoscopic techniques despite their safety in expert hands. Furthermore, there are reports of increased severity of peptic ulcer symptoms and complications during pregnancy [22,68,199,284], especially in association with toxaemia [164,199]. In addition, quiescent ulcers may erupt [68], especially in the puerperium [13,61,164,199,279].

Presentation may be acute with massive haemorrhage [13,57,313] and perforation [9,279,313]. The interrelation between duodenal and gastric ulceration, *Helicobacter pylori* (initially termed *Campylobacter pylori*), gastritis and pregnancy is not known.

Diagnosis relies on a high index of suspicion. Prodromal symptoms of pain exacerbated after meals may be absent or confused with simple dyspepsia. Physical examination may be normal or reveal minimal abdominal tenderness despite severe peptic ulceration, perforation and peritonitis. Upper oesophagogastroduodenoscopy (endoscopy) is safe in pregnancy and, in experienced hands, can be carried out in many instances with only topical anaesthesia to the nasopharynx. Unfortunately, experience in pregnancy is very limited. Out of 3300 questionnaires sent to the members of the American Society for Gastrointestinal Endoscopy only 73 fibreoptic examinations (three of the oesophagus, 70 of the stomach) were carried out in pregnancy [311]. The average age of the mother was 26 years, and of the fetus 18.3 weeks. Vomiting was listed as an indication in 41 (56.2 per cent) cases including 15 with frank haematemesis. Oesophagitis was found most commonly (34.2 per cent) but peptic ulceration was diagnosed in seven cases [311].

Haemorrhage and perforation of peptic ulcer are uncommon in late pregnancy and the puerperium but under-recognized and may be fatal [13,279]. Mistaken diagnoses have included perforated pyometra [296] and gastric carcinoma [76].

Management

General principles are unchanged by pregnancy [164]. Conservative measures include prohibition of smoking, bed rest and regular antacids [157,158]. Indications for surgery and outcome, including mortality, are similar to the non-pregnant state [22,164]. Prompt resuscitation of the mother may be followed by surgery and, if necessary, delivery by caesarean section [164].

ANTI-ULCER THERAPY

Antacids remain the mainstay of therapy. There is sufficient evidence from studies in the non-pregnant that adequate dosage can achieve the same rates of healing of duodenal ulcers as cimetidine [158]. Relapse rates also are not significantly faster or greater in patients receiving antacids compared to cimetidine therapy for duodenal ulcers [158]. The specific interactions of anti-ulcer therapy and pregnancy are considered above.

Coeliac disease

Gluten-sensitive enteropathy is an abnormality of the small intestinal mucosa caused by the ingestion of gluten-containing substances in susceptible individuals. In most cases, histology from a jejunal and duodenal biopsy shows subtotal villous atrophy. Withdrawal of gluten from the diet results in marked clinical and histological improvement. The histopathological appearances may remain abnormal for months.

Epidemiology

The prevalence of coeliac disease in the West has been estimated at 0.03 per cent [58]. The incidence varies considerably from one in 6500 of the general population in Sweden [41] and one in 890 in Switzerland to between one in 2000 to 8000 in the UK [45]. The highest recorded incidence is one in 300 for western Ireland [231]. The true incidence may be higher because reports tend to reflect early studies with the classical, more florid presentations (see below). Coeliac disease probably occurs worldwide but histological documentation in developing countries is limited. The preponderance of females [32,132,379] has been matched by an equal sex ratio [64,219] in other reports.

Up to 80 per cent are positive for the histocompatibility antigen HLA-B8 [981] and there is a familial link [213,261]. Symptomless relatives may have biochemical abnormalities suggesting malabsorption such as a low serum folate, low xylose excretion and elevated faecal fats making coeliac disease a likely diagnosis [91]. The onset of coeliac disease may be prevented, or delayed for many months, with extended breast feeding in infants with a strong family history, independent of their concurrent ingestion of gluten [17].

Clinical features

Coeliac disease can present at any age [45,132]. The classical features are diarrhoea, malabsorption, anorexia and weight loss. Importantly, many patients, especially adults [32,64,132,261,379], present with only mild and non-specific gastrointestinal symptoms. Presentation to departments other than gastroenterology is frequent, especially for haematological disorders such as megaloblastic and iron-deficiency anaemias, particularly in pregnancy [64,90,91,132]. Diarrhoea and steatorrhoea may be absent. Other presentations include bone pain from osteoporosis and osteomalacia and, rarely, tetany [64,132] secondary to malabsorption of calcium and vitamin D [167]. Neurological manifestations range from generalized muscle weakness to peripheral neuropathies, encephalopathy, syndromes associated with deficiencies of vitamins B_6 and B_{12} and psychiatric illnesses, including psychoses. Changes in the skin and mucous membranes are common. Coeliac disease may present with glossitis, cheilosis, stomatitis, aphthous ulceration, pigmentation, dermatitis herpetiformis and oedema [32,64,132,219].

Effects on fertility

Female. Untreated disease is associated with delayed menarche, oligomenorrhoea and involuntary infertility but pathogenetic mechanisms remain unclear. Outcome improves with restoration of normal gut histology following withdrawal of gluten and correction of any nutritional deficiencies.

Most studies [132,252] of untreated disease show that menarche is delayed by about 1 year and that amenorrhoea is prevalent. In an Italian study [252] based on 54 consecutive women with untreated disease and control women (healthy and with irritable bowel syndrome) matched for age and sexual behaviour, amenorrhoea was significantly more common in untreated coeliacs (38.8 per cent) than controls (9.2 per cent). The numbers of pregnancies and live births were similar among the 38 coeliacs and matched controls who did not use contraceptive measures. Infertility has been reported in males with untreated disease; impotence was reported in 18 per cent, with sperm motility impaired in 75 percent [101,102]. Abnormal sperm forms recorded in 46 per cent, improved after gluten withdrawal [101,102].

Male. In the untreated male, dysfunction of the hypothalamic–pituitary axis has been implicated to account for the elevations in plasma levels of testosterone and luteinizing hormone [102] and serum prolactin [348] found in some cases. Infertility was reversible on treatment in one study [23].

Effects in pregnancy

Maternal outcome. In known coeliacs, exacerbation of symptoms can occur during pregnancy and the puerperium [271]. Data relating to histological relapse, intercurrent infection and dietary factors are lacking. Recall of gastrointestinal symptoms in childhood is common for women who present in pregnancy. Symptoms may resolve around puberty despite persistently abnormal histology [258] and recur during pregnancy [90,91,219], surgery [100], stress and intercurrent infection [47,88,89].

Fetal outcome. In the Italian study [252] spontaneous abortions were more common in the untreated coeliacs (26 cases) compared with controls (10 cases) and this agrees with previous reports [165,271]. Cumulative data link untreated coeliac disease with recurrent abortion [165,252,271]. In the Italian study of untreated coeliacs, recurrent spontaneous abortion occurred independent of severity and duration of clinical disease and unspecified biochemical abnormalities [270]. Spontaneous abortion has also been linked with megaloblastic anaemia [90,91, 219] secondary to folic acid deficiency [221]. In Sweden between 1952 and 1961, five of 39 women with coeliac disease had megaloblastic anaemia documented in a previous pregnancy [90]. In a later study of 32 women diagnosed more than 10 years previously as having megaloblastic anaemia in pregnancy, 41 per cent had low levels of serum folate compared with healthy matched controls (10 per cent) and 27 per cent of patients had elevated levels of faecal fat suggesting malabsorption [90,91]. Folic acid deficiency is particularly relevant to the current concern relating to neural tube defect [80] (see below).

A study was carried out at the Hammersmith Hospital between 1965 and 1973 on 25 women (60 pregnancies) with jejunal histology consistent with coeliac disease and supplemented during pregnancy with carbohydrates and vitamins [271]. In untreated disease, eight of 38 pregnancies (21 per cent) ended in first trimester abortion compared to only one of 22 who adhered strictly to a gluten-free diet [271]. The number of small-for-dates infants was higher than normal and similar between non-compliant coeliacs (16 per cent) and those who adhered strictly to their gluten-free diets (19 per cent).

Overall, study samples have been too small to assess the impact of treated and untreated coeliac disease, and related vitamin deficiencies, on fetal outcome, including congenital abnormalities.

Diagnosis

This requires a high index of suspicion in clinical practice. Investigation for suspected folate and B_{12} deficiency (see below) should be carried out before indiscriminate prescription of vitamins. Women with suspected disease who present during pregnancy require full investigation. Duodenal biopsy via fibre-optic gastroduodenoscopy is safe in expert hands. Jejunal biopsy with a capsule and radiological imaging is not recommended in pregnancy. In the West less common causes of a flat jejunal biopsy include Crohn's disease, tropical sprue and intolerance to cows' milk protein [384] and soy protein [3]. The main differential diagnosis is from other small bowel disorders such as Crohn's disease, infestations and infections such as *Campylobacter*, *Giardia* and HIV.

Management

A known coeliac should be encouraged to adhere strictly to a gluten-free diet if pregnancy is planned [257,271]. Careful attention should be paid to deficiencies of vitamin B_{12} [74], folic acid [75,305], iron and trace metals such as zinc [290,291] with supplementation through pregnancy and lactation. Serum levels of folate fall progressively through pregnancy and the fetus accumulates folic acid regardless of the maternal stores [74] (see Chapter 2).

There is no universal agreement on the exact daily requirement of folate. Daily intakes above 4000 μg during pregnancy and lactation would comply with recommendations by an expert panel reporting to the Department of Health in the UK [80]. These recommendations are based on results of a single dose study carried out by the Medical Research Council (MRC) [238] in apparently healthy high risk pregnant women with a previous baby affected by a neural tube defect. Prevention of neural tube defects was less convincing for low risk women without a previously affected child in a case control study [245]. Folic acid given as 4 ml (4000 μg) daily resulted in a protective effect of 72 per cent for recurrent neural tube defect [238]. Minimum daily intakes above 0.37 ml (370 μg) have been shown to reduce the risk of recurrent neural tube defects if commenced before conception [340] but this aspect was not addressed in the MRC study. The recommendations by the MRC are considerably higher than average daily intakes (around 150–220 μg total folate) found for healthy pregnant women in the first trimester [305] and general population in the UK in 1990 [238] and 10 times higher than the recommended dietary allowance for folic acid in pregnancy in the USA.

In all patients with gastrointestinal diseases, regardless of their compliance to diet, serial monitoring is essential throughout pregnancy and lactation. Supplements of folate may have to be increased considerably to achieve satisfactory serum and red cell levels. Severe zinc deficiency may occur in acrodermatitis enteropathica and is an established cause of congenital malformation, particularly neural tube defects [290,291].

Failure to respond to a gluten-free diet and clinical relapse should be investigated as in the non-pregnant with attention to dietary indiscretion, inadvertent ingestion of gluten-containing drugs [40], intercurrent infection and infestations such as giardiasis (see below), inflammatory bowel diseases and associated disorders including autoimmune diseases and malignancy. Dyspepsia and dysphagia occurring in coeliac disease should be taken seriously. Upper endoscopy should be carried out in view of the association between oesophageal malignancy and coeliac disease. Follow-up of coeliac disease should be lifelong. All coeliacs, including those who adhere strictly to a gluten-free diet, remain at significant risk of gastrointestinal malignancies, particularly intestinal lymphoma (>50 per cent of malignancies) and oesophageal carcinoma [354].

Infections and infestations

Infections and infestations of the gastrointestinal tract cause significant morbidity worldwide (Box 10.1). Studies to detect pathogens and their effects and management in pregnancy, including safety of any antimicrobial therapy, are few. In an infectious diseases department in Sweden a prospective survey was carried out between 1975 and 1984 on 303 women admitted post-partum with suspected infections linked to gastroenteritis. A pathogenic organism (four bacterial, two parasitic,

Box 10.1. Gastrointestinal infections and infestations

- Bacterial-specific
  - *Escherichia coli*
  - *Salmonella* spp.
  - *Shigella* spp.
  - *Staphylococcus* spp.
  - *Campylobacter* spp.
  - *Cholera*
  - *Listeria* spp.
  - *Aeromonas hydrophilia*
  - *Plesiomonas shigelloides*
  - *Balantidium coli*
  - *Cryptosporidium* spp.
  - *Clostridium difficile*
- Viral infections
  - Rotaviruses
  - Norwalk-like viruses
- Protozoa
  - *Giardia lamblia*
  - *Entamoeba histolytica*
  - *Isospora belli*
- Nematodes (roundworms)
  - *Trichinella spiralis*
  - *Enterobius vermicularis*
  - *Trichuris trichiura*
  - *Ascaris lumbricoides*
  - *Strongyloides stercoralis*
  - *Ancylostoma duodenale*
  - *Necator americanus*
- Cestodes (tapeworms)
  - *Taenia* spp.
  - *Echinococcus* spp.
  - *Hymenolepis nana*

two viral) was found in only eight of 33 (24 per cent) with overt gastroenteritis; a viral aetiology was suspected in half the remaining cases [129].

Bacterial infections

Travellers' diarrhoea

Acute diarrhoea associated with abdominal cramps, bloating, nausea, fever and malaise is well known to travellers. Symptoms typically begin abruptly, occur during travel or shortly after return, usually are self-limiting and require no specific therapy [262]. Infection occurs through ingestion of food and water contaminated with organisms and their toxins. Enterotoxigenic *Escherichia coli* accounts for 40–70 per cent of cases. Other organisms such as the genus *Shigella* may be isolated from the stools in 5–20 per cent of cases. Less commonly isolated organisms include the *Vibrio cholerae*, the genus *Campylobacter, Staphylococcus, Salmonella* and *Clostridium difficile* [262], *Aeromonas hydrophilia* and *Plesiomonas shigelloides*. Occasional causes of travellers' diarrhoea include viruses such as rotaviruses, Norwalk-like viruses and parasites including *Giardia lamblia, Entamoeba histolytica, Strongyloides stercoralis, Isospora belli, Balantidium coli* and the genus *Cryptosporidium*.

HIV, acquired immunodeficiency syndrome (AIDS) and the gastrointestinal tract

(see also Chapter 17)

The impact of HIV infection in the gut relates to the propensity to develop persistent opportunistic infections [390]. Studies specifically in pregnancy are lacking. There is no evidence to believe that the spectrum of infection will differ significantly from non-pregnant HIV seropositive subjects. Oral manifestations include ulcers from herpes simplex virus and *Candida albicans*. Dysphagia can arise from *C. albicans*, cytomegalovirus and Kaposi's sarcoma. The small bowel typically can become infected with various species of *Cryptosporidium, Salmonella, Strongyloides, Isospora* and *Mycobacterium avium intracellulare* and which manifest as watery diarrhoea [390]. Infections of the large bowel typically occur with cytomegalovirus and species of *Shigella* and *Campylobacter*. HIV infection must be considered in all cases of unexplained bowel dysfunction and in the differential diagnosis of IBD and coeliac disease.

Most of the drug therapies recommended [390] are containdicated in pregnancy. However, oral acyclovir has been used safely in pregnant women with severe genital ulcers due to herpes simplex and helps prevent transmission to the neonate [202]. Close consultation with the microbiologist and virologist is essential.

HIV infection predisposes to several malignancies affecting the gastrointestinal tract, including Kaposi's sarcoma, non-Hodgkin's lymphoma and rectal carcinoma [390].

Management principles

Acute diarrhoea lasting < 72 hours often can be managed conservatively with attention to rehydration with clear fluids and without recourse to drugs. Common remedies such as kaolin, pectin and hydrated aluminium silicate act to reduce stool frequency by absorbing water. There is no evidence to show a reduction in water loss by the gut [126].

Controlled prospective trials in non-pregnant subjects using charcoal, preparations containing kaolin, pectin and diphenoxylate showed no influence on outcome and speed of resolution of symptoms (72 hours) compared with controls receiving simple fluid replacement [2]. Occasionally, these preparations may exacerbate symptoms and delay the excretion of organisms such as *Shigella* [126].

Diarrhoea lasting > 72 hours should be investigated. Fresh stools should be sent directly for microscopic examination for ova, cysts and parasites and microbial culture (see Box 10.1). Flexible fibre-optic endoscopy with biopsy is safe in pregnancy in careful expert hands.

ANTIMICROBIAL THERAPY

Controlled studies have indicated that doxycycline, trimethoprim–sulfamethoxazole or trimethoprim alone when taken prophylactically are consistently effective in reducing the incidence of travellers' diarrhoea by up to 90 per cent in certain areas [262]. None, however, is recommended for use in pregnancy. Trimethoprim is a folate antagonist [169] and also may be teratogenic [51] and there is no information on the safety of doxycycline in pregnancy. The injudicious use of antibiotics has led to problems such as increasing microbial resistance which may limit their efficacy. Furthermore, the widespread use of antimicrobial agents such as clindamycin [357], lincomycin, tetracyclines, erythromycin, ampicillin and some cephalosporins [11,236], amongst many others, has led to an increase in pseudomembranous colitis [200].

The diagnosis of antibiotic-associated colitis should be considered in any pregnant patient with diarrhoea complicating recent or previous antimicrobial therapy, even after a single dose [236]. Severity is independent of dose, duration of treatment and route of administration. Nosocomial spread has been reported, in which three women from the same ward treated with cefoxitin as prophylaxis prior to caesarean section, developed diarrhoea [11]. All had *C. difficile* grown from fresh stool culture [11]. Sigmoidoscopy may reveal the characteristic yellow–white plaques, copious mucus and erythematous mucosa. Fresh specimens of stool should be sent for detection of the toxin [11,200]. Therapy includes withdrawal of all antimicrobial agents and administration of vancomycin orally 125–250 mg every 6 hours [11,176]. Vancomycin is poorly absorbed but serum levels should be monitored to prevent damage to the fetal VIIIth cranial nerve [349].

Campylobacteriosis

This is a common, underrecognized cause of acute diarrhoea. In a general survey of acute diarrhoea in adults and children in west Scotland between 1986 and 1987, *Campylobacter* spp. were the second most commonly identified cause after *Salmonella* spp. [330]. *Campylobacter* spp. are found in the faeces of the majority of chickens examined in the UK and USA [52,129] and are a major cause of sterility and abortion in cattle and sheep. In probably the first published report of septicaemia in human pregnancy in 1947, the mother had drunk milk from an aborting cow [378]. *C. fetus* is divided into subspecies *C. jejuni* (*C. coli*) and the more severe *C. fetus* (*C. intestinalis*).

In a review of the literature between 1977 and 1986 there were 97 (19 *C. fetus*) documented cases associated with pregnancy [399]. The 78 cases of *C. jejuni* resulted in 13 babies with meningitis; eight of these also had documented septicaemia [399]. Still-birth occurred in eight cases [399]. In a retrospective study of enteric infections in pregnancy in Canada between 1984 and 1988, *Campylobacter* spp. were the most commonly identified pathogenic organisms being detected in 10 out of 24 000 pregnancies [333], most (eight cases) occurring in the third trimester. Nine proceeded to full-term normal delivery; one baby of a well mother developed *C. jejuni* enterocolitis 3 days later. The 10th pregnancy was complicated by pre-term labour at 28 weeks, neonatal sepsis and death [333].

Infection with *C. fetus* is more serious than with *C. jejuni*. In a retrospective review of seven women, there were three cases of pre-term labour and stillbirth and a further baby died of neonatal sepsis [133]. The mothers had a febrile illness with respiratory symptoms. Although one woman pursued a fulminating course, two others were symptomless [133]. *C. fetus* was isolated from cultures of blood, fetal spleen, brain and placenta. The placenta showed necrosis, infarction and abscess formation. The sources of infection were never identified. In neonatal meningitis and enteritis the source probably is faeco-oral from mothers with diarrhoea at delivery [171,355].

DIAGNOSIS

Gastrointestinal infection in pregnancy with *Campylobacter* can cause abdominal pain, fever and often bloody diarrhoea [133]. *Campylobacter* spp. can cause diarrhoea in HIV seropositive subjects [390]. The typical presentation in an HIV seronegative mother is with a respiratory tract infection with fever [333,378]. Neonatal infection including septicaemia has been reported despite seemingly well mothers [133,333]. These Gram-negative bacilli can be grown from cultures of blood, stool and placenta but may require prolonged incubation under selective media with microaerophilic conditions [37,117,133,171,376]. Blood cultures are preferred to stool cultures which often give false negative results [399].

Analysis and culture of multiple samples of blood, fresh stool and cervical swabs are essential for suspected campylobacter enteritis especially near delivery [6,133,355]. Appropriate cultures, especially of blood, should also be taken from the fetus in cases of septic abortion [133,166], intrauterine death [100] and neonatal gastroenteritis [6]. Samples should be delivered directly to the laboratory without refrigeration. *Campylobacter* infection should be included in the differential diagnosis of toxic megacolon [288].

MANAGEMENT

The advice to avoid unpasteurized milk and to cook poultry thoroughly should be re-inforced in pregnancy. Treatment for maternal gastroenteritis consists of 4 weeks of oral erythromycin base or stearate. Addition of gentamicin and chloramphenicol should be considered for suspected systemic infection [133,399]. Prompt instigation of antimicrobial therapy should be considered because cultures may require extended time for growth. Susceptibility to the β lactam antibiotics such as ampicillins and cephalosporins varies [399]. Relapses are common with shorter courses. Erythromycin is used extensively in pregnancy, especially for genital mycoplasmal infections. Erythromycin crosses the placenta but fetal blood levels remain low [233]. Abnormal levels of serum AST (SGOT) can occur. Erythromycin estolate is contraindicated because of potential hepatotoxicity.

Microbial surveillance, particularly blood cultures, is essential in seemingly healthy neonates born to mothers who excrete campylobacter at delivery [133]. Breast feeding can be allowed with adherence to strict hygiene to prevent cross-infection. Erythromycin is first line therapy for suspected neonatal infection. CT and MRI scanning of the brain and, possibly, lumbar puncture should be considered in neonates with suspected meningitis and intracerebral haemorrhage and infarction [399].

Outbreaks from cross-infection are rare but high standards of hygiene are important, especially the thorough washing of hands and disposal of faeces and contaminated fomites. In suspected maternal gastroenteritis, delivery is best carried out under conditions of nursing isolation [133].

Listeriosis (see also Chapter 16)

The number of cases reported in the general population has increased significantly since 1987. Data from the Public Health Laboratory Service and Communicable Disease Surveillance Centre for the UK [80,345] reflect similar rises elsewhere in Europe [112] and the USA [59,254]. Pregnant women and the immunocompromised are at special risk. Maternofetal listeriosis is uncommon within the

UK; only 24 cases were confirmed out of over 700 000 births in England and Wales in 1990. Nevertheless, awareness of the potentially serious outcome in pregnancy has led to guidelines being published by the Department of Health. All pregnant women are advised to avoid high risk foods such as soft, ripened cheeses and all types of pâté. Sporadic cases have been associated with ingestion of hot-dogs [320] and outbreaks with Mexican-style cheeses [210]. Re-heated food such as cooked–chilled food and pre-cooked poultry should be eaten only if heated thoroughly to piping hot. Refrigeration should be maintained and raw foods separated from cooked foods.

DIAGNOSIS

This requires a high index of suspicion because there are no specific features. Listeriosis should be considered in all cases of febrile illness and flu-like symptoms although even fever may be absent, particularly in neonates. Listeriosis should be excluded in all cases of mid-trimester abortion and pre-term labour and in patients with suspected immunodeficiency, including HIV infection. Definitive diagnosis relies on cultures of blood and meconium-stained liquor sent to the laboratory without delay and without refrigeration. Direct microscopy for Gram-positive bacilli should be carried out on meconium-stained liquor in all cases of pre-term labour with a live baby. Prompt instigation of antibiotic therapy can improve neonatal outcome. The microbiologist should be alerted to screen for listeria. Microbial growth may require selective media.

MANAGEMENT

There are no published results from clinical trials on the choice of antibiotics in pregnancy. Results from isolated reports favour intravenous therapy with ampicillin, amoxycillin or erythromycin. Resistance to cephalosporins is common. Therapy should be instigated without delay and reviewed following results of cultures.

Typhoid and paratyphoid fever, shigellosis and their carriers

Historically, typhoid fever was implicated in up to 3 per cent of cases of spontaneous abortion and pre-term labour [129] but this is a rare cause in the West except in the HIV seropositive subject [390]. These acute infections run a course which is similar to that in the non-pregnant although transplacental infection has been recorded [86,113,310]. Amoxycillin 1 g every 6 hours remains the first line antibiotic in pregnancy [287a,322,324], although resistance of *Salmonella* and *Shigella* spp. is increasing, especially in developing countries [4,218]. Nosocomial outbreaks are uncommon but reported more frequently for *Salmonella* than *Shigella* spp. [129,346]. Breast feeding can continue for mothers complying with strict standards of hygiene.

Delivery of symptomless carriers of *Salmonella* and *Shigella* spp. should be carried out under conditions of isolation. Antibiotic therapy should be instigated in the newborn for symptoms and positive stool cultures. The choice of antibiotic should be anticipated in advance and will depend on expert advice and local microbiological surveillance. Ciprofloxacin and other synthetic quinolones pass into breast milk and have been shown to cause damage to joints and cartilage in growing animals and are not recommended in pregnancy or with breast feeding.

Immunization with typhoid vaccine is contraindicated in pregnancy. There are insufficient data regarding the safety of the parenteral vaccines of *S. typhi* containing either purified Vi polysaccharide antigen Ty2 or the conventional heat-killed, whole organism.

Miscellaneous

The treatment of bacterial overgrowth, tropical sprue and Whipple's disease (*Tropheryma whippelii*) traditionally involves tetracyclines but these are contraindicated in pregnancy. There are no specific guidelines for their management in pregnancy. HIV seropositive patients can present with clinical features indistinguishable from Whipple's disease [390].

Intestinal parasites and infestations

Up to half of pregnant women from developing countries carry worms and other infestations. Intestinal helminths can persist for years in immigrants from highly endemic countries [63]. The prevalence increases with congenital immunodeficiency syndromes and AIDS [390]. Common species are hookworm (*Ancylostoma duodenale, Necator americanus*), whipworm (*Trichuris trichiura*), dwarf tapeworm (*Hymenolepis nana*), roundworm (*Ascaris lumbricoides*), threadworm (*Enterobius vermicularis*) and tapeworm (*Taenia saginata, T. solium*) [282].

Intestinal parasites were found in 44 per cent [72,377] and 65 per cent [300] of women from south-east Asia and Mexico during pregnancy. The infestations are often multiple [377]. The most common infestations are hookworm (37–47 per cent), *Trichuris trichiura* (21 per cent), giardiasis (17 per cent) and ascaris (14.5 per cent) [72,300,377].

Maternal aspects

Pregnancy adversely affects parasite burden and clearance in many animal models but data are lacking in humans. Intrauterine growth retardation is associated with multiple infestations and maternal malnutrition. Purgation should be avoided. Treatment for most parasites can be delayed until after delivery. Maternal malnutrition should be corrected and the diet supplemented with iron, folic acid and other vitamins.

Treatment should only be considered for intractable symptoms and, if possible, deferred until the third trimester. Important exceptions are symptomatic infections with *E. histolytica* significant *G. lamblia*, ascariasis and malaria which should be treated prior to delivery (see below).

Fetal outcome

The outcomes for the well-nourished mother and child are favourable. Treatment is rarely required except in the presence of malnutrition and multiple infestations [377]. An infested group of south-east Asians when compared to those without detectable parasites on stool analysis showed no significant difference between mean maternal haemoglobin levels, mean gestational age at delivery or birthweights of the babies [300]. However, multiple infestations may account for about 10 per cent of intrauterine growth retardation and reduced birthweight in developing countries in association with malnutrition and heavy parasite burden [377].

Congenital and neonatal infection is uncommon although there have been isolated reports of *A. lumbricoides*, South American and African type trypanosomiasis, *E. histolytica* and *G. lamblia* [194]. Faecal contamination at birth is responsible for most cases.

Helminthic infestations

Most infestation can be managed conservatively. Re-infection with hookworm is high in crowded circumstances such as refugee camps. Therapy with pyrantel pamoate or a single dose (5 g) of bephenium is reserved for very heavy worm burdens. Relapses are common in the puerperium. Irradication of sporadic cases of hookworm in an urban society is usually successful after delivery since there is no intermediate host to sustain the reservoir of infection. Anaemia from hookworm may require supplementation with iron. Piperazine can be given for roundworm and threadworm but should be reserved for large worm burdens in pregnancy and not used concurrently with pyrantel which antagonizes its action. Abdominal discomfort, dyspepsia and diarrhoea from taeniasis is usually tolerated in pregnancy. Quinacrine (for *T. solium*) and niclosamide (for *T. saginata*) should be given only after delivery. Whipworm and mixed helminth infestations can be treated with mebendazole or albendazole but these should be avoided in early pregnancy because of suspected teratogenicity. Purgation using laxatives such as senna and liquid paraffin should also be avoided in pregnancy (see below). Breast feeding is permitted with quinacrine but should be avoided when the mother is being treated with mebendazole, thiabendazole, albendazole and niclosamide [282,300]. Maternal ascariasis should be treated with pyrantel pamoate prior to delivery. Treatment reduces the risk of the parasite migrating into the trachea which has been a cause of several obstetric deaths in the USA [300]. Therapy should be continued immediately after delivery even for mild symptoms to prevent neonatal acquisition of worms, and breast feeding is permitted.

Trematodes

Shistosomiasis affects over 200 million individuals worldwide with a particularly high prevalence in Africa, Egypt and South America. *Shistosoma mansoni* and *S. japonicum* affect the gastrointestinal tract (acute phase) and liver (chronic phase) predominantly, whereas *S. haematobium* affects the urinogenital system. *Chlonorchis sinensis*, a common liver fluke in the East, was found in 20 per cent of pregnant refugees from south-east Asia [300] and can present with cholecystitis, obstructive jaundice and biliary problems. The course of the disease with these parasites is not affected adversely by pregnancy. Therapy can often be withheld until the puerperium. In sporadic cases in urban populations in the West, spread of infection is uncommon because there is no intermediate host. All drugs used in the treatment of shistosomiasis, such as oxamniquine, praziquantel, niridazole and hycanthone, are effective but very toxic. Caesarean section may be necessary because of scarring of the cervix in chronic disease.

Shistosomiasis should be considered in the differential diagnosis of bloody diarrhoea, hepatosplenomegaly and portal hypertension. Diagnosis of shistosomiasis is by microscopic examination of stools and rectal biopsy material for eggs. Sigmoidoscopic examination should be carried out to exclude the possible association of carcinoma of the colon. Cholecystitis due to *Clonorchis* should be treated with praziquantel but therapy delayed, if possible, to post-partum. Breast feeding is contraindicated in mothers receiving drug therapy.

Entamoeba histolytica

This may cause dysenteric or non-dysenteric colitis, amoebic appendicitis, amoeboma or hepatic abscess. *E. histolytica* is endemic in the tropics and subtropics but also occurs in the UK, Europe and North America, especially amongst immigrants from developing countries. Amoebiasis can mimic and coexist with other diarrhoeal illnesses such as bacillary dysentery, hookworm, schistosomiasis, giardiasis [72] and colonic IBD. These should be considered in the differential diagnosis by regular examination of fresh stools and careful flexible sigmoidoscopy in all patients with a dysenteric illness. A positive antibody test using enzyme linked immunosorbent assay (ELISA) may be helpful but a positive result does not correlate with parasite burden, or with the presence of cysts in stool.

Amoebiasis in pregnancy is reported to follow a severe course [201,394]. The neonate may acquire the infection from faecal contamination at birth [300] although clinical sequelae are uncommon in breast-fed communities since antibodies to amoeba are present in breast milk [119]. In the general population, metronidazole (800 mg three times daily) for 5 days has been used to treat intestinal and hepatic amoebiasis. Earlier reports of infants born with craniofacial abnormalities to mothers who were treated in the first trimester for amoebiasis [56] have not been confirmed. More recent evaluation has shown no detrimental effect on mother or foetus in over 800 pregnancies, including in 300 where it was used in the first trimester [208]. Tinidazole may be more effective than metronidazole in the treatment of amoebiasis [289] but it has not been evaluated in pregnancy. An alternative drug is paromomycin which has been used in pregnancy and in post-partum women who were breast feeding [300]. Diloxanide furoate (500 mg three times daily) for 14 days has been used to increase elimination of parasites from the bowel [363] but again it should be reserved for use post-partum; breast feeding is safe [300].

Giardiasis

G. lambilia (*G. intestinalis*) is one of the most common causes of travellers' diarrhoea and malabsorption. It is endemic in Europe, the UK and the USA. Infestation is especially common in developing countries [159,377] and amongst immigrants resident in the West. In two studies of intestinal infestations in south-eastern Asian [72] and Mexican [377] women during pregnancy, where 44 per cent had intestinal parasites, giardiasis (17–25 per cent) was second only to hookworm (47 per cent) [72] and tapeworm (35.2 per cent) [377].

This infestation may occur *de novo* but susceptibility to infection is increased with achlorhydria, hypogammaglobulinaemia, coeliac disease, chronic pancreatitis and protein malnutrition. Clinical features include nausea, headache, abdominal discomfort and diarrhoea with steatorrhoea and malabsorption. Unlike amoebic and bacillary dysentery, bloody diarrhoea and fever are uncommon. *G. lamblia* infests a variety of mammals including cattle, horses, rabbits, cats and dogs. Transmission is by the faeco-oral route and ingestion of water contaminated by introduction of animal excreta and untreated sewage. Giardia can spread directly from person to person and this route may explain the high prevalence of infection amongst homosexual men [347]. Diagnosis is confirmed by isolation of parasites or cysts from the stool but duodenal aspirates and small intestinal biopsy may improve diagnostic yields. Metronidazole or paromomycin remain the treatments of choice for symptomatic infections in pregnancy (see below). Quinacrine is a cheap alternative for developing countries [347] but should be reserved for post-partum therapy (see taeniasis above). Tinidazole and furazolidone also may be used [347] although their safety in pregnancy has not been established.

Viral gastroenteritis

Acute diarrhoea and vomiting attributed to a virus is a common diagnosis in pregnancy but identification of the offending pathogen is rare [129,346]. Rotavirus has been detected in stool and by serology (ELISA) in individual women with diarrhoea at delivery [346] but is more common in children, especially in the West. Occasional reports have implicated adenovirus, Norwalk-like virus, the astroviruses and coronaviruses. The concern in obstetrics is the potential cause of outbreaks of infection, including gastroenteritis, amongst neonates in nurseries. Attention to hygiene, especially washing hands thoroughly between handling babies, is important in limiting spread. Attendants with suspected gastroenteritis should be excluded from obstetrical wards and nurseries.

Inflammatory bowel disease (IBD)

The incidence and prevalence of IBD, which describes ulcerative colitis, Crohn's disease and non-specific colitis and proctitis, have risen in the last 40 years [43,116,178,196,226,246,304,309,325]. IBD is common in North America, the UK and Scandinavia with annual prevalence rates per 100 000 population reported as high as 40–100 for ulcerative colitis and four to six for Crohn's disease [183]. The incidence of Crohn's disease in the USA rose fourfold from 1.9 to 6.6/100 000 between 1935 and 1979 [325]. Similar increases for Crohn's disease were reported for Wales [226] and Israel [116,309] but not for Scotland and Sweden [196]. IBD is reported as uncommon in areas such as Morocco and Saudi Arabia [183] and amongst blacks rather than whites [326]. IBD is more common amongst Jews than non-Jews [43,267a]. There is a small familial tendency for IBD.

IBD can become manifest at any age with bimodal peaks between 15 and 20 [304] and 55 and 60 [183] years and with an equal sex ratio.

Effects of disease on pregnancy (see Box 10.2)

FEMALE FERTILITY

Early studies suggested a higher rate of involuntary female infertility than in the normal population. However, data were weakened by insufficient numbers [77] and omission of relevant factors such as fertility of the partner, voluntary infertility of the couple, nutritional status [78,108,148,246] and psychological problems with sexual dysfunction, particularly after resective surgery [136], and with chronic disease [115,241].

Ulcerative colitis

Several studies suggest that involuntary fertility is not affected adversely for quiescent disease and little altered for all but severely active disease. Crohn *et al.* [70] and Korelitz [191] found no impairment in fertility for well-controlled disease. In later studies [396] with variable disease activity, the number of involuntarily infertilities was comparable (around 10–15 per cent) to that for the general

Box 10.2. Effects of inflammatory bowel disease (IBD) on pregnancy and management plan

- Effects
  - Overall, no deleterious effect
  - Fertility is normal in well-controlled IBD
  - Full-term, normal delivery and fetal outcome if IBD:
    - is quiescent at conception
    - preceded pregnancy and is quiescent
  - No deleterious effect on subsequent pregnancies
  - Increased fetal loss if IBD:
    - is first manifest in pregnancy and severe
    - is colonic rather than small bowel alone
    - occurs after previous surgery
    - is severe and being treated by current surgery
- Plan
  - Postpone pregnancy if disease is active
  - Drugs for IBD safe in pregnancy

population [152,191,358]. Voluntary infertility can be high (21–45 per cent), especially in patients with previous surgery [152] (see below).

Crohn's disease

Amenorrhoea and involuntary infertility correlate with disease activity. Normal fertility can be anticipated in well-controlled disease including after surgical resection [78,152,191]. Data from Oxford [179] and north-east Scotland [152] show similar rates of involuntary infertility (11–14 per cent) to the general population [358]. Voluntary infertility was high, especially amongst those with previous surgery (23–36 per cent) [152] (see below).

The effect of the anatomical extent of disease is not clearly defined and would require very large studies for proper elucidation. Two groups found that conception was less frequent in women with Crohn's colitis (67 per cent) compared with small bowel disease alone [108], or with ileitis and ileocolitis [78]. In contrast, in another study [148], only women with small intestinal disease had lower than normal fertility rates. In a case control study by the European Collaborative Group of infertility in Crohn's disease [227] subfertility (46 versus 29 per cent control group) and number of children (0.4 versus 0.7 per family) were independent of disease site.

Drug therapy

No direct data are available for salazopyrine and female fertility. Salazopyrine (sulphasalazine) is an important, reversible cause of male infertility [206, 274]. This is due probably to the sulphapyridine component and is associated with a reduced sperm count and high proportion of abnormal forms [274]. Infertility can be reversed by stopping therapy or transferring to 5-aminosalicylic acid alone [55,274, 328]. However, infertility is not invariable with salazopyrine [274].

There is no evidence that corticosteroids cause infertility. The safety of azathioprine, used occasionally for severe IBD [152], is discussed in Chapter 7.

Deficiencies of trace metals also may contribute to infertility. Low serum levels of zinc and chromium have been reported in Crohn's disease associated with hypogonadism [232].

SPONTANEOUS ABORTION

Several early reports stressed the detrimental effect of IBD [19,26,27,31,103,181,224,295,317]. More recent data show that the rates of spontaneous abortion with pre-existing ulcerative colitis (7–16 per cent) [78,107,152,193,214,215,216,235,266,396] and Crohn's disease (6–18 per cent) [69,78,108,148, 152,266,269] are not significantly different from the normal population [137,246,358].

ACTIVE IBD AT CONCEPTION

Only the coexistence of severely active disease, particularly at conception, seems detrimental to mother and fetus. Such women tend to avoid conception [152]. By contrast most authorities [1,24,70, 152,267] have reported normal deliveries and good fetal outcome in more than 80 per cent of those who have quiescent disease around conception. This optimistic outcome persists despite subsequent relapse during pregnancy and for first presentations during pregnancy and the puerperium [1,24,70,152].

In the Scottish study, IBD became clinically quiescent in more than half the patients with active disease at conception [152].

PRESENTATION IN PREGNANCY AND THE PUERPERIUM

Poor outcome [1,24,69,224] is not invariable [70,152]. Abramson *et al.* [1] reported fetal loss in three of five pregnancies for ulcerative colitis. Crohn *et al.* [69] reported a fetal loss in two of three pregnancies for presentations with terminal ileitis. In a later study [224] of 11 pregnancies in 10 women with Crohn's disease presenting during pregnancy, there was a 55 per cent fetal loss; four fetal deaths occurred in the six women requiring surgery during pregnancy. By contrast, Crohn *et al.* [70] reported only one fetal death amongst 19 pregnancies for ulcerative colitis presenting during pregnancy. In the Scottish study, one of three first presentations of Crohn's disease in pregnancy was particularly severe [152] and associated with spontaneous pre-term labour at 30 weeks. The baby survived but the mother required an ileocaecal resection 2 days later [152]. The 10 presentations in pregnancy with ulcerative colitis were uneventful as were all eight presentations (five Crohn's disease, three ulcerative colitis) in the puerperium [152].

PREVIOUS SURGERY FOR IBD

In a large retrospective community survey of 409 women with IBD extending over 20 years in north-east Scotland [152], involuntary infertility was higher (20–30 per cent) than normal following surgery, especially for ulcerative colitis, and less likely to be resolved than in patients without prior surgery. Voluntary infertility also was high (see above).

ILEOSTOMY AND COLOSTOMY

Involuntary infertility following resective surgery has not been considered directly in most studies. Women with an ileostomy from a previous colectomy and quiescent disease have a fair chance of a full-term normal vaginal delivery and healthy infant (see below).

Fetal outcome is less good for previous surgery and current severely active disease [152] and for severe IBD requiring surgical resection during pregnancy (see below).

Effects of pregnancy on disease

These remain controversial. Conflicting results can be explained in part by changing management over a follow-up period which spans 60 years from 1931. The outcome of more recent cases has been influenced by earlier diagnosis and improved control of inflammatory activity both by drugs and resective surgery. In 1931, Barnes and Hayes [27] reported two maternal and two fetal deaths in three women who developed ulcerative colitis post-partum. This report led to the initial, pessimistic conclusion that women with pre-existing ulcerative colitis should avoid pregnancy. During the period 1950–56 there were several reports of pregnant women with pre-existent ulcerative colitis who experienced an increase in the number of relapses during pregnancy and, particularly, post-partum [1,70,365]. The course was also stormy and maternal prognosis poor. Several maternal deaths were recorded for first presentations of ulcerative colitis in pregnancy and post-partum. Many later studies have shown a high relapse rate (between 30 and 40 per cent per annum) regardless of pregnancy for ulcerative colitis [78,152,266,396] and Crohn's disease [69,78,108,148,152,267,269]. Clinical relapse may occur at any time during pregnancy but tends to be particularly common in the first trimester [69,108,152,267].

Although results remain conflicting [179], there is general agreement that patients with Crohn's disease seemingly limited to the terminal ileum, fare better in pregnancy and post-partum than those with colonic Crohn's disease or ulcerative colitis. More precise data are needed on disease site, extent and inflammatory activity, rather than relying on clinical scores.

Summary

Most women with pre-existing IBD should expect normal fertility and a full-term normal delivery [170,266,267,396] with no additional risk to the fetus. Rates of involuntary infertility and spontaneous abortion are similar to those for the general population for ulcerative colitis and Crohn's disease. Fertility is impaired and fetal outcome less good for patients with IBD who have undergone previous surgery and have active disease [170]. Relapses are frequent during pregnancy [1], especially in the first trimester for ulcerative colitis and in the puerperium for Crohn's disease [170].

The impact on the mother who first presents in pregnancy and the puerperium remains unclear. Severe courses have been reported [1,69] but these are not invariable [24,69,70,266], especially for ulcerative colitis [152].

Management

Women with known IBD should be encouraged to become pregnant during clinically quiescent disease [396] and whilst taking minimum medication. Medical management is the same as for the non-pregnant patient [246,374,396]. There have been reports [21, 249,267,396] of a higher incidence of fetal complications when a woman requires active treatment during pregnancy. The current consensus is that this outcome is more likely to reflect severe disease activity rather than the direct effect of drugs.

Acute severe disease

The pregnant patient should be admitted to hospital and fresh stools taken for culture for pathogenic micro-organisms and detection and analysis of their toxins (see above) [37,129,133,282,340,376]. Stools should be screened for parasites, including *Entamoeba histolytica* and *Strongyloides stercoralis* (see above) prior to treatment, particularly with corticosteroids, since the latter may cause disseminated parasitosis. HIV infection can cause problems in the differential diagnosis (see above). In general, treatment consists of bed rest, oral corticosteroids such as prednisolone 20–60 mg/day, rectal corticosteroids, oral salazopyrine (sulphasalazine) (3–4 g/day), nil by mouth, and intravenous fluids.

In a moderately severe attack of colonic IBD, initial treatment is with topical corticosteroid enemas [309a], oral salazopyrine (1 g twice daily) and oral prednisolone up to 20 mg/day. In colitis predominantly confined to the left side, therapy with 5-aminosalicylic acid [54,285] seems to be effective though this drug has not been fully evaluated in pregnancy (see below).

DRUG THERAPIES

Corticosteroids remain the single, most effective drug for active IBD [180,351]. Symptoms typically improve using clinical disease activity scores. Inflammatory activity lessens on sigmoidoscopy and by laboratory indices including serum albumin, erythrocyte sedimentation rate (ESR) and the C reactive protein [96]. Oral feeding usually may be resumed within 48 hours. The daily dose of prednisolone may be reduced from 30 to 20 mg/day after 7 days, and below 20 mg, in small, step-wise reductions [95]. Eventually corticosteroid therapy should be withdrawn completely; continued therapy does not prevent relapse [336,351].

Before 1980 there were no reports of pregnancy in women given steroids for IBD. Current information is reassuring regarding their safety in IBD in pregnancy [246,249,266,374,396]. The overall safety of corticosteroids in pregnancy is discussed in Chapter 1. The indications for the use of corticosteroids in acute, active IBD are the same as in the non-pregnant patient [396]. Breast feeding is probably safe even with nursing mothers taking up to 50 mg/day prednisolone for asthma [208,366].

Salazopyrine (sulphasalazine) is valuable in the treatment of colonic IBD in the non-pregnant [337, 351] and pregnant patient [147,235,249]. This drug has been studied extensively in randomized controlled double-blind clinical trials. Salazopyrine is superior to placebo for ulcerative colitis and Crohn's disease using the oral [337,351] or rectal form [251,275]. Salazopyrine, a pro-drug, is split (azo-reduction) by colonic bacteria into the components sulphapyridine and 5-aminosalicylic acid (5-ASA) [186,285]. The therapeutic efficacy of salazopyrine depends on the ability of colonic bacteria to split the parent compound into 5-ASA and sulphapyridine and to deliver 5-ASA to the colon [186]. Clinical efficacy is related to the 5-ASA component [187] and general toxicity to the sulphapyridine and acetylator status (drug clearance). Sulphapyridine, unlike its parent pro-drug. is almost totally absorbed and responsible for many of the common side-effects including skin rashes and headaches [187]. Salazopyrine generally is considered safe for use throughout pregnancy and the puerperium [21,235, 249] and also during breast feeding [160,396]. Sulphapyridine has been replaced by *p*-amino-hippurate in the formulation ipsalazide, by 4-aminobenzoyl-β-alanine in balsalazide, and by polymers in poly-ASA and dimers (disodium azodisalicylate). These oral preparations require an intact gut without bacterial contamination of small bowel and a normal transit time [186]. Specific data relating to pregnancy are lacking.

Salazopyrine and its components cross the placenta. Salazopyrine and sulphapyridine reach a concentration in cord blood and breast milk of approximately half that in maternal serum [18] but levels are not considered detrimental to the fetus [21]. The ability of sulphapyridine to displace bilirubin from albumin binding sites [142] has been overemphasized [186,208]. Salazopyrine impairs absorption, transport and metabolism of dietary folic acid necessitating additional supplementation (see above).

The component 5-ASA is unstable but believed to be the major active principle in the treatment of IBD [84,186,187]. More than 25 per cent of 5-ASA is absorbed from the colon. The principal mode of action is believed to be topical because more than half can be recovered from faeces. In colitis, rectal preparations including suppositories [285] are as effective as rectal and oral preparations of salazopyrine. Retention enemas are more effective than those containing hydrocortisone in inducing clinical, sigmoidoscopic and histological remission in left-sided moderately severe ulcerative colitis [54]. Because of the safety of salazopyrine 5-ASA should be safe for use in pregnancy but trials of the coated preparation (mesalazine), and the related olsalazine, are lacking.

Azathioprine and its component, 6-mercaptopurine (6-MP), have been reserved for use in the non-pregnant patient with severe Crohn's disease considered unresponsive to corticosteroids and salazopyrine [190,203,292,338,351]. Long-term studies with azathioprine and 6-MP have shown benefit with minimal toxicity in the non-pregnant population with severe IBD [190,270,292]. There is extensive experience of the use of azathioprine in pregnancy from renal transplant patients (see Chapter 7). In the short term the drug is safe though there is concern about potential effects on fertility of female fetuses exposed to azathioprine *in utero* (see Chapter 7).

Other treatments for acute IBD found to be safe during pregnancy include total parenteral nutrition (see below) for small bowel Crohn's disease and the penicillin antibiotics. Metronidazole has been used extensively in the non-pregnant population for trichomoniasis [302], giardiasis and amoebiasis (see above). The safety of metronidazole in early pregnancy and during breast feeding remain to be proven. No data are available for the use of elemental diets [182,183] and levamisole [374] in pregnant patients with IBD.

Chronic disease

Assessment of nutritional status is important. Supplementation with folic acid above the daily dose (400 μg) recommended by the MRC study group [238] is advisable in all pregnant patients with IBD. Vitamin B_{12} is essential for ileal Crohn's disease and following ileal resection (see below). In theory, measurement and assessment of trace elements including chromium, zinc and copper as well as vitamins should be carried out regularly during pregnancy and through lactation but this is not practical. Osteomalacia and vitamin D deficiency syndromes are well recognized in Crohn's disease and require early therapeutic intervention (see Chapter 14). Additional supplementation with iron (see Chapter 2) may be required for chronic blood loss. The use of antimotility agents and stool thickeners such as codeine phosphate and diphenoxylate with atropine (Lomotil) should be kept to a minimum. Many of the antimotility and anti-spasmodic compounds contain anticholinergic agents such as atropine, hyoscine and barbiturates. These can adversely affect fetal heart rate and have been associated with congenital abnormalities (reviewed in [95,208]). Their use is therefore contra-indicated during pregnancy and lactation. In any case the severity of diarrhoea can be better assessed when such preparations are withheld. Emphasis should focus on treating the underlying inflammatory activity and any infection rather than treatig symptoms alone.

Constipation may impair the efficiency of action of oral salazopyrine on the left colon ('constipated colitis'). All patients should be encouraged to take adequate fluids, a high fibre diet if strictures are excluded, and, if necessary, poorly absorbed processed hydrophilic agents [123]. Magnesium hydroxide and lactulose are preferred to many complex commercial laxatives (see below).

Salazopyrine (2–4 g/day) is superior to placebo in maintenance of remission of chronic ulcerative colitis. Results for chronic Crohn's disease are less convincing.

Emergency surgery

In general, resective surgery may be required for up to 25 per cent of patients with fulminating ulcerative colitis [65,182] and up to 50 per cent with Crohn's disease affecting the small bowel or ileocolitis complicated by obstruction, fistulae and abdominal suppuration [182]. Prior to surgery, total parenteral nutrition (see below) should be considered [385], including provision for a long-term, indwelling intravenous line for post-operative feeding. Surgery for severe colonic IBD involves a single stage colectomy and ileostomy with or without preservation of the rectal stump [182] (see Ileostomy and colostomy below). In late pregnancy, a total colectomy may prove difficult. A partial colectomy with ileostomy may need to suffice until after delivery [385]. In Crohn's disease, limited gut resection with end-to-end anastomosis is preferred to bypass procedures and extensive resections. Clinical relapse and disease recurrence of the site of previous resective surgery for Crohn's disease occurs in over 90 per cent of patients regardless of disease site, severity of inflammation and extent of resection [182]. Bypass procedures are discouraged today because the problems remain of the residual inflammation, potential blind-loop and bacterial overgrowth and increased risk of carcinoma [182].

Early papers, often of individual cases, report a poor outcome for mother and fetus for fulminating IBD requiring resective surgery [19,152,179,224, 231,266,267,295,317]. In a later series Mogadam *et al.* [249] followed 178 women with ulcerative colitis and 146 with Crohn's disease through pregnancy. Bowel resection was required rarely (seven colectomies and ileostomies for ulcerative colitis; one iliectomy and one ileal ascending colostomy for Crohn's disease). Although there were no maternal deaths, only four (three for ulcerative colitis; one for Crohn's disease) of the nine fetuses survived [249]. Fulminating IBD during pregnancy is uncommon in more recent studies, probably reflecting earlier diagnosis and successful medical intervention for maintenance therapy and treatment of active disease [39,65,246,266,374,396]. Nevertheless the rates of spontaneous abortion and still-birth for emergency resective surgery during pregnancy may be as high as 66 per cent [19,179,224,231,246,247,317].

Mogadam *et al.* [249] reported no maternal deaths amongst seven of 178 pregnant women with severe ulcerative colitis who required resection and an ileostomy (five total colectomy, two colonic diversion). Three of the fetuses survived (three spontaneous abortions, one pre-term labour).

A normal delivery and fetal outcome are possible after total proctocolectomy for fulminating ulcerative colitis during pregnancy [65]. In a review of 33 cases of free perforation in Crohn's disease [172], one was a woman in her third month of pregnancy who was treated with resection and diversion and subsequently had a full-term, normal delivery.

Ileostomy and colostomy

In general, loss of up to 50 per cent of small bowel and/or colon is well tolerated in the non-pregnant patient. Adaptation in the ileostomy occurs with time. More extensive small and large bowel resection can result in complex metabolic and neuroendocrine dysfunction [49,66,109,134,248].

Pregnancy is not contraindicated in patients with an ileostomy or colostomy carried out for urinary or alimentary diversion.

The pregnant woman with an ileostomy or massive gut resection may develop malabsorption of fat, fat-soluble vitamins, vitamin B_{12}, water and electrolyte imbalance, hyperoxaluria and cholelithiasis. Complications such as obstruction of ureters and of fallopian tubes with pyosalpinx, and effects of surgery on subsequent fertility and sexual function, should also be anticipated. Adhesions, fistulae and infections add to the general morbidity [29, 108,148,151,152].

Pregnancy may interfere with function of the ileostomy, especially after the first trimester with mechanical displacement of the bowel.

Intestinal obstruction is a serious complication in pregnancy (see below). The diagnosis can be mistaken for hyperemesis gravidarum or abruptio placentae with a tender uterus, shock and absent fetal heart sounds. Less serious, but more common problems, include cracking of the skin and bleeding around the area of the stoma.

IBD

The majority of women with a stoma and quiescent disease will have full-term, normal vaginal deliveries [24,29,70,78,151,193,235,256,324]. In one large review [151] based on questionnaires from the Ileostomy Society, 75 women were followed through 89 pregnancies. All had had an ileostomy carried out at some time prior to pregnancy for vesicovaginal fistula following previous obstetric trauma or colectomy for IBD. Pregnancy was uneventful to term in 84 instances and a normal vaginal delivery was achieved in 71 per cent. The increase in use of forceps occurred from impaired ability to push. Caesarean section was carried out in 16 cases for obstetrical reasons and in one case only for ileal prolapse. One maternal death in the UK reported between 1985 and 1987 occurred at 33 weeks in a patient with a previous total colectomy for ulcerative colitis. She died from a massive haemorrhage through the ileostomy resulting from erosion of bowel by the placenta in an abdominal pregnancy which was not suspected despite 3 months of amenorrhoea [79].

Intestinal obstruction was reported in 10 per cent of pregnant women with ileostomies with one maternal death following a caesarean section and one spontaneous abortion [151]. Details of disease activity and anatomical site were not given.

The ileal pouch–anal anastomosis aims to provide continence. Experience in pregnancy is limited but encouraging. Out of 92 women who underwent proctocolectomy and fashioning of a J-shaped anastomosis for IBD between 1981 and 1983 at the Mayo Clinic, four of six conceptions resulted in normal vaginal deliveries [240]. Stool frequency increased slightly in the third trimester. Anal function returned to baseline post-partum. Caesarean section was considered unnecessary except for cephalopelvic disproportion [240].

Appendicitis

This is the most common non-obstetric condition requiring surgery during pregnancy [400] and is reported as occurring in one in 2500 to one in 3500 deliveries [28,170]. In a retrospective analysis of acute appendicitis during pregnancy in Brazil between 1959 and 1988 there were seven cases out of 18 065 deliveries [28]. Gestational age was 11–27 weeks.

Maternal outcome

Abdominal complications, especially perforation, wall abscess and adynamic ileum are common [28]. In a retrospective review of the literature [217], of 713 maternal cases of confirmed appendicitis since 1960, rupture had occurred in one-quarter; there were five maternal deaths.

Fetal outcome

Pre-term labour and perinatal mortality occur in about 20 per cent of cases with perforation [28,209, 217].

Clinical course and management

The literature suggests that acute appendicitis during pregnancy shows an aggressive evolution. Whether this reflects delays in diagnosis and the bias of reporting severe cases, remains unclear. Twenty-four pregnant women with acute appendicitis received exploratory laparotomy during an 8-year period [209]. Abdominal pain with rebound tenderness accompanied by nausea and vomiting were the most common features. A peripheral blood leucocytosis above 15 000/mm^3 and granulocytes >87 per cent were risk factors for perforation.

Routine use of high resolution ultrasonography has significantly improved diagnostic accuracy in suspected appendicitis and reduced the negative laparotomy rate. In a prospective study of 121 German women of childbearing age with suspected appendicitis [321], the criteria for diagnosis included visualization of a non-compressible aperistaltic appendix, with a target-like appearance in transverse view and a diameter ⩾7 mm. The overall accuracy was 96.7 per cent: 82.6 per cent sensitivity and 100 per cent specificity. Of 27 patients 24 (89 per cent) with appendiceal rupture (incidence 20.8 per cent) were correctly diagnosed with ultrasound.

A McBurney's incision and regional anesthesia should be considered for appendectomy during pregnancy. In cases of uncomplicated appendicitis, tocolytic agents and antibiotics are not used routinely.

Intestinal obstruction

This is a serious complication in pregnancy. The incidence in healthy pregnant women seems to be rising and is approaching that of appendicitis (one in 2500–3500 deliveries) [170]. This relates to the rising number of laparotomies in young women carried out for appendicitis and gynaecological disorders and is independent of age and parity [73]. Intestinal obstruction was reported in 10 per cent of pregnant women with ileostomies with one maternal death following a caesarean section and one spontaneous abortion [246]. Causes other than adhesions and appendiceal abscesses include inflammatory bowel disease, caecal volvulus [99], pseudo-obstruction of the colon (Ogilvie's syndrome), endometriosis, multiple pregnancy and abdominal malignancies [85].

Intestinal volvulus

Sigmoid, and less commonly, caecal, volvulus account for about one-quarter of cases of intestinal obstruction in pregnancy [335]. Presentation typically is in the third trimester when the uterus enlarges sufficiently to displace the viscera. Constipation and previous abdominal surgery may play a role. Caecal volvulus and pseudo-obstruction of the colon are recognized complications of caesarean section [99,303].

Differential diagnosis

The differential diagnosis in pregnancy of abdominal pain, nausea and vomiting is wide. Apart from intestinal obstruction, appendicitis and ruptured tubal and abdominal pregnancy, the list includes peptic ulceration, renal infections, many liver disorders such as hepatitis, abscess, cholecystitis, pancreatitis and gastrointestinal infestations (see above). In obstetric practice such presentations are mistaken for hyperemesis gravidarum, preeclamptic toxaemia and abruption with a tender uterus, shock and absent fetal heart sounds [73,402]. A ruptured ectopic pregnancy or ruptured spleen may be difficult to exclude especially with bloody ascites.

Management

This requires a high index of suspicion and close collaboration between surgeons, radiologists and physicians.

Non-surgical measures should include correction of fluid and electrolyte imbalance and nasogastric suction. Endoscopic decompression may be successful in colonic pseudo-obstruction. In Ogilvie's syndrome, a plain abdominal radiograph shows dilatation of the caecum with or without dilatation in the ascending and transverse colon and no distal air. Serial abdominal radiography is essential and requires close monitoring for continued caecal distension and possible perforation [303]. MRI has been reported in one pregnant women with colonic obstruction due to a tumour [327]. Surgery should be considered for a caecum diameter of ⩾9 cm because the possibility of perforation is high. Surgical intervention depends on local expertise. Successful outcomes have been reported with puncture decompression or caecostomy.

Two pregnant women with small bowel obstruction due to Crohn's disease improved with an elemental diet without recourse to surgery [356].

Abdominal complications of tubal pregnancy

Four of 16 maternal deaths in the UK from ruptured tubal pregnancy between 1985 and 1987 had significant involvement of the bowel [79]. Gastrointestinal complications included spontaneous perforation of the bowel, suspected gastroenteritis and abdominal pregnancy with erosion of the placenta into the bowel. Tubal pregnancy typically was not suspected until late; typical presentations were with non-specific abdominal pain and vomiting. A maternal death in an ileostomy patient caused by erosion of bowel by the placenta is considered above.

Total parenteral nutrition (hyperalimentation)

This is recommended for any condition in pregnancy where there is maternal protein–calorie malnutrition [141,222]. Successful outcomes in pregnancy have been reported for severe IBD, massive gut resection, small bowel fistula, radiation enteritis, prolonged post-operative ileus, severe pancreatitis and protracted hyperemesis [407]. In a normal pregnancy adequate nutrition results in a healthy fetus and placenta [308]. A paradox arises in protein–calorie malnutrition and semi-starvation whereby, on re-feeding, there is preferential uptake by maternal rather than fetal tissues to replete maternal body stores [308]. Although most studies have been limited to animal models, there is some evidence that this also holds true for humans [336]. During the famine in Holland in 1944–45, a 10 per cent reduction in fetal weight was associated with only a 3 per cent loss in maternal weight in the second and third trimesters [308]. Guidelines for adequate replacement of nutrients in pregnancy are lacking [222]. Current experience is limited to individual case reports [222,299,361].

Insertion of the indwelling catheter must be carried out under strict aseptic technique, preferably in theatre. Although lipid-containing solutions (emulsions) have been shown to damage the placenta in experimental animals [141] they seem to be safe in human pregnancy [407]. Lipid emboli were not found in the placenta after giving solutions containing up to 50 per cent lipid emulsions [222, 407]. Concern continues to be expressed over the effects to the fetus of continual use of glucose-containing solutions from early in pregnancy. Whether these create a state of continuous hypertonicity, akin to the situation in a poorly controlled diabetic pregnancy, is not known.

Maternal monitoring

Serial blood levels of glucose, electrolytes, trace elements and minerals, vitamins, amino acids should be estimated throughout pregnancy and lactation [299]. Maternal levels may be compared with those in cord blood taken simultaneously at delivery. The optimal daily nutritional requirements of calories, nitrogen and trace elements and vitamins in a pregnant woman receiving total parenteral nutrition are not known. More information on maternal/fetal ratios is urgently needed. Deficiencies of fat soluble vitamins, pyridoxine (vitamin B_6) and other group B vitamins, calcium, iron, free fatty acids amongst many other essential nutrients are common despite supplementation. Wernicke–Korsakoff syndrome due to thiamine deficiency has developed in one patient with a twin pregnancy who received total parenteral nutrition with B vitamins for a previous jejuno-ileal bypass [299].

Fetal outcome

The expected weight can be maintained provided total parenteral nutrition is commenced early and is adequate for fetal and maternal needs. Frequent serial monitoring of fetal growth using ultrasonography is essential. Pre-term labour is a recognized complication of maternal nutritional deprivation and may occur despite evidence of satisfactory fetal growth [222,361]. Neural tube defects have been related to deficiency of folic acid [143] at the time of conception and supplements should be given prior to, and through, pregnancy and lactation [146] (see above).

Jejuno-ileal bypass

A successful outcome to pregnancy has been

reported in a few women who previously had undergone jejuno-ileal bypass surgery for morbid obesity [156,299,316], including after total parenteral nutrition [299]. One study reported normal frequency (no diarrhoea) of bowel function during pregnancy in four women with a jejuno-ileal bypass and normal fetal outcomes including normal birthweights [273]. This study supports the concept of delayed small bowel transit in pregnancy (see below). In contrast other studies report a poor fetal outcome from still-birth [156], congenital defects [316] and small-for-dates babies [156]. Total parenteral nutrition should be considered early in this situation (see above).

Constipation

Constipation is difficult to define. Most authorities agree to a definition of less than three stools in 1 week [140,220,315]. Reduced stool frequency typically is accompanied with daily weights below 35 g, and more than 25 per cent of the time in defaecation spent as straining [315]. Women, especially of childbearing age, have been shown to have a more constipated bowel habit than men [140].

The few studies on constipation in pregnancy have yielded conflicting results. Evaluation of patterns of bowel habit in one series of 1000 healthy Israeli women during pregnancy showed a reduction in stool frequency in only 11 per cent; 1.5 per cent required laxatives. In over half, there was no change in bowel habit and about one-third showed an increase in stool frequency [207].

Physiology

Constipation is often considered a common consequence of the physiological effects of pregnancy although difficulties in definition and lack of objective data may be misleading.

There are few studies on intestinal motility in pregnancy and they are mostly confined to the small bowel [278,278a]. Parry *et al.* assessed transit time in the small bowel (stomach to caecum) using mercury-loaded capsules in 22 healthy pregnant women between the 12th and 20th week and in 12 non-pregnant female controls. Mean stomach-to-caecum transit times were 57.9 hours compared to 51.7 hours in the non-pregnant group. Transit times in over one-third of the pregnant women exceeded 60 hours. In the small bowel of non-pregnant women, mouth-to-caecum transit time is increased during the luteal phase (days 18–20) compared with follicular phase, of the menstrual cycle [380]. This delay has been attributed to elevated serum levels of progesterone [380], and, possibly, its inhibitory action on motilin amongst other gut hormones [60].

Direct studies on colonic motility have not been carried out in pregnant women. Water and sodium absorption in the colon during pregnancy was increased in one study [278a] and attributed to reduced colonic activity. Effects of hormones were not assessed directly.

Delays in whole gut transit times have been found in non-pregnant women of normal bodyweight with gallstones [139,140]. Slow colonic transit may favour increased absorption of deoxycholic acid to account for the increase in lithogenic bile and predisposition to form biliary sludge and gallstones in pregnancy [139].

The influence of diet was not considered directly but plays an important role in patterns of bowel habit. In a survey by Anderson *et al.* [7,8] in Cambridge, UK, a detailed dietary questionnaire was taken of 18 women in the third trimester, nine of whom complained of severe constipation. No significant difference was found between the two matched groups for diet, including fibre content (around 18 g daily). Dietary intake of fibre of women who claimed to have increased their intake was similar to that of the general British population (20 g daily) [7,8].

IDIOPATHIC SLOW TRANSIT CONSTIPATION

Severe constipation resistant to therapeutic manoevres such as high fibre diets is recognized especially in young women [140]. In one study, this condition was diagnosed in 64 non-pregnant young women on the basis of delayed elimination of barium markers on radiographic studies in the presence of a structurally normal radiograph [293]. The aetiology is unknown but it may have a hormonal basis.

Management

Every patient with 'constipation' requires detailed consideration and, if necessary, a full investigation to exclude other disorders especially hypothyroidism. A thorough enquiry should include details of the patient's definition, dietary and laxative habits and drug therapy. General measures include education about the normal, variable pattern of bowel activity. Emphasis should focus on the importance of an adequate fluid intake and, in the absence of bowel strictures, inclusion of a high intake of dietary fibre.

Constipation was reduced significantly by supplementing the daily fibre intake (average 20 g daily in the UK at that time) by only an additional 7 g/day [7,8]. This amounted to an increase in wholemeal bread eaten daily from an average of 2.5 to six slices. The equivalent number of calories was maintained by reducing intake of fat [7]. Common complications are backache, faecal impaction and haemorrhoids (see below).

STOOL BULKING AGENTS AND LAXATIVES

The choices in pregnancy include processed hydrophilic stool bulking agents such as methyl celllulose, ispaghula, sterculia and unprocessed (Miller's) bran with a high fluid intake [122,123], magnesium hydroxide tablets (4–6 tablets daily; see above for side-effects), lactulose or Senokot. Magnesium hydroxide causes increased osmotic retention of fluid in the colon. Although up to 20 per cent of magnesium salts are absorbed, no adverse effects have been reported in pregnancy. Lactulose, a synthetic disaccharide (fructose and galactose), is widely prescribed in pregnancy and seems to be safe. Lactulose in a dose of 30 ml daily for 15 days resulted in normalization of stool habit in 87 per cent of pregnant women with constipation and was well tolerated [197]. Direct information is lacking regarding any passage across the placenta and also into breast milk [208]. Lactulose is contraindicated in lactose intolerance and galactosaemia.

Senokot, an anthraquinone, is widely used in pregnancy and the puerperium [95,331,332]. Senna glycosides, the active principles, are released into the colon after bacterial breakdown and undergoing an enterohepatic circulation. Senna metabolites can pass into breast milk but have not been detected invariably. Controlled studies have shown no adverse effect on infants [24,331,392]. Senokot is of particular value in the prevention of constipation in the puerperium. In one study, 2 Senokot tablets given daily during the first 4 days post-partum reduced the requirement for an enema from 83 per cent to 1 per cent without any adverse effects [331]. Senna can colour urine leading to the erroneous estimation of urinary oestrogens.

Senokot is safe in pregnancy and the puerperium but other anthraquinone laxatives such as aloe and danthron have been associated with congenital malformations [263]. Dorbanex (co-danthramer, danthron/poloxamer) was withdrawn from the market in 1987 by the Committee of Safety of Medicines after concern that chronic, high doses of danthron in rats and mice were associated with gastrointestinal and liver tumours. No adverse reports have been documented in humans. Liquid paraffin and lubricants such as mineral oil are contraindicated in pregnancy. These impair absorption of fat-soluble vitamins, namely vitamins D and K, and may lead to neonatal coagulation defects with haemorrhage. Vomiting increases the risk of maternal aspiration with lipoid pneumonia. Seepage through the anal sphincter may cause pruritus. These agents, castor oil and soap enemas are outdated and should not be used in current obstetric practice [339,404]. The polyphenolic laxatives include phenolphthalen, oxyphenacetin and bisacodyl (Dulcolax). Phenolphthalein is excreted in breast milk and should not be used in pregnancy or during lactation; 1 g given to mothers who were breast feeding resulted in infant colic [367]. Bisacodyl has been safely used in pregnancy [353] in enema form and as suppositories but has been superseded by oral lactulose.

Irritable bowel syndrome

This includes a heterogeneous group of conditions characterized by intermittent abdominal pain — 'spastic colon' — altered bowel habit, incomplete evacuation of stool and passage of clear mucus per rectum [393]. The causes are unknown. Physiological changes in non-pregnant patients show abnormal myoelectrical activity throughout the gastrointestinal tract [341]. Studies in pregnancy are lacking.

Management

Diagnosis is by exclusion of many other causes of altered bowel habit. Patients require a full enquiry and investigation. Inflammatory bowel disease, laxative abuse, gut infections and infestations, bile salt malabsorption, coeliac disease, lactose intolerance and hormone-secreting tumours (those secreting vasoactive inhibitory polypeptide and calcitonin, amongst others) should be excluded especially for presentations with diarrhoea. Hypothyroidism is an important exclusion for constipation.

Therapies are empirical and depend on the predominant symptoms. Bulking agents are preferred to unprocessed bran which may exacerbate symptoms and cause bloating [393]. Fluid intake should be encouraged. Antispasmodic agents such as hyoscine and dicyclomine (anticholinergic) and mebeverine, alverine and peppermint oil (smooth muscle relaxant) are used widely in the non-pregnant patient with abdominal pain. Such antispasmodic agents and antidiarrhoeal agents such as loperamide are contraindicated in pregnancy.

Anorectal and perineal disorders

Haemorrhoids, tears of the anal sphincter resulting from obstetric injury and fissure *in ano* can cause considerable discomfort. Perianal fistulae in Crohn's disease and vaginal discharge following proctocolectomy in ulcerative colitis [395] can add to the morbidity of IBD. Dyspareunia is common in patients with IBD and the frequency more than doubles (12–27 per cent) following proctocolectomy [395].

Haemorrhoids

These are extremely common in pregnancy and post-partum. They can be exacerbated by constipation and straining during labour and infection following episiotomy resulting in thrombosis, strangulation and rectal prolapse. In a study of 40 patients studied in the puerperium with anorectal disorders, 95 per cent had external haemorrhoids and, in 37.5 per cent, these were accompanied by internal haemorrhoids [14]. Prolapse and thrombosis was found in 20 per cent and fissure *in ano*, in 5 per cent [14]. Women prone to develop haemorrhoids commonly present during pregnancy and there is an increased incidence in multiparous patients [14].

Pathogenetic mechanisms remain unclear. Suggestions include high pressure in the pelvic veins and undefined hormonal factors acting on the unique haemorrhoidal plexus [359,360].

Common presentations of anorectal disorders include pruritus, rectal bleeding and perineal pain. Mucoid and purulent discharge may occur with secondary inflammation and infection. Uncomplicated haemorrhoids are said not to cause pruritus [114] its presence warrants investigation for underlying causes (see below). Haemorrhoidectomy has been carried out for severe symptoms during pregnancy [312].

Sphincter injuries

In a survey of 20 500 women with episiotomies, 1040 (5 per cent) had third and fourth degree extensions, including some with a perianal tear [375]. In 101 (10 per cent) of these severe injuries, the episiotomy wound had disrupted. Complications included anal ulcer and abscess, disruption of the sphincter and rectovaginal fistula [375]. Surgical intervention was successful in most cases.

Assessment by manometric and endosonographic techniques of patients with faecal incontinence resulting from obstetric injury is useful to assess quantitatively the degree of sphincter dysfunction and may help to assess those who should benefit from surgery [111,265,286,301]. Use of ultrasound and pulsed electromagnetic energy therapies for perineal trauma following delivery showed no benefit in a randomized placebo-controlled trial [130].

Herpes simplex

Rectal and perianal ulcers can occur with herpes simplex virus, typically type II. Some success has been reported following oral acyclovir and this should be considered in late pregnancy to prevent transmission to the newborn [202].

Papillomaviruses and warts

Flat condylomata of the cervix and anogenital area are common and occur in up to 2 per cent of women of childbearing age [239]. Many result from transmission of human papillomaviruses (HPV) and are as common a sexually transmitted disease as herpes genitalis and gonorrhoea [239]. Some HPVs, such as HPV-6 and HPV-11 are considered of low oncogenic potential and are associated with condyloma acuminata [260] whereas HPV-16 and HPV-18 carry high risk and are associated with squamous cell carcinoma of the vulva and cervical intraepithelial neoplasia [212,260].

Condyloma acuminata are associated with promiscuity and other sexually transmitted diseases, diabetes mellitus, corticosteroid therapy and depression of cell-mediated immunity [212]. At least half of vestibular warts will be accompanied by warts detectable on the cervix, and 70 per cent of those with perianal warts also will have rectal warts [212]. Condyloma acuminata may grow rapidly during pregnancy. Caesarean section may have to be considered since anal warts have been associated with development of laryngeal papillomata in the infant [212]. Treatment is with podophyllin as a 25 per cent solution in tincture of benzoic acid although cryosurgery may be preferable for small lesions in pregnancy.

Gastrointestinal malignancies

Malignancy discovered during a normal pregnancy poses a considerable problem for the patient and her health-care attendants. Less than 20, often single, case reports of primary adenocarcinoma of the stomach were reported before 1980 [334] and just over 20 cases of primary [25,82,131,294,352,386] and metastatic [264,364,387] carcinoma of the large intestine have been recorded up to 1986. The true incidence of gastrointestinal malignancy complicating pregnancy is unknown. Carcinoma of the stomach (one case) and rectum (one case) accounted for two of the nine cases of malignancy causing fortuitous deaths in the report into maternal deaths in the UK between 1985 and 1987 [79].

Colonic and colorectal carcinoma

Less than 40 cases of colonic cancer have been reported up to 1993 concurrent with pregnancy [401].

Colonic carcinoma is a risk for patients with colonic IBD. Patients considered most at risk are those with extensive disease, typically of more than 10 years' duration [198]. Colonic malignancy presenting in pregnancy in association with IBD remains a rare possibility and should be considered in the differential diagnosis of diarrhoea and rectal bleeding.

About 200 cases of colorectal carcinoma have been recorded in the literature up to 1985 [120,264]. In a review of the literature up to 1986, one-third of patients diagnosed during pregnancy were less than 21 years of age [364]. Diagnosis was most frequent (two-thirds) during the third trimester. Typically, this was late in the natural history of the disease (Duke's grade C) and the outcome was poor [264, 364]. Metastatic spread is common, and occurs more often to the ovaries in pregnancy (24 per cent) compared to the non-pregnant population (4–6 per cent) [264]. An elevated level of carcinoembryonic antigen (CEA) may be useful in diagnosis but usually indicates late disease. Malignancy should be considered in patients presenting with iron-deficiency anaemia resulting from occult blood loss [371].

Colonic resection with rectal anastomosis is possible up to the third trimester. Bilateral salpingo-oophorectomy should be avoided because spontaneous abortion occurs frequently despite hormone replacement. Surgery for colorectal carcinoma diagnosed after the 20th week should be delayed until after delivery of a viable fetus. Vaginal delivery is usually feasible. Colorectal carcinoma in the young adult has a familial association [264] and family members should be screened for treatable underlying conditions such as familial polyposis and IBD among others.

The general consensus, however, is that pregnancy does not seem to have an adverse effect on the carcinoma *per se* or vice versa. All authors stress the need to exclude gastrointestinal malignancy in the differential diagnosis of common symptoms of pregnancy. Unexplained nausea, vomiting, altered bowel habit and rectal bleeding require investigation, including use of fibre-optic and occasionally radiological imaging [264,334,364].

Acknowledgement

This chapter is dedicated to Sir Francis Avery-Jones. Dr Fagan is supported by fellowships from the Wellcome Trust and British Digestive Foundation, London, UK and Abbott Laboratories, North Chicago, USA.

References

1 Abramson D, Jankelson IR *et al*. Pregnancy in idiopathic ulcerative colitis. *American Journal of Obstetrics and Gynecology* 1951; **61**: 121–9.

2 Alestig K, Trollfors B *et al*. Acute non-specific diarrhoea: studies on the use of charcoal, kaolin–pectin and diphenoxylate. *Practitioner* 1979; **222**: 859–62.

3 Ament ME & Rubin CE. Soy Protein — another cause of a flat intestinal lesion. *Gastroenterology* 1972; **62**: 227–34.

4 Anand AC, Kataria VK *et al*. Epidemic multiresistant enteric fever in eastern India. *Lancet* 1990; **i**: 352.

5 Anand S & Van Thiel DH. Prenatal and neonatal exposure to cimetidine results in gonadal and sexual dysfunction in adult males. *Science* 1982; **218**: 493–4.

6 Anders BJ, Lauer BA *et al*. Campylobacter gastroenteritis in neonates. *American Journal of Diseases of Children* 1981; **135**: 900–2.

7 Anderson AS. Dietary factors in the aetiology and treatment of constipation during pregnancy. *British Journal of Obstetrics and Gynaecology* 1986; **93**: 245–9.

8 Anderson AS & Whichelow M. Constipation during pregnancy: dietary fibre intakes and the effect of fibre supplementation. *Human Nutrition, Applied Nutrition* 1985; **39A**: 202–7.

9 Anderson GW. Pregnancy complicated by acute perforated peptic ulcer. *American Journal of Obstetrics and Gynecology* 1942; **43**: 883–7.

10 Antoon JW & Miller RL. Apthous ulcers — a review of the literature on etiology, pathogenesis, diagnosis and treatment. *Journal of the American Dental Association* 1980; **101**: 803–8.

11 Arsura EL, Fazio RA *et al*. Pseudomembranous colitis following prophylactic antibiotic use in Caesarian section. *American Journal of Obstetrics and Gynecology* 1985; **151**: 87–9.

12 Aselton P, Jick H *et al*. Pyloric stenosis and maternal Bendectin exposure. *American Journal of Epidemiology* 1984; **120**: 251–6.

13 Aston NO, Kalaichandran S *et al*. Duodenal ulcer hemorrhage in the puerperium. *Canadian Journal of Surgery* 1991; **34**: 482–3.

14 Atkinson RE & Hudson CH. Ano-rectal and perineal disorders of pregnancy and the puerperium. *Practitioner* 1970; **205**: 789–90.

15 Atlay RD, Gillison EW *et al*. A fresh look at pregnancy heartburn. *Journal of Obstetrics and Gynaecology of the British Commonwealth* 1973; **80**: 63–6.

16 Atlay RD & Weekes AR. The treatment of gastrointestinal disease in pregnancy. *Clinics in Obstetrics and Gynaecology* 1986; **13**: 335–47.

17 Auricchio S, Follo D *et al*. Does breast feeding protect against the development of clinical symptoms of celiac disease in children? *Journal of Pediatric Gastroenterology* 1983; **2**: 428–33.

18 Azad Khan AK & Truelove SC. Placental and mammary transfer of sulphasalazine. *British Medical Journal* 1979; **ii**: 1553.

19 Babson WW. Terminal ileitis with obstruction and abscess complicating pregnancy. *New England Journal of Medicine* 1946; **235**: 544–7.

20 Baimbridge ET, Nicholas SD *et al*. Gastro-oesophageal reflux in pregnancy. Altered function of the barrier to reflux in asymptomatic women during early pregnancy. *Scandinavian Journal of Gastroenterology* 1984; **19**: 85–9.

21 Baiocco PJ & Korelitz BI. The influence of inflammatory bowel disease and its treatment on pregnancy and fetal outcome. *Journal of Clinical Gastroenterology* 1984; **6**: 211–16.

22 Baird RM. Peptic ulceration in pregnancy. Report of a case with perforation. *Canadian Medical Association Journal* 1966; **94**: 861–2.

23 Baker PG & Read AE. Reversible infertility in male coeliac patients. *British Medical Journal* 1975; **ii**: 316–17.

24 Banks BM, Korelitz BI *et al*. The course of nonspecific ulcerative colitis: review of twenty years experience and late results. *Gastroenterology* 1957; **32**: 983–1012.

25 Banner EA, Hunt AB *et al*. Pregnancy associated with carcinoma of the large bowel. *Surgery, Gynecology and Obstetrics* 1945; **80**: 211–16.

26 Bargen JA, Nunez CJ *et al*. Pregnancy associated with chronic ulcerative colitis. *American Journal of Obstetrics and Gynecology* 1939; **38**: 146–8.

27 Barnes CS & Hayes HM. Ulcerative colitis complicating pregnancy and the puerperium. *American Journal of Obstetrics and Gynecology* 1931; **22**: 907–12.

28 Barros F de C & Kunzle JR *et al*. Apendicite aguda na gravidez (Acute appendicitis in pregnancy). *Revue Paulo Medicina* 1991; **109**: 9–13.

29 Barwin BN & Hartley JMG *et al*. Ileostomy and pregnancy. *British Journal of Clinical Practice* 1974; **28**: 256–8.

30 Bassey OO. Pregnancy heartburn in Nigerians and Caucasians with theories about aetiology based on manometric recordings from the oesophagus and

stomach. *British Journal of Obstetrics and Gynaecology* 1977; **84**: 439–43.
31 Bauman F. Ulcerative colitis complicated by a pregnancy. *American Journal of Obstetrics and Gynecology* 1931; **22**: 944–5.
32 Benson GD, Kowlessar OD *et al*. Adult celiac disease with emphasis upon response to the gluten-free diet. *Medicine (Baltimore)* 1964; **43**: 1–40.
33 Bergin PS & Harvey P. Wernicke's encephalopathy and central pontine myelinolysis associated with hyperemesis gravidarum. *British Medical Journal* 1992; **305**: 517–18.
34 Berkowitz RS & Goldstein DP. Pathogenesis of gestational trophoblastic neoplasms. *Pathobiology Annual* 1981; **11**: 391–411.
35 Bifarini G, Favetta P *et al*. Prevenzione farmacologica della sindrome di Mendelson. Studio clinico controllato (Pharmacologic prevention of Mendelson syndrome. A controlled clinical trial). *Minerva Anestesiologie* 1992; **58**: 95–9.
36 Biggs JSG & Vesey EJ. Treatment of gastrointestinal disorders of pregnancy. *Drugs* 1980; **19**: 70–6.
37 Blaser MJ, Berkowitz ID *et al*. Campylobacter enteritis: clinical and epidemiologic features. *Annals of Internal Medicine* 1979; **91**: 179–85.
38 Bober SA, McGill AC *et al*. Thyroid function in hyperemesis gravidarum. *Acta Endocrinologica (Copenhagen)* 1986; **111**: 404–10.
39 Bohe MG, Ekelund GR *et al*. Surgery for fulminating colitus during pregnancy. *Diseases of the Colon and Rectum* 1983; **26**: 199–22.
40 Booth CC. The enterocyte in coeliac disease. *British Medical Journal* 1970; **iv**: 14–17.
41 Borgfors N & Selander P. The incidence of coeliac disease in Sweden. *Acta Paediatrica Scandinavica* 1968; **57**: 260.
42 Bouillon R, Naesens M *et al*. Thyroid function in patients with hyperemesis gravidarum. *American Journal of Obstetrics and Gynecology* 1982; **143**: 922–6.
43 Brahme F, Lindstrom C *et al*. Crohn's disease in a defined population. An epidemiological study of incidence, prevalence, mortality and secular trends in the city of Malmo, Sweden. *Gastroenterology* 1975; **69**: 342–51.
44 Briggs GG, Bodendorfer TW *et al*. (eds), *Drugs in Pregnancy and Lactation: a Reference Guide to Fetal and Neonatal Risk*. Williams & Wilkins, Baltimore, 1983.
45 *British Medical Journal* editorial. Coeliac disease. *British Medical Journal* 1970; **iv**: 1–2.
46 Brock-Utne JG, Dow TGB *et al*. Gastric and lower oesophageal sphincter pressures in early pregnancy. *British Journal of Anaesthesia* 1981; **53**: 381–4.
47 Brooks FP, Powell KC *et al*. Variable clinical course of adult celiac disease. *Archives of Internal Medicine* 1966; **117**: 789–94.
48 Bruin T & Kristoffersen K. Thyroid function during pregnancy with special reference to hydatidiform mole and hyperemesis. *Acta Endocrinologica (Copenhagen)* 1978; **88**: 383–9.
49 Bryant MG & Bloom SR. Distribution of the gut hormones in the primate intestinal tract. *Gut* 1979; **20**: 653–9.
50 Burrow GN & Ferris TF (eds) *Medical Complications during Pregnancy*. WB Saunders & Co., Philadelphia, 1975.
51 Bushby SRM & Hitchings GH. Trimethoprim, a sulphonamide potentiator. *British Journal of Pharmacology* 1968; **33**: 72–90.
52 Butzler JP & Skirrow MB. *Campylobacter* enteritis. *Clinics in Gastroenterology* 1979; **8**: 737–65.
53 Byrne JJ. Diagnostic evaluation of patients with intestinal problems. *Clinics in Obstetrics and Gynaecology* 1972; **15**: 473–83.
54 Campieri M, Lanfranchi GA et al. Treatment of ulcerative colitis with high-dose 5-aminosalicylic acid enemas. *Lancet* 1981; **ii**: 270–1.
55 Cann PA & Holdsworth CD. Reversal of male infertility on changing treatment from sulphasalazine to 5 aminosalicylic acid. *Lancet* 1984; **i**: 1119.
56 Cantu JM & Garcia-Cruz D. Midline facial defect as a teratogenic effect of metronidazole. *Birth Defects* 1982; **18**: 85–8.
57 Carangelo J & Efstation TD. Massive gastric hemorrhage in pregnancy. *American Journal of Obstetrics and Gynecology* 1948; **56**: 191–4.
58 Carter CO, Sheldon W *et al*. Coeliac disease. *Annals of Human Genetics* 1959; **23**: 266.
59 Centers for Disease Control (CDC). Foodborne listeriosis — United States, 1988–1990. *Journal of the American Medical Association* 1992; **267**: 2446–8.
60 Christofides ND, Ghalei MA *et al*. Decreased plasma motilin concentrations in pregnancy. *British Medical Journal* 1982; **285**: 1453–4.
61 Clark DH. Pregnancy and peptic ulcer in women. *British Medical Journal* 1953; **i**: 1254–7.
62 Cohen S & Harris LD. Does hiatus hernia affect competence of the gastro esophageal sphincter? *New England Journal of Medicine* 1971; **284**: 1053–6.
63 Constantine G, Arundell L *et al*. Helminth infestations in Asian women attending an antenatal clinic in England. *British Journal of Obstetrics and Gynaecology* 1988; **95**: 493–6.
64 Cooke WT, Peeney ALP *et al*. Symptoms, signs and diagnostic features of idiopathic steatorrhoea. *Quarterly Journal of Medicine* 1953; **22**: 59–77.
65 Cooksey G, Gunn A *et al*. Case report. Surgery for acute ulcerative colitis and toxic megacolon during pregnancy. *British Journal of Surgery* 1985; **72**: 547.
66 Cosnes J, Hecketsweiler P *et al*. Consequences of extensive bowel resections in Crohn's disease: a study of 53 cases. *Gastroenterologie Clinique et Biologique (Paris)* 1981; **5**: 198–206.
67 Cotton BR & Smith G. The lower oesophageal sphincter and anaesthesia. *British Journal of Anaesthesia* 1984; **56**: 37–46.
68 Crisp WE. Pregnancy complicating peptic ulcer. *Post-*

graduate Medicine 1960; **27**: 445–7.
69 Crohn BB, Yarnis H *et al*. Regional ileitis complicating pregnancy. *Gastroenterology* 1956; **31**: 615–28.
70 Crohn BB, Yarnis H *et al*. Ulcerative colitis and pregnancy. *Gastroenterology* 1956; **30**: 391–403.
71 Crosby WH. Clay ingestion and iron deficiency. *Annals of Internal Medicine* 1982; **97**: 456.
72 D'Alauro F, Lee RV *et al*. Intestinal parasites and pregnancy. *Obstetrics and Gynecology* 1985; **66**: 639–43.
73 Davis MR & Bohon CJ. Intestinal obstruction in pregnancy. *Clinics in Obstetrics and Gynecology* 1983; **26**: 832–42.
74 Davis RE. Clinical chemistry of vitamin B_{12}. *Advances in Clinical Chemistry* 1985; **24**: 163–216.
75 Davis RE. Clinical chemistry of folic acid. *Advances in Clinical Chemistry* 1986; **25**: 233–94.
76 Davis JL & Chen MD. Gastric carcinoma presenting as an exacerbation of ulcers during pregnancy. A case report. *Journal of Reproductive Medicine* 1991; **36**: 450–2.
77 De Dombal FT, Watts JM *et al*. Ulcerative colitis and pregnancy. *Lancet* 1965; **ii**: 599–602.
78 De Dombal FT, Burton IL *et al*. Crohn's disease and pregnancy. *British Medical Journal* 1972; **iii**: 550–3.
79 Department of Health (DOH). *Report on Confidential Enquiries into Maternal Deaths in the United Kingdom 1985–87*. HMSO, London, 1991: 54–8.
80 Department of Health (DOH). Folic acid and the prevention of neural tube defects. *Report from an Expert Advisory Group*. 1992; CNO (92) 12 and addendum.
81 Depue RH, Bernstein L *et al*. Hyperemesis gravidarum in relation to estradiol levels, pregnancy outcome, and other maternal factors: a seroepidemiologic study. *American Journal of Obstetrics and Gynecology* 1987; **156**: 1137–41.
82 Der Brucke MG. Intestinal obstruction due to malignancy complicating pregnancy. *American Journal of Obstetrics and Gynecology* 1949; **40**: 307–11.
83 Desmond PV & Watson KJ. Metoclopramide — a review. *Medical Journal of Australia* 1986; **144**: 366–9.
84 Dew MJ, Hughes P *et al*. Maintenance of remission in ulcerative colitis with oral preparation of 5-aminosalicylic acid. *British Medical Journal* 1982; **285**: 1012–13.
85 Dgani R, Rozenman D *et al*. Ovarian malignancies in pregnancies complicated by colonic perforation. *Israeli Journal of Medical Science* 1988; **24**: 241–4.
86 Diddle AW & Stephens RL. Typhoid fever in pregnancy. Probable intrauterine transmission of the disease. *American Journal of Obstetrics and Gynecology* 1939; **38**: 300–5.
87 Dodds WJ, Dent J *et al*. Pregnancy and the lower esophageal sphincter. *Gastroenterology* 1978; **74**: 1334–6.
88 Ebbs JH. Coeliac disease. *Canadian Medical Association Journal* 1956; **75**: 885–93.
89 Ebbs JH, Thompson M *et al*. Etiologic factors in celiac disease. *American Journal of Diseases of Children* 1950; **79**: 936–7.
90 Ek B. Studies on idiopathic sprue. On the familiar incidence of idiopathic sprue and the significance of pregnancy and partial gastrectomy for the manifestation of the symptoms. *Acta Medica Scandinavica* 1967; **181**: 125–6.
91 Ek B. Studies on idiopathic sprue. Familial incidence and relation to pregnancy and partial gastrectomy. *Acta Medica Scandinavica* 1969; **185**: 463–4.
92 Elbourne D, Mutch L *et al*. Debendox revisited. *British Journal of Obstetrics and Gynaecology* 1985; **92**: 780–5.
93 Eskenazi B & Bracken MB. Bendectin (Debendox) as a risk factor for pyloric stenosis. *American Journal of Obstetrics and Gynecology* 1982; **144**: 919–24.
94 Evans AJ, Li CT *et al*. Morning sickness and thyroid function. *British Journal of Obstetrics and Gynaecology* 1986; **93**: 520–2.
95 Fagan EA & Chadwick VS. Drug treatment of gastrointestinal disorders in pregnancy. In: Lewis P (ed), *Clinical Pharmacology in Obstetrics*. Wright PSG, Bristol, 1983: 114–37.
96 Fagan EA, Dyck RF *et al*. Serum levels of C-reactive protein in Crohn's disease and ulcerative colitis. *European Journal of Clinical Investigation* 1982; **12**: 351–9.
97 Fairweather DV. Nausea and vomiting during pregnancy. *Obstetrics and Gynecology Annual* 1978; **7**: 91–105.
98 Falchuk ZM, Rogentine GN *et al*. Predominance of histocompatibility antigen HLA B8 in patients with gluten-sensitive enteropathy. *Journal of Clinical Investigation* 1972; **51**: 1602–5.
99 Fanning J & Cross CB. Post-cesarean section cecal volvulus. *American Journal of Obstetrics and Gynecology* 1988; **158**: 1200–2.
100 Farrell DJ & Harris MJ. A case of intrauterine fetal death associated with maternal *Campylobacter* coli bacteraemia. *Australia and New Zealand Journal of Obstetrics and Gynaecology* 1992; **32**: 172–7.
101 Farthing MJC, Edwards CRW *et al*. Male gonadal function in coeliac disease. I. Sexual dysfunction, infertility and semen quality. *Gut* 1982; **23**: 608–14.
102 Farthing MJC, Rees LH *et al*. Male gonadal function in coeliac disease. II. Sex hormones. *Gut* 1983; **24**: 127–35.
103 Feder IA. Chronic ulcerative colitis: An analysis of 88 cases. *American Journal of Digestive Diseases* 1938; **5**: 239–45.
104 *Federal Register*. Food and Safety Administration (on Bendectin). *Federal Register* 1979; **44**: 41 068.
105 Feeney JG. Leading article. Heartburn in pregnancy. *British Medical Journal* 1982; **284**: 1138–9.
106 Feldman MD. Pica: current perspectives. *Psychosomatics* 1986; **27**: 519–23.
107 Felsen J & Wolarsky W. Chronic ulcerative colitis and

pregnancy. *American Journal of Obstetrics and Gynecology* 1948; **56**: 751–5.
108 Fielding JF & Cooke WT. Pregnancy and Crohn's disease. *British Medical Journal* 1970; **ii**: 76–7.
109 Filipsson S, Hulten L *et al*. The metabolic consequences of surgery in Crohn's disease. *Scandinavian Journal of Gastroenterology* 1978; **13**: 471–9.
110 Fischer-Rassmussen W, Kjaer SK *et al*. Ginger treatment of hyperemesis gravidarum. *European Journal of Obstetrics and Gynecology and Reproduction Biology* 1990; **38**: 19–24.
111 Fleshman JW, Dreznik Z *et al*. Anal sphincter repair for obstetric injury: manometric evaluation of functional results. *Diseases of the Colon and Rectum* 1991; **34**: 1061–7.
112 Frederiksen B & Samuelsson S. Feto-maternal listeriosis in Denmark 1981–1988. *Journal of Infection* 1992; **24**: 277–87.
113 Freedman ML, Christopher P *et al*. Typhoid carriage in pregnancy with infection of neonate. *Lancet* 1970; **i**: 310–11.
114 Gallagher DM. Pruritus ani. *Modern Treatment* 1971; **8**: 963–70.
115 Gazzard BG, Price HL *et al*. The social toll of Crohn's disease. *British Medical Journal* 1978; **ii**: 1117–19.
116 Gilat T & Rozen P. Epidemiology of Crohn's disease and ulcerative colitis: etiologic implications. *Israeli Journal of Medical Science* 1979; **15**: 305–8.
117 Gilbert GL, Davoren RA *et al*. Midtrimester abortion associated with septicaemia caused by *Campylobacter jejuni*. *Medical Journal of Australia* 1981; **1**: 585–6.
118 Gillet GB, Watson JD *et al*. Ranitidine and single-dose antacid therapy as prophylaxis against acid aspiration syndrome in obstetric practice. *Anaesthesia* 1984; **39**: 638–44.
119 Gillon FD, Reiner DS *et al*. Human milk kills intestinal protozoa. *Science* 1983; **221**: 1290–2.
120 Girard RM, Lamarche J *et al*. Carcinoma of the colon associated with pregnancy: a report of a case. *Diseases of the Colon and Rectum* 1981; **24**: 473–5.
121 Glade G, Saccar CL *et al*. Cimetidine in pregnancy: apparent transient liver impairment in the newborn. *American Journal of Diseases of Children* 1980; **134**: 87–8.
122 Godding EW. Constipation and allied disorders. *Pharmaceutical Journal* 1976; **2**: 8.
123 Godding EW. Constipation and allied disorders. *Pharmaceutical Journal* 1976; **5**: 17.
124 Godsey RK & Newman RB. Hyperemesis gravidarum. A comparison of single and multiple admissions. *Journal of Reproductive Medicine* 1991; **36**: 287–90.
125 Golding J, Vivian S *et al*. Maternal anti-nauseants and clefts of lip and palate. *Human Toxicology* 1983; **2**: 63–73.
126 Gorbach SL. Travelers' diarrhea. *New England Journal of Medicine* 1982; **307**: 881–3.
127 Gorlin RJ & Goldman HM (eds) Hyperplastic gingivitis. In: *Thoma's Oral Pathology*, 6th edn, Volume 1. CV Mosby Co., St Louis, 1970: 400–2.
128 Goyal RK & Rattan S. Neurohumeral, hormonal and drug receptors for the lower esophageal sphincter. *Gastroenterology* 1978; **74**: 598–619.
129 Grandien M, Sterner G *et al*. Management of pregnant women with diarrhoea at term and of healthy carriers of infectious agents in stools at delivery. *Scandinavian Journal of Infectious Diseases* 1990; **71** (suppl): 9–18.
130 Grant A, Sleep J *et al*. Ultrasound and pulsed electromagnetic energy treatment for perineal trauma. A randomized placebo-controlled trial. *British Journal of Obstetrics and Gynaecology* 1989; **96**: 434–9.
131 Green LK, Harris RE *et al*. Cancer of the colon during pregnancy. A review of the literature and report of a case associated with ulcerative colitis. *Obstetrics and Gynecology* 1975; **46**: 480–3.
132 Green PA & Wollaeger EE. The clinical behavior of sprue in the United States. *Gastroenterology* 1960; **38**: 399–418.
133 Gribble MJ, Salit IE *et al*. Campylobacter infections in pregnancy. Case report and literature review. *American Journal of Obstetrics and Gynecology* 1981; **140**: 423–6.
134 Griffin GE, Fagan EA *et al*. Enteral therapy in the management of massive gut resection complicated by chronic fluid and electrolyte depletion. *Digestive Diseases and Sciences* 1982; **27**: 902–8.
135 Gross S, Librach C *et al*. Maternal weight loss associated with hyperemesis gravidarum: a predictor of fetal outcome. *American Journal of Obstetrics and Gynecology* 1989; **160**: 906–9. (Comment in: *American Journal of Obstetrics and Gynecology* 1990; **162**: 1349.)
136 Gruner O-PN, Naas R *et al*. Marital status and sexual adjustment after colectomy. *Scandinavian Journal of Gastroenterology* 1977; **12**: 193–7.
137 Harlap S, Shiono PH *et al*. A prospective study of spontaneous fetal losses after induced abortions. *New England Journal of Medicine* 1979; **301**: 677–81.
138 Harrington RA, Hamilton CW *et al*. Metoclopramide: an updated review of its pharmacological properties and clinical use. *Drugs* 1983; **25**: 451–94.
139 Heaton KW, Emmett PM *et al*. An explanation for gallstones in normal-weight women: slow intestinal transit. *Lancet* 1993; **341**: 8–10.
140 Heaton KW, Radvan J *et al*. Defecation frequency and timing, and stool form in the general population: a prospective study. *Gut* 1992; **33**: 818–24.
141 Heller L. Parenteral Nutrition in Obstetrics and Gynaecology. In: Greep JM, Soeters PB, Wesdorp RIC *et al* (eds), *Current Concepts in Parenteral Nutrition*. Nyhoff Medical Division, The Hague, 1977: 179–86.
142 Hensleigh PA & Kauffman RE. Maternal absorption and placental transfer of sulphasalazine. *American Journal of Obstetrics and Gynecology* 1977; **127**: 443–4.
143 Hibbard ED & Smithells RW. Folic acid metabolism and human embryopathy. *Lancet* 1965; **i**: 1254.

144 Hill RM & Tennyson LM. Drug-induced malformations in humans. In: Stern L (ed), *Drug Use in Pregnancy*. ADIS Health Science Press, Sydney, 1984: 99–133.

145 Hogan WJ, de Andrade SRV *et al*. Ethanol-induced acute esophageal motor function. *Journal of Applied Physiology* 1972; **32**: 755–60.

146 Holmes-Siedle M, Lindenbaum RH *et al*. Vitamin supplementation and neural tube defects (letter). *Lancet* 1982 **i**: 276.

147 Holtermuller KH & Weis HJ. Gastroenterologishe Erkrankungen in der Schwangershaft. *Gynakologe* 1979; **12**: 35–51.

148 Homan WP & Thorbjarnarson NB. Crohn's disease and pregnancy. *Archives of Surgery* 1976; **111**: 545–7.

149 Hoos PC & Hoffman LH. Effective histamine receptor antagonists and indomethacin on implantation in the rabbit. *Biology and Reproduction* 1983; **29**: 833–40.

150 Horner RD, Lackey CJ *et al*. Pica practices of pregnant women. *Journal of the American Dietetic Association* 1991; **91**: 34–8.

151 Hudson CN. Ileostomy in pregnancy. *Proceedings of the Royal Society of Medicine* 1972; **62**: 281–3.

152 Hudson M, Flett G *et al*. Fertility and pregnancy in inflammatory bowel disease — a community study of 409 patients in North East Scotland. *Quarterly Journal of Medicine* 1993 (in press).

153 Huff PS. Safety of drug therapy for nausea and vomiting of pregnancy. *Journal of the Family Practitioner* 1980; **ii**: 969–70.

154 Hunt JN & Murray FA. Gastric function in pregnancy. *Journal of Obstetrics and Gynaecology of the British Empire* 1958; **65**: 78–83.

155 Hytten FE. The alimentary system. In: Hytten F & Chamberlain G (eds), *Clinical Physiology in Obstetrics*. Blackwell Scientific Publications, Oxford, 1991: 137–49.

156 Ingardia CJ & Fischer JR. Pregnancy after jejunoileal bypass and the SGA infant. *Obstetrics and Gynecology* 1978; **52**: 215.

157 Ippoliti AF & Sturdevant RAL. Cimetidine versus intensive antacid therapy for duodenal ulcer. *Gastroenterology* 1978; **74**: 393–5.

158 Ippoliti AF, Elashoff J *et al*. Recurrent ulcer after successful treatment with cimetidine or antacid. *Gastroenterology* 1983; **85**: 875–8.

159 Islam A, Stoll BJ *et al*. The prevalence of *Entamoeba histolytica* in lactating women and in their infants in Bangladesh. *Transactions of the Royal Society of Tropical Medicine and Hygiene* 1988; **82**: 99–103.

160 Jarnerot G & Into-Malmberg MB. Sulphasalazine treatment during breast feeding. *Scandinavian Journal of Gastroenterology* 1979; **14**: 869–71.

161 Jarnfelt-Samsioe A, Eriksson B *et al*. Some new aspects in emesis gravidarum. Relations to clinical data, serum electrolytes, total protein and creatinine. *Gynecologic and Obstetric Investigation* 1985; **19**: 174–86.

162 Jarnfelt-Samsioe A, Samsioe G *et al*. Nausea and vomiting in pregnancy — a contribution to its epidemiology. *Gynecologic and Obstetric Investigation* 1983; **16**: 221–9.

163 Jeffcoate WJ & Bain C. Recurrent pregnancy-induced thyrotoxicosis presenting as hyperemesis gravidarum. Case Report. *British Journal of Obstetrics and Gynaecology* 1985; **92**: 413–15.

164 Jones PF, McEwan AB *et al*. Haemorrhage and perforation complicating peptic ulcer in pregnancy. *Lancet* 1969; **iii**: 350–1.

165 Joske RA & Martin JD. Coeliac disease presenting as recurrent abortion. *Journal of Obstetrics and Gynaecology of the British Commonwealth* 1971; **78**: 754–8.

166 Jost PM, Galvin MC *et al*. Campylobacter septic abortion. *Southern Medical Journal (Birmingham, Alabama)* 1984; **77**: 924.

167 Juergens JL, Scholz DA *et al*. Severe osteomalacia associated with occult steatorrhoea due to nontropical sprue. *Archives of Internal Medicine* 1956; **98**: 774–82.

168 Juras N, Banovac K *et al*. Increased serum reverse triiodothyronine in patients with hyperemesis gravidarum. *Acta Endocrinologica (Copenhagen)* 1983; **102**: 284–7.

169 Kahn SB, Fein SA *et al*. Effects of trimethoprim on folate metabolism in man. *Clinical Pharmacology and Therapeutics* 1968; **9**: 550–60.

170 Kammerer WS. Non-obstetric surgery during pregnancy. *Medical Clinics of North America* 1979; **63**: 1157–64.

171 Karmali MA & Tan YC. Neonatal Campylobacter enteritis. *Canadian Medical Association Journal* 1980; **122**: 192–7.

172 Katz S, Schulman N *et al*. Free perforation in Crohn's disease: a report of 33 cases and review of literature. *American Journal of Gastroenterology* 1986; **81**: 38–43.

173 Kauppila A, Huhtaniemi I *et al*. Raised serum human chorionic gonadotrophin concentrations in hyperemesis gravidarum. *British Medical Journal* 1979; **ii**: 1670–1.

174 Kauppila A, Heikinheimo M *et al*. Human chorionic gonadotrophin and pregnancy-specific beta-1-glycoprotein in predicting pregnancy outcome and in association with early pregnancy vomiting. *Gynecologic and Obstetric Investigation* 1984; **18**: 49–53.

175 Kaye MD & Showalter JP. Pyloric incompetence in patients with symptomatic gastroesophageal reflux. *Journal of Laboratory and Clinical Medicine* 1974; **83**: 198–206.

176 Keighley MRB, Burdon DW *et al*. Randomised controlled trial of vancomycin for pseudomembranous colitis and post operative diarrhoea. *British Medical Journal* 1978; **ii**: 1667.

177 Kerr AM. Unprecedented rise in incidence of infantile hypertrophic pyloric stenosis. *British Medical Journal* 1980; **281**: 714–15.

178 Kerwenter J, Hulten L *et al*. The relationship and

epidemiology of acute terminal ileitis and Crohn's disease. *Gut* 1974; **15**: 801–4.

179 Khosla R & Willoughby CP. Crohn's disease and pregnancy. *Gut* 1984; **25**: 52–6.

180 Kirsner JB. Observations on the medical treatment of inflammatory bowel disease. *Journal of the American Medical Association* 1980; **243**: 557–64.

181 Kirsner JB, Palmer WL *et al*. Clinical course of chronic nonspecific ulcerative colitis. *Journal of the American Medical Association* 1948; **137**: 922–8.

182 Kirsner JB & Shorter RG. Recent developments in 'non-specific' inflammatory bowel disease, part 1. *New England Journal of Medicine* 1982; **306**: 775–85.

183 Kirsner JB & Shorter RG. Recent developments in nonspecific inflammatory bowel disease, part 2. *New England Journal of Medicine* 1982; **306**: 837–48.

184 Klebanoff MA, Koslowe PA *et al*. Epidemiology of vomiting in early pregnancy. *Obstetrics and Gynecology* 1985; **66**: 612–16.

185 Klebanoff MA & Mills JL. Is vomiting during pregnancy teratogenic? *British Medical Journal* 1986; **292**: 724–6.

186 Klotz U. Clinical pharmacokinetics of sulphasalazine, its metabolites and other prodrugs of 5-aminosalicylic acid. *Clinical Pharmacokinetics* 1985; **10**: 285–302.

187 Klotz U, Maier K *et al*. Therapeutic efficacy of sulphasalazine and its metabolites in patients with ulcerative colitis and Crohn's disease. *New England Journal of Medicine* 1980; **26**: 1499–502.

188 Koch KL, Stern RM *et al*. Gastric dysrhythmias and nausea of pregnancy. *Digestive Diseases and Sciences* 1990; **35**: 961–9.

189 Korelitz BI. From Crohn to Crohn's disease: 1979. An epidemiologic study in New York city. *Mount Sinai Journal of Medicine* 1979; **46**: 533–40.

190 Korelitz BI. Therapy of inflammatory bowel disease including use of immunosuppressive agents. *Clinics in Gastroenterology* 1980; **9**: 331–49.

191 Korelitz BI. Pregnancy, fertility and inflammatory bowel disease. *American Journal of Gastroenterology* 1985; **80**: 365–70.

192 Kornman KS & Loesche WJ. The subgingival microbial flora during pregnancy. *Journal of Periodontal Research* 1980; **15**: 111–22.

193 Krawitt EL. Ulcerative colitis and pregnancy. *Obstetrics and Gynecology* 1959; **14**: 354–61.

194 Kreutner AK, Del Bene VE *et al*. Giardiasis in pregnancy. *American Journal of Obstetrics and Gynecology* 1981; **140**: 895–901.

195 Kullander S & Kallen B. A prospective study of drugs and pregnancy. *Acta Obstetricia et Gynecologica Scandinavica Supplement* 1976; **55**: 105–11.

196 Kyle J & Stark G. Fall in the incidence of Crohn's disease. *Gut* 1980; **21**: 340–3.

197 Lachgar M & Morer I. Efficiency and tolerance of lactulose in constipation in pregnant women. *Revue Francaise De Gynecologie et D'Obstetrique* 1985; **80**: 663–5.

198 *Lancet* editorial. Colorectal carcinoma in ulcerative colitis. *Lancet* 1986; **ii**: 197–8.

199 Langmade CF. Epigastric pain in pregnancy toxaemias. *Western Journal Surgery* 1956; **64**: 540–4.

200 Larson HE & Price AB. Pseudomembranous colitis: presence of clostridial toxin. *Lancet* 1977; **ii**: 1312–14.

201 Lawson JB & Stewart DB (eds), *Obstetrics and Gynaecology in the Tropics*. Edward Arnold, London, 1967: 52–9.

202 Ledward RS, Hawkins DF *et al*. (eds), *Drug Treatment in Obstetrics*. Chapman & Hall Medical, London, 1991: 155–7.

203 Lennard-Jones JE & Powell-Tuck J. Drug treatment of inflammatory bowel disease. *Clinics in Gastroenterology* 1979; **8**: 187–217.

204 Lenz W. Malformations caused by drugs in pregnancy. *American Journal of Diseases of Children* 1966; **112**: 99–106.

205 Lenz W & Knapp K. Thalidomide embryopathy. *Deutsche Medizinische Wochenschrift* 1962; **87**: 1232–42.

206 Levi AJ, Fisher AM *et al*. Male infertility due to sulphasalazine. *Lancet* 1979; **ii**: 276–8.

207 Levy N, Lemberg E *et al*. Bowel habit in pregnancy. *Digestion* 1971; **4**: 216–22.

208 Lewis JH & Weingold AB. The use of gastrointestinal drugs during pregnancy and lactation. *American Journal of Gastroenterology* 1985; **80**: 912–23.

209 Liang C-C, Hsieh T-T *et al*. Appendicitis during pregnancy. *Chang Keng I Hsueh*. 1989; **12**: 208–14.

210 Linnan MJ, Mascola L *et al*. Epidemic of listeriosis associated with Mexican-style cheese. *New England Journal of Medicine* 1988; **319**: 823–8.

211 Loe H & Silness J. Periodontal disease in pregnancy. *Acta Odontica Scandinavica* 1963; **21**: 533–51.

212 Lynch PJ. Condylomata acuminata (anogenital warts). *Clinics in Obstetrics and Gynecology* 1985; **28**: 142–51.

213 MacDonald WC, Dobbins WO *et al*. Studies of the familial nature of celiac sprue using biopsy of the small intestine. *New England Journal of Medicine* 1965; **272**: 448–56.

214 MacDougall I. Ulcerative colitis and pregnancy. *Lancet* 1956; **271**: 641–3.

215 Machella TE. Problems in ulcerative colitis. *American Journal of Medicine* 1952; **13**: 760–76.

216 Maddix BL. Ulcerative colitis and pregnancy. *Minnisota Medicine* 1962; **45**: 1097–2011.

217 Mahmoodian S. Appendicitis complicating pregnancy. *Southern Medical Journal* 1992; **85**: 19–24.

218 Mandal BK. Modern treatment of typhoid fever (editorial). *Journal of Infection* 1991; **22**: 1–4.

219 Mann JG, Brown WR *et al*. The subtle and variable clinical expressions of gluten-induced enteropathy (adult coeliac disease, nontropical sprue). An analysis of twenty-one consecutive cases. *American Journal of Medicine* 1970; **48**: 357–66.

220 Martelli H, Duguay C *et al*. Some parameters of large bowel motility in normal man. *Gastroenterology* 1978; **75**: 612–18.

221 Martin JD & Davis RE. Serum folic acid activity and vaginal bleeding in early pregnancy. *Journal of Obstetrics and Gynaecology of the British Commonwealth* 1964; **71**: 400–3.

222 Martin R, Trubow M *et al*. Hyperalimentation during pregnancy: a case report. *Journal of Parenteral and Enteral Nutrition* 1985; **9**: 212–15.

223 Martin RH, Harper TA *et al*. Serum folic acid in recurrent abortions. *Lancet* 1965; **i**: 670–2.

224 Martinbeau PN, Welch JS *et al*. Crohn's disease and pregnancy. *American Journal of Obstetrics and Gynecology* 1975; **122**: 746–9.

225 Masson GM, Antony F *et al*. Serum choriogonadotrophin, schwangerschaftsprotein 1 (SP1), progesterone and oestradiol levels in patients with nausea and vomiting in early pregnancy. *British Journal of Obstetrics and Gynaecology* 1985; **92**: 211–15.

226 Mayberry J, Rhodes J *et al*. Incidence of Crohn's disease in Cardiff between 1934 and 1977. *Gut* 1979; **20**: 602–8.

227 Mayberry JF & Weterman IT. European Survey of fertility and pregnancy in women with Crohn's disease: a case control study by the European Collaborative Group. *Gut* 1986; **27**: 821–5.

228 McBride WG. Thalidomide and congenital abnormalities. *Lancet* 1961; **ii**: 1358.

229 McBride WG. An aetiological study of drug ingestion by women who gave birth to babies with cleft palate. *Australian, New Zealand Journal of Obstetrics and Gynaecology* 1969; **9**: 103–4.

230 McCartan BE & Sullivan A. The association of menstrual cycle, pregnancy and menopause with recurrent oral apthous stomatitis: a review of critique. *Obstetrics and Gynecology* 1992; **80**: 455–8.

231 McCarthy CF, Mylotte M *et al*. Family studies on coeliac disease in Ireland. *Proceedings of the Second International Coeliac Symposium, Coeliac Disease*. Stenfert Kroese, Leiden, 1974.

232 McClain C, Soutor C *et al*. Zinc deficiency: A Complication of Crohn's disease. *Gastroenterology* 1980; **78**: 272–9.

233 McCormack WM, George H *et al*. Hepatotoxicity of erythromycin estolate during pregnancy. *Antimicrobial Agents and Chemotherapy* 1977; **12**: 630–5.

234 McCrae WM, Eastwood MA *et al*. Neglected coeliac disease. *Lancet* 1975; **i**: 187–90.

235 McEwen HP. Ulcerative colitis in pregnancy. *Proceedings of the Royal Society of Medicine* 1972; **65**: 279–81.

236 McNeeley SG, Anderson GD *et al*. *Clostridium difficile* colitis associated with single-dose cefazolin prophylaxis. *Obstetrics and Gynecology* 1985; **66**: 737–8.

237 Medalie JH. Relationship between nausea and/or vomiting in early pregnancy and abortion. *Lancet* 1957; **ii**: 117–19.

238 Medical Research Council (MRC) Vitamin Study Group. Prevention of neural tube defects: results of the Medical Research Council Vitamin Study. *Lancet* 1991; **238**: 131–7.

239 Meisels A & Morin C. Human papillomavirus and cancer of the uterine cervix. *Gynecologic Oncology* 1981; **12**: 5111.

240 Metcalf A, Dozois RR *et al*. Pregnancy following ileal pouch-anal anastomosis. *Diseases of the Colon and Rectum* 1985; **28**: 859–61.

241 Meyers S, Walfish JS *et al*. Quality of life after surgery for Crohn's disease: a psychosocial survey. *Gastroenterology* 1980; **78**: 1–6.

242 Midwinter A. Causes of vomiting in pregnancy. *Practitioner* 1971; **206**: 743–50.

243 Mihaly GW, Jones DB *et al*. Placental transfer and renal elimination of cimetidine in maternal and fetal sheep. *Journal of Pharmacology and Experimental Therapeutics* 1983; **227**: 441–5.

244 Mikovich L & Van den Berg BJ. An evaluation of the teratogenicity of certain antinauseant drugs. *American Journal of Obstetrics and Gynecology* 1976; **125**: 244–8.

245 Mills JL, Tuomilehto *et al*. Maternal vitamin levels during pregnancies producing infants with neural tube defects. *Journal of Pediatrics* 1992; **120**: 863–71.

246 Miller JP. Inflammatory bowel disease in pregnancy: a review. *Journal of the Royal Society of Medicine* 1986; **79**: 221–5.

247 Mitchell AA & Shapiro S. Bendectin (Debendox) and congenital diaphragmatic hernia. *Lancet* 1983; **i**: 930 (letter).

248 Mitchell JE, Breuer RI *et al*. The colon influences ileal resection diarrhoea. *Digestive Diseases and Sciences* 1980; **25**: 33–41.

249 Mogadam M, Dobbins WO *et al*. Pregnancy in inflammatory bowel disease: effect of sulphasalazine and corticosteroids on fetal outcome. *Gastroenterology* 1981; **80**: 72–6.

250 Moir DD. Cimetidine, antacids and pulmonary aspiration. *Anesthesiology* 1983; **59**: 81–3.

251 Moller C, Kiviluoto O *et al*. Local treatment of ulcerative proctitis with salicylazosulphapyridine (salazopyrin) enema. *Clinical Trials Journal (London)* 1978; **15**: 199–203.

252 Molteni N, Bardella MT *et al*. Obstetric and gynecological problems in women with untreated celiac sprue. *Journal of Clinical Gastroenterology* 1990; **12**: 37–9.

253 Morali GA & Braverman DZ. Abnormal liver enzymes and ketoneuria in hyperemesis gravidarum. A retrospective review of 80 patients. *Journal of Clinical Gastroenterology* 1990; **12**: 303–5.

254 *Morbidity Mortality Weekly Report* (MMWR) Update: foodborne listeriosis — United States 1988–1990. *Morbidity Mortality Weekly Report* 1992: **41**: 251, 257–8.

255 Mori M, Amino N *et al*. Morning sickness and thyroid

function in normal pregnancy. *Obstetrics and Gynecology* 1988; **72**: 355–9.

256 Morowitz DA & Kirsner JB. Ileostomy in ulcerative colitis: a questionnaire study of 1803 patients. *American Journal of Surgery* 1981; **141**: 370–5.

257 Morris JS, Ajdukiewicz AB *et al*. Coeliac infertility: an indication for dietary gluten restriction? *Lancet* 1970; **i**: 213–14.

258 Mortimer PE, Stewart JS *et al*. Follow-up study of Coeliac disease. *British Medical Journal* 1968; **iii**: 7–9.

259 Multicenter study of the use of drugs during pregnancy in Spain — III. Drugs used during the first pregnancy trimester. DUP workshop of Spain (Estudio multicentrico sobre el uso de medicamentos durante el embarazo en Espana — III. Los farmacos utilizados durante el primer trimestre de la gestacion. Grupo de Trabajo DUP Espana. *Medical Clinics of Barcelona* 1991; **96**: 52–7.

260 Munger K, Scheffner M *et al*. Interactions of HPV E6 and E7 oncoproteins with tumour suppressor gene products. *Cancer Surveys* 1992; **12**: 197–217.

261 Mylotte MJ, Egan-Mitchell B *et al*. Familial coeliac disease. *Quarterly Journal of Medicine* 1972; **41**: 527–8.

262 National Institutes of Health (NIH) Consensus Conference. Travelers diarrhea. *Journal of the American Medical Association* 1985; **253**: 2700–4.

263 Nelson MM & Forfar JO. Associations between drugs administered during pregnancy and congenital abnormalities of the foetus. *British Medical Journal* 1971; **i**: 523–7.

264 Nesbitt JC, Moise KJ *et al*. Colorectal carcinoma in pregnancy. *Archives of Surgery* 1985; **120**: 636–40.

265 Nielsen MB, Hauge C *et al*. Anal endosonographic findings in the follow-up of primarily sutured sphincteric ruptures. *British Journal of Surgery* 1992; **79**: 104–6.

266 Nielsen OH, Andreasson B *et al*. Pregnancy in ulcerative colitis. *Scandinavian Journal of Gastroenterology* 1983; **18**: 735–42.

267 Nielsen OH, Andreasson B *et al*. Pregnancy in Crohn's disease. *Scandinavian Journal of Gastroenterology* 1984; **19**: 724–32.

267a Niv Y & Abukasis G. Prevalence of ulcerative colitis in the Israeli kibbutz population. *Journal of Clinical Gastroenterology* 1991; **13**: 98–101.

268 Norman RJ, Green-Thompson RW *et al*. Hyperthyroidism in gestational trophoblastic neoplasia. *Clinical Endocrinology* 1981; **15**: 395–401.

269 Norton RA & Patterson JF. Pregnancy and regional enteritis. *Obstetrics and Gynecology* 1972; **40**: 711–12.

270 O'Donoghue DP, Dawson AM *et al*. Double blind withdrawal trial of azathioprine as maintenance treatment for Crohn's disease. *Lancet* 1978; **ii**: 955–7.

271 Ogborn ADR. Pregnancy in patients with coeliac disease. *British Journal of Obstetrics and Gynaecology* 1975; **82**: 293–6.

272 Ogorek CP & Cohen S. Gastroesophageal reflux disease: new concepts in pathophysiology. *Gastroenterology Clinics of North America* 1989; **18**: 275–92.

273 Olow B, Akesson BA *et al*. Pregnancy after jejunoileostomy because of obesity. *Acta Chirurgica Scandinavica* 1976; **142**: 82–6.

274 O'Morain C, Smethurst P *et al*. Reversible male infertility due to sulphasalazine: studies in man and rat. *Gut* 1984; **25**: 1078–84.

275 Palmer KR, Goepel JR *et al*. Sulphasalazine retention enemas in ulcerative colitis: a double-blind trial. *British Medical Journal* 1981; **282**: 1571–3.

276 Parbhoo SP & Johnston IDA. Effect of oestrogens and progestagens on gastric secretion in patients with duodenal ulcer. *Gut* 1966; **7**: 612–18.

277 Parker S, Schade RR *et al*. Prenatal and neonatal exposure of male rat pups to cimetidine but not ranitidine adversely affects subsequent adult sexual functioning. *Gastroenterology* 1984; **86**: 675–80.

278 Parry E, Shields R *et al*. The effect of pregnancy on the colonic absorption of sodium, potassium and water. *Journal of Obstetrics and Gynaecology of the British Commonwealth* 1970; **77**: 616–19.

278a Parry E, Shields R *et al*. Transit time in the small intestine in pregnancy. *Journal of Obstetrics and Gynaecology of the British Commonwealth* 1970; **77**: 900–1.

279 Parry GK. Perforated duodenal ulcer in the puerperium. *New Zealand Medical Journal* 1974; **80**: 448–9.

280 Patterson D. Congenital deformities (letter). *Canadian Medical Association Journal* 1969; **101**: 175–6.

281 Patterson D. Congenital deformities associated with Bendectin. *Canadian Medical Association Journal* 1977; **116**: 1348.

282 Pawlowski ZS. Intestinal helminthiases. *Medicine International* 1992; **108**: 4535–42.

283 Pearl M & Boxt LM. Radiographic findings in congenital lead poisoning. *Radiology* 1980; **136**: 83–4.

284 Peden NR, Boyd EJS *et al*. Women and duodenal ulcer. *British Medical Journal* 1981; **282**: 866.

285 Peppercorn MA. Sulphasalazine. Pharmacology, clinical use, toxicity and related new drug development. *Annals of Internal Medicine* 1984; **101**: 377–86.

286 Perry RE, Blatchford GJ *et al*. Manometric diagnosis of anal sphincter injuries. *American Journal of Surgery* 1990; **159**: 112–16, discussion 116–17.

287 Philipson EH, Rossi KQ *et al*. Glucose, insulin, gastric inhibitory polypeptide, and pancreatic polypeptide responses to polycose during pregnancy. *Obstetrics and Gynecology* 1992; **79**: 592–6.

287a Pillay N, Adams EB *et al*. Comparative trial of amoxycillin and chloramphenicol in treatment of typhoid fever in adults. *Lancet* 1975; **ii**: 333–4.

288 Pockros PJ, Weiss JB *et al*. Toxic megacolon complicating *Campylobacter* enterocolitis (letter). *Journal of Clinical Gastroenterology* 1986; **8**: 318–19.

289 Prakash C, Bansal BC *et al*. A comparative study of tinidazole and metronidazole in symptomatic

intestinal amoebiasis. *Journal of the Association of Physicians of India* 1974; **22**: 527–9.
290 Prasad AS. Zinc deficiency in human subjects. *Progress in Clinical and Biological Research* 1983; **129**: 1–33.
291 Prasad AS. Clinical manifestations of zinc deficiency. *Annual Review of Nutrition* 1985; **5**: 341–63.
292 Present DH, Korelitz BI *et al*. Treatment of Crohn's disease with 6-mercaptopurine: A long-term, randomised, double-blind trial. *New England Journal of Medicine* 1980; **302**: 981–7.
293 Preston DM & Lennard-Jones JE. Severe chronic constipation of young women: 'idiopathic slow-transit constipation'. *Gut* 1986; **27**: 41–8.
294 Putzki PS, Scully JH *et al*. Carcinoma of the colon producing acute intestinal obstruction during pregnancy. *American Journal of Surgery* 1949; **77**: 749–54.
295 Raffensperger EC. Recurrence of regional terminal ileitis associated with pregnancy. *Gastroenterology* 1948; **10**: 1010–17.
296 Rasmussen KL, Knudsen TA *et al*. Perforation of a pyometra mimicking a perforated peptic ulcer. *Archives of Gynecological Obstetrics* 1991; **248**: 211–12.
297 Riezzo G, Pezzolla F *et al*. Gastric myoelectrical activity in the first trimester of pregnancy: a cutaneous electromyographic study. *American Journal of Gastroenterology* 1992; **87**: 702–7.
298 Riley AJ, Crowley P *et al*. Transfer of ranitidine to biological fluids; milk and serum. In: Misiewicz JJ & Wormsley KG (eds), *The Clinical Use of Ranitidine. The Second International Symposium on Ranitidine*. Medicine Publishing Foundation, Oxford, 1982: 78–81.
299 Rivera-Alsina ME, Saldana LR *et al*. Fetal growth sustained by parenteral nutrition in pregnancy. *Obstetrics and Gynecology* 1984; **64**: 138–41.
300 Roberts NS, Copel JA *et al*. Intestinal parasites and other infections during pregnancy in southeast Asian refugees. *Journal of Reproductive Medicine* 1985; **30**: 720–5.
301 Roberts PL, Coller JA *et al*. Manometric assessment of patients with obstetric injuries and fecal incontinence. *Diseases of the Colon and Rectum* 1990; **33**: 16–20.
302 Rodin P & Hass G. Metronidazole and pregnancy. *Journal of Venereal Diseases* 1966; **42**: 210–12.
303 Rodriguez Ballesteros R, Torres Bautista A *et al*. Ogilvie's syndrome in the postcesarean section patient. *International Journal of Gynaecology and Obstetrics* 1989; **28**: 185–7.
304 Rogers BHG, Clark LM *et al*. The epidemiologic and demographic characteristics of inflammatory bowel disease: An analysis of a computerized file of 1400 patients. *Journal of Chronic Disease* 1971; **24**: 743–73.
305 Rogozinski H, Ankers C *et al*. Folate nutrition in early pregnancy. *Human Nutrition, Applied Nutrition* 1983; **37**: 357–64.
306 Rooney PJ, Dow TGB *et al*. Immunoreactive gastrin and gestation. *American Journal of Obstetrics and Gynecology* 1975; **122**: 834–6.
307 Rosenthal FD, Jones C *et al*. Thyrotoxic vomiting. *British Medical Journal* 1976; **ii**: 209–11.
308 Rosso P. Nutrition and maternal–fetal exchange. *American Journal of Clinical Nutrition* 1981; **34**: 744.
309 Rozen P, Zonis J *et al*. Crohn's disease in the Jewish population of Tel-Aviv, Yafo: epidemiologic and clinical aspects. *Gastroenterology* 1979: **76**: 25–30.
309a Ruddell WSJ, Dickinson RJ *et al*. Treatment of distal ulcerative colitis (proctosigmoiditis) in relapse: comparison of hydrocortisone enemas and rectal hydrocortisone foam. *Gut* 1980; **21**: 885–9.
310 Ruderman JW, Stroller KP et al. Bloodstream invasion with *Shigella sonnei* in an asymptomatic newborn infant. *Pediatric Infectious Diseases* 1986; **5**: 379–80.
311 Rustgi VK, Cooper JN *et al*. Endoscopy in the pregnant patient. In: Rustgi VK & Cooper JN (eds), *Gastrointestinal and Hepatic Complications in Pregnancy*. J Wiley & Sons, New York, 1986: 104–23.
312 Saleeby RG, Rosen L *et al*. Hemorrhoidectomy during pregnancy: risk or relief? *Diseases of the Colon and Rectum* 1991; **34**: 260–1.
313 Sandweiss DJ, Podolsky HM *et al*. Deaths from perforation and hemorrhage of gastroduodenal ulcer during pregnancy and the puerperium. *American Journal of Obstetrics and Gynecology* 1943; **45**: 131–6.
314 Santos A & Datta S. Prophylactic use of droperidol for control of nausea and vomiting during spinal anaesthesia for Cesarean section. *Anaesthesia and Analgesia* 1984; **63**: 85–7.
315 Sarna SK. Physiology and pathophysiology of colonic motor activity, part 2. *Digestive Diseases and Sciences* 1991; **36**: 998–1018.
316 Savel LE, Simon SR *et al*. Pregnancy after jejunoileal bypass. *Obstetrics and Gynecology* 1978; **52**: 585.
317 Schofield PF, Turnbull RB *et al*. Crohn's disease and pregnancy. *British Medical Journal* 1970; **ii**: 364.
318 Schulze-Delrieu K. Drug Therapy: metoclopramide. *New England Journal of Medicine* 1981: **305**: 28–33.
319 Schuster K, Bailey LB *et al*. Morning sickness and vitamin B_6 status of pregnant women. *Human Nutrition, Clinical Nutrition* 1985; **39C**: 75–9.
320 Schwartz B, Ciesielski CA *et al*. Association of sporadic listeriosis with consumption of uncooked hot dogs and undercooked chicken. *Lancet* 1988; **ii**: 779–82.
321 Schwerk WB, Wichtrup B *et al*. Ultrasonography in the diagnosis of acute appendicitis: a prospective study. *Gastroenterology* 1989; **97**: 630–9.
322 Scioli C, Fiorentino F *et al*. Treatment of *Salmonella typhi* carriers with intravenous ampicillin. *Journal of Infectious Diseases* 1972; **125**: 170–3.
323 Scott NM & Deutsch DL. The esophagus during pregnancy. *American Journal of Gastroenterology* 1955; **24**: 305–13.
324 Scragg JN & Rubidge CJ. Amoxycillin in the treatment of typhoid fever in children. *American Journal of*

Tropical Medicine and Hygiene 1975; **24**: 860–5.

324a Scudamore HH, Rogers AG *et al*. Pregnancy after ileostomy for ulcerative colitis. *Gastroenterology* 1957; **32**: 295–303.

325 Sedlack RE, Whisnant J *et al*. Incidence of Crohn's disease in Olmsted County Minnesota 1935–1975. *American Journal of Epidemiology* 1980; **112**: 759–63.

326 Segal I, Tim LO *et al*. The rarity of ulcerative colitis in South African Blacks. *American Journal of Gastroenterology* 1980; **74**: 332–6.

327 Seidman DS, Heyman Z *et al*. Use of magnetic resonance imaging in pregnancy to diagnose intussusception induced by colonic cancer. *Obstetrics and Gynecology* 1992; **79**: 822–3.

328 Shaffer JL, Kershaw A *et al*. Sulphasalazine-induced infertility reversed on transfer to 5-aminosalicylic acid. *Lancet* 1984; **i**: 1240.

329 Shapiro S, Heinonen OP *et al*. Antenatal exposure to doxylamine succinate and dicyclomine hydrochloride (Bendectin) in relation to congenital malformations, perinatal mortality rate, birthweight and intelligence quotient score. *American Journal of Obstetrics and Gynecology* 1977; **128**: 480–5.

330 Shepherd RC & Sinha GP. Cryptosporidiosis in the west of Scotland. *Scottish Medical Journal* 1988; **33**: 365–8.

331 Shelton MG. Standardized senna in the management of constipation in the puerperium: a clinical trial. *South African Medical Journal* 1980; **57**: 78–80.

332 Sichel MS. Postpartum and postoperative bowel function. *Northwest Medicine* 1961; **60**: 708–9.

333 Simor AE & Ferro S. *Campylobacter jejuni* infection occurring during pregnancy. *European Journal of Clinical Microbiology and Infectious Diseases* 1990; **9**: 142–4.

334 Sims EH, Schlater TL *et al*. Obstructing gastric carcinoma complicating pregnancy. *Journal of the National Medical Association* 1980; **72**: 21–3.

335 Singer AJ & Brandt LJ. Pathophysiology of the gastrointestinal tract during pregnancy. *American Journal of Gastroenterology* 1991; **86**: 1695–712.

336 Singleton JW, Law DH *et al*. National Cooperative Crohn's Disease Study: adverse reactions to study drugs. *Gastroenterology* 1979; **77**: 870–82.

337 Singleton JW, Summers RW *et al*. A trial of sulphasalazine as adjunctive therapy in Crohn's disease. *Gastroenterology* 1979; **77**: 887–97.

338 Sleisenger MH. How should we treat Crohn's disease? *New England Journal of Medicine* 1980; **302**: 1024–6.

339 Smith D. Severe anaphylactic reaction after a soap enema. *British Medical Journal* 1967; **iv**: 215.

340 Smithells RW, Sheppard S *et al*. Apparent prevention of neural tube defects by periconceptional vitamin supplementation. *Archives of Diseases of Childhood* 1981; **56**: 911–18.

341 Snape WJ, Carlson GM *et al*. Colonic myometric activity in the irritable bowel syndrome. *Gastroenterology* 1976; **70**: 326–30.

342 Solanki DR, Suresh M *et al*. The effects of intravenous cimetidine and metoclopramide on gastric volume and pH. *Anaesthesia and Analgesia* 1984; **63**: 599–602.

343 Starks GC. Pregnancy-induced hyperemesis (hyperemesis gravidarum). A reassessment of therapy and proposal of a new etiologic theory. *Missouri Medicine* 1984; **81**: 253–6.

344 Stather JW, Muirhead CR *et al*. *Health effects models developed from the 1988 UNSCEAR report*. Chilton NRPB-R226, 1988, HMSO, London.

345 Sterling N. The diagnosis and treatment of suspected listeriosis in pregnancy. *Report of a Working Group. Department of Health Standing Medical Advisory Committee*, 1992.

346 Sterner G, Granstrom G *et al*. Management of pregnant women with contagious infections at delivery. *Scandinavian Journal of Infectious Diseases* 1988; **20**: 463–73.

347 Stevens DP. Selective primary health care: strategies for control of disease in the developing world. XIX. Giardiasis. *Reviews of Infectious Diseases* 1985; **7**: 530–5.

348 Stevens FM & Craig A. Prolactin and coeliac disease. *Irish Journal of Medical Science* 1981; **150**: 329–31.

349 Stirrat GM & Beard RW. Drugs to be avoided or given with caution in the second or third trimesters of pregnancy. *Prescribers Journal* 1973; **13**: 135–40.

350 Soules MR, Hughes CL *et al*. Nausea and vomiting of pregnancy: role of human choriogonadotrophin and 17 hydroxyprogesterone. *Obstetrics and Gynecology* 1980; **55**: 696–700.

351 Summers RW, Switz DM *et al*. National Cooperative Crohn's Disease Study: results of drug treatment. *Gastroenterology* 1979; **77**: 847–69.

352 Swartley WB, Newton ZB *et al*. Perforated carcinoma of large intestine complicating pregnancy: successful operative management. *Annals of Surgery* 1947; **125**: 251–6.

353 Sweeney WJ. Use of bisacodyl suppositories as a routine laxative in post partum patients. *American Journal of Obstetrics and Gynecology* 1963; **85**: 908–11.

354 Swinson CM, Lavin GS *et al*. Coeliac disease and malignancy. *Lancet* 1983; **i**: 111–15.

355 Tabak MA, Hart MD *et al*. *Campylobacter* enteritis: prenatal and perinatal implications. *American Journal of Obstetrics and Gynecology* 1983; **147**: 845–6.

356 Teahon K, Pearson M *et al*. Elemental diet in the management of Crohn's disease during pregnancy. *Gut* 1991; **32**: 1079–81.

357 Tedesco FJ, Stanley RJ *et al*. Diagnostic features of clindamycin-associated pseudomembranous colitis. *New England Journal of Medicine* 1974; **290**: 841–3.

358 Templeton A, Fraser C *et al*. The epidemiology of infertility in Aberdeen. *British Medical Journal* 1990; **301**: 148–52.

359 Thomson H. Piles: their nature and management.

Lancet 1975; **ii**: 494–5.
360 Thulesius O & Gjores JE. Arterio-venous anastomoses in the anal region with reference to the pathogenesis and treatment of haemorrhoids. *Acta Chirurgica Scandinavica* 1973; **139**: 476–8.
361 Tresadern JC, Falconer GF *et al.* Maintenance of pregnancy in a home parenteral nutrition patient. *Journal of Parenteral and Enteral Nutrition* 1984; **8**: 199–202.
362 Truelove SC. Stilboestrol, phenobarbitone and diet in chronic duodenal ulcer. *British Medical Journal* 1960; **ii**: 559–66.
363 Trussell RR & Beeley L. Infestations. *Clinical Obstetrics and Gynecology* 1981; **8**: 333–40.
364 Tsukamoto N, Uchino H *et al.* Carcinoma of the colon presenting as bilateral ovarian tumors during pregnancy. *Gynecologic Oncology* 1986; **24**: 386–91.
365 Tumen HJ & Cohn EM. Pregnancy and chronic ulcerative colitis. *Gastroenterology* 1950; **16**: 1–11.
366 Turner ES & Greenberger PA. Management of the pregnant asthmatic patient. *Annals of Internal Medicine* 1980; **93**: 905–8.
367 Tyson RM, Shrader EA *et al.* Drugs transmitted through breast milk. Part I: Laxatives. *Journal of Pediatrics* 1937; **11**: 824–32.
368 Van Kruiningen HJ, Coloubel JF *et al.* An in-depth study of Crohn's disease in two French families. *Gastroenterology* 1993; **104**: 351–60.
369 Van Thiel DH, Gavaler JS *et al.* Heartburn of pregnancy. *Gastroenterology* 1977; **72**: 666–8.
370 Van Thiel DH & Wald A. Evidence refuting a role for increased abdominal pressure in the pathogenesis of the heartburn associated with pregnancy. *American Journal of Obstetrics and Gynecology* 1981; **140**: 420–2.
371 Van Voorhis B & Cruikshank DP. Colon carcinoma complicating pregnancy. A report of two cases. *Journal of Reproductive Medicine* 1989; **34**: 923–7.
372 Varadi S. Pernicious anaemia and infertility. *Lancet* 1967; **ii**: 1305.
373 Vella L, Francis D *et al.* Comparison of the antiemetics metoclopramide and promethazine in labour. *British Medical Journal* 1985; **290**: 1173–5.
374 Vender RJ & Spiro HM. Inflammatory bowel disease and pregnancy. *Journal of Clinical Gastroenterology* 1982; **4**: 231–49.
375 Venkatesh KS, Ramanujam PS *et al.* Anorectal complications of vaginal delivery. *Diseases of the Colon and Rectum* 1989; **32**: 1039–41.
376 Vesikari T, Huffunen L *et al.* Perinatal *Campylobacter fetus* ss. *jejuni* enteritis. *Acta Pediatrica Scandinavica* 1981; **70**: 261–3.
377 Villar J, Klebanoff M *et al.* The effect on fetal growth of protozoan and helminthic infection during pregnancy. *Obstetrics and Gynecology* 1989; **74**: 915–20.
378 Vinzent R, Dumas J *et al.* Septicemie grave au couride la grossesse due a un vibrion avortement consecutif. *Bulletin de l'Acadamie National Medical (Paris)* 1947; **131**: 90.
379 Visakorpi JK, Immonen P *et al.* Malabsorption syndrome in childhood. The occurrence of absorption defects and their clinical significance. *Acta Pediatrica Scandinavica* 1967; **56**: 1–9.
380 Wald A, Van Thiel DH *et al.* Gastrointestinal transit: the effect of the menstrual cycle. *Gastroenterology* 1981; **80**: 1497–500.
381 Waldmann CS, Verghese C *et al.* The evaluation of domperidone and metoclopramide as antiemetics in day care abortion patients. *British Journal of Clinical Pharmacology* 1985; **19**: 307–10.
382 Waldum HL, Straume BK *et al.* Serum group I pepsinogens (PG1) during pregnancy. *Scandinavian Journal of Gastroenterology* 1980; **15**: 61–3.
383 Walker AR, Walker BF, *et al.* Nausea and vomiting and dietary craving and aversions during pregnancy in South African women. *British Journal of Obstetrics and Gynaecology* 1985; **92**: 484–9.
384 Walker-Smith JA, Harrison M *et al.* Cow's milk-sensitive enteropathy. *Archives of Diseases of Childhood* 1978; **53**: 375–80.
385 Warsof SL. Medical and surgical treatment of inflammatory bowel disease in pregnancy. *Clinics in Obstetrics and Gynecology* 1983; **26**: 822–31.
386 Waters EG & Fenimore ED. Perforated carcinoma of cecum in pregnancy. *Obstetrics and Gynecology* 1954; **3**: 263–7.
387 Watson R & Kennedy JH. An unusual case of maternal death. *Scottish Medical Journal* 1980; **25**: 241–2.
388 Weigel MM & Weigel RM. The association of reproductive history, demographic factors, and alcohol and tobacco consumption with the risk of developing nausea and vomiting in early pregnancy. *American Journal of Epidemiology* 1988; **127**: 562–70.
389 Weigel RM & Weigel MM. Nausea and vomiting of early pregnancy and pregnancy outcome. A meta-analytical review. *British Journal of Obstetrics and Gynaecology* 1989; **96**: 1312–18.
390 Weller IVD. AIDs and the gut. *Scandinavian Journal of Gastroenterology* 1985; **20** (suppl 114): 77–81.
391 Wells CN. Treatment of hyperemesis gravidarum with cortisone. *American Journal of Obstetrics and Gynecology* 1953; **66**: 598–601.
392 Werthmann MW & Kress SV. Quantitative excretion of Senokot in human breast milk. *Medical Annals of the District of Columbia* 1973; **42**: 4–5.
393 Whorwell PJ. Irritable bowel syndrome. *Prescribers' Journal* 1992; **32**: 152–6.
394 Wig JD, Bushnurmath SR *et al.* Complications of amoebiasis in pregnancy and puerperium. *Indian Journal of Gastroenterology* 1984; **3**: 37–8.
395 Wikland M, Jansson I *et al.* Gynaecological problems related to anatomical changes after conventional protocolectomy and ileostomy. *International Journal of Colorectal Diseases* 1990; **5**: 49–52.
396 Willoughby CP & Truelove SC. Ulcerative colitis and

pregnancy. *Gut* 1980; **21**: 469–74.

397 Wilson JT, Brown RD *et al*. Drug excretion in human breast milk: principles, pharmacokinetics and projected consequences. *Clinical Pharmacokinetics* 1980; **5**: 1–66.

398 Winship DH. Gastrointestinal diseases. In: Burrow GN & Ferris TF (eds), *Medical Complications during Pregnancy*. WB Saunders & Co., Philadelphia, 1975: 275–350.

399 Wong SN, Tam AY *et al*. *Campylobacter* infection in the neonate: a case report and review of the literature. *Pediatric Infectious Disease Journal* 1990; **9**: 665–9.

400 Woodhouse DR & Haylen B. Gallbladder disease complicating pregnancy. *Australian and New Zealand Journal of Obstetrics and Gynaecology* 1985; **25**: 233–7.

401 Woods JB, Martin JN *et al*. Pregnancy complicated by carcinoma of the colon above the rectum. *American Journal of Perinatology* 1992; **9**: 102–10.

402 Yaron Y, Lessing JB *et al*. Abruptio placentae associated with perforated appendicitis and generalized peritonitis. *American Journal of Obstetrics and Gynecology* 1992; **166**: 14–15.

403 Ylikorkala O, Kauppila A *et al*. Follicle stimulating hormone, thyrotropin, human growth hormone and prolactin in hyperemesis gravidarum. *American Journal of Obstetrics and Gynecology* 1976; **83**: 528–33.

404 Young JF, Cave D *et al*. Enema shock in Hirschsprung's disease. *Diseases of the Colon and Rectum* 1968; **11**: 391–5.

405 Zegarelli EV, Kutscher AH & Hyman GA. *Diagnosis of the Mouth and Jaws*. Lea & Febiger, Philadelphia, 1978: 73.

406 Zhang J & Cai W-W. Severe vomiting during pregnancy: antenatal correlates and fetal outcomes. *Epidemiology* 1991; **2**: 454–7.

407 Zibell-Frisk D, Jen KL *et al*. Use of parenteral nutrition to maintain adequate nutritional status in hyperemesis gravidarum. *Journal of Perinatology* 1990; **10**: 390–5.

408 Zierler S & Rothman KJ. Congenital heart disease in relation to maternal use of Bendectin and other drugs in early pregnancy. *New England Journal of Medicine* 1985; **313**: 347–52.

Further reading

Baldwin WF. Drugs in pregnancy. Senna — clinical study of senna administered to nursing mothers: assessment of effects on infant bowel habits. *Canadian Medical Association Journal* 1963; **89**: 566–8.

Beeley L. Adverse effects of drugs in later pregnancy. In: Wood SM & Beeley L (eds), *Prescribing in Pregnancy. Clinics in Obstetrics and Gynaecology*. WB Saunders Co., London, 1981: 281.

Berkowitz RL, Constan DR *et al*. *Handbook for Prescribing Medications during Pregnancy*. Little, Brown & Co., Boston, 1981: 22–3.

Boyes BE, Woolf IL *et al*. Treatment of gastric ulceration with a bismuth preparation. *Postgraduate Medical Journal* 1975; **51** (suppl 5): 29–33.

Clark DH & Tankel HI. Gastric acid and plasma histaminase during pregnancy. *Lancet* 1954; **ii**: 886.

Connon JJ. De Nol, an effective drug in the therapy of duodenal ulceration. *Journal of the Irish Medical Association* 1977; **70**: 206–7.

Croese J. Coeliac disease. Haematological features and delay in diagnosis. *Medical Journal of Australia* 1979; **2**: 335–8.

Department of Health (DOH). Management and prevention of listeriosis and other food-borne infections in pregnancy. 1992; PL/CMO (92) 13 and 19.

Department of Health and Social Security (DHSS). *Recommended Daily Amounts of Food Energy and Nutrients for Groups of People in the UK*. Report of the Health Society, No. 15. 1979 HMSO, London.

Drug and Therapeutics Bulletin. *Helicobacter pylori* infection — when and how to treat. *Drug and Therapeutic Bulletin* 1993; **31**: 13–15.

Farmer RG, Michener WM *et al*. Studies of family history among patients with inflammatory bowel disease. *Clinical Gastroenterology* 1980; **9**: 271–8.

Finkelstein W & Isselbacher KJ. Medical Intelligence: Drug Therapy Cimetidine. *New England Journal of Medicine* 1978; **299**: 992–6.

Fisher RS, Roberts GS *et al*. Altered lower esophageal sphincter function during early pregnancy. *Gastroenterology* 1978; **74**: 1233–7.

Gonsoulin W, Mason B *et al*. Colon cancer in pregnancy with elevated maternal serum alpha-fetoprotein level at presentation. *American Journal of Obstetrics and Gynecology* 1990; **163**: 1172–3.

Guttmacher AF. Hyperemesis. In: Guttmacher AF & Rovinsky JJ (eds), *Medical, Surgical and Gynecological Complications of Pregnancy*. Williams & Wilkins, Baltimore, 1960: 166–9.

Hall M & Davidson RJL. Prophylactic folic acid in women with pernicious anaemia pregnant after periods of infertility. *Journal of Clinical Pathology* 1968; **21**: 599–602.

Helzer JE, Chammas S *et al*. A study of the association between Crohn's disease and psychiatric illness. *Gastroenterology* 1984; **86**: 324–30.

Howard FM & Hill JM. Drugs in pregnancy. *Obstetrical and Gynecological Survey* 1979; **34**: 643–53.

Jackson IMD, Doig WB *et al*. Pernicious anaemia as a cause of infertility. *Lancet* 1967; **ii**: 1159–60.

Jarnfelt-Samsoie A, Bremme K *et al*. Steroid hormones in emetic and non-emetic pregnancy. *European Journal of Obstetrics, Gynecology and Reproductive Biology* 1986; **21**: 87–99.

Korelitz BI, Glass JL *et al*. Long-term immunosuppressive therapy of ulcerative colitis: continuation of personal series. *American Journal of Digestive Diseases* 1973; **18**: 317–22.

Kumar PJ. Reintroduction of gluten in adults and children with treated coeliac disease. *Gut* 1979; **20**: 743–9.

Langman MJ, Henry DA *et al*. Cimetidine and ranitidine in duodenal ulcer. *British Medical Journal* 1980; **281**: 473–4.

Monk JP & Clissold SP. Misoprostol. A preliminary review of its pharmacodynamic and pharmacokinetic properties, and therapeutic efficacy in the treatment of peptic ulcer disease. *Drugs* 1987; **33**: 1–30.

Poulantzas J, Polymeropoulos PS *et al*. Double-blind evaluation of the effect of tri-potassium di-citrato-bismuthate in peptic ulcer. *British Journal of Clinical Practice* 1978; **32**: 147–8.

Ryan JP & Bhojwani A. Effect of ovariectomy, sex steroid hormones, and pregnancy. *American Journal of Physiology* 1986; **14**: G46–50.

Sealy DP & Shuman SH. Endemic giardiasis and daycare. *Pediatrics* 1983; **72**: 154–8.

Shiono PH & Klebanoff MA. Bendectin and human congenital malformations. *Teratology* 1989; **40**: 151–5. Erratum appears in *Teratology* 1990; **41**: 250–1.

Smithells RW & Sheppard S. Fetal malformation after Debendox in early pregnancy. *British Medical Journal* 1978; **i**: 1055–6.

Srikantia SG & Reddy V. Megaloblastic anaemia of infancy and vitamin B_{12}. *British Journal of Haematology* 1967; **13**: 949–53.

Webb MJ & Sedlack RE. Ulcerative colitis in pregnancy. *Medical Clinics of North America* 1974; **58**: 823–7.

Witter FR & King TM. Drugs and the management of chronic diseases in the pregnant patient. In: Stern L (ed), *Drug Use in Pregnancy*. ADIS Health Science Press, Sydney, 1984: 190–211.

11

Diabetes

Michael Maresh & Richard Beard

Terminology, 424
Potential diabetes
Gestational diabetes mellitus
Established diabetes mellitus
Physiology and pathophysiology, 425
Maternal glucose homeostasis
Abnormalities of maternal glucose homeostasis
Fetal glucose homeostasis
Fetal haematology
Glycosylated (glycated) haemoglobin and other glycated proteins
Effect of diabetes on the fetus, 429
Congenital malformations
Spontaneous miscarriage
Perinatal mortality in established diabetes
Unexplained fetal death *in utero*
Perinatal mortality in GDM
Neonatal morbidity
Abnormalities of growth
Respiratory dysfunction
Hypoglycaemia
Polycythaemia and jaundice
Hypocalcaemia and hypomagnesaemia
Hypertrophic cardiomyopathy
Summary of causes of neonatal morbidity
Diagnosis of diabetes in pregnancy, 436
Screening, 437
Medical management, 438
Pre-pregnancy care
The joint pregnancy diabetic clinic
Principles of treatment
Inpatient versus outpatient care
Management of IDDM
Management of IGT and GDM
Treatment by diet alone
Treatment by diet and insulin therapy
Control of blood glucose during labour
Postnatal management
Pregnancy in diabetic women with renal or vascular complications
Obstetric management, 445
First trimester
Second trimester
Third trimester
Indices of fetal well-being
Pregnancy complications
Timing and route of delivery
Contraception, 450
Oral contraceptives
Intrauterine contraceptive device
Other methods
Sterilization

Management of the pregnant woman with diabetes continues to present a challenge to the physician, obstetrician and paediatrician. Before insulin was available, those women with juvenile diabetes who survived to the age of reproduction and were able to become pregnant had less than a 50 per cent chance of having a living child. The problems now are different but nonetheless taxing. The recognition that diabetes results in a disturbance of the environment of the fetus that may seriously interfere with organogenesis and development has led to the acknowledgement that normoglycaemia (Fig. 11.1) is an important objective in diabetic control. Until this can be achieved before conception and throughout the early part of pregnancy, there seems little likelihood that it will be possible to reduce the increased incidence of congenital malformation that threatens the pregnancy of every woman with established diabetes. Unexplained fetal death *in utero* remains increased in diabetic pregnancy, but further research yet again points to links with the failure to obtain normoglycaemia. Macrosomia, hypoglycaemia, respiratory problems and severe jaundice of the newborn remain as unacceptable complications of diabetes in pregnancy again probably related to poor diabetic control in the mother. These conditions rather than perinatal mortality are being used increasingly as sensitive indices of the management of diabetic pregnancy.

Much has changed in recent years that has dramatically improved the prognosis for the diabetic pregnancy. In the past, a great deal of the evidence upon which management was based was speculative, but it is now clear that with better

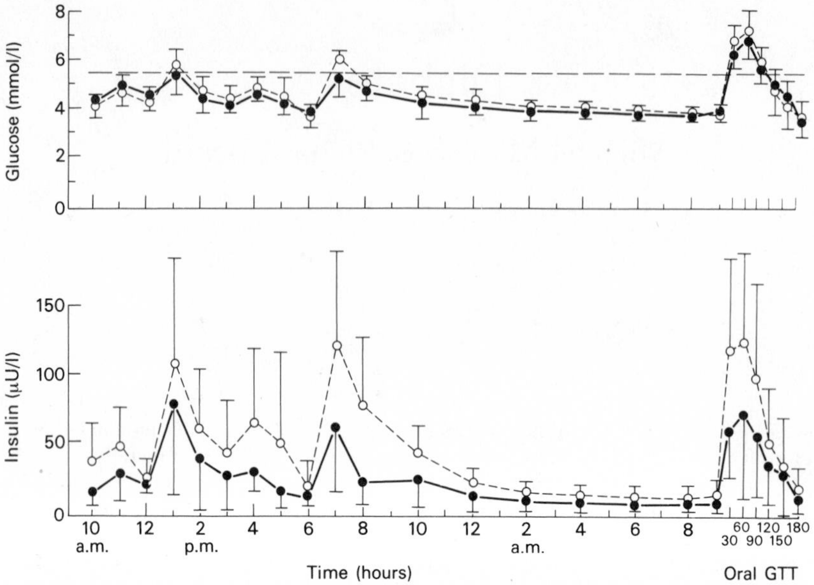

Fig. 11.1. Plasma glucose and insulin concentrations over a 24-hour period and during an oral glucose tolerance test (GTT) in nine women studied in early and late pregnancy [51]. Figures are mean ± SD. ● Early pregnancy (12–22 weeks); ○ late pregnancy (32–35 weeks).

control of diabetes, close monitoring of the fetus in late pregnancy, and the outstanding achievements in the care of the newborn, management of the pregnant diabetic mother and her fetus needs to be reviewed.

Terminology

Over the years a variety of descriptive terms have entered the literature concerning diabetes in pregnancy and it is important that the reader should have a clear idea of their meaning.

Potential diabetes

The term is applied to pregnant women who have certain features in their family or medical or obstetric history which predispose them to an increased possibility of developing diabetes in pregnancy. Potential diabetic features are: (a) diabetes in a first degree relative (e.g. mother, sister); (b) maternal obesity (>120 per cent ideal bodyweight); (c) previous large baby (>4 kg); (d) previous unexplained still-birth; or (e) previous abnormal glucose tolerance. To these features identified at booking can be added glycosuria (more than one occasion) and hydramnios. The prevalence of potential diabetes depends considerably on the population surveyed and figures ranging from 8.5 per cent [63] to 35 per cent [54] have been reported.

Gestational diabetes mellitus (GDM)

Gestational diabetes is a term which is widely used, but not in a consistent manner. Strictly speaking GDM is defined as carbohydrate intolerance that arises in pregnancy and disappears after delivery, but this definition is of little practical value for a number of reasons. It is rarely possible to be certain that these women did not have undiagnosed diabetes before becoming pregnant. In addition, many women who are diagnosed as having diabetes for the first time in pregnancy continue after pregnancy with an abnormal glucose tolerance test (GTT), and those with a normal GTT at this time have an increased risk of developing one in the future. Finally, and most important, the classification is irrelevant to the fetus since all that matters is that maternal glucose tolerance is abnormal. Accordingly for those women diagnosed for the first time, or who were known to be normal prior to pegnancy, but then became abnormal during pregnancy, classification should be based on their GTT in pregnancy. If the GTT is frankly diabetic then they should be classified as GDM. If the GTT shows only impaired glucose tolerance (IGT) then it would seem more logical to use the term gestational impaired glucose tolerance (GIGT) [92]. Precise definitions with regard to the GTT values are discussed below. In addition, the conditions are often subdivided according to whether fasting hyperglycaemia is present or not.

Established diabetes mellitus

Established diabetes is a term used to describe the condition when diabetes is known to have been present for a variable time before pregnancy. In the USA, the term pre-gestational diabetes is often used. The vast majority of these women will have type 1 insulin-dependent diabetes (IDDM), the remainder having type 2 non-insulin dependent diabetes (NIDDM). The White classification, devised by Dr Priscilla White from Boston, USA, has been used widely in Europe and the US and has subsequently been revised [67,195]. Diabetes is graded from A to F/R according to the severity as judged by the age of onset, duration and the presence or absence of complications of the disease. This classification, which is not in general use in the UK, provides a useful system for comparison of results from different centres and has the advantage that the outcome of this pregnancy can be related to the severity of the disease. In practice, data are usually classified by the presence of vascular complications (groups F and R) or not (groups B, C and D).

Physiology and pathophysiology

Pregnancy itself induces profound metabolic alterations in every woman, regardless of whether or not she has diabetes, which tend to become more marked with advancing gestational age. It seems likely that these changes are adaptive, ensuring the optimal environment for fetal growth and development. A knowledge of these changes is essential if an understanding of the principles of care of the diabetic mother and her baby is to be achieved.

Maternal glucose homeostasis

Figure 11.1 shows the remarkably stable concentration of plasma glucose that is maintained by the normal mother over a 24-hour period. Both in early and late pregnancy the glucose concentration stays constant between 4 and 4.5 mmol/l, except after meals. This degree of homeostasis is only maintained by doubling the secretion of insulin from the end of the first to the third trimester of pregnancy (Fig. 11.1). In general, the relative normality or otherwise of a diurnal profile is reflected by the GTT. Although there is some disagreement as to whether glucose tolerance decreases as normal pregnancy advances, longitudinal studies have shown glucose concentrations to be increased postprandially and decreased with fasting as pregnancy continues.

Insulin resistance develops although the aetiology remains uncertain. Studies of insulin receptor binding in normal pregnancy have been conflicting, but the review by Kuhl [86] concluded that pregnancy-induced insulin resistance was likely to be a post-receptor defect. The effect is likely to be mediated by the increased production of one or more of the pregnancy-associated hormones or of free cortisol which is elevated in pregnancy. Changes in insulin activity result in the other effects on intermediary metabolism. Withholding food from pregnant women results in a much earlier recourse to breakdown of triglyceride, leading to increased concentration of circulatory free fatty acids and ketone bodies, described by Freinkel as 'accelerated starvation' [46].

Abnormalities of maternal glucose homeostasis

Both β cell insufficiency and an increase in insulin resistance may contribute to the development of GIGT and GDM. The initiating factor is likely to be the increased peripheral insulin resistance of normal pregnancy. Those with severe β cell insufficiency will not be able to increase their insulin secretion adequately, and will tend to show hyperglycaemia and hypo- or normo-insulinaemia as described by Gillmer *et al.* [51]. Other studies [99,105] have shown women with a more heterogeneous picture ranging from hypo- to hyperinsulinaemia, resulting in abnormal glucose tolerance. Those with a normal or increased plasma insulin concentration are likely to have a marked increase in peripheral resistance to insulin which results in hyperglycaemia. A further cause of abnormal glucose homeostasis in pregnancy occurs when pregnancy intervenes in the prodromal stage of IDDM. This occurs about once in 8000 deliveries [17] so that a typical obstetric unit in the UK could anticipate one case every 2 or 3 years.

The decrease in insulin activity in GDM and IGT is associated with changes in more than just glucose concentration. The concentrations of glycerol, free fatty acids, ketone bodies and branched chain amino acids have all been found to be elevated in untreated women [99,105,143]. Figure 11.2 is a striking demonstration of the development of abnormal glucose tolerance during pregnancy [123]. The mean diurnal plasma glucose has increased over the 15 weeks between the measurements by about 3 mmol/l whereas the insulin secretion has increased very little. This failure of the normal increased secretion of insulin is evidence of pancreatic β cell insufficiency. The established diabetic woman who has had the disease for some years before becoming pregnant usually has complete loss of endogenous insulin secretion as determined by plasma C peptide concentration. The use of measurable C peptide as an additional subclassification in IDDM is being investigated.

Fetal glucose homeostasis

The plasma glucose concentration of the fetus closely follows that of the mother, with the normal maternal–fetal difference in glucose concentration being about 0.5 mmol/l in favour of the mother. Oakley *et al.* [124] showed that, with an increase in glucose concentration in the mother, the maternal–fetal difference increases until the system of 'facilitated diffusion' by which glucose crosses the

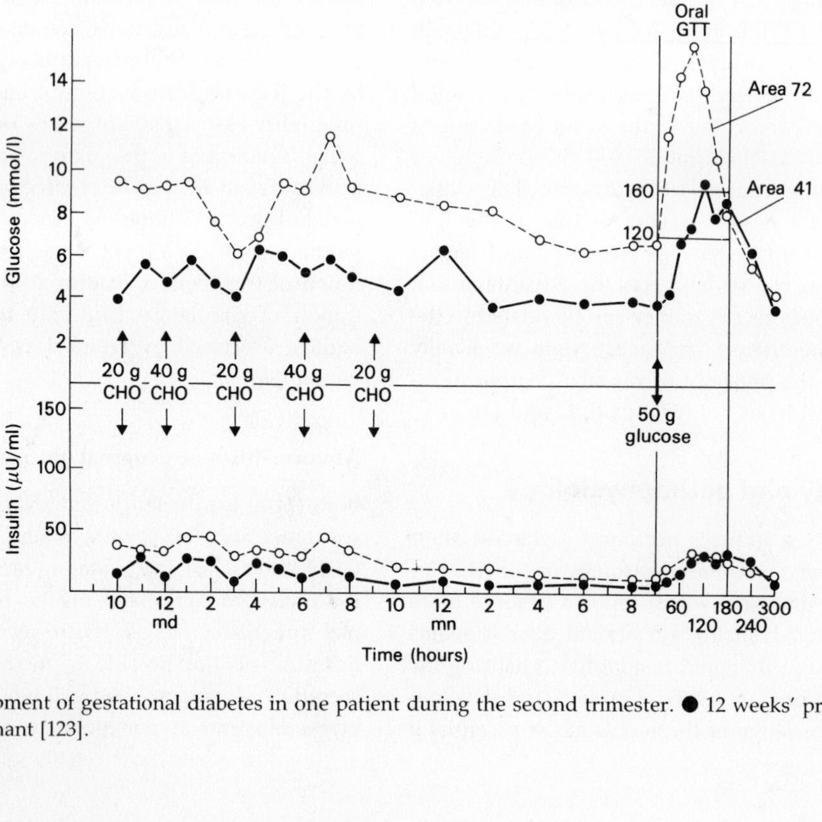

Fig. 11.2. Development of gestational diabetes in one patient during the second trimester. ● 12 weeks' pregnant; ○ 27 weeks' pregnant [123].

placenta appears to be saturated at a maternal value of about 11–13 mmol/l. After this, despite a considerable increase in maternal hyperglycaemia, it is not possible to increase the fetal concentration further. This phenomenon is present in diabetic as well as non-diabetic mothers and can be viewed as a protective mechanism for the fetus to avoid the damaging effects of severe hyperglycaemia. Recent data obtained by cordocentesis at term has confirmed this close relationship [156].

Insulin appears in the fetal circulation as early as 10 weeks' gestational age. Unpublished data obtained through cordocentesis have suggested that fetal insulin concentrations in diabetic pregnancy are elevated by the second trimester. There is agreement that insulin does not cross the placenta at physiological concentrations. The β cell pancreatic response of the fetus to a maternal glucose infusion is sluggish [110,124] and in the fetus of the non-diabetic mother insulin plays no part in the regulation of glucose homeostasis, its role being more likely as a growth promoting hormone. Figure 11.3 compares the difference between the maternal and fetal glucose and insulin responses to a glucose load in a non-diabetic and a diabetic woman. The difference in the maternal–fetal glucose concentration increases as the mother becomes more hyperglycaemic. This effect is the same for the diabetic as for the non-diabetic woman. The brisk fetal insulin response in the diabetic is in marked contrast to the sluggish response in the fetus of the non-diabetic mother. The fetus can also secrete insulin from the pancreas in response to amino acids [109].

Observations such as these have led to an increasing acceptance of the 'hyperglycaemic hyperinsulinism' theory of Pedersen [134]. Stated simply, this proposes that the fetal hyperglycaemia resulting from maternal hyperglycaemia stimulates fetal pan-

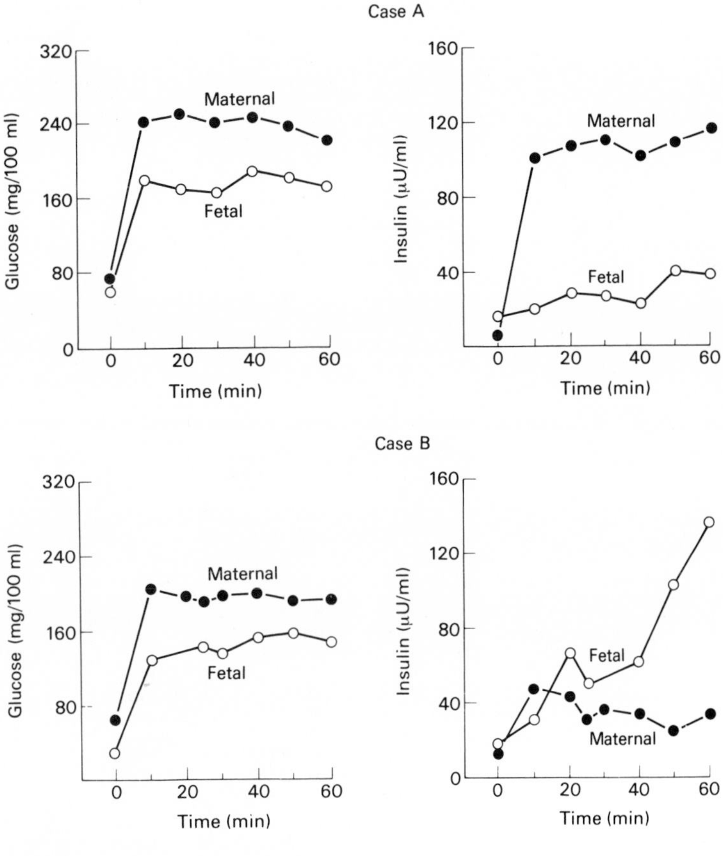

Fig. 11.3. Examples of glucose and insulin response following 60 min of glucose infusion in a non-diabetic (case A) and a gestational diabetic (case B) (for conversion of glucose to mmol/l divide by 18) [124].

creatic β cell hypertrophy resulting in an inappropriate release of insulin. This theory has gained wide acceptance because it convincingly explains the aetiology of much of the fetal pathology found in diabetic pregnancy. An expanded hypothesis is shown in Fig. 11.4. These observations are of particular clinical significance because they indicate the possibility that normalization of the glucose environment of the fetus of the diabetic mother will diminish the tendency to hyperinsulinaemia and hence lead to a diminution of many perinatal problems.

It has been shown that if growth is restricted *in utero* as indicated by being born light for gestational age, then the fetus will have fewer β cells [189]. In later life other studies have shown that if adults who were light at birth then become overweight, they will have increased insulin resistance and are more likely to develop IGT or type 2 diabetes, than their counterparts who were of average birth weight [65,146]. Thus, intrauterine effects on the fetal pancreas may have profound long-term effects.

Fetal haematology

Studies on cord blood at delivery have reported increased erythropoietin and haemoglobin concentrations [198] and suggested a relationship with maternal glucose control [199]. Now data obtained antenatally by cordocentesis have confirmed that the incidence of fetal polycythaemia is increased and that this relates to maternal diabetic control [155]. Concentrations of erythropoietin in the fetus could not be related to maternal glucose control [157] but erythropoeitin levels are very variable. The erythropoietin concentration could be raised because of the effects of insulin on both erythropoietin production and erythropoiesis itself or alternatively through poor tissue oxygenation. Fetal thrombocytopenia has also been demonstrated in association with maternal diabetes and the most likely cause is increased platelet consumption through aggregation [155].

Glycosylated (glycated) haemoglobin and other glycated proteins

Glycosylated haemoglobin (HbA_{1c}) is a normally occurring moiety of haemoglobin which in non-

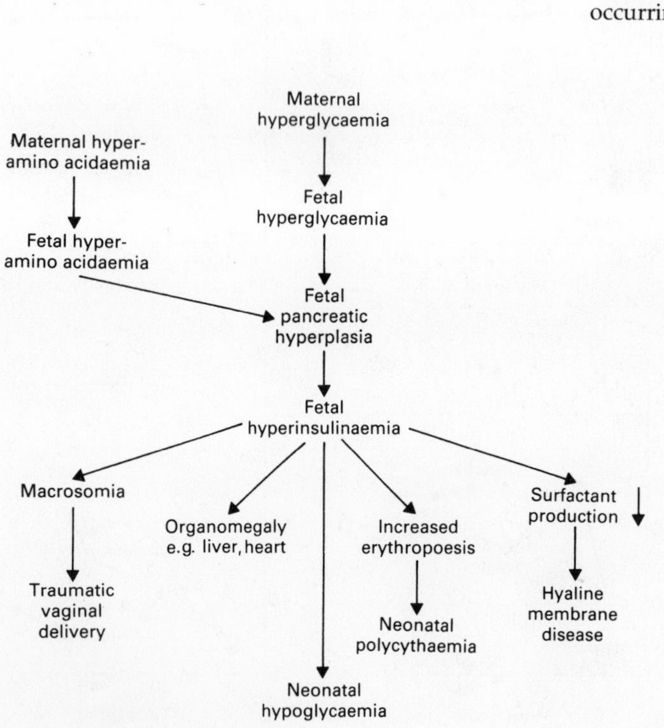

Fig. 11.4. An expanded modification of the Pedersen hypothesis [134].

pregnant normoglycaemic women is fairly constant at 5–6 per cent of the total haemoglobin mass. The glucose is bound irreversibly to the red cell and the measurement of the percentage of HbA_1 which has been glycosylated gives an indication of the plasma glucose concentrations to which the current red cells have been exposed. Accordingly, the HbA_{1c} percentage gives a retrospective estimate of mean plasma glucose concentration over the preceding 2 months. With the increased erythropoiesis of early pregnancy, the HbA_{1c} value should drop slightly as the proportion of young erythrocytes increases. Other compounds are also glycosylated and measurement of glycosylated serum proteins, e.g. albumen, are used as an alternative to HbA_{1c}. This provides a retrospective picture of glucose concentrations over the preceding month.

Effect of diabetes on the fetus

Congenital malformations

There is an increased incidence of congenital malformations amongst the offspring of mothers with established diabetes, varying from 2.7 per cent [28] to 11.9 per cent [162]. The variation is probably due to: (a) methodological differences in assessing malformations; (b) differing susceptibility of populations studied; (c) variations in the severity of the diabetes and its control; (d) different policies with regard to screening for malformations and termination of pregnancy; and (e) different time periods studied. The results from the UK Survey of Diabetic Pregnancy [10] reported an incidence of 5.7 per cent amongst 664 mothers with established diabetes. The consensus is that there is about a threefold increase over the rate for non-diabetic pregnancy. However, in some centres the malformation rate is decreasing. For example, in Copenhagen it is 2.7 per cent, less than in earlier reports [28] and less than twice as much as in the normal population.

Both minor and major malformations are increased in maternal diabetes. Specific abnormalities are cardiac and neural tube defects and the caudal regression syndrome (absence or hypoplasia of caudal structures), the last mentioned of which is otherwise very rare [85].

How does diabetes so unpredictably disrupt fetal organogenesis? In 1964, the Copenhagen group reported an association between malformation and maternal diabetic vascular disease [117]. They subsequently showed an association between malformation rate and poor diabetic control, i.e. a rate of 7 per cent in 363 class B–F diabetics whose diabetes had been well controlled before pregnancy compared to a rate of 14 per cent in 284 women with diabetes of similar severity who had been poorly controlled [136]. Leslie *et al.* [90] suggested that the malformation rate was higher amongst the offspring of mothers with established diabetes who had a higher than normal glycosylated haemoglobin in early pregnancy. This has subsequently been confirmed by others [106,149,177,202]. However, in a large American study, no relationship was found between glycaemic control assessed 21 days post-conception and congenital malformation rate [107], but the women were moderately well controlled and few had the degree of elevation of glycosylated haemoglobin found in the studies mentioned previously. Their finding of a decreased malformation rate in those women seen early, in contrast to those seen later (4.9 versus 9.0 per cent), is in accord with studies that have shown that women seen in pre-pregnancy clinics are less likely to have babies with congenital malformations than those not seen [48, 171]. These findings suggest that there may be a critical concentration of blood glucose above which fetal malformations are more likely to develop. However, the relationship is not so simple as it first appears, since there is a considerable overlap between glucose control and glycosylated haemoglobin values of women bearing abnormal babies and those with unaffected babies.

It has long been known that malformations can be induced in animals by exposing the fetus at the time of organogenesis to high concentrations of glucose [30], and Lewis *et al.* [91] suggested that ketonaemia potentiates this effect. Work in rats [6,39] has shown that lumbosacral defects in the fetus could only be induced if the mother was hyperglycaemic in the first days of pregnancy, the period when organogenesis is occurring. If the rat mothers were made diabetic after the first week of pregnancy or insulin treatment was given, the defects did not appear. The exact mechanism is uncertain, but Eriksson has suggested that free oxygen radicals generated by embryonic mitochondria may be responsible [38]. Hypoglycaemia has also been investigated in rats *in vivo* and a slight increase in congenital malformations has been reported [1,16]. To date no clinical evidence supports such a relationship with hypoglycaemia in the human [107,172]. Women with gestational diabetes do not have an increased incidence of malformations in their offspring [97] presumably because the metabolic disturbance of diabetes does not appear in the mother until later in pregnancy when organogenesis is complete.

To date, attention has been directed mainly at malformations that are detected at or shortly after birth. Therefore the rate is likely to be underestimated since many malformations are overlooked in the neonatal period, only becoming apparent in childhood. In addition, little is known about the 'malformation' rate in organ systems such as the brain where a relatively minor disruption of organogenesis might cause significant behavioural abnormalities in later life. A study from Denmark of 740 children of diabetic mothers [204] showed that 36 per cent had some form of cerebral dysfunction. Although this study was uncontrolled, it serves as a reminder of how seriously one should regard the potential damaging effects of uncontrolled diabetes in early pregnancy. A number of other studies have looked at the development of the child and attempted to correlate this with maternal metabolic control. For example Churchill *et al.* [20] and Stehbens *et al.* [174] in the USA linked ketonuria with subsequent intellectual impairment, but reanalysis of Churchill's data did not support this [121]. More recent detailed studies have investigated second and third trimester maternal metabolism and correlated this with intellectual development in the offspring [150]. An inverse relationship was demonstrated between intellectual development and ketone and free fatty acids levels, but not with markers of glucose control. This is discussed later with regard to management.

Spontaneous miscarriage

Uncontrolled studies had suggested an increased incidence of miscarriage amongst women known to have diabetes before pregnancy [113], possibly related to poor diabetic control during embryogenesis as determined by glycosylated haemoglobin measurement at 8–9 weeks [114]. By contrast, no difference was found in a large prospective American study in diabetic compared with control women seen by 21 days post-conception [108]. However, those with diabetes who did miscarry had higher fasting and postprandial glucose concentration and glycosylated haemoglobin than those with continuing pregnancies. Women who attend for pre-pregnancy counselling have also been shown to have no increased miscarriage rate [32]. Poorly controlled diabetes does appear to be associated with an increased risk of miscarriage.

Perinatal mortality in established diabetes

The perinatal mortality rate (PNMR) amongst women with established diabetes has always been higher than that for the population as a whole. However, rates have been falling consistently as can be seen from the figures from King's College Hospital, London, shown in Table 11.1. Gillmer *et al.* [55] quoting the Swedish data for 1973–78 point out that the PNMR was falling in the whole obstetric population over this period, so that it is unwise to attribute the fall solely to the provision of better diabetic control. Care must also be taken when considering PNMR to ensure that a correction has not been made for fatal malformations. The Swedish figures suggest that the major improvement can be ascribed to both better diabetic and obstetric care before delivery since the still-birth rate has fallen more steeply amongst women who have diabetes compared to those who do not.

Another factor that has to be taken into account when considering perinatal mortality figures, such as those in Table 11.1, is that most reports come from centres with a special interest in diabetic pregnancy. In fact, the PNMR for the whole UK is higher, as is shown by the figure of 61 per 1000 for mothers with established diabetes in Britain in 1979–80 [10] compared to 37 per 1000 for 1971–80 and 18 per 1000 for 1981–90 at King's College Hospital. The wide variation between different maternity units in PNMR is likely to be due to variation in the quality of medical and obstetric care. For example, Persson *et al.* [142] reported a fourfold difference in PNMR in favour of a centre with a particular interest in diabetes in pregnancy when compared to the rate in three adjacent hospitals.

Table 11.1 shows the changes in PNMR relative to the cause of death. It can be seen that deaths due to obstetric disaster, complications of diabetes, respiratory distress and 'unknown' have all fallen, whereas death rates due to congenital malformation remained unaltered until they too started falling in the 1980s. The fact that, if malformations are removed from the figures, PNMR would be essentially the same as for a non-diabetic population emphasizes the effects of improved obstetric and diabetic care.

Unexplained fetal death *in utero*

Despite improvement in diabetic care, unexplained fetal deaths *in utero* still accounted for 51 per cent of the perinatal mortality in the 1979–80 UK survey [94]. Occasionally perinatal deaths are also still reported from major centres using careful fetal monitoring programmes [15,187]. The aetiology is almost certainly multifactorial but hyperglycaemia is likely to be important. Initially, much of the evidence had to be obtained from post-mortem samples, amniotic fluid and cord blood taken at delivery and from animal studies. Data obtained by direct blood sampling of the fetus are now giving more insight. A number of factors are now considered.

Placental blood supply. Early radio-isotope studies had suggested a decrease in flow of between 35 and 40 per cent in maternal diabetes [122]. Initial Doppler flow measurements had produced data which were difficult to interpret, but more recent studies indicate that values are within the normal range unless growth retardation or pre-eclampsia is present [72,160]. No relationship was found between diabetic control and umbilical artery velocity waveforms [72]. Additional data on six women with nephropathy, i.e. diabetic vascular disease, showed no evidence of impaired placental perfusion [159].

Placental abnormalities. Fox reviewed the subject [43] and concluded that placental changes were not specific to diabetes and did not relate to the severity of the diabetes or its control. In addition, the evidence suggests that the placental area available for maternal–fetal exchange is increased. Accordingly, it seems unlikely that the placenta is a relevant factor in unexplained fetal death.

Placental oxygen transfer. This has been comprehensively reviewed by Madsen [96]. Although there is an increase in maternal red blood cell 2,3-diphosphoglycerate (DPG) content in diabetic pregnancy throughout all trimesters, increasing concentration of maternal glycosylated haemoglobin was found to be associated with a small but significant decrease in arterial oxygen saturation. The women studied did not have poorly controlled diabetes (HbA_1c median 7.8 per cent with a maximum of 9.9 per cent) and with poor control the red cell oxygen release is likely to be further impaired. Women who smoke have a smaller increase in red cell 2,3-DPG and are, therefore, likely to have further impairment of oxygen release. In addition, in patients recovering from ketoacidosis there is a marked reduction in red cell oxygen release which

Table 11.1. Perinatal mortality rates and causes of death amongst 1449 diabetic babies born to diabetic mothers over a 40-year period at King's College Hospital, London. (J.M. Brudenell, personal communication.)

			Causes of death				
	n	Perinatal deaths (per (1000)	Obstetric	Diabetic	Congenital malformations	Respiratory distress	Unknown
1951–60	318	72(226)	26	5	6	17	18
1961–70	389	39(100)	9	2	5	8	15
1971–80	352	13(37)	3	1	6	1	2
1981–90	390	7(18)	0	0	4	0	3

may account for the poor fetal prognosis in this situation.

Fetal acid–base balance. In 1975, it was reported that in sheep hyperglycaemia was of no significance to a well-oxygenated fetus, but with mild hypoxia, there was a rapid fall in pH with hyperglycaemia [164]. Cordocentesis in fetuses of diabetic women in the third trimester has demonstrated relatively normal blood Po_2 concentrations, but a tendency to mild acidaemia with increased lactate concentrations [156]. In addition, an inverse relationship between fetal pH and glucose concentration was demonstrated as in the sheep studies (Fig. 11.5). These findings suggest the fetus of the diabetic mother has a tendency towards metabolic acidosis, that increasing glucose concentrations adversely affect it and that this can occur in the absence of hypoxaemia. As there is a correlation between fetal pH and Po_2 one can speculate that sudden rises in maternal glucose could be enough to cause fetal acidaemia and mild hypoxaemia. Extrapolating from animal work [164] this mild hypoxaemia might be sufficient to cause an irreversible pH decline and fetal demise.

Fetal metabolic demand. The organomegaly induced by hyperinsulinaemia [179] in the fetus of the diabetic mother will result in an increased oxygen demand as has been shown in animal experiments [19].

Fetal thrombosis. As mentioned in the section on fetal haematology there is both polycythaemia and thrombocytopenia [155], the latter probably due to platelet aggregation. The fetus is likely to be at increased risk of thrombotic episodes and this has been documented in post-mortem studies [125].

In conclusion, a number of factors are likely to be relevant to the pathogenesis of intrauterine death, but a common factor is that of poor diabetic control.

Perinatal mortality in GDM

There is still controversy as to whether PNMR is raised in pregnancy complicated by GDM or IGT [9,70]. It has been claimed that there is an increased incidence of previous perinatal deaths in women with GDM [49,102]. The inference is that in their previous pregnancy the condition was unrecognized and untreated, resulting in increased mortality. However, in a study using controls matched for age, parity and ethnic group no significant difference was found in the number of previous perinatal deaths in women with IGT whilst there was an increase when contrasted with the general obstetric population [98]. Much of the controversy relates to the degree of abnormality. Abnormalities of glucose tolerance vary in severity from the individual with a mild disturbance of carbohydrate metabolism to the mother who develops symptomatic diabetes requiring insulin as pregnancy progresses. It is, therefore, reasonable to assume that if the PNMR is raised, it will be higher in this latter group.

With regard to the current pregnancy, O'Sullivan *et al.* [129] found a fourfold increase in perinatal mortality in women with untreated gestational diabetes compared with controls, although this increase was confined to the older more obese group. Similar results were reported from a study in Pima Indian women where those with IGT had an increased PNMR by contrast with controls with normal glucose tolerance [145]. The only large randomized trial of treatment of GDM versus routine antenatal care demonstrated a non-significant increase in PNMR in the untreated group (8.5 versus 3.6 per cent) [126]. It would no longer be possible to perform such studies in most developed countries. Further data may come from less well-developed countries where patients are more reluctant to accept treatment. However, on balance it seems likely that PNMR is increased when abnormalities of glucose tolerance are untreated, the worse the abnormality the greater the risk.

Neonatal morbidity

The concern about perinatal mortality has meant that until recently little attention has been paid to reducing the neonatal morbidity commonly associated with maternal diabetes. The expanded Pedersen hypothesis shown in Fig. 11.4 can be used to explain much of the neonatal morbidity that follows a diabetic pregnancy. Guthberlet and Cornblath [61] reported an incidence of 30–50 per

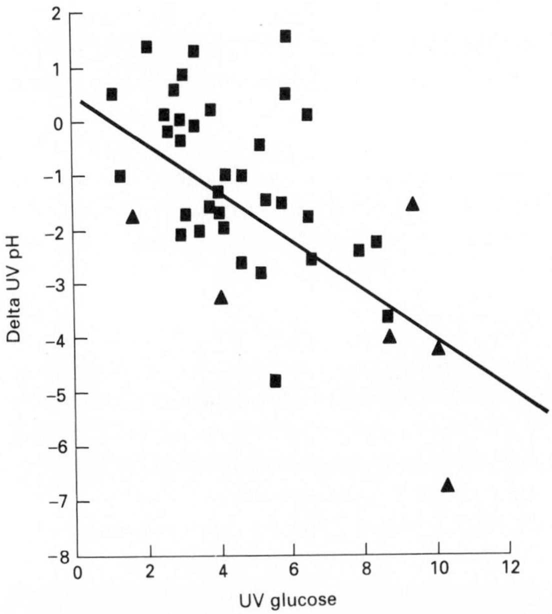

Fig. 11.5. Relationship between umbilical venous (UV) pH and umbilical cord blood glucose obtained from antenatal cordocentesis in diabetic pregnancy. Six women had nephropathy and hypertension (▲). Value of Δ pH is in SD from normal mean for gestational age. $r = 0.603$, $P < 0.0001$ [156].

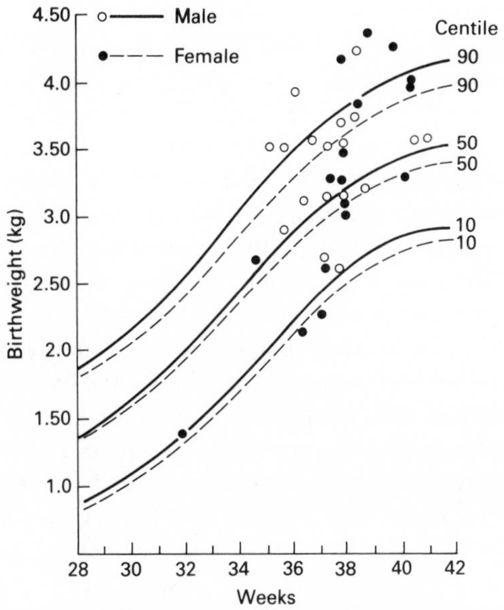

Fig. 11.6. Birthweight and gestation distribution for infants of insulin dependent diabetic mothers 1985–86 at St Mary's Hospital, Manchester. ○ Males; ● females. Percentile charts [111]. (M. Maresh, unpublished observations.)

cent morbidity amongst babies of mothers with established diabetes. A more recent review by Hod *et al.* [68] still shows unacceptably raised morbidity rates both in GDM and established diabetes.

Abnormalities of growth

IDDM is associated with an increased incidence of infants who are both large and small for gestational age, both conditions being associated with increased perinatal morbidity. The distribution of birthweight from a typical population with established diabetes is shown in Fig. 11.6. Typically, between 25 and 40 per cent of infants of mothers with established diabetes have birthweights over the 90th percentile. Excessive fetal growth rarely becomes apparent before 28 weeks gestation, although one longitudinal ultrasound study has suggested it may not be so rare when assessed by abdominal circumference measurement at 24 weeks gestation [79]. The macrosomic baby of the diabetic mother is characteristically fat and plethoric, with all organs, with the exception of the brain, being enlarged due to an increase in cytoplasmic mass. There is much evidence to support the Pederson hypothesis [134] (see Fig. 11.4) that birthweight is increased through fetal pancreatic hyperplasia and hyperinsulinism. Using the hyperinsulinaemic, normoglycaemic monkey model Susa and Schwartz [179] showed that it is hyperinsulinaemia which is responsible for these changes. In the human fetus, subcutaneous fat is markedly increased, the amount being directly related to the maternal plasma glucose concentration in the third trimester of pregnancy [196] and to glycosylated haemoglobin [178]. In addition, analysis of amniotic fluid C peptide concentrations and the insulin/glucose ratio in fetal plasma obtained by cordocentesis have shown correlations with large for gestational age babies [41, 156]. Furthermore, morphological studies of the fetus of the diabetic mother have shown that the greater the percentage area of total pancreatic tissue occupied by insulin-secreting islet cells, the bigger the baby [18].

Whilst fetal hyperinsulinaemia is clearly associated with excessive fetal growth, the growth itself could be mediated through insulin-like growth factors (IGFs) and their binding proteins (IGFBPs) [192]. However, a longitudinal study in normal and diabetic pregnancy has not shown a relationship between IGF-1 or IGFBP-1 with ultrasound determined fetal growth or birthweight [197].

The clinical importance of fetal macrosomia, which is often associated with hydramnios, is that it is a useful sign of poor diabetic control and accordingly of increased risk of perinatal mortality. Whilst more common in the established diabetic woman it may also occur with GDM. In addition, excessive fetal growth increases the risk of trauma during vaginal delivery particularly from shoulder impaction. This is an exceedingly dangerous complication because of the rapid onset of fetal hypoxia at a time when, so often, individuals with experience in dealing with this complication are not available.

It has been suggested by Jarrett [70] that the increased birthweight of babies in GDM may be accounted for by the tendency for these women to be older and fatter than normal. However, these women had their diabetes treated [98]. If they had not been treated, the babies might have been fatter than would have been expected from their mothers' age and obesity. Regardless of the cause of the increase in birthweight, the baby of the mother with abnormal glucose tolerance is still at increased risk of disproportion and trauma at delivery.

Respiratory dysfunction

Respiratory distress syndrome of the newborn is a known complication of maternal diabetes. It is suggested that fetal hyperinsulinism reduces pulmonary phospholipid production, particularly phosphatidyl glycerol, leading to surfactant deficiency [14]. There is evidence to associate poor diabetic control with an inadequate amniotic fluid phospholipid profile [147]. Prediction of subsequent neonatal respiratory distress syndrome can be improved by the measurement of the phospholipid profile in addition to the lecithin/sphingomyelin ratio [69].

Respiratory distress syndrome is becoming less common due to less pre-term elective delivery and better diabetic control. It is being replaced by transient tachypnoea of the newborn, which is thought to be due to delayed removal of fetal lung liquid and is seen quite commonly especially after caesarean section. This is characterized by a rapid respiratory rate and transient cyanosis usually disappearing within 24–36 hours of birth.

Hypoglycaemia

This is usually asymptomatic in the newborn of the diabetic woman. Plasma glucose concentrations of <2 mmol/l without evidence of systemic disturbance are quite common. The condition is caused by endogenous hyperinsulinism developing in fetal life that becomes clinically apparent only when the fetus is separated from its maternal supply of glucose. In addition, the combination of reduced hepatic phosphorylase activity and diminished glucagon and catecholamine release results in decreased output of glucose from the liver of these babies [78].

It is fortunate that the symptomatic variety is less common because it carries an increased likelihood of cerebral damage for the baby. It is preceded by jitteriness and convulsions, or simply by limpness or an abnormal cry [50]. The concentration of plasma glucose in the newborn correlates inversely with the degree of carbohydrate intolerance of the mother in the third trimester of pregnancy [52] and also with maternal glycosylated haemoglobin [203]. By encouraging early feeding and by performing regular glucose estimations in the newborn after birth, the condition can be detected and treated before symptoms develop. A value <1 mmol/l is an indication for the intravenous administration of glucose because of the risk of brain damage.

Polycythaemia and jaundice

Polycythaemia is more common in infants of diabetic mothers. A venous haematocrit >65 per cent is considered abnormal and was detected in 29 per cent of infants of diabetic mothers by contrast with 6 per cent of controls [112]. In GDM the frequency increases with greater degrees of abnormality [98]. Cordocentesis has also demonstrated a relationship between maternal diabetic control and fetal polycythaemia [155]. Animal work suggests that fetal hyperinsulinism results in elevated levels of erythropoietin, leading to increased haematopoiesis. The erythropoietin concentration in the umbilical vein has been found to be higher in women with established diabetes than in those with GDM or in controls [198]. The clinical consequence of the polycythaemia is an increase in blood viscosity leading to increased cardiac work and microcirculatory disturbances. Hyperviscosity within the pulmonary bed may be a contributory factor to respiratory distress. It might also explain the increased incidence of renal vein thrombosis and necrotizing enterocolitis. The destruction of many cells and the relative immaturity of the liver enzyme systems of the newborn which handle bilirubin, predispose to the high prevalence of jaundice in these babies. The rate of jaundice varies between series, but typically about 19 per cent would have bilirubin values exceeding 15 mg/dl [82]. These complications led Persson *et al.* [141] to recommend early clamping of the umbilical cord and exchange transfusion if the haematocrit exceeds 70 per cent.

Hypocalcaemia and hypomagnesaemia

The incidence of hypocalcaemia is increased in infants of diabetic mothers. Whilst an incidence of 50 per cent is often quoted [185] this is likely to be an overestimate and a frequency of between 5 per cent [142] and 22 per cent [82] is more likely. In addition, hypomagnesaemia appears more frequently [186]. Reduced parathyroid hormone concentrations have been noted in pregnancy associated with normal calcium concentrations. The exact mechanism of these changes is uncertain, but again there is a relationship with diabetic control. In view of the possibility of neonatal fits associated with these metabolic changes careful surveillance of the neonates is necessary.

Hypertrophic cardiomyopathy

It has been claimed that about 30 per cent of infants of mothers with IDDM have cardiomegaly and 10 per cent have evidence of cardiac dysfunction [89]. The characteristic abnormality which is best demonstrated by echocardiography [59] is asymmetric septal hypertrophy. This is similar to that seen in familial obstructive cardiomyopathy, except that it is reversible over a period of weeks if the infant survives [66] and that fibre disarray is not a prominent feature [66,89]. The animal work of Susa and Schwartz [179] suggests that the cardiomegaly is caused by hyperinsulinism and clinical data again show a link with the degree of maternal diabetic control [60].

Summary of causes of neonatal morbidity

As mentioned above it seems likely that fetal hyperinsulinism is an important factor causing some or all of these complications and that anything which can reduce this is likely to diminish the neonatal complication rate in diabetic pregnancy. Guthberlet and Cornblath [61] showed that the incidence of neonatal complications after birth was lower amongst mothers with mild diabetes. Maresh *et al.* [98] showed in a controlled study of women with IGT that the incidence of admission to the special care baby unit for more than 48 hours and of polycythaemia related directly to the severity of the maternal glucose abnormality. These facts, and the demonstrable relationship between GTT in the last trimester of pregnancy and the neonatal plasma glucose concentration, strongly suggest that normalization of maternal plasma glucose in the latter part of pregnancy is likely to reduce neonatal morbidity.

Added weight is given to this view by the five surveys of neonatal morbidity following pregnancy in women with established diabetes shown in Table 11.2. The figures of Larsson and Ludvigsson (1974) [88] were obtained from some Swedish hospitals where diabetic control was known to be poor with a correspondingly high mortality and morbidity rate. The UK survey [10] was carried out 10 years later when diabetic control was probably better and the rate of associated neonatal complications — except for respiratory distress — was much less. The surveys from Drury [35] and Jovanovic *et al.* [73] are characterized by the provision of diabetic care by a single individual with much greater attention being paid to obtaining good diabetic control throughout pregnancy. This is particularly so in the case of Jovanovic *et al.* [73], in which normoglycaemia in

Table 11.2. Comparison of perinatal morbidity and mortality amongst women with diabetic pregnancy. A, Swedish Hospitals 1974 [88]; B, UK National Survey of Diabetic Pregnancy 1979–80 [10]; C, Dublin, reported in [35]; D, New York, reported in [73]; E, Israel 1980–9 reported in [68]

	A ($n = 157$)	B ($n = 664$)	C ($n = 285$)	D ($n = 55$)	E ($n = 132$)
Respiratory distress (%)	10	12	3	0	2
Jaundice (%)	30	20	15	0	17
Hypoglycaemia (%)	48	15	11	<2	8
Macrosomia (%)	43	29	—	0	25
PNM (per 1000)	220	61	45	0	0

the mother was maintained for the greater part of pregnancy so that neonatal morbidity virtually disappeared.

Diagnosis of diabetes in pregnancy

In non-pregnant individuals, it is common practice to leave untreated minor degrees of carbohydrate intolerance, whereas in pregnancy such deviations in the metabolism of the mother may be critical to the normal development of the fetus [9]. Diagnostic criteria and therapeutic goals must, of necessity, be more demanding in pregnancy.

GDM is diagnosed on the basis of an abnormal GTT. One standard (and very arbitrary) approach to defining abnormal glucose tolerance in pregnancy is to take the limit of 2 SDs above the mean for a group of non-diabetic pregnant women [131]. Until recently there have been no agreed criteria for defining abnormality because of such variables as whether an oral or intravenous test is performed, the amount of glucose that is given and the variety of methods used for glucose assay. The criteria of O'Sullivan *et al.* [132] were generally regarded as being most acceptable because of the careful long-term follow-up of the women following the pregnancy during which they had their initial GTT. They used a 100 g load of glucose administered orally following prior dietary preparation and collected venous blood every 30 min over 3 hours. They defined an abnormal result as two or more venous whole-blood glucose values exceeding the following limits: fasting 5 mmol/l, 1 hour 9.2 mmol/l, 2 hours 8.1 mmol/l and 3 hours 6.9 mmol/l. Subsequent recommendations for venous plasma are 5.8, 10.6, 9.2 and 8.1 mmol/l respectively [183].

Alternatively, Gillmer *et al.* [51,52] have used a 50 g oral load followed by a 3-hour GTT. This group utilized the known tendency in diabetic pregnancy for the newborn to become hypoglycaemic after birth, and showed a relationship between the GTT of the mother and the 2-hour plasma glucose of her baby. By defining neonatal hypoglycaemia 2 hours after birth as a plasma glucose concentration of 1.7 mmol/l or less, they determined the upper limit of normal glucose tolerance in the mother. They found that critical values differed little from those of O'Sullivan *et al.* [132]. The best predictor in the mother of neonatal hypoglycaemia proved to be the total area under the curve. For a 3-hour test this is calculated by adding together half of the fasting value and half of the 3-hour value to all the remaining 30-min values. For the 50 g oral glucose test a measurement of 43 or more was considered as abnormal. The World Health Organization (WHO) [201], in an attempt to standardize the GTT, have recommended a 75 g oral load and have given cut-offs for the fasting and 2-hour value in non-pregnant subjects. A diagnosis of diabetes is made if the fasting plasma glucose is ≥8 mmol and/or the 2-hour value is ≥11 mmol/l. Alternatively, a diagnosis of impaired glucose tolerance is made if the fasting plasma glucose is <8 mmol/l and the 2-hour level is <11 mmol/l and ≥8 mmol/. These criteria were based on complications of diabetes recorded from long-term follow-up studies of men and non-pregnant women. A large multicentre pregnancy study was conducted by Lind [92]. This confirmed earlier suggestions that a 2-hour value ≥8 mmol/l was common after a 75 g GTT, being found in about 10 per cent of women. He recommended raising the 2-hour cut-off to 9 mmol/l and combining this with the 95 percentile value for the 1-hour value which was 10.5 mmol/l.

Although there are methodological problems with the data, these criteria should be accepted, i.e. abnormal glucose tolerance should be defined on the basis of a 1-hour blood glucose of 10.5 mmol/l and 2 hours of 9 mmol/l following a 75 g load. Lind also recommended the use of the term GIGT for this group, GDM being reserved for those with a frankly diabetic GTT (WHO criterion).

Screening

Attempts to detect unrecognized diabetes in pregnancy are a part of established practice in every antenatal clinic in this country. The justification for this is the possible increased risk of perinatal death amongst women who have an abnormal GTT in pregnancy. The success of these efforts varies widely because of the generalized lack of any consistent and systematic approach to the problem. If screening is to be effective it must be comprehensive. The accepted practice in antenatal clinics, of only performing a GTT on a mother if she has one of the features of potential diabetes, is both time-consuming and incomplete. Screening studies of entire obstetric populations have shown that only 45 per cent of women found to have carbohydrate intolerance have defined features of potential diabetes [132]. The traditional method of waiting for glycosuria to appear has a low pick-up rate and, as such, is of little value. Sutherland *et al.* [181]. found that 11 per cent of an unselected obstetric population of 1418 women had random glycosuria but <1 per cent of those with glycosuria had an abnormal GTT. Most women have glycosuria if all urine samples are tested throughout pregnancy whilst, in contrast, many women with GDM never have glycosuria detected when they visit the antenatal clinic.

Many screening systems have been advocated but few are worthy of consideration for the reasons given above. The most comprehensive and practical method of screening for diabetes in pregnancy is that advocated by O'Sullivan *et al.* [132]. The method has a sensitivity of 79 per cent and a specificity of 83 per cent (see Table 11.3). When a mother first attends the antenatal clinic (not fasting), she is given a fruit-flavoured drink containing 50 g glucose. One hour later, blood is taken for glucose assay along with other routine screening blood tests. If the value is ≥7.8 mmol/l (>2 SD of the mean for an unselected obstetric population), a full GTT is done. If the GTT is negative or the patient has one of the features of potential diabetes, the screening procedure is repeated at 28 weeks gestation because of the diabetogenic effect of pregnancy which will unmask incipient diabetes as pregnancy advances. The cost can be halved by confining the screening test to women aged 25 or over, with only a small reduction in diagnostic sensitivity from 79 to 74 per cent. The saving in time, patient and staff involvement, and cost, would seem to justify this modification. The screening system is shown in a flow diagram in Fig. 11.7 [8]. Of all the pregnant women tested at their first visit, 6.3 per cent had a positive screening value, of whom 17 per cent had an abnormal GTT. Overall, the incidence of mothers with abnormal GTT values by the beginning of the third trimester was 1.5 per cent, two-thirds of whom had been picked up in the booking clinic and one-third by repeating the screen at 28 weeks gestation.

The Copenhagen group have used a screening system which combines potential diabetic features with the fasting glucose concentration [119]. A fasting blood glucose cut-off of 4.1 mmol/l produced a sensitivity of over 90 per cent. Applying these criteria Jowett [77] also found a sensitivity of 92 per cent with a specificity of 49 per cent. This method appears to warrant further evaluation.

Random glucose measurement has been encouraged as a simple way to screen for abnormal glucose tolerance [93]. A positive cut-off was taken as 6.4 mmol/l if taken <2 hours after a meal and 5.8 mmol/l if >2 hours. However, subsequently sensitivity and specificity data were obtained [77,120] which showed this to be a poor method of screening (see Table 11.3).

Glycosylated haemoglobin has been extensively investigated. As a one-sample blood screening test with no preparation it could have many advantages. However, most studies have shown it to be not specific or sensitive enough [4,5,24,47,101,163]. Only one study which used a specific affinity chromatographic assay in women between 10 and 15 weeks gestation has produced high sensitivity and specificity [118]. Likewise glycosylated proteins which

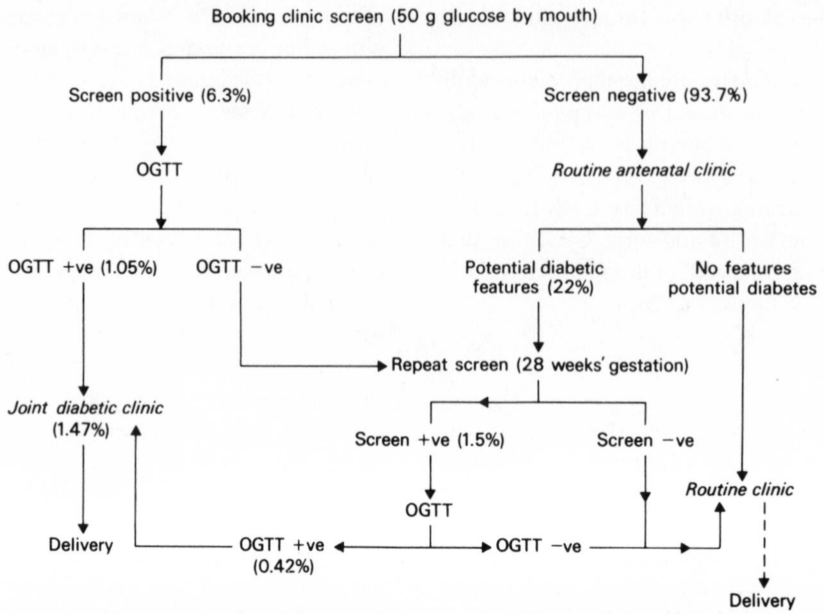

Fig. 11.7. Flow diagram depicting the screening programme and management of patients screened at St Mary's Hospital, London. All percentages are expressed as a proportion of the original booking clinic population screened [8].

reflect glucose concentrations over the preceding few weeks have been investigated using the fructosamine method. The initial encouraging results [151] have not been substantiated in further studies [101,152,154].

The justification for any screening system is that it should be cost-effective and also acceptable to the patient. A full oral GTT, apart from being expensive, is time-consuming and unpleasant for pregnant women. Equally, limiting the test to potential diabetics is not justified because of the relatively lower pick-up rate (see Table 11.3). From Table 11.3, the system originally proposed by O'Sullivan *et al.* [132] (Fig. 11.7) is the best screening method.

Table 11.3. Comparison of screening methods for impaired glucose tolerance

	Sensitivity (%)	Specificity (%)
Potential diabetic features*	50	66
Random glucose†	40	90
Glucose load*	79	83
Glycated Hb*	40	90

* Positive outcome being an abnormal GTT as defined by O'Sullivan [113].

† Positive outcome being an abnormal GTT as defined by WHO, impaired glucose tolerance [115].

Medical management

Pre-pregnancy care

To be effective, medical management of established diabetes must start well before pregnancy. All affected teenage girls should be warned of the risks of pregnancy to them and their babies and that their diabetic control should be good when they become pregnant. Attention to general health, contraception and good metabolic control are subjects that must be discussed by physicians, general practitioners, diabetic liaison nurses, health visitors and by youth workers and indeed by all who have contact with diabetics. The trend towards managing diabetes in special centres and the increasing use of diabetic liaison nurses will enable advice to be given more readily to some of the younger women who need it most.

Whether a specific pre-pregnancy clinic is necessary remains controversial [36,58,81,170]. Although some have achieved very high attendance rates, with about 60 per cent of pregnant women having been seen prior to conception [171], this is the exception. What is required is easy access to a knowledgeable person; whether that person is a physician or obstetrician, specialist nurse or midwife is irrelevant. Similarly, whether a clinic is established or whether there is an alternative method of access is again irrelevant.

In general, the establishment of a pre-pregnancy counselling service in centres with a large diabetic clinic population is sensible. The major objective is to ensure that good diabetic control prevails at the time of conception and embryogenesis. Those who were counselled before pregnancy were found to have lower HbA_{1c} values [171], lower glucose values [48] in the first trimester and fewer congenital malformations amongst their babies [48,171] than those who did not. Pre-conception care gives the opportunity for a change to insulin for all diabetic women on oral hypoglycaemic drugs. Apart from the possible problems of transplacental drug passage, the major reason for changing to insulin is the tighter diabetic control that can be achieved. The complications of diabetes and its interrelations with pregnancy also need discussing before pregnancy. Any retinopathy should be treated prior to pregnancy. In cases of severe nephropathy it may be necessary to discourage pregnancy for the health of the woman. In addition, to improving diabetic control, the opportunity may be taken to give general advice regarding the importance of being as healthy as possible at the start of the pregnancy — stopping smoking, reducing alcohol intake and achieving an ideal bodyweight, being obvious examples. Furthermore, contraceptive or fertility advice may be required and rubella immunity status can be checked.

The joint pregnancy diabetic clinic

The pregnant diabetic woman is best managed in a special antenatal clinic where all those with the necessary expertise can work together. Few obstetricians and diabetic physicians in the UK are likely to care for more than two cases of IDDM a year. Care should be centred on one obstetrician and physician within each maternity unit. There is also a need for a referral unit which would take some of the more difficult cases in a health region with 40 000–60 000 births year. The midwife, should not be relegated solely to helping in the organization of the clinic, but can use her skills to complement those of the obstetrician. With the trend towards outpatient care throughout pregnancy (see below) the specialist diabetic midwife or nurse has a major role in teaching women blood glucose home monitoring and how to adjust their insulin regimes themselves. The presence of a dietitian is essential for initiating the treatment of GDM and unravelling some of the more difficult problems presented in IDDM. Medical and obstetric problems in diabetic pregnancy are often interdependent and are best managed by an obstetrician and physician working together.

Principles of treatment

The major objective of medical management is to attain normoglycaemia or as near to normoglycaemia as is practical. The non-diabetic woman maintains a plasma glucose in pregnancy within the range of 3.5–4.5 mmol/l [1] rarely exceeding 5.5 mmol/l except immediately after meals. However, this is a blood glucose concentration which is considerably lower than most people with established diabetes are used to in the non-pregnant state and it may initially lead to attacks of hypoglycaemia. Whilst this is distressing for up to 2 weeks, normoglycaemia usually can be achieved with support and encouragement from all those caring for her. As pregnancy advances, insulin requirements increase eventually reaching a plateau and sometimes decreasing near term. The female IDDM patient, therefore, requires considerable attention to the dosage regime. Women with NIDDM established before pregnancy usually require insulin to achieve normoglycaemia during pregnancy. Some with GDM may need to transfer from diet to insulin at some time during pregnancy for adequate control, although many can achieve acceptable normoglycaemia by restrictive dietary advice alone.

The objective of diabetic control in pregnancy

is to maintain normoglycaemia at all times. The authors' experience has been that three paired pre- and postprandial glucose measurements around the main meals during the day (the glucose profile) are useful in adjusting insulin dosage or in deciding on whether to commence a woman on insulin. Many IDDM patients are able to adjust these insulin dosages according to their results without the need for hospital advice. Outcomes such as birth-weight correlate better with postprandial than with preprandial values [21,75]. The use of blood glucose measurement strips (Dextrostix, B-M stix) with or without reflectance meters has made this easier to achieve and home monitoring of blood glucose is now widely practised by pregnant women. In general, visits to the clinic should be made every 2 weeks up until about 28 weeks and then weekly. It is wise to obtain a random blood glucose estimation using a reflectance meter at each visit and to measure the glycosylated haemoglobin or an alternative glycosylated protein monthly, as an additional safeguard. Studies of how patients record their meter glucose values in their diaries have shown that there is a trend towards omitting or lowering high values [100].

Dietary advice is an essential part of the management of all diabetic women whether insulin dependent or not. Dietary compliance can be monitored by regular weighing of the woman as well as by observation of glucose concentrations. The major problems tend to be with NIDDM. A diet which is designed to achieve normoglycaemia should also produce a static bodyweight and any increase in weight suggests that the diet is not being adhered to.

If blood glucose concentration is to be well regulated, thought must be given to the effect of daily events on insulin requirements. Emotional lability is a potent factor in inducing hyperglycaemia and marked diurnal fluctuations in blood glucose. Many diabetic women do not alter their lifestyle when they become pregnant and may continue to do stressful jobs. When this occurs, considerable difficulty may be experienced in controlling the diabetes. An example of this was a nurse whose diabetes failed to respond to a number of changes in insulin regime until it was found that she was working an 8-hour shift in an intensive care unit, often missing meals and getting home exhausted. Transfer to less arduous nursing duties resulted in a significant improvement in her diabetic control.

Inpatient versus outpatient care

In the 1970s when it was realized that improved control of blood glucose in the third trimester led to better results, the philosophy of full inpatient care of pregnant diabetics from 32 weeks was advocated [40]. However, with the advent of home monitoring of blood glucose using reagent strips with or without reflectance meters it became possible to decrease hospital admissions, so that in 1984 Gillmer *et al.* [53] reported that one-third of their female IDDM patients were not admitted at any time during pregnancy prior to delivery. This trend has increased.

The advantages of being an inpatient were said to be that tighter diabetic control could be achieved and that closer fetal surveillance could be obtained. Leaving aside the latter which will be discussed below, it is perfectly possible for a woman to measure as many glucose values at home as would be done in hospital. Furthermore, it is also possible for home results to be checked in the laboratory using either the original blood samples or the original paper strips. Hospital admission will decrease physical activity and normoglycaemia achieved in hospital may lead to hypoglycaemia on returning home to more activity. It has been claimed that outpatient management leads to better control through involving the mother in the care of her diabetes [168]. Clearly outpatient care is easier for the rest of the family. Comparisons of glucose control [176] and neonatal outcome [140] in women who have had inpatient as opposed to outpatient care have shown no significant differences.

The routine now is outpatient care, admission being reserved for cases where good diabetic control is not being achieved as an outpatient or if fetal or maternal complications are developing.

Management of IDDM

To achieve normoglycaemia throughout the 24 hours, short and longer acting insulins are required.

Since the introduction of pen-type syringes, these have become increasingly used, and now are the standard method of administration in our practices. Three doses of short-acting insulin are given preprandially combined with one dose of a long acting insulin such as Ultratard at night or with two doses of a medium acting insulin such as protophane before breakfast and before retiring at night. Continuous subcutaneous insulin infusion (CSII) has been used in pregnancy, but it appears to offer no advantage to most diabetic pregnant women and can only be used if there is a well supported CSII service already established for the non-pregnant. In view of the state of 'accelerated starvation' found in pregnancy, ketoacidosis will develop more rapidly than in the non-pregnant state should there be pump failure and an intrauterine death has been reported [173].

A method of giving insulin known as 'the maximum tolerated dose' was pioneered by Roversi *et al.* [153]. Soluble insulin dosages were increased daily until symptomatic hypoglycaemia resulted and the dosage was then reduced to that of the previous day. Although Roversi's results were good, women on the regime found it distressing and there was a higher than expected rate of fetal growth retardation so that this method is not widely used nowadays.

Management of IGT and GDM

Though there is no consensus view, in the UK most women with IGT and GDM are initially managed with dietary advice alone. If control is deemed inadequate insulin is added until delivery. The indication for the addition of insulin remains controversial. The view of Persson *et al.* [144], that if fasting concentrations are persistently above 7 mmol/l (14 per cent of their cases), insulin should be commenced, seems sensible. However, a study is needed to investigate which is the best management to achieve normoglycaemia and whether this is necessary.

Oral hypoglycaemic agents have never been widely used and should not be used if compliance with insulin injection can be achieved. Drugs such as chlorpropamide cross the placenta and induce fetal hyperinsulinism [180] although the experience of the Aberdeen group which has used hypoglycaemic agents extensively reveals that whilst neonatal hypoglycaemia is more prevalent than amongst the insulin-treated group, it was still uncommon. Coetzee and Jackson [22] from South Africa have reported similarly good results.

Treatment by diet alone

This can be a most effective way of reducing blood glucose as can be seen in Fig. 11.8. Dieting has not only decreased postprandial hyperglycaemia, but also fasting concentrations. The effect of diet is to make insulin more efficient, as demonstrated by a decrease in the insulin/glucose ratio [99]. The general recommendations of the British Diabetic Association are that 50 per cent of energy should be obtained from carbohydrate and this should also apply to pregnancy. The total calories in the diet should be between 1800 and 2000 daily. In the obese this should be restricted further so that these women will put on little or no weight. Such 'hypocaloric diets' are controversial in the USA, but the recommendations of the Third International Workshop Conference on Gestational Diabetes Mellitus in 1990 [183] did advise a weight gain of only 7 kg in the obese (body mass index $>29\,kg/m^2$).

The British Diabetic Association also advised that maximal fibre intake is beneficial in pregnancy in order to reduce the degree of postprandial hyperglycaemia [45]. Persuading the diabetic mother to keep to her diet is usually easier in pregnancy because of the incentive to benefit her baby. However, cultural factors play a part which are sometimes difficult to resolve; for example, Indian women believe that it is important to keep the baby well fed and their mothers-in-law will insist on a high calorie intake, regardless of the advice of the doctor!

Restrictive dietary advice leads to an increase in ketonaemia. Although there is wide individual variation it is generally accepted that ketonaemia in pregnancy tends to increase with gestation [99,200]. Figure 11.8 shows that dietary treatment of women with gestational diabetes does not increase significantly, the 24-hour concentration of β hydroxybutyrate. Also ketonaemia can be reduced further

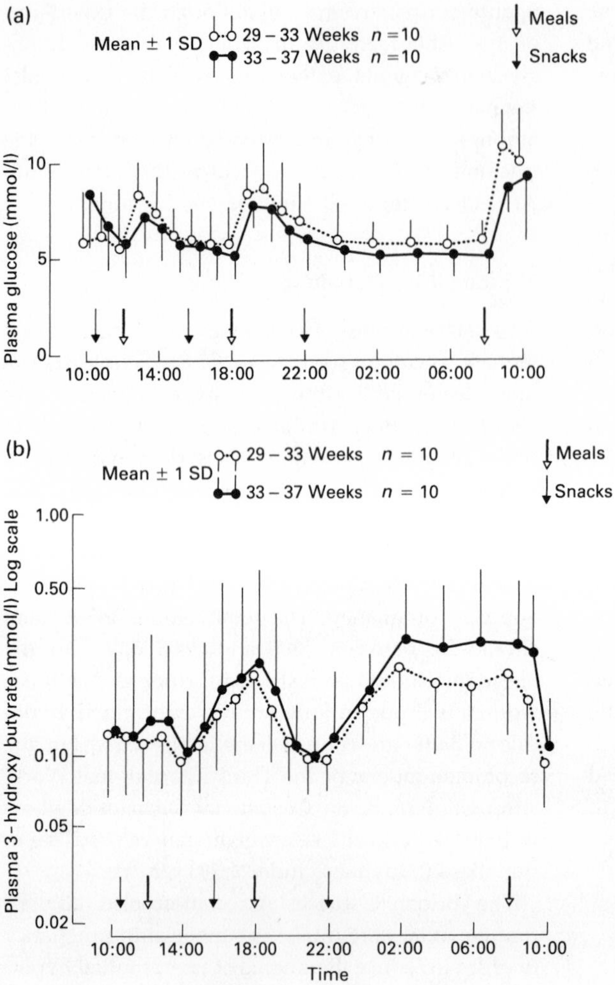

Fig. 11.8. Twenty-four hour metabolic profiles (mean ± 1 SD) in 10 women with abnormal glucose tolerance studied between 29 to 33 weeks and again between 33 to 37 weeks [99]. ○ Before dietary restriction; ● After dietary restriction for 4 weeks. A, Plasma glucose; B, plasma 3-hydroxybutyrate.

by high fibre diets [44] which were not used in the data illustrated. However, it is because of concern about possible long-term effects of ketonaemia on the fetus (see above) that in the USA tight dietary restrictive advice is not routinely given.

Treatment by diet and insulin therapy

Although there have been advocates for the routine use of insulin [26], the usual view is to reserve insulin for those who, despite keeping to their diet, have fasting hyperglycaemia. The only doubt is at what level to commence therapy (see above). As with established diabetes, patients can give themselves short acting insulin three times a day before each main meal starting at 6 units and using a pen syringe. Alternatively, they can use an insulin régime of twice daily biphasic insulin, i.e. a combination of a short and medium acting insulin with a starting dose of 20 units a day which can be altered to obtain control. Whilst insulin therapy has not been associated with clinical or biochemical evidence of hypoglycaemia in reported series, the management should be conducted by the same team who look after those with IDDM. Insulin therapy must be combined with restrictive dietary advice because if it is not the insulin will lead to excessive deposition of fat. This will increase the peripheral resistance to insulin, with the result that, despite increasing doses of insulin, hyperglycaemia persists.

Control of blood glucose during labour

Avoidance of hyper- or hypoglycaemia in the mother is essential if the fetus is to withstand the stress of labour. Insulin requirement in labour tends to be low [74], but the dose will need adjustment because of fluctuations in blood glucose due, for example, to the pain of uterine contractions. Normoglycaemia is best achieved in both the established diabetic and the insulin-requiring GDM patient by the intravenous administration of both glucose and insulin and this is estimated to be the current practice in 87 per cent of hospitals in the UK [205]. However, with increasing desire for mobilization in labour, in a well-organized unit and with highly motivated women with well-controlled diabetes, multiple subcutaneous injections of insulin could be considered.

The following regime is outlined as a guide to the practical management of the diabetic mother during labour. When the mother is admitted in spontaneous labour or prior to induction of labour, an intravenous infusion of 10 per cent dextrose solution should be commenced. The infusion rate should be adjusted to provide 1 l of fluid every 8 hours. Twenty units of soluble insulin (0.2 ml of 100 units/ml) should be mixed in 19.8 ml of normal saline in a 20 ml syringe which is then administered intraenously by infusion pump at a final concentration of 1 unit per ml.

The plasma glucose concentration should be estimated prior to deciding whether to start an insulin infusion. It is useful to have a glucose reflectance meter on the delivery unit for this purpose provided there are staff familiar with its use. Alternatively, if the woman has her own then she or her partner can use that. Blood glucose concentrations can be adjusted by altering either the glucose or insulin infusion rates. If the initial blood glucose is <7 mmol/l and >3.5 mmol/l then the insulin infusion should be given at a rate of 1 unit/hour; if it exceeds 7 mmol/l, then the infusion should commence at 2 units/hour. Glucose estimations should initially be repeated at hourly intervals and the insulin infusion rate increased or decreased by 1 unit/hour until a stable blood glucose concentration of between 4.5 and 5.5 mmol/l has been achieved. If the concentration falls below 3.5 mmol/l the glucose infusion rate should be increased and insulin should be stopped. After a rise in early labour, the glucose concentration tends to fall as labour progresses so that eventually it may be necessary to stop insulin administration and even to give extra glucose intravenously.

Women with impaired glucose tolerance require intravenous insulin if glucose concentrations (which should be checked every 2 hours) are persistently >7 mmol/l.

Should any additional intravenous fluids be necessary during labour such as oxytocin, then isotonic saline or Hartmann's solution should be used. Additional potassium is only advisable if labour is prolonged (e.g. >12 hours) and then potassium chloride should be added to the infusate (e.g. 20 mmol/l). Prior to any operative procedure requiring an anaesthetic, the obstetrician should discuss blood glucose control with the anaesthetist to avoid hypoglycaemia and also the inadvertent use of glucose-containing fluids intravenously.

Should problems arise with glucose control with this regime the usual causes are staff unfamiliarity with glucose measurements, the infusion pump being accidentally turned off or disconnected, or oxytocin being infused in a glucose solution.

Postnatal management

Immediately after delivery, insulin and glucose infusions should be discontinued. If this is not done hypoglycaemia is likely to occur as a consequence of the increase in insulin sensitivity following the delivery of the placenta. For the insulin-dependent woman it is simplest to revert to the insulin regime she was taking before pregnancy and to wait until breast feeding is established before attempting more precise diabetic control. Women with GDM or IGT who have been treated with insulin during pregnancy usually do not require any form of treatment, but should have blood glucose measurements made before leaving hospital to check that hyperglycaemia has not persisted.

Breast feeding should be encouraged, but because

of increased nutritional demands, an extra 50 g of carbohydrate a day in the dietary intake is recommended [194]. An alternative philosophy is to reduce the insulin dosage [2]. If oral hypoglycaemic agents are used, breast feeding is not advised because of their possible transfer to the fetus in breast milk.

Women who have had IGT or GDM should have a glucose tolerance test done about 6–12 weeks after delivery. If this is normal they should be warned that the condition is likely to re-occur in a subsequent pregnancy. Thus, all women who have had IGT or GDM particularly those who are overweight (>120 per cent of bodyweight) should be encouraged to either reduce their weight or maintain it if they are within the range of their ideal bodyweight. This can often be achieved by a visit to the dietitian who advised them during pregnancy. There is now good evidence to show that more than 50 per cent of women who have had GDM will develop type 2 (NIDDM) diabetes. The data are summarized in Table 11.4. The longest follow-up was by O'Sullivan [127] who has shown that in women whose glucose tolerance reverts to normal after pregnancy there was a 50 per cent risk of developing diabetes at 22–28 years of follow-up. O'Sullivan has also demonstrated the importance of avoiding obesity as in one study 47 per cent of the obese, but only 28 per cent of the non-obese showed abnormality at follow-up [127]. In conclusion, the predictive power of IGT in pregnancy for subsequent diabetes is such that one can argue strongly for routine screening of all pregnant women for this reason alone. If one extrapolates from the studies of Sartor *et al.* [161] it seems likely that women with IGT and GDM can diminish this risk by attention to diet.

Pregnancy in diabetic women with renal or vascular complications

These women fortunately represent a small proportion of diabetic women who become pregnant. They deserve separate mention because their problems require special consideration.

Diabetic nephropathy (see Chapter 7)

The condition is manifested by increasing proteinuria, hypertension and fluid retention — all with

Table 11.4. Follow-up studies on the incidence of diabetes or impaired glucose tolerance following a previous gestational diabetic pregnancy. Modified from [128]

Location	Year	Diagnostic criteria GDM	Follow-up period (years)	% diabetic or IGT	Reference
Sweden	1960	FBG > 11.2 mmol/l	1–7	62.0	[64]
Los Angeles, USA	1972	2 FBG >5 mmol/l	0–5	55.6	[103]
Leningrad, Russia	1974	Abnormal OGTT	0–6	44.2	[84]
Belfast, UK	1979	Local criteria	10	2.0	[62]
		2 hour > 7.2 mmol/l	10	87.5	
Phoenix, USA	1980	Abnormal OGTT	4–8	45.5	[145]
Aberdeen, UK	1985	Abnormal IVGTT	<22	35.0	[175]
Chicago, USA	1985	Abnormal OGTT &	1		[104]
		FBS <5.9 mmol/l		38.0	
		FBS 5.9–7.3 mmol/l		67.0	
		FBS > 7.3 mmol/l		95.0	
Melbourne, Australia	1986	Abnormal OGTT	1–12	18.8	[57]
Stockholm, Sweden	1987	Abnormal OGTT	<3	65.0	[37]
Copenhagen, Denmark	1989	Abnormal OGTT	2–10	34.0	[29]
Boston, USA	1989	Abnormal OGTT	<28	49.9	[127]
Trinidad, West Indies	1990	Abnormal OGTT	3–7	78.3	[3]
Lost Angeles, USA	1990	Abnormal OGTT	<2	40.0	[83]
London, UK	1990	Abnormal OGTT	6–12	64.0	[34]

IVGTT, intravenous glucose tolerance test; FBS, fasting blood glucose.

or without evidence of diminishing renal function. It may worsen in pregnancy and management must be determined according to the risk to the mother and fetus. If renal function is seriously impaired before pregnancy then termination must be considered in early pregnancy, particularly if hypertension is an associated complication. In the series of Steel *et al.* [172] a good outcome was achieved in ongoing pregnancies when creatinine clearance was >40 ml/min in the first trimester.

Renal function must be closely monitored throughout pregnancy as it may deteriorate at any time and may require interruption of the pregnancy. Fortunately renal function does not deteriorate in the majority of cases [80]. Occasionally a severe transient diabetic nephrotic syndrome may develop [12,133,193]. Distinguishing this from pre-eclampsia is difficult and requires a renal biopsy which is best avoided in pregnancy. Fetal growth retardation is a common accompaniment of diabetic nephropathy presumably due to the impaired ability of the utero-placental blood vessels to accommodate the increasing blood flow required to support the growing fetus. Antenatal fetal blood sampling in six women with diabetic nephropathy and hypertension showed the fetal pH to be below the fifth centile in all cases [159]. Antenatal fetal surveillance in the third trimester accordingly must be very close (see below). Birthweight, as expected is inversely related to maternal blood pressure and directly to creatinine clearance in the third trimester [80].

Diabetic retinopathy

Almost all women will have features of background diabetic retinopathy after about 15 years of diabetes. With further time proliferative retinopathy may develop, so during the 9 months of pregnancy new cases may appear. Most series of diabetes in pregnancy report a few cases of developing proliferative retinopathy [31,42,76,115,148]. The incidence may be as high as 22 per cent [42]. Provided proliferative retinopathy (whether new or pre-existing) is actively treated there appears to be no deterioration in visual acuity after pregnancy.

Background retinopathy may appear to deteriorate during pregnancy through impaired diabetic control leading to an ischaemic retinopathy [42]. These changes usually resolve spontaneously.

In conclusion, all juvenile onset diabetic women should be examined carefully before an intended pregnancy to exclude renal and vascular complications. If pregnancy continues in any woman with juvenile diabetes then fundoscopy should be performed at least twice and treatment given as necessary. Retinopathy should not be regarded as a contraindication to pregnancy.

Autonomic neuropathy

Neuropathy can be demonstrated in diabetic women in pregnancy, but it is uncommon as a clinical problem. It can occasionally present with gastric symptoms of severe and continued vomiting leading to metabolic disturbance. This can be associated with fetal loss [95].

Obstetric management

There is a certain artificiality in attempting to distinguish between obstetric and medical management of diabetic pregnancy when there are so many problems that require a joint approach. The distinction is further blurred by the interests of the individuals undertaking care of diabetic mothers. In some centres the obstetricians may be responsible for the total management of these women, whereas in others it may be a physician or even a paediatrician who decides on how and when the diabetic mother should be delivered. Nevertheless, although, as has been repeatedly emphasized in this chapter, the most important contribution to management is good control of maternal blood glucose, there are numerous issues which only the obstetrician can decide upon. As the guardian of the fetus he or she has a responsibility to ensure that fetal development is proceeding satisfactorily from the time of conception until delivery. For instance, in early pregnancy congenital malformations should be excluded, whilst in later pregnancy, detection of excessive fetal growth and/or hydramnios is often evidence that diabetic control needs to be improved.

The management decisions with which the obstetrician is faced can be considered sequentially according to the duration of pregnancy.

First trimester

As soon as pregnancy is confirmed, the diabetic mother should attend hospital and preferably a joint clinic for antenatal care. An ultrasound examination at this time is essential for dating the pregnancy. Pedersen and Molsted-Pedersen [137,138] have suggested that the finding of delayed growth from measurement of the crown–rump length is peculiar to diabetic pregnancy and that it is evidence of future growth retardation and likely congenital malformation. Other authors have been unable to substantiate this observation [25]. If there is any concern at all about the quality of diabetic control, admission to hospital is advised. This provides a good opportunity to educate the mother. She may need to be advised on nutrition and to be convinced of the importance of achieving normoglycaemia in the interests of her baby. Hopefully, the mother will already be familiar with measuring her own blood glucose at home, but if not, she should be taught at this stage.

The mother who is found to have GDM needs particularly careful counselling so that she understands that, although the diabetes may disappear after pregnancy, attention to diabetic control is essential if the risk to the fetus is to be minimized. All these women will be treated by some dietary restriction whether or not they take additional insulin. They will need to be motivated to accept the discipline this requires in the interests of their babies. Effective counselling takes time and, if the woman is not admitted to hospital, the midwife, dietitian and diabetic health visitor should be prepared to spend plenty of time with her at the first visit or ideally perform a home visit.

Second trimester

From the little that is known of intrauterine life in diabetic pregnancy, it appears that the second trimester is a time of relative security for the fetus of the woman with well-controlled diabetes. Organogenesis is virtually complete and excessive growth due to fetal hyperinsulinism appears to only manifest itself after 26 weeks gestation. Ultrasound screening for congenital malformations should be discussed with all mothers and is best done at 18–20 weeks' gestation. If the glycosylated haemoglobin fraction in early pregnancy is high (>10 per cent) then a detailed cardiac scan should be done at about 20 weeks because of the higher incidence of cardiac abnormalities associated with diabetes. Scanning should also aim to exclude a neural tube defect and sacral agenesis which are known to be increased in diabetic pregnancy [94]. If maternal serum α fetoprotein screening is performed care is needed with interpretation since the values are lower in diabetic pregnancy [190]. The incidence of Down's syndrome is not increased, but if serum marker screening is being used again care is needed with interpretation [191].

The frequency of antenatal visits can be determined in general by the degree of blood glucose control which has been achieved. Should proteinuria occur, protein and creatine excretion should be measured over 24 hours along with plasma urea, urate and creatinine. Many obstetricians and physicians like to have baseline renal function tests done as early as possible in pregnancy in all diabetic mothers whether or not they have proteinuria. Ultrasound measurements of head and abdominal circumference should start at 24–26 weeks to act as a baseline for the serial assessment of growth of the fetus in the remainder of the pregnancy.

Third trimester

The last 12 weeks of pregnancy is the time when the combination of good medical and obstetric care is likely to have the greatest impact on fetal health. Complications such as pregnancy-induced hypertension, hydramnios and fetal macrosomia, preterm labour and perinatal death are increased in the poorly controlled diabetic. Good control achieved in the earlier months of pregnancy has to be maintained in the face of increasing insulin requirements. The obstetrician must be constantly on the lookout for any problems, in particular the development of maternal hypertension or hydramnios or of fetal macrosomia.

Indices of fetal well-being

Ultrasound

Most studies have shown that the head size in diabetic pregnancy remains within normal limits [87]. This is not surprising since brain size has not been reported to be increased in diabetic pregnancy and head size is a poor indicator of fetal weight. The measurement of abdominal circumference of the fetus is a better index of fetal weight in the pregnant diabetic [139] and should be performed every 2 weeks in the third trimester along with an assessment of amniotic fluid volume. Examples of two abnormal growth patterns are shown in Fig. 11.9. Umbilical artery Doppler flow velocity waveforms have been used widely in diabetic pregnancy. Early promising results in their ability to differentiate the at risk pregnancy have not been substantiated [72,160]. The consensus view is that abnormal results tend to be only found in cases where growth retardation has already been detected. Accordingly, there is no point in their routine use in all diabetic pregnancies; the technique should be reserved for helping in the management of the growth retarded fetus.

Antenatal fetal heart rate (FHR) monitoring

FHR monitoring is a useful means of assessing fetal health irrespective of whether maternal diabetes is present. Curet and Olson [27] in a study of a heterogenous population, found that perinatal death was six times higher amongst those with an abnormal contraction stress test than if the test was normal. Conversely a normal non-stress test can be used to allow pregnancy to continue. If the test is performed two or three times a week from 36 weeks gestation onwards, many who would be delivered before 38 weeks of gestation because of the obstetrician's anxiety about the possibility of intrauterine death, can be allowed to progress nearer to term. This is now the most widely accepted practice. Teramo *et al.* [182] found a significant correlation between abnormal non-stress tests and poor metabolic control. This is in agreement with the findings that

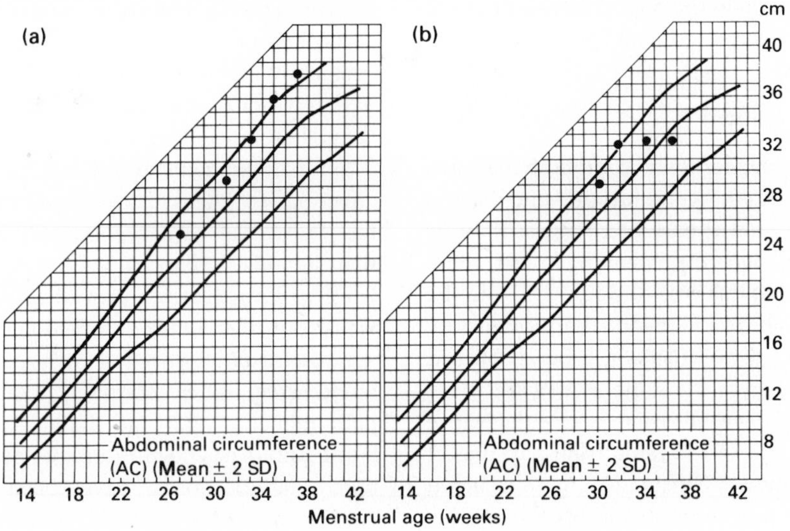

Fig. 11.9. Abnormal fetal abdominal circumference growth patterns in diabetic pregnancy: (a), Excessive fetal growth. Diabetes not optimally controlled, induced at 38 weeks, shoulder dystocia. 4340 g female infant. (b), Excessive fetal growth with superimposed growth retardation. Spontaneous labour at 37 weeks, late decelerations, fetal acidosis, emergency caesarean section. 2580 g female infant. (M. Maresh, unpublished observations.)

FHR variation correlates well with the degree of fetal acidaemia in diabetic pregnancy [158]. However, six of 12 fetuses in this study with a pH below the fifth centile had normal heart rate variability.

Great care must be taken in deciding how frequently tests of fetal well-being and growth should be done and also in their interpretation. This can only be conducted by experienced staff who are aware of the details of the case, and are either a part of or have good liaison with the obstetric/diabetic team. In the well-controlled woman with permanent normoglycaemia, FHR monitoring may be unnecessary [76].

Biophysical profile

The biophysical profile has been proposed as part of routine care [33,71]. However, there is no evidence to support the addition of ultrasound detection of fetal breathing, movement and tone to a surveillance programme of standard ultrasound and cardiotocography. Salvesen *et al.* [158] noted a correlation between fetal acidaemia and the biophysical profile score, but nine of 12 fetuses with a pH below the fifth centile had normal scores. The biophysical profile does not appear to have a role in routine care and even in the high risk case a normal result should be interpreted with care.

Pregnancy complications

In the past, the incidence of complications such as pregnancy-induced hypertension, ante-partum haemorrhage and urinary tract infection was thought to be increased in diabetic pregnancy. In fact, there is little evidence that this is so nowadays [23]. In the UK Survey of Diabetic Pregnancy the incidence of pre-eclampsia — 12 per cent amongst the established diabetic mothers — was the same as that for those with GDM [10]. However, what is of significance is the increased risk to the fetus from any one of these complications of pregnancy in association with diabetes. Pre-eclampsia and pyelonephritis have a prominent place in Pedersen's classification of prognostically bad signs of pregnancy in diabetics [135]. The appearance of a potentially life-threatening complication of pregnancy to the fetus is an indication for hospital admission and possibly delivery within a short time.

Pre-term labour

In diabetic pregnancies the incidence of pre-term delivery (<37 completed weeks of gestation) is increased. Molsted-Pedersen [116] reported a threefold increase in women with mild diabetes for which there are two main reasons. In the UK Survey of Diabetic Pregnancy [10], 50 per cent of women with established diabetes were delivered before 38 weeks of gestation. Approximately two-thirds of these women were induced or were delivered by elective caesarean section, either because of suspected fetal compromise or because of established routine management. The remaining third went into spontaneous labour for reasons that are unknown, but some early deliveries were likely to have been associated with hydramnios. The effect of pre-term delivery on the baby of the diabetic mother is likely to be more serious than on that the non-diabetic because of the known predisposition of the former to complications such as respiratory distress.

Tocolytic drugs, which prevent pre-term labour by suppressing uterine contractions, and glucocorticoids administered to the mother to achieve premature maturation of the fetal lungs also induce hyperglycaemia and can cause diabetes to become completely uncontrolled precipitating ketoacidosis. β sympathomimetic drugs have a gluconeogenic effect whilst glucocorticosteroids antagonize insulin. Individual case reports [13] have suggested that steroids and tocolytics can safely be used in women with diabetes providing blood glucose is well controlled with intravenous insulin. Intravenous insulin is needed in large concentrations immediately after starting parenteral β sympathomimetics and an initial starting dose of 5 units/hour has been recommended [13] although much larger doses have been required [7]. Additional potassium, at a rate of about 100 mmol every 24 hours, is recommended to counteract the drug induced hypokalaemia [7].

This form of treatment is obviously only suitable for a short period, usually 24 hours, while the simultaneously administered steroids are having their effect. There is little place for delaying delivery more than 24 hours to increase the maturity of the fetus if phosphatidyl glycerol concentrations in the amniotic fluid show pulmonary maturity. In addition, the treatment is potentially dangerous to the mother and fetus. Hyperglycaemia has usually been caused by failing to realize that the insulin infusion pump was not working.

Timing and route of delivery

In the past, unexpected still-birth was a relatively common event near term in the pregnant diabetic woman. This led to a policy of delivery at a gestational age when the fetus was considered to have a reasonable chance of extrauterine survival [184] usually between 36 and 38 weeks. As a result, the incidence of hyaline membrane disease rose. Usher *et al.* [188] demonstrated that a policy of early intervention leads to pre-term delivery and to the increased use of caesarean section. Delayed pulmonary maturation of the fetus is a feature of diabetic pregnancy [14]. This is thought to be primarily due to a deficiency of one of the important constituents of pulmonary surfactant — phosphatidyl glycerol. Measurement of phosphatidyl glycerol in the amniotic fluid is a useful index of whether the baby is likely to develop respiratory distress but it involves an amniocentesis near term. Fortunately, improved diabetic control and the recent tendency to allow an increasing number of women to go into spontaneous labour has diminished the need for amniocentesis for phosphatidyl glycerol measurement. Ideally it should be measured prior to elective caesarean section if there is any doubt about the fetal maturity, and in cases of pre-term labour if there is any doubt about whether or not to suppress labour. Unfortunately, being rarely used it may be difficult to find a laboratory prepared to do the test.

A policy of delivery between 36 and 38 weeks of gestation for women with established diabetes is common in the UK and is often applied as well to those with GDM. Table 11.5 shows that the incidence of delivery by caesarean section was as high as 58 per cent amongst mothers with established diabetes in the UK. Even amongst the GDM group, the incidence was 33 per cent.

Now that it is accepted that good diabetic control improves the prognosis for the baby, it seems reasonable to intervene less and to allow more women to go into spontaneous labour near term. There is increasing evidence of the safety of waiting for the onset of spontaneous labour, providing that the diabetes is well controlled and the pregnancy is uncomplicated. Drury [35] in Dublin has reported on a series of 285 pregnant women with established diabetes (Table 11.5). His practice was to assume that diabetic women would go into spontaneous labour unless complications supervened. His results are in marked contrast with those of the Survey of Diabetic Pregnancy in the UK (1979–80) [10], with the incidence of pre-term delivery and the caesarean section rate being much lower in Dublin because of a less interventionist policy. When perinatal mortality is considered, the two studies are not strictly comparable for perinatal mortality because it is likely that diabetic control was considerably better overall in the Dublin series, due to the individual care provided by one physician. Nevertheless the important point that can still be

Table 11.5. Comparison of the incidence of caesarean section, pre-term labour and perinatal mortality amongst mothers with established diabetes from the National Maternity Hospital, Dublin [35] and the UK Survey of Diabetic Pregnancy [10]

		Caesarean section rate			
	n	Elective (%)	Intrapartum (%)	Gestation <38 weeks (%)	PNM (per 1000)
UK Survey	664	43	15	51	61
NMH Dublin	285	19	7	18	45

made is that there was no obvious adverse fetal or neonatal outcome from less interventionist obstetric management.

These results underline one of the basic tenets of modern obstetric practice. 'Across the board' policies on such an important issue as the route and timing of delivery are no longer acceptable — each case should be assessed on its merits which in the case of maternal diabetes includes diabetic control and fetal well-being. If the fetus is in good condition and normally grown, the mother's pregnancy is uncomplicated with her diabetes well controlled, there is no cause for intervention. Nor is there any obvious reason to repeat a caesarean section if the indications for the operation in a previous pregnancy were non-recurrent. However, elective caesarean section may be indicated for a number of valid reasons, such as demonstrable fetal compromise or a baby which, on clinical and ultrasound assessment, is so large that traumatic vaginal delivery is a serious hazard. It needs to be stressed that whilst a much more liberal view about allowing vaginal delivery can be taken nowadays, this approach must be accompanied by careful antenatal assessment by an experienced obstetrician, good control of the blood glucose of the mother and the use of cardiotocography and fetal pH estimation if required, throughout labour.

Intrapartum monitoring

The fetus of the gestational and of the established diabetic should always be regarded as being at particular risk during labour no matter how well controlled the diabetes is. Fetal asphyxia and disproportion are particular hazards, and apart from close surveillance required during labour with good control of blood glucose and fetal monitoring, the presence of an experienced obstetrician is required at the delivery.

There is no good evidence that the well-recognized FHR abnormalities and acidosis — which are diagnostic of fetal asphyxia in the non-diabetic — are in any way different in the case of diabetes. The most common cause of an abnormal FHR pattern in labour is secondary to maternal hyperglycaemia so the first step in the management of an abnormal FHR is to ensure normoglycaemia is present.

Contraception

Advice on contraception before and after pregnancy is an important part of the present day care of diabetic women during the reproductive years. The subject is difficult because of the adverse effects of some methods of contraception on metabolic and circulatory systems. Equally, diabetes may interfere with the effectiveness of contraceptives. The various methods are now discussed but for a comprehensive review the reader is referred to Skouby *et al.* [167].

Oral contraceptives (OC)

There is well-documented evidence that the combined OC interferes with the metabolism of women with subclinical diabetes [11], with a trend towards worsening glucose tolerance and rising triglycerides. The current consensus is that in combined preparations, it is the progestogenic component which is mainly responsible for the diabetogenic effect of oral contraceptives.

Steel and Duncan [169] observed an increase in insulin requirements in only 17 out of 88 diabetics who had started OC and there was no difference between 30 and 50 μg oestrogen preparations. If, as seems likely, deterioration of glucose tolerance in diabetics is the product of increasing insulin resistance, then those women who have presented with GDM during pregnancy would be more liable to remain diabetic if they took OC after pregnancy. However in general, women with previous GDM were shown by Skouby *et al.* [166] not to have had a worsening of their glucose tolerance when contrasted to controls when given low dose OC, although, the insulin response to glucose increased significantly. Effects on lipid profile have been investigated and reviewed [167]; in general current preparations do not appear to have effects with the possible exceptions of the monophasic ethinyloestradiol/norethisterone preparations. Little data have been published on the metabolic effects of the newer progestrogens such as gestodene, but what is available suggests no change in glycaemic control [167].

An increased risk of thrombotic or thromboembolic lesions in diabetic women on OCs has long been postulated. The combination of proliferative intimal vascular lesions which are known to occur as a complication of diabetes, and an increase in platelet aggregation induced by OCs, sets the scene for thrombus formation. Steel and Duncan [169] reported an alarming incidence of near fatal lesions in insulin-requiring diabetic women aged below 30 years on OCs compared with a similar group not on OCs. These ranged from cerebral ischaemia to myocardial infarction. These authors have argued that because it is the oestrogen component of the OC that induces the abnormal clotting, it is logical to use a 'progestogen-only' OC. The disadvantages of this method of contraception are an increased failure rate (six per 100 woman years) and a 50 per cent rate of menstrual irregularity.

Intrauterine contraceptive device (IUCD)

This should be an ideal method of contraception for women with diabetes. It has been suggested that copper-bearing devices are rendered ineffective more frequently in insulin-requiring diabetic women as compared with non-diabetic, by the tendency for the copper to become encrusted with sulphur and chloride, and to be eroded [56]. However, in a large series the failure rate for copper IUCDs was not found to be increased in diabetic women [165] and the corrosive process was no different from that found in controls and was purely time dependent.

Other methods

Whilst mechanical methods (male and female condom and diaphragm) are currently unfashionable they remain effective alternatives without the disadvantages of the pill in particular.

Sterilization

Sterilization is particularly indicated when there is evidence of progressive vascular degeneration and/or nephropathy but should only be performed after full consultation with the diabetic woman and her partner. All diabetic women should consider some limitation of their family. Laparoscopic sterilization, as a day case, is the method of choice because it involves minimal disturbance of diabetic control and care of the baby.

Pregnancy may have such disastrous consequences for the diabetic woman with severe nephropathy or progressive retinopathy that occasionally it is necessary to advise termination of pregnancy. In such cases sterilization should obviously be discussed with the diabetic woman and her partner.

References

1 Akazawa AM, Hashimoto M *et al*. Effects of hypoglycaemia on early embryogenesis in rat embryo organ culture. *Diabetologia* 1987; **30**: 791–6.

2 Alban Davies H, Clark JDA, Dalton KJ & Edwards OM. Insulin requirements of diabetic women who breast feed. *British Medical Journal* 1989; **298**: 1357–8.

3 Ali Z & Alexis SD. Occurrence of diabetes mellitus after gestational diabetes mellitus in Trinidad. *Diabetes Care* 1990; **13**: 527–9.

4 Artal R, Mosley GM & Dorey FJ. Glycohemoglobin as a screening test for gestational diabetes. *American Journal of Obstetrics and Gynecology* 1984; **148**: 412–14.

5 Bacigalupo G, Langner K & Saling E. Glycosylated haemoglobin (HbA_1), glucose tolerance and neonatal outcome in gestational diabetic and non diabetic mothers. *Journal of Perinatal Medicine* 1984; **12**: 137–45.

6 Baker L, Egler JM, Klein SH & Goldman AS. Meticulous control of diabetes during organogenesis prevents congenital lumbo-sacral defects in rats. *Diabetes* 1981; **30**: 955–9.

7 Barnett AH, Stubbs SM & Mander AM. Management of premature labour in diabetic pregnancy. *Diabetologia* 1980; **18**: 365–8.

8 Beard RW, Gillmer MDG, Oakley NW & Gunn PJ. Screening for gestational diabetes. *Diabetes Care* 1980; **3**: 468–71.

9 Beard RW & Hoet JJ. Is gestational diabetes a clinical entity? *Diabetologia* 1982; **23**: 307–12.

10 Beard RW & Lowy C. The British Survey of Diabetic Pregnancies. Commentary. *British Journal of Obstetrics and Gynaecology* 1982; **89**: 783–6.

11 Beck P. The effect of oral anticonceptual drugs on diabetes mellitus. In: Camerini-Davalos RA & Cole HS (eds), *Early Diabetes in Early Life. Proceedings of the Third International Symposium, Madeira, 1974*. Academic Press, London, 1975: 349–52.

12 Biesenbach G & Zazgornik J. Incidence of transient nephrotic syndrome during pregnancy in diabetic women with and without pre-existing microalbuminuria. *British Medical Journal* 1989; **299**: 366–7.

13 Borberg C, Gillmer MDG, Beard RW & Oakley NW. Metabolic effects of beta-sympathomimetic drugs and dexamethasone in normal and diabetic pregnancy. *British Journal of Obstetrics and Gynaecology* 1978; **85**: 184–9.

14 Bourbon JR & Farrell PM. Fetal lung development in

the diabetic pregnancy. *Pediatric Research* 1985; **19**: 253–67.

15 Bradley RJ, Brudenell JM & Nicolaides KH. Chronic fetal hypoxia in diabetic pregnancy. *British Medical Journal* 1988; **296**: 790.

16 Buchanan TA, Schemmer JK & Freinkel N. Embryotoxic effects of brief maternal insulin-hypoglycemia during organogenesis in the rat. *Journal of Clinical Investigation* 1986; **78**: 643–9.

17 Buschard K, Buck I, Molsted-Pedersen L, Hougaard P & Kuhl C. Increased incidence of true type I diabetes acquired during pregnancy. *British Medical Journal* 1987; **294**: 275–9.

18 Cardell BA. Hypertrophy and hyperplasia of the pancreatic islets in new born infants. *Journal of Pathology and Bacteriology* 1953; **66**: 335–8.

19 Carson BS, Phillips AF & Simmons MA. Effects of a sustained insulin infusion upon glucose uptake and oxygenation of the ovine fetus. *Pediatric Research* 1980; **14**: 147–52.

20 Churchill JA, Berendes HW & Nemore J. Neuropsychological deficits in children of diabetic mothers. *American Journal of Obstetrics and Gynecology* 1969; **105**: 257–67.

21 Combs CA, Gunderson E, Kitzmiller JL, Gavin LA & Main EK. Relationship of fetal macrosomia to maternal postprandial glucose control during pregnancy. *Diabetes Care* 1992; **15**: 1251–7.

22 Coetzee EJ & Jackson WPU. Metformin in management of pregnant insulin-dependent diabetes. *Diabetologia* 1979; **16**: 241–5.

23 Cousins L. Pregnancy complications among diabetic women: review 1965–85. *Obstetrical and Gynecological Survey* 1987; **42**: 140–9.

24 Cousins L, Dattel BJ, Hollingsworth DR & Zettner A. Glycosylated hemoglobin as a screening test for carbohydrate intolerance in pregnancy. *American Journal of Obstetrics and Gynecology* 1984; **150**: 455–60.

25 Cousins L, Key TC, Schorzman L & Moore TR. Ultrasonographic assessment of early fetal growth in insulin-treated diabetic pregnancies. *American Journal of Obstetrics and Gynecology* 1988; **159**: 1186–90.

26 Coustan DR & Lewis SB. Insulin therapy for gestational diabetes. *Obstetrics and Gynecology* 1978; **51**: 306–10.

27 Curet LB & Olson RW. Oxytocin challenge tests and urinary oestriols in the management of high risk pregnancies. *Obstetrics and Gynecology* 1980; **55**: 296–300.

28 Damm P & Molsted-Pederson L. Significant decrease in congenital malformations in newborn infants of an unselected population of diabetic women. *American Journal of Obstetrics and Gynecology* 1989; **161**: 1163–7.

29 Damm P, Molsted-Pedersen L & Kühl C. High incidence of diabetes mellitus and impaired glucose tolerance in women with previous gestational diabetes. *Diabetologia* 1989; **32**: 479A (abstract).

30 Deuchar EM. Culture *in vitro* as a means of analysing the effect of maternal diabetes on embryonic development in rats. In: Elliott K & O'Conner M (eds), *Pregnancy Metabolism Diabetes and the Fetus*. Ciba Foundation Symposium, No. 63. Excerpta Medica, Amsterdam, 1979: 181–97.

31 Dibble CM, Kochenour NK, Worley RJ, Tyler FH & Swartz M. Effect of pregnancy on diabetic retinopathy. *Obstetrics and Gynecology* 1982; **59**: 699–704.

32 Dicker D, Feldberg D, Samuel N, Yeshaya A, Karp M & Goldman JA. Spontaneous abortion in patients with insulin-dependent diabetes mellitus: The effect of preconceptional diabetic control. *American Journal of Obstetrics and Gynecology* 1988; **158**: 1161–4.

33 Dicker D, Feldberg D, Yeshaya A, Peleg D, Karp M & Goldman JA. Fetal surveillance in insulin-dependent diabetic pregnancy: Predictive value of the biophysical profile. *American Journal of Obstetrics and Gynecology* 1988; **159**: 800–4.

34 Dornhorst A, Bailey PC, Anyaoku V, Elkeles RS, Johnston DG & Beard RW. Abnormalities of glucose tolerance following gestational diabetes. *Quarterly Journal of Medicine* 1990; **284**: 1219–28.

35 Drury MI. Management of the pregnant diabetic — are the pundits right? *Diabetologia* 1986; **29**: 10–12.

36 Drury PL & Doddridge M. Pre-pregnancy clinics for diabetic women. *Lancet* 1992; **340**: 919.

37 Efendic S, Hansson U, Persson B, Wajngot A & Luft R. Glucose tolerance, insulin release, and insulin sensitivity in normal-weight women with previous gestational diabetes mellitus. *Diabetes* 1987; **36**: 413–19.

38 Eriksson UJ & Borg LAH. Diabetes and embryonic malformations: role of substrate-induced free-oxygen radical production for dysmorphogenesis in cultured rat embryos. *Diabetes* 1993; **42**: 411–19.

39 Eriksson UJ, Dahlstrom E & Hellerstrom C. Diabetes in pregnancy. Skeletal malformations in the offspring of diabetic rats after intermittent withdrawal of insulin in early gestation. *Diabetes* 1983; **32**: 1141–5.

40 Essex NL, Pyke DA, Watkins PJ, Brudenell JM & Gamsu HR. Diabetic pregnancy. *British Medical Journal* 1973; **iv**: 89–93.

41 Fallucca F, Gargiulo P *et al*. Amniotic fluid insulin, C peptide concentrations, and fetal morbidity in infants of diabetic mothers. *American Journal of Obstetrics and Gynecology* 1985; **153**: 534–40.

42 Forrester JV, Towler HMA & Pearson DWM. Pregnancy and diabetic retinopathy. In: Sutherland HW, Stowers JM & Pearson DWM (eds), *Carbodydrate Metabolism in Pregnancy and the Newborn*, Volume IV. Springer-Velag, Berlin, Heidelberg, 1989: 189–200.

43 Fox H. The placenta in diabetes mellitus. In: Sutherland HW, Stowers JM & Pearson DWM (eds), *Carbodhydrate Metabolism in Pregnancy and the Newborn*, Volume IV. Springer-Verlag, Berlin, Heidelberg,

1989: 109–17.

44 Fraser RB. High fibre diets in pregnancy. In: Campbell DM & Gillmer MDG (eds), *Nutrition in Pregnancy*. Royal College of Obstetricians and Gynaecologists, London, 1983: 269–77.

45 Fraser RB, Ford FA & Milner RDG. A controlled trial of a high dietary fibre intake in pregnancy — effects on plasma glucose and insulin levels. *Diabetologia* 1983; **25**: 238–41.

46 Freinkel N. Effects of the conceptus on maternal metabolism during pregnancy. In: Leibel NBA & Wrenshall GA (eds), *On the Nature and Treatment of Diabetes*. Excerpta Medica Foundation, Amsterdam, 1965.

47 Frisoli G, Naranjo L, Shehab N. Glycohemoglobins in normal and diabetic pregnancy. *American Journal of Perinatology* 1985; **2**: 183–7.

48 Fuhrmann K, Reiher H, Semmler K, Fischer F, Fischer M & Glockner E. Prevention of congenital malformations in infants of insulin dependent diabetic mothers. *Diabetes Care* 1983; **6**: 219–23.

49 Gabbe SG, Mestman JH, Freeman RK, Anderson GV & Lowensohn RI. Management and outcome of class A diabetes mellitus. *American Journal of Obstetrics and Gynecology* 1977; **127**: 465–9.

50 Gentz J, Persson B & Zetterstrom R. On the diagnosis of symptomatic neonatal hypoglycaemia. *Acta Paediatrica Scandinavica* 1969; **58**: 449–59.

51 Gillmer MDG, Beard RW, Brooke FM & Oakley NW. Carbohydrate metabolism in pregnancy. Part I. Diurnal plasma glucose profile in normal and diabetic women. *British Medical Journal* 1975; **iii**: 399–402.

52 Gillmer MDG, Beard RW, Brooke FM & Oakley NW. Carbohydrate metabolism in pregnancy. Part II. Relation between maternal glucose tolerance and glucose metabolism in the newborn. *British Medical Journal* 1975; **iii**: 402–4.

53 Gillmer MDG, Holmes SM *et al*. Diabetes in pregnancy: obstetric management 1983. In: Sutherland HW & Stowers JM (eds), *Carbohydrate Metabolism in Pregnancy and the Newborn*. Churchill Livingstone, Edinburgh, 1984: 102–18.

54 Gillmer MDG, Oakley NW, Beard RW, Nithyanawthan R & Cawston M. Screening for diabetes during pregnancy. *British Journal of Obstetrics and Gynaecology* 1980; **87**: 377–82.

55 Gillmer MDG, Oakley NW & Persson B. Diabetes mellitus and the fetus. In: Beard RW & Nathanielsz PW (eds), *Fetal Medicine and Physiology*. Marcel-Dekker, New York, 1984: 211–54.

56 Gosden C, Ross A, Steel J & Springbett A. Intrauterine contraceptive devices in diabetic women. *Lancet* 1982; **i**: 530–5.

57 Grant PT, Oats JN & Beischer NA. The long-term follow-up of women with gestational diabetes. *Australia and New Zealand Journal of Obstetrics and Gynaecology* 1986; **26**: 17–22.

58 Gregory R & Tattersall RB. Are diabetic pre-pregnancy clinics worthwhile? *Lancet* 1992; **340**: 656–8.

59 Gutgesell HP, Mullins CE, Gillette PC, Speer M, Rudolph AJ & McNamara DG. Transient hypertrophic subaortic stenosis in infants of diabetic mothers. *Journal of Pediatrics* 1976; **89**: 120–5.

60 Gutgesell HP, Speer MG & Rosenburg HS. Characterization of the cardiomyopathy in infants of diabetic mothers. *Circulation* 1980; **61**: 441–50.

61 Guthberlet RL & Cornblath M. Infants born to diabetic women. In: Gellis SS & Kagan BM (eds), *Current Pediatric Therapy*. WB Saunders, Philadelphia, 1973: 327–9.

62 Hadden DR. Asymptomatic diabetes in pregnancy. In: Sutherland HW & Stowers JM (eds), *Carbohydrate Metabolism in Pregnancy and the Newborn*. Springer-Verlag, Berlin, 1979: 407–24.

63 Hadden DR. Screening for abnormalities of carbohydrate metabolism in pregnancy 1966–1977: the Belfast experience. *Diabetes Care* 1980; **3**: 440–6.

64 Hagbard L & Svanborg A. Prognosis of diabetes mellitus with onset during pregnancy. *Diabetes* 1960; **9**: 296–302.

65 Hales CN, Barker DJP *et al*. Fetal and infant growth and impaired glucose tolerance at age 64. *British Medical Journal* 1991; **303**: 1019–22.

66 Halliday HL. Hypertrophic cardiomyopathy in infants of poorly-controlled diabetic mothers. *Archives of Disease in Childhood* 1981; **56**: 258–63.

67 Hare JW & White P. Gestational diabetes and White classification. *Diabetes Care* 1980; **3**: 394.

68 Hod M, Merlob P, Friedman S, Schoenfeld A & Ovadia J. Gestational diabetes mellitus: a survey of perinatal complications in the 1980s. *Diabetes* 1991; **40** (suppl 2): 74–8.

69 James DK, Chiswick ML, Harkes A, Williams M & Tindall VR. Maternal diabetes and neonatal respiratory distress. II. Prediction of fetal lung maturity. *British Journal of Obstetrics and Gynaecology* 1984; **91**: 325–9.

70 Jarrett RJ. Gestational diabetes: a non-entity. *British Medical Journal* 1993; **306**: 37–8.

71 Johnson JM, Lange IR, Harman CR, Torchia MG & Manning FA. Biophysical profile scoring in the management of the diabetic pregnancy. *Obstetrics and Gynecology* 1988; **72**: 821–6.

72 Johnstone FD, Steel JM, Haddad NG, Hoskins PR, Greer IA & Chambers S. Doppler umbilical artery flow velocity waveforms in diabetic pregnancy. *British Journal of Obstetrics and Gynaecology* 1992; **99**: 135–40.

73 Jovanovic L, Druzin M & Peterson CM. Effect of euglycaemia on the outcome of pregnancy in insulin-dependent diabetic women as compared with normal control subjects. *American Journal of Medicine* 1981; **71**: 921–7.

74 Jovanovic L & Peterson CM. Insulin and glucose requirements during the first stage of labour in

insulin-dependent diabetic women. *American Journal of Medicine* 1983; **75**: 607–12.
75 Jovanovic-Peterson L, Peterson CM *et al*. Maternal postprandial glucose levels and infant birth weight: The Diabetes in Early Pregnancy Study. *American Journal of Obstetrics and Gynecology* 1991; **164**: 103–11.
76 Jovanovic R & Jovanovic L. Obstetric management when normoglycaemia is maintained in diabetic pregnant women with vascular compromise. *American Journal of Obstetrics and Gynecology* 1984; **149**: 617–23.
77 Jowett NI, Samanta AK & Burden AC. Screening for diabetes in pregnancy: Is a random blood glucose enough? *Diabetic Medicine* 1987; **4**: 160–3.
78 Kalhan SC, Savin SM & Adam PAJ. Attenuated glucose production rate in newborn infants of insulin-dependent diabetic mothers. *New England Journal of Medicine* 1977; **296**: 375–6.
79 Keller JD, Metzger BE, Dooley SL, Tamura RK, Sabbagha RE & Freinkel N. Infants of diabetic mothers with accelerated fetal growth by ultrasonography: Are they all alike? *American Journal of Obstetrics and Gynecology* 1990; **163**: 893–7.
80 Kitzmiller JL, Brown ER *et al*. Diabetic nephropathy and perinatal outcome. *American Journal of Obstetrics and Gynecology* 1981; **141**: 741–51.
81 Kitzmiller JL, Buchanan T & Coustan D. Pre-pregnancy clinics for diabetic women. *Lancet* 1992; **340**: 919–20.
82 Kitzmiller JL, Cloherty JP *et al*. Diabetic pregnancy and perinatal morbidity. *American Journal of Obstetrics and Gynecology* 1978; **131**: 560–80.
83 Kjos SL, Buchanan TA, Greenspoon JS, Montoro M, Bernstein GS & Mestman JH. Gestational diabetes mellitus: the prevalence of glucose intolerance and diabetes mellitus in the first two months post partum. *American Journal of Obstetrics and Gynecology* 1990; **163**: 93–8.
84 Konradi LI & Matveeva OF. Prognostic value of disorders of glucose tolerance in pregnant women. *Problemy Endokrinologii* 1974; **20**: 10–13.
85 Kucera J. Rate and type of congenital anomalies among offspring in diabetic women. *Journal of Reproductive Medicine* 1971; **7**: 61–70.
86 Kuhl C. Aetiology of gestational diabetes. In: Oats JN (ed.), *Diabetes in Pregnancy*. Baillière's Clinical Obstetrics and Gynaecology. WB Saunders, London, 1991: 279–92.
87 Landon MB, Mintz MC & Gabbe SG. Sonographic evaluation of fetal abdominal growth: Predictor of the large-for-gestational-age infant in pregnancies complicated by diabetes mellitus. *American Journal of Obstetrics and Gynecology* 1989; **160**: 115–21.
88 Larsson Y & Ludvigsson J. Perinatal dodlighet vid diabetes-graviditet. *Lakartidningen* 1974; **71**: 155–7.
89 Leslie J, Shen SC & Strauss L. Hypertrophic cardiomyopathy in a midtrimester fetus born to a diabetic mother. *Journal of Pediatrics* 1982; **100**: 631–2.
90 Leslie RDG, Pyke DA, John PN & White JM. Haemoglobin A_1 in diabetic pregnancy. *Lancet* 1978; **ii**: 958–9.
91 Lewis NJ, Akazawa S & Freinkel N. Teratogenesis from B-hydroxybutyrate during organogenesis in rat embryo organ culture and enhancement by subteratogenic glucose. *Diabetes* 1983; **2** (suppl 1): 11A.
92 Lind T. A prospective multicentre study to determine the influence of pregnancy upon the 75 g oral glucose tolerance test. In: Sutherland HW, Stowers JM & Pearson DWM (eds), *Carbohydrate Metabolism in Pregnancy and the Newborn*, Volume IV. Springer-Verlag, Berlin, Heidelberg, 1989: 209–26.
93 Lind T & Anderson J. Does random blood glucose sampling outdate testing for glycosuria in the detection of diabetes during pregnancy? *British Medical Journal* 1984; **289**: 1569–71.
94 Lowy C, Beard RW & Goldschmidt J. Congenital malformations in babies of diabetic mothers. *Diabetic Medicine* 1986; **3**: 458–62.
95 Macleod AF, Smith SA, Sönksen PH & Lowy C. The problem of autonomic neuropathy in diabetic pregnancy. *Diabetic Medicine* 1990; **7**: 80–2.
96 Madsen H. Fetal oxygenation in diabetic pregnancy. *Danish Medical Bulletin* 1986; **33**: 64–74.
97 Malins J. Fetal anomalies related to carbohydrate metabolism. The epidemiological approach. In: Sutherland HW & Stowers JM (eds), *Carbohydrate Metabolism in Pregnancy and the Newborn*. Springer-Verlag, Berlin, 1979: 229–46.
98 Maresh MJA, Beard RW, Bray CS, Elkeles RS & Wadsworth J. Factors predisposing to and outcomes of gestational diabetes. *Obstetrics and Gynecology* 1989; **74**: 342–6.
99 Maresh MJA, Gillmer MDG, Beard RW, Alderson CS, Bloxham BN & Elkeles RS. The effect of diet and insulin on metabolic profiles of women with gestational diabetes mellitus. *Diabetes* 1985; **34** (suppl 2): 880–93.
100 Mazze RS, Shamoon H *et al*. Reliability of blood glucose monitoring by patients with diabetes mellitus. *American Journal of Medicine* 1984; **77**: 211–17.
101 McFarland KF, Murtiashaw M & Baynes JW. Clinical value of glycosylated serum protein and glycosylated haemoglobin levels in the diagnosis of gestational diabetes mellitus. *Obstetrics and Gynecology* 1984; **64**: 516–18.
102 Merkatz IR, Duchon MA, Yamashita TS & Houser HB. A pilot community-based screening programme for gestational diabetes. *Diabetes Care* 1980; **3**: 453–7.
103 Mestman JH, Anderson GV & Guadalupe V. Follow-up study of 360 subjects with abnormal carbohydrate metabolism during pregnancy. *Obstetrics and Gynecology* 1972; **39**: 421–5.
104 Metzger BE, Bybee DE, Freinkel N, Phelps RL, Radvany RM & Vaisrub N. Gestational diabetes mellitus. Correlations between the phenotypic and

genotypic characteristics of the mother and abnormal glucose tolerance during the first year postpartum. *Diabetes* 1985; **34** (suppl 2): 111–15.

105 Metzger BE, Phelps RL, Freinkel N & Navickas IA. Effects of gestational diabetes on diurnal profiles of plasma glucose, lipids, and individual amino acids. *Diabetes Care* 1980; **3**: 402–9.

106 Miller E, Hare JW *et al*. Elevated maternal haemoglobin A_{1C} in early pregnancy and major congenital anomalies in infants of diabetic mothers. *New England Journal of Medicine* 1981; **304**: 1331–4.

107 Mills JL, Knopp RH *et al*. Lack of relation of increased malformation rates in infants of diabetic mothers to glycemic control during organogenesis. *The New England Journal of Medicine* 1988; **318**: 671–6.

108 Mills JL, Simpson JL *et al*. Incidence of spontaneous abortion among normal women and insulin-dependent diabetic women whose pregnancies were identified within 21 days of conception. *New England Journal of Medicine* 1988; **319**: 1617–23.

109 Milner RDG, Ashworth MA & Barson AJ. Insulin release from human fetal pancreas in response to glucose, leucine and arginine. *Journal of Endocrinology* 1972; **52**: 497–505.

110 Milner RDG & Hales CN. Effect of intravenous glucose on concentration of insulin in maternal and umbilical cord plasma. *British Medical Journal* 1965; **i**: 284–6.

111 Milner RDG & Richards B. An analysis of birthweight by gestational age of infants born in England and Wales, 1967–1971. *Journal of Obstetrics and Gynaecology of the British Commonwealth* 1974; **81**: 956–67.

112 Mimouni F, Miodovnik M, Siddiqi TA, Butler JB, Holroyde J & Tsang RC. Neonatal polycythemia in infants of insulin-dependent diabetic mothers. *Obstetrics and Gynecology* 1986; **68**: 370–2.

113 Miodovnik M, Lavin JP, Knowles HC, Holroyde J & Stys SJ. Spontaneous abortion among insulin-dependent diabetic women. *American Journal of Obstetrics and Gynecology* 1984; **150**: 372–6.

114 Miodovnik M, Mimouni F, Tsang RC, Ammar E, Kaplan L & Siddiqi TA. Glycemic control and spontaneous abortion in insulin-dependent diabetic women. *Obstetrics and Gynecology* 1986; **68**: 366–9.

115 Moloney JBM & Drury MI. The effect of pregnancy on the natural course of diabetic retinopathy. *American Journal of Ophthalmology* 1982; **93**: 745–56.

116 Molsted-Pedersen L. Preterm labour and perinatal mortality in diabetic pregnancy. Obstetric considerations. In: Sutherland HW & Stowers JM (eds), *Carbohydrate Metabolism in Pregnancy and the Newborn*. Springer-Verlag, Berlin, 1979: 392–406.

117 Molsted-Pedersen L, Tygstrup I & Pedersen J. Congenital malformations in newborn infants of diabetic women. Correlation with maternal diabetic vascular complications. *Lancet* 1964; **i**: 1124–6.

118 Morris MA, Grandis AS & Litton J. Glycosylated hemoglobin: A sensitive indicator of gestational diabetes. *Obstetrics and Gynecology* 1986; **68**: 357–61.

119 Mortensen HB, Molsted-Pedersen L, Kuhl C & Backer P. A screening procedure for diabetes in pregnancy. *Diabete et Metabolisme* 1985; **ii**: 249–53.

120 Nasrat AA, Johnstone FD & Hasan SAM. Is random plasma glucose an efficient screening test for abnormal glucose tolerance in pregnancy? *British Journal of Obstetrics and Gynaecology* 1988; **95**: 855–60.

121 Naeye RL & Chez RA. Effects of maternal acetonuria and low pregnancy weight gain on childrens' psychomotor development. *American Journal of Obstetrics and Gynecology* 1981; **139**: 189–93.

122 Nylund L, Lunell NO, Lewander R, Persson B, Sarby B & Thornström S. Uteroplacental blood flow in diabetic pregnancy: Measurements with indium 113m and a computer-linked gamma camera. *American Journal of Obstetrics and Gynecology* 1982; **144**: 298–302.

123 Oakley NW. The management of diabetes in pregnancy. In: Rooth G & Bratteby L-E (eds), *Perinatal Medicine. Proceedings of the Fifth European Congress, Uppsala, June, 1976*. Almquist & Wiksell International, Stockholm, 1976: 92–7.

124 Oakley NW, Beard RW & Turner RC. Effect of sustained maternal hyperglycaemia on the fetus in normal and diabetic pregnancies. *British Medical Journal* 1972; **i**: 466–9.

125 Oppenheimer EH & Esterly JR. Thrombosis in the newborn: comparison between diabetic and nondiabetic mothers. *Journal of Pediatrics* 1965; **67**: 549.

126 O'Sullivan JB. Prospective study of gestational diabetes and its treatment. In: Stowers JM & Sutherland HW (eds), *Carbohydrate Metabolism in Pregnancy and the Newborn*. Churchill Livingstone, Edinburgh, 1975: 195–204.

127 O'Sullivan JB. The Boston gestational diabetes studies: review and perspectives. In: Sutherland HW, Stowers JM & Pearson DWM (eds), *Carbohydrate Metabolism in Pregnancy and the Newborn*. Springer-Verlag, London, 1989: 287–94.

128 O'Sullivan JB. Diabetes mellitus after GDM. *Diabetes* 1991; **40** (suppl 2): 131–5.

129 O'Sullivan JB, Charles D, Mahon CM & Dandrow RV. Gestational diabetes and perinatal mortality rate. *American Journal of Obstetrics and Gynecology* 1973; **11**: 901–4.

130 O'Sullivan JB, Gellis SS, Dandrow RV & Tenney BO. The potential diabetic and her treatment in pregnancy. *Obstetrics and Gynecology* 1966; **27**: 683–9.

131 O'Sullivan JB & Mahan CM. Criteria for the oral glucose tolerance test in pregnancy. *Diabetes* 1964; **13**: 278–85.

132 O'Sullivan JB, Mahan CM, Charles D & Dandrow RV. Screening criteria for high risk gestational diabetic patients. *American Journal of Obstetrics and Gynecology* 1973; **116**: 895–900.

133 Paterson KR, Lunan CB & MacCuish AC. Severe

transient nephrotic syndrome in diabetic pregnancy. *British Medical Journal* 1985; **291**: 1612.
134 Pedersen J. *The Pregnant Diabetic and her Newborn — Problems and Management*. Munksgaard, Copenhagen, 1977.
135 Pedersen J & Molsted-Pedersen L. Prognosis of the outcome of pregnancies in diabetics. A new classification. *Acta Endocrinologica* 1965; **50**: 70–4.
136 Pedersen J & Molsted-Pedersen L. Congenital malformations: the possible role of diabetes care outside pregnancy. In: Elliott K & O'Connor M (eds), *Pregnancy, Metabolism, Diabetes and the Fetus, Ciba Symposium No. 63*. Excerpta Medica, Amsterdam, 1979: 265–81.
137 Pedersen J & Molsted-Pedersen L. Early growth retardation in diabetic pregnancy. *British Medical Journal* 1979; **i**: 18–19.
138 Pedersen J & Molsted-Pedersen L. Early fetal growth delay detected by ultrasound marks increased risk of congenital malformations in diabetic pregnancy. *British Medical Journal* 1981; **283**: 269–71.
139 Pedersen J & Molsted-Pedersen L. Sonographic estimation of fetal weight in diabetic pregnancy. *British Journal of Obstetrics and Gynaecology* 1992; **99**: 475–8.
140 Persson B, Bjork O, Hansson U & Stangenberg M. Neonatal management 1983. In: Sutherland HW & Stowers JM (eds), *Carbohydrate Metabolism in Pregnancy and the Newborn*. Churchill Livingstone, Edinburgh, 1984: 133–43.
141 Persson B, Gentz J & Lunell NO. Diabetes in pregnancy. In: Scarpelli EM & Cosmi EV (eds), *Reviews in Perinatal Medicine*. Raven Press, New York, 1978; **2**: 1–55.
142 Persson B, Gentz J & Stangenberg M. Neonatal problems. In: Sutherland HW & Stowers JM (eds), *Carbohydrate Metabolism in Pregnancy and the Newborn*. Springer-Verlag, Berlin, 1979: 376–91.
143 Persson B & Lunell NO. Metabolic control in diabetic pregnancy. *American Journal of Obstetrics and Gynecology* 1975; **122**: 737–45.
144 Persson B, Stangenberg M, Hansson U & Nordlander E. Gestational diabetes mellitus (GDM): comparative evaluation of two treatment regimes, diet versus insulin and diet. *Diabetes* 1985; **34** (suppl 2): 101–5.
145 Pettitt DJ, Knowler WC, Baird HR & Bennett PH. Gestational diabetes: infant and maternal complications of pregnancy in relation to third-trimester glucose tolerance in the Pima Indians. *Diabetes Care* 1980; **3**: 458–64.
146 Phipps K, Barker DJP, Hales CN, Fall CHD, Osmond C & Clark PMS. Fetal growth and impaired glucose tolerance in men and women. *Diabetologia* 1993; **36**: 225–8.
147 Piper JM & Langer O. Does maternal diabetes delay fetal pulmonary maturity? *American Journal of Obstetrics and Gynecology* 1993; **168**: 783–6.
148 Price JH, Hadden DR, Archer DB & Harley JMcDG. Diabetic retinopathy in pregnancy. *British Journal of Obstetrics and Gynaecology* 1984; **91**: 11–17.
149 Reid M, Hadden D, Harley JMG, Halliday HL & McClure BG. Fetal malformation in diabetics with high haemoglobin A_{1c} in early pregnancy. *British Medical Journal* 1984; **289**: 1001.
150 Rizzo T, Metzger BE, Burns WJ & Burns K. Correlations between antepartum maternal metabolism and intelligence of offspring. *New England Journal of Medicine* 1991; **325**: 911–16.
151 Roberts AB, Baker JR, Court DJ, James AG, Henley P & Ronayne ID. Fructosamine in diabetic pregnancy. *Lancet* 1983; **ii**: 998–9.
152 Roberts AB, Baker JR, Metcalf P & Mullard C. Fructosamine compared with a glucose load as a screening test for gestational diabetes. *Obstetrics and Gynecology* 1990; **76**: 773–5.
153 Roversi GD, Gargiulo M *et al*. A new approach to the treatment of diabetic pregnant women: 479 cases (1963–75). *American Journal of Obstetrics and Gynecology* 1979; **135**: 567–76.
154 Ryan EA, Stark R, Crockford PM & Suthijumroon A. Assessment of value of glycosylated albumin and protein in detection of gestational diabetes. *Diabetes Care* 1987; **10**: 213–16.
155 Salvesen DR, Brudenell MJ & Nicolaides KH. Fetal polycythemia and thrombocytopenia in pregnancies complicated by maternal diabetes mellitus. *American Journal of Obstetrics and Gynecology* 1992; **166**: 1287–93.
156 Salvesen DR, Brudenell JM, Proudler AJ, Crook D & Nicolaides KH. Fetal pancreatic β-cell function in pregnancies complicated by maternal diabetes mellitus: Relationship to fetal acidemia and macrosomia. *American Journal of Obstetrics and Gynecology* 1993; **168**: 1363–9.
157 Salvesen DR, Brudenell JM, Snijders RJM, Ireland RM & Nicolaides KH. Fetal plasma erythropoietin in pregnancies complicated by maternal diabetes mellitus. *American Journal of Obstetrics and Gynecology* 1993; **168**: 88–94.
158 Salvesen DR, Freeman J, Brudenell JM & Nicolaides KH. Prediction of fetal acidaemia in pregnancies complicated by maternal diabetes mellitus by biophysical profile scoring and fetal heart rate monitoring. *British Journal of Obstetrics and Gynaecology* 1993; **100**: 227–33.
159 Salvesen DR, Higueras MT, Brudenell JM, Drury PL & Nicolaides KH. Doppler velocimetry and fetal heart rate studies in nephropathic diabetics. *American Journal of Obstetrics and Gynecology* 1992; **167**: 1297–303.
160 Salvesen DR, Higueras MT, Mansur CA, Freeman J, Brudenell JM & Nicolaides KH. Placental and fetal Doppler velocimetry in pregnancies complicated by maternal diabetes mellitus. *American Journal of Obstetrics and Gynecology* 1993; **168**: 645–52.

161 Sartor G, Schersten B, Carlstrom S, Melander A & Persson G. Ten year follow up of subjects with impaired glucose tolerance; prevention of diabetes by tolbutamide and diet regulation. *Diabetes* 1980; **29**: 41–9.

162 Schneider JM, Curet LB, Olson RW & Stay G. Ambulatory care of the pregnant diabetic. *Obstetrics and Gynecology* 1980; **56**: 144–9.

163 Shah BD, Cohen AW, May C & Gabbe SG. Comparison of glycohaemoglobin determination and the one hour oral glucose screen in the identification of gestational diabetes. *American Journal of Obstetrics and Gynecology* 1982; **144**: 774–7.

164 Shelley HJ, Bassett JM & Miller RDG. Control of carbohydrate metabolism in the fetus and newborn. *British Medical Bulletin* 1975; **31**: 37–43.

165 Skouby SO, Molsted-Pedersen L & Kosonen A. Consequences of intrauterine contraception in diabetic women. *Fertility and Sterility* 1984; **42**: 568–73.

166 Skouby SO, Molsted-Pedersen L & Kuhl C. Low dosage oral contraception in women with previous gestational diabetes. *Obstetrics and Gynecology* 1982; **59**: 325–8.

167 Skouby SO, Molsted-Pedersen L & Petersen KR. Contraception for women with diabetes: an update. In: Oats JN (ed.), *Diabetes in Pregnancy*. Baillière's Clinical Obstetrics and Gynaecology. WB Saunders, London, 1991: 493–503.

168 Sonksen PH, Judd SL & Lowy C. Home monitoring of blood glucose. Method for improving diabetic control. *Lancet* 1978; **i**: 729–32.

169 Steel JM & Duncan LJP. Contraception for the insulin-dependent diabetic woman: the view from one clinic. *Diabetes Care* 1980; **3**: 557–60.

170 Steel JM & Johnstone FD. Pre-pregnancy clinics for diabetic women. *Lancet* 1992; **340**: 918–19.

171 Steel JM, Johnstone FD, Hepburn DA & Smith AF. Can prepregnancy care of diabetic women reduce the risk of abnormal babies? *British Medical Journal* 1990; **301**: 1070–4.

172 Steel JM, Johnstone FD & Smith AF. Prepregnancy preparation. In: Sutherland HW, Stowers JM & Pearson DWM (eds), *Carbohydrate Metabolism in Pregnancy and the Newborn*, Volume IV. Springer-Verlag, Berlin, Heidelberg, 1989: 129–39.

173 Steel JM & West CP. Intrauterine death during continuous subcutaneous infusion of insulin. *British Medical Journal* 1985; **290**: 1787.

174 Stehbens JA, Baker GL & Kitchell M. Outcome at ages 1, 3 and 5 years of children born to diabetic women. *American Journal of Obstetrics and Gynecology* 1977; **127**: 408–13.

175 Stowers JM, Sutherland HW & Kerridge DF. Long-range implications for the mother. The Aberdeen experience. *Diabetes* 1985; **34** (suppl 2): 106–10.

176 Stubbs SM, Brudenell JM, Pyke DA & Watkins PJ. Management of the pregnant diabetic: Home or hospital, with or without meters? *Lancet* 1980; **i**: 1122–4.

177 Stubbs SM, Doddridge MC, John PN, Steel JM & Wright AD. Haemoglobin A_1 and congenital malformation. *Diabetic Medicine* 1987; **4**: 156–9.

178 Stubbs SM, Leslie RDG & John PN. Fetal macrosomia and maternal diabetic control in pregnancy. *British Medical Journal* 1981; **282**: 439–40.

179 Susa JB & Schwartz R. Effects of hyperinsulinaemia in the primate fetus. *Diabetes* 1985; **34** (suppl 2): 36–41.

180 Sutherland HW, Bewsher PD *et al*. The effect of moderate dosage of chlorpropamide in pregnancy on fetal outcome. *Archives of Disease in Childhood* 1974; **49**: 283–91.

181 Sutherland HW, Stowers JM & McKenzie C. Simplifying the clinical problem of glycosuria in pregnancy. *Lancet* 1970; **i**: 1069–71.

182 Teramo K, Ammala P, Ylinen K & Raivio KO. Pathological fetal heart rate associated with poor metabolic control in diabetic pregnancies. *Obstetrics and Gynecology* 1983; **61**: 559–65.

183 Third International Workshop Conference on Gestational Diabetes Mellitus, Chicago 1990. Summary and recommendations. *Diabetes* 1991; **40** (suppl 2): 197–201.

184 Titus RS. Diabetes and pregnancy from the obstetric point of view. *American Journal of Obstetrics and Gynecology* 1937; **33**: 386–92.

185 Tsang RC, Kleinman LI, Sutherland JM & Light IJ. Hypocalcemia in infants of diabetic mothers. *Journal of Pediatrics* 1972; **80**: 384–95.

186 Tsang RC, Strub R, Brown DR, Steichen J, Hartman C & Chen I-W. Hypomagnesemia in infants of diabetic mothers: Perinatal studies. *Journal of Pediatrics* 1976; **89**: 115–19.

187 Tyrrell SN. Doppler studies in diabetic pregnancy. *British Medical Journal* 1988; **296**: 428.

188 Usher RM, Allen AC & Maclean FH, Risk of respiratory distress syndrome related to gestational age, route of delivery and maternal diabetes. *American Journal of Obstetrics and Gynecology* 1971; **111**: 826–9.

189 Van Assche FA & Aerts L. The fetal endocrine pancreas. *Contributions to Gynecology and Obstetrics* 1979; **5**: 44–57.

190 Wald NJ, Cuckle H, Boreham J, Stirrat GM & Turnbull AC. Maternal serum alpha-fetoprotein and diabetes mellitus. *British Journal of Obstetrics and Gynaecology* 1979; **86**: 101–5.

191 Wald NJ, Cuckle HS, Densem JW & Stone RB. Maternal serum unconjugated oestriol and human chorionic gonadotrophin levels in pregnancies with insulin-dependent diabetes: implications for screening for Down's syndrome. *British Journal of Obstetrics and Gynaecology* 1992; **99**: 51–3.

192 Wang HS & Chard T. The role of insulin like growth factor-1 and insulin-like growth factor-binding protein-1 in the control of human fetal growth. *Journal of Endocrinology* 1992; **132**: 11–19.

193 Weinstock RS, Kopecky RT, Jones DB & Sunderji S. Rapid development of nephrotic syndrome, hypertension, and hemolytic anemia early in pregnancy in patients with IDDM. *Diabetes Care* 1988; **11**: 416–21.

194 Whichelow MJ & Doddridge MC. Lactation in diabetic women. *British Medical Journal* 1983; **287**: 649–50.

195 White P. Pregnancy and diabetes. Medical aspects. *Medical Clinics of North America* 1965; **49**: 1015–24.

196 Whitelaw A. Subcutaneous fat in newborn infants of diabetic mothers: an indication of quality of diabetic control. *Lancet* 1977; **i**: 15–18.

197 Whittaker PG, Stewart MO, Taylor A, Howell RJS & Lind T. Insulin-like growth factor 1 and its binding protein 1 during normal and diabetic pregnancies. *Obstetrics and Gynecology* 1990; **76**: 223–9.

198 Widness JA, Susa JB *et al*. Increased erythropoiesis and elevated erythropoietin in infants born to diabetic mothers and in hyperinsulinaemic rhesus fetuses. *Journal of Clinical Investigation* 1981; **67**: 637–42.

199 Widness JA, Teramo K & Clemons GK. Direct relationship of anterpartum glucose control and fetal erythropoietin in human type I (insulin-dependent) diabetic pregnancy. *Diabetologia* 1990; **33**: 378–83.

200 Williamson DH. Regulation of the utilisation of glucose and ketone bodies by brain in the perinatal period. In: Camerini-Davalos RA & Cole HS (eds), *Early Diabetes in Early Life*. New York: Academic Press, 1975: 200.

201 World Health Organization. *Expert Committee: Diabetes Mellitus Technical Report Series* 1980: 646.

202 Ylinen K, Aula P, Stenman UH, Kesaniemi-Kuokkanen T & Teramo K. Risks of minor and major fetal malformations in diabetics with high haemoglobin A_{1c} values in early pregnancy. *British Medical Journal* 1984; **289**: 345–6.

203 Ylinen K, Raivio K & Teramo K. Haemoglobin A_{1c} predicts the perinatal outcome in insulin-dependent diabetic pregnancies. *British Journal of Obstetrics and Gynaecology* 1981; **88**: 961–7.

204 Yssing M. Long term prognosis of children born to mothers diabetic when pregnant. In: Camerini-Davalos RA & Cole HS (eds), *Early Diabetes in Early Life*. Proceedings of the 3rd International Symposium, Madeira. New York: Academic Press, 1975: 575–86.

205 Yudkin JS & Knopfler A. Glucose and insulin infusions during labour. *Lancet* 1992; **339**: 1479.

12

Thyroid Disease

Ian Ramsay

Normal thyroid physiology, 459
Effect on pregnancy of thyroid physiology
Thyroid function in the fetus
Relationship of maternal to fetal pituitary–thyroid axis
Thyroid disease in pregnancy, 463
Endemic goitre
Sporadic goitre
Hypothyroidism
Thyrotoxicosis
Fetal and neonatal thyrotoxicosis
Post-partum thyroiditis
Thyroid nodules

In most developed countries thyroid disease is relatively uncommon in pregnancy, only about two per 1000 pregnancies being associated with hyperthyroidism and nine per 1000 being complicated by hypothyroidism [133]. In these countries the problems are that the obstetrician is usually unfamiliar with thyroid disease and the physician may be unaware of the ways in which the pregnant state may modify the clinical presentation of these diseases and may alter the results of thyroid function tests. However, in many parts of the Third World the major thyroid problem in pregnancy is that of iodine deficiency and endemic goitre. It is estimated that throughout the world 800 million people live in areas of iodine deficiency [67], up to 250 million suffer from endemic goitre [143] and, in some regions, 10 per cent or more of the children are born as cretins [170]. This terrible toll could be totally prevented by the prophylactic intramuscular injection of iodized oil every 4 or 5 years, at a cost of between 3 and 4 pence per head of the population each year or by the annual administration of oral iodized oil [175]. It is almost impossible to measure what effect this proportion of retarded and crippled beings has upon the productivity of people whose economic status is already very low.

No excuse, therefore, is made for including a section on the effect of endemic goitre in pregnancy but, before discussing thyroid disease, it is necessary to consider the normal physiology of the thyroid gland and the ways in which it is altered by pregnancy, the physiology of the fetal thyroid and the relationship between the thyroid status of mother and fetus.

Normal thyroid physiology

The thyroid gland produces two hormones thyroxine (T_4) and tri-iodothyronine (T_3). Although T_3 is secreted by the thyroid gland, a large proportion of it (70–80 per cent) is produced by the peripheral monodeiodination of T_4. It is thought that, functionally, T_3 is a more important hormone than T_4. In order to make T_4 and T_3 it is essential for the thyroid gland to have an adequate supply of iodine. Dietary iodide, absorbed from the gut into the blood stream is actively trapped by the follicular cells of the thyroid which can concentrate it 20 times more than in the perfusing blood. Between 100 and 200 μg of iodide are taken up by the thyroid each day.

The iodide in the thyroid is oxidized to iodine which then iodinates tyrosyl residues present in thyroglobulin to form monoiodotyrosine (MIT) and di-iodotyrosine (DIT). MIT and DIT molecules combine and form either T_4 (tetra-iodothyronine) or T_3 (Fig. 12.1).

Once the thyroid hormone has been formed it is joined to thyroglobulin and stored in the colloid of the follicle. In order for thyroid hormones to be

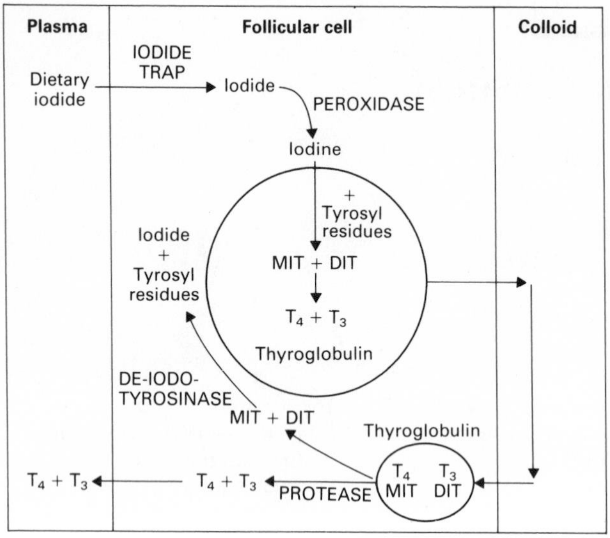

Fig. 12.1. The synthesis of thyroid hormones. MIT, monoiodotyrosine; DIT, di-iodotyrosine; T_4, thyroxine; T_3, tri-iodothyronine.

released, colloid droplets are taken up by the apical border of the follicular cell. Lysosomes cause the release of T_4, T_3, MIT and DIT: MIT and DIT are deiodinated and the iodide is largely stored in the thyroid in order to be used again. Some of it passes into the blood. T_4 and T_3 are secreted in a ratio of 5:1. Of the T_4 30–40 per cent is deiodinated peripherally to form T_3. An even greater proportion (50 per cent) is converted to an inactive hormone called reverse T_3 (rT_3) [18].

Thyroid hormones circulate in the blood almost entirely bound to plasma proteins. Of the bound T_4 85 per cent is attached to a specific protein called T_4 binding globulin (TBG). The rest is bound either to T_4 binding pre-albumin or to albumin itself [185]. Only 0.05 per cent of T_4 is in the free, unbound, form. T_3 is bound to TBG to a lesser extent, so that 0.5 per cent of the hormone circulates in the free state. The half-life of T_4 in the blood is about 1 week but that of T_3 is only 1–1.5 days.

The synthesis and secretion of thyroid hormones is controlled by thyroid stimulating hormone (TSH or thyrotrophin), synthesized in the pituitary, which binds to receptors on the thyroid follicular cell membrane. This binding to TSH receptors activates adenylcyclase which catalyses the formation of cyclic adenosine monophosphate (cAMP) from adenosine triphosphate (ATP). TSH binding also increases cytosol calcium and causes increased synthesis of prostaglandins. All three mechanisms seem to play a part in thyroid hormone synthesis.

The amount of TSH stimulation of the thyroid depends upon how much is synthesized and released from the pituitary gland. This is controlled largely by the negative feedback of thyroid hormones on the pituitary, though the sensitivity of this feedback mechanism is modulated by a hypothalamic hormone called thyrotrophin releasing hormone (TRH) which passes down the portal vessels of the pituitary stalk and renders the pituitary thyrotroph cells more sensitive to the feedback mechanism. Increased amounts of TSH are present in situations when thyroid hormone levels are low, as in hypothyroidism. Conversely, TSH is suppressed when thyroid hormone levels are high, as in hyperthyroidism. The net result in hypothyroidism is an enhanced basal release of TSH by the pituitary which can be increased even further by the administration of TRH [135]. In hyperthyroidism the secretion of TSH is inhibited and cannot be increased by TRH [60].

Thyroid hormones are important physiologically because of their major role in energy production. The hormones are bound to cell mitochondria which produce the high energy bonds of ATP. Small amounts of thyroid hormone encourage the formation of ATP but large amounts, as in hyperthyroidism, have a converse effect, causing a reduction in the amount of ATP and bringing about a waste of energy as heat. Two other important actions of thyroid hormones are their effect upon the stimulation of protein synthesis and upon growth in children.

Effect on pregnancy of thyroid physiology

Before the 12th week of pregnancy there is evidence of a reduction in the renal tubular absorption of iodide which probably occurs because of the increased glomerular filtration rate (Chapter 7). As a result the urinary excretion of iodide doubles, the plasma level falls, and the thyroid gland is forced to triple its uptake of iodine from the blood [3]. In situations where there is already at least a partial deficiency of iodine in the diet, the thyroid gland hypertrophies in order to be able to manufacture a sufficient amount of thyroid hormone. Thus, in Aberdeen, Crooks *et al.* [25] found that 70 per cent of pregnant women, when examined carefully, had a goitre. In a part of Belgium where there is a marginally low iodine intake goitre was found in 9 per cent of women at term [56]. In an area of Italy with moderate iodine deficiency goitres increased in size during pregnancy and this could be prevented by the prophylactic administration of iodine [152]. Crooks *et al.* [25] carried out a survey in Iceland, where the dietary intake of iodine is high, and found that there was no increase in the prevalence of goitre during pregnancy. Similarly in the USA, where domestic salt is almost always iodized, iodine balance was not found to be compromised during pregnancy [36] and goitre was no commoner in the pregnant than in the non-pregnant female population [94]. Thus it seems that most cases of pregnancy goitre could be prevented by an adequate intake of iodine.

How the compensatory increase in thyroid size comes about is, at the moment, unknown. Theoretically the hypertrophy should be brought about by an increased secretion of TSH, but so far there is no general agreement that this occurs in pregnancy. Human chorionic gonadotrophin (HCG) has thyroid-stimulating properties during the first trimester of pregnancy which may be sufficient to suppress serum TSH concentrations and prevent a rise in TSH following TRH administration [56,58,184]; amounts such as are found in hydatidiform mole or choriocarcinoma may even cause hyperthyroidism [21,65, 66,85,136,144,176]. A chorionic thyrotrophin has been described but its existence is doubtful and all placental thyroid-stimulating properties are thought to be due to HCG [65,154]. Thyrotrophin-releasing hormone has been isolated from the placenta [53,159]. Any effect this might have on the thyroid would have to be mediated by TSH.

The second major effect of pregnancy upon thyroid metabolism is that of increased placental oestrogen secretion upon the synthesis of TBG by the liver. By the 12th week of pregnancy the serum concentration of TBG has doubled [100,125]. The result is that increased amounts of both T_4 and T_3 are bound and this is reflected in increased total concentrations of thyroid hormones in the blood. It is possible to measure the amount of binding of thyroid hormones to TBG by means of tests such as the T_3 resin uptake test, and from this and the total amount of hormone to calculate a free T_4 or free T_3 index. Unfortunately in situations such as pregnancy or oestrogen medication, the high TBG levels tend to make the estimation of free hormone a little erroneous [14], the derived free hormone levels tending to be higher than those obtained by their direct measurement. Measurement of actual free T_4 and free T_3 shows slight falls of both hormones below the normal non-pregnant range in the second trimester and more marked reductions in the third trimester (see Fig. 12.4), though there are some discordant results in the literature [76,138,144].

Figure 12.2 shows values of total T_4, T_3 resin uptake (RU) and free T_4 index (FTI) in normal pregnancy at term and also normal non-pregnant ranges. Free T_4 (Fig. 12.3) measured by equilibrium dialysis shows a close approximation to non-pregnant levels though it is apparent that mean values are slightly less than in the normal non-pregnant female. Free T_3 concentrations (Fig. 12.3) are appreciably lower than the normal non-pregnant range. The normal ranges for free T_4 and free T_3 throughout pregnancy are shown in Fig. 12.4.

The highly sensitive immunoradiometric assay (IRMA) for TSH [16] provides the most accurate information about thyroid status in pregnancy. Values below normal will suggest thyrotoxicosis or autonomous thyroid function; this occurs in

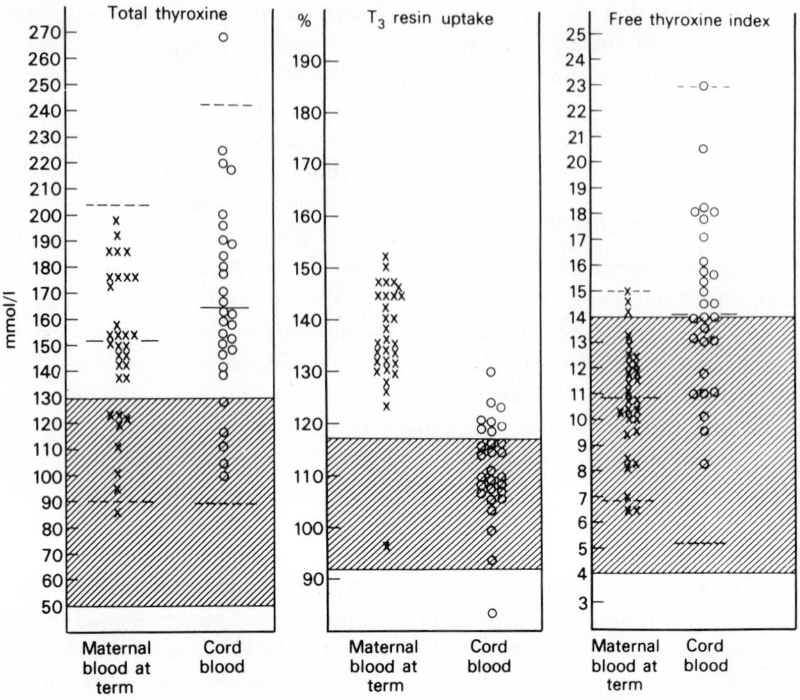

Fig. 12.2. Total T_4, T_3 resin uptake and free T_4 index in maternal blood at term and in cord blood. The mean values are indicated by a solid line and 2 SD from the mean by broken lines. The shaded areas indicate the normal adult non-pregnant ranges. (Data from [147].)

approximately 40 per cent of patients with multinodular goitre. The only likely error of interpretation will be in the first trimester of pregnancy when the high HCG levels stimulate the thyroid and tend to suppress TSH [56,58]. IRMA TSH levels will be raised in primary hypothyroidism.

Thyroid function in the fetus

The fetal thyroid begins to secrete T_4 by the 12th week of intrauterine life and at the same time TSH is just detectable in fetal blood. Concentrations of TSH, total and free T_4, total and free T_3 and TBG increase steadily until term [9,173]. The fetal TSH at term is higher than that of the mother: the total T_4 is about the same or marginally greater (see Fig. 12.2). Although fetal TBG is increased, owing to the effects of placental oestrogen [35] its concentration is not as high as in the mother. Consequently the fetal FTI at term is higher than in the mother [158] (see Fig. 12.2). Fetal free T_4 is also significantly higher at term than in the mother [150] (Fig. 12.3). Fetal total T_3 is very much lower than in the mother, being about one-third of the value: free T_3 is also lower [39] (Fig. 12.3). However, the inactive hormone, reverse T_3 is increased in the fetus [19]. It is likely that the low free T_3 levels are responsible for the slightly elevated amounts of TSH in fetal blood [91].

Within 30 min of birth, neonatal TSH levels rise sharply to a mean peak level of 86 μU/ml [43] and this is followed within a few hours by rises in total T_4 and T_3 [4,39]. Indeed, a state of physiological hyperthyroidism takes place, so that blood sampled a day or two after birth will be in the adult thyrotoxic range. It is probable that this surge of TSH and physiological hyperthyroidism is an adaptive phenomenon brought about by the immediate drop in ambient temperature consequent upon birth, though it is possible that more general 'stress' may play a part [43]. After 72 hours [43] the TSH has

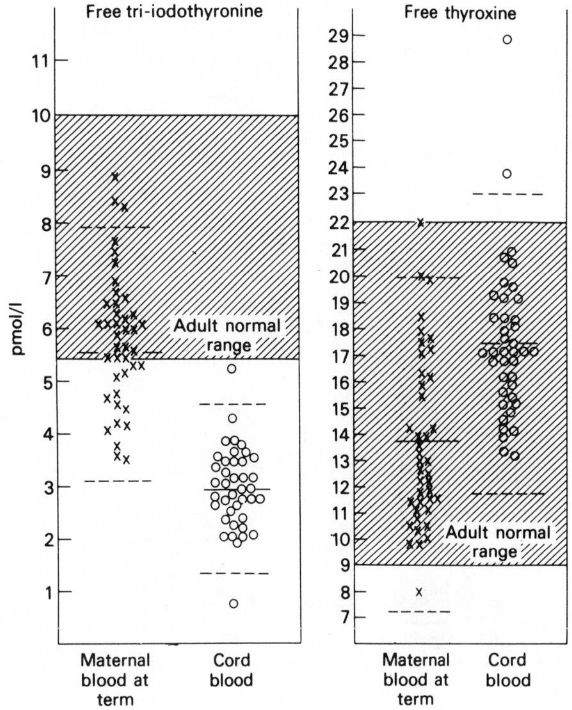

Fig. 12.3. Free T_3 and free T_4 in maternal blood at term and in cord blood measured by equilibrium dialysis. Mean values are indicated by solid lines and 2 SD from the mean by broken lines. The shaded areas indicate the normal adult non-pregnant ranges. (Data from [147].)

returned virtually to normal. Total T_3 returns to normal values in the same length of time [39], but total T_4 takes about a week to return to normal. However, free hormone levels are raised for longer periods [39]. These factors must be borne in mind when testing thyroid function in the neonate.

For fuller accounts and further information about intrauterine and neonatal thyroid function see [9,44,47,173].

Relationship of maternal to fetal pituitary–thyroid axis

The control of the thyroid in mother and fetus is almost entirely separate, though it is probable that the fetus is totally dependent upon the mother for supplies of thyroid hormone during the first 3 months of intrauterine life [38,67]. Thyroid hormones do cross the placenta, in amounts that produce about 25–50 per cent of normal T_4 concentrations in athyrotic fetuses at term [45,93,178]. In addition, pharmacological doses of iodine [51] and ingested antithyroid drugs or other goitrogens will cross the placenta and may cause both a goitre and hypothyroidism in the fetus. A full list of potential goitrogenic agents is shown in Box 12.1. It is important to avoid giving any of these substances to a pregnant woman and, if it is necessary (as in the treatment of maternal hyperthyroidism), the dose should be kept to the minimum necessary for the control of the disease. A difficult problem is self-medication, usually by iodine-containing proprietary cough preparations, of which the doctor may be unaware [51].

Thyroid disease in pregnancy

Endemic goitre

Up to 800 million people throughout the world are affected by iodine deficiency, and of these 250 million have a goitre [85,92,143]. The prevalence of goitre may vary from area to area because of other factors, such as goitrogens in food and water, auto-

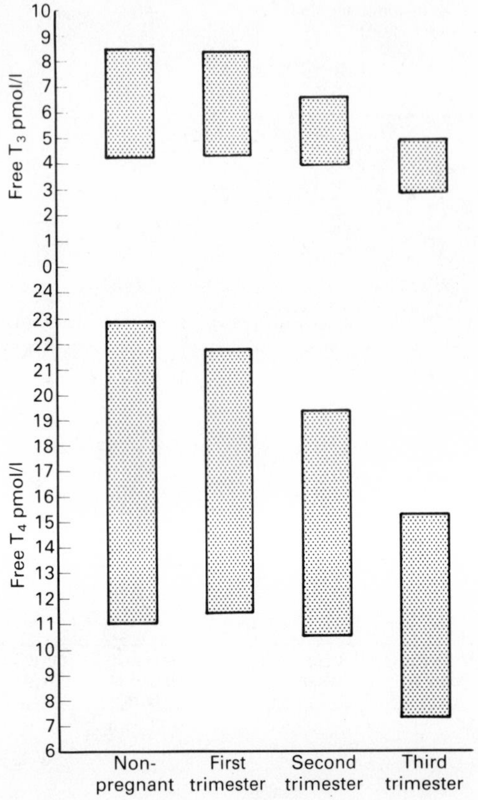

Fig. 12.4. Free T_3 in normal (upper panel) pregnancy measured by Amerlex kit. Free T_4 in normal pregnancy measured by Amerlex kit (lower panel). (Data from [138].)

Box 12.1. Potential goitrogens. Those which have been shown to produce fetal goitre are printed in bold. The others do not normally cause goitre in the fetus but may possibly be goitrogenic in areas of endemic iodine deficiency [41,50,57,111,149]

- Drugs used in the treatment of thyrotoxicosis
  - **Carbimazole**
  - **Methimazole**
  - **Propyl thiouracil**
  - **Methyl thiouracil**
  - **Potassium perchlorate**
  - **Iodides** in doses as low as 12 mg/day
  - Radioactive iodine may cause fetal hypothyroidism but not goitre
- **Iodine**-containing drugs:
  - **Idoxuridine ophthalmic solution** 18 mg of iodine per drop

Continued

Box 12.1. (*Continued*)

- **Amiodarone** 75 mg of iodine per 200 mg tablet
  - **Iodine tincture** 40 mg of iodine per ml
  - **Povidone iodine** 10 mg/ml
  - **Renografin** 370 mg/ml
  - **Iopanoic acid (Telepaque)** 333 mg/tablet
  - **Iodized oil (Lipiodol)** 370–480 mg/ml
- Drugs used for other conditions
  - Acetazolamide
  - Aminoglutethimide
  - Antihistamines
  - Cobalt-containing drugs
  - Ethionamide
  - Lithium
  - Methylxanthines
  - Para-aminobenzoic acid
  - Phenylbutazone
  - Resorcinol
  - Sulphonamides
  - Sulphonylureas
  - Thiocyanate
- Foodstuffs
  - Cassava, Maize, Sorghum, Sweet potatoes } contain cyanogenic glycosides which may be converted to thiocyanate
  - Cabbage
  - Cauliflower
  - Brussels sprouts
  - Piñon nuts
  - Rutabagas
  - Turnips
- Other dietary factors
  - Calcium
  - *Escherichia coli* in drinking water
  - Fluoride
  - Nitrate
  - Rubidium
  - Sulphurated hydrocarbons (from sedimentary rocks) in drinking water

immune disorders [13] and genetic susceptibility. The areas most affected now are the Andes in South America, the Himalayan region, south-east Asia, Papua New Guinea and central Africa. In these areas up to 100 per cent of the female population may have a goitre [88], so clearly a goitre will frequently be present in a pregnant woman. In most patients with endemic goitre, frank hypothyroidism is not present because the fall in T_4 levels due to iodine deficiency leads to a compensatory rise in TSH. This stimulates the growth of the thyroid, leads to an increased uptake of iodine by the gland and causes the thyroid to secrete T_3 in preference to T_4. This is of advantage to the individual since each molecule of T_3 only requires three iodine atoms instead of the four necessary for T_4; T_3 is also the more important of the two hormones.

However, the presence of endemic goitre has a deleterious effect on the outcome of the pregnancy. In patients whose thyroid has not managed to compensate and who are hypothyroid, the fetal wastage will be about 30 per cent [112] due to miscarriages, still-births and congenital abnormalities [72]. Even in mothers who are euthyroid, the iodine deficiency during the first 3 months of pregnancy may lead to failure of proper development of the fetal central nervous system so that the baby is born with neurological cretinism. The baby is usually clinically euthyroid, but may have biochemical hypothyroidism, more often than not has a goitre, and is suffering from mental retardation, deafness and spasticity. This type of cretinism, which is due more to iodine deficiency than to fetal hypothyroidism, is the type usually found in South America and Papua New Guinea [143]. It does not respond to any form of treatment.

When iodine deficiency leads to fetal hypothyroidism in the second and third trimester of pregnancy, the baby is born as a hypothyroid cretin. The baby is lethargic, has a large tongue, a hoarse cry, dry coarse skin, a pot belly and sometimes an umbilical hernia. Neonatal jaundice may be prolonged, the infant feeds badly, is constipated and has weak muscles. Goitre is less commonly present than in neurological cretins and this may be due to thyroid growth blocking immunoglobulin [13]. This type of cretinism responds to iodine supplementation [176a] or to thyroid hormone replacement, the efficacy of which is directly related to how soon after birth it is started. The hypothyroid type of cretinism occurs commonly in central Africa and affects up to 11 per cent of all babies born [143,170]. It is not known for certain why some areas of iodine deficiency have mainly cretins of the neurological variety whilst other areas have hypothyroid cretins. It is thought that, in the latter case, dietary ingestion of goitrogens, such as occur in cassava (a starchy root vegetable) may play some part.

Both forms of cretinism and the effects of maternal hypothyroidism on the outcome of pregnancy can be prevented by treatment with iodine before the pregnancy occurs. This can be done either by the use of iodized salt or by the intramuscular injection of 2–4 ml of iodized oil every 4 or 5 years [68]. Both forms of treatment are very cheap, the former costing 3–5 US cents per person per year and the latter 10–15 US cents per person per year [90]. More recently it has been shown that oral administration of iodized oil gives protection for at least 1 year [175]. It is important for doctors practising in areas of endemic goitre to press for money to prevent this avoidable disease.

Sporadic goitre

Most Western developed countries have eliminated endemic goitre by the use of iodized salt (e.g. Switzerland and the USA), but there nevertheless remains a residuum of patients who have a goitre. These patients are described as having 'sporadic goitre'. In patients with non-toxic goitre it is difficult to know what factors are important in aetiology. In California amongst the 6 per cent of pregnant teenagers who had a goitre 50 per cent had a simple non-toxic goitre, 28 per cent had autoimmune thyroid disease and 22 per cent had subacute thyroiditis [94]. Clearly relative iodine deficiency or ingested goitrogens may play a part in the genesis of non-toxic goitre, or there may be a partial defect in one of the enzymes necessary for the formation of thyroid hormones. Autoimmune thyroiditis, as evidenced by the presence of significant titres of thyroid antibodies, is much more common than was thought previously, and in one series, accounted for two out of every three young girls presenting with what appeared to be a 'simple goitre' [59]. A 'thyroid growth stimulating immunoglobulin', has been described by Drexhage *et al.* [35]; the presence of this immunoglobulin may account for the growth of a goitre in those patients who have no other obvious cause.

During pregnancy pre-existing sporadic goitres tend to become bigger, possibly because of the effects of iodine deficiency or because of HCG stimulation in the first trimester. In Aberdeen, 70 per cent of pregnant women were shown to have a goitre, whereas in Iceland and the USA, countries with a high iodine intake, there was no increase in the prevalence of goitre in pregnancy compared with the non-pregnant state [25,26,94].

It would seem sensible to promote an adequate iodine intake during pregnancy in a woman who has a simple goitre. This can be done simply by the use of iodized salt in cooking and at the table. One part of iodine per 40 000 of salt will give an average daily intake of 700 μg, which is adequate.

If there is evidence of thyroiditis (e.g. positive thyroid microsomal antibodies) or of a possible partial enzyme defect (elevated TSH level with or without normal thyroid hormone levels and no thyroid antibodies), it is reasonable either to monitor thyroid function on a monthly basis or to give the patient replacement T_4 during pregnancy to obviate the possibility of sub-clinical hypothyroidism and further growth of the goitre. A useful guide to dosage is 2 μg of T_4 per kilogram of bodyweight per day. An adequate amount has been given when the TSH has been suppressed into the normal range. Excessive dosage can be avoided by checking the free T_4, though note that it tends to fall below the normal non-pregnant range as pregnancy progresses [76,138] (see Fig. 12.4).

Hypothyroidism

Severe hypothyroidism leads to an increased conversion of oestradiol to oestriol which interferes with hypothalamic feedback and causes anovulation [171]. Some patients with hypothyroidism have hyperprolactinaemia secondary to increased hypothalamic release of TRH, and this causes amenorrhoea [171]. Patients with less severe hypothyroidism may suffer from menorrhagia due to acyclical shedding of the endometrium due to chronic unopposed oestrogen stimulation [171].

Previously undiagnosed hypothyroidism was found on screening in three per 1000 pregnant women [94]. Frank hypothyroidism diagnosed pre-pregnancy or during pregnancy occurs in nine per 1000 white and three per 1000 black women [133].

It is important to diagnose hypothyroidism in pregnancy since abortion and still-birth rates are twice as high in hypothyroid women as in controls [133,171]. In one study of 16 pregnancies in untreated hypothyroid women, maternal complications included anaemia (31 per cent), pre-eclampsia (44 per cent), placental abruption (19 per cent) and post-partum haemorrhage [29]. Birth-weight of <2 kg occurred in 31 per cent and the fetal death rate was 12 per cent [29]. Although one review suggested that even in treated hypothyroid patients the congenital anomaly rate was three times normal [171], a community-based case-controlled study showed no increased risk in hypothyroid patients, whether or not they had received thyroid hormone [86]. Even the presence of thyroid antibodies in pregnant euthyroid women seems to have some adverse effect on the outcome, the spontaneous abortion rate being two to four times greater than in women with no antibodies [56,163].

In one 7-year follow-up study of the children of women who were hypothyroid during pregnancy, their intelligence quotient was only 91.1 compared with 104.5 for children whose mothers received adequate amounts of thyroid hormone replacement during pregnancy [99]. However, a more recent study has shown no evidence of intellectual or physical disability in babies born of hypothyroid mothers [122]. Nevertheless, because the fetus is totally dependent upon maternal thyroid hormone during the first 12 weeks of intrauterine life, it would seem logical to optimize thyroid hormone replacement throughout the whole of pregnancy.

The symptoms which should draw one's attention to the possible diagnosis of hypothyroidism are fatigue, hair loss, dry skin [29], excessive weight gain despite a poor appetite and cold intolerance (a feature which is unusual in pregnancy). Muscle aches and stiffness and pain or tingling in the median nerve distribution due to the carpal tunnel syndrome, may be additional features. The pulse rate may be inappropriately slow for pregnancy and there may be delayed relaxation of the tendon reflexes ('hung-up jerks') [29]. A goitre may be present in patients with thyroiditis or enzyme defects but will be absent in primary atrophic hypothyroidism.

Thyroid function should be measured in any pregnant woman in whom there is the least suspicion of hypothyroidism. The T_4 will be inappropriately low for pregnancy, but note that it may be in the normal range for non-pregnant women (Fig. 12.5). This is because of the doubling of TBG concentration during pregnancy. A measurement of thyroid hormone binding, such as the T_3 test, will show a very large number of vacant binding sites because of the high TBG and the low T_4. From the T_4 and the T_3RU the FTI can be calculated and will be low, though it may still be in the normal non-pregnant range, since in situations where the TBG is high the FTI may overestimate the true value for free T_4 [14,162]. Again, actual measurement of free T_4 should provide a much more accurate index of thyroid function in pregnancy. Measurement of free T_4 shows a fall below normal values in the second and third trimesters of euthyroid pregnancy [138] so values must always be compared to the normal pregnancy range for that trimester (see Fig. 12.4.) In patients with a low or low–normal free T_4, a TSH level should be done. In primary hypothyroidism this will be elevated. However, it is important to be sure that the immunoassay used is specific for TSH, since in some of the older radioimmunoassays the high HCG of pregnancy will cross-react and will give rise to falsely elevated 'TSH' concentrations. The more modern immunoradiometric assays do not cross-react with HCG.

It has already been mentioned that pre-eclampsia is a common complication of untreated hypothyroid pregnancy [29]. However, hypothyroidism may present in pregnancy with hypertension, oedema and proteinuria, which may closely mimic pre-eclampsia [139]. There is therefore a case for measuring free T_4 and TSH in all such patients until more data are available concerning the frequency with which hypothyroidism causes some of the clinical features of pre-eclampsia.

Once hypothyroidism has been diagnosed, treatment should be instituted without delay. So long as the pregnant woman has no evidence of other, particularly heart, disease, replacement therapy can be instituted rapidly. T_4 can be given in an initial dose of 0.1 mg every morning for a week and then

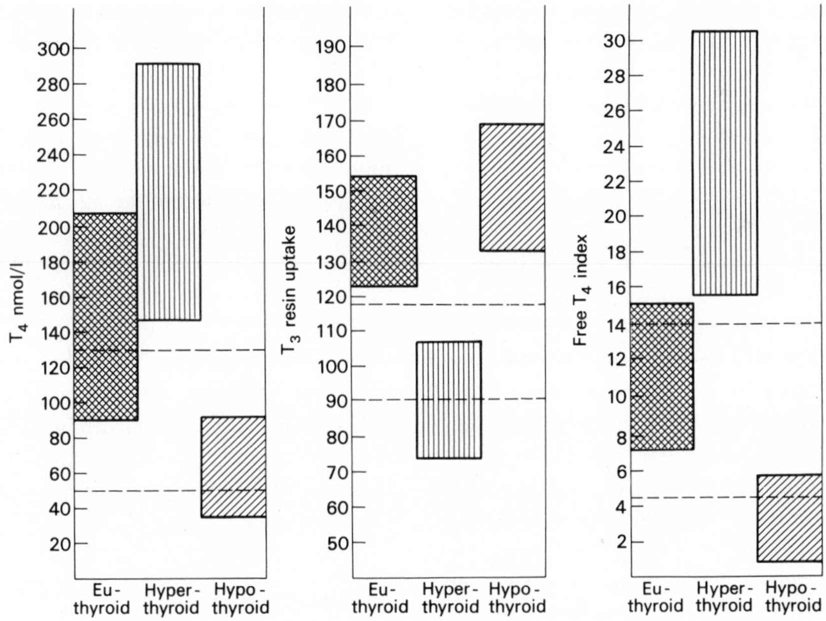

Fig. 12.5. Diagrammatic representation of the ranges of total T_4, T_3RU and free T_4 index which may be found in euthyroid, hyperthyroid and hypothyroid pregnant patients. The normal non-pregnant ranges are indicated by the broken lines. It should be emphasized that the values will vary between laboratories.

adjusted according to the patient's weight. A replacement dose of 2 μg/kg bodyweight provides a rough guide. After a month on this dosage, the free T_4 and the TSH can be re-checked and the dosage altered if both results are not in the normal range. It is wise to continue to check the hormone levels monthly during the rest of pregnancy, because as the patient gains more weight, the dosage of T_4 may need to be increased. Although some have thought that no increase in T_4 dosage in pregnancy is needed [55], others have found it to be necessary [101]. The author's patients have on average required 28 μg more T_4 per day by term compared with the pre-pregnancy requirements. Since the average daily T_4 replacement in an adult is 2 μg/kg, this increase in dosage corresponds closely to the normal weight gain in pregnancy.

Following childbirth, if the mother wishes to do so, there is no contraindication to breast feeding just because she is taking T_4. Usually the dose of T_4 will need to be reduced post-partum because of the loss of weight.

Although babies should all have a routine neonatal thyroid screen, it is wise in the baby of a mother with hypothyroidism to measure free T_4 and TSH on the cord blood, because the mother may have a variety of thyroid-blocking antibodies which pass across the placenta and cause either intrauterine or temporary neonatal hypothyroidism [34,106,164,186]; (see above).

Fetal and neonatal hypothyroidism

For many years now in the developed world neonates have been screened for hypothyroidism and, with prompt treatment, the results of early studies into intellectual and physical development seemed to be good [78,129]. However, there was a suggestion that not all children were achieving their full potential and that some may suffer from minor deficits [129] in motor visuospatial and language areas, particularly those who had evidence of fetal hypothyroidism [155].

More recently attention has therefore focused on fetal hypothyroidism with a view to diagnosis and treatment *in utero*. Of live infants born to mothers with chronic thyroiditis during pregnancy, a quarter of whom were hypothyroid, 23 per cent showed evidence of minor neurological abnormality, with an IQ of less than 80 [104]. The risk seems to be greatest in those mothers with atrophic thyroiditis rather than Hashimoto's thyroiditis with goitre, since three out of 12 of the former had babies with neonatal hypothyroidism, whereas none of the 92 mothers with Hashimoto's thyroiditis delivered other than euthyroid babies. All the mothers with atrophic thyroiditis and hypothyroid babies had positive TSH binding inhibiting immunoglobulins [160] and TSH receptor blocking antibodies [166,168]. There might therefore seem to be a case for measuring these antibodies in pregnant women with hypothyroidism, or at least in those without goitres.

Other fetuses at risk for hypothyroidism are those conceived of parents known to be suffering from defects in enzymes necessary for thyroid hormone synthesis [69], those fetuses of mothers being treated for thyrotoxicosis in pregnancy with large amounts of antithyroid drugs [29] or those exposed to any other potential goitrogen (Box 12.1). The chance finding of a goitre on fetal ultrasound [29,141] might also prompt an attempt to diagnose fetal hypothyroidism.

Amniotic fluid sampling to assess fetal thyroid hormone levels has generally been disappointing [73,156], though in a recent case it demonstrated a raised TSH concentration in a fetus subsequently shown to have neonatal hypothyroidism [69]. But, more recently percutaneous umbilical cord sampling has been found to be an effective way of assessing fetal thyroid function [9,29,141,172,173]. The risks of sampling are fetal bleeding, bradycardia, infection [109] and death [27] and occur in 0.5–1 per cent of procedures.

Once the diagnosis of fetal hypothyroidism has been made the intra-amniotic injection of 500 μg of L-thyroxine every 2 weeks can improve fetal thyroid status [69] or even normalize it [141] and may reduce the size of a fetal goitre, thus making delivery easier.

Thyrotoxicosis

Thyrotoxicosis causes an increased hepatic production of sex hormone binding globulin (SHBG) and leads to a reduced free oestradiol concentration.

This interferes with both negative and positive hypothalamic feedback control of gonadotrophin secretion and results in anovulation and amenorrhoea [82]. Thus severely thyrotoxic patients do not generally become pregnant. However, mildly thyrotoxic patients may do so, though just over 25 per cent of these patients will abort [118].

Thyrotoxicosis occurs in 2.2 per 1000 pregnant white and in 1.7 per 1000 pregnant black women [72,80,121,133]. In the majority of instances the disease has been diagnosed before pregnancy and the patient is taking treatment; however, in about 0.5 per 1000 pregnancies [31] the hyperthyroidism may develop during pregnancy. The most common time for it to occur is between 10 and 15 weeks of pregnancy [7]: in a few it may supervene later in pregnancy, though this is most unusual.

In 95 per cent of cases the thyrotoxicosis is due to Graves' disease, which is caused by TSH receptor stimulating antibodies [82]. Occasionally it may be due to a solitary toxic adenoma or to an autonomously functioning multinodular goitre. Rarely it occurs early on in de Quervain's thyroiditis (see above) or in association with hyperemesis gravidarum, hydatidiform mole and choriocarcinoma (see also above and Chapter 10).

The disease should be suspected in any pregnant patient who fails to gain weight satisfactorily despite a good appetite, and who has either exophthalmos or lid lag and persistent tachycardia. Many of the features of hyperthyroidism such as heat intolerance, palpitations, emotional lability, palmar erythema, goitre and thyroid bruit may also occur in normal pregnancy and thus are not of much diagnostic help. However, a family history of autoimmune thyroid disease is found in about 50 per cent of patients with Graves' disease and should increase one's diagnostic suspicion.

The T_4 will be inappropriately elevated even for normal pregnancy (Fig. 12.5), but the T_3RU will not be so 'hypothyroid' as normally occurs in pregnancy. The resultant FTI will be elevated, but remember that minor elevations of FTI may be found spuriously in pregnancy because of the high TBG levels [14,164]. Much better tests are either the measurement of free T_4 or free T_3, elevated levels of which will determine whether the patient is hyperthyroid, especially when accompanied by a suppressed TSH measured by radioimmunometric assay [16]. This has now obviated the need for thyrotropin releasing hormone tests for the diagnosis of thyrotoxicosis [135].

It is important to treat thyrotoxicosis during pregnancy since, without treatment, the fetal mortality may be as high as 48 per cent [52]. For example, in association with maternal hyperthyroidism, Davis *et al.* [31] described 24 per cent still-births and 53 per cent premature deliveries with only 18 per cent being born alive at term [31]. One group has noted a significantly increased risk of congenital malformation [119], though this is disputed [86]. The untreated pregnant thyrotoxic woman has a 21 per cent chance of a thyroid crisis ('thyroid storm') at the time of delivery [31]. This is a very exaggerated form of thyrotoxicosis with confusion, psychotic behaviour or coma, accompanied by tachycardia, cardiac failure and fever [61]. Heart failure complicated labour in five of eight patients in one series who presented with untreated thyrotoxicosis [31]. Thyroid crisis is considered in detail above.

Antithyroid drugs

The most convenient method of treatment is by means of antithyroid drugs, the commonly used ones being carbimazole (or its metabolite methimazole) and propylthiouracil.

If thyrotoxicosis is newly diagnosed during pregnancy it should be controlled as quickly as possible. This can usually be achieved in 4 or 5 weeks by carbimazole in a dosage of 15 mg 8-hourly or by propylthiouracil 150 mg 8-hourly. The dose is then progressively lowered so that the maintenance dose of carbimazole is 15 mg/day or less and that of propylthiouracil 150 mg/day or less. The ability to use a fairly low maintenance dose is helped by a tendency for TSH receptor stimulating antibodies to fall during pregnancy [118] and for Graves' disease to ameliorate particularly during the last trimester of pregnancy. It is necessary to use the lowest dose of antithyroid drug possible because these agents pass across the placenta very readily and may cause goitre and hypothyroidism in the fetus.

The mother must be seen at least monthly during

pregnancy, preferably by an endocrinologist, for a clinical evaluation and for measurements of free T_4 and TSH. In this way the dose of antithyroid drugs can be adjusted more precisely. Only one-third of the amount of propylthiouracil seems to cross the placenta as carbimazole or methimazole [102] and thus it should have less effect on fetal thyroid function. Propylthiouracil is also favoured by some because it has an effect on reducing the peripheral conversion of T_4 to T_3 [72]. However, in practice there seems to be little difference between the two drugs in the therapeutic effect on mother or fetus [118,120,121].

Early reports of scalp defects (aplasia cutis) in nine infants whose mothers received carbimazole or its metabolite methimazole during pregnancy [115] have not been substantiated by population studies [177] or by extensive clinical experience [119].

Drug rashes or urticaria, more rarely fever or arthralgia occur in 1–5 per cent of patients taking carbimazole or propylthiouracil [22]. The patient should be switched to the alternative preparation in the equivalent dose.

A much rarer complication, agranulocytosis, occurs in 0.2–0.5 per cent of patients [22]. If a patient develops a sore throat or mouth ulcers, the drug should be stopped and a white cell count done. If it is low or absent the patient should be barrier nursed and given intravenous antibiotics. If the condition is caught early the bone marrow should recover in a week or so.

Some physicians try to stop antithyroid drugs completely during the last trimester of pregnancy because of a possible diminution in the activity of Graves' disease at this time. This manoeuvre has the advantage of avoiding the effects of the drug on the fetal thyroid, but necessitates very careful supervision of the mother in case she does become toxic again. This happens in over 60 per cent of patients 2–4 months post-partum [6,7], when it may be overlooked, since weight loss and emotional disturbances are so common at that time.

Graves' disease, however, is a fluctuating condition [102]: these variations in disease activity are probably brought about by changes in the level of thyroid-stimulating antibodies [124]. It is therefore possible for the dose of antithyroid drug, based on the results of thyroid function studies one month, to be inappropriately high or low by the time of the next month's clinical evaluation, so that the patient has become either hypothyroid or thyrotoxic. For this reason some authorities favour the addition of physiological replacement doses of T_4 (see above) to the antithyroid drug [48,158]. In this way the fluctuations in maternal thyroid status are smoothed out and patient management becomes easier. Recent evidence suggests that significant amounts of T_4 cross the placenta [178]. This may help to keep the fetus euthyroid and might explain the reduced risk of goitre in babies whose mothers had received antithyroid drugs plus supplementary T_4 [147]. Critics of this method of treatment object to it because of the need for slightly higher doses of antithyroid drugs than when these drugs are being used alone without supplementary T_4 [10,62,82,114]. However, a comparison of the two methods of treatment shows that the combination of antithyroid drug with T_4 produces less neonatal goitres and cretinism than are produced by the use of antithyroid drugs alone [147].

In my own series [147] of 20 babies whose mothers were treated with a combination of antithyroid drugs and T_4, all of them had normal total and/or free thyroid hormone concentrations in cord blood, whereas, in a study by Mamotani *et al.* [120] of 43 babies, whose mothers had received antithyroid drugs alone, 40 per cent had a cord blood free T_4 below normal and 46.5 per cent had elevated TSH levels. In a later series Momotani and Ito [118] published improved figures showing that in mothers treated with methimazole or propylthiouracil the cord blood free T_4 was below normal in 33 per cent and the TSH was elevated in 29 per cent. They found no correlation between daily drug doses and cord blood free T_4 levels and noted that high TSH values occurred in babies whose mothers were taking 100 mg or less of propylthiouracil per day.

In a series of 11 mothers treated with propylthiouracil, seven of whom also received thyroid supplements (T_4 and T_3), Cheron *et al.* [17a] found a reduction of T_4 and free T_4 index in the cord blood of their babies, compared with controls. They found no differences in the cord hormone levels of the four treated with propylthiouracil alone, compared with those receiving thyroid supplements. A large randomized trial of antithyroid drugs alone versus antithyroid drugs plus T_4 is needed to settle the issue finally. It is my feeling, however, that good results are likely to be achieved by either method if the mother is closely observed during pregnancy and if the doses of drugs are adjusted according to the results of thyroid function tests.

The offspring of thyrotoxic mothers controlled successfully with antithyroid drugs are born at term but tend to be slightly lighter than control babies [113,147]; there is no evidence of an increased risk of congenital malformation [119]. Subsequent growth and both physical and mental development is normal [108,113].

At the time of delivery, cord blood should be taken for free T_4 and TSH concentrations and the paediatricians should be asked to examine the baby to make sure that it has neither goitre, hypothyroidism nor neonatal thyrotoxicosis (see below).

Since antithyroid drugs are excreted in breast milk [181], mothers taking these drugs have been advised not to breast feed. Recent work [83,96] has suggested that the amount of propylthiouracil present in breast milk is insufficient to materially affect neonatal thyroid function. The excretion of methimazole, the active metabolite of carbimazole, appears to be greater than that of propylthiouracil [96], but further studies suggest that no abnormalities of thyroid function appear in neonates whose mothers are taking 15 mg or less of carbimazole per day or 150 mg or less of propylthiouracil per day [57]. If mothers do breast feed while taking antithyroid drugs, thyroid function should be checked periodically in the infant.

β adrenergic receptor blocking drugs

Over the last 20 years or so, there has been a vogue for the use of these drugs in the treatment of thyrotoxicosis, in order to ameliorate the sympathetically mediated symptoms, such as tremor and tachycardia [77,103]. Some people have advocated their use in the treatment of thyrotoxicosis in pregnancy [92].

β blockers relieve mainly the symptoms of thyrotoxicosis, and not the metabolic derangement [84]. Propranolol has been shown to decrease the peripheral conversion of T_4 to T_3 [95,169] and, since the drug crosses the placenta [23], it would seem likely to have this effect on the fetus also, in a situation where circulating T_3 is already low [46]. The other possible side-effects of β adrenergic blockade — intrauterine growth retardation, acute fetal distress in labour, and hypoglycaemia in the neonate — are discussed in Chapter 6. Although the incidence of side-effects is low, it would seem wise to continue to use the already well-established antithyroid drugs as the mainstay of therapy and to only use β adrenergic blockers, such as propranolol, in situations such as thyrotoxic crisis or in severe hyperthyroidism, where there is a very rapid heart rate.

Surgery

Some authors recommend surgery as the treatment of choice for thyrotoxicosis in pregnancy [64], preferably carried out during the middle trimester. However, the general consensus of opinion amongst endocrinologists is that it is unnecessary, since young women with mild to moderate thyrotoxicosis are the very group who are most likely to go into remission after a course of antithyroid drugs. Moreover, since up to 25 per cent of patients become temporarily hypothyroid during the first 6 months after partial thyroidectomy [174], all women treated by surgery will have to be monitored as frequently during their pregnancy as if they were thyrotoxic, so that they can be treated with T_4 as necessary.

There is no doubt, however, that surgery is indicated in certain pregnant women. If the goitre is very large and causing pressure symptoms, if there is any suspicion of malignancy, if the patient is allergic to all antithyroid drugs or if the patient is uncooperative in the taking of antithyroid medication, then surgery would be justified. The latter group of patients, however, continue to be a problem because they frequently do not attend postoperative follow-up appointments and, if they need to be put on T_4, they often either do not take it or take it infrequently.

Radioactive iodine

Radioactive iodine should never be given in pregnancy. It is concentrated in the fetal thyroid from the 12th week on, but 10 times more avidly than in the mother's thyroid. The result will be fetal thyroid destruction and hypothyroidism. There is very little chance of inducing carcinoma of the thyroid in the future since a therapeutic dose of radioactive iodine will ablate the fetal thyroid.

Thyroid crisis

Thyroid crisis or 'storm' is a rapid worsening of the thyrotoxicosis brought about by stresses such as infection, labour, caesarean section or any other type of surgery. Fever is a prominent feature, accompanied by tachycardia or rapid atrial fibrillation and the patient can either be extremely nervous and restless or psychotic and, when *in extremis*, may lapse into coma [117].

This condition should not occur in patients who have been properly controlled with antithyroid drugs during pregnancy, but has been described in 21 per cent of patients whose thyrotoxicosis has been untreated [31]. Treatment must be instituted immediately, for this is a life-threatening condition [61], the mortality being about 10 per cent. Therefore treatment of the mother is the most important consideration, notwithstanding any possible effects of this aggressive therapy on the fetus.

Propylthiouracil is the drug of choice because it not only inhibits thyroid hormone synthesis but also decreases the conversion of T_4 to T_3 peripherally. It should be given orally in large doses of 1000 mg initially, followed by 200 mg 6-hourly. If the patient is unconscious the drug can be introduced via a nasogastric tube [117]. In patients with post-operative ileus methimazole can be administered rectally as a suppository [127]. An hour or two after the antithyroid drug has been administered, and not before, sodium or potassium iodide 500 mg should be given by infusion every 8 hours or by mouth every 6 hours to inhibit the release of thyroid hormone. Dexamethasone 2 mg every 6 hours for the first day has an effect on decreasing the peripheral conversion of T_4 to T_3. So long as there is no evidence of heart failure propranolol can be given for tachyarrhythmias, a 0.5 mg intravenous stat. dose, followed as necessary by 0.5 mg/min up to a maximum of 5 mg, or orally in a dose of 80 mg three times daily. Propranolol also has a beneficial effect on T_4 to T_3 conversion. Reduction of fever can be achieved by tepid sponging or by covering in a wet sheet and using an electric fan. Chlorpromazine has a hypothermic effect and will also be useful for sedation in a dose of 25–50 mg orally or intravenously 6–8-hourly. Aspirin should not be used as a temperature lowering agent since it displaces thyroid hormones from TBG and thus increases the free hormone concentrations.

Intravenous fluids need to be monitored carefully since the patient is losing a large amount of water through the skin. Energy requirements are very high, so glucose should be given.

Heart failure due to rapid atrial fibrillation should be treated in the usual manner with digoxin and diuretics, though the dose of digoxin needs to be higher than normal in a thyrotoxic patient, since the rate of degradation is increased.

Fetal and neonatal thyrotoxicosis

Neonatal hyperthyroidism was first described in 1910 by Ochsner and Thompson in a baby whose mother had exophthalmos and a goitre [134]. Although this condition is considered to be very rare, occurring in only 1 per cent of women with a current or past history of Graves' disease [15], the author has found it in 10 per cent of the babies of mothers with Graves' disease in pregnancy, or with a previous history of Graves' disease [148]. Recent publications indicate that the prevalence is indeed of this order, or even greater. Tamaki *et al.* [168] found it in 9.6 per cent of 104 patients. Mortimer *et al.* [131] in Brisbane found an overall figure of 8 per cent in all women suffering from Graves' disease in pregnancy, but this rose to 22 per cent in the babies of those mothers who had to continue antithyroid drugs to term.

Matsuura *et al.* [105] in Japan had a 25 per cent prevalence of neonatal thyrotoxicosis in untreated mothers and in France 20 per cent of babies developed neonatal thyrotoxicosis in a group of 35 mothers with either active Graves' disease in pregnancy, or a previous history of Graves' disease [20].

Neonatal thyrotoxicosis is due to the transplacental passage of thyroid-stimulating antibodies (TSab). If the mother is euthyroid, following a partial thyroidectomy or is hypothyroid and on replacement T_4, the fetus has no protection from these stimulating antibodies and so may develop thyrotoxicosis *in utero*. The same may happen to the fetus of a thyrotoxic woman who is receiving insufficient antithyroid medication during pregnancy.

The first TSab to be discovered was long-acting thyroid stimulator (LATS); this was detected by its ability to stimulate prolonged uptake of radioactive iodine by the thyroids of guinea-pigs and mice [2,110] — but not in humans [1], though as a marker it is predictive in a mother for the subsequent development of neonatal thyrotoxicosis in her baby [32].

More recently a radioreceptor assay for these stimulating antibodies has been developed which measures TSH receptor binding inhibiting antibodies (TBII) [160]. This assay also measures TSH receptor blocking antibodies but, as these are not normally present in Graves' disease, any TBII activity is assumed to be stimulatory [148]. It is also possible to measure TSab using human thyroid cells in a monolayer culture [97] and there seems to be a good correlation between TBII and TSab measured by this method [20,105,165].

TBII measurements in maternal blood at the time of delivery correlate well with the mean third trimester maternal free T_4 index, indicating that it is a good indicator of maternal thyroid overactivity [123], as are maternal measurements of TSab after birth [167,168]. Measuring the maternal antibodies by either of these methods will predict which babies are at risk *in utero* and in the neonatal period [105]. Measuring TBII is the simpler procedure and a commercial kit is available. Matsuura *et al.* [105] found that all babies with neonatal thyrotoxicosis had maternal TBII concentrations >37 per cent, whereas others have found levels >70 per cent [123]. The author quoted figures >60 per cent [148], but recently has seen a case whose mother had a TBII of 36 per cent.

Fetal thyrotoxicosis

It is suggested therefore that all women with active Graves' disease in pregnancy or with a past history of treated Graves' disease should have TBII measured at the time of booking and possibly also at the start of the third trimester. In those with TBII >60 per cent, or possibly even >36 per cent (see above) the fetus should be screened for hyperthyroidism. Ultrasound should be carried out to see if the fetus is small and suffering from intrauterine growth retardation [17] and to detect the presence of a goitre [140]. The fetal heart rate should also be monitored — a rate of more than 160/min is suggestive of thyrotoxicosis. Amniotic fluid sampling as a diagnostic tool has generally proved disappointing [73,140,156], though Maxwell *et al.* [107] found inappropriately high levels of rT3 in their case. Percutaneous umbilical cord sampling should prove to be an effective way of assessing fetal thyroid function [9,141,172,173], though the risk of this procedure should not be forgotten (see above).

Once a diagnosis of fetal thyrotoxicosis has been made, it is imperative to treat it immediately, since without treatment the mortality is 50 per cent [140] because of intrauterine death, still-birth and neonatal death [137,146]. An additional danger is accelerated skeletal maturation with craniosynostosis and abnormal mental function [11,29,42,71,75,107]. If the mother is already being treated with antithyroid drugs for active Graves' disease in pregnancy, the dosage should be increased until the fetal heart rate falls into the normal range of 120–160/min, or if percutaneous umbilical cord sampling is being done, the fetal free T_4 has become normal [173] for that period of gestation. The dosage is then lowered in order to keep the fetal heart rate (and possibly the cord free T_4) in the normal range [24,151]. If on the other hand the mother is hypothyroid following previous treatment for Graves' disease, antithyroid drugs are added to the mother's T_4 [17,98,146]. Occasionally following previous partial thyroidectomy a mother may be euthyroid but still have very high levels of TSab; her baby is at risk for fetal thyrotoxicosis [20]. The fetus will respond to maternal antithyroid drug therapy, but the mother will probably become hypothyroid and so will need replacement T_4 in addition.

With careful monitoring and regulation of the doses of antithyroid drugs it is possible to control fetal thyrotoxicosis and for the baby to be born both normal and euthyroid [17,24,142,146]. Umbilical cord blood free T_4 and TSH should be measured.

Neonatal thyrotoxicosis

As soon as the baby is born and the umbilical cord is cut, it is deprived of maternal antithyroid drugs, which have a short half-life in blood (75 min for propylthiouracil or 6–8 hours for methimazole [22], though the duration of action in the thyroid gland is 12–24 hours for propylthiouracil and considerably longer for methimazole [22]. In most babies whose mothers have high TBII levels neonatal thyrotoxicosis will develop in 1 day to 1 week after birth [24,142,146], but rarely the onset may be considerably delayed [98,188]. This is thought to be due to the presence of another IgG immunoglobulin in the baby which temporarily inhibits the action of the TSab [187,188]. For this reason early discharge from hospital of an at risk baby is to be discouraged and the baby should be seen frequently in the paediatric outpatient department for the first 2 weeks of life at least.

The physical features of neonatal thyrotoxicosis are weight loss (which is greater than is usually found in a neonate), irritability, jitteriness, avid (but sometimes poor) feeding, tachycardia, goitre, exophthalmos, splenomegaly and petechiae.

Once diagnosed, treatment should be started immediately, even before the blood test results are back, since without therapy the mortality of neonatal thyrotoxicosis is 12–16 per cent [74,157] usually from congestive cardiac failure [15]. A dose of 0.75 mg three times daily of carbimazole or propylthiouracil 10 mg/kg in divided doses is usually sufficient and need only be given for a few weeks in diminishing doses since the half-life of thyroid stimulating antibodies is between 5 and 20 days [183]. Occasionally in severe cases, Lugol's iodine, one drop three times per day, may need to be used in addition to antithyroid drugs. Exchange transfusion has proved of benefit in two babies [126,182]. Rarely treatment has had to be continued up to 20 weeks of life, when TBIIs with more prolonged half-lives have been found [123]. Propranolol in a dosage of 2 mg/kg/day is useful if there are tachyarrhythmias, but should be used with caution if there is heart failure, when digoxin and diuretics will be needed.

Post-partum thyroiditis

At least 11 per cent of all women develop post-partum thyroid dysfunction [130,132,179] and recent evidence suggests that the prevalence may be nearly as high as 17 per cent [49]. The diagnosis may be missed because the condition often starts after the time of the usual postnatal examination.

Ginsberg and Walfish [54] showed that a condition of painless thyroiditis started 1–3 months post-partum with an episode of hyperthyroidism. This could be distinguished from the thyroid overactivity of Graves' disease by the finding (in non-breast feeding women) of a low thyroid uptake of radioactive iodine or technetium, due to the fact that the raised thyroid hormone concentrations are caused by abnormal release from the gland, secondary to autoimmune destruction, rather than by hyperfunction of the gland induced by thyroid stimulating antibodies. The thyrotoxic phase starts quite suddenly, but the clinical features are not pronounced and indeed fatigue and palpitations are the only two symptoms which are more common than in normal post-partum women [6]. A goitre is present in half the patients and 80–85 per cent [96] have positive antithyroid antibodies [6]. Evidence of lymphocytic thyroiditis is found on fine needle biopsy [79,81,130].

The thyrotoxicosis is usually mild, but, if symptomatic, can be controlled by β adrenergic receptor blocking drugs such as propranolol. The use of antithyroid drugs (carbimazole and propylthiouracil) is inappropriate and likely to accelerate the development of hypothyroidism by inhibiting thyroid hormone synthesis.

In two-thirds of the affected women [6] the transient thyrotoxicosis goes into remission after 2–3 months and the patient remains euthyroid. However, the remaining one-third of the patients pass into a hypothyroid phase 4–6 months post-partum [6].

Another group of patients with post-partum thyroid dysfunction, perhaps a quarter of the total, appear to go straight into a hypothyroid phase [6], though a mild, evanescent, phase of thyrotoxicosis may have been overlooked.

Virtually all patients who become hypothyroid post-partum recover, only about 3.5 per cent remaining permanently hypothyroid [6], though the others are at risk of thyroid problems in years to come (see below). If symptoms of hypothyroidism are minor the patient can be left untreated in the expectation that they will recover. Severe symptoms warrant treatment with T_4. After about 6 months the T_4 should be withdrawn to see whether or not the patient is permanently hypothyroid.

Patients who have had post-partum thyroiditis must be regarded as being at risk for future thyroid disease, since half continue to have a goitre, a third have antimicrosomal antibodies and there is evidence of lymphocytic thyroiditis on fine needle biopsy of the thyroid [131]. TSH levels may remain above normal, implying a reduced thyroid reserve which may lead to overt hypothyroidism in the future [131]. Othman *et al.* [136] found overt hypothyroidism in 23 per cent of post-partum thyroiditis patients 3–5 years after delivery. Ten to twenty five per cent of women who have had post-partum thyroiditis develop it following subsequent pregnancies [136,179].

Of patients with post-partum thyroiditis 20–25 per cent have a first degree relative with autoimmune disease [40]. Patients more commonly have the HLA combinations B8, DR3 or A1, B8, DR3 than do a control population [89,146]. The presence of microsomal antibodies in a titre of >1 in 1600 during the first trimester of pregnancy makes a patient's chances of developing postpartum hypothyroidism greater [5,6,8,10,43,80a].

It is well recognized that other autoimmune diseases may remit during pregnancy but show an exacerbation following delivery [8]. In patients with autoimmune thyroid disease levels of TSab (as in Graves' disease) or of microsomal antibodies (as in thyroiditis) may be high at the end of the first trimester of pregnancy, but decline or disappear during the second and third trimester, only to rebound to high levels during the first 4 months following delivery [5,8,43,185]. The result is either a relapse of Graves' disease or the initiation of thyroiditis and occasionally the development of the former followed by the latter. In patients with thyroiditis fine needle biopsy of the thyroid reveals an increase in β lymphocytes and a decrease in suppressor cytotoxic T cells [81], findings similar to those in patients with Hashimoto's thyroiditis [81].

Thyroid nodules

Solitary thyroid nodules [63,161] occur in about 1–2 per cent of women of reproductive age and have a cancer risk of 15–29 per cent [70]. The risk is greater in those with a history of radiation to neck or chest in childhood and in those with voice change, fixation of the lump, lymphadenopathy or Horner's syndrome. Free T_3, free T_4 and TSH by the immunoradiometric method should be carried out to exclude a hyperfunctioning adenoma. An ultrasound examination of the thyroid should be performed. If the lesion is cystic and <4 cm in diameter it is more likely to be benign [116]; it can be aspirated and the fluid sent for cytology. If the ultrasound examination shows that the nodule is solid, then a fine needle [37,180] or drill biopsy of the thyroid should be performed. Malignant lesions can be operated on in the second or third trimesters and then the patient should be put on doses of T_4 sufficient to suppress TSH, since any residual tumour not removed by surgery is likely to be TSH dependent. Residual tumour and metastases can then be treated with radioactive iodine in the post-partum period.

In patients who have already been treated pre-pregnancy and with no residual disease, pregnancy seems to have no adverse effect [70]. Pregnancy does however seem to increase the prevalence of thyroid cancer and in about 20 per cent of patients seems to increase the rate of growth of the tumour [153].

Other investigations which may modify one's diagnostic approach to an apparently solitary thyroid nodule in pregnancy include the finding of an inappropriately low free T_4, a raised TSH, and strongly positive thyroid antibodies – in which case the diagnosis is Hashimoto's thyroiditis. If the appearance of the nodule has been preceded by sore throat and systemic upset, and if the nodule is tender, a markedly raised ESR may indicate subacute (de Quervain's, viral) thyroiditis and fine needle biopsy may reveal multinucleated giant cells. Thyroid function tests done early on may indicate mild thyrotoxicosis; later temporary hypothyroidism may occur and this should be adequately treated during pregnancy. Post-partum T_4 can be reduced and stopped. Recovery from de Quervain's thyroiditis virtually always takes place, though there are occasional exceptions.

References

1 Adams DD & Kennedy TH. Evidence to suggest that LATS-protector stimulates the human thyroid gland. *Journal of Clinical Endocrinology and Metabolism* 1971; **33**: 47–51.

2 Adams DD & Purves HD. Abnormal responses in the assay of thyrotrophin. *Proceedings of the University of Otago Medical School* 1956; **34**: 11.

3 Aboul-Khair SA, Crooks J, Turnbull AC & Hytten FE. The physiological changes in thyroid function during pregnancy. *Clinical Science* 1964; **27**: 195–207.

4 Abuid J, Klein AH, Foley TP Jr & Larsen PR. Total and free triiodothyronine and thyroxine in early infancy. *Journal of Clinical Endocrinology and Metabolism*, 1974; **39**: 263–8.

5 Amino N, Iwatani Y, Tamaki H, Mori H, Miyai K & Tanizawa O. Mechanism of post-partum thyroid disease. In: Labrie F & Proulx LG (eds), *Endocrinology, Proceedings of the 7th International Congress of Endocrinology, Quebec City, 1–7 July*. Excerpta Medica, Amsterdam, 1984: 461–4.

6 Amino N, Mori H *et al*. High prevalence of transient post-partum thyrotoxicosis and hypothyroidism. *New England Journal of Medicine* 1982; **306**: 849–52.

7 Amino N, Tanizawa O *et al*. Aggravation of thyrotoxicosis in early pregnancy and after delivery in Graves' disease. *Journal of Clinical Endocrinology and Metabolism* 1982; **55**: 108–12.

8 Amino N & Miyai. Postpartum autoimmune endocrine syndrome. In: Davies TF (ed), *Autoimmune Endocrine Disease*. John Wiley and Sons, New York, 1983: 247–70.

9 Ballabio M, Nicolini V, Jowett T, Ruiz De Elvira MC, Ekins RP & Rodeck CH. Maturation of thyroid function in normal human fetuses. *Clinical Endocrinology (Oxford)* 1989; **31**: 505–71.

10 Becks GP & Burrow GN. Thyroid disease and pregnancy. *Medical Clinics of North America* 1991; **75**: 121–50.

11 Blackett PR, Seely JR & Altmiller DH. Neonatal thyrotoxicosis following maternal hypothyroidism. *Journal of Pediatrics* 1978; **92**: 159–60.

12 Bober SA, McGill AC & Tunbridge WMG. Thyroid function in hyperemesis gravidarum *Acta Endocrinologica* 1986; **111**: 404–10.

13 Boyages SC, Halpern J-P *et al*. Endemic cretinism: possible role for thyroid autoimmunity. *Lancet* 1989; **ii**: 529–32.

14 Burr WA, Evans SF, Lee J, Prince HP & Ramsden DB. The ratio of thyroxine to thyroxine-binding globulin in the assessment of thyroid function. *Clinical Endocrinology* 1979; **11**: 333–42.

15 Burrow GN. Thyroid diseases. In: Burrow GN & Ferris TF (eds), *Medical Complications during Pregnancy*. WB, Saunders, Philadelphia, 1988: 224–53.

16 Caldwell G, Kellett HA & Gow SM. A new strategy for thyroid function testing. *Lancet* 1985; **i**: 1117–19.

17 Check JH, Rezvani I, Goodner D & Hopper B. Prenatal treatment of thyrotoxicosis to prevent intrauterine growth retardation. *Obstetrics and Gynecology* 1982; **60**: 122–4.

17a Cheron RG, Kaplan MM, Larsen PR, Selenkow HA & Crigler JF Jr. Neonatal thyroid function after propylthiouracil therapy for maternal Graves' diseases. *New England Journal of Medicine* 1981; **304**: 525–8.

18 Chopra IJ. An assessment of daily production and significance of thyroidal secretion of 3,3,5'-triiodothyronine (reverse T_3) in man. *Journal of Clinical Investigation* 1976; **58**: 32–40.

19 Chopra IJ, Sack J & Fisher DA. 3,3,5'-triiodothyronine (reverse T_3) and 3,3,5'-triiodothyronine (T_3) in fetal and adult sheep: studies of metabolic clearance rates, production rates, serum binding, and thyroidal content relative to thyroxine. *Endocrinology* 1975; **97**: 1080–8.

20 Clavel S, Madec AM, Bornet H, Deviller P, Stefanutti A & Orgiazzi J. Anti TSH-receptor antibodies in pregnant patients with autoimmune thyroid disorder. *British Journal of Obstetrics and Gynaecology* 1990; **97**: 1003–8.

21 Cohen JD & Utiger RD. Metastatic choriocarcinoma associated with hyperthyroidism. *Journal of Clinical Endocrinology and Metabolism* 1970; **30**: 423–9.

22 Cooper DS. Treatment of thyrotoxicosis. In: Braverman LE & Utiger RD (eds) *Werner and Ingbar's The Thyroid, a Fundamental and Clinical Text*. JB Lippincott, Philadelphia, 1991: 887–916.

23 Cottrill CM, McAllister RG Jr, Gettes L & Noonan JA. Propranolol therapy during pregnancy, labor and delivery: evidence for transplacental drug transfer and impaired neonatal drug disposition. *Journal of Pediatrics* 1977; **91**: 812–14.

24 Cove DH & Johnston P. Fetal hyperthyroidism: experience of treatment in four siblings. *Lancet* 1985; **i**: 430–2.

25 Crooks J, Aboul-Khair SA, Turnbull AC & Hytten FE. The incidence of goitre during pregnancy. *Lancet* 1964; **ii**: 334–6.

26 Crooks J, Tulloch MI, Turnbull AC, Davidsson D, Skulason T & Snaedal G. Comparative incidence of goitre in pregnancy in Iceland and Scotland. *Lancet* 1967; **ii**: 625–7.

27 Daffos F. Fetal blood sampling. *Annual Review of Medicine* 1989; **40**: 319–29.

28 Daneman D & Howard NJ. Neonatal thyrotoxicosis: intellectual impairment and craniosynostosis in later years. *Journal of Pediatrics* 1980; **97**: 257–9.

29 Davidson KM, Richards DS, Schatz DA & Fisher DA. Successful *in utero* treatment of fetal goiter and hypo-

thyroidism. *New England Journal of Medicine* 1991; **324**: 543–6.

30 Davis LE, Leveno KJ & Cunningham FG. Hypothyroidism complicating pregnancy. *Obstetrics and Gynecology* 1988; **72**: 108–12.

31 Davis LE, Lucas MJ, Hankins GDV, Roark ML & Cunningham FG. Thyrotoxicosis complicating pregnancy. *American Journal of Obstetrics and Gynecology* 1989; **160**: 63–70.

32 Dirmikis SM & Munro DS. Placental transmission of thyroid-stimulating immunoglobulins. *British Medical Journal* 1975; **ii**: 665–6.

33 Dowling JT, Freinkel N & Ingbar SH. The effect of oestrogens upon the peripheral metabolism of thyroxine. *Journal of Clinical Investigation* 1960; **39**: 1119–30.

34 Drexhage HA, Bottazo GF, Bitensky L, Chayen J & Doniach D. Thyroid growth blocking antibodies in primary myxoedema. *Nature* 1981; **289**: 594–6.

35 Drexhage HA, Bottazzo GF, Doniach D, Bitensky L & Chayen J. Evidence for thyroid-growth-stimulating immunoglobulins in some goitrous thyroid diseases. *Lancet* 1980; **ii**: 287–92.

36 Dworkin HJ, Jacquez JA & Beierwaltes WH. Relationship of iodine ingestion to iodine excretion in pregnancy. *Journal of Clinical Endocrinology and Metabolism* 1966; **26**: 1329.

37 Einhorn J & Franzen S. Thin-needle biopsy in the diagnosis of thyroid disease. *Acta Radiologica (Stockholm)* 1962; **58**: 321–36.

38 Ekins R. Roles of serum thyroxine-binding proteins and maternal thyroid hormones in fetal development. *Lancet* 1985; **i**: 1129–32.

39 Erenberg A, Phelps DL, Lam R & Fisher DA. Total and free thyroid hormone concentrations in the neonatal period. *Pediatrics* 1974; **53**: 211–16.

40 Farid NR & Bear JC. Autoimmune endocrine disorders and the major histocompatibility complex. In: Davies TF (ed.), *Autoimmune Endocrine Disease*. John Wiley and Sons, New York, 1983: 59–91.

41 Farrehi C. Accelerated maturity in fetal thyrotoxicosis. *Clinical Pediatrics* 1968; **7**: 134.

42 Fisher DA. In: Werner SC & Ingbar SH (eds), *The Thyroid, a Fundamental and Clinical Text*. Harper & Row, Hagerstown, Maryland, 1978: 955.

43 Feldt-Rasmussen U, Hoier-Madsen M, Rasmussen NG, Hegedus L & Hornnes P. Anti-thyroid peroxidase antibodies during pregnancy and postpartum. Relation to postpartum thyroiditis. *Autoimmunity* 1990; **6**: 211–14.

44 Fisher DA & Polk DH. Development of the thyroid. In: Jones CT (ed.) *Perinatal Endocrinology*. Baillière's Clinical Endocrinology and Metabolism 1989; **3**: 627–57.

45 Fisher DA, Lehman H & Lackey C. Placental transport of thyroxine. *Journal of Clinical Endocrinology and Metabolism* 1964; **24**: 393–400.

46 Fisher DA, Dussault JH, Hobel CJ & Lam R. Serum and gland triiodothyronine in the human fetus. *Journal of Clinical Endocrinology and Metabolism* 1973; **36**: 397–400.

47 Fisher SA & Klein AH. Thyroid development and disorders of thyroid function in the newborn. *New England Journal of Medicine* 1981; **304**: 702–11.

48 Fraser R & Wilkinson M. Simplified method of drug treatment for thyrotoxicosis using a uniform dosage of methyl thiouracil and added thyroxine. *British Medical Journal* 1953; **i**: 481–4.

49 Fung HYM, Kologlu M *et al*. Postpartum thyroid dysfunction in mid-Glamorgan. *British Medical Journal* 1988; **296**: 241–4.

50 Gaitan E. Goitrogens in the etiology of endemic goiter. In: Stanbury JB & Hetzel BS (eds) *Endemic Goiter and Endemic Cretinism*. John Wiley & Sons, New York, 1980: 219–36.

51 Galina MP, Avnet NL & Einhorn A. Iodides during pregnancy. An apparent cause of neonatal death. *New England Journal of Medicine* 1962; **267**: 1124–7.

52 Gardiner-Hill H. Pregnancy complicating simple goitre and Graves' disease. *Lancet* 1929; **i**: 120–4.

53 Gibbons JM, Mitnik M & Chieffo V. *In-vitro* biosynthesis of TSH- and LH-releasing factors by the human placenta. *American Journal of Obstetrics and Gynecology* 1975; **121**: 127.

54 Ginsberg J & Walfish PG. Post-partum transient thyrotoxicosis with painless thyroiditis. *Lancet* 1977; **i**: 1125–8.

55 Girling JC & de Swiet M. Thyroxine dosage during pregnancy in women with primary hypothyroidism. *British Journal of Obstetrics and Gynaecology* 1992; **99**: 368–70.

56 Glinoer D, Soto MF *et al*. Pregnancy in patients with mild thyroid abnormalities: maternal and neonatal repercussions. *Journal of Clinical Endocrinology and Metabolism* 1991; **73**: 421–30.

57 de Groot LJ. Thyroid physiology: endocrine and neural relationships. In: de Groot LJ *et al*. (eds) *Endocrinology*, Volume 1, Grune & Stratton, New York, 1979: 381–2.

58 Guillaume J, Schussler GC & Goldman J. Components of the total serum thyroid hormone concentrations during pregnancy: high free thyroxine and blunted thyrotropin (TSH) response to TSH-releasing hormone in the first trimester. *Journal of Clinical Endocrinology and Metabolism* 1985; **60**: 678–84.

59 Gutteridge DH & Crell SR. Non-toxic goitre: diagnostic role of aspiration cytology, antibodies and serum thyrotropin. *Clinical Endocrinology* 1978; **9**: 505–14.

60 Hall R, Evered DC & Tunbridge WMG. The role of TSH and TRH in thyroid disease. In: Walker G. (ed.) *9th Symposium on Advanced Medicine*. Pitman Medical, London, 1973: 15–26.

61 Halpern SH. Anaesthesia for Caesarian section

in patients with uncontrolled hyperthyroidism. *Canadian Journal of Anaesthesia* 1989; **36**: 454–9.

62 Hamburger JL. Management of the pregnant hyperthyroid. *Obstetrics and Gynecology* 1972; **40**: 114–17.

63 Hara T, Tamai H, Mukata T, Fukata S & Kuma K. The role of thyroid stimulating antibody (TSAb) in the thyroid function of patients with post-partum hypothyroidism. *Clinical Endocrinology* 1992; **36**: 69–74.

64 Hawe P & Francis HH. Pregnancy and thyrotoxicosis. *British Medical Journal* 1962; **ii**: 817–23.

65 Hershman JM. Role of human chorionic gonadotropin as a thyroid stimulator (editorial). *Journal of Clinical Endocrinology and Metabolism* 1992; **74**: 258–9.

66 Hershman JM & Higgins HP. Hydatidiform mole — A cause of clinical hyperthyroidism. *New England Journal of Medicine* 1971; **284**: 573–7.

67 Hetzel BS & Mano MT. A review of experimental studies of iodine deficiency during fetal development. *Journal of Nutrition* 1989; **119**: 145.

68 Hetzel BS, Thilly CH, Fierro-Benitez R, Pretell EA, Buttfield IH & Stanbury JB. Iodised oil in the prevention of endemic goiter and cretinism. In: Stanbury JB & Hetzel BS (eds) *Endemic Goiter and Endemic Cretinism. Iodine Metabolism in Health and Disease.* John Wiley & Sons, New York, 1980: 513–32.

69 Hirsch M, Josefsberg Z *et al.* Congenital hereditary hypothyroidism — prenatal diagnosis and treatment. *Prenatal Diagnosis* 1990; **10**: 491–6.

70 Hod M, Sharony R, Friedman S & Ovadia J. Pregnancy and thyroid carcinoma: a review of incidence, course and prognosis. *Obstetrics and Gynecological Survey* 1989; **44**: 774–9.

71 Hollingsworth DR. Hyperthyroidism in pregnancy. In: Ingbar SH & Braverman LE (eds) *Werner's The Thyroid*. JB Lippincott, Philadelphia, 1986: 1043–63.

72 Hollingsworth DR. Endocrine disorders of pregnancy. In: Creasy RK & Resnik R (eds) *Maternal–Fetal Medicine: Principles and Practice*, 2nd edn. WB Saunders Co., Philadelphia, 1989: 989–1031.

73 Hollingsworth DR & Alexander NM. Amniotic fluid concentrations of iodothyronines and thyrotropin do not reliably predict fetal thyroid status in pregnancies complicated by maternal thyroid disorders or anencephaly. *Journal of Clinical Endocrinology and Metabolism* 1983; **57**: 349–55.

74 Hollingsworth DR & Mabry CC. Congenital Graves' disease: four familial cases with long-term follow-up and perspective. *American Journal of Diseases of Children* 1976; **130**: 148–35.

75 Hollingsworth DR, Mabry CC & Eckerd JM. Hereditary aspects of Graves' disease in infancy and childhood. *Journal of Pediatrics* 1972; **81**: 446–59.

76 Hopton MR, Ashwell K, Scott IV & Harrop JS. Serum free thyroxine concentration and free thyroid hormone indices in normal pregnancy. *Clinical Endocrinology* 1983; **18**: 431–7.

77 Howitt G & Rowlands DJ. Beta-sympathetic blockade in hyperthyroidism. *Lancet* 1966; **i**: 628–31.

78 Hulse JA, Grant DB, Jackson D & Clayton BE. Growth, development and reassessment of hypothyroid infants diagnosed by screening. *British Medical Journal* 1982; **284**: 1435–7.

79 Inada M, Nishikawa M, Naito K, Ishii H, Tanaka K & Imura H. Reversible changes of the histological abnormalities of the thyroid in patients with painless thyroiditis. *Journal of Clinical Endocrinology and Metabolism* 1981; **52**: 431–5.

80 Jansson R, Tötterman TH, Sällström J & Dahlberg PA. Thyroid-infiltrating T lymphocyte subsets in Hashimoto's thyroiditis. *Journal of Clinical Endocrinology and Metabolism* 1983; **56**: 1164–8.

80a Jansson R, Bernander S, Karlsson A, Levin K & Nilsson G. Autoimmune thyroid dysfunction in the postpartum period. *Journal of Clinical Endocrinology and Metabolism* 1984; **58**: 681–7.

81 Jansson R, Tötterman TH, Sällström J & Dahlberg PA. Intra-thyroidal and circulating lymphocyte subsets in different stages of autoimmune postpartum thyroiditis. *Journal of Clinical Endocrinology and Metabolism* 1984; **58**: 942–6.

82 Johnson MR & McGregor AM. Endocrine disease and pregnancy. In: Franks S (ed.) *Endocrinology of Pregnancy*. Baillière's Clinical Endocrinology and Metabolism 1990; **4**: 313–32.

83 Kampmann JP, Johansen K, Hansen JM & Helweg J. Propyl thiouracil in human milk: revision of a dogma. *Lancet* 1980; **i**: 736–8.

84 Kaur S, Krassas G & Ramsay I. Sotalol in hyperthyroidism. *Clinical Endocrinology* 1981; **15**: 627–34.

85 Kenimer JG, Hershman JM & Higgins HP. The thyrotropin in hydatidiform moles is human chorionic gonadotropin. *Journal of Clinical Endocrinology and Metabolism* 1975; **40**: 482–91.

86 Khoury MJ, Becerra JE & d'Almada PJ. Maternal thyroid disease and the risk of birth defects in offspring: a population-based case-control study. *Paediatric and Perinatal Epidemiology* 1989; **3**: 402–20.

87 Klein RZ, Haddow JE *et al.* Prevalence of thyroid deficiency in pregnant women. *Clinical Endocrinology (Oxford)* 1991; **35**: 41–6.

88 Kochupillai N, Ramalingaswami V & Stanbury JB. South East Asia. In: Stanbury JB & Hetzel BS (eds) *Endemic Goiter and Endemic Cretinism. Iodine Nutrition in Health and Disease*. John Wiley & Sons, New York, 1980: 101–21.

89 Kologlu M, Fung H, Darke C, Richards CJ, Hall R & McGregor AM. Postpartum thyroid dysfunction and HLA status. *European Journal of Clinical Investigation* 1990; **20**: 56–60.

90 *Lancet* editorial. Prevention and control of iodine deficiency disorders. *Lancet* 1986; **ii**: 433–4.

91 *Lancet* editorial. Thyroid dysfunction *in utero*. *Lancet* 1992; **339**: 155.

92 Langer A, Hung CT, McA'nulty JA, Harrigan JT

& Washington E. Adrenergic blockade — a new approach to hyperthyroidism during pregnancy. *Obstetrics and Gynecology* 1974; **44**: 181–6.

93 Larsen PR. Maternal thyroxine and congenital hypothyroidism. *New England Journal of Medicine* 1984; **321**: 44–6.

94 Long TJ, Felice ME & Hollingsworth DR. Goiter in pregnant teenagers. *American Journal of Obstetrics and Gynecology* 1985; **152**: 670–4.

95 Lotti G, Delitala G, Devilla L, Alagna S & Masala A. Reduction of plasma triiodothyronine (T_3) induced by propranolol. *Clinical Endocrinology* 1977; **6**: 405–10.

96 Low LCK, Lang J & Alexander WD. Excretion of carbimazole and propylthiouracil in breast milk. *Lancet* 1979; **ii**: 1011.

97 Madec AM, Laurent MC *et al*. Thyroid stimulating antibodies: an aid to the strategy of treatment of Graves' disease? *Clinical Endocrinology* 1984; **21**: 247–55.

98 Maisey MN & Stimmler L. The role of long acting thyroid stimulator in neonatal thyrotoxicosis. *Clinical Endocrinology* 1972; **1**: 81–90.

99 Man EB. Maternal hypothyroxinaemia: development of 4 and 7 year old offspring. In: Fisher DA & Burrow GN (eds) *Perinatal Thyroid Physiology and Disease*. Raven Press, New York, 1975: 117.

100 Man EB, Reid WA, Hellegers AF & Jones WS. Thyroid function in human pregnancy, III, Serum thyroxine-binding prealbumin (TBPA) and thyroxine-binding globulin (TBG) of pregnant women aged 14 through to 43 years. *American Journal of Obstetrics and Gynecology* 1969; **103**: 338.

101 Mandel SJ, Larsen PR, Seely EW & Brent GA. Increased need for thyroxine during pregnancy in women with primary hypothyroidism. *New England Journal of Medicine* 1990; **323**: 91–6.

102 Marchant B, Brownlie BEW, McKay Hart D, Horton PW & Alexander WD. The placental transfer of propyl thiouracil, methimazole and carbimazole. *Journal of Clinical Endocrinology and Metabolism* 1977; **45**: 1187–93.

103 Marsden CD, Gimlette TMD, McAllister RG, Owen DAI & Miller TN. Effect of β-adrenergic blockade on finger tremor and Achilles reflex time in anxious and thyrotoxic patients. *Acta Endocrinologica (København)* 1968; **57**: 353–62.

104 Matsuura N & Konishi J. Transient hypothyroidism in infants born to mothers with chronic thyroiditis — a nationwide study of twenty-three cases. *Endocrinologia Japonica* 1990; **37**: 369–79.

105 Matsuura N, Fujieda K *et al*. TSH-receptor antibodies in mothers with Graves' disease and outcome in their offspring. *Lancet* 1988; **i**: 14–17.

106 Matsuura N, Yamada Y *et al*. Familial neonatal transient hypothyroidism due to maternal TSH-binding inhibitor immunoglobulins. *New England Journal of Medicine* 1980; **303**: 738–41.

107 Maxwell KD, Kearney KK, Johnson JWC, Eagan JW & Tyson JE. Fetal tachycardia associated with intrauterine fetal thyrotoxicosis. *Obstetrics and Gynecology* 1980; **55** (suppl): 18–22.

108 McCarroll AM, Hutchinson M, McAuley R & Montgomery DAD. Long-term assessment of children exposed *in utero* to carbimazole. *Archives of Disease in Childhood* 1976; **51**: 532–6.

109 McColgin SW, Hess LW, Martin RW, Martin JN Jr & Morrison JC. Group B streptococcal sepsis and death *in utero* following funipuncture. *Obstetrics and Gynecology* 1989; **74**: 464–5.

110 McKenzie JM. Delayed thyroid response to serum from thyrotoxic patients. *Endocrinology* 1958; **62**: 865.

111 McLaren EH & Alexander WD. Goitrogens. *Clinics in Endocrinology and Metabolism* 1979; **8**: 129–44.

112 McMichael AJ, Potter JD & Hetzel BS. Iodine deficiency, thyroid function, and reproductive failure. In: Stanbury JB & Hetzel BS (eds) *Endemic Goiter and Endemic Cretinism. Iodine Nutrition in Health and Disease*. John Wiley & Sons, New York, 1980: 445–60.

113 Messer PM, Hauffa BP, Olbricht T, Benker G, Kotulla P & Reinwein D. Antithyroid drug treatment of Graves' disease in pregnancy: long-term effects on somatic growth, intellectual development and thyroid function of the offspring. *Acta Endocrinologica (Copenhagen)* 1990; **123**: 311–16.

114 Mestman JH. Thyroid disease in pregnancy. *Clinics in Perinatology* 1985; **12**: 651–67.

115 Milham S Jr. Scalp defects in infants of mothers treated for hyperthyroidism with methimazole or carbimazole during pregnancy. *Teratology* 1985; **32**: 321.

116 Miller JM, Zafar SU & Karo JJ. The cystic thyroid nodule: recognition and management. *Radiology* 1974; **110**: 257–61.

117 Molitch ME. Endocrine emergencies in pregnancy. In: Burger AG & Philippe J (eds) *Endocrine Emergencies*. Baillière's Clinical Endocrinology and Metabolism 1992; **6**: 167–91.

118 Momotani N & Ito K. Treatment of pregnant patients with Basedow's disease. *Experimental and Clinical Endocrinology* 1991; **97**: 268–74.

119 Momotani N, Ito K, Hamada N, Ban Y, Nishikawa Y & Mimura T. Maternal hyperthyroidism and congenital malformation in the offspring. *Clinical Endocrinology* 1984; **20**: 695–700.

120 Momotani N, Noh J, Oyanagi H, Ishikawa N & Ito K. Antithyroid drug therapy for Graves' disease in pregnancy. *New England Journal of Medicine* 1986; **315**: 24–8.

121 Montgomery DAD & Harley JMG. Endocrine disorders. *Clinics in Obstetrics and Gynaecology* 1977; **4**: 339–70.

122 Montoro M, Collea JV *et al*. Successful outcome of pregnancy in women with hypothyroidism. *Annals of*

Internal Medicine 1981; **94**: 31–4.
123 Mortimer RH, Tyack SA, Galligan JP, Perry-Keene DA & Tan YM. Graves' disease in pregnancy: TSH receptor binding inhibiting immunoglobulins and maternal and neonatal thyroid function. *Clinical Endocrinology* 1990; **32**: 141–52.
124 Mukhtar ED, Smith BR, Pyle GA, Hall R & Vice P. Relation of thyroid-stimulating immunoglobulins to thyroid function and effects of surgery, radioiodine, and antithyroid drugs. *Lancet* 1975; **i**: 713–15.
125 Mulaisho C & Utiger RD. Serum thyroxine-binding globulin: determination by competitive ligand-binding assay in thyroid disease and pregnancy. *Acta Endocrinologica (København)* 1977; **85**: 314.
126 Munro DS, Cooke ID *et al*. Neonatal thyrotoxicosis. *Quarterly Journal of Medicine* 1976; **45**: 689–90.
127 Nabil N, Miner DJ & Amatruda JM. Methimazole: an alternative route of administration. *Journal of Clinical Endocrinology and Metabolism* 1982; **54**: 180–1.
128 Nagataki S, Mizuno M *et al*. Thyroid function in molar pregnancy. In: Robbins J & Braverman LE (eds) *Thyroid Research*. Excerpta Medica, Amsterdam, 1976: 535.
129 New England Congenital Hypothyroidism Collaborative. Characteristics of infantile hypothyroidism discovered on neonatal screening. *Journal of Pediatrics* 1984; **104**: 539–44.
130 Nicolai TF, Brosseau J, Kettrick MA, Roberts R & Beltaos E. Lymphocytic thyroiditis with spontaneously resolving hyperthyroidism (silent thyroiditis). *Archives of Internal Medicine* 1980; **140**: 478–82.
131 Nicolai TF, Coombs GJ & McKenzie AK. Lymphocytic thyroiditis with spontaneously resolving hyperthyroidism and subacute thyroiditis – a long-term follow-up. *Archives of Internal Medicine* 1981; **141**: 1455–8.
132 Nicolai TF, Turney SL, Roberts RC. Postpartum lymphocyctic thyroiditis. *Archives of Internal Medicine* 1987; **147**: 221–4.
133 Niswander KR & Gordon M. *Women and Their Pregnancies*. WB Saunders, Philadelphia, 1972: 246.
134 Ochsner AJ & Thompson RL. *The Surgery and Pathology of the Thyroid and Parathyroid Glands*. CV Mosby, St Louis; 1910: 192.
135 Ormston BJ, Garry R, Cryer RJ, Besser GM & Hall R. Thyrotrophin-releasing hormone as a thyroid-function test. *Lancet* 1971; **ii**: 10–14.
136 Othman S, Phillips DI *et al*. A long-term follow-up of postpartum thyroiditis. *Clinical Endocrinology (Oxford)* 1990; **32**: 559–64.
137 Page DV, Brady K, Mitchell J, Pehrson J & Wade G. The pathology of intrauterine thyrotoxicosis: two case reports. *Obstetrics and Gynecology* 1988; **72**: 479–81.
138 Parker JH. Amerlex free triiodothyronine and free thyroxine levels in normal pregnancy. *British Journal of Obstetrics and Gynaecology* 1985; **92**: 1234–8.
139 Patel A, Robinson S, Bidgood RJ & Edmonds CJ. A pre-eclamptic-like syndrome associated with hypothyroidism during pregnancy. *Quarterly Journal of Medicine* 1991; **79**: 435–41.
140 Pekonen F, Teramo K, Mäkinen T, Ikonen E, Osterlund K & Lamberg B-A. Prenatal diagnosis and treatment of fetal thyrotoxicosis. *American Journal of Obstetrics and Gynecology* 1984; **150**: 893–4.
141 Perelman AH, Johnson RL, Clemons RD, Finberg HJ, Clewell W & Trujillo L. Intrauterine diagnosis and treatment of fetal goitrous hypothyroidism. *Journal of Clinical Endocrinology and Metabolism* 1990; **71**: 618–21.
142 Petersen S & Serup J. Neonatal thyrotoxicosis. *Acta Paediatrica Scandinavica* 1977; **66**: 639–42.
143 Pharoah P, Delange F, Fierro-Benitez R & Stanbury JB. Endemic cretinism. In: Stanbury JB & Hetzel BS (eds) *Endemic Goiter and Endemic Cretinism, Iodine Metabolism in Health and Disease*. John Wiley and Sons, New York, 1980: 395–421.
144 Price A, Griffiths H & Morris BW. A longitudinal study of thyroid function in pregnancy. *Clinical Chemistry* 1989; **35**: 275–8.
145 Ramsay I. Attempted prevention of neonatal thyrotoxicosis. *British Medical Journal* 1976; **ii**: 1110.
146 Ramsay I. Post-partum thyroiditis; an under-diagnosed disease. *British Journal of Obstetrics and Gynaecology* 1986; **93**: 1121–3.
147 Ramsay I, Kaur S & Krassas G. Thyrotoxicosis in pregnancy: results of treatment by antithyroid drugs combined with T_4. *Clinical Endocrinology* 1983; **18**: 75–85.
148 Ramsay I. Fetal and neonatal hyperthyroidism. *Contemporary Reviews in Obstetrics and Gynaecology* 1991; **3**: 74–8.
149 Rey E, Bachrach LK & Burrow GN. Iodides in pregnancy and the perinatal period. *Medicine North America* 1986; **38**: 5609–15.
150 Robin NI, Refetoff S, Gleason RE & Selenkow HA. Thyroid hormone relationships between maternal and fetal circulations in human pregnancy at term; a study of patients with normal and abnormal thyroid function. *American Journal of Obstetrics and Gynecology* 1970; **108**: 1269–76.
151 Robinson PL, O'Mullane NM & Alderman B. Prenatal treatment of fetal thyrotoxicosis. *British Medical Journal* 1979; **i**: 383–4.
152 Romano R, Jannini EA *et al*. The effects of iodoprophylaxis on thyroid size during pregnancy. *American Journal of Obstetrics and Gynecology* 1991; **164**: 482–5.
153 Rosen IB & Walfish PG. Pregnancy as a predisposing factor in thyroid neoplasia. *Archives of Surgery* 1986; **121**: 1287–90.
154 Roti E, Gnudi A & Braverman LE. The placental transport, synthesis and metabolism of hormones and drugs which affect thyroid function. *Endocrine Reviews* 1983; **4**: 131–49.

155 Rovet J, Ehrlich R & Sorbara D. Intellectual outcome in children with fetal hypothyroidism. *Journal of Pediatrics* 1987; **110**: 700–4.

156 Sack J, Fisher DA, Hobel CJ & Lam R. Thyroxine in human amniotic fluid. *Journal of Pediatrics* 1975; **87**: 364–8.

157 Samuel S, Pildes RS, Lewison M & Rosenthal IM. Neonatal hyperthyroidism in an infant born of an euthyroid mother. *American Journal of Diseases of Children* 1971; **121**: 440.

158 Selenkow HA, Birnbaum MD & Hollander CS. Thyroid function and dysfunction during pregnancy. *Clinical Obstetrics and Gynecology* 1973; **16**: 66–108.

159 Shambaugh G III, Kubek M & Wilber JF. Thyrotropin-releasing hormone activity in the human placenta. *Journal of Clinical Endocrinology and Metabolism* 1979; **48**: 483–6.

160 Shewring G & Smith BR. An improved radioreceptor assay for TSH receptor antibodies. *Clinical Endocrinology* 1982; **17**: 409–17.

161 Shigemasa C, Mitani Y *et al*. Development of postpartum spontaneously resolving transient Graves' hyperthyroidism followed immediately by transient hypothyroidism. *Journal of Internal Medicine* 1990; **228**: 23–8.

162 Souma JA, Niejadlik DC, Cottrell S & Rankel S. Comparison of thyroid function in each trimester of pregnancy with the use of triiodothyronine uptake, thyroxine iodine-free thyroxine, and free thyroxine index. *American Journal of Obstetrics and Gynecology* 1973; **116**: 905–10.

163 Stagnaro-Green A, Roman SH, Cobin R, El-Harazy E, Alvarez-Marfany M & Davies TF. Detection of at-risk pregnancy by means of highly sensitive assays for thyroid autoantibodies. *Journal of the American Medical Association* 1990; **264**: 1422–5.

164 Takasu N, Naka M, Mori T & Yamada T. Two types of thyroid function blocking antibodies in autoimmune atrophic thyroiditis and transient neonatal hypothyroidism due to maternal IgG. *Clinical Endocrinology* 1984; **21**: 345–55.

165 Tamaki H, Amino N *et al*. Universal predictive criteria for neonatal overt thyrotoxicosis requiring treatment. *American Journal of Perinatology* 1988; **5**: 152–8.

166 Tamaki H, Amino N *et al*. Effective method for prediction of transient hypothyroidism in neonates born to mothers with chronic thyroiditis. *American Journal of Perinatology* 1989; **6**: 296–303.

167 Tamaki H, Amino N *et al*. Evaluation of TSH receptor antibody by 'natural in vivo human assay' in neonates born to mothers with Graves' disease. *Clinical Endocrinology* 1989; **30**: 493–503.

168 Tamaki H, Amino N *et al*. Prediction of later development of thyrotoxicosis or central hypothyroidism from the cord serum thyroid-stimulating hormone level in neonates born to mothers with Graves' disease. *Journal of Pediatrics* 1989; **115**: 318–21.

169 Theilade P, Hansen JM *et al*. Propranolol influences serum T_3 and reverse T_3 in hyperthyroidism. *Lancet* 1977; **ii**: 363.

170 Thilly CH, Delange F *et al*. Fetal hypothyroidism and maternal thyroid status in severe endemic goiter. *Journal of Clinical Endocrinology and Metabolism* 1978; **47**: 354–60.

171 Thomas R & Reid RL. Thyroid disease and reproductive dysfunction: a review. *Obstetrics and Gynecology* 1987; **70**: 789–98.

172 Thorpe-Beeston JG, Nicolaides KH, Gosden CM & McGregor AM. Thyroid function in fetuses with chromosomal abnormalities. *British Medical Journal* 1991; **302**: 628.

173 Thorpe-Beeston JG, Nicolaides KH, Felton CV, Butler J & McGregor AM. Maturation of the secretion of thyroid hormone and thyroid-stimulating hormone in the fetus. *New England Journal of Medicine* 1991; **324**: 532–6.

174 Toft AD, Irvine WJ, Sinclair I, McIntosh D, Seth J & Cameron EHD. Thyroid function after surgical treatment of thyrotoxicosis. *New England Journal of Medicine* 1978; **298**: 643–7.

175 Tonglet R, Bourdoux P, Minga T & Ermans A-M. Efficacy of low oral doses of iodised oil in the control of iodine deficiency in Zaire. *New England Journal of Medicine* 1992; **326**: 236–41.

176 Uchimura H, Nagataki S, Tabuchi T, Mizuno M & Ito K. The thyroid stimulating activity of highly purified preparations of human chorionic gonadotrophin. In: Robbins J & Braverman LE (eds), *Thyroid Research*. Excerpta Medica, Amsterdam, 1976: 37.

176a Vanderpas JB, Rivera-Vanderpas MT *et al*. Reversibility of severe hypothyroidism with supplementary iodine in patients with endemic cretinism. *New England Journal of Medicine* 1986; **315**: 791–5.

177 Van Dijke CP, Heyendael RJ & De Kleine MJ. Methimazole, carbimazole and congenital skin defects. *Annals of Internal Medicine* 1987; **106**: 60–1.

178 Vulsma T, Gons MH & de Vijlder JJM. Maternal–fetal transfer of thyroxine in congenital hypothyroidism due to a total organification defect or thyroid agenesis. *New England Journal of Medicine* 1989; **321**: 13–16.

179 Walfish PG & Chan JYC. Postpartum hypothyroidism. In: *Clinics in Endocrinology and Metabolism*, Volume 14, No. 2. WB Saunders Co, London, 1985: 417–47.

180 Walfish PG, Miskin M, Rosen IB & Strawbridge HTG. Application of special diagnostic techniques in the management of nodular goitre. *Canadian Medical Association Journal* 1976; **115**: 35–40.

181 Williams RH, Kay GA & Jandorf BJ. Thiouracil. Its absorption, distribution and excretion. *Journal of Clinical Investigation* 1944; **23**: 613–27.

182 Wit JM, Gerards LJ, Vermeulen-Meiners C & Bruinse HW. Neonatal thyrotoxicosis treated with exchange transfusion and Lugol's iodine. *European Journal of Pediatrics* 1985; **143**: 317–19.

183 Wit JM, Rees-Smith B *et al*. Thyroid stimulating immunoglobulins and thyroid function tests in two siblings with neonatal thyrotoxicosis. *European Journal of Pediatrics* 1986; **145**: 143–7.

184 Yoshimura M, Nishikawa M *et al*. Mechanism of thyroid stimulation by human chorionic gonadotropin in sera of normal pregnant women. *Acta Endocrinologica (Copenhagen)* 1991; **124**: 173–8.

185 Zakarija M & McKenzie JM. Pregnancy-associated changes in the thyroid-stimulating antibody of Graves' disease and the relationship to neonatal hyperthyroidism. *Journal of Clinical Endocrinology and Metabolism* 1983; **57**: 1036–40.

186 Zakarija M, McKenzie JM & Eidson MS. Transient neonatal hypothyroidism: characterization of maternal antibodies to the thyrotropin receptor. *Journal of Clinical Endocrinology and Metabolism* 1990; **70**: 1239–46.

187 Zakarija M, McKenzie JM & Hoffman WH. Prediction and therapy of intrauterine and late-onset neonatal hyperthyroidism. *Journal of Clinical Endocrinology and Metabolism* 1986; **62**: 368–71.

188 Zakarija M, McKenzie JM & Munro DS. Immunoglobulin G inhibitor of thyroid-stimulating antibody is a cause of delay in the onset of neonatal Graves' disease. *Journal of Clinical Investigation* 1983; **72**: 1352–6.

Further reading

Bech K, Hertel J *et al*. Effect of maternal thyroid autoantibodies and post-partum thyroiditis on the fetus and neonate. *Acta Endocrinologica (Copenhagen)* 1991; **125**: 146–9.

Chin RKH, Lao TTH, Cockram CS, Swaminathan R & Panesar NS. Transient hyperthyroidism in pregnancy. Case report. *British Journal of Obstetrics and Gynaecology* 1987; **941**: 483–4.

Dozeman R, Kaiser FE, Cass O & Pries J. Hyperthyroidism appearing as hyperemesis gravidarum. *Archives of Internal Medicine* 1983; **143**: 2202–3.

Ekins RP & Ellis SM. The radioimmunoassay of free thyroid hormones in serum. In: Robbins J & Braverman LE (eds), *Thyroid Research. Proceedings of the Seventh International Thyroid Conference, Boston, Massachusetts, June 9–13, 1975*. Excerpta Medica, Amsterdam, 1976: 597–600.

Fisher DA & Odell WD. Acute release of thyrotropin in the newborn. *Journal of Clinical Investigation* 1969; **48**: 1670–7.

Glinoer D, de Nayer P *et al*. Regulation of maternal thyroid during pregnancy. *Journal of Clinical Endocrinology and Metabolism* 1990; **71**: 276–87.

Hardisty CA & Munro DS. Serum long acting thyroid protector in pregnancy complicated by Graves' disease. *British Medical Journal* 1983; **286**: 934–5.

Jeffcoate WJ & Bain C. Recurrent pregnancy-induced thyrotoxicosis presenting as hyperemesis gravidarum. *British Journal of Obstetrics and Gynaecology* 1985; **92**: 413–15.

Lamberg B-A, Ikonen E *et al*. Antithyroid treatment of maternal hyperthyroidism during lactation. *Clinical Endocrinology* 1984; **21**: 81–7.

Volpé R, Ehrlich R, Steiner G & Row VV. Graves' disease in pregnancy years after hypothyroidism with recurrent passive-transfer neonatal Graves' disease in offspring. *American Journal of Medicine* 1984; **77**: 572–8.

Volpé R, Farid NR, von Westarp C & Row VV. The pathogenesis of Graves' disease and Hashimoto's thyroiditis. *Clinical Endocrinology* 1974; **3**: 239–61.

Wilkin TJ, Swanson Beck J, Crooks J, Isles TE & Gunn A. Time and tides in Graves' disease: their implications in predicting outcome of treatment. *British Medical Journal* 1979; **i**: 88–9.

Woeber KA & Ingbar SH. The contribution of thyroxine-binding prealbumin to the binding of thyroxine in human serum, as assessed by immunoabsorption. *Journal of Clinical Investigation* 1968; **47**: 1710–21.

13

Diseases of the Pituitary and Adrenal Gland

Michael de Swiet

Pituitary gland, 483
Pituitary tumours
Hyperprolactinaemia
Acromegaly
Cushing's syndrome
Hypopituitarism
Diabetes insipidus
Adrenal gland, 495
Addison's disease
Acute adrenal failure
Congenital adrenal hyperplasia

Pituitary gland

During pregnancy, diseases of the pituitary gland may manifest themselves either because of the associated endocrine disturbance or because a tumour arising from the pituitary gland causes local pressure; an effect which either specifically damages the optic nerve or generally causes a rise in intracerebral pressure. Secretion of one or more of the hormones produced by the gland may be increased (usually as a result of a tumour) or decreased. Since underactivity may also be due to the local pressure of a pituitary tumour or its treatment, the presentation of patients with these tumours can be very varied. Nevertheless, there are specific clinical syndromes associated with pituitary disease.

Pituitary tumours

Pituitary tumours comprise 10 per cent of all cerebral tumours [135a]. They may secrete any or a mixture of the hormones of the anterior pituitary: prolactin, growth hormone, adrenocorticotrophic hormone (ACTH), follicle-stimulating hormone (FSH), luteinizing hormone (LH) or thyroid-stimulating hormone (TSH). However, only tumours secreting the first three hormones are at all common clinically, and these will be considered in this chapter. In the past, pituitary tumours have been classified on the basis of their reactions with haemotoxylin and eosin stains. Prolactin and growth hormone secreting tumours may be chromophobic or acidophilic; ACTH-secreting tumours are basophilic [48]. However, pituitary tumours are now classified on the basis of the hormones that they produce.

Hyperprolactinaemia

For general reviews see [44a,75,86a,48,112,60b]. About 12 per cent of non-pregnant women with secondary amenorrhoea during their reproductive life have the pituitary prolactinoma syndrome [74a]; this proportion rises to 50 per cent if galactorrhoea is also present [74a,82]. Hyperprolactinaemia may be due to drugs which interfere with dopamine function (e.g. reserpine, methyldopa, phenothiazines), renal or liver disease, hypothyroidism, or disease of the pituitary gland itself. This may be a macroadenoma (>10 mm in diameter) which can extend beyond the pituitary fossa, or a microadenoma (<10 mm in diameter) [48]. In the absence of any other cause, hyperprolactinaemia is usually considered to be due to pituitary disease, even if the lesion cannot be demonstrated radiologically [155].

The standard technique for the anatomical diagnosis of pituitary tumours used to be tomography of the pituitary fossa, with air encephalography in suspicious cases, to demonstrate upward or lateral expansion of the tumour. Considerable expertise was needed to interpret the subtle changes that may be seen in tomographs [37,155], and doubt has been cast on their relevance since similar changes may be seen in the pituitary fossae of other patients, who have no clinical or laboratory evidence of pituitary tumour [151a].

The advent of computerized tomography (CT), with or without contrast enhancement [77a,107a,170] has markedly improved discrimination, and this in turn is being superseded by magnetic resonance imaging (MRI) which does not involve ionizing radiation and gives better definition. An alternative approach in those with doubtful or negative pituitary tomography was to consider the absolute level of prolactin. A normal level is up to 1000 mU/l (30 ng/ml) [75]. A basal level in excess of 1500 mU/l (45 ng/ml) is suggestive of pituitary tumour, though patients with tumours may have lower levels than this [74]. It is also believed that patients with adenomata are less likely to show a further rise in prolactin when challenged with thyrotrophin-releasing hormone (TRH) or metoclopramide [27]; however, the value and specificity of these tests has been questioned [97] and in general they have been replaced by the availability of CT and MRI.

The effect of pregnancy on prolactin-secreting tumours

The pituitary prolactinoma syndrome can be treated in over 80 per cent of women by bromocriptine [170], thus these patients frequently become pregnant. They may also become pregnant spontaneously [22]. The main problem in their management in pregnancy is that, under the influence of oestrogen stimulation, the pituitary adenoma (if present) may enlarge — threatening vision or even life. (Increase in prolactin concentration and episodes of visual loss in patients with a prolactin-secreting adenoma, while taking an oestrogen-containing contraceptive, has also been reported [44,111]).

Before bromocriptine therapy and prolactin estimations were available, it was possible to achieve pregnancy in about 80 per cent of patients with amenorrhoea and galactorrhoea, using gonadotropin, and Gemzell [47] reported the outcome of pregnancy in 250 of 700 anovulatory women who became pregnant with pituitary stimulation. In the light of modern knowledge, it is likely that the 250 women who did succeed in becoming pregnant would have included a number with hyperprolactinaemia. In only four of these pregnancies (1.5 per cent) were there symptoms of tumour expansion in pregnancy, and only one patient required neurosurgery. Thorner *et al.* [155] cited literature reports of 32 cases of visual field defects in patients with tumours around the pituitary fossa, and a number of unreported cases. Of the 32 cases, 29 had pituitary tumours, and the remainder had a craniopharyngioma or a meningioma. Some of these 32 cases have been reported to the manufacturers, who have given details of over 800 pregnancies achieved with the aid of bromocriptine [58]. There was evidence of pituitary tumour in 116 completed pregnancies, and amongst these are nine tumour-related complications (7.8 per cent). Gemzell and Wang [48], on the basis of a questionnaire sent to interested doctors, suggest that the risk of tumour-related complications in pregnant patients with previously untreated microadenomata is 5.5 per cent; however, in 56 pregnancies with previously untreated macroadenomata, they found an incidence of tumour-related complications in 37.5 per cent. In a more recent review based on 246 pregnancies in the literature, Molitch [112] estimated that the overall risk of symptomatic tumour expansion in pregnancy is 1.6 per cent; this increases to 4.5 per cent if asymptomatic enlargement shown by CT scanning is taken into account. The data of Gemzell and Wang [48] suggest that patients who have macroadenomata are much more likely to suffer from expansion of their tumours in pregnancy than those who have microadenomata and this was confirmed by Molitch [112] who found that symptomatic tumour expansion occurred in 15 per cent of such patients. However, Lamberts *et al.* [95] believe that it is not possible to predict which tumours will enlarge sufficiently in pregnancy to cause symptoms. This may possibly be related to the varied prolactin response that was found by White *et al.* [161] when they gave oestrogen (oestradiol benzoate) to women with prolactinomata. Nevertheless, the patients with the largest tumours studied by White *et al.* [161] did appear to increase their prolactin levels most when given oestrogen.

Other studies of prolactin-secreting tumours in pregnancy with minimal or zero tumour-related complications are those of Zarate *et al.* [169], Jewelwicz and Van de Wiele [76] and Hancock *et al.* [61]. The response of women with prolactin-secreting tumours in successive pregnancies can be quite varied [48], although Thorner *et al.* [155] found that, in women with visual field defects in one pregnancy, the defects increased in succeeding pregnancies.

If the risk of tumour-related complications in pregnancy is considered to be greater in those with macroadenomata than in those with micro-adenomata, the question arises whether they should be managed differently before they become pregnant.

First, all patients with hyperprolactinaemia who are treated with bromocriptine should be warned of the risks of tumour expansion if they become pregnant. As we have seen, these risks vary depending on whether or not there is a demonstrable tumour, and how large it is. In the past, a number of treatments have been used for the pituitary prolactinaemia syndrome, including both external [155] and internal radiation with yttrium^{-90} [24] and surgery [62]. It was particularly advocated that 'definitive' treatment be performed before pregnancy, because of the risk of tumour complications in pregnancy. However, more recently, the consensus of opinion is that the dopamine agonist bromocriptine can be used to decrease prolactin secretion and the size of the tumour in all patients with the pituitary prolactinoma syndrome [98]. If tumour-related complications do develop in pregnancy, they can usually be treated with further bromocriptine (see below). Patients with macroadenomata should defer pregnancy until their tumours have been shown to shrink by CT or MRI scanning following bromocriptine therapy and the risk of tumour-related complications in pregnancy is lower. Some authors including Molitch [112] have argued that patients with macroadenomata with suprasellar extension should be treated surgically before pregnancy, citing evidence that such patients who are treated are less likely to have tumour expansion in pregnancy than those treated by bromocriptine alone. The arguments against surgery in general are given below; furthermore Tan and Jacobs [152] have convincingly challenged the data that suggest that treatment with bromocriptine alone is associated with a higher risk of tumour expansion: it is not clear whether ovulation was induced by pituitary stimulation rather than bromocriptine in those patients whose tumours expanded and also tumour size was not shown to have regressed before pregnancy was embarked on [69]. I, therefore, agree that bromocriptine should be used before pregnancy in all patients with prolactinomata regardless of size and that surgery should be reserved for the few cases where bromocriptine has failed to reduce tumour size. Although other dopamine agonists such as pergolide [86] and CV205–502 [69] have been used to reduce prolactin levels in hyperprolactinaemic women, bromocriptine is preferable in those considering pregnancy because of its extensive safety record (see below). It may be administered vaginally in those who suffer from unpleasant gastrointestinal side-effects [49].

Alternative forms of therapy, such as radiation, are unpleasant for the patient, and surgery is not always effective in treating the condition [22,45,145] or in preventing complications in pregnancy [95]; it may also result in permanent hypopituitarism [45,62,160]; recurrence of hyperprolactinaemia may occur in 25–50 per cent of patients at a mean follow-up time of 6 years after trans-sphenoidal microsurgery [144] although others have reported better results particularly following more extensive resection [139,153]. More recent surgical series have also reported more favourable outcomes in pregnancy [133,137].

Although external irradiation has enthusiastic advocates [60] it has been reported to cause sarcoma and damage to other intracerebral structures, i.e. loss of vision [64] and bone necrosis. There is also a 1–5 per cent chance of developing a second brain tumour in patients treated with radiotherapy and followed up to 20 years. This is a ninefold increase in risk compared to the general population [15]. In addition external irradiation may also be ineffective in preventing tumour complications in pregnancy, particularly if the tumour is large [96].

Pituitary tumours may remit in up to 40 per cent of patients following bromocriptine-induced pregnancy [31,113]. The larger the tumour, the less likely this is to occur.

The effect of prolactin-secreting tumours on pregnancy

The overall incidence of the specific complications of prolactin-secreting tumours in pregnancy has been considered above. The most common and clearly documented complication is a visual field defect, typically bitemporal hemianopia. Patients may also complain of headache, due presumably to raised intracerebral pressure. Very occasionally diabetes insipidus or pituitary apoplexy [117] occurs. All these complications are more likely after 30 weeks' gestation, but they have been reported in the first months of pregnancy [117,155]. They almost invariably regress after delivery.

The incidence of spontaneous abortion is between 13 and 32 per cent of pregnancies that have been confirmed by elevated human chorionic gonadotrophin (HCG) levels [11,48,155]. This is rather higher than the 10 per cent suggested by Lewellyn-Jones [104] possibly due to the inhibiting effect of prolactin on progesterone synthesis [108]. However, it must be remembered that the majority of these women will have been infertile before taking bromocriptine; pregnancy is more likely to be diagnosed early; and therefore there will be very few cases of abortion that are 'missed'. The incidence of abortion is also about 25 per cent in pregnancies following clomiphene or pergonal treatment for other causes of ovulatory failure.

Kelly *et al.* [82] found a high incidence of operative delivery in their series of patients with pituitary tumour, but the indications for intervention were varied, and they, and others, have not found any specific complication of pregnancy. Assuming that there is not a miscarriage, there are no specific fetal complications.

MANAGEMENT OF PREGNANCY IN PATIENTS WITH HYPERPROLACTINAEMIA

All patients with previous hyperprolactinaemia should be followed carefully in pregnancy, since tumour expansion has occurred in some patients where there was no previous radiological abnormality [78]. Patients have usually conceived while taking bromocriptine although some conceive with no treatment [22]. They should have been shown before pregnancy to have otherwise normal anterior pituitary function. Alternatively, the appropriate therapy for hypopituitarism with thyroxine and/or cortisone should have been started (see below). When the pregnancy is confirmed, bromocriptine should be discontinued [76] except in the unlikely event that a patient with a large pituitary tumour conceives without prior therapy. Here, I believe, the risk of tumour-related complication is so much higher (see above) that bromocriptine should be continued throughout pregnancy [32].

There is considerable experience in the use of bromocriptine in pregnancy, and no association with congenital abnormalities has been documented in up to 1973 pregnancies [58,112]. The long-term development of the children also appears to be normal [32]. At one time [24], bromocriptine was even continued for the first 12 weeks of pregnancy, because of the suggestion that prolactin depressed progesterone levels. In the series by Child *et al.* [24] there was no excess teratogenicity, confirming the safety of bromocriptine in early pregnancy. This experience has been repeated by Konopka *et al.* [89] who also used bromocriptine throughout 10 pregnancies.

At least every month in patients with macroadenomata the visual field should be plotted by an experienced observer. This objective documentation is helpful, although most patients know when their visual acuity or visual fields are deteriorating. In patients with microadenomata, history and clinical examination by direct confrontation are probably sufficient to exclude any expansion of the tumour. Particular note should be taken of any headaches (raised intracerebral pressure) or thirst (diabetes insipidus): these symptoms are an indication for further investigation if necessary, by CT or MRI scanning. Some clinicians have followed serum prolactin levels in an attempt to monitor tumour activity during pregnancy [35]. However, prolactin levels rise rather variably during pregnancy, and the within-patient, hour-to-hour variability is also much greater in pregnancy than in the non-pregnant state [164]. Reported values for prolactin in normal pregnancy are shown in Table 13.1. The considerable variability is evident in the large standard deviations. Also tumour expansion is not necessarily associated with a rise in prolactin level

Table 13.1. Serum prolactin levels in 20 normal pregnancies [164] and in the non-pregnant state [148a]. Conversion from mg/l to mU/l according to MRC standard 75/504 [22]. Data are ranges or means ± SD

	Pregnant			
Non-pregnant	3 weeks	12 weeks	25 weeks	36 weeks
mg/l 2–15	7 ± 3	20 ± 9	106 ± 39	147 ± 65
mmol/l 0.08–6.0	0.28 ± 0.13	0.82 ± 0.38	4.25 ± 1.55	5.90 ± 2.62
μm/l 60–450	210 ± 98	612 ± 285	3185 ± 1161	4426 ± 1962

[33]. Therefore, there is little if any value in routine estimation of prolactin levels [112].

If there is evidence of tumour expansion during pregnancy, the patient should restart bromocriptine therapy [11]. Injectable bromocriptine has been used in patients unable to take oral therapy because of vomiting [101]. Additional treatment that may be indicated includes therapeutic abortion, early delivery, the use of dexamethasone [77] or hydrocortisone [95] and pituitary surgery [95]. Also, those centres that use yttrium^{90} implants have successfully controlled tumour expansion in pregnancy in this way [24]. Whether any of these additional measures is necessary depends on the severity of the condition, and which treatment is used depends on the maturity of the fetus. Blindness in early pregnancy would be an indication for abortion, followed probably by surgery, although very severe visual field abnormalities [35,111] and pituitary apoplexy have been treated successfully surgically without interruption of the pregnancy. Deteriorating visual fields at 38 weeks gestation could be managed by early delivery [154] since visual field defects regress after delivery [154]. Diabetes insipidus has responded to intranasal synthetic vasopressin, and it also usually regresses after delivery [11].

No special precautions are necessary in labour in the majority of cases. However, patients with macroadenomata or complications of tumour expansion should be delivered electively by forceps because of the rise in intracerebral pressure caused by maternal effort [117]. Labour itself proceeds normally, despite the possible interruption of the pathways from the hypothalamus to the posterior pituitary [82], and possible interference with oxytocin release. Breast feeding is possible [76,82] and should be encouraged; there is no evidence that breast feeding causes pituitary tumours to enlarge. Presumably they are insensitive to the stimuli which, in normal women, cause a further rise in prolactin during the first few weeks of lactation. Certainly prolactin levels do not rise on suckling in these patients [35]. The risk of tumour expanding during lactation is likely to be considerably less than the already small risk of expansion during pregnancy [112].

CONTRACEPTION

Because of the remote risk of tumour expansion caused by the oestrogen component of oral contraception [111], barrier methods are theoretically preferable. In practice, many patients have used oral contraceptives without any problems. The low dose combined preparations where progesterone may antagonize the effect of oestrogen are particularly suitable [44]. The risk of tumour expansion is greater with high dose prolonged oestrogen treatment [12].

Acromegaly

In normal individuals, growth hormone secretion is inhibited by somatostatin, and stimulated by a peptide growth hormone releasing factor. Acromegaly is caused by excess secretion of growth hormone from the anterior pituitary, most commonly because of the presence of an adenoma, but possibly because of loss of hypothalamic control [103]. Some mixed tumours may secrete both growth hormone and prolactin [115] and prolactin may be elevated in patients with tumours that only produces growth hormone because of the mechanical effect causing loss of hypothalamic control.

Estimation of growth hormone in pregnancy is complicated by possible cross-reaction with human placental lactogen [71]. However, Yen *et al.* [157] using a specific antiserum to human growth hormone, showed that growth hormone levels were no different in pregnancy compared to the non-pregnant state. Nevertheless, the placenta also secretes a growth hormone and in the second half of pregnancy this is the dominant variety of growth hormone present in the placenta. Since the placental secretion of growth hormone is non-pulsatile, growth hormone levels in the second half of pregnancy are steady and do not fluctuate as they do in the non-pregnant state [39]. The diagnosis of growth hormone excess is made by demonstration of elevating fasting levels, above 4 μmol/l (2 ng/ml) [170] which are not suppressed by a glucose load of 1 g/kg bodyweight [103]. In the non-pregnant state measurement of insulin growth factor 1 levels correlates better with disease activity than does isolated growth hormone determinations [6] but the normal rise in insulin growth factor 1 in pregnancy precludes its use for diagnosis in pregnancy.

Before puberty and epiphyseal fusion, hypersecretion by growth hormone causes giantism; after puberty it causes coarsening of the features, acromegaly. Acromegaly may also be associated with diabetes mellitus and hypertension; patients frequently complain of headache. The pituitary tumour, like the prolactinoma, can cause hypopituitarism by compression of other pituitary cells, visual field defects and symptoms and signs of raised intracranial pressure.

The same forms of treatment are used as have been used in the treatment of prolactinomata: transsphenoidal microsurgery [165], internal and external irradiation [38] and bromocriptine [159]. In addition somatostatin analogues have been used [94], without complication when given in early pregnancy in one case [102].

Patients with acromegaly whether treated or not rarely become pregnant [43]. For example, in the series of Gemzell and Wang [48] there were only three women with growth hormone or ACTH-secreting adenomata amongst 187 patients with pituitary adenoma. These three had each had their tumours treated before pregnancy, which was subsequently uncomplicated. Not only are growth hormone secreting tumours rarer than prolactinomata, but ovulation is also suppressed, either because of pressure effects on other pituitary cells or because of concomitant hyperprolactinaemia. Therefore acromegaly has been diagnosed for the first time in pregnancy on only a few occasions [167].

During pregnancy in treated patients, the tumour may expand or symptoms may recur [118]. These complications should be managed in the same way as tumour expansion in prolactinomata, with the resumption of bromocriptine therapy, irradiation or surgery.

To ensure that the mother is not hyperglycaemic, it is advisable to perform a blood sugar profile at 12 weeks gestation or on presentation, and repeat it at 28 and 36 weeks gestation. If the patient has more than one blood glucose in excess of 8 mmol/l, or two between 7.5 and 8 mmol/l, she should be managed as a diabetic (Chapter 11). The infants may be growth retarded [118] or macrosomic [43], possibly because of maternal hyperglycaemia. Growth hormone does not cross the placenta [85]. However, pregnancy is usually normal, producing an appropriately sized infant.

The fetal growth occurs normally even in the absence of growth hormone, either in the mother or in the fetus [134], possibly due to the presence of human placental lactogen, the 'growth hormone of pregnancy'. Those patients with isolated growth hormone deficiency (sexual ateliosis) also lactate normally.

Cushing's syndrome

Cushing's syndrome is the clinical condition caused by excess cortisol or cortisol-like substances. There are a number of causes. Cushing's syndrome has been included in the pituitary rather than the adrenal section of this chapter, because of the findings that in 80 per cent of non-pregnant cases the primary pathology is in the pituitary gland (Cushing's disease) or possibly the hypothalamus [170]. A pituitary adenoma secretes excess ACTH which inappropriately stimulates the adrenal glands to produce glucocorticoids. ACTH production by the pituitary is in part controlled by corticotrophin-releasing hormone (CRH) itself produced in the hypothalamus. In pregnancy, levels of CRH are markedly elevated because of CRH production by the placenta [51]. An autonomous non-ACTH dependent benign or malignant tumour in the adrenal cortex is the other major cause of Cushing's syndrome. Primary pathology in the adrenal gland is considerably more common in Cushing's syndrome in pregnancy than in the non-pregnant state. In pregnancy, only 44 per cent of cases are of pituitary origin, 56 per cent are of adrenal origin and of these 21 per cent (12 per cent of all pregnant women with Cushing's syndrome) are due to adrenal cancer [127]. The reason why adrenal causes of Cushing's syndrome should be more common in pregnancy is not clear. However, pregnancy itself often mimics a mild form of hypercortisolism and it may be that the milder forms of Cushing's syndrome which are typically the pituitary forms, pass undetected. Adrenal tumours and particularly adrenal carcinoma are much more florid and are more likely to be detected in pregnancy.

Neoplasms arising outside the hypothalamo-pituitary–adrenal axis and producing ACTH may also cause Cushing's syndrome, but this is very uncommon in pregnancy. It has been recognized in one case of ovarian teratoma coincidental with pregnancy [130]. Treatment with corticosteroid drugs, obesity and alcoholism can also reproduce the clinical features of Cushing's syndrome.

Cushing's syndrome is exceedingly rare in pregnancy. Even amongst 187 patients with microadenomata of the pituitary in pregnancy, there were at most three ACTH-producing tumours [48] and about 50 cases of Cushing's syndrome in pregnancy have been reported in the world literature [3,48,127].

Because of the associated infertility, patients do not usually present with Cushing's syndrome *de novo* in pregnancy. More commonly the condition has been diagnosed before pregnancy and only partially treated, or a relapse has occurred during pregnancy [142].

Cushing's syndrome has been reported to appear in pregnancy, and then remit after delivery [5,20, 92]; it is not clear to what extent pregnancy is a specific risk factor in the development of Cushing's syndrome [142].

The clinical features of Cushing's syndrome in women include bruising, myopathy, hypertension, plethora, oedema, hirsutism, red striae, menstrual irregularity, truncal obesity, headaches, acne, general obesity and impaired glucose tolerance. The presence of these does not necessarily indicate that the patient has Cushing's syndrome; the first three are the most powerful discriminators [135]. Some of these features occur in normal pregnancy.

The diagnosis of Cushing's syndrome in pregnancy, as in the non-pregnant state, depends on imaging and the results of biochemical tests, the choice of imaging depending on what biochemical abnormalities are found. All relevant biochemical parameters are changed in pregnancy [46,132]; the normal pregnant woman has total cortisol levels similar to those seen in Cushing's syndrome; this is partly due to the oestrogen-mediated increase in cortisol binding globulin [34], but there is also an increase in plasma free cortisol. Normal values for total and free plasma cortisols, free urinary cortisol and ACTH in pregnancy and the non-pregnant state are given in Table 13.2. Note the higher levels at 9.00 a.m. than those at midnight, i.e. diurnal variation persists despite the higher total levels of plasma cortisol. Table 13.2 also shows the normal range for 24-hour urinary free cortisol in pregnancy. This is an estimate of the daily cortisol production rate. If, as is likely, there are not the facilities for estimation of plasma free cortisol, urinary cortisol estimation should be performed, particularly in pregnancy, because of varying levels of cortisol binding globulin. Alternatively estimation of salivary glucocorticoid and aldosterone levels gives a good estimate of their free plasma concentrations [42] though note that aldosterone levels are markedly variable in pregnancy [150].

In light of the above information, the biochemical investigation of a woman with suspected Cushing's syndrome in pregnancy can be considered as follows.

Random estimations of cortisol are very variable and affected by stress. In addition total cortisol levels increase in pregnancy. Therefore arrange two 24-hour urine estimations of free cortisol and confirm the completion of collection by also measuring 24-hour urine creatinine (should be 0.13–0.22 mmol/kg bodyweight/day). The two figures for 24-hour free cortisol should agree to within 10 per cent [121] and if clearly elevated

Table 13.2. Morning and evening plasma cortisol, urinary free cortisol and plasma ACTH in pregnancy and the non-pregnant state. Values are mean ± SD or (range)

		Non-pregnant	Second trimester	Third trimester	Labour‡ Onset	Labour‡ Delivery
Total cortisol*	9.00 a.m.	324 ± 100		1029 ± 200	1490 ± 630	2120 ± 65
nmol/l	midnight	103 ± 76		470 ± 124		
Free cortisol*	9.00 a.m.	18 ± 9		38 ± 12		
nmol/l	midnight	6 ± 4		17 ± 5		
Urinary free cortisol*						
nmol/day		103 (13–256)		348 (229–680)		
ACTH ng/ml		(15–70)	30 (20–70)**	50 (20–120)**		

* [46]
** [132]
‡ [60a]

(Table 13.2) indicate hypercortisolism in pregnancy and not stress. If in doubt give dexamethasone 0.5 mg every 6 hours for 48 hours (2 mg suppression test) and collect urinary free cortisol for the last 24 hours and plasma cortisol 6 hours after the last dose. In normal patients these values will be <230 nmol/day and 300 nmol/l respectively. Note that normal pregnant women do not suppress fully following dexamethasone 1 mg (Table 13.3 [3]).

If hypercortisolism is confirmed, distinguish ACTH dependency (pituitary tumour, ectopic ACTH) from ACTH independency (adrenal tumour) by the 8 mg high dose dexamethasone suppression test. Give dexamethasone 2 mg every 6 hours for 48 hours. Collect 24-hour urinary free cortisol and plasma cortisol as in the 2 mg dexamethasone suppression test. Suppression of these values to <230 nmol/day and 300 nmol/l indicates an ACTH dependent cause. If there are facilities for measurement of ACTH, this will be elevated in ACTH dependent causes. The ACTH will fall following high dose dexamethasone in pituitary adenoma and may or may not fall in ectopic ACTH syndrome.

In the non-pregnant state the response of cortisol production to exogenous CRH has been used to distinguish amongst the various forms of Cushing's syndrome. Patients with pituitary tumour show a rise in cortisol (plasma or 24-hour urinary) following CRH whereas those with adrenal tumour or ectopic ACTH production do not [99]. However, this test is unlikely to be helpful in pregnancy because of the very high endogenous CRH levels due to placental production of CRH [51].

On the basis of biochemical tests, the diagnosis is likely to be a pituitary or adrenal tumour (more likely adrenal in pregnancy).

If an adrenal tumour is suspected the best imaging technique is MRI and this should be arranged. If MRI is unavailable, ultrasound may demonstrate the tumour. If a pituitary cause is suspected, MRI

Table 13.3. Plasma cortisol — diurnal variation and response to dexamethasone, 1 mg in normal late pregnancy. Values given are means with range in parentheses (data from [3])

	Control 8.00 a.m.	After dexamethasone 8.00 a.m.	After dexamethasone 5.00 p.m.
Normal pregnant nmol/l	830 (560–1070)	520 (360–600)	450 (320–560)
Non-pregnant nmol/l	(200–700)	(100–400)	

scanning of the pituitary should be arranged. If a tumour is found, definitive treatment can be considered (see below). If a pituitary tumour is not found, further investigation can be postponed until after delivery. This is in contrast to the situation concerning adrenal tumour where because of the high maternal and fetal morbidity and mortality treatment in pregnancy is essential.

The treatments that have been employed have been best evaluated in non-pregnant patients and depend on the primary cause of the condition. For pituitary tumour, bilateral adrenalectomy entails lifelong corticosteroid therapy. Also because there is considerable morbidity associated with the procedure, and because of the subsequent possible development of ACTH-secreting pituitary adenomata (Nelson's syndrome) it is becoming less popular [170] and is now rarely used. Irradiation of the pituitary fossa is not always successful in curing the condition [170]. Therefore, pituitary microsurgery is the optimal treatment for those with pituitary-dependent Cushing's syndrome where an adenoma can be demonstrated [52,156], although the results vary from centre to centre [18]. It may be safely performed in pregnancy.

If pituitary surgery is not performed, either because the diagnosis is not certain, or because of reluctance to operate in pregnancy, and the patient needs to be treated, cyproheptadine, a serotonin antagonist which decreases ACTH activity is the alternative. Kasperlik-Zaluska *et al.* [80] reported two pregnancies in a patient after treatment with cyproheptadine. Griffith and Ross [57] have also reported a successful case following cyproheptadine therapy.

Cushing's syndrome due to adrenal tumour should be treated surgically in pregnancy. These patients invariably develop hypertension which is often severe [127,130] leading to pulmonary oedema and death [88]. In addition there is the worry that 21 per cent of the adrenal tumours are malignant [127]. Metastasis following resection of adrenal carcinoma may respond to the adrenal cytotoxic agent mitotane [105] but the pregnancy should be terminated first. Post-operatively the patient may become temporarily cortisone deficient and this will require hydrocortisone replacement therapy.

Although metyrapone therapy has been used successfully in one pregnancy [54] to decrease cortisol synthesis, in another [26] its use was associated with severe hypertension, possibly due to increased 11-deoxycorticosterone (DOC) levels. Therefore, metyrapone should only be used with considerable caution and where other forms of therapy are deemed unsuitable.

In addition the fetal outcome is not good in Cushing's syndrome, with fetal loss of 10 of 25 cases (400 per 1000), where pregnancy was not interrupted [3]. The reason for this high fetal loss rate is not known but, since there were four still-births, maternal hyperglycaemia may also be a factor. Certainly the fetus may be macrosomic, as in non-Cushing's diabetic pregnancy [3].

Another possible cause of fetal and neonatal mortality is suppression of the fetal hypothalamo-pituitary–adrenal axis [2]. Kreines and Devaux [91] reported marked hypoplasia of the fetal zone of the adrenal cortex in two still-born babies born to mothers with Cushing's syndrome. Although neonatal adrenal insufficiency appears to be a risk in these circumstances, it is exceptionally rare in the neonates to patients taking therapeutic steroids in pregnancy, occurring in only one of 260 cases studied by Bongiovanni and McPadden [13] (see Chapter 1). Since the elevated levels of cortisol binding globulin which are present in pregnancy limit placental transfer of cortisol, the mechanism of suppression of the fetal hypothalamopituitary–adrenal axis may be other than simple transference of glucocorticoids across the placenta.

If pregnancy does continue in the presence of Cushing's syndrome, treated or not, patients should be checked for hyperglycaemia, as in acromegaly (see above) and for hypertension. If there is any possibility of a pituitary tumour, the visual fields should be checked regularly. The newborn infant should be carefully watched for adrenal failure.

Lactation has been discouraged [80] because of: (a) the possibility of permanent galactorrhoea [3]; (b) the justifiable concern that drugs such as cyproheptadine may be secreted in breast milk; and (c) the unjustified concern that lactation will maintain the 'cushingoid state of pregnancy'.

Hypopituitarism

The classical studies of Sheehan have shown that the pituitary gland is very vulnerable during pregnancy and the puerperium and that severe post-partum haemorrhage can cause permanent hypopituitarism by avascular necrosis [146–8]. The vulnerability of the anterior pituitary during pregnancy is presumably related to its two- to threefold increase in size at this time. Several hundred cases of Sheehan's syndrome have been reported, with 39 subsequent pregnancies in 19 well-documented cases reviewed by Grimes and Brooks [59]. Almost invariably it is the anterior pituitary that is affected by post-partum haemorrhage, possibly because its blood supply is via the superior hypophyseal artery, whereas the posterior pituitary and hypothalamus are supplied by the inferior hypophyseal artery and the circle of Willis [9]. Only two cases of diabetes insipidus following post-partum haemorrhage have been reported [9,25]. Hypopituitarism may follow pregnancy in which there has not been overt post-partum haemorrhage and in these patients in particular, the condition may only affect some functions of the pituitary gland [50]. Other rare causes of hypopituitarism in pregnancy are the pressure effect of pituitary tumours — either adenoma (see above) or craniopharyngioma [157] and eosinophilic granuloma, histiocytosis X or Hand–Schueller–Christian disease [1,119]. More recently, lymphocytic hypophysitis has been described as an autoimmune condition affecting the anterior pituitary after delivery (see Chapter 15). Occasionally no cause can be found [55].

Ante-partum pituitary infarction has also been described in eight cases but only in insulin-dependent diabetics [36]. The patient develops a severe headache, usually in the third trimester, and her insulin requirements decrease markedly. She is then very liable to hypoglycaemic episodes. After delivery, she does not lactate, and has other features of hypopituitarism, most frequently lack of growth hormone and gonadotropins.

In those cases of Sheehan's syndrome presenting during the puerperium, there is usually a history of severe post-partum haemorrhage and hypotension, followed by lack of lactation. The patients rapidly become apathetic and are often thought to be depressed. Subsequently, there is persistent amenorrhoea, with loss of axillary and pubic hair, and the symptoms and signs of hypothyroidism and adrenocortical insufficiency. The diagnosis is rarely made during the puerperium, but any patient with a history of severe post-partum haemorrhage and impaired lactation should be followed for at least 1 year with this complication in mind. However, in one series assessment of 17 women who had had severe blood loss from abruption did not show any cases of impaired pituitary function [116] 1 week after delivery. Therefore severe blood loss alone is a poor predictor of hypopituitarism at least as assessed in the puerperium.

The diagnosis of hypopituitarism is confirmed by demonstrating impaired secretion by the pituitary target organs (low thyroxine and plasma cortisol, etc.) with low levels of the pituitary hormones (TSH, ACTH, FSH, LH and growth hormone) that do not rise on provocative stimulation. The provocative tests that have been used include administration of LH- and TSH-releasing hormones (LHRH and TRH). The ability of the hypothalamopituitary axis to secret ACTH, growth hormone and prolactin is tested by insulin-induced hypoglycaemia. The dose of insulin is 0.1 unit/kg bodyweight, or 0.05 unit/kg if hypopituitarism is strongly suspected. Insulin hypoglycaemia is not without risk, since patients who are deficient in glucocorticoids, either because of adrenal or pituitary failure, can have very severe hypoglycaemic reactions. The test should not be performed unless an intravenous infusion has already been set up for subsequent emergency administration of glucose and hydrocortisone. Occasionally metyrapone, which is a metabolic inhibitor of cortisol synthesis, may be used to test ACTH secretion by the hypothalamopituitary axis.

Diabetes insipidus is diagnosed by demonstrating a high urine volume with low osmolality, which is maintained as the plasma osmolality increases with water deprivation. Pituitary-dependent diabetes insipidus is reversed by giving a synthetic analogue of vasopressin, DDAVP (deamino-D-arginine vasopressin); nephrogenic diabetes insipidus is not (see diabetes insipidus, below).

Since patients may have a wide spectrum of disease, with only one or all pituitary hormones affected, each aspect of pituitary function should be studied as far as possible. Any patient who is considered to have hypopituitarism should have an assessment of the visual fields, CT or preferably MRI to exclude pituitary tumour.

Most patients with hypopituitarism become pregnant with the diagnosis already made; pregnancy without treatment is unusual. However, the condition can present in pregnancy for the first time even if, in retrospect, it is clear that the patient had some evidence of prior hypopituitarism [59]; this is particularly likely if the syndrome is incomplete [138,149].

Most indices of pituitary function have now been tested in pregnancy in patients with hypopituitarism. Grimes and Brooks [59] demonstrated levels of TSH that were not elevated despite subnormal thyroxine values. It is said that the pituitary is more sensitive to TRH in pregnancy than in the non-pregnant state [19]. Low ACTH levels [14], which did not rise above 20 pg/ml (normal range 10–70 pg/ml) during ante-partum haemorrhage, have also been reported [59] — the assumption being that the hypothalamopituitary axis was unable to react to the stress of hypotension. It has been suggested that the response to metyrapone is blunted in pregnancy [10]. However, the outcome of the test was judged by a relative lack of increase in urinary steroids rather than the direct assay of ACTH. In early pregnancy, the cortisol and ACTH response to insulin hypoglycaemia (0.1 unit/kg) is similar to that in non-pregnant individuals [81].

In patients with hypopituitarism diagnosed and treated before pregnancy the outcome of pregnancy is good (Table 13.4). Where treatment is absent or inadequate the mother is at risk, and three fatalities have been reported [72,149]. Apart from glucocorticoid deficiency (hypopituitarism, Addison's disease) the differential diagnosis of hypoglycaemia in pregnancy includes hypothyroidism, insulinoma [143], and self-administration of insulin; thyroxine and insulin levels should be measured to exclude these conditions. Other causes of hypoglycaemia such as liver failure (acute fatty liver of pregnancy, see Chapter 9) are usually obvious. Overwhelming infection with falciparum malaria treated with quinine is a recently described cause of hypoglycaemia in pregnancy ([162], see Chapter 16).

For patients with anterior pituitary deficiency, replacement therapy with hydrocortisone up to 30 mg/day, and thyroxine up to 300 μg/day should be sufficient. It may be necessary to start this therapy, particularly hydrocortisone, before a precise diagnosis is made. It is unlikely to cause any harm, and may be life-saving [149]. In contrast to patients with Addison's disease, these patients usually secrete sufficient mineralocorticoid not to need fludrocortisone. Additional parenteral hydrocortisone 100 mg 6-hourly should be given to cover the acute stresses of labour and intercurrent illness. However, parenteral treatment may also be necessary in more chronic conditions, such as hyperemesis. Exogenous gonadotrophin may be necessary before pregnancy to stimulate ovulation, but once the patient is pregnant, replacement gonadotrophin, oestrogen and progesterone will not be necessary because of their production by the fetoplacental unit.

Table 13.4. Outcome of pregnancy in patients with Sheehan's syndrome. The figures in parenthesis are the proportions (per cent) of the total number of pregnancies in each case (data from [59])

	Without therapy	With therapy
Pregnancies	24	15
Live births	13 (54)	13 (87)
Spontaneous abortion	10 (42)	2 (13)
Still-birth	1 (4)	0
Maternal death	3 (12)	0

Abortion is the major fetal risk in untreated hypopituitarism (Table 13.4). Still-birth has also been reported [140]. Lactation may also be impaired because of prolactin deficiency [59].

Diabetes insipidus

Diabetes insipidus may also be present in pregnancy when it can be a sign of tumour expansion — either pituitary adenoma (see above) or craniopharyngioma [66,157]. It may also be caused by skull trauma which has occurred in pregnancy [126] and it may be idiopathic [126]. Hime and Richardson [67] have reviewed the subject and commented on 67 cases of diabetes insipidus in pregnancy in the world literature. Patients with pre-existing, isolated diabetes insipidus have no impairment of fertility and the incidence of the disease in pregnancy is about the same as in the general population, i.e. one in 15 000 [67]. Hime and Richardson [67] found that, in 67 cases, 58 per cent deteriorated in pregnancy, 20 per cent improved, and 15 per cent remained the same. There were inadequate data to assess the remaining 7 per cent. A number of reasons have been put forward why diabetes insipidus should deteriorate in pregnancy; these include the increase in glomerular filtration rate (Chapter 7), the production of vasopressinase from the placenta and the possibility that certain eicosanoids related to increased renal prostaglandin production may also antagonize vasopressin [7]. Similar reasons have been entertained to account for the phenomenon of transient diabetes insipidus which may occur in pregnancy [5,53,65,73] or immediately post-partum [131]. Barron *et al.* [5] suggest that this is most likely to be due to resistance to vasopressin; however, some of these patients undoubtedly do have excess vasopressinase [37] and there may well be other factors involved since impaired liver function has also been noted in several of these cases [5,53]; diabetes insipidus has also been seen in overt acute fatty liver of pregnancy [21] (see Chapter 9). Transient diabetes insipidus usually regresses within a few days of delivery. It has been suggested that patients with transient diabetes insipidus are particularly susceptible to epileptic seizures and that these seizures are resistant to conventional treatment for eclampsia (magnesium and diazepam).

Diabetes insipidus presents with excessive thirst and polyuria. After exclusion of diabetes mellitus, diagnosis is made as above. However, to achieve maximum urine concentration, fluid deprivation is necessary for 22 hours [110] which is very distressing for the patient. The synthetic analogue of vasopressin DDAVP is therefore frequently used for primary diagnosis [70]. DDAVP is metabolized by vasopressin and therefore the response to DDAVP is not usually altered in transient diabetes insipidus. Hutchon *et al.* [70] have compared the responses to DDAVP (20 μg intranasally) and 15-hour fluid deprivation. Although the 15-hours of fluid deprivation was a greater stimulus to urine concentration in the non-pregnant state, DDAVP was an equally effective stimulus in pregnancy, and these authors conclude that this should be the method of choice for diagnosis of diabetes insipidus in pregnancy. The maximum urine concentration achieved in normals was about 1000 mosmol/kg. Any value over 700 mosmol/kg in the 11 hours after instillation of DDAVP should be considered normal [70].

A possible risk of DDAVP late in pregnancy for the diagnosis of diabetes insipidus is premature labour, even though it has minimal oxytocic action (see below). Van Der Wilt *et al.* [157] infused 1 μg in one patient at 36 weeks' gestation, and noted a marked increased in uterine contractility. The patient went into labour 3 days later. A further theoretical risk is that of thrombosis since DDAVP increases the levels of clotting factors, particularly Factor VIII and has been used for the therapy of acquired and congenital bleeding conditions. However, no excess cases of thrombosis have been reported to the manufacturers, nor has there been any difference in the thrombosis rate in meta-analysis of the controlled trials where DDAVP has been used to reduce bleeding [107].

Treatment of diabetes insipidus in pregnancy should be with DDAVP [120,136]. The drug is given as intranasal drops 10–20 μg, two to three times daily. Its particular advantage in pregnancy is that it has 75 times less oxytocic action than preparations of arginine vasopressin [158]. However, Van Der Wilt *et al.* [157] did find that DDAVP caused some uterine contraction when given at 36 weeks' gestation (see above). DDAVP is also less likely to cause abdominal pain than vasopressin which, in turn, can cause rhinitis and allergic pulmonary lesions [17]. Patients with some residual pituitary function, and those with nephrogenic diabetes insipidus, have been treated with chlorpropamide [4]. This drug increases the renal responsiveness to endogenous vasopressin, but it should not be used in pregnancy because of the risk of fetal hypoglycaemia (Chapter 11). Carbamazepine acts in a similar way [109], and is reasonably safe in pregnancy (Chapter 15).

Labour proceeds normally in patients with diabetes insipidus; breast feeding is usually successful [119,136,157].

Adrenal gland (see also Conn's syndrome, Chapter 6)

Addison's disease

Addison's disease is characterized by atrophy of the adrenal cortex and subsequent lack of glucocorticoid and mineralocorticoid activity. The clinical picture — of weight loss, vomiting, hypotension and weakness with hyperpigmentation due to excess ACTH secretion — is well known, although less florid cases are often not diagnosed. At one time, the commonest cause was tuberculosis, with autoimmune destruction of the adrenal gland accounting for a minority of cases. The situation is now reversed and patients may have other autoimmune conditions such as pernicious anaemia [141].

Interestingly the autoantigens in immune Addison's disease have been identified as key enzymes in steroid biosynthesis, 21-hydroxylase in patients with adult type late onset disease [166] and 17-hydroxylase in early onset disease (type 1 polyendocrine autoimmunity syndrome) [93].

The most comprehensive historical account of the interaction between Addison's disease and pregnancy was given by Davis and Plotz [30]. Before hormone therapy was possible, there were 18 cases reported with a maternal mortality of 77 per cent; when extracts of the adrenal cortex became available, there were 17 cases with a maternal mortality of 30 per cent. Once deoxycorticosterone could be used, the mortality dropped to 11 per cent in 34 cases. Now that we have experience of the use of full steroid replacement therapy, pregnancy should not be any risk in cases with previously diagnosed Addison's disease, and there should be no excess maternal mortality [84]. Patients are at risk from the nausea and vomiting of early pregnancy, from labour (when they will not be able to increase their output of steroids from the adrenal glands), and during the puerperium when the physiological diuresis may cause profound hypotension. All of these complications can be treated with extra parenteral hydrocortisone, and with intravenous saline if there is any question of hypovolaemia. Labour should be managed with intramuscular hydrocortisone 100 mg 6-hourly; because of the risk of hypovolaemia in the puerperium, this dose should be reduced only slowly in the first 6 days following delivery.

The only consistently recorded fetal complication is intrauterine growth retardation [122]. Baum and Chantler [8] reported one case of fetal hyperinsulinism which they thought was due to fetal hypoglycaemia secondary to a temporary Addisonian state, caused by transplacental passage of maternal antibodies.

The diagnosis of Addison's disease in pregnancy is difficult, because so many of the features of Addison's disease may be associated with normal pregnancy (vomiting, syncope, weakness, hyperpigmentation). However, persistence of nausea and vomiting after 20 weeks gestation and weight loss should be considered abnormal. The diagnosis will be made on the basis of high levels of endogenous ACTH and low plasma cortisol levels (see above) which do not rise 30 min after the patient is given intramuscular synacthen 0.25 mg. Fortunately, most patients with undiagnosed Addison's disease usually tolerate pregnancy well. The diagnosis is often made when they suffer Addisonian collapse after delivery [16] or following an obstetric catastrophe such as abruption [141] (see Chapter 4 for causes of collapse).

Patients who are being treated with corticosteroids for other reasons such as bronchial asthma (Chapter 1) or systemic lupus erythematosus (Chapter 8) should be managed during labour or in other crises in the same way as patients with Addison's disease. They do not require increased steroid medication for the same period after delivery; 24 hours is usually sufficient.

Acute adrenal failure

This is a rare complication, not necessarily associated with Addison's disease, which is said to result from thrombosis or haemorrhage in the adrenal glands. It normally follows some obstetric catastrophe, such as eclampsia or post-partum haemorrhage. The patient presents with rigors, abdominal pain, circulatory collapse and vomiting. It is almost invariably fatal. The largest review is that of MacGillivray [106] which describes nine patients who died, all with haemorrhage of the adrenal glands. It may well be that acute adrenal failure is not a specific entity, but another manifestation of disseminated intravascular coagulation (Chapter 3).

Congenital adrenal hyperplasia

This term covers a group of inborn errors of metabolism affecting glucocorticoid and mineralocorticoid synthesis. Due to the absence or reduced levels of these hormones, the pituitary gland produces large quantities of ACTH which stimulates the adrenal gland to produce excessive quantities of alternative steroid hormones; these have virilizing and hypertensive actions. For management and diagnostic purposes, the level of 17-hydroxyprogesterone is usually monitored. In 90 per cent of cases there is a deficiency of 21-hydroxylase; other causes are 11-hydroxylase, 3β-hydroxysteroid dehydrogenase and 17-hydroxylase deficiencies [79]. This condition is inherited as an autosomal recessive. If a woman has had one child with congenital adrenal hyperplasia, she has a one in four chance that subsequent pregnancies will be affected. If the patient herself has the condition and her husband is a carrier (risk of one in 200 to one in 400) there is a one in two chance that her children will be affected [19]. Prenatal diagnosis has been helped by the finding that HLA and complement genes are closely linked to those involved with congenital adrenal hyperplasia [128]. If the fetus has the same HLA and complement status as its previously affected sibling, it is likely that it will also have congenital adrenal hyperplasia. In addition advances have been made in the molecular genetics of these conditions [163] and it is now possible to make a prenatal diagnosis with a battery of gene probes [151] on material obtained by chorionic villous sampling.

In addition couples are understandably anxious to test for zygosity of the unaffected partner, if one partner has congenital adrenal hyperplasia. About 30 per cent of heterozygotes have a gene deletion abnormality that can be detected easily, but unfortunately the remaining 70 per cent have point mutations which arise *de novo* and these mutations are mimicked by a 'pseudogene' that is present in normal individuals. So even if the laboratory detects the mutation it is not certain whether this is significant or not. Nevertheless the absence of the gene deletion reduces the *a priori* risk of heterozygosity from one in 50 to one in 70 which some couples find helpful. An alternative approach has been to study the levels of various adrenal steroids following corticotrophin stimulation. Peter *et al.* [125] claim that it is possible to detect all congenital adrenal hyperplasia heterozygotes by such specific steroid analysis, without examining the index case.

The diagnosis is usually made in infancy, either because of the presence of ambiguous genitalia in a female child, or because the child becomes acutely ill due to hyponatraemia. Children [68] and perhaps adults are also at risk from hypoglycaemia. Treatment is with glucocorticoids and sometimes mineralocorticoid replacement with sodium supplementation as indicated. This reduces pituitary secretion of ACTH and subsequent formation of alternative steroid hormones. In addition, reconstructive plastic surgery may be necessary for the ambiguous female genitalia.

The occurrence of congenital adrenal hyperplasia in one child raises the possibility of prenatal diagnosis in subsequent pregnancies with a view to intrauterine treatment, not only to prevent masculinization of the genitalia of a female fetus but also because of worries about the female child's subsequent gender orientation (see below). The majority of this work has been performed in fetuses at risk for 21-hydroxylase deficiency. Antenatal diagnosis cannot be made by estimation of 17-hydroxyprogesterone and androgen levels in amniotic fluid or HLA typing of cultured amniotic cells until about 17 weeks. Earlier diagnosis is now available at about 10 weeks by chorionic villous sampling but even by this age masculinization of the genitalia of a female fetus may have occurred (differentiation at 9–16 weeks). David and Forest [28] have therefore suggested treating all pregnancies subsequent to one in which the infant has been affected by congenital adrenal hyperplasia. Both hydrocortisone and dexamethasone have been given [28,29,40], the rationale being that in contrast to prednisone [40] (see Chapter 1) these steroids will cross the placenta and suppress excessive fetal ACTH production, thus removing the cause of fetal masculinization. The effectiveness of such therapy in suppressing fetal (and maternal) steroid production, although disputed [23], has been demonstrated by depression of maternal oestriol (and cortisol) levels [40]. Dexamethasone has been preferred to hydrocortisone because of its greater effect in suppressing ACTH production in adults with congenital adrenal hyperplasia [83]. Current recommendations [100,124] are to start dexamethasone 1.5 mg/day not later than the fifth week of gestation. Maternal compliance should be checked by showing depressed urinary cortisol and oestriol levels. Fetal material should be obtained as early in gestation as possible preferably by chorionic villous sampling at 8–10 weeks rather than amniocentesis at 16 weeks. Such material should be analysed for HLA status, fetal sex and zygosity for 21α hydroxylase deficiency. If these investigations suggest congenital adrenal hyperplasia and if the fetus is female, treatment should be continued until delivery to avoid possible neuroendocrine effects of excess androgens as well as late masculinization of female genitalia. Since congenital hyperplasia is less serious in the male, such treatment should be discontinued if the fetus is shown to be male or if it is not thought to be affected. In pregnancies where dexamethasone treatment is continued, amniocentesis should be performed at mid-gestation and if 17-hydroxyprogesterone and androgen levels are elevated, the dose of dexamethasone should be increased.

Extra steroid therapy, intravenous hydrocortisone 100 mg 6-hourly, will be necessary to cover the stress of labour. The fetus will require glucocorticoid therapy after delivery, not only as treatment for its presumed metabolic defect, but also because its adrenal glands will have been suppressed *in utero*. In the first 15 female affected pregnancies in which intrauterine suppressive therapy was reported, five of the girls had normal genitalia [124]. In six there was partial virilization and in the remaining four there was a marked virilization. The degrees of virilization did not appear to be related to the degree of suppression which appeared complete even in some of the severe failures [124]. Suppression of the fetal pituitary–adrenal axis is therefore not the only factor controlling masculinization of the female fetus. This form of intrauterine therapy is still very much in its infancy and further studies must be performed concerning the prenatal diagnosis of congenital adrenal hyperplasia and the dose, timing, route and monitoring of steroid therapy. The informed consent of the mother is particularly important in such cases [40].

Effect on pregnancy

In two series [87,56] menarche was delayed by about 2 years compared to normal girls. Although the incidence of regular menstruation is related to the degree with which the condition is controlled by hormone replacement therapy, this rule is not invariable, since some patients do not menstruate, despite adequate biochemical control. The fertility of these patients is therefore reduced. Klingensmith *et al.* [87] found that of 14 patients who wished to become pregnant, six were unable to do so. Grant *et al.* [56] reported a lower proportion, four of 53 patients. However, the necessity for plastic surgery is not a bar to pregnancy. For example, Andersen *et al.* [2] studied one individual who was originally named as a boy and then, after hormone therapy and construction of an artificial vagina, had a successful pregnancy. In a recent study of 80 women with 21-hydroxylase deficiency, Mulaikal *et al.* [114] identified the following reasons for the low fertility rate of only 13 (16 per cent) normal pregnancies.

1 Presence of the salt-losing variety (only one pregnancy in 40 patients and that terminated) which was associated with marked masculinization and the necessity for major plastic surgery. Despite this, the vaginal introitus was inadequate for intercourse in 35 per cent of patients.

2 Poor compliance with endocrine therapy (25 per cent).

3 Irregular or no menstruation (39 per cent).

4 The majority (68 per cent) were single.

5 Infrequent heterosexual intercourse.

It is quite clear that these patients have serious physical and emotional difficulties preventing successful pregnancy. Both these factors may relate to the women's intrauterine exposure to sex hormones [41].

The outcome of pregnancy, where it has been reported, is shown in Table 13.5. Since there has only been a total of 38 pregnancies reported, it is difficult to be certain about the likely outcome of pregnancy in patients with congenital adrenal hyperplasia. There is no reason to believe that the

Table 13.5. Outcome of pregnancy in 38 patients with congenital adrenal hyperplasia

	Normal pregnancy	Abortion	Termination	Comments	Total
[87]	8	3	2	1 premature and spastic 1 multiple congenital abnormalities	15
[56]	4		1	1 eclampsia	6
[2]	1				1
[114]	13	1	2	79% LSCS rate	16
Total	26	4	5	3	38

steroid replacement therapy with prednisolone, hydrocortisone or fludrocortisone is teratogenic (see Chapter 1).

Management of pregnancy

In patients who are not pregnant, the dose of steroid replacement therapy is usually based on clinical judgement, and assay of serum 17-hydroxyprogesterone; the aim being to achieve a level of 17-hydroxyprogesterone <10 nmol/l, without the patient becoming cushingoid; however, if this cannot be achieved, levels of 20–40 nmol/l are probably acceptable. During pregnancy, the level of 17-hydroxyprogesterone is unreliable as an estimate of adrenal suppression, but Klingensmith *et al.* [87] did not find it necessary to change the dose of steroid replacement, and this has also been the author's experience [129].

It has been reported that fetal congenital adrenal hyperplasia due to the rare deficiency of desmolase may be associated with low maternal oestriol levels [63]. This is of importance where oestriol levels are still used for assessment of fetal well-being since it adds to the other causes, anencephaly, sulphatase deficiency and maternal steroid therapy where low oestriol levels do not indicate fetal asphyxia. It may also be important for prenatal diagnosis not only of congenital adrenal hyperplasia but also of Down's syndrome where maternal serum oestriol is used as a marker for the 'at risk' patient.

Some of these patients may be hypertensive, and can require antihypertensive therapy. Despite this, one of our patients developed post-partum eclampsia, but her lack of cooperation may also have contributed [129]. Another of our patients lost a pregnancy because of severe intrauterine growth retardation. My impression is that these are very high risk patients.

Labour should be covered by increased and parenteral steroid medication. Our usual practice in these and all patients who may have depression of the hypothalamopituitary axis is to give intramuscular hydrocortisone 100 mg 6-hourly, while the patient is in labour. This will also contain sufficient mineralocorticoid activity if the patient is also taking fludrocortisone at other times.

There is controversy concerning the need for caesarean section in these patients; Klingensmith *et al.* [87] reported nine caesarean sections for disproportion, possibly due to the presence of an android pelvis caused by the masculinizing influence of abnormal hormone secretion. Grant *et al.* [56] reported only one caesarean section (for severe pre-eclampsia), but they only studied six pregnancies in four women. Mulaikal *et al.* [114] observed a 79 per cent caesarean section rate in 16 pregnancies.

References

1 Almeida OD, Menderson J & Kitay DZ. Hand–Schueller–Christian disease and pregnancy. *American Journal of Obstetrics and Gynecology* 1984; **149**: 906–7.

2 Andersen M, Andreasen E, Jest P & Larsen S. Successful pregnancy in a woman with severe congenital 21-hydroxylase deficiency of the salt losing type. *Pediatric and Adolescent Gynecology* 1983; **1**: 47–52.

3 Anderson KJ & Walters WAW. Cushing's syndrome and pregnancy. *Australian and New Zealand Journal of Obstetrics and Gynaecology* 1976; **14**: 225–30.

4 Arduino F, Ferrar FPJ & Rodrigues J. Antidiuretic action of chlorpropamide in idiopathic diabetes insipidus. *Journal of Clinical Endocrinology and Metabolism*

1966; **26**: 1325–8.
5 Aron DC, Schnall AM & Sheeler LR. Spontaneous resolution of Cushing's syndrome after pregnancy. *American Journal of Obstetrics and Gynecology* 1990; **162**: 472–4.
6 Barkan AL, Beitins R & Kelch RP. Plasma insulin-like growth factor-1/somatomedin-C in acromegaly: correlation with the degree of growth hormone hypersecretion. *Journal of Clinical Endocrinology* 1988; **67**: 69–73.
7 Barron WM, Cohen LM *et al*. Transient vasopressin-resistant diabetes insipidus of pregnancy. *New England Journal of Medicine* 1984; **310**: 442–4.
8 Baum JD & Chantler C. Hyperinsulinaemic child of mother with Addison's disease. *Proceedings of the Royal Society of Medicine* 1968; **61**: 1261–2.
9 Bayliss PH, Milles JJ, London DR & Butt WR. Post partum cranial diabetes insipidus. *British Medical Journal* 1980; **280**: 20.
10 Beck P, Eaton CJ, Young K & Upperman HS. Metyrapone response in pregnancy. *American Journal of Obstetrics and Gynecology* 1968; **100**: 327–30.
11 Bergh T, Nillius SJ & Wide L. Clinical course and outcome of pregnancies in amenorrhoeic women with hyperprolactinaemia and pituitary tumours. *British Medical Journal* 1978; **i**: 875–80.
12 Bevan JS, Sussman J *et al*. Development of an invasive macroprolactinoma: a possible consequence of prolonged oestrogen replacement. Case report. *British Journal of Obstetrics and Gynaecology* 1989; **96**: 1440–4.
13 Bongiovanni AM & McPadden AJ. Steroids during pregnancy and possible fetal consequences. *Fertility and Sterility* 1960; **11**: 181–6.
14 Bowers JH & Jubiz W. Pregnancy in a patient with hormone deficiency. *Archives of Internal Medicine* 1974; **133**: 312–14.
15 Brada M, Ford D *et al*. Risk of second brain tumour after conservation surgery and radiotherapy for pituitary adenoma. *British Medical Journal* 1992; **304**: 1343–6.
16 Brent F. Addison's disease in pregnancy. *American Journal of Surgery* 1950; **79**: 645.
17 *British Medical Journal* editorial. Diabetes insipidus — turning off the tap. *British Medical Journal* 1977; **i**: 1050.
18 Burch W. A survey of results with transsphenoidal surgery in Cushing's disease. *New England Journal of Medicine* 1983; **308**: 103–4.
19 Burrow GN. Adrenal, pituitary and parathyroid disorders. In: Burrow G & Ferris TF (eds), *Medical Complications during Pregnancy*. WB Saunders, Philadelphia, 1975.
20 Calodney L, Eaton RP, Black W & Cohn F. Excerbation of Cushing's disease during pregnancy. Report of a case. *Journal of Clinical Endocrinology and Metabolism* 1973; **36**: 81–6.
21 Cammu H, Velkeniers B *et al*. Idiopathic acute fatty liver of pregnancy associated with transient diabetes insipidus. Case report. *British Journal of Obstetrics and Gynaecology* 1987; **94**: 173–8.
22 Ch'ng JL, Rosenstock J, Mashiter K & Joplin GF. Pregnancy in untreated hyperprolactinaemic women. *Journal of Obstetrics and Gynaecology* 1983; **3**: 258–61.
23 Charnvises S, Fenci M de M *et al*. Adrenal steroids in maternal and cord blood after dexamethasone administration at mid-term. *Journal of Clinical Endocrinology and Metabolism* 1985; **61**: 1220–2.
24 Child DF, Gordon H, Mashiter K & Joplin GF. Pregnancy, prolactin and pituitary tumours. *British Medical Journal* 1975; **ii**: 87–9.
25 Collins ML, O'Brien P & Cline A. Diabetes insipidus following obstetric shock. *Obstetrics and Gynecology* 1979; **53** (suppl): 16S–17.
26 Connell JMC, Cordiner J *et al*. Pregnancy complicated by Cushing's syndrome: potential hazard of metyrapone therapy. Case report. *British Journal of Obstetrics and Gynaecology* 1985; **92**: 1192–5.
27 Cowden EA, Thomson JA *et al*. Tests of prolactin secretion in diagnosis of prolactinomas. *Lancet* 1979; **i**: 1156–8.
28 David M & Forest MG. Prenatal treatment of congenital adrenal hyperplasia resulting from 21-hydroxylase deficiency. *Journal of Pediatrics* 1984; **105**: 799–803.
29 David M, Forest MG & Betuel M. Prenatal treatment of congenital adrenal hyperplasia (CAH): Further studies in mothers and CAH unaffected infants. *Pediatric Research* 1985; **19**: 617.
30 Davis ME & Plotz E. Hormonal inter-relationship between maternal adrenal, placental and fetal adrenal functions. *Obstetrics and Gynecology* 1956; **2**: 1.
31 Daya S, Shewchuk AB & Bryceland N. The effect of multiparity on intrasellar prolactinomas. *American Journal of Obstetrics and Gynecology* 1984; **148**: 512–15.
32 De Wit W, Bennink HJTC & Gerards LJ. Prophylactic bromocriptine treatment during pregnancy in women with macroprolactinomas: report of 13 pregnancies. *British Journal of Obstetrics and Gynaecology* 1984; **91**: 1059–69.
33 Divers WM & Yen SSC. Prolactin-producing microadenomas in pregnancy. *Obstetrics and Gynecology* 1983; **62**: 426–9.
34 Doe RP, Fernandez R & Seal US. Measurement of corticosteroid-binding globulin in man. *Journal of Clinical Endocrinology and Metabolism* 1964; **24**: 1029–39.
35 Dommerholt HBR, Assies J & Van Der Werf. Growth of a prolactinoma during pregnancy. Case report and review. *British Journal of Obstetrics and Gynaecology* 1981; **88**: 62–70.
36 Dorfman SG, Dillaplain RP & Gambrell RD. Ante partum pituitary infarction. *Obstetrics and Gynecology* 1979; **53** (suppl): 12S–24.
37 Doyle F & Mclachlan M. Radiological aspects of

pituitary-hypothalamic disease. *Clinics of Endocrinology and Metabolism* 1977; **6**: 53–81.

37a Durr JA, Hoggard JG, Hunt JM & Schrier RW. Diabetes insipidus in pregnancy associated with abnormally high circulating vasopressinase activity. *New England Journal of Medicine* 1987; **316**: 1070–4.

38 Eastman RC, Gorden P & Roth J. Conventional supervoltage irradiation is an effective treatment for acromegaly. *Journal of Clinical Endocrinology and Metabolism* 1979; **48**: 931–40.

39 Eriksson L, Frankenne F *et al*. Growth hormone 24-h serum profiles during pregnancy — lack of pulsatility for the secretion of the placental variant. *British Journal of Obstetrics and Gynaecology* 1989; **96**: 949–53.

40 Evans MI, Chrousos GP *et al*. Pharmacologic suppression of the fetal adrenal gland *in utero*. Attempted prevention of abnormal external genital masculinization in suspected congenital adrenal hyperplasia. *Journal of the American Medical Association* 1985; **253**: 1015–20.

41 Federman DD. Psychosexual adjustment in congenital adrenal hyperplasia. *New England Journal of Medicine* 1987; **316**: 209–11.

42 Few JD, Paintin DB & James VHT. The relation between aldosterone concentrations in plasma and saliva during pregnancy. *British Journal of Obstetrics and Gynaecology* 1986; **93**: 928–32.

43 Fisch RO, Prem KA, Feinberg SB & Gehrz RC. Acromegaly in a gravida and her infant. *Obstetrics and Gynecology* 1974; **43**: 861–5.

44 Franks S. Regulation of prolactin secretion by oestrogens: physiological and pathological significance. *Clinical Science* 1983; **65**: 457–62.

44a Franks S. Modern management of pituitary prolactinomas. *Current Obstetrics and Gynaecology* 1991; **1**: 84–92.

45 Franks S, Jacobs HS *et al*. Management of hyperprolactinaemic amenorrhoea. *British Journal of Obstetrics and Gynaecology* 1977; **84**: 241–53.

46 Galvao-Teles A & Burke CW. Cortisol levels in toxaemic and normal pregnancy. *Lancet* 1973; **i**: 737–40.

47 Gemzell C. Induction of ovulation in infertile women with pituitary adenoma. *American Journal of Obstetrics and Gynecology* 1975; **121**: 311–15.

48 Gemzell C & Wang CF. Outcome of pregnancy in women with pituitary adenoma. *Fertility and Sterility* 1979; **31**: 363–72.

49 Ginsburg J, Hardiman P & Thomas M. Vaginal bromocriptine. *Lancet* 1991; **338**: 1205–6.

50 Giustina G, Zuccato F, Salvi A & Candrina R. Pregnancy in Sheehan's syndrome corrected by adrenal replacement therapy. Case report. *British Journal of Obstetrics and Gynaecology* 1985; **92**: 1061–2.

51 Goland RS, Wardlaw SL *et al*. High levels of corticotropin-releasing hormone immunoactivity in maternal and fetal plasma during pregnancy. *Journal of Clinical Endocrinology and Metabolism* 1986; **63**: 1199–203.

52 Gold EM. The Cushing syndrome: Changing views of diagnosis and treatment. *Annals of Internal Medicine* 1979; **90**: 829–44.

53 Goodman M, Sachs BP, Phillippe M & Moore T. Transient nephrogenic diabetes insipidus. *American Journal of Obstetrics and Gynecology* 1984; **149**: 910–12.

54 Gormley MJJ, Madden DR *et al*. Cushing's syndrome in pregnancy — treatment with metyrapone. *Clinical Endocrinology* 1982; **16**: 283–93.

55 Gossain VV, Rhodes CE & Rovner DR. Pregnancy in hypothalamic hypopituitarism. *Obstetrics and Gynecology* 1980; **56**: 762–6.

56 Grant D, Muram D & Dewhurst J. Menstrual and fertility patterns in patients with congenital adrenal hyperplasia. *Journal of Adolescent Gynecology* 1983; **1**: 97–103.

57 Griffith DN & Ross EJ. Pregnancy after cyproheptadine treatment for Cushing's disease. *New England Journal of Medicine* 1981; **305**: 893–4.

58 Griffith RW, Turkalj I & Braun P. Pituitary tumours during pregnancy in mothers treated with bromocriptine. *British Journal of Clinical Pharmacology* 1979; **7**: 393–6.

59 Grimes HG & Brooks MH. Pregnancy in Sheehan's syndrome. Report of a case and review. *Obstetrical and Gynecological Survey* 1980; **35**: 481–8.

60 Grossman A, Cohen BL *et al*. Treatment of prolactinomas with megavoltage radiotherapy. *British Medical Journal* 1984; **288**: 1105–9.

60a Haddad PF & Morris NF. Maternal plasma cortisol levels during labour. *Journal of Obstetrics and Gynaecology* 1986; **6**: 158–61.

60b Hammond CB, Haney AF et al. The outcome of pregnancy in patients with treated and untreated prolactin-secreting pituitary tumors. *American Journal of Obstetrics and Gynecology* 1983; **147**: 148–57.

61 Hancock KW, Scott JS *et al*. Conservative management of pituitary prolactinomas: evidence of bromocriptine-induced regression. *British Journal of Obstetrics and Gynaecology* 1980; **87**: 523–9.

62 Hardy J, Baeuregard H & Robert F. Prolactin-secreting pituitary adenomas: transsphenoidal microsurgical treatment. In: Rolyn C & Harter M (eds), *Progress in Prolactin Physiology and Pathology*. Elsevier North-Holland Biomedical Press, Amsterdam, 1978: 361–70.

63 Hardy MJ, Ragbeer MS & Goodwin JW. Low maternal blood oestriol levels resulting from congenital adrenal hyperplasia in a female baby. *Journal of Obstetrics and Gynaecology* 1984; **5**: 84–6.

64 Harries JR & Levene MB. Visual complications following irradiation for pituitary adenomas and craniopharyngiomas. *Radiology* 1976; **120**: 167–71.

65 Harrower ADB & Galloway RK. Transient diabetes insipidus in pregnancy. *British Medical Journal* 1984; **289**: 162.

66 Hiett AK & Barton JR. Diabetes insipidus associated with craniopharyngioma in pregnancy. *Obstetrics and Gynecology* 1990; **76**: 982–4.
67 Hime MC & Richardson JA. Diabetes insipidus and pregnancy. A case report, incidence and review of literature. *Obstetrical and Gynecological Survey* 1978; **33**: 375–9.
68 Hinde FRS & Johnstone DI. Hypoglycaemia during illness in children with congenital adrenal hyperplasia. *British Medical Journal* 1984; **289**: 1603–4.
69 Homburg R, West C *et al*. A double-blind study comparing a new non ergot, long acting dopamine agonist CV205–502 in women. *Clinical Endocrinology* 1990; **32**: 565–72.
70 Hutchon DJR, Van Zijl JAWM, Campbell-Brown BM & McFayden IR. Desmopressin as a test of urinary concentrating ability in pregnancy. *Journal of Obstetrics and Gynaecology* 1982; **2**: 206–9.
71 Hytten FE & Lind T. *Diagnostic Indices in Pregnancy*. Documenta Geigy, Basle, 1973.
72 Israel SL & Conston AS. Unrecognised pituitary necrosis (Sheehan's syndrome). A cause of sudden death. *Journal of the American Medical Association* 1952; **148**: 189–93.
73 Iwaski Y, Oiso Y *et al*. Aggravation of subclinical diabetes insipidus during pregnancy. *New England Journal of Medicine* 1991; **324**: 522–4.
74 Jacobs HS, Franks S *et al*. Clinical and endocrine features of hyperprolactinaemic amenorrhoea. *Clinical Endocrinology* 1976; **5**: 439–54.
74a Jeffcoate SL. Diagnosis of hyperprolactinaemia. *Lancet* 1978; **ii**: 1245–7.
75 Jeffcoate SL. The pituitary prolactinoma syndrome and the mythology of hyperprolactinaemia. *Clinical Reproduction and Fertility* 1982; **1**: 209–17.
76 Jewelwicz R & Van de Wiele RL. Clinical course and outcome of pregnancy in twenty-five patients with pituitary microadenomas. *American Journal of Obstetrics and Gynecology* 1980; **136**: 339–43.
77 Jewelwicz R, Zimmerman EA & Carmel PW. Conservative management of pituitary tumour during pregnancy following induction of ovulation with gonadotrophins. *Fertility and Sterility* 1977; **28**: 35–40.
77a Jung RT, White MC *et al*. CT abnormalities of the pituitary in hyperprolactinaemic women with normal or equivocal sellae radiologically. *British Medical Journal* 1982; **285**: 1078–81.
78 Kajtar T & Tomkin GH. Emergency hypophysectomy in pregnancy after induction of ovulation. *British Medical Journal* 1971; **iv**: 88–90.
79 Kaplan SA. Disorders of the adrenal cortex. *Pediatric Clinics of North America* 1979; **26**: 77.
80 Kasperlik-Zaluska A, Migdalska B *et al*. Two pregnancies in a woman with Cushing's syndrome treated with cyproheptadine. Case report. *British Journal of Obstetrics and Gynaecology* 1980; **87**: 1171–3.
81 Kauppila A, Ylikorkalama O, Jarvinen PA & Haapalahti J. The function of the anterior pituitary-adrenal cortex axis in hyperemesis gravidarum. *British Journal of Obstetrics and Gynaecology* 1976; **83**: 11–16.
82 Kelly WF, Doyle FH *et al*. Pregnancies in women with hyperprolactinaemia: clinical course and obstetrics complications of 41 pregnancies in 27 women. *British Journal of Obstetrics and Gynaecology* 1979; **86**: 698–705.
83 Khalid BAK, Burke CW *et al*. Steroid replacement in Addison's disease and in subjects adrenalectomized for Cushing's disease: Comparison of various glucocorticoids. *Journal of Clinical Endocrinology and Metabolism* 1982; **55**: 551.
84 Khunda S. Pregnancy and Addison's disease. *Obstetrics and Gynecology* 1972; **39**: 431–4.
85 King KC, Adam PAJ, Schwartz R & Teramo K. Human placental transfer of human growth hormone. *Pediatrics* 1971; **48**: 534–9.
86 Kleinberg DL, Boyd AE III & Wardlaw S. Pergolide for the treatment of pituitary tumours secreting prolactin or growth hormone. *New England Journal of Medicine* 1983; **309**: 704–9.
86a Klibanki A & Zervas NT. Diagnosis and management of hormone-secreting pituitary adenomas. *New England Journal of Medicine* 1991; **324**: 822–31.
87 Klingensmith GJ, Garcia SC *et al*. Glucocorticoid treatment of girls with congenital adrenal hyperplasia: Effects of height, sexual maturation and fertility. *Journal of Pediatrics* 1977; **90**: 996–1004.
88 Koerten JM, Morales WJ, Washington SR & Castaldo TW. Cushing's syndrome in pregnancy: A case report and literature review. *American Journal of Obstetrics and Gynecology* 1986; **154**: 626–8.
89 Konopka P, Raymond JP, Merceron RE & Seneze J. Continuous administration of bromocriptine in the prevention of neurological complications in pregnant women with prolactinomas. *American Journal of Obstetrics and Gynecology* 1983; **146**: 935–8.
90 Kreiger DT, Amorosa L & Linick F. Cyproheptadine-induced remission of Cushing's disease. *New England Journal of Medicine* 1975; **293**: 893–6.
91 Kreines K & Devaux WD. Neonatal adrenal insufficiency associated with maternal Cushing's syndrome. *Pediatrics* 1971; **47**: 516–19.
92 Kreines K, Perin E & Salzer R. Pregnancy in Cushing's syndrome. *Journal of Clinical Endocrinology and Metabolism* 1964; **24**: 75.
93 Krohn K, Uibo R *et al*. Identification by molecular cloning of an autoantigen associated with Addison's disease as steroid 17-hydroxylase. *Lancet* 1992; **339**: 770–3.
94 Lamberts SWJ. The role of somatostatin in the regulation of anterior pituitary hormone secretion and the use of its analogs in the treatment of human pituitary tumours. *Endocrinology Review* 1988; **9**: 417–36.
95 Lamberts SWJ, Klijen JGM *et al*. The incidence of complication during pregnancy after treatment of

hyperprolactinaemia with bromocriptine in patients with radiologically evident pituitary tumours. *Fertility and Sterility* 1979; **31**: 614–19.

96 Lamberts SWJ, Seldenlath JH, Kwa HG & Birkenhager JC. Transient bitemporal hemianopia during pregnancy after treatment of galactorrhoea-amenorrhoea syndrome with bromocriptine. *Journal of Clinical Endocrinology and Metabolism* 1977; **44**: 180–4.

97 *Lancet* editorial. PG-synthetase inhibition in obstetrics and after. *Lancet* 1980; **ii**: 185–6.

98 *Lancet* editorial. Prolactinomas: bromocriptine rules OK? *Lancet* 1982; **i**: 430–1.

99 Lancet editorial. CRH test in the 1990s. *Lancet* 1990; **336**: 1416.

100 Lancet editorial. Prenatal treatment of congenital adrenal hyperplasia. *Lancet* 1990; **335**: 510–11.

101 Landolt AM, Del Pozo E & Mayek J. Injectable bromocriptine to treat acute oestrogen-induced swelling of invasive prolactinoma. *Lancet* 1984; **ii**: 111.

102 Landolt AM, Schmid J, Karlsson ERC & Boerlin V. Successful pregnancy in a previously infertile woman treated with SMS-201–995 for acromegaly. *New England Journal of Medicine* 1989; **320**: 671–2.

103 Lawrence AM, Goldfine ID & Kirstens L. Growth hormone dynamics in acromegaly. *Journal of Clinical Endocrinology and Metabolism* 1970; **31**: 239–47.

104 Lewellyn-Jones D. *Fundamentals of Obstetrics and Gynaecology*. Faber and Faber, London, 1969: 157.

105 Luton JP, Cerdas S *et al*. Clinical features of adrenocortical carcinoma, prognosis factors, and the effect of mitotane therapy. *New England Journal of Medicine* 1990; **322**: 1195–201.

106 MacGillivray I. Acute suprarenal insufficiency in pregnancy. *British Medical Journal* 1951; **ii**: 212.

107 Mannucci PM & Lusher JM. Desmopressin and thrombosis. *Lancet* 1989; **ii**: 675–6.

107a McGregor AM, Scanlon MF, Hall R & Hall K. Effects of bromocriptine on pituitary tumour size. *British Medical Journal* 1979; **ii**: 700–3.

108 McNeilly AS. Prolactin and human reproduction. *British Journal of Hospital Medicine* 1974; **12**: 57–62.

109 Meinders AE, Cejka V & Robertson GL. The antidiuretic action of carbamazepine in man. *Clinical Science* 1974; **47**: 289–99.

110 Miles BE, Paton A & de Wardener HE. Maximum urine concentration. *British Medical Journal* 1954; **ii**: 901–4.

111 Mills RP, Harris AB, Heinrichs L & Burry KA. Pituitary tumor made symptomatic during hormone therapy and induced pregnancy. *Annals of Ophthalomology* 1979; **11**: 1672–6.

112 Molitch ME. Pregnancy and the hyperprolactinaemic woman. *New England Journal of Medicine* 1985; **312**: 1364–9.

113 Mornex R & Hugues B. Remission of hyperprolactinemia after pregnancy. *New England Journal of Medicine* 1991; **324**: 60.

114 Mulaikal RM, Migeon CJ & Jock JA. Fertility rates in female patients with congenital adrenal hyperplasia due to 21-hydroxylase deficiency. *New England Journal of Medicine* 1987; **316**: 178–82.

115 Nabarro JDN. Pituitary prolactinomas. *Clinical Endocrinology* 1982; **17**: 129–55.

116 Norman RJ, Joubbert SM & Mobbs CM. Effects of severe postpartum haemorrhage on puerperal pituitary function. *Journal of Obstetrics and Gynaecology* 1987; **7**: 197–200.

117 O'Donovan PA, O'Donovan PJ *et al*. Apoplexy in a prolactin secreting macroadenoma during early pregnancy with successful outcome. Case report. *British Journal of Obstetrics and Gynaecology* 1986; **93**: 389–91.

118 O'Herlihy C. Pregnancy in an acromegalic after bromocriptine therapy. *Irish Journal of Medical Science* 1980; **149**: 281–2.

119 Ogburn PL, Cefalo RC, Nagel T & Okagaki T. Histiocytosis X and pregnancy. *Obstetrics and Gynecology* 1981; **58**: 513–51.

120 Oravec D & Lichardus B. Management of diabetes insipidus in pregnancy. *British Medical Journal* 1972; **iv**: 114–15.

121 Orth DN. Differential diagnosis of Cushing's syndrome. *New England Journal of Medicine* 1991; **325**: 957–9.

122 Osler M. Addison's disease and pregnancy. *Acta Endocrinologica* 1962; **4**: 67.

123 Pang S, Levine LS & Cederquist LL. Amniotic fluid concentrations of delta 5 and delta 4 steroids in fetuses with congenital adrenal hyperplasia due to 21-hydroxylase deficiency and anencephalic fetuses. *Journal of Clinical Endocrinology and Metabolism* 1980; **51**: 223–9.

124 Pang S, Pollack M, Marshall RN & Immken L. Prenatal treatment of congenital adrenal hyperplasia to 21-hydroxylase deficiency. *New England Journal of Medicine* 1990; **322**: 111–15.

125 Peter M, Sippell WG *et al*. Improved test to identify heterozygotes for congenital adrenal hyperplasia without index case examination. *Lancet* 1990; **335**: 1269–99.

126 Phelan JP, Guay AT & Newman C. Diabetes insipidus in pregnancy. *American Journal of Obstetrics and Gynecology* 1978; **130**: 365–6.

127 Pickard J, Jochen AL, Sadur CN & Hofeldt FD. Cushing's syndrome in pregnancy. *Obstetrical and Gynecological Survey* 1990; **45**: 87–93.

128 Pollack MS, Levine LS & Pang S. Prenatal diagnosis of congenital adrenal hyperplasia (21-hydroxylase deficiency) by HLA typing. *Lancet* 1979; **i**: 1107–8.

129 Porter RJ & de Swiet M. Pregnancy in a patient with congenital adrenal hyperplasia. *Pediatric and Adolescent Gynecology* 1983; **1**: 39–45.

130 Pricolo VE, Monchik JM *et al*. Management of Cushing's syndrome secondary to adrenal adenoma during pregnancy. *Surgery* 1990; **108**: 1072–8.

131 Raziel A, Rosenberg T *et al*. Transient postpartum diabetes insipidus. *American Journal of Obstetrics and Gynecology* 1991; **164**: 616–18.

132 Rees LH, Lowry PJ. ACTH and related peptides. In: James FVT, Serio M, Guisli G & Martini L (eds), *Endocrine Function of the Human Adrenal Cortex*. Academic Press, London, 1978: 330.

133 Richards AM, Bullock MRR *et al*. Fertility and pregnancy after operation for a prolactinoma. *British Journal of Obstetrics and Gynaecology* 1986; **93**: 495–502.

134 Rimoin DL, Holzman GB *et al*. Lactation in the absence of human growth hormone. *Journal of Clinical Endocrinology and Metabolism* 1968; **28**: 1183–8.

135 Ross EJ & Linch DC. Cushing's syndrome — killing disease: discriminatory value of signs and symptoms during early diagnosis. *Lancet* 1983; **ii**: 646–9.

135a Russell DS & Rubenstein LJ. *Pathology of Tumours of the Nervous System*. Edward Arnold, London, 1971.

136 Sack J, Friedman E, Katznelson D & Frenkel Y. Long-term treatment of diabetes insipidus with a synthetic analog of vasopressin during pregnancy. *Israel Journal of Medical Science* 1980; **16**: 406–7.

137 Samann NA, Leavens ME *et al*. The effects of pregnancy on patients with hyperprolactinaemia. *American Journal of Obstetrics and Gynecology* 1984; **148**: 466–73.

138 Satterfield RG & Williamson HO. Isolated ACTH deficiency and pregnancy. *Obstetrics and Gynecology* 1976; **48**: 693–6.

138a Scammell GE, McGarrick G, Chamberlain GVP & Jeffcoate SL. The significance of hyperprolactinaemia: 2 years experience. *Journal of Obstetrics and Gynaecology* 1982; **2**: 249–51.

139 Scanlon MF, Peters JR *et al*. Management of selected patients with hyperprolactinaemia by partial hypophysectomy. *British Medical Journal* 1985; **291**: 1547–50.

140 Schneeberg NG, Perloff WH & Israel SL. Incidence of unsuspected Sheehan's syndrome. Hypopituitarism after postpartum haemorrhage and/or shock — clinical and laboratory study. *Journal of the American Medical Association* 1960; **172**: 20–7.

141 Seaward PGR, Guidozzi F & Sonnendecker EWW. Addisonian crisis in pregnancy. Case report. *British Journal of Obstetrics and Gynaecology* 1989; **96**: 1348–50.

142 Semple CG, McEwan M *et al*. Recurrence of Cushing's disease in pregnancy. Case report. *British Journal of Obstetrics and Gynaecology* 1985; **92**: 295–8.

143 Serrano-Rios M, Cifuentes J *et al*. Insulinoma in a pregnant woman. *Obstetrics and Gynecology* 1976; **47**: 361–4.

144 Serri O, Rasio E *et al*. Recurrence of hyperprolactinaemia after selective transsphenoidal adenomectomy in women with prolactinoma. *New England Journal of Medicine* 1983; **309**: 280–3.

145 Shearman RP & Fraser K. Impact of the new diagnostic methods on the differential diagnosis and treatment of secondary amenorrhoea. *Lancet* 1977; **i**: 1195–7.

146 Sheehan HL. Post partum necrosis of the anterior pituitary. *Journal of Pathology and Bacteriology* 1937; **45**: 189–214.

147 Sheehan HL. The pathology of hyperemesis and vomiting of late pregnancy. *Journal of Obstetrics and Gynaecology of the British Empire* 1939; **46**: 685.

148 Sheehan HL & Murdoch R. Post partum necrosis of the anterior pituitary: pathological and clinical aspects. *Journal of Obstetrics and Gynaecology of the British Empire* 1938; **45**: 456–89.

148a Sinha YA, Salby FW, Lewis VJ *et al*. A homologous radioimmunoassay for human prolactin. *Journal of Clinical Endocrinology and Metabolism* 1973; **36**: 509.

149 Smallridge RC, Corrigan DF, Thomason AM & Blue PW. Hypoglycemia in pregnancy. *Archives of Internal Medicine* 1980; **140**: 564–5.

150 Stevens KJ, Paintin DB & Few JD. Aldosterone is secreted intermittently during pregnancy. *British Journal of Obstetrics and Gynaecology* 1989; **96**: 80–7.

151 Strachan T, Sinnott PJ *et al*. Prenatal diagnosis of congenital adrenal hyperplasia. *Lancet* 1987; **ii**: 1272–3.

151a Swanson HA & Du Boulay G. Borderline variations of the normal pituitary fossa. *British Journal of Radiology* 1975; **48**: 366–9.

152 Tan SL & Jacobs HS. Management of prolactinomas. *British Journal of Obstetrics and Gynaecology* 1986; **93**: 1025–9.

153 Thomson JA, Teasdale GM *et al*. Treatment of presumed prolactinoma by transsphenoidal operation: early treatment and results. *British Medical Journal* 1985; **291**: 1550–3.

154 Thorner MO, Besser GM *et al*. Bromocriptine treatment of female infertility: report of 13 pregnancies. *British Medical Journal* 1975; **iv**: 694–7.

155 Thorner MO, Edwards CRW *et al*. Pregnancy in patients presenting with hyperprolactinaemia. *British Medical Journal* 1979; **ii**: 771–4.

156 Tyrell JB, Brooks RM *et al*. Cushing's disease: selective trans-sphenoidal resection of pituitary microadenomas. *New England Journal of Medicine* 1978; **298**: 753–8.

157 Van Der Wilt B, Drayer JIM & Eskes TAB. Diabetes insipidus in pregnancy as a first sign of a craniopharyngioma. *European Journal of Obstetrics, Gynecology and Reproductive Biology* 1980; **10**: 269–74.

158 Vavra IM, Machova A *et al*. Effects of synthetic analogue of vasopressin in animals and in patients with diabetes insipidus. *Lancet* 1968; **i**: 948–51.

159 Wass JAH, Mpult PJA *et al*. Reduction of pituitary-tumour size in patients with prolactinomas and acromegaly treated with bromocriptine with or without radiotherapy. *Lancet* 1979; **i**: 66–9.

160 Werder KV, Fahlbusch R *et al*. Treatment of patients

with prolactinomas. *Endocrinological Investigation* 1978; **1**: 47–58.

161 White MC, Anapliotu M *et al*. Heterogenity of prolactin response to oestradiol benzoate in women with prolactinomas. *Lancet* 1981; **i**: 1394–6.

162 White NJ, Warrell DA *et al*. Severe hypoglycaemia and hyperinsulinemia in falciparum malaria. *New England Journal of Medicine* 1983; **309**: 61–6.

163 White PC, New MI & Dupont B. Congenital adrenal hyperplasia. *New England Journal of Medicine* 1987; **316**: 1580–6.

164 Whittaker PG, Wilcox T & Lind T. The effect of stress upon serum prolactin concentrations in pregnant and non-pregnant women. *Journal of Obstetrics and Gynaecology* 1982; **2**: 149–52.

165 Wilson CB & Dampsey LC. Transsphenoidal removal of 250 pituitary adenomas. *Journal of Neurosurgery* 1978; **48**: 13–22.

166 Winqvist O, Karlsson FA & Kampe O. 21-hydroxylase, a major autoantigen in idiopathic Addison's disease. *Lancet* 1992; **339**: 1559–62.

167 Yap AS, Clouston WM, Mortimer RH & Drake RF. Acromegaly first diagnosed in pregnancy: The role of bromocriptine therapy. *American Journal of Obstetrics and Gynecology* 1990; **163**: 477–8.

168 Yen SSC, Saman N & Pearson H. Growth hormone levels in pregnancy. *Journal of Clinical Endocrinology and Metabolism* 1967; **27**: 1341–7.

169 Zarate A, Canales ES *et al*. The effect of pregnancy and lactation on pituitary prolactin-secreting tumours. *Acta Endocrinologica* 1979; **92**: 407–12.

170 Zervas NT & Martin JB. Management of hormone-secreting pituitary adenomas. *New England Journal of Medicine* 1980; **302**: 210–14.

14

Bone Disease, Disease of the Parathyroid Glands and Some Other Metabolic Disorders

Barry N.J. Walters & Michael de Swiet

Bone structure and function, 505
- Calcium and phosphate
- Hormonal regulation of calcium, phosphate and bone

Changes in bone, calcium and phosphate homeostasis during pregnancy, 509
- Bone density

Metabolic bone disease, 513
- Nutritional osteomalacia
- Rickets
- Gastrointestinal and hepatic osteomalacia
- Renal bone disease
- Drug-induced osteopenia
- Anticonvulsants
- Parathyroid disease
- Osteoporosis of pregnancy and the puerperium

Other inherited skeletal and metabolic disorders, 520
- Osteogenesis imperfecta
- Achondroplasia
- Marfan's syndrome
- Homocystinuria
- Pseudoxanthoma elasticum
- Phenylketonuria
- Hyperxanthinuria, hyperglycinaemia, hypertyrosinaemia
- Glycogen storage diseases (Gaucher's disease, Forbe's disease)
- Hereditary angioneurotic oedema
- Porphyria
- Ornithine carbamoyltransferase deficiency

The association of pregnancy with bone disease is by no means common in the Western world. Nevertheless, there are very real changes in bone physiology and calcium and phosphate homeostasis in pregnancy. An understanding of these changes and their derangements is necessary for a full appreciation of the problems that occur from time to time in pregnancy. The initial part of this chapter is devoted first, to a consideration of normal physiology in the non-pregnant state; second, to the changes seen in pregnancy; and third, to the relevant clinical problems that may be seen. The second part of the chapter is concerned with various inherited metabolic and skeletal disorders of significance in pregnancy.

Bone structure and function

The skeletal framework of the body is in a state of constant metabolic activity. Simultaneous processes of new bone formation and dissolution of older bone achieve remodelling of individual bones in response to changing needs.

Further, bone acts as the major repository for calcium and phosphate in the body. Regulation of the plasma concentration of these ions is effected largely through changes in bone mediated by certain hormones.

Bone is composed of bone cells, protein matrix and mineral. The matrix comprises about half of the bone volume, and bone cells only about 3 per cent. Osteoblasts synthesize and mineralize bone. Osteocytes are osteoblasts incorporated in the bony matrix they have secreted. The osteoclast, probably of macrophage origin, appears as a multinucleate cell responsible for bone resorption.

After epiphyseal closure, the cellular activity of bone represents a dynamic balance between resorption and resynthesis. Remodelling begins when osteoblasts and osteoclasts appear at a focus on the bone's surface. The osteoclasts dissolve bone, leaving a bay (Howship's lacuna), into which the osteoblasts nestle and deposit new bone matrix, which later undergoes mineralization. This organic matrix (osteoid) is 90–95 per cent collagen but also contains mucopolysaccharides and lipids. Mineralization is part of the function of the osteoblast and involves deposition of calcium and phosphorus as amorphous salts. Over days, these assume a more crystalline structure resembling dyhydroxyapatite, $Ca_{10}(PO_4)_6(OH)_2$, the dominant mineral found in mature bone. The majority of the mineral phase is accommodated in spaces interspersed throughout the collagen fibrils.

Osteoblasts are rich in alkaline phosphatase. Its level rises in the blood when their activity increases as in conditions of rapid bone turnover. It is possible that alkaline phosphatase locally inactivates inhibitors of precipitation (such as inorganic pyrophosphate) resulting in the formation of crystals.

Calcium and phosphate

The total body calcium content is 25–30 mol (1000–1500 g) and 99 per cent of this is incorporated in bone crystals. This pool is in equilibrium with the extracellular fluid calcium. Total exchange of the ions of extracellular fluid occurs several times daily. Bone deposition, and resorption, which also contribute to calcium economy, proceed much more slowly.

The daily dietary intake of calcium averages 25 mmol (1 g). Of this, only 6 mmol is absorbed by active transport in the proximal small bowel. Under normal circumstances, 98 per cent of calcium filtered by the kidney is re-absorbed in the proximal tubule. Calcium economy is effected by adjustments in this tubular re-absorption.

Total serum calcium includes protein bound (45 per cent) and free ionized fractions. A small amount is present as diffusible complexes. Binding is largely to albumin and variations in albumin concentration will lead to misinterpretation of effective calcium concentration unless corrective calculations are performed. The biological activity of calcium relates to its free ionized concentration and a low serum calcium may be due to a low albumin concentration, in which event serum ionized calcium should be normal.

The normal serum calcium in the non-pregnant state, after correction for albumin concentration, is 2.25–2.65 mmol/l. The normal ionized calcium is 1.1–1.4 mmol/l. Many clinical laboratories now measure ionized calcium directly. If this cannot be measured, it can be derived from the total serum calcium, albumin and globulin concentrations by the following equations:

$$\% \text{ protein bound calcium} = 0.8 \times \text{albumin (g/l)} + 0.2 \times \text{globulin (g/l)} + 3$$

$$\% \text{ ionized calcium} = 100 - \% \text{ protein bound calcium.}$$

It should be noted that the accuracy of the first equation in pregnancy has not been established.

Of the total body phosphorus, 85 per cent is in the skeleton and the remainder is inside cells elsewhere. One-third of the plasma phosphorus is present as inorganic phosphate (0.8–1.4 mmol/l), whilst two-thirds is in phospholipid form. In contrast to calcium, about 88 per cent of inorganic phosphate is free and not protein bound. Phosphate concentration is labile and alters from hour to hour. After eating, plasma phosphate falls because phosphate enters the cells with glucose under the influence of insulin. For these reasons samples for phosphate estimation should be taken early in the morning with the patient fasting.

Phosphate is abundant in normal foods. Its absorption is very efficient and dietary privation, short of actual starvation, does not lead to deficiency. Even so, non-absorbable antacids, if taken in large amounts, can interfere with phosphate absorption by binding it in the gut lumen. Under normal circumstances, the daily requirement of 40 mmol is easily satisfied by gastrointestinal absorption.

The kidney plays a major role in regulating phosphate balance. After glomerular filtration, 80–90 per cent of phosphate is re-absorbed in the proximal convoluted tubule. A rise in plasma phosphate is countered by increased renal excretion. Parathyroid hormone (PTH) achieves this by inhibiting proximal tubular phosphate re-absorption. Bone uptake and release of phosphate also contribute to homeostasis, but the renal mechanism predominates.

Hormonal regulation of calcium, phosphate and bone

The functions of bone, kidney and gut in calcium and phosphate homeostasis are regulated by hormones, chiefly PTH and vitamin D. Thyroid and adrenal hormones, as well as glucagon, growth hormone and sex steroids also have influence. The place of calcitonin in this system has not been fully characterized.

Vitamin D

The healing effect of ultraviolet light on rachitic bone lesions was recognized in 1919. Soon after, it was demonstrated that sunlight activates a sterol in the skin to become the antirachitic agent. This is the photochemical conversion of 7–dehydrocholesterol to cholecalciferol or vitamin D_3 (Fig. 14.1). To a lesser extent, the diet contributes to the body stores of vitamin D but about 90 per cent of circulating vitamin D is skin derived [4]. Natural dietary sources include fish oils, eggs, butter and liver and these yield both vitamin D_3 and vitamin D_2 (ergocalciferol). Absorption from the proximal small intestine is aided by bile salts as for other fat-soluble vitamins.

Vitamin D is transported to the liver bound to a specific vitamin D binding globulin. In the liver, its first metabolic activation step yields 25-hydroxycholecalciferol (25-OHD) — the dominant circulating form of the vitamin. The serum concentration of 25-OHD is an index of vitamin D nutritional status. The same transport protein conveys 25-OHD to the kidney, the only known site of the 1α-hydroxylase enzyme in the non-pregnant state, though there are extrarenal sites in pregnancy, the placenta in particular [72,203]. Hydroxylation at either the C_1 or C_{24} position takes place in cells of the proximal convoluted tubule producing 1α'25-OHD and 24, 25-OHD. 24, 25-OHD is elaborated when vitamin D, calcium and phosphate are abun-

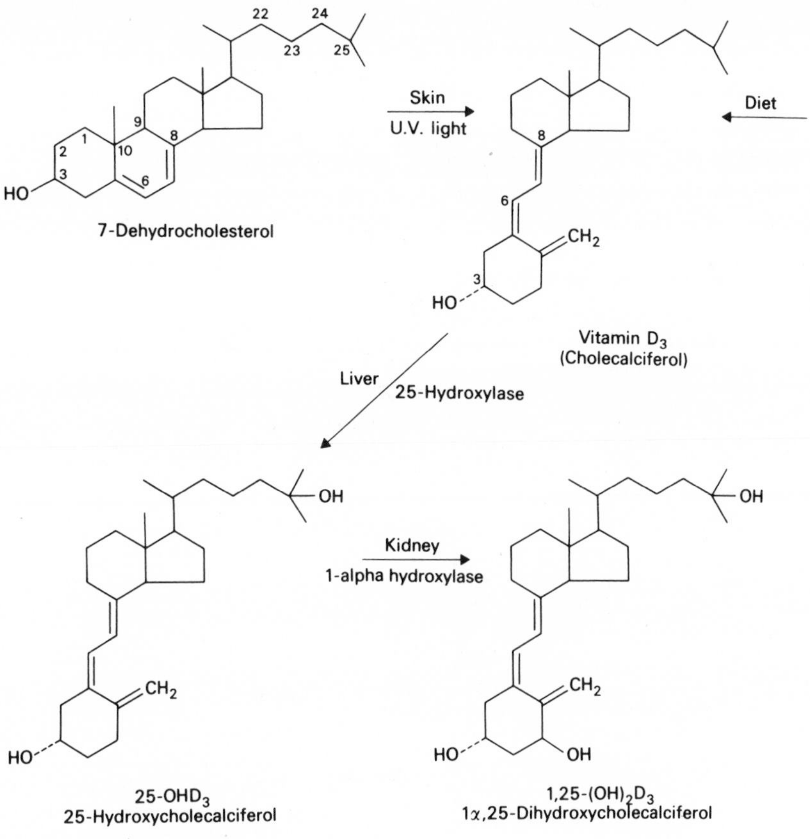

Fig. 14.1. Metabolic activation of vitamin D to 1,25-OHD. In addition the kidney also synthesizes 24,25-OHD, but its function is uncertain.

dant. It is a major vitamin D metabolite, second to 25-OHD but its biological importance is not settled. It may have a role in bone mineralization as its synthesis is favoured by hypercalcaemia, which inhibits 1,25-OHD formation. The reverse situation pertains when serum calcium is low [66]. However, 1,25-OHD clearly has a very significant role and is the most potent vitamin D metabolite. Its serum concentration (30–40 pg/ml) is a thousand times less than that of 25-OHD (20–30 ng/ml) but, in its absence, the complete syndrome of vitamin D deficiency develops. As it is synthesized in the kidney, secreted into the blood stream, and exerts its chief effects elsewhere in the body, it can correctly be regarded as a hormone. Several other vitamin D metabolites of weaker activity exist, but will not be considered here.

The prime function of 1,25-OHD is to sustain plasma levels of calcium and phosphate. This permits mineralization of newly forming bone. The vitamin acts on at least three target organs: gut, bone and kidney (Fig. 14.2). Its major function is in the small intestine where it induces synthesis of brush border proteins which bind calcium and phosphate, promoting their active transport from lumen to blood stream. In the absence of vitamin D, gut absorption of these ions virtually ceases.

In the kidney, the action of vitamin D is uncertain in significance, although a direct action on the proximal convoluted tubule leads to enhanced calcium and phosphate re-absorption. However, even in the absence of vitamin D, 99 per cent of all calcium filtered at the glomerulus can still be re-absorbed. In X-linked familial hypophosphataemia, where the tubule does not respond to vitamin D, phosphate is lost in the urine and rickets results.

Although vitamin D clearly has effects on the skeleton, its action is complex.

The various metabolites have disparate effects and no explanation is yet available to integrate them all. 1,25-OHD is a potent direct stimulator of bone absorption [87,158], but the physiological effect of this is not established. Vitamin D is also essential for normal growth and mineralization of the skeleton. Whether it has a direct growth promoting action or acts only indirectly by providing the optimum milieu for bone growth is not certain. Production of 1,25-OHD is enhanced at times of rapid growth, pregnancy and lactation which are accompanied by an increased need for calcium and phosphorus.

Hypocalcaemia, by stimulating PTH secretion, activates renal 1,α-hydroxylase. This increases

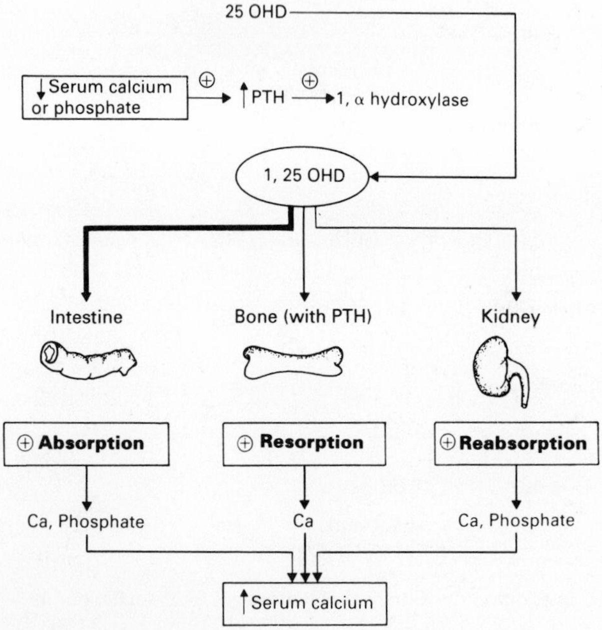

Fig. 14.2. Actions of 1,25-dihydroxyvitamin D. Hypocalcaemia stimulates PTH secretions which activates renal 1,α-hydroxylase, thus increasing production of 1,25-OHD. The actions of 1,25-OHD on intestine, bone and renal tubule are directed at returning serum calcium to normal range (⊕= stimulant effect).

production of 1,25-OHD synthesis (but without the mediation of PTH). This reduces phosphate excretion. The gonadal steroids, growth hormone, human placental lactogen and prolactin as well as PTH and phosphate deficiency all have the capacity to stimulate 1,α-hydroxylase [20,183].

PTH

PTH is the second major hormone influencing calcium balance and bone. Its effects are mediated by intracellular cyclic adenosine monophosphate (cAMP) and its physiological function is to sustain, within narrow limits, extracellular fluid calcium concentration. Any fall in ionized calcium is countered by secretion of PTH. The fall in calcium is checked by the direct effects of PTH on bone and kidney, and its indirect stimulation of calcium absorption from the gut mediated by 1,25-OHD.

In bone, PTH stimulates the activity of osteoclasts and osteoblasts causing bone resorption with calcium and phosphate mobilization. As it stimulates secretion of osteoclast collagenases and similar lytic enzymes, it acts to accomplish metabolic destruction of the bony matrix. This is reflected in increased urinary and plasma hydroxyproline. In general, remodelling activity is stimulated, but osteoclast function predominates. However, the action of PTH on bone is more complex than this and not yet fully elucidated.

In the kidney, PTH acts initially to inhibit phosphate re-absorption by the proximal tubule. Phosphate released from bone is thereby rapidly excreted with resulting hypophosphataemia and hyperphosphaturia in states of PTH excess. By a different mechanism, probably operating distally in the tubule, PTH tends to increase calcium re-absorption. Nevertheless, the flood of calcium from bone exceeds the capacity for calcium re-absorption so that hypercalciuria ensues. PTH also inhibits proximal tubular re-absorption of bicarbonate so that states of PTH excess are often accompanied by a mild metabolic acidosis.

Calcitonin

In the absence of thyroid and parathyroid glands, the response to an intravenous calcium load is blunted and the return to normocalcaemia delayed. This observation suggested the existence of an hypocalcaemic factor, which is now known to be the hormone calcitonin. It is secreted by the parafollicular C cells of the thyroid. Its output is stimulated by a rise in ionized calcium concentration but also by the gut hormones gastrin and cholecystokinin. Hypocalcaemia has the opposite effect. The effect of calcitonin in lowering serum calcium is accompanied by a fall in serum phosphate and both probably result from a direct inhibition of bone breakdown. Also calcitonin inhibits the bone reabsorption produced by a number of substances, including PTH and vitamin D metabolites. The role of calcitonin in the complex system of calcium balance is not yet certain. In medullary carcinoma of the thyroid, where there is hypersecretion of this hormone, there are no overt bony changes and no disturbances of calcium or phosphate levels. An intriguing observation has been that of osteopetrosis in the newborn babies of women with medullary carcinoma, but this may represent genetic linkage of two disorders rather than causation [197].

Changes in bone, calcium and phosphate homeostasis during pregnancy

The requirements for many nutrients and minerals increase during pregnancy, therefore this is a time of increased demand on maternal calcium stores. The fetus is known to accumulate nearly 30 g of calcium and half as much phosphorus in its own tissues [91] and all of this must be maternally derived. Of the calcium accumulation 70 per cent occurs in the third trimester when fetal skeletal growth is maximal. Without an anticipatory rise in calcium absorption, the necessary calcium would be drawn from the maternal skeleton. Furthermore, lactation prolongs the calcium demand. Human milk contains 6–9 mmol of calcium per litre [48] (two to three times the maternal serum level) and the intake of a normal 3 kg infant is 2–3 l/week, increasing with age. Furthermore, there may even be a need for increased bone deposition to provide the added structural support made necessary by the increased bodyweight of pregnancy. What then are the physiological changes which have evolved in pregnancy and how are they achieved?

Early in pregnancy gut absorption of calcium increases. It has doubled by the beginning of the third trimester and remains elevated in the puerperium during lactation [82,177]. The increment in calcium absorption must exceed fetal and maternal needs, as it is accompanied by an increase in urinary loss of calcium in the postprandial state. The 24-hour calcium excretion increases sharply in early pregnancy and may exceed hypercalciuric levels in the third trimester [61].

The explanation for the enhanced calcium absorption may lie in the rise in plasma 1,25-OHD that occurs early and continues through pregnancy [61,102,159,206] (Fig. 14.3). After delivery in the lactating mother, the level falls promptly but remains slightly higher than in non-pregnant women. The concentration of 1,25-OHD in cord blood is appreciably lower than in maternal blood [102,119,209] but, by 24 hours of age, has risen significantly [185]. This can be seen as an adaptive response by the baby to the new need to absorb calcium from the intestinal lumen.

The gestational increase in 1,25-OHD activity suggests that maternal 1,α-hydroxylase activity is stimulated. The cause of this remains enigmatic. It is tempting to postulate that the initial stimulus is a slight fall in ionized calcium which causes PTH release, thus stimulating the enzyme. This is unlikely. Whether PTH rises in pregnancy [38,148] or is unchanged [61,206] has been disputed. A recent study, however, showed a mild but definite increase in PTH bioactivity in late pregnancy [2] supporting the previous notion of a state of mild physiological 'hyperparathyroidism' in pregnancy [38]. However, the timing of the demonstrated rise in PTH, where this has been found, does not coincide with the onset of enhanced calcium absorption. Moreover, after delivery, 1,25-OHD levels fall rapidly to non-pregnant levels within 3 days of delivery [123,159] whilst PTH levels decline slowly to normal levels [119]. Urinary cAMP levels remain normal during pregnancy [61].

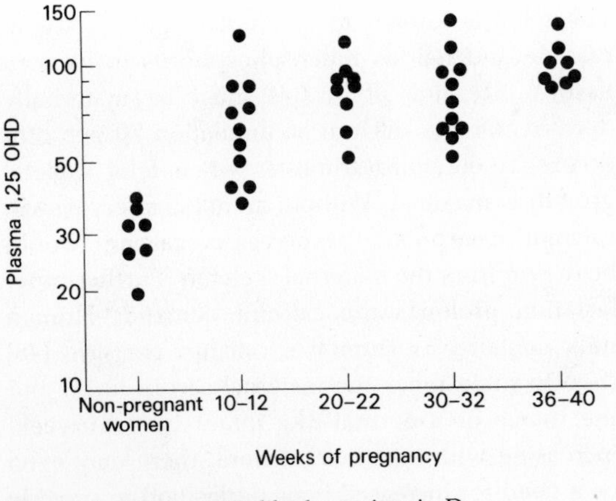

Fig. 14.3. Plasma 1,25-dihydroxyvitamin D concentrations in control women and during pregnancy [206]. Units are ng/l.

However, there is no need to invoke PTH as the sole cause of the rise in 1,25-OHD levels. There are several other stimulators of renal 1,α-hydroxylase activity (see above). Oestrogens are known to do this, at least in post-menopausal osteoporotic women [58,142] and egg-laying birds [24]. The stimulatory effect in the bird is fortified by the presence of progesterone [190]. Both these hormones of course are high in pregnancy, and fall promptly after delivery. Prolactin or human placental lactogen (HPL) may be involved or even growth hormone [20] which bears structural similarity to HPL. Another potent stimulator of the enzyme is lowered plasma phosphate (see below).

Furthermore, the increase in biologically active 1,25-OHD in pregnancy may come from synthesis of the hormone by the placenta itself [203].

In summary, the enhanced calcium absorption of pregnancy is probably due to activation of renal 1,α-hydroxylase. This results in rising concentrations of 1,25-OHD. The initiating stimulus has not been identified.

Total serum calcium and phosphorus fall in pregnancy (Fig. 14.4). The fall in calcium continues from soon after conception until at least the middle of the third trimester [61] but there may be a slight rise thereafter [148]. Phosphates fall in the first trimester and then falls even further to reach low levels in the third trimester [61] but Newman, in 1957 [140], found the level to rise near term. It is likely that the fall in serum proteins accounts for the decline in calcium and the closely parallel patterns for calcium and albumin support this. Furthermore, it has been

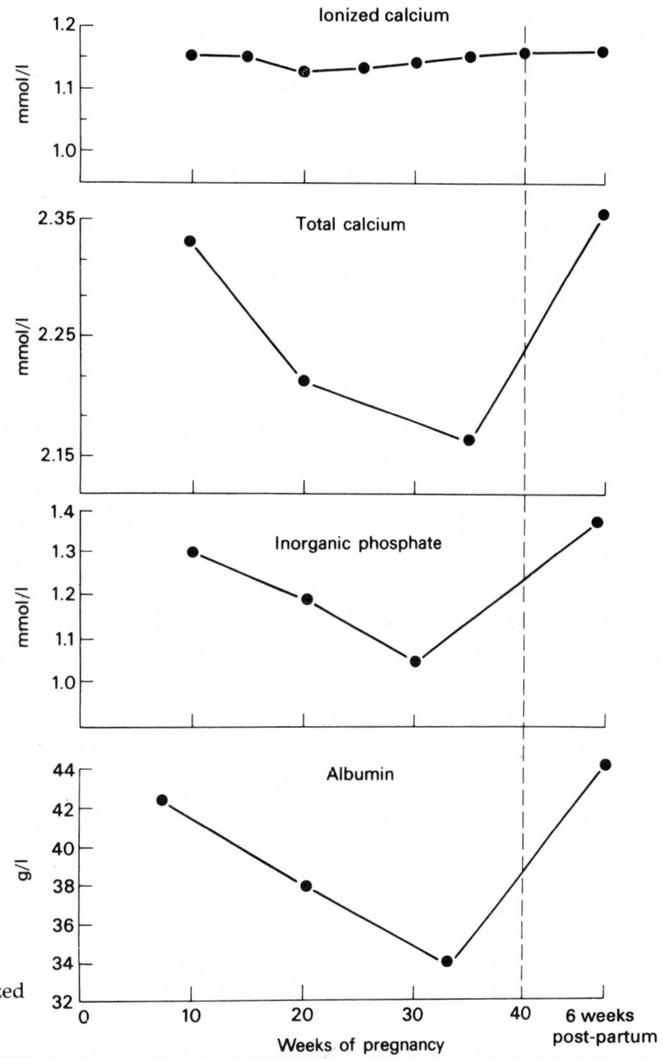

Fig. 14.4. Maternal serum concentrations of ionized calcium, total calcium, inorganic phosphate and albumin during and after pregnancy [148].

demonstrated in longitudinal studies that the fall must be due to the protein bound fraction as ionized calcium either rises very slightly [51] or remains quite constant [61,148], with a minimal decline near delivery [125].

Early in gestation fetal serum calcium is lower than maternal serum calcium [135,204]. At term, however, fetal levels exceed maternal by 0.25–0.5 mmol/l both for total serum calcium [135,209] and free ionic calcium [125]. This has been confirmed to occur from early in the third trimester by direct fetal blood sampling [135]. The existence of a placental active transport mechanism seems likely. Experimental data lend support to this idea [207]. Further circumstantial evidence lies in the observation that serum calcium levels fall promptly in the newborn after separation from placental supply [185,195]. Perhaps maternal 1,25-OHD stimulates a carrier protein to accomplish transplacental passage in the same way that it stimulates transmucosal importation of calcium from the gut lumen.

It is also likely that the fetus can control its calcium influx. This may be through fetal production of 1,25-OHD and there is evidence for this in an umbilical arteriovenous concentration gradient for 1,25-OHD [103,209] with higher arterial levels.

A study in sheep, however, has suggested that it is PTH which promotes the active transport of calcium from mother to fetus and that the calcium pump cannot function in its absence, even where 1,25-OHD levels are sustained [23]. This was also postulated in a human study which showed high fetal levels of bioactive PTH [2].

The state of vitamin D nutrition is conveniently assessed by the plasma level of 25-OHD. This is no different in pregnancy from the non-pregnant range, at least in Caucasian women [42,121,206]. However, levels fluctuate seasonally [31]. A careful longitudinal study [121] (Fig. 14.5) demonstrated a fall during the third trimester when it occurred in winter (January–March). The implication was that, in normal Caucasian women, vitamin D levels are maintained in pregnancy except when the period of greatest demand (third trimester) coincides with the time of least supply (winter). Thus the major determinant is exposure to sunlight and this has been confirmed in Finland [98], North America [86] and Saudi Arabia [175,189], where local customs of dress lead to reduced exposure. In these studies, neonatal 25-OHD levels reflect maternal levels and low levels can be clinically significant as discussed below.

The linear relationship between maternal and cord blood concentrations of 25-OHD suggests direct transfer across the placenta [17,85,121]. On the other hand, 1,25-OHD is significantly lower in the newborn baby than in maternal blood at delivery and bears no relationship to it [85]. This certainly implies that it does not cross the placenta freely.

A definite rise in calcitonin secretion can be detected during pregnancy and lactation [186,206]. Bearing in mind the considerable ability of calcitonin to inhibit bone resorption, even that caused by PTH and vitamin D, it is possible that it has a role in protecting the maternal skeleton from demineralization. The newborn baby also has high calcitonin levels [100,167].

Bone density

The net effect of pregnancy and lactation on skeletal mineral content is not finally established. A retrospective study of Bantu and Caucasian women showed no radiological evidence of bone loss after multiple pregnancies and long lactations [200]. In other studies, bone mass tended to increase with parity [65,141]. Conti[illegible]ng results from photon scanning of the femur [illegible] 10 lactating women suggested mineral losses of 2.2 per cent over 100 days [7]. Distal bone mass in the forearm, assessed by single photon densitometry, was nearly 20 per cent lower in a long-term lactation group (three to four children averaging 11 months lactation) than in a short lactation group [201]. Furthermore, there is evidence that some adolescent mothers demonstrate bone demineralization after 16 weeks of lactation, perhaps because of low dietary intake of calcium and phosphorus [25].

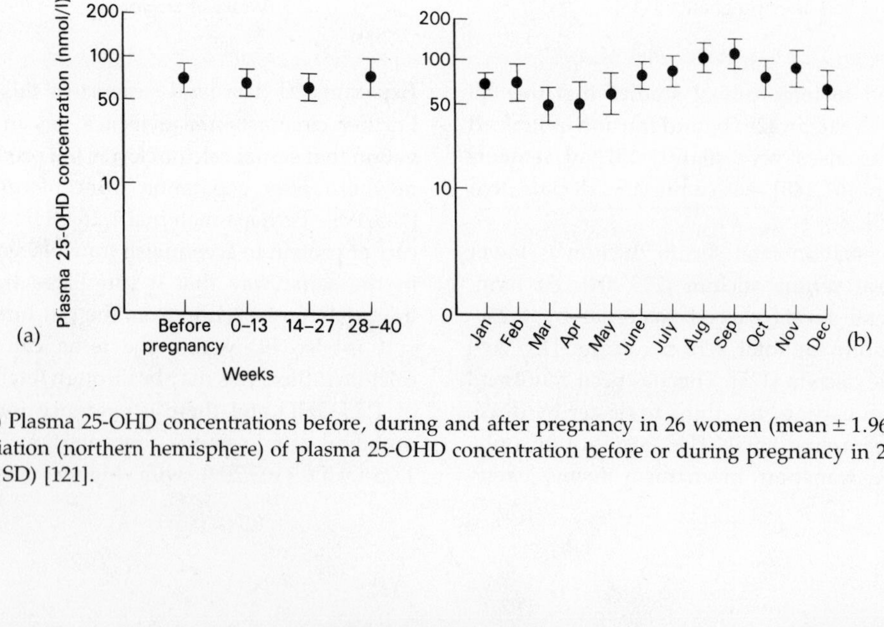

Fig. 14.5. (a) Plasma 25-OHD concentrations before, during and after pregnancy in 26 women (mean ± 1.96 SD). (b) Seasonal variation (northern hemisphere) of plasma 25-OHD concentration before or during pregnancy in 26 women (mean ± 1.96 SD) [121].

X-ray spectrophotometry was used in a prospective investigation [105] and showed a small but significant loss of mineral from trabecular but not cortical bone during pregnancy. Part of this diversity in findings can be attributed to the variety of methods used to assess bone mineral content. Nevertheless, in normal pregnancy there is probably no great change in maternal bone content. Perhaps this is what one would expect as the calcium content of a term infant is <5 per cent of that of its mother and maternal absorption of calcium spread over a 40-week period should be more than adequate to provide for this under normal circumstances. During lactation, however, adequate dietary intake of calcium and phosphorus is important to prevent bone loss.

Table 14.1 summarizes the changes in normal pregnancy discussed above. There is a possibility that there are changes in end organ responsiveness to these hormones in pregnancy, but this has not been taken into account. If this were so, there could be changes in metabolism without quantifiable changes in serum levels of the hormones.

Metabolic bone disease

Metabolic bone diseases are those that affect the whole skeleton, though often the involvement is not uniform. We will discuss here a number of disorders which are important in pregnancy and which can be understood on the basis of aberrations in normal functions considered above. Complete descriptions of each clinical entity in the non-pregnant state can be found elsewhere. For a woman with any of the following disorders, prepregnancy counselling to explain the clinical significance, obstetric and genetic implications of her medical problem is highly desirable.

Rickets and osteomalacia has been classified by Harrison [80] into two types. Type I is secondary to deficiency of 1,25-OHD and an important feature is secondary hyperparathyroidism. Type II rickets (and osteomalacia) is the result of hypophosphataemia, most commonly due to impaired renal tubular phosphate re-absorption. Secondary hyperparathyroidism is not a prominent feature. The pathological disorders within each type are listed in Box 14.1. Most of them are discussed here.

Nutritional osteomalacia

Delay in or failure of bone mineralization is the hallmark of osteomalacia. If it occurs in childhood before closure of the epiphyses, it results in the characteristic disorder of rickets. The rachitic epiphysis, with widened growth plate and distorted architecture, demonstrates hyperosteoidosis, i.e. the presence of excess unmineralized osteoid. The same histopathological features are seen in adults with osteomalacia, but in different sites. The epiphyses having closed, changes can be seen throughout the skeleton wherever remodelling occurs.

There are many causes of osteomalacia, but all exert their pathological effects through abnormalities in vitamin D metabolism or through hypophosphataemia (Table 14.1). The biochemical triad of low serum calcium and phosphate combined with high alkaline phosphatase (heat labile or bone component to be distinguished in pregnancy) is

Table 14.1. Mineral metabolism: changes in serum concentrations in normal pregnancy. Values are representative means from the literature. Individual studies show wide variation and are referenced in square brackets

	Non-pregnant	Third trimester
Total calcium (mmol/l)	2.48[196a]	2.34[31,196a]
Ionized calcium (mmol/l)	1.18[51]	1.22[51]
Urinary calcium (mg/24 hours)	90[61]	300[61]
Total phosphate (mmol/l)	1.24[196a]	1.05[31,196a]
25-OHD (μg/l)	14[43,59]	15[43,159]
1,25-OHD (ng/l)	50[61,206]	120[61,206]

Box 14.1. Classification of rickets and osteomalacia [80]

- Type I
  - Vitamin D deficiency
    - sunlight deficiency
    - dietary deficiency
  - Vitamin D malabsorption
  - Liver disease
  - Drug-induced
    - anticonvulsants
    - corticosteroids
    - heparin
  - Renal insufficiency
- Type II
  - Fanconi's syndrome
  - Renal tubular acidosis
    - cystinosis
    - tyrosinosis
    - idiopathic
  - Familial primary hypophosphataemia
  - Acquired primary hypophosphataemia

generally seen with osteomalacia. Urinary hydroxyproline is almost always raised. The diagnosis of nutritional osteomalacia, however, should also include low plasma 25-OHD and high PTH concentrations (reflecting secondary hyperparathyroidism). X-ray features will not be discussed here.

In pregnant Asians in Britain, nutritional osteomalacia seems to be common, though often unrecognized. The appearance of clinical osteomalacia with fractures in a pregnant woman may be a presenting feature of vitamin D deficiency [39,146] as may be the birth of a baby with rickets [53,134] or hypocalcaemia in the first week of life [83]. Enamel defects may develop in the teeth later in life [31,154], particularly after neonatal hypocalcaemic tetany.

In an investigation of maternal factors relevant to neonatal hypocalcaemia, Watney *et al.* [202] demonstrated lower serum calcium levels in Asian women than in Caucasian women at booking, 36 weeks and 6 weeks after delivery. The Asian babies had lower serum calcium levels on the sixth day of life. Elsewhere, it was shown prospectively that 25-OHD levels in Asians were lower than in Caucasians at every occasion when they were sampled throughout late pregnancy [44] (Fig. 14.6). Brooke *et al.* [18] showed that vegetarian Asians had significantly lower levels on each occasion studied and 70 per cent of them had undetectable 25-OHD levels after pregnancy (compared with 12 per cent of non-vegetarians). Nearly half of the babies of vegetarian women had hypocalcaemia whilst none of the other babies developed the problem. These studies supported the findings of a number of previous investigations into the vitamin D and calcium status of pregnant Asian women in the UK [17,43,83,150].

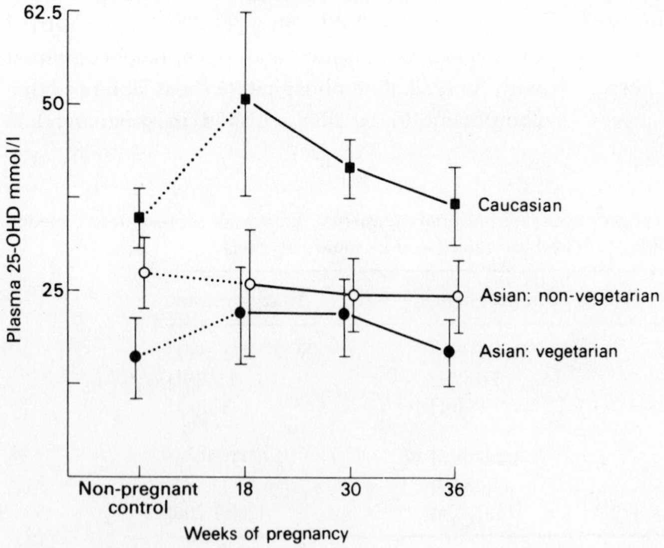

Fig. 14.6. Plasma 25-OHD concentrations in non-pregnant women and during pregnancy [43].

Studies from Pakistan [157] and India [160] have shown a high prevalence of subclinical and even overt osteomalacia in pregnant women. In Saudi Arabia, many women and their babies have very low levels of 25-OHD and serum calcium [175, 189] indicating vitamin D deficiency. This is chiefly attributed to lack of exposure to sunlight owing to the traditional custom of women being entirely covered by their clothes.

Certainly vitamin D supplementation in pregnancy can ameliorate these changes. If pregnant Asians are given 1000 units daily, the 25-OHD level in cord blood is higher than after unsupplemented pregnancy. Even so there was no difference in bone mineral content of neonatal forearms as assessed by photon absorptiometry [34]. The conclusion was that fetal mineralization is not impaired by maternal vitamin D deficiency. Unfortunately, as neither maternal 1,25-OHD nor 25-OHD were measured this conclusion may not be justified. In a similar study [41], 25-OHD levels were higher in both cord and maternal serum after supplementation in pregnancy but there was no attempt to assess neonatal bone density.

Others also have disputed that pregnancy leads to an increased requirement for vitamin D. Dent and Gupta [43] showed that 25-OHD levels were low in a group of Asian women and remained so throughout pregnancy without further fall. They argued that this suggested there was no increased need for vitamin D in pregnancy.

Nevertheless the association between pregnancy and osteomalacia, at least in Asians [127,210] is undeniable. It may be that pregnancy brings a vitamin D deficient woman to medical attention for the first time by coincidence rather than causation. What is still unknown is whether women with very low vitamin D levels can furnish the normal pregnancy rise in 1,25-OHD concentration. If there is a tendency for pregnancy to unmask latent osteomalacia, it may be explicable on this basis.

It is established that low maternal 25-OHD levels are associated with neonatal morbidity [31,83,202] and impaired first year growth in some groups [19]. This underlies the recommendation that vitamin D supplements be given routinely to all Asian women in the UK from the Indian subcontinent or East Africa during pregnancy. A dose of 400 IU daily from 20 weeks or 1000 IU from 30 weeks is probably sufficient [19]. The basis for their deficiency seems to lie in dietary inadequacy (even in non-vegetarians, the diet usually contains little vitamin D) and equally, if not more so, in lack of skin exposure to sunlight. Of course indoor dwelling, northern latitudes, poor diet and the winter season all tend to aggravate the problem in many patients and a valid argument can be made for supplementing all women in these circumstances.

The World Health Organization [208] and National Academy of Sciences [52] recommend 400 IU (10 μg) of vitamin D daily during pregnancy and lactation. In the absence of widespread milk supplementation with vitamin D, as practised in the USA, prescription of vitamin D by doctors is necessary. In a controlled trial [31] 400 IU of ergocalciferol was as effective at preventing, neonatal problems as 1000 IU has been [17]. The preferred dose would, therefore, seem to be 400 IU. Moreover, it is of great interest that perhaps even a single dose of vitamin D at the beginning of the third trimester will suffice. In a French study this was the case, with maternal and cord 25-OHD levels being no lower than after daily supplementation [122].

The added loss of calcium in milk in the puerperium makes the consumption of either 0.6–1.2 l (1–2 pints) of milk per day, supplemental calcium or a high calcium diet advisable in all lactating women.

Rickets

Childhood rickets results in stunting of bone growth so that the pelvis may not attain normal size and structure. This often results in reduction of the pelvic diameters. In particular the anteroposterior diameter of the brim is reduced (Fig. 14.7). Subsequent mechanical problems in vaginal delivery are well established. Whilst the bone structure cannot be improved in the short term, it remains essential that these women receive vitamin D during pregnancy as the fetus is at risk of bone disease.

Gastrointestinal and hepatic osteomalacia

Osteomalacia due to vitamin D and calcium deficiency may complicate any disorder of intestinal

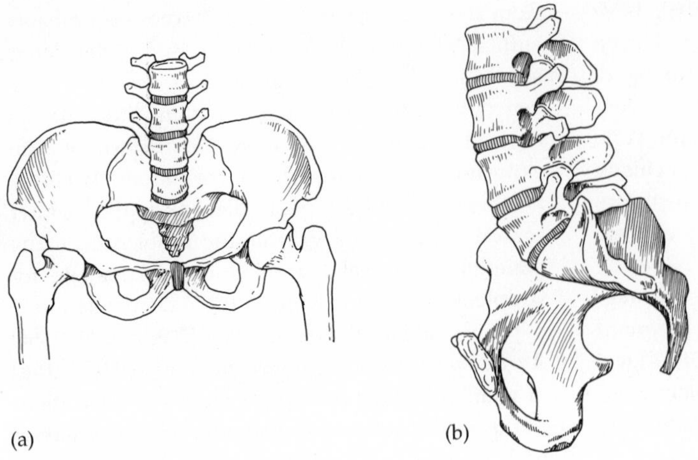

Fig. 14.7. (a) Rachitic flat pelvis. (b) Sagittal section of rachitic flat pelvis with false promontory and reduced diameter of pelvic inlet.

absorptive function (see Chapters 9 and 10) for an account of these conditions). Patients with inflammatory bowel disease, particularly Crohn's disease after intestinal resection, are at high risk. Seventy per cent of patients with Crohn's disease in an American series had subnormal 25-OHD levels [60]. Moreover, these patients may need very high doses of vitamin D (20 000–50 000 IU) to reverse the bone disease [44], probably because little of the administered dose is absorbed. Vitamin D may be given weekly due to its long duration of action. Patients may also have osteoporosis related to corticosteroid therapy and complex metabolic disturbances, as well as osteomalacia. Despite these potential problems, neither bony complications nor hypocalcaemia in mother or baby have been noticed in pregnancies complicated by Crohn's disease [133]. Nevertheless, it is advisable to monitor calcium and phosphate levels of women who have had bowel resection and thus may be subject to malabsorption. Vitamin D should be given in the usual recommended dose and a larger dose, which may be monitored by serum 25-OHD levels should be given if the mother has had prior evidence of vitamin D deficiency. Also the infant should be monitored for hypocalcaemia. One study of Asian mothers who did not have inflammatory bowel disease [202] indicated that elevated maternal heat labile alkaline phosphatase and lowered serum phosphate are predictors of neonatal hypocalcaemia. These findings may be relevant to the pregnant patient with Crohn's disease.

Depression of serum 25-OHD, possibly temporary, has been seen in 33–60 per cent of patients after jejuno-ileal bypass for morbid obesity, in spite of supplementation with 800 IU of vitamin D/day [172,191] and bone loss also occurs in these patients. A larger number of such women are now becoming pregnant and supplementation is warranted, with monitoring of mother and baby as detailed.

Gluten-sensitive enteropathy (coeliac disease) also affects vitamin D absorption [5] and osteomalacia is a risk. There is a suggestion that 25-OHD may be better absorbed than vitamin D itself in this condition. Of course, the first prerequisite of care must be the obsessional adherence to a gluten-free diet. Such dietary treatment can reverse infertility and normal pregnancies have been reported [137] (see Chapter 10).

Modern treatment of cystic fibrosis of the pancreas allows increasing numbers of women to successfully conceive and complete pregnancy (see Chapter 1). Whilst bone disease is far from the most serious problem, it can exist and low 25-OHD levels with decreased bone mass have been detected, even after dietary vitamin D supplementation [77]. Exocrine pancreatic enzyme replacement must be continued throughout pregnancy, and vitamin D may have to be given parenterally.

As the liver is the site of synthesis of 25-OHD,

liver diseases are often associated with low serum 25-OHD concentrations. However, osteomalacia is seen more frequently with cholestatic liver disorders than with hepatocellular disease. This probably reflects lack of bile salts in the intestinal lumen rendering vitamin D absorption inadequate. Even so, malabsorption is not the sole problem since, even if vitamin D is given parenterally, large doses (100 000 IU/month) are required to elevate 25-OHD levels in patients with primary biliary cirrhosis [178].

The only cholestatic disease seen with any frequency in pregnancy is idiopathic cholestasis of pregnancy (Chapter 9). Although a temporary deficit of 25-OHD might be expected in this condition, it has not been reported.

Renal bone disease

Bone lesions are common in long-standing kidney disease. They are seen in two different clinical settings. First, osteomalacia with retardation of growth in children, resulting from conditions causing renal tubular acidosis. There may also be renal calculi and nephrocalcinosis. The bone lesions probably result from calcium and phosphate loss in the urine, but may be related to the acidosis itself, causing osteolysis with liberation of calcium.

Second, in the presence of chronic renal failure, the pathogenesis of osteomalacia is related to deficiency of 1,25-OHD. There is phosphate retention and hypocalcaemia causing secondary hyperparathyroidism in chronic renal failure. Treatment includes administration of vitamin D and calcium, and lowering of phosphate absorption from the gut using non-absorbable antacids. The more potent forms of vitamin D (e.g. calcitriol) are needed and careful monitoring is necessary to avoid hypercalcaemia from these cases.

Pregnancy is occasionally encountered in women with chronic renal failure (see Chapter 7). Congenital rickets has been reported as a complication in their babies [170]. Certainly, vitamin D should be administered (and calcitriol is preferred), but the exact dose is not yet established and monitoring of maternal calcium is essential.

Drug-induced osteopenia

Drugs that affect bone which may be used in pregnancy are the anticonvulsants, heparin and corticosteroids. Steroids will not be discussed here, since steroid-induced bone disease is rarely a problem in pregnancy; heparin-induced osteopenia is considered in Chapter 4.

Anticonvulsants

Anticonvulsant osteomalacia results from drug-induced disturbance of vitamin D metabolism, and disordered mineral ion transport in bone and intestine. Most of the currently used anticonvulsants have been implicated and the changes are dose dependent.

Most anticonvulsants stimulate activity of the hepatic microsomal oxidase enzymes, thereby converting vitamin D and 25-OHD to inactivate metabolites [76]. Furthermore, phenytoin may also inhibit transintestinal calcium transport [75]. Phenytoin and phenobarbitone can inhibit bone resorption caused by PTH and 25-OHD [92]. The usual manifestations of this are a slightly low serum calcium and a distinctly low serum 25-OHD level, often with elevated alkaline phosphatase [76]. Bone loss can be detected by radiology, by photon absorption, and of course, by bone biopsy. Only in the most severe cases will the complete picture of osteomalacia (or rickets in children) develop.

Christiansen *et al.* [28] found that the bone content of epileptic gravidae was 86 per cent of that of age-matched controls at 18 weeks. This difference persisted at 8 days and at 6 months post-partum. The bone content of the babies was no different from a control group. It is noteworthy that all epileptics and controls received vitamin D supplements throughout. Fleischman *et al.* [50] reported reduced 25-OHD levels in epileptic mothers and their babies, and hypocalcaemia in one infant. These findings were reproduced in a longitudinal study of epileptic women in pregnancy. Those on phenytoin had lower 25-OHD and 1,25-OHD values than controls, both in maternal and cord serum, but the levels in carbamazepine treated mothers tended to be intermediate [124]. All mothers had received

400 IU of vitamin D_3 daily. None of the women or their babies had clinical evidence of hypocalcaemia or bone disease.

It is regarded as advisable, at least in the UK, to give supplements to all women on anticonvulsant drugs [16] in a dose of 400 IU daily from early in the second trimester, or 1000 IU daily in the third trimester. It is established that supplements of this dose are safe, and do not cause hypercalcaemia of infancy which may have resulted from the much higher doses used some decades ago [113].

Parathyroid disease

Primary hyperparathyroidism

The use of multichannel analysers has led to a great increase in the detection of patients with asymptomatic hypercalcaemia, many of whom have primary hyperparathyroidism. It should be remembered that the total serum calcium is lowered in pregnancy and a corrective factor for the low albumin concentration should be applied. Thus total calcium levels within the normal non-pregnant range may represent hypercalcaemia in a pregnant woman.

Hyperparathyroidism in pregnancy is a serious condition associated with a high rate of fetal loss and increased perinatal morbidity and mortality. Several literature reviews [101,117,176,211] have reiterated the high risks which comprise neonatal tetany, still-birth, neonatal death and abortion. In fact maternal hyperparathyroidism is occasionally diagnosed only after suspicion provoked by tetany in her newborn baby [10].

Wagner *et al.* [199] found the presence of maternal bone disease (osteitis fibrosa or bone cysts) to be a worrying feature as perinatal deaths came from this group in their study. Conversely, pregnancy outcome was not correlated with renal involvement.

Neonatal hypocalcaemia is a result of parathyroid suppression by high ambient calcium levels during intrauterine life. Recovery of normal parathyroid gland function appears to take a considerable time in these infants and hypocalcaemia may continue for many weeks [10]. Intrauterine death may relate to severe hypercalcaemia, as fetal calcium levels exceed maternal [185] because of transplacental active transport of calcium.

Most women with hyperparathyroidism tolerate pregnancy well. In fact pregnancy may offer some protection against hypercalcaemia because of the low serum albumin and calcium transfer to the fetus. Even so, there are several reports of hypercalcaemic crisis in pregnancy [29,192,205]. What might seem more likely is post-partum crisis; but this has been reported only three times [126,165,171]. One case was fatal [126]. The nausea and vomiting of hypercalcaemia may be confused with hyperemesis gravidarum and a case of this, caused by hyperparathyroidism, has been reported [68]. Hyperparathyroidism may also be complicated by acute pancreatitis (see Chapter 9). There is no doubt that the definitive treatment of hyperparathyroidism is surgical. Moreover, neck exploration has proven a relatively safe procedure in pregnancy. In 16 cases reported by Shangold, operation was performed during pregnancy with only one stillbirth, at 26 weeks [205]. The remaining 27 of the 28 fetal losses described occurred in the absence of surgical treatment, as did all of the 35 cases of neonatal tetany. The reviews of Kristoffersson *et al.* [101] and Wilson *et al.* [211] have also concluded that there is a higher risk of fetal and neonatal complications when parathyroidectomy is not performed antenatally. For the fetus, therefore, maternal parathyroidectomy seems to be the best course of action. Ultrasound may successfully locate a parathyroid adenoma. Isotope studies are contraindicated in pregnancy and often the adenoma or hyperplasia is not located until surgery. If for any reason neck exploration cannot be performed, medical treatment with low calcium diet, high fluid intake and oral phosphate should be commenced. Montoro *et al.* [136] reported success with this therapy. Of course women with mild asymptomatic hypercalcaemia may be followed throughout pregnancy without operation and with good outcome [117].

Hypoparathyroidism

In young women this usually represents a complication of thyroid surgery. Rarely, it is part of an autoimmune disorder where antibodies are directed against adrenal, thyroid, gastric and ovarian tissue as well. Treatment is intended to maintain serum calcium within normal limits with vitamin D and oral calcium supplements. In pregnancy the requirement for vitamin D has been seen to increase two- to threefold, as its behaviour in normal pregnancy might suggest [164,166]. For the fetus, the consequences of untreated maternal hypoparathyroidism are serious. There is evidence that severe hypocalcaemia is associated with mid-trimester abortion [46]. Also, intrauterine parathyroid overactivity has been reported [63,106,168] and neonatal rickets may occur [69]. In those cases where the maternal condition has been undiagnosed or inadequately treated, maternal hypocalcaemia leads to fetal hypocalcaemia, secondary parathyroid hyperplasia and bone demineralization [106,168].

Maternal therapy with oral vitamin D and calcium prevents deleterious effects in the fetus [71]. The successful use of oral 1,25-OHD has been reported [144,164], but this must be monitored carefully as one baby showed increased density of skull and long bones consistent with excessive mineralization [166]. Frequent estimation of maternal calcium and phosphate is necessary and vitamin D is safest given as 1,α-OHD or 1,25-OHD. These have the shortest half-life (6–8 hours) thereby allowing titration of dose against response. As mentioned, it will usually be necessary to increase the dose to maintain normocalcaemia as pregnancy progresses. However, there is also the danger of provoking hypercalcaemia, particularly if using the potent synthetic analogue of vitamin D, dihydrotachysterol [93] or calcitriol. Moreover continuation of these high doses into the puerperium is hazardous. When the dose is not decreased after delivery, serious maternal hypercalcaemia may ensue and has also been reported in a breast-feeding infant. Calcium monitoring is indicated.

In pseudohypoparathyroidism there is end-organ resistance to the actions of PTH resulting in hypocalcaemia and renal resistance to the phosphaturic effect of PTH. The implications for pregnancy are the same as in hypoparathyroidism [62,144]. The therapy is identical although patients have been described in whom prior vitamin D dependency disappeared in pregnancy without treatment, suggesting placental production of 1,25-OHD.

Osteoporosis of pregnancy and the puerperium

Significant osteoporosis is rare in pregnant women, but three forms have been recognized, including that associated with heparin (see Chapter 4). The two major varieties are detailed here.

1 Post-pregnancy spinal osteoporosis presents with severe back pain and loss of height due to vertebral compression fractures, possibly at a number of levels in late pregnancy or the puerperium. Over three decades at least 27 cases have been documented [42,73,116,143,182]. Most of these have had full investigation, including bone biopsy, with no cause for osteoporosis having been found. In all cases subsequent pregnancy was uneventful, with no further fractures, but lactation was usually proscribed. This is rational as lactation is associated with bone loss [96a]. Fortunately, elevated bone formation, in excess of resorption, seems to follow weaning allowing restoration of bone mass. Calcium intake of at least 1200 mg daily is necessary. Other studies of normal lactating women suggest that bone turnover is accelerated [74] but that significant bone loss usually does not occur. It may occur, however, in adolescents or in women with an as yet undefined propensity to osteoporosis. It is postulated that such women develop osteoporosis of pregnancy. The existence of this entity has been disputed by Dent and Friedman [42] whose contention was that the association with pregnancy is coincidental. They believed that women with idiopathic osteoporosis had developed fractures consequent to the weight gain of normal pregnancy and that it was unlikely that the physiological changes of normal pregnancy were of sufficient magnitude to cause significant bone loss in an otherwise healthy woman. Calcitriol normally falls dramatically postpartum.

2 Transient hip osteoporosis of pregnancy. This was described by Curtiss and Kincaid in 1959 [37a]. The neck of the femur is also susceptible to osteoporosis in pregnancy. Many women complain of pain in the hip, but radiographical studies are seldom performed in pregnancy. Some of these patients may have osteoporosis as described by Longstreth *et al.* [115]. Apropos of this observation, severe hip pain in late pregnancy was studied recently by bone mineral content estimation. In six women with severe pain undergoing six femoral bone density studies each (three on each femur), 33 per cent of the densities were decreased. Conversely in 20 normal women studied, only 10 per cent of the bone densities were decreased. Many other cases have been reported with symptoms limited to pregnancy and the puerperium [14a,43a]. The pain may be in one or both hips, worse with weight bearing and usually begins around 35 weeks gestation. Radiology may demonstrate pronounced loss of cortical bone in the hip joint but spontaneous recovery is usual. Prudence dictates cessation of lactation although no studies have proven this. Calcitonin has been used to reduce bone resorption.

The progression of femoral head necrosis is very uncommon, and resembles that seen after steroid ingestion. There are some cases occurring in pregnancy where no cause was apparent [96,217]. These women complain of increasingly severe pain in the hip which may be of sudden onset.

In summary, the diagnosis of osteoporosis should be considered in any woman with persistent and severe back or hip pain in late pregnancy or the puerperium, who has appropriate radiological findings. A complete search for other causes is necessary before ascribing a diagnosis of idiopathic osteoporosis of pregnancy.

Other inherited skeletal and metabolic disorders

Osteogenesis imperfecta

This is a generalized disorder affecting connective tissue. The most common variety (tarda) has autosomal dominant inheritance with very variable penetrance and expression. Less common is osteogenesis imperfecta congenita which is inherited as an autosomal recessive but which is lethal with death occurring *in utero* or in the immediate neonatal period. Second trimester diagnosis of osteogenesis imperfecta congenita by ultrasound is now an established technique in pregnancies at risk [130]. Pope *et al.* [151] have characterized a deletion within a collagen gene in four cases of lethal congenital osteogenesis imperfecta which makes it likely that prenatal diagnosis from chorion biopsy material will soon be available [181]. In osteogenesis imperfecta tarda, the basic defect is not known but the fully developed syndrome involves blue sclerae, deafness from otosclerosis, multiple fractures, joint laxity and heart valve abnormalities. Metabolic abnormalities include impaired platelet function and hyperpyrexia during general anaesthesia [161].

The bones are porotic and fragile and repeated fractures leave the sufferer with skeletal deformity. The pelvis is often misshapen with subsequent cephalopelvic disproportion. Ultrasound or radiography of the fetus should be performed before delivery. If the baby is affected, it is best to minimize birth trauma and this usually means delivery by caesarean section.

Because of the potential complications of general anaesthesia (hyperpyrexia, skeletal injury to the unconscious patient, respiratory embarrassment from kyphoscoliosis), a lumbar epidural is the anaesthesia of choice, although accurate needle placement may be difficult due to bony deformity [153].

Scoliosis is the most common deformity. If severe, it is accompanied by diminished lung volume, as in the case of Sengupta *et al.* [174]. Despite the fact that respiratory difficulties have not been prominent in the reported cases, pulmonary function should be monitored.

No therapy is of proven benefit in this disorder. Even so, all patients should be given calcium supplements as a propensity for hypocalcaemia in pregnancy has been demonstrated [56].

Achondroplasia

Inheritance is autosomal dominant, but many cases represent new mutations. Women with this bony disorder tend to have an early menopause. They have an increased prevalence of uterine fibroids.

During pregnancy, cardiorespiratory compromise due to restriction of lung volume is a risk as the fetus grows larger. All women with achondroplasia require caesarean section because of pelvic contraction. Moreover, general anaesthesia should be used because spinal stenosis is usual in these patients making epidural anaesthesia technically difficult. Furthermore, particular care must be taken in manipulating the neck during tracheal intubation because of cervical spinal stenosis [78]. Fetal achondroplasia may be diagnosed by ultrasound, even early in the second trimester [70,104], with detection of abnormal limbs.

Other rare, inherited bone disorders

There are a number of very rare bone dysplasias. They will not be discussed here but details can be found in the articles of Hall [78] and Allanson and Hall [1].

Marfan's syndrome (see also Chapter 5 for Ehlers–Danlos syndrome)

This generalized disorder of connective tissue displays autosomal dominant inheritance. It has recently been shown that Marfan's syndrome is due to a defect in fibrillin synthesis. In Marfan's syndrome (but not in some other marfanoid conditions such as contractural arachnodactyly) this defect is due to mutations of a fibrillin gene on chromosome 15 [196]. Definitive diagnosis in the index case and prenatal diagnosis in fetuses of patients with Marfan's disease is now possible in many families.

The chief defects in Marfan's syndrome are in the skeletal, ocular and cardiovascular systems. The cardiovascular problems are dominant particularly in pregnancy and these are considered in Chapter 5.

There is an increase in length of the tubular bones and there are weak yielding ligaments leading to joint laxity and kyphoscoliosis. These abnormalities usually cause no problem in pregnancy; neither is there any severe structural problem with the pelvis. Women with Marfan's syndrome have an increased risk of spontaneous abortion with low birthweight babies [155] and also of pre-term labour [112]. Spontaneous uterine inversion in association with Marfan's syndrome has been reported [156] and so has the formation of rectovaginal fistula [114].

Homocystinuria

Homocystinuria is a condition in which deficiency of cystathionine β synthase results in increased plasma levels of homocysteine and methionine and decreased plasma cysteine. It is inherited as an autosomal recessive but there is considerable heterogeneity in its expression since some patients, more severely affected, do not respond to pyridoxine whilst others do. The major clinical effects are mental retardation and seizures, dislocation of the optic lens, osteoporosis and thromboembolism, the last being the most frequent cause of mortality [138]. The mechanism of thromboembolism is not known. Treatment is by methionine restriction and pyridoxine administration in those patients responsive to pyridoxine.

The condition has been reviewed in 629 patients on the basis of an international questionnaire by Mudd *et al.* [138]. These authors also discussed 108 pregnancies amongst 47 homocystinuric women [138]. The majority (88 per cent) occurred in pyridoxine-responsive women, either because of their higher intelligence and better general health, or because of some undefined factor acting against fertility in pyridoxine-resistant patients. The overall poor results (40 per cent pregnancy loss rate), are dominated by three patients who between them lost 22 pregnancies. These women may also represent a subset with a specific abnormality mitigating against successful pregnancy. However, patients with modestly elevated homocysteine levels who are heterozygotes for homocystinuria also have high perinatal mortality rate [22] and recurrent abortion and placental abruption have been reported in association with hyperhomocysteinaemia in general [184]. (Homocysteine levels may also be elevated because of abnormalities in folate and vitamin B_{12} metabolism.) Hyperhomocysteinaemia is a known risk factor for premature vascular disease [30]. Therefore by analogy with patients with the cardiolipin syndrome (see Chapter 8) who are also at risk from still-birth and thromboembolism, the abnormality in homocystinuria may cause extensive placental infarction though this suggestion remains speculative.

Thromboembolism is the other cause for concern. In non-pregnant patients thromboembolism is a major cause of mortality and it may also occur postoperatively [138]. There have been at least two cases of cerebrovascular disease reported in pregnancy; one a fatal case in a woman with a poor obstetric history [35] and the other occurring in a heterozygote following caesarean section [131]. Yet Brenton *et al.* [14] have reviewed seven pregnancies under their care which were all uncomplicated. The patients were able to maintain normal methionine levels taking pyridoxine with no change in their biochemical control during pregnancy.

So the decision concerning thromboprophylaxis in pregnancy is difficult. Standard 'high risk' prophylaxis would involve giving heparin throughout pregnancy but this would increase the risk of osteoporosis (see Chapter 4) to which these patients are already exposed. The cases of thromboembolism which have occurred have both been after delivery. Perhaps the best compromise would be antenatal low dose aspirin (75 mg/day). This has been used in the non-pregnant state [138] in homocystinuria and also may improve the fetal outcome (see above and Chapter 8). At delivery they could be treated with low dose subcutaneous heparin continuing for at least 1 week post-partum with a further 5 weeks of subcutaneous heparin or warfarin (see Chapter 4). Patients who have already had thromboembolism, who have a poor family history, who have ultrasound evidence of preexisting vascular disease [163] or who are unable to maintain normal methionine levels may need to consider subcutaneous heparin treatment throughout prenancy.

Pseudoxanthoma elasticum

Pseudoxanthoma elasticum is inherited as an autosomal recessive condition although dominant inheritance has been reported. It is characterized by degeneration and calcification of elastic tissue causing characteristic skin which is very lax and appears prematurely aged particularly around the neck. In addition abnormalities may be seen in the retina on fundoscopy (angioid streaks) and are present in blood vessels leading to premature cerebral, coronary and peripheral vascular disease. Hypertension was present in 22 per cent of 200 cases [47]. Weakness of splanchnic arteries may lead to gastrointestinal bleeding. Mitral valve prolapse is common [108]. Until 1987 there had been about 28 pregnancies reported in 11 women [8,107]. Haematemesis was common and often required blood transfusion. It was clearly the major risk in pregnancy although patients are not necessarily more susceptible to haemorrhage in pregnancy than in the non-pregnant state. Because many patients have hypertension and because they are at risk from cerebrovascular disease, any additional hypertension due to pre-eclampsia should be treated aggressively [107]. However, in 1987 a large study was reported from South Africa concerning pseudoxanthoma elasticum in 54 pregnancies [198]. The risk of haemorrhage was not confirmed although the risk of hypertension was. First trimester miscarriage and the cosmetic problems of lax abdominal skin in multigravidae were additional features.

Phenylketonuria

Classical phenylketonuria is an inborn error of metabolism, inherited as an autosomal recessive, whereby phenylalanine is not metabolized to tyrosine because of the absence of phenylalanine hydroxylase. Its metabolic precursor, phenylpyruvic acid, is then excreted in the urine. It is usually diagnosed in the newborn by the Guthrie test, which detects the excess of phenylalanine in the blood; the diagnosis is confirmed by quantifying the high level of phenylalanine and low level of tyrosine. If left untreated, the condition is associated with severe retardation in the growing child. The presence of the phenylketonuria gene in the fetus seems unlikely to affect the fetal outcome, at least in a comparison of phenylketonuria and non-phenylketonuria siblings from a woman with untreated phenylketonuria in pregnancy [110].

Since phenylalanine is present in nearly all proteins, dietary treatment consists of virtual elimination of natural proteins, and substitution of an hydrolysate of amino acid with very low phenylalanine content. Children can often continue the diet for the first years of life and if they do their subsequent development is nearly normal. Neonatal screening and early dietary intervention are so efficient that it is very unusual to see children with severe mental handicap from phenylketonuria [129]. However, when the children return to a normal diet, at between 4 and 8 years of age, blood levels of phenylalanine rise again. Many such girls previously treated in childhood are now reaching reproductive age. In addition some individuals with milder forms of previously underdiagnosed hyperphenylalaninaemia are also being detected in screening programmes [90]. It is now realized that phenylketonuria is quite a heterogeneous condition. More than 40 different mutations of the phenylalanine hydroxylase gene have been identified [99] resulting in a range of phenylalanine levels from only just over those found in heterozygotes to 20 times the normal level.

The importance of these observations is that maternal hyperphenylalaninaemia >1.2 mmol/l ('classical phenylketonuria') is associated with a very high incidence of abortion, intrauterine growth retardation, fetal congenital abnormalities, almost exclusively congenital heart disease [109] and in particular tetralogy of Fallot [36], and also microcephaly and mental retardation [90,111,120,214]. The risk of microcephaly and mental retardation appears to be 75 per cent in the infants of women with phenylalanine levels between 0.96 and 1.2 mmol/l [109]. The association is not complete. Some normal infants have been born to mothers with documented hyperphenylalaninaemia in pregnancy [212] but the chance of producing a normal infant in these circumstances is very low. The exact mechanism of fetal damage is not known but the ability of the placenta to concentrate phenylalanine on the fetal side may be a major factor. More recently Levy and Waisbren [111] have revised their recommendations concerning maternal phenylalanine levels and subsequent mental status of the offspring. Although they found that the child's IQ was proportional to both maternal IQ and maternal phenylalanine level, with one exception amongst 53 children they only found mental retardation where the maternal phenylalanine level was >1.1 mmol/l [111]. However, as others have pointed out [21,97] in the data of Levy and Waisbren [111] there was a steady decline of IQ levels with increasing maternal phenylalanine >0.4 mmol/l. In addition, Hyanek *et al.* [90] have shown a mild degree of retardation in the offspring of women with serum phenylalanine concentrations >0.25 mmol/l. However, it is clear that if dietary therapy is to be effective, it must be started before conception [45]. In the above studies, the timing of blood sampling in relation to the beginning of pregnancy is not always stated.

The re-introduction of dietary therapies can certainly improve the fetal prognosis [6,40] even if started in the third trimester [215] though the latter has been disputed [149]. However, abnormal babies have been born to women taking adequate dietary therapy [173,180], including one case of congenital heart disease in a woman who started a diet at 6 weeks' gestation [12]. The most recent collaborative international study of 64 pregnancies [45] indicates that the fetus will not be grossly affected if the maternal diet results in a phenylalanine concentration $<600\,\mu$mol/l at the time of conception and if this diet is maintained through pregnancy. This at least should be the target of dietary therapy in the estimated 500 fertile women with phenylketonuria that there will be in the UK by the year 2000 [45]. However, from the data of Hyanek *et al.* [90] cited above, it appears that optimal results will only be obtained at normal levels of maternal phenylalanine (50–150 μmol/l) [179,193].

Since there is some suggestion that low maternal tyrosine levels may also harm the fetus [9], dietary tyrosine supplementation has also been used [40,193]. The diet will also require supplementation with glucose, vitamins and minerals [40]. Since the re-introduction of a low phenylalanine diet is unpleasant, and, since conception may be unexpected, girls should be encouraged to continue the diet from the time of first diagnosis, until after they stop having children [139].

Some children with phenylketonuria may be lost to follow-up and, because of the evidence that moderate elevations of phenylalanine in the blood do not cause phenylketonuria but are still harmful to the fetus [90], there is a case for a routine screening test in pregnancy [194]. Ideally, the test should be for hyperphenylalaninaemia [90]. The Guthrie test has been used [173] as have urine screening tests [6]. Since the maximum gain appears to be from treatment instituted before conception, such a screen should really be part of a pre-pregnancy or pre-marital screening service [118,173]. Nevertheless, the yield of such screening tests is low: one in 10 000 Guthrie tests performed in pregnancy in Glasgow [173]. Screening may be more worthwhile in populations where the risk of phenylketonuria is greater. Hyanek *et al.* [90] found nine cases of abnormal amino acid metabolism in 15 000 women screened by blood paper chromatography in Czechoslovakia. Screening for maternal phenylketonuria should be part of the investigation of any microcephalic infant or fetus.

There are no specific pregnancy complications in maternal phenylketonuria, apart from the slight excess of intrauterine growth retardation. However, the emotional strain put on the mother, both by worrying about the fetal outcome and by having to follow an unpleasant diet, may be considerable. It would be sensible to perform a detailed scan of the fetus early in gestation to exclude lethal congenital heart disease [36]. Breast feeding can be allowed, since the increased dietary load of phenylalanine in breast milk will not cause hyperphenylalaninaemia in the newborn [40]. In the future, transfer of normal genes for phenylalanine hydroxylase to liver cells may allow patients to maintain normal phenylalanine levels without dietary therapy [129].

Hyperxanthinuria, hyperglycinaemia, hypertyrosinaemia

In the few cases of hyperxanthinuria reported in pregnancy there has been no evidence of excess fetal abnormalities [37,128]. Nevertheless, one patient lost two out of three pregnancies, both associated with prematurity [37]. Mothers are at risk from the formation of xanthine urinary stones. Maternal uric acid levels — which are helpful in the management of hypertensive disease in pregnancy (see Chapter 6) — cannot be relied upon because of the impairment of uric acid formation which is part of the metabolic block [37].

Hyanek *et al.* [90] report that one of two cases of maternal hyperglycinaemia was associated with mental retardation in the newborn. Two children from a woman with hypertyrosinaemia were normal.

Glycogen storage diseases (Gaucher's disease, Forbe's disease)

The glycogen storage diseases are characterized by various abnormalities in the synthesis of glycogen. The abnormal glycogens are deposited in the monocytes and macrophages of the reticulo-endothelial system so that affected patients suffer chronic ill-health due to abnormalities of the liver, spleen and bone marrow. The glycogen storage diseases are much more common in Ashkenazy Jews and prenatal diagnosis is usually available to detect homozygotes [64].

Gaucher's disease is an autosomal recessive disorder in which there is a deficit of acid β-glucosidase. The genetic basis of the disease has now been characterized and it is possible to detect heterozygotes for counselling and homozygotes for prenatal diagnosis [132]. Enzyme therapy is available at the staggering cost of US$550 000 per year [11]; in the near future gene replacement therapy is likely to be a realistic option [11].

Goldblatt and Beighton [64] have reviewed 21 pregnancies in their personal series of more than 50 patients. They conclude that there is no evidence that pregnancy affects the course of Gaucher's disease or that fertility is affected by Gaucher's disease. Potential problems in pregnancy relate to haematological and orthopaedic complications and the worry about splenic rupture. Most patients have a mild chronic anaemia. This may become more obvious in pregnancy but apart from giving extra folate and iron, no specific therapy is necessary; transfusion is very rarely indicated [64]. Thrombocytopenia is more worrying because it has been associated with post-partum haemorrhage in seven pregnancies in two patients of the South African series [64]. Prophylactic crossmatching and early transfusion are indicated. Platelet transfusion is generally unhelpful because the platelets are rapidly destroyed by the enlarged spleen. Similar results in pregnancy have been reported in 47 pregnancies from Jerusalem [216].

Although there may be considerable skeletal deformities in Gaucher's disease, these do not usually affect the pelvis and only one patient in the South African series required delivery by caesarean section for cephalopelvic disproportion [64]. Splenomegaly which may become more marked in pregnancy is obviously of concern because of the possibility of rupture [213]. However, there have been no cases of splenic rupture in association with labour and Goldblatt and Beighton [64] conclude that the only indication for splenectomy should be haematological [162]; if elective splenectomy is to be performed in pregnancy, the second trimester is preferred [64].

In Forbe's disease, the abnormality is a deficiency of amylo-1,6-glucosidase. In addition to the problems above, Confino *et al.* [33] have drawn attention to the associated problems with glucose metabolism which may be exaggerated by pregnancy. It is not clear whether such patients are particularly at risk of developing diabetes but whether they are or not, their pregnancies have the potential for being complicated by gestational diabetes as does any other pregnancy. If they do require insulin for blood glucose control, they are particularly likely to develop hypoglycaemia because their metabolic abnormalities impair glucose release from glycogen. In some forms of glycogen storage disease (e.g. von Gierke's disease) cornstarch may be preferable as a source of carbohydrate in pregnancy [94] since by contrast with glycogen, glucose can be released by debranching enzymes.

Hereditary angioneurotic oedema

Hereditary angioneurotic oedema is inherited as an autosomal dominant. The inheritance of recurrent attacks of abdominal pain and oedema of the extremities, face and larynx was first described by Osler [145]. Laryngeal oedema may be fatal. More recently it has been demonstrated that the condition is due to an abnormality of the serum inhibitor of the activated first component of complement (C1-esterase inhibitor). If C1 esterase inhibitor is either reduced in concentration (common form) or abnormal in function (variant form) the complement cascade can be activated by mild and often undetected trigger factors causing angioneurotic oedema. Attacks of abdominal pain are thought to be due to oedema of the intestines. Alteration of C1-inhibitor genes in both common [188] and variant forms have been reported but it is not clear to what extent these spectacular advances in the 'new biology' should be applied to antenatal diagnosis of a condition compatible with normal lifespan.

The first treatment used to prevent attacks was ε aminocaproic acid (EACA) which inhibits the fibrinolytic system in general and also inhibits C1 activation [55]. However, such treatment has been limited by muscle pain, weakness and the potential for thromboembolism [55] and the last would be of particular concern in pregnancy. EACA therapy has largely been superseded by androgens, particularly danazol, since they have been shown to reduce the frequency of attacks and increase the plasma level of C1 esterase inhibitor [59]. More recently concentrates of C1 esterase inhibitor have been made available and although these are very expensive and must be given intravenously, they should be used to treat acute attacks [57]. Fresh frozen plasma may be used [54] if the concentrate is unavailable. Corticosteroid therapy and adrenaline are not effective. In life-threatening episodes endotracheal intubation or tracheostomy should be used.

There is no consensus concerning the interaction between pregnancy and hereditary angioneurotic oedema in the cases that have been reported [26,27,49,55,79,88,147,152,187]. It has been suggested that studies of the molecular form of high molecular weight kininogen present in pregnancy may predict the 'at risk' patient [27] but this remains to be confirmed. If there is any tendency, pregnancy decreases the frequency of attacks [55] and that has certainly been our experience in one patient. However, in another the attacks became more frequent. Nevertheless danazol therapy should be discontinued because of the risk of masculinization of a female fetus.

Clinicians should be aware that abdominal pain in pregnancy may or may not be due to the condition. As always, history is of vital importance. One of our patients who had a concealed accidental haemorrhage was able to indicate that the pain had a different character from that of her usual attacks of abdominal pain thus facilitating her treatment. Although trauma may initiate attacks of hereditary angioneurotic oedema and one patient has died from laryngeal oedema following vaginal delivery [152], it does not seem that vaginal delivery is associated with any greater risk of angio-oedema [187]. On this basis caesarean section should be reserved for the usual obstetric indications. Epidural anaesthesia is preferred to general anaesthesia since intubation may itself precipitate an attack of laryngeal angio-oedema [147]. Patients should be given prophylactic treatment with C1 esterase inhibitor concentrate or failing that, 2 units of fresh frozen plasma before any abdominal surgery. There is no reason why such patients should not breast feed.

Porphyria

The porphyrias are disorders of haem synthesis which may be inherited or acquired. Porphyrins are intermediates in the haem synthetic pathway formed from δ aminolevulinic acid and porphobilinogen and different porphyrins accumulate in the various disorders.

The chief clinical manifestations are acute attacks of neurological dysfunction (the acute porphyrias) or chronic cutaneous photosensitivity (the cutaneous porphyrias).

The acute porphyrias, acute intermittent porphyria (AIP), variegate porphyria (VP) and hereditary coproporphyria (HC) are of significance in pregnancy. Each of these may present acutely with abdominal pain, fever and leucocytosis which may mimic other intra-abdominal conditions. Labile hypertension and tachycardia are further confusing features and some patients have symptoms of nervous system involvement such as neuropathy or psychiatric disturbance. Neuropathy typically follows the abdominal symptoms by at least 3 days.

A review in 1971 [89] described 72 cases in pregnancy with a 27 per cent mortality rate. However, a later study of 50 women with acute porphyria recorded only one death [15]. Fetal loss was 13 per cent in this study. Just over half of the women with AIP had an attack during pregnancy and the babies from these pregnancies weighed an average of 800 g less than in pregnancies free from attack. About 25 per cent of the attacks occurred after delivery and frequently were precipitated by intrapartum barbiturate therapy. The effects of pregnancy on HC and VP were less pronounced with only 25 and 33 per cent respectively having attacks.

The activity of erythrocyte porphobilinogen deaminase activity in AIP is not affected by pregnancy [169]. However, the incidence of acute porphyric attacks is increased in pregnancy, and both oestrogens and progestogens are known to provoke attacks in non-pregnant women. Attacks can also be precipitated by alcohol excess and fasting, and many drugs may activate an acute attack. Some drugs which may be met in obstetric practice and should be avoided are listed in Table 14.2. Before the use of any drug in a patient with porphyria it is strongly advisable to seek assistance from a specialist in the field. Kantor and Rolbin [95] have discussed the drugs used in anaesthesia.

Treatment of the acute attack is firstly supportive with careful monitoring of fluid and electrolyte balance. Intravenous glucose at a rate of 20 g/hour is recommended and, if no improvement within 48 hours is seen, an intravenous infusion of haematin may be tried though this improves the biochemical abnormalities more than the clinical features [67,84]. β blockade is used for tachycardia and hypertension. Of course close fetal monitoring is necessary when a woman has an acute attack.

Ornithine carbamoyltransferase deficiency

This is a rather rare X-linked disorder of urea synthesis which usually presents to paediatricians when newborn boys die from hyperammonaemic coma. But it has recently been reported that female carriers are also susceptible to cortical impairment varying from subtle abnormalities of cognitive thinking to fatal coma; and that coma is particularly likely to occur after delivery [3]. Arn [3] described five such women who between them had six episodes of coma, four of which occurred between 3 and 8 days post-partum and two of which were

Table 14.2. Drugs which may precipitate an acute porphyric attack

Barbiturates	Lignocaine
Carbamazepine	Methyldopa
Chlordiazepoxide	Metoclopramide
Chlormethiazole	Metronidazole
Clonidine	Nitrazepam
Danazol	Oral contraceptives
Dimenhydrinate	Oestrogens
Ergot derivatives	Pancuronium
Erythromycin	Phenytoin
Ethanol	Progesterone
Frusemide	Ranitidine
Halothane	Steroids
Hydralazine	Sulphonamides
	Theophylline

fatal. In each post-partum case the fetus was not affected so perhaps the fetus had been providing ureagenic activity for its mother. The condition should be considered in any woman who becomes comatose for no obvious reason after delivery. There may be decorticate posturing and raised intracranial pressure. The diagnosis is suggested by elevated ammonia levels in the presence of normal liver function and confirmed by high levels of glutamine and low levels of citrullin and arginine. Treatment is with intravenous sodium benzoate, sodium phenylacetate and arginine hydrochloride [3]. A biochemical screening test using allopurinol is available for screening female carriers [81].

References

1 Allanson JC & Hall JG. Obstetric and gynecologic problems in women with chondrodystrophies. *Obstetrics and Gynecology* 1986; **67**: 74–8.

2 Allgrove J, Adami S, Manning RM & O'Riordan JLH. Cytochemical bioassay of parathyroid hormone in maternal and cord blood. *Archives of Disease in Childhood* 1985; **60**: 110–15.

3 Arn PH, Hauser ER *et al*. Hyperammonemia in women with a mutation at the ornithine carbamoyltransferase locus. *New England Journal of Medicine* 1990; **322**: 1652–5.

4 Arnaud SB, Matthusen M, Gilkinson JB & Goldsmith RS. Components of 25-hydroxy-vitamin D in serum of young children in upper midwestern United States. *American Journal of Clinical Nutrition* 1977; **30**: 1082–6.

5 Arnaud SB, Newcomer AD *et al*. Serum 25-OHD and the pathogenesis of osteomalacia in patients with non-tropical sprue. *Gastroenterology* 1977; **72**: 1025.

6 Arthur LJG & Hulme SRD. Intelligent, small-for-dates baby born to oligophrenic phenylketonuric mother after low phenylalanine diet during pregnancy. *Pediatrics* 1970; **46**: 235–9.

7 Atkinson PJ & West RR. Loss of skeletal calcium in lactating women. *Journal of Obstetrics and Gynaecology of the British Commonwealth* 1970; **77**: 555–60.

8 Berde C, Willis DC & Sandberg EC. Pregnancy in women with pseudoxanthoma elasticum. *Obstetrical and Gynecological Surgery* 1983; **38**: 332–44.

9 Bessman SP, Williamson ML & Koch R. Diet, genetics and mental retardation interaction between phenylketonuric heterozygous mother and fetus to produce non-specific diminution of IQ: evidence in support of the justification hypothesis. *Proceedings of the National Academy of Sciences USA* 1978; **75**: 1562–6.

10 Better O, Levi J *et al*. Prolonged neonatal parathyroid suppression: A sequel to asymptomatic maternal hyperparathyroidism. *Archives of Surgery* 1973; **106**: 722–4.

11 Beutler E. Gaucher's disease. *New England Journal of Medicine* 1991; **325**: 1354–60.

12 Bouvierre-Lapierre M, Saint-Dizier C *et al*. Deux enfants nés de mère phenylcetonurique. Echec d'un regime pauvre en phenylalanine instite pendant la deuxieme grossesse. *Pediatrie* 1974; **29**: 51–72.

13 Boyle IT, Gray RW & DeLuca F. Regulation by calcium of *in vivo* synthesis of 1,25 dihydroxycholecalciferol and 21, 25 dihydroxycholecalciferol. *Proceedings of the National Academy of Sciences USA* 1971; **68**: 2131–4.

14 Brenton DP, Cusworth DC *et al*. Pregnancy and homocystinuria. *Annals of Clinical Biochemistry* 1977; **14**: 161–2.

14a Brodell JD, Burns JE & Heiple KG. Transient osteoporosis of the hip of pregnancy. *Journal of Bone and Joint Surgery* 1989; **71A**: 1252–7.

15 Brodie MJ, Moore MR *et al*. Pregnancy and the acute porphyrias. *British Journal of Obstetrics and Gynaecology* 1977; **84**: 726–31.

16 Brooke OG. Vitamin D supplements in pregnancy. *Journal of Maternal and Child Health* 1981; **1**: 18–20.

17 Brooke OG, Brown IRF *et al*. Vitamin D supplements in pregnant Asian women: effects on calcium status and fetal growth. *British Medical Journal* 1980; **i**: 751–4.

18 Brooke OG, Brown IRF, Cleeve HJW & Sood A. Observations of the vitamin D state of pregnant Asian women in London. *British Journal of Obstetrics and Gynaecology* 1981; **88**: 18–26.

19 Brooke OG, Butters F & Wood C. Intrauterine vitamin D nutrition and postnatal growth in Asian infants. *British Medical Journal* 1981; **283**: 1025.

20 Brown DJ, Spanos E & MacIntyre I. Role of pituitary hormones in regulating renal vitamin D metabolism in man. *British Medical Journal* 1980; **280**: 277–8.

21 Buist NRM, Tuerck J, Lis E & Penn R. Effects of untreated maternal phenylketonuria and hyperphenylalaninemia on the fetus. *New England Journal of Medicine* 1984; **311**: 52–3.

22 Burke G, Robinson K *et al*. Intrauterine growth retardation, perinatal death, and maternal homocysteine levels. *New England Journal of Medicine* 1992; **326**: 69–77.

23 Care AD, Caple IW, Abbas SK & Pickard DW. The effect of fetal thyro-parathyroidectomy on the transport of calcium across the ovine placenta of the fetus. *Placenta* 1986; **7**: 417–24.

24 Castillo L, Tanaka Y *et al*. Production of 1,25-dihydroxyvitamin D3 and formation of medullary bone in the egg-laying hen. *Endocrinology* 1979; **104**: 1598–601.

25 Chan GM, Slater P *et al*. Bone mineral status of lactating mothers of different ages. *American Journal of Obstetrics and Gynecology* 1982; **144**: 438–41.

26 Chappatte O & de Swiet M. Hereditary angioneurotic

oedema and pregnancy. Case reports and review of the literature. *British Journal of Obstetrics and Gynaecology* 1988; **95**: 938–42.

27 Chhibber G, Cohen A *et al*. Immunoblotting of plasma in a pregnant patient with hereditary angioedema. *Journal of Laboratory and Clinical Medicine* 1990; **115**: 112–21.

28 Christiansen C, Brandt NJ *et al*. Bone mineral content during pregnancy in epileptics on anticonvulsant drugs and in their newborns. *Acta Obstetricia et Gynecologica Scandinavica* 1981; **60**: 501–3.

29 Clark D, Seeds JW & Cefalo RC. Hyperparathyroid crisis and pregnancy. *American Journal of Obstetrics and Gynecology* 1981; **140**: 840–2.

30 Clarke R, Daly L *et al*. Hyperhomocysteinemia: An independent risk factor for vascular disease. *New England Journal of Medicine* 1991; **324**: 1149–55.

31 Cockburn F, Belton NR *et al*. Maternal vitamin D intake and mineral metabolism in mothers and their newborn infants. *British Medical Journal* 1980; **281**: 11–14.

32 Cohen LF, di Sant'Agnese PA & Friedlander J. Cystic fibrosis and pregnancy. *Lancet* 1980; **ii**: 842–4.

33 Confino E, Pauzner D *et al*. Pregnancy associated with amylo-1,6-glucosidase deficiency (Forbe's disease) Case report. *British Journal of Obstetrics and Gynaecology* 1984; **91**: 494–7.

34 Congdon P, Horsman A *et al*. Mineral content of the forearms of babies born to Asian and white mothers. *British Medical Journal* 1983; **286**: 1233–5.

35 Constantine G & Green A. Untreated homocystinuria: a maternal death in a woman with four pregnancies. *British Journal of Obstetrics and Gynaecology* 1987; **94**: 803–6.

36 Copel JA, Pilu G & Kleinman CS. Congenital heart disease and extracardiac anomalies: Associations and indications for fetal echocardiography. *American Journal of Obstetrics and Gynecology* 1986; **154**: 1121–32.

37 Curiel P & Bandinelli R. Pregnancy in a woman with xanthinuria: study of amniotic fluid uric acid. *American Journal of Obstetrics and Gynecology* 1979; **134**: 721–2.

38 Curtiss PH & Kincaid WE. Transitory demineralization of the hip in pregnancy: a report of three cases. *Journal of Bone and Joint Surgery* 1959; **41**: 1327–30.

38a Cushard WG, Creditor S, Canterbury MJ & Reiss E. Calcium, magnesium, phosphorus and parathyroid hormone interrelationships in pregnancy and newborn infants. *Journal of Clinical Endocrinology and Metabolism* 1972; **34**: 767–71.

39 Dandona F, Okonofua F & Clements RV. Osteomalacia presenting as pathological fractures during pregnancy in Asian women of high socioeconomic class. *British Medical Journal* 1985; **290**: 837–8.

40 Davidson DC, Isherwood DM, Ireland JT & Rae PG. Outcome of pregnancy in a phenylketonuric mother after low phenylalanine diet introduced from the ninth week of pregnancy. *European Journal of Pediatrics* 1981; **137**: 45–8.

41 Delvin EE, Salle BL *et al*. Vitamin D supplementation during pregnancy: effect on neonatal calcium homeostasis. *Journal of Pediatrics* 1986; **109**: 328–34.

42 Dent CE & Friedman M. Pregnancy and idiopathic osteoporosis. *Quarterly Journal of Medicine* 1965; **34**: 314–57.

43 Dent CE & Gupta MM. Plasma 25-hydroxyvitamin D levels during pregnancy in Caucasians and in vegetarian and non-vegetarian Asians. *Lancet* 1975; **ii**: 1057–60.

43a Drinkwater BL & Chesnut CH. Bone density changes during pregnancy and lactation in active women: a longitudinal study. *Bone and Mineral* 1991; **14**: 153–60.

44 Driscoll RH, Meredith S, Wagonfeld J & Rosenfeld I. Bone histology and vitamin D status in Crohn's disease: assessment of vitamin D therapy. *Gastroenterology* 1977; **72**: 1051.

45 Drogani E, Smith I, Beasley M & Lloyd JK. Timing of strict diet in relation to fetal damage in maternal phenylketonuria. *Lancet* 1987; **ii**: 927–30.

46 Eastell R, Edmonds CJ, de Chayal RCS & McFadyen IR. Prolonged hypoparathyroidism presenting eventually as second trimester abortion. *British Medical Journal* 1985; **291**: 955–6.

47 Eddy DD & Farber EM. Pseudoxanthoma elasticum. Internal manifestations: A report of cases and a statistical review of the literature. *Archives of Dermatology* 1962; **86**: 729.

48 Feeley RM, Eitenmiller RR, Jones JB & Barnhart H. Calcium, phosphorus, and magnesium contents of human milk during early lactation. *Journal of Pediatric Gastroenterology and Nutrition* 1983; **2**: 262–7.

49 Ferlazzo B, Barrile A *et al*. Clinical contribution to the problem of correlations between hereditary angioneurotic edema and pregnancy. *Istituto de Patologia Medica e Medicina Mediterranea* 1990; **42**: 351–6.

50 Fleischman AR, Rosen JF & Nathenson G. 25-hydroxyvitamin D. Serum levels and oral administration of calciferol in neonates. *Archives of Internal Medicine* 1978; **138**: 869–73.

51 Fogh-Anderson N & Schultz-Larsen P. Free calcium ion concentration in pregnancy. *Acta Obstetricia et Gynecologica Scandinavica* 1981; **60**: 309–12.

52 Food and Nutrition Board. *Recommended Dietary Allowances*, 9th edn. *National Research Council, National Academy of Sciences, Washington DC*, 1979.

53 Ford JA, Davidson DC *et al*. Neonatal rickets in Asian immigrant population. *British Medical Journal* 1973; **iii**: 211–12.

54 Frank MM, Gelfand JA & Atkinson JP. Hereditary angioedema: The clinical syndrome and its management. *Annals of Internal Medicine* 1976; **4**: 580.

55 Frank MM, Sergent JS, Kane MA & Alling DW. Epsilon aminocaproic acid therapy of hereditary angioedema. *New England Journal of Medicine* 1972; **286**: 803.
56 Freda VJ, Vosburgh GJ & Di Liberti C. Osteogenesis imperfecta congenita. *Obstetrics and Gynecology* 1961; **18**: 535–47.
57 Gadek JE, Mosea SW & Gelfand JA. Replacement therapy of hereditary angioedema. Successful treatment of acute episodes of angioedema with partly purified CI-INH. *New England Journal of Medicine* 1980; **302**: 542.
58 Gallagher JC, Riggs BL *et al*. Effect of estrogen therapy on calcium absorption and vitamin D metabolism in postmenopausal osteoporosis. *Clinical Research* 1987; **26**: 415A.
59 Gelfand JA, Sherins RJ, Alling DW & Frank MM. Treatment of hereditary angioedema with danazol. Reversal of clinical and biochemical abnormalities. *New England Journal of Medicine* 1976; **95**: 1444.
60 Genant HK, Mall JC *et al*. Skeletal demineralisation and growth retardation in inflammatory bowel disease. *Investigative Radiology* 1976; **11**: 541–9.
61 Gertner JM. Coustan DR *et al*. Pregnancy as a state of physiologic absorptive hypercalciuria. *American Journal of Medicine* 1986; **81**: 451–6.
62 Glass EJ & Barr DG. Transient neonatal hyperparathyroidism secondary to maternal pseudo-hypoparathyroidism. *Archives of Disease in Childhood* 1981; **56**: 566–8.
63 Goldberg E, Winter ST, Better OS & Berger A. Transient neonatal hyperparathyroidism associated with maternal hypoparathyroidism. *Israel Journal of Medical Sciences* 1976; **12**: 199–201.
64 Goldblatt J & Beighton P. Obstetric aspects of Gaucher's disease. *British Journal of Obstetrics and Gynaecology* 1985; **92**: 145–9.
65 Goldsmith NF & Johnston JO. Bone mineral: Effects of oral contraceptives, pregnancy and lactation. *Journal of Bone and Joint Surgery* 1975; **57A**: 657–68.
66 Goodwin D, Noff D & Edelstein S. 24,25-Dihydroxyvitamin D is a metabolite of vitamin D essential for bone formation. *Nature* 1978; **276**: 517.
67 Gorchein A & Webber R. Delta-aminolaevulinic acid in plasma, cerebrospinal fluid, saliva and erythrocytes: studies in normal, uraemic and porphyric subjects. *Clinical Science* 1987; **72**: 103–12.
68 Gould CS, O'Malley BP & MacVicar J. Endocrine hyperemesis — the need for a high index of clinical suspicion. *Journal of Obstetrics and Gynaecology* 1984; **4**: 191–2.
69 Gradus D, Le Roith D *et al*. Congenital hyperparathyroidism and rickets secondary to maternal hypoparathyroidism and vitamin D deficiency. *Israel Journal of Medical Sciences* 1981; **17**: 705–9.
70 Graham D, Tracey J *et al*. Early second trimester sonographic diagnosis of achondrogenesis. *Journal of Clinical Ultrasound* 1983; **11**: 336–8.
71 Graham WP, Gordon GS *et al*. Effect of pregnancy and of the menstrual cycle on hypoparathyroidism. *Journal of Clinical Endocrinology and Metabolism* 1964; **24**: 512–16.
72 Gray TK, Lester GE & Lorenc RS. Evidence for extrarenal 1-hydroxylation of 25-hydroxyvitamin D_3 in pregnancy. *Science* 1979; **204**: 1311–13.
73 Gutteridge DH, Doyle FH, Joblin GF & Brenton DP. Two types of osteoporosis in younger women — natural history and relationship to pregnancy and lactation. *Calcified Tissue International* 1986; **39** (suppl 2): A133.
74 Gutteridge DH, Price RI *et al*. Bone turnover, renal phosphate handling and forearm bone density during peak human lactation. *Calcified Tissue International* 1986; **39** (suppl 2): A132.
75 Hahn TJ & Halstead LR. Anticonvulsant drug-induced osteomalacia: alterations in mineral metabolism and response to vitamin D_3 administration. *Calcified Tissue International* 1979; **27**: 13–18.
76 Hahn TJ, Hendin BA *et al*. Effect of chronic anticonvulsant therapy on serum 25-hydroxycalciferol levels in adults. *New England Journal of Medicine* 1972; **287**: 900–3.
77 Hahn TJ, Squires AE, Halstead LR & Strominger DB. Reduced serum 25-hydroxyvitamin D concentration and disordered mineral metabolism in patients with cystic fibrosis. *Journal of Pediatrics* 1979; **94**: 38–42.
78 Hall JG. Disorders of connective tissue and skeletal dysplasia. In: Simpson JL & Shulman JD (eds), *Genetic Disorders in Pregnancy*. Academic Press, New York, 1981: 57–87.
79 Hardy F, Ngwingtin L, Bazin C & Babinet P. Hereditary angioneurotic edema and pregnancy. *Journal de Gynecologie, Obstetrique et Biologie de la Reproduction* 1990; **19**: 65–8.
80 Harrison HE. Vitamin D, the parathyroid and the kidney. *Johns Hopkins Medical Journal* 1979; **144**: 180–91.
81 Hauser ER, Finkelstein JE, Valle D & Brusilow SW. Allopurinol-induced orotidinuria. A test for mutations at the ornithine carbamyltransferase locus in women. *New England Journal of Medicine* 1990; **322**: 1641–5.
82 Heaney RP & Skillman TG. Calcium metabolism in normal human pregnancy. *Journal of Clinical Endocrinology and Metabolism* 1971; **33**: 661–70.
83 Heckmatt JZ, Peacock M *et al*. Plasma 25-hydroxyvitamin D in pregnant Asian women and their babies. *Lancet* 1979; **ii**: 546–9.
84 Herrick AL, McColl KEL *et al*. Controlled trial of haem arginate in acute hepatic porphyria. *Lancet* 1989; **i**: 1295–7.
85 Hillman LS & Haddad JG. Human perinatal vitamin D metabolism. I. 25-hydroxyvitamin D in maternal and cord blood. *Journal of Pediatrics* 1974; **84**: 742–9.
86 Hillman LS & Haddad JG. Perinatal vitamin D

metabolism. III: Factors influencing late gestational human serum 25-hydroxyvitamin D. *American Journal of Obstetrics and Gynecology* 1976; **125**: 196–200.

87 Holtrop ME, Cox KA *et al.* 1,25-Dihydroxycholecalciferol stimulates osteoclasts in rat bones in the absence of parathyroid hormone. *Endocrinology* 1981; **108**: 2293–301.

88 Hopkinson RB & Sutcliffe AJ. Hereditary angioneurotic oedema. *Anaesthesia* 1979; **34**: 183–6.

89 Hunter DJ. Acute intermittent porphyria and pregnancy. *Journal of Obstetrics and Gynaecology of the British Commonwealth* 1971; **78**: 746–50.

90 Hyanek J, Homolka J *et al.* Results of screening for phenylalanine and other amino acid disturbances among pregnant women. *Journal of Inherited Metabolic Disease* 1979; **2**: 59–63.

91 Hytten FE & Leitch I. *The Physiology of Human Pregnancy*, 2nd edn. Blackwell Scientific Publications, Oxford, 1971: 383.

92 Jenkins MV, Harris M & Wills MR. The effect of phenytoin on parathyroid extract and 25-hydroxycholecalciferol-induced bone reabsorption. *Calcified Tissue Research* 1974; **16**: 163–7.

93 Jensen LP, Ras G & Boes EG. Hypercalcaemia in pregnancy. A case report. *South African Medical Journal* 1980; **57**: 712–13.

94 Johnson MP, Compton A, Drugan A & Evans MI. Metabolic control of von Gierke disease (glycogen storage disease type Ia) in pregnancy: maintenance of euglycamia with cornstarch. *Obstetrics and Gynecology* 1990; **75**: 507–10.

95 Kantor G & Rolbin SH. Acute intermittent porphyria and caesarean delivery. *Canadian Journal of Anaesthesia* 1992; **39**: 282–5.

96 Kay NRM, Park WM & Bark M. The relationship between pregnancy and femoral head necrosis. *British Journal of Radiology* 1972; **45**: 828–31.

96a Kent GN, Price RI *et al.* Human lactation: forearm trabecular bone loss, increased bone turnover, and renal conservation of calcium and inorganic phosphate with recovery of bone mass following weaning. *Journal of Bone and Mineral Research* 1990; **5**: 361–9.

97 Kirkman HW & Hicks RE. More on untreated maternal hyperphenylalaninemia. *New England Journal of Medicine* 1984; **311**: 1125.

98 Kokkonen J, Koivisto M & Kirkinen P. Seasonal variation in serum-25-OHD_3 in mothers and newborn infants in Northern Finland. *Acta Paediatrica Scandinavica* 1983; **72**: 93–6.

99 Konecki DS & Lichter-Konecki V. The phenylketonuria locus: current knowledge about defects and mutations of the phenylalanine hydroxylase gene in various populations. *Human Genetics* 1991; **87**: 377–88.

100 Kovarik J, Woloszczuk W, Linkesch W & Pavelka R. Calcitonin in pregnancy. *Lancet* 1980; **i**: 199–200.

101 Kristoffersson A, Dahlgren S, Lithner F & Jarhult J. Primary hyperparathyroidism in pregnancy. *Surgery* 1985; **97**: 326–30.

102 Kumar R, Cohen WR, Silva P. Epstein FH. Elevated 1,25-dihydroxyvitamin D plasma levels in normal human pregnancy and lactation. *Journal of Clinical Investigation* 1979; **63**: 342–4.

103 Kuoppala T, Tiumala R, Parviainen M & Koskinen T. Can the fetus regulate its calcium uptake? *British Journal of Obstetrics and Gynaecology* 1984; **91**: 1192–6.

104 Kurtz AB, Filly RA *et al. In utero* analysis of heterozygous achondroplasia: variable time of onset as detected by femur length measurements. *Journal of Ultrasound in Medicine* 1986; **5**: 137–40.

105 Lamke B, Brundin J & Moberg P. Changes of bone mineral content during pregnancy and lactation. *Acta Obstetricia et Gynecologica Scandinavica* 1977; **56**: 217–19.

106 Landing BH & Kamoshita S. Congenital hyperparathyroidism secondary to maternal hypoparathyroidism. *Journal of Pediatrics* 1970; **77**: 842–7.

107 Lao TT, Walters BNJ & de Swiet M. Pseudoxanthoma elasticum and pregnancy. A report of two cases. *British Journal of Obstetrics and Gynaecology* 1984; **91**: 1049–50.

108 Lebwohl MG, Distefano D *et al.* Pseudoxanthoma elasticum and mitral valve prolapse. *New England Journal of Medicine* 1982; **307**: 228–31.

109 Lenke RR & Levy HL. Maternal phenylketonuria and hyperphenylalaninemia. An international survey of the outcome of untreated and treated pregnancies. *New England Journal of Medicine* 1980; **303**: 1202–8.

110 Levy HL, Lobbregt D, Sansaricq C & Snyderman SE. Comparison of phenylketonuric and nonphenylketonuric sibs from untreated pregnancies in a mother with phenylketonuria. *American Journal of Genetics* 1992; **44**: 439–42.

111 Levy ML & Waisbren SE. Effects of untreated maternal phenylketonuria and hyperphenylalaninemia on the fetus. *New England Journal of Medicine* 1983; **309**: 1269–74.

112 Liang ST. Marfan syndrome, recurrent preterm labour and grandmultiparity. *Australian and New Zealand Journal of Obstetrics and Gynaecology* 1985; **25**: 288–9.

113 Lightwood R. Idiopathic hypercalcaemia with failure to thrive: nephrocalcinosis. *Proceedings of the Royal Society of Medicine* 1952; **45**: 401.

114 Lind J & Hoynck-van-Papendrecht HP. Obstetrical complications in a patient with the Marfan syndrome. *European Journal of Obstetrics, Gynecology and Reproductive Biology* 1984; **18**: 161–8.

115 Longstreth PL, Malinak LR & Hill CS. Transient osteoporosis of the hip in pregnancy. *Obstetrics and Gynecology* 1973; **41**: 563–9.

116 Lose G & Lindholm P. Transient painful osteoporosis of the hip in pregnancy. *International Journal of Gynaecology and Obstetrics* 1986; **24**: 13–16.

117 Lowe DK, Orwoll ES *et al.* Hyperparathyroidism in pregnancy. *American Journal of Surgery* 1983; **145**: 611–14.

118 Luke B & Keith LG. The challenge of maternal phenylketonuria screening and treatment. *Journal of Reproductive Medicine* 1990; **35**: 667–73.

119 Lund B & Selnes A. Plasma 1,25-dihydroxyvitamin D levels in pregnancy and lactation. *Acta Endocrinologica* 1979; **92**: 330–5.

120 Mabry CC, Denniston JC & Coldwell JG. Mental retardation in children of phenylketonuric mothers. *New England Journal of Medicine* 1966; **275**: 1331–6.

121 MacLennan WJ, Hamilton JC & Darmady JM. The effects of season and stage of pregnancy on plasma 25-hydroxyvitamin D concentrations in pregnant women. *Postgraduate Medical Journal* 1980; **56**: 75–9.

122 Mallet E, Gugi B *et al.* Vitamin D supplementation in pregnancy. A controlled trial of two methods. *Obstetrics and Gynecology* 1986; **68**: 300–4.

123 Markestad T, Ulstein M *et al.* Vitamin D metabolism in normal and hypoparathyroid pregnancy and lactation. Case report. *British Journal of Obstetrics and Gynaecology* 1983; **90**: 971–6.

124 Markestad T, Ulstein M *et al.* Anticonvulsant drug therapy in human pregnancy: effects on serum concentrations of vitamin D metabolites in maternal and cord blood. *American Journal of Obstetrics and Gynecology* 1984; **150**: 254–8.

125 Martinez ME, Sanchez C *et al.* Ionic calcium levels during pregnancy, at delivery and in the first hours of life. *Scandinavian Journal of Clinical Laboratory Investigation* 1986; **46**: 27–30.

126 Mattias GSH, Helliwell TR & Williams A. Postpartum hyperparathyroid crisis. Case report. *British Journal of Obstetrics and Gynaecology* 1987; **94**: 807–10.

127 Maxwell JP. Further studies in adult rickets (osteomalacia) and foetal rickets. *Proceedings of the Royal Society of Medicine* 1934; **28**: 265–300.

128 McKeran RO. Xanthinuria and pregnancy. *Lancet* 1977; **ii**: 86–7.

129 Medical Research Council Working Party on Phenylketonuria. Phenylketonuria due to phenylalanine hydroxylase deficiency: an unfolding story. *British Medical Journal* 1993; **306**: 115–19.

130 Merz E & Goldhofer W. Sonographic diagnosis of lethal osteogenesis imperfecta in the second trimester. Case report and review. *Journal of Clinical Ultrasound* 1986; **14**: 380–3.

131 Minkhorst AG, van Dongen PW, Boers GH & de Wit PH. Cerebral infarction after caesarean section due to heterozygosity for homocystinuria; a case report. *European Journal of Obstetrics' Gynecology and Reproductive Biology* 1991; **40**: 241–3.

132 Mistry PK, Smith SJ *et al.* Genetic diagnosis of Gaucher's disease. *Lancet* 1992; **339**: 889–92.

133 Mogadam M, Dobbins WO, Korelitz BI & Ahmed SW. Pregnancy in inflammatory bowel disease: Effect of sulphasalazine and corticosteroids on fetal outcome. *Gastroenterology* 1981; **80**: 72–6.

134 Moncrief MW & Fadahunsi TO. Congenital rickets due to maternal vitamin D deficiency. *Archives of Disease in Childhood* 1974; **49**: 810–11.

135 Moniz DF, Nicolaides KM, Bamford FJ & Rodeck CH. Normal reference ranges for biochemical substances relating to renal, hepatic, and bone function in fetal and maternal plasma throughout pregnancy. *Journal of Clinical Pathology* 1985; **38**: 468–72.

136 Montoro MN, Collea JV & Mestman JH. Management of hyperparathyroidism in pregnancy with oral phosphate therapy. *Obstetrics and Gynecology* 1980; **65**: 431–4.

137 Morris JDS, Adjukiewicz AB & Read AE. Coeliac infertility: an indication for dietary gluten restriction. *Lancet* 1970; **i**: 213–14.

138 Mudd SH, Skovby F *et al.* The natural history of homocystinemia due to cystathionine β-synthetase deficiency. *American Journal of Human Genetics* 1985; **37**: 1–31.

139 Murphy D & Troy EM. Maternal phenylketonuria. *Irish Journal of Medical Science* 1979; **48**: 310–13.

140 Newman RL. Serum electrolytes in pregnancy, parturition and the puerperium. *Obstetrics and Gynecology* 1957; **10**: 51–5.

141 Nilsson BE. Parity and osteoporosis. *Surgery, Gynecology and Obstetrics* 1969; **129**: 27–8.

142 Nordin BEC, Heyburn PJ *et al.* Osteoporosis and osteomalacia. *Clinics of Endocrinology and Metabolism* 1980; **9**: 177–205.

143 Nordin BEC & Roper A. Post-pregnancy osteoporosis, a syndrome? *Lancet* 1955; **i**: 431–4.

144 O'Donnell D, Costa J & Meyers AM. Management of pseudohypoparathyroidism in pregnancy. Case report. *British Journal of Obstetrics and Gynaecology* 1985; **92**: 639–41.

145 Osler W. Hereditary angio-neurotic edema. *American Journal of Medical Sciences* 1888; **95**: 362.

146 Parr JH & Ramsay I. The presentation of osteomalacia in pregnancy. Case report. *British Journal of Obstetrics and Gynaecology* 1984; **91**: 816–18.

147 Peters M, Ryley D & Lockwood C. Hereditary angioedema and immunoglobulin A deficiency in pregnancy. *Obstetrics and Gynecology* 1988; **72**: 454–5.

148 Pitkin RM, Reynolds WA, Williams GA & Haryis GK. Calcium metabolism in normal pregnancy. A longitudinal study. *American Journal of Obstetrics and Gynecology* 1979; **133**: 781–91.

149 Platt LD, Koch R *et al.* Maternal phenylketonuria collaborative study, obstetric aspects and outcome: the first 6 years. *American Journal of Obstetrics and Gynecology* 1992; **166**: 1150–60.

150 Polanska N, Dale RA & Wills MR. Plasma calcium levels in pregnant Asian women. *Annals of Cinical Biochemistry* 1976; **13**: 339–44.

151 Pope FM, Cheam KSE *et al.* Lethal osteogenesis

imperfecta and a 300 base pair deletion for an (I)-like collagen. *British Medical Journal* 1984; **288**: 431–4.

152 Postnikoff IM & Pritzker KPH. Hereditary angioneurotic edema: an unusual cause of maternal mortality. *Journal of Forensic Sciences* 1979; **24**: 473–8.

153 Price J & Reynolds F. Management of pregnancy complicated by severe osteogenesis imperfecta. *Journal of Obstetrics and Gynaecology* 1987; **7**: 178–80.

154 Purvis RJ, Barrie WJM *et al*. Enamel hypoplasia of the teeth associated with neonatal tetany; a manifestation of maternal vitamin D deficiency. *Lancet* 1973; **ii**: 811–14.

155 Pyeritz RE. Maternal and fetal complications of pregnancy in the Marfan syndrome. *American Journal of Medicine* 1981; **71**: 784–90.

156 Quinn RJ & Mukerjee B. Spontaneous uterine inversion in association with Marfan's syndrome. *Australian and New Zealand Journal of Obstetrics and Gynaecology* 1982; **22**: 163–4.

157 Rab SM & Baseer A. Occult osteomalacia amongst healthy and pregnant women in Pakistan. *Lancet* 1976; **ii**: 1211–13.

158 Raisz LG, Trummel CL, Holick MF & DeLuca HF. 1,25-Dihydroxycholecalciferol: a potent stimulator of bone reabsorption in tissue culture. *Science* 1972; **175**: 786–9.

159 Reddy GS, Norman AW *et al*. Regulation of vitamin D metabolism in normal human pregnancy. *Journal of Clinical Endocrinology and Metabolism* 1983; **56**: 363–70.

160 Risvi SNA & Vaishnava H. Occult osteomalacia in pregnant women in India. *Lancet* 1977; **i**: 1102.

161 Roberts JM & Solomons CC. Management of pregnancy in osteogenesis imperfecta: new perspectives. *Obstetrics and Gynecology* 1975; **45**: 168–70.

162 Rose JS, Grabowski GA, Barnett SM & Desnick RJ. Accelerated skeletal deterioration after splenectomy in Gaucher type I disease. *American Journal of Roentgenology* 1982; **139**: 1202–4.

163 Rubba P, Faccenda F, Strisciuglio P & Andria G. Ultrasonographic detection of arterial disease in treated homocystinuria. *New England Journal of Medicine* 1989; **321**: 1759–60.

164 Sadeghi-Nejad A, Wolfsdorf JI & Senior B. Hypoparathyroidism and pregnancy: treatment with calcitriol. *Journal of the American Medical Association* 1980; **243**: 254–5.

165 Salam R & Taylor S. Hyperparathyroidism in pregnancy. *British Journal of Surgery* 1979; **66**: 648–50.

166 Salle BL, Berthezene F *et al*. Hypoparathyroidism during pregnancy: treatment with calcitriol. *Journal of Clinical Endocrinology and Metabolism* 1981; **52**: 810–12.

167 Samaan NA, Anderson GD & Adam-Mayns ME. Immunoreactive calcitonin in the mother, neonate, child and adult. *American Journal of Obstetrics and Gynecology* 1975; **121**: 622–5.

168 Sann L, David L *et al*. Congenital hyperparathyroidism and vitamin D deficiency secondary to maternal hypoparathyroidism. *Acta Paediatrica Scandinavica* 1976; **65**: 381–5.

169 Sassa S & Kappas A. Lack of effect of pregnancy or hematin therapy on erythrocyte porphobilinogen deaminase activity in acute intermittent porphyria. *New England Journal of Medicine* 1989; **321**: 192–3.

170 Savdie E, Caterson RJ *et al*. Successful pregnancies in women treated by haemodialysis. *Medical Journal of Australia* 1982; **2**: 9.

171 Schenker J & Kallner B. Fatal postpartum hyperparathyroid crisis. *Obstetrics and Gynecology* 1965; **25**: 705–9.

172 Schoen MS, Lindenbaum J, Roginsky MS & Holt PR. Significance of serum level of 25-hydroxycholecalciferol in gastro-intestinal disease. *American Journal of Digestive Disease* 1978; **23**: 137–42.

173 Scott TM, Morton Fyfe W & McKay Hart D. Maternal phenylketonuria: abnormal baby despite low phenylalanine diet during pregnancy. *Archives of Disease in Childhood* 1980; **55**: 634–9.

174 Sengupta BS, Sivapragasam S *et al*. Osteogenesis imperfecta: its physiopathology in pregnancy. *Journal of the Royal College of Surgeons of Edinburgh* 1977; **22**: 358–64.

175 Serenius F, Elidrissy ATH & Dandona P. Vitamin D nutrition in pregnant women at term and in newly born babies in Saudi Arabia. *Journal of Clinical Pathology* 1984; **37**: 444–7.

176 Shangold MM, Dor N *et al*. Hyperparathyroidism and pregnancy: A review. *Obstetrical and Gynecological Survey* 1982; **37**: 217–28.

177 Shenolikar IS. Absorption of dietary calcium in pregnancy. *American Journal of Clinical Nutrition* 1970; **23**: 63–7.

178 Skinner RK, Sherlock S, Long RG & Willis MR. 25-hydroxylation of vitamin D in primary biliary cirrhosis. *Lancet* 1977; **i**: 720–1.

179 Smith I, Glossop J & Beasley M. Fetal damage due to maternal phenylketonuria: effects of dietary treatment and maternal phenylalanine concentrations around the time of conception (an interim report from the UK Phenylketonuria Register). *Journal of Inherited Metabolic Disease* 1990; **13**: 651–7.

180 Smith J, Macartney FJ *et al*. Fetal damage despite low-phenylalanine diet after conception in a phenylketonuric woman. *Lancet* 1979; **i**: 17–18.

181 Smith R. Osteogenesis imperfecta. *British Medical Journal* 1984; **289**: 394–6.

182 Smith R, Stevenson JC *et al*. Osteoporosis in pregnancy. *Lancet* 1985; **i**: 1178–80.

183 Spanos E, Pike JW *et al*. Circulating 1 alpha, 25 dihydroxyvitamin D in the chicken: enhancement by injection of prolactin and during egg laying. *Life Sciences* 1976; **19**: 1751–6.

184 Steegers-Theunissen RPM, Boers GHJ *et al*. Hyper-

homocysteinaemia and recurrent spontaneous abortion or abruptio placentae. *Lancet* 1992; **i**: 1122–3.

185 Steichen JJ, Tsang RC *et al*. Vitamin D homeostasis in the perinatal period. *New England Journal of Medicine* 1980; **302**: 315–19.

186 Stevenson JC, Hillyard CJ *et al*. A physiological role for calcitonin: Protection of the maternal skeleton. *Lancet* 1979; **ii**: 769–70.

187 Stiller RJ, Kaplan BM & Andreoli JW. Hereditary angioedema and pregnancy. *Obstetrics and Gynecology* 1984; **64**: 133–5.

188 Stoppa-Lyonnet D, Tosi M *et al*. Inhibitor genes in type 1 hereditary angioedema. *New England Journal of Medicine* 1987; **317**: 1–6.

189 Taha SA, Dost SM & Sedrani SH. 25-Hydroxyvitamin D and total calcium: extraordinary low plasma concentrations in Saudi mothers and their neonates. *Pediatric Research* 1984; **18**: 739–41.

190 Tanaka Y, Castillo L, Wineland MJ & DeLuca HF. Synergistic effect of progesterone, testosterone, and estradiol in the stimulation of chick renal 25-hydroxyvitamin D-1 alpha-hydroxylase. *Endocrinology* 1978; **103**: 2035–9.

191 Teitelbaum SL, Halverson JD *et al*. Abnormalities of circulating 25-OH vitamin D after jejunoileal bypass for obesity and evidence of an adaptive response. *Annals of Internal Medicine* 1977; **86**: 289–93.

192 Thomason JL, Sampson MB, Farb HF & Spellacy WN. Pregnancy complicated by concurrent primary hyperparathyroidism and pancreatitis. *Obstetrics and Gynecology* 1981; **57**: 345–65.

193 Thompson GN, Francis DE, Kirby DM & Compton R. Pregnancy in phenylketonuria: dietary treatment aimed at normalising maternal plasma phenylalanine concentration. *Archives of Disease in Childhood* 1991; **66**: 1346–9.

194 Tolmie JL, Harvie A & Cockburn F. The teratogenic effects of undiagnosed maternal hyperphenylalaninaemia: a case for prevention? *British Journal of Obstetrics and Gynaecology* 1992; **99**: 347–8.

195 Tsang R, Abrams L *et al*. Ionised calcium in neonates in relation to gestational age. *Journal of Pediatrics* 1979; **94**: 126–9.

196 Tsipouras P, Del Mastro R *et al*. Genetic linkage of the Marfan syndrome, ectopia lentis and congenital contractural arachnodactyly to the fibrillin genes on chromosomes 15 and 5. *New England Journal of Medicine* 1992; **326**: 905–9.

196a Turton CWG, Stanley P, Stamp TC, Maxwell JD. Altered vitamin D metabolism in pregnancy. *Lancet* 1977; **i**: 222–5.

197 Verdy M, Beaulieu R *et al*. Plasma calcitonin activity in a patient with thyroid medullary carcinoma and her children with osteopetrosis. *Journal of Clinical Endocrinology* 1971; **32**: 216–21.

198 Viljoen DL, Beatty S & Beighton P. The obstetric and gynaecological implications of pseudoxanthoma elasticum. *British Journal of Obstetrics and Gynaecology* 1987; **94**: 884–8.

199 Wagner G, Transbol I & Melchior J. Hyperparathyroidism and pregnancy. *Acta Endocrinologica* 1964; **47**: 549–64.

200 Walker ARP, Richardson B & Walker F. The influence of numerous pregnancies and lactations on bone dimensions in South African Bantu and Caucasian mothers. *Clinical Science* 1972; **42**: 189–96.

201 Wardlaw GM & Pike AM. The effect of lactation on peak adult shaft and ultra-distal forearm bone mass in women. *American Journal of Clinical Nutrition* 1986; **44**: 283–6.

202 Watney PJ, Chance GW, Scott P & Thompson JM. Maternal factors in neonatal hypocalcaemia: a study in three ethnic groups. *British Medical Journal* 1971; **ii**: 432–6.

203 Weisman Y, Harell A *et al*. 1,25-dihydroxyvitamin D3 and 24, 25 dihydroxyvitamin D_3 *in vitro* synthesis by human placenta and decidua. *Nature* 1979; **281**: 317–19.

204 Westin B, Kaiser IH *et al*. Some constituents of umbilical venous blood of previable human fetuses. *Acta Paediatrica Scandinavica* 1959; **48**: 609–13.

205 Whalley P. Hyperparathyroidism and pregnancy. *American Journal of Obstetrics and Gynecology* 1963; **86**: 517–21.

206 Whitehead M, Lane G *et al*. Interrelations of calcium regulating hormones during normal pregnancy. *British Medical Journal* 1981; **283**: 10–12.

207 Whitsett JA & Tsang RC. Calcium uptake and binding by membrane fractions of human placenta: ATP-dependent calcium accumulation. *Pediatric Research* 1980; **14**: 769–75.

208 WHO. *Nutrition in Pregnancy and Lactation. Report of a WHO Expert Committee*. World Health Organization Technical Report Series, 1965; **302**: 37.

209 Wieland P, Fischer JA *et al*. Perinatal parathyroid hormone, vitamin D metabolites and calcitonin in man. *American Journal of Physiology* 1980; **239**: E385–90.

120 Wilson DC. The incidence of osteomalacia and late rickets in Northern India. *Lancet* 1931; **ii**: 10–12.

211 Wilson DT, Martin T *et al*. Hyperparathyroidism in pregnancy: case report and review of the literature. *Canadian Medical Association Journal* 1983; **129**: 986–9.

211a Wilson SG, Retallack RW *et al*. Serum free 1,25-dihydroxyvitamin D index during a longitudinal study of human pregnancy and lactation. *Clinical Endocrinology* 1990; **32**: 613–22.

212 Woolf LI, Ounsted C *et al*. Atypical phenylketonuria in sisters with normal offspring. *Lancet* 1961; **ii**: 464–5.

213 Young KR & Payne MJ. Obstetric aspects of Gaucher's disease. *British Journal of Obstetrics and Gynaecology* 1985; **92**: 993.

214 Yu JS & O'Halloran MT. Children of mothers with

phenylketonuria. *Lancet* 1970; **i**: 210–12.
215 Zaleski A, Casey RE & Zaleski W. Maternal phenylketonuria: dietary treatment during pregnancy. *Canadian Medical Association Journal* 1979; **121**: 1591–4.
216 Zlotogora J, Sagi M, Zeigler M & Bach G. Gaucher disease type I and pregnancy. *American Journal of Medical Genetics* 1989; **32**: 475–7.
217 Zolla-Pazner S, Pazner SS, Lanyi V & Meltzer M. Osteonecrosis of the femoral head during pregnancy. *Journal of the American Medical Association* 1980; **244**: 689–90.

15

Neurological Disorders

James O. Donaldson

Diagnostic tests, 535
Epilepsy, 536
Oral contraception
Pregnancy
Epilepsy and the fetus
Birth defects
Counselling and management
Cerebrovascular disease, 539
Ischaemic stroke
Cerebral venous thrombosis
Subarachnoid haemorrhage
Eclamptic hypertensive encephalopathy
Tumours, 543
Choriocarcinoma
Pituitary adenoma
Lymphocytic hypophysitis
Pseudotumour cerebri, 545
Hydrocephalus, 545
Multiple sclerosis, 545
Headache, 546
Muscle contraction headache
Classic migraine
Neuropathy, 546
Bell's palsy
Carpal tunnel syndrome
Meralgia paraesthetica
Intra-partum lumbosacral plexopathy
Guillain–Barré syndrome
Muscle disease, 547
Polymyositis
Myasthenia gravis
Myotonic muscular dystrophy
Paraplegia, 548
Chorea gravidarum, 549

Active obstetricians each year encounter women with some major or minor neurological condition, and during a lifetime of active practice will participate in the care of women with many of the disorders discussed in this chapter. However, most obstetricians do not have an extensive experience with any one neurological disorder and must rely upon the collective experience in order to answer questions concerning diagnostic procedures, management and prognosis. In some instances all concerned are thrust into a complex medical, ethical and legal situation, such as the fate of the fetus after a woman has lost function of her cerebrum and brain stem due to a disastrous car accident [5,51]. Although obstetricians have an important role in preventing and detecting neurological conditions in the fetus, this chapter focuses upon the more common maternal neurological disorders.

Diagnostic tests

Before considering specific neurological conditions it is important to mention neurodiagnostic procedures during pregnancy. The best, most important and cheapest procedure is a probing history and a detailed examination by a skilled neurologist. The neurologist's task is to localize the lesion which *per se* often limits the list of diagnostic possibilities. Thereafter, additional studies may be needed to define the diagnosis. Only after an accurate diagnosis has been secured can physicians properly advise a pregnant woman and her family concerning the management and prognosis of her condition.

Electromyography (EMG) and electroencephalography (EEG) are without risk. Pregnancy alters neither the composition of cerebrospinal fluid (CSF) nor the indications for examination of CSF [17].

However, far too often the author has been presented with cases in which treating physicians have shied away from neuroradiological procedures just because the patient was pregnant, only to have found themselves in a quandary when something unexpected later endangered the patient. Pregnancy is not an absolute contraindication for any neuroradiological study, although it is prudent to limit fetal X-ray exposure, especially during the first trimester. An increased risk of malformation can be detected with fetal exposure to more than 0.015 Gy

(1.5 rad). The absolute risk of malformation is increased 1 per cent with exposure to more than 0.1 Gy (10 rad). Compare this to background fetal radiation exposure of 0.75 mGy (75 mrad). Abdominal lead shielding reduces fetal radiation from plain X-ray and computed tomography (CT) of the head and neck to right angle scatter, approximately 0.01 mGy (1 mrad). Transfemoral cerebral angiography adds exposure during fluoroscopy which can be limited if the procedure is performed by an experienced angiographer with 'good hands'. Plain films of the thoracic and lumbar spine expose the fetus to 5 mGy (500) and 10 mGy (1000 mrad), respectively. Lumbar myelography involves at least 0.015 Gy (1.5 rad) plus fluoroscopy time plus (often) lumbar CT, another 7 mGy (700 mrad).

Magnetic resonance imaging (MRI) has no radiation exposure and apparently little, if any, risk to the fetus. Thus in most instances MRI is preferred during pregnancy for imaging of the thoracic and lumbar spine.

Epilepsy

Epilepsy occurs in one of 200 women of childbearing age and is the most common major neurological disorder to be encountered by obstetricians. A unit delivering 3000 mothers a year will have about 15 pregnant women with epilepsy on their books at any one time. Although much has been learned about the complex interactions amongst the different types of epilepsy, anticonvulsant metabolism, birth defects, genetics and socioeconomic and environmental factors, much of this immense literature is contradictory and controversies abound. The following is my assimilation of that literature and my current approach to this clinical situation.

Oral contraception

Although oestrogens can lower seizure threshold and aggravate the condition of some women with intractable epilepsy, oral contraceptives can be used by almost all epileptic women. Some women with epilepsy become unexpectedly pregnant while taking conventional doses of oral contraceptives because most first choice anticonvulsants, with the probable exception of valproic acid, induce hepatic hydroxylating enzymes and thereby accelerate oestrogen catabolism [52]. Thus, breakthrough bleeding and pregnancy are more likely to occur if a low oestrogen-containing contraceptive is used.

Pregnancy

The effect of pregnancy upon epilepsy can be estimated according to the degree of control achieved beforehand. The longer a woman has been seizure free, the less likely she will convulse during pregnancy. Almost all women with an average seizure frequency of >1 per month will worsen during pregnancy, whereas only 25 per cent who did not convulse in the 9 months preceding pregnancy will convulse during pregnancy [44]. Sleep deprivation in the last month of pregnancy may induce seizures, even in well-controlled epilepsy [76]. An epileptic woman has a 1 per cent chance of convulsing during labour with hyperventilation as a probable factor. Aggravation of epilepsy by lactation is extremely rare.

Pregnancy-induced change in anticonvulsant metabolism is the most important manageable factor affecting the course of epilepsy during pregnancy [38,48]. In the era before blood levels of anticonvulsants could be easily monitored, approximately 50 per cent of patients deteriorated during pregnancy [23]. If daily dosages are adjusted so as to maintain blood levels within a range found to be therapeutic before pregnancy, only approximately 10 per cent will experience more seizures during pregnancy.

The course of pregnancy is unaffected by epilepsy for most women. Other maternal diseases, parity, socioeconomic status and the quality of prenatal care are more important factors. The rate of spontaneous abortion is not increased [3]. Although the risk of almost any complication can be found to be increased in one survey or another, maternal epilepsy is not consistently associated with any obstetric complication of pregnancy with the possible exception of third trimester bleeding, which may be secondary to anticonvulsant-induced folate deficiency [36]. Maternal epilepsy is rarely an indication for caesarean section unless either a seizure occurs during the second stage of labour or the patient can not cooperate with vaginal delivery.

Epilepsy and the fetus

The fetus is remarkably tolerant of isolated maternal *grand mal* convulsions although it can be assumed that the hypoxia and lactic acidosis which accompany a seizure cannot be good for it. Fetal bradycardia occurs during and for 20 min after a maternal convulsion. In rare instances fetal death and intraventricular haemorrhages have been attributed to a maternal convulsion. However, the effect of maternal convulsions may be remote, and only detected in intellectual performance years later as Gaily *et al.* [32] suggest. Status epilepticus is a certain threat to both mother and fetus with a doubling of risk of maternal death and a 50 per cent chance of fetal wastage.

Neonatal coagulopathy

A neonatal bleeding disorder due to a deficiency of vitamin K dependent clotting factors has been reported with maternal use of phenytoin, phenobarbital and primidone. Maternal coagulation studies are usually normal.

Birth defects

Birth defects are not unusual, and occur in 3–5 per cent of all babies depending upon methodology and the population studied. The risk of some malformation increases, perhaps doubles, for the offspring of women with treated epilepsy. The largest controlled series, a Norwegian study with 3879 infants in each group, found the absolute risk increased from 3.5 to 4.4 per cent if the mother was epileptic [7]. The risk of birth defects increases with the number of anticonvulsants used. However, a fundamental problem is difficulty distinguishing the risk of congenital malformation due to the severity of the maternal trait of epilepsy from the risk due to treatment.

Orofacial clefts

Orofacial clefting is the most common major malformation which has been attributed to anticonvulsants, particularly phenytoin. The relative risk is approximately 5. However, a genetic link between epilepsy and orofacial clefts is suspected because epileptics have twice the expected incidence of orofacial clefts. Furthermore epilepsy is more common than expected in the extended families of children with orofacial clefts [30]. Thus an important part of counselling sessions is taking a detailed family history concerning congenital malformations—especially orofacial clefts, neural tube defects and congenital heart disease.

Neural tube defects

Surveillance studies have found a 1–2 per cent risk of neural tube defects amongst infants exposed *in utero* to valproic acid [59]. The relative risk is approximately 10. More recently a smaller risk has been reported due to carbamazepine [69]. Fortunately prenatal diagnosis of serious neural tube defects can be made in the second trimester. High resolution ultrasonography at 18–19 weeks plus serum α fetoprotein determination will be diagnostic in most instances [19]. Quantitation of α fetoprotein in amniotic fluid is preferred by some centres but the procedure carries a 1 per cent risk of miscarriage.

Dysmorphic features and digital hypoplasia

Craniofacial dysmorphic features plus hypoplasia of fingertips and fingernails have been attributed to all major anticonvulsants [33]. Distal digital hypoplasia and hypertelorism are most strongly associated with phenytoin exposure. It should be emphasized that most babies with these 'minor malformations' regarded as typical of the fetal anticonvulsant syndrome grow out of these features, with the possible exception of hypertelorism.

PATHOGENESIS

The increased risk of congenital malformations in the offspring of epileptic mothers is probably multifactorial. The role of genetics in the 'fetal anticonvulsant syndrome' is well illustrated by the remarkable case of heteroparental dizygotic twins simultaneously exposed to phenytoin throughout gestation [61]. One baby had the syndrome; the other did not. Other aspects sometimes ascribed to the fetal anticonvulsant syndrome may have a genetic basis if families are studied. For instance epicanthus in exposed infants was strongly associated with epicanthus in the mothers [33]. Similar studies of head circumference and stature of the infants of epileptic mothers show genetics to be the major factor [34].

One mechanism could be an inherited deficiency of epoxide hydrolase which in the case of phenytoin could increase arene oxides [9]. Polytherapy can shift metabolism to potentially teratogenic pathways [50]. For instance, the combination of valproic acid plus carbamazepine plus phenobarbitone appears to be associated with an exceptionally high rate of major congenital malformations. Thus monotherapy could lessen the risk of birth defects.

A second proposed teratogenic mechanism is folate deficiency [16]. Folate malabsorption is most commonly associated with phenytoin and phenobarbitone therapy but also occurs with carbamazepine and valproic acid. Therapy with multiple drugs causes the lowest levels. Folic acid supplementation before conception appears to decrease birth defects in children of epileptic and non-epileptic mothers. Folate deficiency could be one way in which socioeconomic status affects the malformation rate. The optimal daily dose of folate has not been determined but 0.5 or 1 mg is reasonable.

Counselling and management

The best management of epilepsy during pregnancy begins with counselling of the prospective parents before conception [19]. First, confirm the diagnosis. Not infrequently patients with syncope, panic attacks, hyperventilation and sometimes more complex pseudoseizures have been mislabelled as epileptics and treated inappropriately with anticonvulsant drugs. In other instances the previous investigation of true seizures may not have been thorough enough to exclude a condition, such as an arteriovenous malformation, which could significantly alter management of both epilepsy and pregnancy. The author recommends measuring erythrocyte folate levels at pre-pregnancy counselling sessions and starting vitamins which typically contain folate before pregnancy occurs. Often women stop oral contraceptives and start prenatal vitamins with folate.

The primary objective is to keep the prospective mother seizure free with the fewest drugs at the lowest dosage that is effective. Monotherapy is recommended if at all possible. The time to change medication is before conception. None of the most commonly used anticonvulsants (carbamazepine, phenytoin, valproic acid and phenobarbitone) is preferred just because pregnancy is contemplated. Trimethadione and paramethadione are strongly teratogenic and best avoided by teenagers and women of childbearing age. A statistically significant comparison of the outcomes of pregnancies of epileptic mothers taking different anticonvulsant drugs in monotherapy has never been done.

The author's first choice for an anticonvulsant drug is dictated by the type of seizure disorder and the patient's potential for compliance. For instance, valproic acid in monotherapy usually completely controls juvenile myoclonic epilepsy, whereas polytherapy in several regimens is often unsuccessful. Thus, the author recommends valproic acid in monotherapy in this situation provided the woman understands the risks. Avoiding high peak blood levels of valproic acid may lessen the risk of neural tube defects and can be accomplished by changing the customary twice daily doses to smaller doses three or four times daily.

Anticonvulsant blood levels should be checked if a convulsion occurs and the author prefers to monitor blood levels approximately each month during pregnancy so that daily dosages can be adjusted in an attempt to kept the level in that patient's pre-determined therapeutic range. Free protein unbound anticonvulsant blood levels are preferred during pregnancy because protein binding decreases during pregnancy. Thus, lower blood levels due to increased metabolism during pregnancy, are partially offset by decreased binding and higher free drug levels. For instance, although total blood phenytoin may drop 56 per cent, free phenytoin declines only 31 per cent. This effect is not as great for carbamazepine, with a 42 per cent decrease in total blood level accompanied by a 28 per cent decrease in the protein unbound amount [92].

Vitamin K_1 should be given during the last month of pregnancy as prophylaxis for the neonatal bleeding disorder reported with maternal use of phenytoin, phenobarbitone and primidone. The lowest effective dose is undetermined, but it is known that 20 mg/day orally will prevent this disorder [18].

If anticonvulsant dosages were increased during pregnancy, remember to decrease the dosage post-partum. Blood levels of phenytoin increase quickly after childbirth. The rebound in carbamazepine and phenobarbitone levels is slower. The pre-pregnancy dosage is usually re-established at 6–8 weeks post-partum.

All anticonvulsants are present in breast milk, but only in some instances with phenobarbitone and the benzodiazepines does the combination of the amount ingested plus slow neonatal metabolism produce sedation. Usually babies cannot ingest enough milk to cause any effect. Beginning at about 1 week after birth, infants of women taking phenobarbitone or primidone can experience withdrawal symptoms if they are not breastfed. These symptoms are hyperexcitability, tremor, high-pitched cry, feeding problems and always seem to be hungry [34]. Withdrawal symptoms may also occur with other anticonvulsant drugs.

Cerebrovascular disease

Cerebrovascular disease is a major cause of maternal mortality and morbidity. Unusual types of cerebrovascular disease are relatively common during pregnancy. For instance, the most common cause of hypertensive encephalopathy is eclampsia. At least 30 per cent of eclamptic deaths are attributed to cerebral pathology. During delivery acute blood loss may infarct the pituitary gland (Sheehan's syndrome), the optic chiasm and cerebral watersheds. Air and amniotic fluid embolisms are dramatic and often fatal. Cerebral venous thrombosis is a rare condition which principally occurs in the puerperium, and is still fatal in 20 per cent. Rupture of a cerebral aneurysm is a more common disaster. Ischaemic stroke is less likely to cause death but can cause significant impairment.

Ischaemic stroke

Both pregnancy and the use of oral contraceptives increase the incidence of transient ischaemic attacks (TIA) and stroke approximately five- to 10-fold [13, 87]. The risk of a cerebral ischaemic event increases with age in both pregnant and non-pregnant young women. Probably less than one-quarter of pregnancy-associated strokes are due to premature atheromatous disease, and these patients are usually women in their thirties with long-standing diabetes mellitus and hypertension who are also at risk for other complications of pregnancy. In another quarter, no underlying cause is said to be found, but that proportion may be reduced by more extensive investigation. The majority of strokes are caused by one of an ever increasing list of relatively unusual causes of cerebral ischaemia including mitral valve prolapse, peri-partum cardiomyopathy, subacute bacterial endocarditis, sickle cell disease, syphilis, vasculitis, thrombotic thrombocytopenic purpura, moya moya disease, fibromuscular dysplasia, carotid artery dissection and choriocarcinoma. Although antiphospholipid antibodies (the 'lupus anticoagulant') are a leading cause of stroke in non-pregnant young women, this and some other hypercoagulable states are associated with fetal wastage due to placental ischaemia and thus are a less frequent cause of stroke during pregnancy than would be expected.

Almost all strokes associated with pregnancy occur in the carotid distribution. In young adults strokes are rarely in the vertebrobasilar system, with the exception of strokes associated with the use of oral contraceptives. Approximately 30 per cent of pregnancy-associated strokes are concentrated during the first week post-partum with equal shares for each in the second and third trimesters. Strokes during pregnancy have a greater than expected incidence of occlusions of a middle cerebral artery, and are sometimes bilateral [13]. This suggests an embolus of cardiac origin. Strokes after delivery have a greater than expected incidence of carotid occlusion. The author suspects that many of these post-partum strokes are caused by paradoxical emboli from peripheral veins and the pelvic venous beds. Transoesophageal echocardiography is superior to trans-sternal echocardiography in both instances and should be used in the investigation of pregnancy-associated cerebral ischaemic events. The physician must be circumspect and should not avoid angiography because the patient is pregnant. Rarities are often found serendipitously during angiography.

Paradoxical embolism is an overlooked diagnosis which should be suspected whenever right atrial pressure is increased, such as following pulmonary embolism [85]. If right atrial pressure exceeds left atrial pressure, an anatomically patent but usually physiologically closed foramen ovale can open, clots can cross to the left side of the heart and thence to the brain, kidneys and peripheral arteries. Sometimes bits of clot trapped in the foramen ovale can intermittently be the source of emboli. A saddle embolus at the carotid bifurcation may be surgically removed sometimes with immediate recovery, if the condition is diagnosed and the embolectomy performed within 4 hours.

Treatment and prognosis depend upon the diagnosis. If anticoagulation is necessary in multiple unexplained transient ischaemic attacks heparin, or preferably low molecular weight heparin is the obvious choice (see Chapters 4 and 5).

A woman who, whilst taking an oral contraceptive or whilst pregnant, had a cerebral ischaemic event which remained unexplained after a thorough evaluation, does not appear to be at greater risk of having another ischaemic event during a subsequent pregnancy.

Cerebral venous thrombosis

Aseptic cerebral venous thrombosis is strongly associated with the use of oral contraceptives and with the puerperium. Most cases of late post-partum eclampsia in the antiquarian literature were probably cerebral venous thromboses [78]. This is a rare condition in western Europe and North America with an incidence of perhaps one per 10 000 deliveries. In these areas the condition typically presents in the second and third weeks post-partum within a range of 4 days to 4 weeks. In India puerperal cerebral venous thrombosis is a public health problem with an incidence of 40–50 per 10 000 deliveries [82]. In most cases, women delivered at home present within days of childbirth. The reason appears to be dehydration because midwives restrict water intake for the first day. Some puerperal cases have been associated with hypercoagulable states including antiphospholipid antibodies (see Chapter 8), protein C deficiency (see Chapter 4), homocystinuria (see Chapter 4) and paroxysmal nocturnal haemoglobinuria (see Chapter 2). Cerebral venous thrombosis may coexist with thrombophlebitis in the legs and pelvis.

The clinical presentation depends upon which veins are occluded and how fast the clot propagates. Sometimes there is a stuttering course for a week before the disease declares itself. Usually a persistent headache or a seizure demand explanation. There are two typical presentations depending upon where the clot starts. In the instance of a cortical vein thrombosis increasingly severe headache precedes focal or generalized convulsions which are followed by aphasia, weakness and other focal neurological signs, in some instances with stupor. The propagation of clot through the cortical veins can provoke more seizures and neurological deficits. The faster the progression the poorer the prognosis because collateral circulation is obstructed and the risk of venous infarction and intracerebral bleeding increases. Increased intracranial pressure may be caused by either the mass effect of intracerebral bleeding or the obstruction of CSF absorption by clot in the superior sagittal sinus.

The second presentation is a thrombosis in the superior sagittal sinus or the right lateral sinus. Headache is due to intracranial hypertension. Sometimes clot spreads into the parasagittal motor cortex causing primarily leg weakness and focal convulsions and into the occipital cortex causing hemianopia or on occasion cortical blindness if both occipital lobes are affected.

The diagnosis is confirmed by neuro-imaging studies. CT is the best method to detect acute intracerebral bleeding. MRI is better able to show established venous clots in cortical veins and sinuses. If there is any doubt, the gold standard is angiography, preferably digital subtraction angiography which can simultaneously study both hemispheres and requires little contrast material.

Treatment consists of hydration, anticonvulsants and anticoagulation. Heparin stops clot formation but adds to the risk of intracerebral bleeding. It use has been controversial, especially in cases in which intracerebral bleeding has already occurred. However, heparin is worth the risk, considering that mortality is 20–30 per cent if not treated. The role of thrombolytic agents is uncertain. Survivors usually do well because the supply of oxygenated blood continues to reach brain tissue. Cerebral venous thrombosis has recurred in subsequent pregnancies but this is extremely rare. Prophylactic anticoagulation during pregnancy is not indicated because this condition is a post-partum phenomenon.

Subarachnoid haemorrhage

Spontaneous subarachnoid haemorrhage complicates only one or two in 10 000 pregnancies but causes as much as 10 per cent of maternal mortality [20,88]. The principal cause of subarachnoid haemorrhage in women under 25 years is an arteriovenous malformation (AVM); most are primigravidas [40,75]. AVMs are more common in Asians than Caucasians. Older women are more likely to have a ruptured berry aneurysm. Cocaine abuse has precipitated rupture of aneurysms and AVMs (see Chapter 18) [55]. Although rupture of a berry aneurysm or an AVM together cause the majority of cases, at all ages approximately one-third of cases are due to other causes including bleeding disorders, vasculitis, subacute endocarditis, sickle haemoglobinopathy and metastatic choriocarcinoma. No cause will be established in approximately 5 per cent. Unless a woman with a subarachnoid haemorrhage is in active labour, she should be evaluated as if she were not pregnant. Four-vessel angiography will be needed in the case of an aneurysm.

The initial haemorrhage of an AVM usually occurs during the second trimester or during childbirth. Oestrogen dilates other arteriovenous shunts, as is clinically apparent in pregnant women and alcoholics with spider naevi and palmar erythema. Blood oestrogen levels reach a plateau during the second trimester. Haemorrhage during childbirth is probably related to haemodynamic abnormalities produced by the Valsalva manoeuvre which accompanies strong labour pains. Venous angiomas, which are now detected frequently by MRI, are not associated with haemorrhage although sometimes a venous angioma is in the vicinity of a cavernous AVM (cavernoma). The morbidity due to the rupture of an AVM is proportional to its size and location. If possible the AVM should be excised during the second trimester. Then the woman can be delivered vaginally without special precautions. Although some studies conclude that vaginal delivery is possible for a woman with an inoperable AVM, the author continues to recommend an elective caesarean section near to term [46].

The initial haemorrhage from berry aneurysms, and aneurysms at other sites throughout the body, increases with each trimester of pregnancy. The peak period is from 32 to 36 weeks. Rarely does an initial haemorrhage occur intra-partum although re-bleeding does occur during labour. The risk of death increases as the patient's stupor increases, and is approximately 20 per cent even if the patient survives the first bleed with little more than a headache and a stiff neck. If possible the offending aneurysm should be clipped or otherwise surgically cured during pregnancy. Hypothermia and controlled hypotension can be used safely during pregnancy [56]. In a few instances a caesarean section has been immediately followed by neurosurgery [89]. If multiple aneurysms exist, as occurs in 10 per cent, the offending aneurysm can be handled during pregnancy and the remainder can be treated several months post-partum, with the possible exception of large aneurysms, with diameters >8–10 mm. If curative surgery is not done, most women are delivered by elective caesarean section. If a multiparous woman with a proven pelvis can avoid bearing down by panting and regional analgesia, vaginal delivery is an option.

Eclamptic hypertensive encephalopathy (see also Chapter 6)

Eclamptic seizures are often preceded by headache, brisk reflexes and the perception of flashing lights. The convulsions are generalized sometimes with superimposed clinical features of multiple foci activated in succession. For example, clonic movements in a leg due to a focus in one hemisphere and aversive eye movements to a focus in the other hemisphere can irregularly punctuate successive seizures or a prolonged eclamptic convulsion.

Eclamptic seizures are caused by patches of small haemorrhages and microinfarctions in the cerebral cortex [78]. Similar lesions in the visual cortex cause visual hallucinations and, if multiple lesions accumulate, cortical blindness. Sometimes multiple petechial haemorrhages are compacted into 'haematomas' in the subcortex, pons, caudate nucleus and other deep central grey matter. Streak haemorrhages occur in the corona radiata. The classic microscopic lesion is a ring haemorrhage about a thrombosed capillary or precapillary. In addition large haematomata, which may be correlated with disseminated intravascular coagulopathy (DIC), often cause sudden coma and need not occur during a convulsion. The mortality associated with eclampsia is greater than that of severe pre-eclampsia, in part because other organs are more seriously involved. Cerebral pathology causes 30–60 per cent of eclamptic and pre-eclamptic deaths.

The onset of brain lesions sometimes precedes the first eclamptic convulsion. The traditional diagnostic criteria for eclampsia excludes both visual hallucinations and cortical blindness even though these are manifestations of lesions in the occipital cortex which are identical to lesions which elsewhere could cause convulsions. The traditional definition also excludes toxaemic women who suddenly become comatose due to a large intracerebral haematoma without convulsing. Furthermore, CT and MRI have demonstrated changes in the brain in toxaemic women who have not convulsed [47].

Neurodiagnostic studies

Neurodiagnostic studies and the input of a neurologist are usually not needed unless the patient has atypical features such as focal deficits, impaired consciousness following a fit, or convulsions occurring more than 24 hours after childbirth [71,80]. In those instances an imaging study is indicated. CT has the advantage of faster scanning, and detects major acute haemorrhages better than MRI [15]. MRI is better than CT in detecting oedema in the cortical mantle and elsewhere in the brain, and gadolinium enhancement denotes breaks in the blood–brain barrier. Both techniques can be normal, show diffuse cerebral oedema with slit-like ventricles, or show regions with decreased density denoting increased brain water [67,71]. Sometimes arcuate bands of oedema course through the internal and external capsules. Cerebral oedema can be apparent on CT immediately after the eclamptic crisis and often disappears in a few days. This timing is compatible with vasogenic cerebral oedema and is unlike the delay of several days in the CT appearance of cytotoxic cerebral oedema following a common ischaemic stroke. Single photon emission computed tomography (SPECT) shows increased perfusion adjacent to abnormal regions on CT and MRI [77].

Special note should be made concerning late post-partum eclampsia, i.e. eclamptic convulsions starting more than 24 or 30 hours after delivery. The differential diagnosis of post-partum convulsions is complex and includes thrombotic thrombocytopenic purpura (see Chapter 3) and cerebral venous thrombosis (see above). Arteriography can suggest the diagnosis of late post-partum eclampsia by demonstrating smooth vasospasm in large and medium calibre cerebral arteries, which resembles spasm following rupture of a berry aneurysm [49,65]. In Europe this entity is called post-partum angiopathy [8].

Other tests usually have a lower priority but can be important in certain instances. CSF pressure is normal or increased [29]. The concentration of protein in CSF is typically 0.5–1.5 g/l. A few red cells or pink-tinged fluid is not unusual. A grossly bloody CSF is a poor prognostic sign. The EEG reflects the status of the patient ranging from mild slowing of the background activity to prominent δ activity in stuporous patients. Slowing is often more prominent in the posterior regions [1]. Recently, transcranial Doppler studies have shown a marked increase in the velocity of flow in the middle cerebral arteries of women who developed post-partum eclampsia.

PATHOGENESIS

In 1928 Oppenheimer and Fishberg [60] understood that the classic form of the eclamptic attack consisted of epileptiform seizures in every way analogous to those occurring in acute glomerulonephritis and included both as causes of hypertensive encephalopathy in usually normotensive young patients [60]. In physiological terms blood pressure has exceeded the zone of blood pressures within which cerebral blood flow remains constant. The upper limit of this cerebral autoregulation is directly dependent upon an individual's customary blood pressure and inversely dependent upon arterial $P\text{CO}_2$. The variability in these functions is probably the reason why obstetricians have difficulty in determining strict blood pressure criteria for various degrees of pre-eclampsia [22].

MANAGEMENT

A corollary of the above concept is that the best prophylaxis for toxaemic hypertensive encephalopathy and eclamptic convulsions is adequate control of hypertension. Some obstetricians do not treat pre-eclamptic women prophylactically with an anti-epileptic drug [11].

If convulsions occur, diazepam is a common choice for immediate control. An intravenous dose of 5 or 10 mg usually stops eclamptic convulsions without any effect upon the fetus [93]. More can interfere with assessment of the level of consciousness and suppress or arrest respiration. Usually the effect of diazepam lasts at least 20 min, long enough to begin antihypertensive treatment and start loading the patient with a longer acting anticonvulsant. The author recommends phenytoin because it can be given intravenously, is non-sedating and has no ill-effect upon the fetus. Several protocols have been devised. All propose less phenytoin than is commonly used for status epilepticus because less phenytoin is protein bound in pregnant women near term — 85 per cent of total serum phenytoin instead of the usual 90 per cent. Thus the effective amount of free phenytoin (i.e. protein unbound phenytoin) is increased by half. Ryan's regimen for pre-eclamptic women is to load initially with 10 mg/kg and then repeat with another 5 mg/kg in 2–6 hours [74]. A therapeutic free blood level can be expected for 24 hours. Therapeutic amounts of phenobarbitone and chlormethiazole will sedate the fetus, and thus are most useful after delivery, if still needed. Although generations of American obstetricians have been wedded to magnesium sulphate as an anticonvulsant for toxaemic women [79], its use is empirical and without scientific support [24]. It must be stressed that no anticonvulsant drug will be 100 per cent effective for eclamptic convulsions unless hypertension is adequately controlled.

The ideal antihypertensive drug for eclamptic hypertensive encephalopathy would lower systemic vascular resistance without affecting cerebral vessels, thereby allowing *pari passu* a decrease in cerebral vasoconstriction by the autoregulatory mechanism. Blood pressure should be lowered rapidly to within the range of autoregulation but in a controlled manner in order to prevent over-shooting that range. The targetted zone of blood pressure can be estimated from knowledge of an individual patient's customary blood pressure. If this is unknown, mean arterial blood pressure should be lowered by 20–25 per cent. Each agent has its advantages and disadvantages. Usually obstetricians use the agent with which they are most familiar.

Mild vasogenic cerebral oedema accompanying eclamptic hypertensive encephalopathy usually abates soon after blood pressure is controlled. In more severe cases with stupor, active management is needed [68]. Hyperventilation appears to be an obvious first measure because it both decreases intracranial pressure and increases the upper limit of autoregulation. Corticosteroid therapy could be effective as it is for vasogenic cerebral oedema surrounding tumours metastatic to brain. If no contraindication exists, dexamethasone therapy is reasonable. In some cases, often eclamptic women with intracerebral haemorrhages, intracranial pressure may need to be monitored and more aggressive treatment may be needed including CSF drainage, hypothermia and barbiturate coma. Surgical evacuation is rarely indicated.

Mannitol can be predicted to be ineffective and sometimes dangerous. The effectiveness of mannitol as an osmotic agent depends upon the integrity of the blood–brain barrier formed by the tight junctions between capillary endothelial cells. Vasogenic cerebral oedema occurs because those junctions are leaky. Leakage of mannitol with its sphere of hydration into brain could worsen patients with widespread vasogenic cerebral oedema.

Tumours

Pregnancy and brain tumours profoundly affect one another. Tumours of virtually every type have been reported to coexist with pregnancy [66]. Yet the coincidence is only 38 per cent of expected, perhaps because libido or fertility are affected by the developing tumour. Nevertheless brain tumours cause approximately 5 per cent of maternal deaths if the first six months post-partum are counted. During pregnancy, tumours grow faster and are more vascular in part in response to stimulation of oestrogen and progesterone receptors which have been found in meningiomata, neurofibromata and some gliomata. After childbirth this can regress, at least temporarily. Symptoms of some benign tumours (e.g. acoustic neuromata and meningiomata) have regressed enough after one pregnancy to escape attention until a recurrence during a subsequent pregnancy.

Exact diagnosis is crucial. Abscess and metastatic cancer should be kept in mind even though they are unlikely. Choriocarcinoma is a special consideration during and for a few years after pregnancy. Fixed guidelines for the management of these cases do not exist because every instance is different. Nevertheless trends emerge. Benign tumours tend to be operated upon after delivery because tumours are smaller and the operative field less bloody. Patients suspected of having a supratentorial astrocytoma presenting during pregnancy usually proceed to diagnostic biopsy and sometimes excision of the tumour. Interruption of an early pregnancy is often recommended for women with malignant gliomata, especially those with uncontrollable convulsions. Childbirth in the face of intracranial hypertension due to a mass lesion is usually accomplished by caesarean section although a few multiparous women have been delivered vaginally.

Choriocarcinoma

Choriocarcinoma is relatively rare in western Europe and North America when compared to Nigeria, the Philippine Islands and elsewhere in the tropics. Patients with choriocarcinoma usually present after miscarriage or a molar pregnancy with uterine enlargement and vaginal bleeding. Approximately 15 per cent occur during or after a normal pregnancy. In some there will be no evidence of tumour in the uterus.

A few patients present with neurological symptoms [43,64]. Most but not all of these cases also have pulmonary spread. Cerebral metastases present in three manners:

1 a solitary mass lesion with or without Jacksonian seizures;

2 single or multiple strokes due to occlusion of arteries of any size including the carotid artery; and

3 haemorrhage into any intracranial compartment.

For instance, the cause of a fatal acute subdural haematoma 9 months following a normal pregnancy was one small nidus of choriocarcinoma. Tumour can also invade the sacral plexus and spine. Serum levels of β human chorionic gonadotrophin (bHCG) may be higher than expected for late pregnancy, and are particularly helpful in diagnosing and following post-partum cases. A serum to cerebrospinal fluid bHCG ratio $< 60:1$ is highly suggestive of a brain metastasis.

Whole-brain irradiation and aggressive chemotherapy can be very successful in what was once a fatal situation.

Pituitary adenoma

Pregnancy induces enlargement of both a normal pituitary gland and pituitary tumours; however only growth of a tumour causes symptoms. Headache typically precedes the constriction of visual fields by 1 month. Large tumours can cause diabetes insipidus and compromise the release of other pituitary hormones. Rarely pituitary apoplexy occurs.

Until the era of CT and MRI allowed the easy detection of microadenomata, many infertile women with small prolactin-secreting adenomata were not diagnosed until after ovulation was induced and pregnancy accomplished. Now women with prolactinomata can be managed according to the size of the tumour [57]. Patients with suprasellar tumours are candidates for surgery before pregnancy. Thirty-five per cent of women with macroadenomata >10 mm in diameter will become symptomatic during pregnancy; whereas only 5 per cent of women with microadenomata will develop symptoms. Thus, bromocriptine therapy is usually discontinued for women with microadenomata once it has permitted a woman to be come pregnant. The management of patients with pituitary tumours is considered in more detail in Chapter 13.

Lymphocytic hypophysitis

Lymphocytic hypophysitis is a rare autoimmune disorder which typically presents post-partum as an intrasellar mass or as hypopituitarism without a history of intra-partum haemorrhage and shock [12].

Pseudotumour cerebri

Pregnancy-associated pseudotumour cerebri (benign intracranial hypertension) usually begins in the third to fifth month of pregnancy and lasts a few months before spontaneously remitting [21]. A few cases persist until the puerperium. Women with pre-existing pseudotumour cerebri typically worsen with the onset of pregnancy. Obesity is characteristic of both pregnant and non-pregnant patients, and rapid excess weight gain is common amongst the pregnant cohort. Headache, often retro-orbital, is the universal presenting complaint. Unless the examining physician is thorough enough to inspect the optic fundi and discover papilloedema, the diagnosis will be missed because these patients can be neurologically normal although some will have diplopia due to abducens palsy. CT or MRI easily rule out hydrocephalus and intracranial space-occupying lesions. CSF pressure is increased. Commonly the CSF level of protein is <0.2 g/l.

Management is aimed at preserving vision. The author weighs the patient, examines the optic fundi and determines visual acuity and visual fields each week. Failing colour vision and visual obscurations are to be reported immediately.

Treatment starts with limitation of weight gain to ordinary increments. Repeated CSF drainage affords some temporary relief. Corticosteroid therapy should be started if visual acuity diminishes or visual fields become restricted when the inferior nasal quadrants may be the first area affected. A reasonable regime would be prednisone 10 mg three times daily in pregnancy. Lumboperitoneal shunting or fenestration of the optic nerve sheath should be considered for recalcitrant cases.

Hydrocephalus

An increasing number of women with indwelling shunts for the treatment of hydrocephalus are becoming pregnant [14,35]. Presumably their offspring are at an increased risk of developing hydrocephalus. Thus, ultrasonography and assays for α fetoprotein are recommended as for the detection of neural tube defects.

Both ventriculoperitoneal and ventriculoatrial shunts have malfunctioned during pregnancy and have required replacement which has been accomplished without special problems. Some patients have received intra-partum prophylactic antibiotics, but whether this is necessary is not clear at present. In the case of shunts to the peritoneal space, caesarean section is recommended only for very definite obstetric indications.

Multiple sclerosis

Disseminated sclerosis is a demyelinating disease of the central nervous system which is characterized by exacerbations and spontaneous remissions. The disease has a propensity to occur in women during their fertile years. With the exception of one dissenting study [31], the only factor which affects the natural history of this disease is pregnancy [6,45]. Both initial episodes and exacerbations are less likely to occur with each successive trimester of pregnancy. However, the relapse rate in the first 3–6 months after delivery is much greater than expected. Retrospective studies which may underestimate this effect generally estimate the risk of a post-partum exacerbation at 40 per cent. Thus the relapse rate for a pregnancy year including the first 3 months of the puerperium is at least equal to if not greater than the risk in a non-pregnancy year. Breast feeding is an indeterminant factor. Antenatal immunosuppression by α fetoprotein has been suggested as a mechanism for this effect of pregnancy and the rebound afterwards [45]. Neither the number of pregnancies nor the timing of those pregnancies *vis-à-vis* the onset of multiple sclerosis appears to affect eventual disability [86].

Multiple sclerosis rarely affects fertility but it profoundly alters family patterns. After the diagnosis of multiple sclerosis has been determined, more women remain unmarried, have more elective abortions, and elect to have either fewer children or no additional children. The divorce rate increases with the degree of disability. Young women with mild disease and no children usually decide to proceed with a pregnancy, whereas older women with children and either significant disability or a progressive course do not.

Uncomplicated multiple sclerosis has little effect on the management of pregnancy. Patients with difficulty walking often experience more problems during the second half of pregnancy. Furthermore, an enlarging uterus can complicate the function of a neurogenic bladder and increase the risk of cystitis. Spasticity often fluctuates during pregnancy. Extensor or flexor spasms can be triggered by labour pains. There is no significant change in the incidence of spontaneous abortion, premature delivery, difficult delivery, toxaemia and still-birth. Nor is the risk of birth defects altered. Experience with epidural analgesia is limited but favourable. Spinal anaesthesia is usually avoided in patients with multiple sclerosis.

Headache

Headache is a common neurological symptom during pregnancy [65]. Headache appearing for the first time should be viewed with suspicion for it can be symptomatic of one of a long list of serious conditions including toxaemia, subarachnoid haemorrhage, tumours, pseudotumour cerebri, cerebral venous thrombosis in addition to more mundane afflictions of sinuses, ears and teeth. Once again a careful history and a neurological examination including inspection of the eye grounds is the important first step in sorting through the list of possibilities.

Muscle contraction headache

The most common headache during pregnancy is muscle contraction headache. This includes bruxism in which increased resting muscle tension exists in the muscles of mastication. Although postural changes predispose some women to generalized muscle contraction headache, the majority are symptomatic of situational stress and depression. The treatment of an occasional acute muscle contraction headache consists of paracetamol, muscle massage and ice packs. Sometimes codeine preparations are needed. Paracetamol is preferred to aspirin for frequent use for chronic headache during pregnancy [73]. Frequent recurrent muscle contraction headache may warrant a psychological assessment and prophylaxis with a tricyclic antidepressant such as amitriptyline or imipramine. Both drugs have been used extensively during pregnancy in psychiatric patients at dosages higher than the 50 or 75 mg which is often effective for these headaches (see Chapter 20).

Classic migraine

Classic migraine is affected by hormonal change, typically oestrogen withdrawal around the time of menstruation [81]. Fortunately 80 per cent of women with classic migraine improve during pregnancy but equally migraine presenting for the first time is a common cause of headache in pregnancy. The first trimester is the usual time for classic migraine to worsen or to present. Not infrequently this is an unusual variety such as hemiplegic migraine, middle cerebral artery migraine or basilar migraine [41,91]. The differential diagnosis can be complicated. During pregnancy, an occasional classic migraine is usually treated with analgesics and, if necessary, an anti-emetic. If classic migraine occurs more than twice monthly, prophylactic therapy can be considered. Aspirin 75 mg daily is the obvious first choice. Propranolol, 40–160 mg daily in divided doses, is also effective and reasonably safe during pregnancy [72] (see Chapter 6). Calcium channel blockers and tricyclic antidepressant agents are third choices. Ergot alkaloids are not used during pregnancy and lactation.

Neuropathy

Bell's palsy

Acute unilateral facial paralysis is 10-fold more common than expected during the third trimester and the first 2 weeks post-partum [37]. This plus the association of Bell's palsy in non-pregnant women with the pre-luteal stage of the menstrual cycle suggests a hormonal mechanism. Cases occurring just before term have an excellent prognosis. A short course of corticosteroid therapy (e.g. prednisone 40 mg/day in divided doses lapsing to zero over 2 weeks) is reasonable for women with complete facial weakness. Bilateral Bell's palsy suggests the Guillain–Barré syndrome, or sarcoid or Lyme disease.

Carpal tunnel syndrome

Nocturnal acroparaesthesia is experienced by one-third of pregnant women [25,54]. Bilateral symptoms are reported by the majority. However, only a few pregnant women develop true entrapment of the median nerve at the wrist, the carpal tunnel syndrome. Progression to weakness of the abductor pollicus brevis is uncommon during pregnancy, but weakness is an indication for surgical division of the transcarpal ligaments. Most pregnant women with carpal tunnel syndrome can expect their symptoms to regress after delivery. Nocturnal splinting of the wrist in mid-position is usually effective although some find an injection of corticosteroid is needed to carry the patient over to the puerperium.

Meralgia paraesthetica

Unilateral or bilateral meralgia paraesthetica develops in the last 10 weeks of pregnancy due to entrapment of the lateral femoral cutaneous nerve at the inguinal ligament by an enlarging abdomen. For most it is a nuisance which remits within 3 months after childbirth if excess weight is lost [53].

Intra-partum lumbosacral plexopathy

Intra-partum entrapment of peripheral nerves with the pelvis can be caused by the fetal head and the application of forceps [27]. The typical patient is a short, overweight primipara with dystocia due to cephalopelvic disproportion.

The most common syndrome is footdrop due to compression of the lumbosacral trunk (L4, L5) against the pelvic brim. Sometimes elements from the S1 root are involved if the point of compression is lower. Although a few bilateral cases have been reported, this syndrome is characteristically unilateral and contralateral to the presentation of the occiput. Footdrop may also be caused by compression of the common peroneal nerve between leg holders and the fibular head.

Femoral (anterior crural) and obturator neuropathies are bilateral in about 25 per cent, with no preference as to right or left side for the unilateral cases. Arrest of labour in a transverse lie is frequent.

The prognosis depends upon the severity of the nerve injury. Complete recovery within 2 months is expected in neuropraxis in which only the myelin sheath has been distorted. If axons have been crushed, improvement is slower and sometimes incomplete. Furthermore, women with axonal lesions are probably at greater risk if nerves are again damaged during a subsequent delivery. Thus, women with EMG evidence of denervation are future candidates for a caesarean section, whereas women with neuropraxis are more likely to have a trial of labour, especially with a smaller fetus.

Guillain–Barré syndrome

The concurrence of acute inflammatory polyneuropathy and pregnancy is coincidental [2]. The course of pregnancy and the fetus are unaffected. Plasmapheresis early in the course of the illness in severely affected patients improves the prognosis by decreasing the duration of assisted ventilation and complications due to immobility. Plasmapheresis has been performed in all three trimesters of pregnancy [84]. Amongst non-pregnant patients intravenous immune globulin is at least as effective as plasmapheresis. There is sufficient experience with the use of immunoglobulin in pregnancy compounded by immune thrombocytopenia (see Chapter 3) to allow its use in Guillain–Barré syndrome also.

Muscle disease

Polymyositis

Polymyositis is a subacute inflammatory disease of multiple aetiologies which typically worsens during pregnancy [70]. Aggressive treatment is warranted. Fetal wastage is approximately 50 per cent. However, infants thrive once removed from the hostile milieu.

Myasthenia gravis

Myasthenia gravis is an autoimmune disease affecting nicotinic acetylcholine receptors of motor endplates of striated muscle. Its severity fluctuates. During pregnancy the chances of worsening, improving or remaining unchanged are approximately equal [28]. The effect of one pregnancy does not predict the effect of the next. In distinction, postpartum exacerbations are common. Previous thymectomy decreases the risk of pregnancy-associated exacerbations [26]. Myasthenic crises have been shortened by plasmapheresis in all three trimesters [84].

Myasthenia gravis does not increase the risk of uterine inertia or uterine involution and usually does not prolong labour and delivery. Smooth muscle and myometrium are not affected. Magnesium sulphate is contraindicated because it can precipitate a myasthenic crisis [4]. Obstetric analgesia and anaesthesia are more complicated. Narcotics should be administered judiciously because they reduce respiratory drive. If an inhalation anaesthetic is needed, ether is usually avoided. Regional anaesthesia is preferred. If the patient is being treated with anticholinesterase agents, large amounts of procaine and related compounds, as used with paracervical and pudendal blocks, should be avoided because their hydrolysis by plasma cholinesterase has been blocked. Lignocaine is recommended because it is metabolized by a different pathway.

Neonatal myasthenia gravis

At least 12 per cent of the offspring of women with generalized myasthenia gravis will develop self-limited neonatal myasthenia gravis [58]. It is important to be aware that symptoms may not present until 4 days after delivery. The condition lasts approximately 3 weeks. Mothers with mild weakness can have severely affected babies, and vice versa. A high maternal titre of antibody to acetylcholine receptor is the best predictor. Antibody titres in maternal blood and cord blood are approximately equal. Unlike other IgG-mediated disorders, there are no manifestations of fetal myasthenia such as polyhydramnios and arthrogryposis. Indeed women report vigorous intrauterine movement. The explanation appears to be α fetoprotein which inhibits the antigen–antibody reaction and protects the infant until its concentration drops.

Myotonic muscular dystrophy

Myotonic muscular dystrophy is the most common inherited disorder of muscle in women of child-bearing age. It is an autosomal dominant disease. A woman can be so mildly affected that her diagnosis may only be established during the evaluation of her floppy baby.

Myotonic dystrophy does affect pregnancy [42]. Polyhydramnios is due to defective fetal swallowing. Smooth muscle and myometrium are also dystrophic. This causes prolonged labours, uterine inertia and delays uterine involution with postpartum haemorrhage. Oxytocin does stimulate contractions. Obstetric anaesthesia is complicated [10]. It is important to be aware that hypoventilation and chronic respiratory acidosis may exist. Regional anaesthesia in preferred. Depolarizing muscle relaxants can precipitate severe spasms and hyperthermia. Curariform agents are preferred.

Paraplegia

Paraplegia does not prevent a young woman from becoming pregnant although orgasm cannot be achieved if both spinothalamic tracts are affected. The manifestations of a spinal cord transection vary with the level of the lesion, and so does its influence upon pregnancy and childbirth [39]. All patients have sacral anaesthesia. Women with lesions of the cauda equina have relaxed perineal muscles. Women with lesions above uterine sensory afferents (T11, T12, L1) have painless labour. Some can time their contractions by a periodic increase in spasticity. Autonomic hyperreflexia occurs if the level is above the splanchnic autonomic outflow (T5/6). In that case the paroxysmal release of catecholamines causes periodic tachycardias, hypertension, flushing and throbbing headache, symptoms which have been mistaken for toxaemia. Both autonomic and somatic hyperreflexia can be treated by interrupting reflex arcs with regional anaesthesia including epidural and spinal anaesthesia.

Paraplegic women are prone to have premature labour; especially those with lesions above T11. Frequent vaginal examinations are warranted during the third trimester in order to detect early cervical dilatation and effacement. Hospitalization is warranted at least 4 weeks before term or if any changes are detected. Sometimes multiparas are admitted after the 30th week even without any cervical changes.

The principal complications are urinary tract infections and compromise of the function of neurogenic bowels and bladder.

Anaemia lowers resistance to pressure sores and is an indication for transfusion at haemoglobin levels which would not ordinarily justify transfusions. Non-absorbable suture material should be used to repair the skin in perineal tears or incisions because buried catgut can cause sterile abscesses.

Chorea gravidarum

Chorea gravidarum is now exceptionally rare even in developing countries and it has become much milder. The obstetrician/gynaecologist is more likely to see chorea subsequent to prescribing the oral contraceptive [63a]. Even in pregnancy chorea is not necessarily of rheumatic origin, but may be the first manifestation of Huntingdon's chorea, or be due to drugs such as the phenothiazines, or be a complication of systemic lupus [89a].

Successful management of the pregnancy and labour complicated by rheumatic chorea depends largely on any associated cardiac lesion. Adequate rest, quiet and reassurance will help the chorea but sedation by a benzodiazepine may be required. Termination of pregnancy is now unlikely to be necessary.

References

1 Aguglia U, Tinuper P *et al*. Electroencephalographic and anatomo-clinical evidences of posterior cerebral damage in hypertensive encephalopathy. *Clinical Electroencephalography* 1984; **15**: 53–60.

2 Ahlberg G & Ahlmark G. The Landry–Guillain–Barré syndrome and pregnancy. *Acta Obstetricia Gynaecologica Scandinavica* 1978; **57**: 377–80.

3 Annegers JF, Baumgartner KB *et al*. Epilepsy, anticonvulsant drugs, and the risk of spontaneous abortion. *Epilepsia* 1988; **29**: 451–8.

4 Bashuk RG & Krendel DA. Myasthenia gravis presenting as weakness after magnesium administration. *Muscle Nerve* 1990; **13**: 708–12.

5 Bernstein IM, Watson M *et al*. Maternal brain death and prolonged fetal survival. *Obstetrics and Gynecology* 1989; **74**: 434–7.

6 Birk K & Rudick R. Pregnancy and multiple sclerosis. *Archives of Neurology* 1986; **43**: 719–26.

7 Bjerkedal T. Outcome of pregnancy in women with epilepsy, Norway, 1967–1978: congenital malformations. In: Janz D, Dam M, Richens A *et al*. (eds), *Epilepsy, Pregnancy and the Child*. Raven Press, New York, 1982: 289–95.

8 Bogousslavsky J, Despland PA *et al*. Postpartum cerebral angiopathy: reversible vasoconstriction assessed by transcranial Doppler ultrasounds. *European Neurology* 1989; **29**: 102–5.

9 Buehler BA, Delimont D *et al*. Prenatal prediction of risk of fetal hydantoin syndrome. *New England Journal of Medicine* 1990; **322**: 1567–72.

10 Camann WR & Johnson MD. Anesthetic management of a parturient with myotonia dystrophica: a case report. *Regional Anesthesia* 1990; **15**: 41–3.

11 Chua S & Redman CWG. Are prophylactic anticonvulsants required in severe pre-eclampsia? *Lancet* 1991; **337**: 250–1.

12 Cosman F, Post KD *et al*. Lymphocytic hypophysitis: report of three new cases and review of the literature. *Medicine* 1989; **68**: 240–56.

13 Cross JN, Castro PO & Jennett WB. Cerebral strokes associated with pregnancy and the puerperium. *British Medical Journal* 1968; **iii**: 214–17.

14 Cusimano MD, Meffe FM *et al*. Ventriculoperitoneal shunt malfunction during pregnancy. *Neurosurgery* 1990; **27**: 969–71.

15 Dahmus MA, Barton JR & Sibai BM. Cerebral imaging in eclampsia: magnetic resonance imaging versus computed tomography. *Obstetrics and Gynecology* 1992; **67**: 935–41.

16 Dansky LV, Rosenblatt DS & Andermann E. Mechanisms of teratogenesis: folic acid and antiepileptic therapy. *Neurology* 1992; **42** (suppl 5): 32–42.

17 Davis LE. Normal laboratory values of CSF during pregnancy. *Archives of Neurology* 1979; **36**: 443.

18 Deblay MF, Vert P *et al*. Transplacental vitamin K prevents haemorrhagic disease of infant of epileptic mother. *Lancet* 1982; **i**: 126–8.

19 Delgado-Escueta AV & Janz D. Consensus guidelines: preconception counseling, management, and care of the pregnant woman with epilepsy. *Neurology* 1992; **42** (suppl 5): 149–60.

20 Dias MS & Selchar LN. Intracranial hemorrhage from aneurysms and arteriovenous malformations during pregnancy and the puerperium. *Neurosurgery* 1990; **27**: 855–66.

21 Digre KB, Varner MW & Corbett JJ. Pseudotumor cerebri and pregnancy. *Neurology* 1984; **34**: 721–9.

22 Donaldson JO. Eclamptic hypertensive encephalopathy. *Seminars in Neurology* 1988; **8**: 230–3.

23 Donaldson JO. *Neurology of Pregnancy*, 2nd edn. WB Saunders, London, 1989.

24 Donaldson JO. The case against magnesium sulfate for

eclamptic convulsions. *International Journal of Obstetrical Anesthesia* 1992; **1**: 159–66.

25 Ekman-Ordeberg G, Salgeback S & Ordebert G. Carpal tunnel syndrome in pregnancy. *Acta Obstetricia et Gynaecologica Scandinavica* 1987; **66**: 233–5.

26 Eymard B, Morel E *et al*. Myasthenie et grossesse: une étude clinique et immunologique de 42 cas (21 myasthenies neonatales). *Revue Neurologique (Paris)* 1989; **45**: 696–70.

27 Feasby TE, Burton SR & Hahn AF. Obstetrical lumbosacral plexus injury. *Muscle Nerve* 1992; **15**: 937–40.

28 Fennell DF & Ringel SP. Myasthenia gravis and pregnancy. *Obstetrical and Gynecological Survey* 1987; **41**: 414–21.

29 Fish SA, Morrison JC *et al*. Cerebral spinal fluid studies in eclampsia. *American Journal of Obstetrics and Gynecology* 1972; **112**: 502–12.

30 Friis ML, Holm NV *et al*. Facial clefts in sibs and children of epileptic patients. *Neurology* 1986; **36**: 346–50.

31 Frith JA & McLeod JG. Pregnancy and multiple sclerosis. *Journal of Neurology, Neurosurgery and Psychiatry* 1988; **51**: 495–8.

32 Gaily EK, Kantola-Sorsa E & Granstrom M-L. Specific cognitive dysfunction in children with epileptic mothers. *Developmental Medicine and Child Neurology* 1990; **32**: 403–14.

33 Gaily E, Granstrom M-L *et al*. Minor abnormalities in offspring of epileptic mothers. *Journal of Pediatrics* 1988; **112**: 520–9.

34 Gaily E & Granstrom M-L. A transient retardation of early postnatal growth in drug-exposed children of epileptic mothers. *Epilepsy Research* 1989; **4**: 147–55.

35 Hassan A & El Mouman AW. Pregnancy and ventriculoperitoneal shunt: Report of a case and literature review. *Acta Obstetricia et Gynaecologica Scandinavica* 1988; **67**: 669–70.

36 Hiilesmaa VK, Bardy A & Terano R. Obstetric outcome in women with epilepsy. *American Journal of Obstetrics and Gynecology* 1985; **152**: 499–504.

37 Hilsinger RL, Adour KK & Doty HE. Idiopathic facial paralysis, pregnancy, and the menstrual cycle. *Annals of Otology, Rhinology and Laryngology* 1975; **84**: 433–42.

38 Hopkins A. Epilepsy and anticonvulsant drugs. *British Medical Journal* 1987; **294**: 497–501.

39 Hughes SJ, Short DJ *et al*. Management of the pregnant woman with spinal cord injuries. *British Journal of Obstetrics and Gynaecology* 1991; **98**: 513–18.

40 Hurton JC, Chambers WA *et al*. Pregnancy and the risk of hemorrhage from cerebral arteriovenous malformations. *Neurosurgery* 1990; **27**: 867–72.

41 Jacobson S-L & Redman CWG. Basilar migraine with loss of consciousness in pregnancy: case report. *British Journal of Obstetrics and Gynaecology* 1989; **96**: 495.

42 Jaffe R, Mock M *et al*. Myotonic dystrophy and pregnancy: a review. *Obstetrical and Gynecological Survey* 1986; **41**: 272–8.

43 Kanazawa K & Takeuchi S. Clinical analysis of intracranial metastases in gestational choriocarcinoma: a series of 15 cases. *Australian and New Zealand Journal of Obstetrics and Gynaecology* 1985; **25**: 16–22.

44 Knight AH & Rhind EG. Epilepsy and pregnancy: A study of 153 pregnancies in 59 patients. *Epilepsia* 1975; **16**: 99–110.

45 Korn-Lubetski I, Kahana E *et al*. Activity of multiple sclerosis during pregnancy and puerperium. *Annals of Neurology* 1984; **16**: 229–31.

46 Laidler JA, Jackson IJ & Redfern N. The management of caesarean sections in a patient with an intracranial arteriovenous malformation. *Anaesthesia* 1989; **44**: 490–1.

47 Lau SPC, Chan FL *et al*. Cortical blindness in toxaemia of pregnancy: findings on computed tomography. *British Journal of Radiology* 1987; **60**: 347–9.

48 Leppik IE & Rask CA. Pharmacokinetics of antiepileptic drugs during pregnancy. *Seminars in Neurology* 1989; **8**: 240–6.

49 Lewis LK, Hinshaw DB *et al*. CT and angiographic correlation of severe neurological disease in toxemia of pregnancy. *Neuroradiology* 1988; **30**: 59–64.

50 Lindhout D. Pharmacokinetics and drug interactions: role in antiepileptic-drug-induced teratogenesis. *Neurology* 1992; **42** (suppl 5): 443–7.

51 Loewy EH. The pregnant brain dead and the fetus. Must we always try to wrest life from death. *American Journal of Obstetrics and Gynecology* 1987; **157**: 1097–101.

52 Mattson RH, Cramer JA *et al*. Use of oral contraceptives by women with epilepsy. *Journal of the American Medical Association* 1986; **256**: 238–40.

53 Massey EW. Mononeuropathies in pregnancy. *Seminars in Neurology* 1988; **8**: 193–6.

54 McLeannan HG, Oats JN & Walstab JE. Survey of hand symptoms in pregnancy. *Medical Journal of Australia* 1987; **147**: 542–4.

55 Mercado A, Johnson G *et al*. Cocaine, pregnancy, and postpartum intracerebral hemorrhage. *Obstetrics and Gynecology* 1989; **73**: 467–78.

56 Minielly R, Yuzde AA & Drake CG. Subarachnoid hemorrhage secondary to ruptured cerebral aneurysm in pregnancy. *Obstetrics and Gynecology* 1979; **53**: 64–70.

57 Molitch ME. Pregnancy and the hyperprolactinemic woman. *New England Journal of Medicine* 1985; **312**: 1364–70.

58 Morel E, Eymard B *et al*. Neonatal myasthenia gravis: a new clinical and immunological appraisal of 30 cases. *Neurology* 1988; **38**: 138–42.

59 Oakeshott P & Hunt GM. Valproate and spina bifida. *British Medical Journal* 1989; **298**: 1300–1.

60 Oppenheimer BS & Fishberg AM. Hypertensive encephalopathy. *Archives of Internal Medicine* 1928; **41**: 264–78.

61 Phelan MC, Pellock MM & Nance EW. Discordant expression of fetal hydantoin syndrome in heteropaternal twins. *New England Journal of Medicine* 1982; **397**: 397–9.

62 Pihl K, Malstrom H & Simonsen E. Choriocarcinoma presenting with cerebral metastases after full-term pregnancy. *Acta Obstetricia et Gynaecologica Scandinavica* 1990; **69**: 433–5.

63 Pulsinelli WA & Hamill RW. Chorea complicating oral contraceptive therapy. *American Journal of Medicine* 1978; **65**: 557–9.

64 Raps EC, Galetta SL *et al*. Delayed peripartum vasculopathy: cerebral eclampsia revisited. *Annals of Neurology* 1993; **33**: 222–5.

65 Reik L. Headaches in pregnancy. *Seminars in Neurology* 1988; **8**: 187–92.

66 Roelvink NCA, Kamphorst W *et al*. Pregnancy-related primary brain and spinal tumors. *Archives of Neurology* 1987; **44**: 209–15.

67 Richards A, Graham D & Bullock R. Clinicopathological study of neurological complications due to hypertensive disorders of pregnancy. *Journal of Neurology, Neurosurgery and Psychiatry* 1988; **51**: 416–21.

68 Richards AM, Moodley J *et al*. Active management of the unconscious eclamptic patient. *British Journal of Obstetrics and Gynaecology* 1986; **93**: 554–62.

69 Rosa FW. Spina bifida in infants of women treated with carbamazepine during pregnancy. *New England Journal of Medicine* 1991; **324**: 674–7.

70 Rosenzweig BA, Rotmensch S *et al*. Primary idiopathic polymyositis and dermatomyositis complicating pregnancy: diagnosis and management. *Obstetrical and Gynecological Survey* 1989; **44**: 162–70.

71 Royburt M, Seidman DS *et al*. Neurologic involvement in hypertensive disease of pregnancy. *Obstetrical and Gynecological Surgery* 1991; **46**: 656–64.

72 Rubin PC. Beta-blockers in pregnancy. *New England Journal of Medicine* 1981; **305**: 1323–6.

73 Rudolph AM. Effects of aspirin and acetaminophen in pregnancy and the newborn. *Archives of Internal Medicine* 1981; **141**: 358–63.

74 Ryan G, Lange IR & Naugler MA. Clinical experience with phenytoin prophylaxis in severe preeclampsia. *American Journal of Obstetrics and Gynecology* 1989; **161**: 1297–304.

75 Sadasivan B, Malik GM *et al*. Vascular malformations and pregnancy. *Surgical Neurology* 1990; **33**: 305–13.

76 Schmidt D, Canger R *et al*. Change of seizure frequency in pregnant epileptic women. *Journal of Neurology, Neurosurgery and Psychiatry* 1983; **46**: 751–5.

77 Schwartz RB, Jones KM *et al*. Hypertensive encephalopathy: findings on CT, MR imaging, and SPECT imaging in 14 cases. *American Journal of Roentgenology* 1992; **159**: 379–83.

78 Sheehan HL & Lynch JB. *Pathology of Toxaemia of Pregnancy*. Churchill Livingstone, Edinburgh, 1973.

79 Sibai BM & Ramanathan J. The case for magnesium sulfate in preeclampsia-eclampsia. *International Journal of Obstetrics and Anesthesia* 1992; **1**: 167–75.

80 Sibai BM, Spinnato JA *et al*. Eclampsia IV. Neurological findings and future outcome. *American Journal of Obstetrics and Gynecology* 1985; **152**: 184–92.

81 Silberstein SD & Merriam GR. Estrogens, progestins, and headache. *Neurology* 1991; **41**: 786–93.

82 Srinivasan K. Puerperal cerebral venous and arterial thrombosis. *Seminars in Neurology* 1988; **8**: 222–5.

83 Steinn AL, Levenick MN & Kletsky OA. Computed tomography versus magnetic resonance imaging for the evaluation of suspected pituitary adenomas. *Obstetrics and Gynecology* 1989; **73**: 996–9.

84 Watson WJ, Katz VL & Bowes WA. Plasmapheresis during pregnancy. *Obstetrics and Gynecology* 1990; **76**: 451–7.

85 Webster MWI, Chancellor AM *et al*. Patent foramen ovale in young stroke patients. *Lancet* 1988; **ii**: 11–12.

86 Weinshenker BG, Hader W *et al*. The influence of pregnancy on disability from multiple sclerosis: a population-based study in Middlesex County, Ontario. *Neurology* 1989; **29**: 1438–40.

87 Wiebers DO. Ischemic cerebrovascular complications of pregnancy. *Archives of Neurology* 1985; **42**: 1106–13.

88 Wiebers DO. Subarachnoid hemorrhage in pregnancy. *Seminars in Neurology* 1988; **8**: 226–9.

89 Whitburn RH, Laishley RS & Jewkes DA. Anaesthesia for simultaneous caesarean section and clipping of intracerebral aneurysm. *British Journal of Anaesthesiology* 1990; **64**: 642–5.

90 Wolfe RE & McBeath JG. Chorea gravidarum in systemic lupus erythematosus. *Journal of Rheumatology* 1985; **12**: 992–3.

91 Wright DS & Patel MK. Focal migraine and pregnancy. *British Medical Journal* 1986; **293**: 1557–8.

92 Yerby MS, Friel PN *et al*. Pharmacokinetics of anticonvulsants in pregnancy: alterations in plasma protein binding. *Epilepsy Research* 1990; **5**: 223–8.

93 Yeh SY, Paul RH *et al*. A study of diazepam during labor. *Obstetrics and Gynecology* 1974; **43**: 363–73.

16

Fever and Infectious Diseases

Dame Rosalinde Hurley

Pathophysiology, 552
Infections associated with pregnancy and the puerperium, 556
Urinary tract infections, 556
Puerperal sepsis and wound infections, 558
Septic abortion and shock, 559
Listeriosis, 560
Toxoplasmosis, 561
Malaria, 562
Viral infections, 562

Pathophysiology

Persistent elevation of the body temperature above those levels that are normal in an individual is defined as fever. Regardless of race or climatic environment, the body temperature usually lies between 37.0 and 37.5°C with diurnal variations so that evening temperatures are 0.5–1.0°C higher than those of the morning. Oral and axillary temperatures are 0.4°C and 1.0°C lower than that of the blood, but both are more reliable recordings than those taken per rectum.

Several explanations have been offered to explain disturbance of temperature regulation in disease. Shifts in body water may interfere with heat production and heat loss, and inadequate hydration causes temperature elevation in the newborn, although *per se* it does not seem to have this effect in adults. Metabolic rate affects body temperature, which is raised in thyrotoxicosis and lowered in myxoedema. Abnormalities of etiocholanolone metabolism occur in some patients with 'periodic fever' and administration of this substance, or of progesterone and some of its congeners, results in fever in humans. Following intravenous injection of purified bacterial endotoxin or killed bacteria such as typhoid vaccine, the body temperature rises after about an hour. The patient feels cold, shivers, and has a rigor lasting some 10–20 min. The skin is pale and cold. As the rigor subsides, the patient feels warmer and complains of feeling feverish as the skin flushes. Profuse sweating begins, and the body temperature starts to fall toward normal. The underlying pathophysiological sequence of events seems to be the rapid removal of endotoxin from the blood stream by the fixed phagocytes of the reticuloendothelial system followed by margination of polymorphonuclear leucocytes along the walls of vessels. These and the fixed phagocytes are activated to release endogenous pyrogen which exists in the cells in inactive form into the circulation. The pyrogen is a protein of low molecular weight produced in response to toxic, immunological or infectious stimuli. Its production is induced through the release of lymphocytic lymphokines arising in response to antigenic recognition, and it acts on the hypothalamic thermoregulatory centre, transmitting information to the vasomotor centre, possibly through local production of prostaglandin. Heat generation is increased, heat loss is prevented and the body temperature rises. The release of endogenous pyrogen by phagocytic cells appears to be the common factor in the pathogenesis of fever, irrespective of its cause (Table 16.1). More detailed accounts of fever are given by Weinstein and Swartz [41] and Dinarello and Wolff [12].

The pattern of the febrile response, be it intermittent (falling to normal each day), remittent (falling each day, but still remaining elevated above the baseline), sustained (without significant diurnal variation), or relapsing (alternating with periods of one or several days of normal temperatures) is not

Table 16.1. Pathogenesis of fever

Endotoxin (or other activator) →	Cell injury (granulocytes, monocytes, macrophages) →	Endogenous pyrogen activation and release
Endogenous pyrogen activation and release →	Stimulation of hypothalamic thermoregulatory centres →	Fever

particularly helpful clinically, although relapsing fever characterizes malaria, relapsing fever itself, rat-bite fever, obstructive infection of the biliary or ureteric tracts, and some cases of Hodgkin's disease ('Pel–Ebstein fever'). Though not strictly a relapsing fever, listeriosis during pregnancy characteristically presents as two or more febrile episodes, the first usually being diagnosed as urinary tract infection (see below).

The perception of fever in individuals varies markedly, some patients, notably those with tuberculosis, being unaware of body temperatures as high as 39°C. Repeated rigors, though typical of septicaemia with pyogenic bacteria, may occur in non-infectious diseases such as lymphoma but are rare in viral infections. Antipyretic drugs themselves may evoke or perpetuate a rigor. Some fevers, especially in pneumococcal and streptococcal infections, malaria, or meningococcal septicaemia are heralded or accompanied by cold sores. Prostration, malaise, backache and headache often accompany infectious fevers, and delirium may occur in bacterial fevers.

Fever is likely to be infectious in origin, its cause depending on the clinical circumstances and variations in locally endemic disease, although drug or serum fever, fever associated with malignant or thromboembolic disease, haemolytic disease or metabolic disorder may have to be considered in its differential diagnosis. Acute febrile illnesses of less than 2 weeks' duration are amongst the most frequent occurrences in medical practice; many are self-limiting, perhaps viral in origin, and definitive aetiological diagnosis is seldom made. However, prolonged febrile illnesses, in which the diagnosis remains obscure for weeks or months, do occur, and in some patients fever is the dominant sign or symptom. Before diagnosis is established, this condition is called pyrexia (or fever) of unknown (or uncertain) origin (FUO, PUO – Boxes 16.1 and 16.2), although the term should be reserved for those patients who have had episodes of fever in excess of 38°C for a period of at least 3 weeks, and who have been investigated for at least 1 week [34].

Any of the acute or chronic specific infectious diseases may be contracted during the course of pregnancy or the puerperium, and conception may occur in women already subject to infection. In labour and in the early part of the puerperium, parturient women are peculiarly susceptible to serious infections of the genital tract, and child-bed fever has always been one of the most important causes of maternal death. Urinary tract infections are common in women, and are frequent during pregnancy and the puerperium [6]. Wound infections, post-operative pneumonia, mastitis and breast abscess and thrombophlebitis may all occur in the puerperium. Most of the conditions enumerated above give rise to fever, and those that are most

Box 16.1. Infectious diseases associated with prolonged fever (Europe and the USA)

- Tuberculosis (Chapter 1)
- Systemic mycoses (Chapter 1)
- Cholecystitis, cholangitis and empyema of the gallbladder (Chapter 9)
- Subphrenic hepatic and other intra-abdominal abscess
- Appendicitis and diverticulitis
- Pelvic inflammatory disease
- Some types of urinary tract infection, e.g. ureteric obstruction (Chapter 7)
- Retroperitoneal infection
- Septicaemias – meningococcal, gonococcal, listeria, vibriosis, brucellosis
- Infective endocarditis (Chapter 5)
- Epstein–Barr, cytomegalovirus and coxsackie B virus disease
- Q-fever and psittacosis
- Parasitic infestations – malaria, amoebiasis, trichinosis
- Leptospirosis and relapsing fever
- Toxoplasmosis

Box 16.2. Non-infectious disease associated with prolonged fever

- Neoplasms
  - Metastatic carcinoma
  - Melanoma
  - Lymphomata — Hodgkin's disease
  - Leukaemias (Chapter 2)
  - Retroperitoneal sarcoma
  - Tumours of lung, kidney, pancreas, liver, heart
- Connective tissue disease
  - Rheumatic fever (Chapter 5)
  - Systemic lupus erythematosus (Chapter 8)
  - Rheumatoid arthritis (Chapter 8)
- Miscellaneous
  - Drug fever
  - Embolic disease (Chapter 4)
  - Sarcoidosis (Chapter 1)
  - Haemolytic disease (Chapter 2)

likely to occur in temperate climates are listed in Boxes 16.3 and 16.4. Charles [9], Monif [32] and Gilstrap and Faro [15] give good accounts of these diseases.

Casual or chance infections occurring during pregnancy range from mild illnesses to the major microbial diseases. In the Far East and in other parts of Asia, Africa and South America, pregnant women may be exposed to epidemic disease such as cholera, plague, the dysenteries (amoebic and bacillary) and enteric fevers. Pandemic influenza may also occur. In parts of Africa and in the Americas, systemic fungal infections (Table 16.2) such as coccidioidomycosis, histoplasmosis, and North and South American blastomycosis occur, and fever characterizes certain parasitic infestations (Table 16.3).

Box 16.3. Non-specific bacterial infections with fever complicating pregnancy or the puerperium

- Urinary tract infection (Chapter 7)
  - Acute lower urinary tract infection
  - Acute pyelonephritis
  - Chronic pyelonephritis
- Puerperal or postabortal sepsis
  - Endometritis
  - Peritonitis
  - Pelvic abscess
  - Thrombophlebitis (Chapter 4)
  - Intraperitoneal abscess
- Septicaemia
- Mastitis and breast abscess
- Wound infection
- Infective endocarditis (Chapter 5)

Box 16.4. Special bacterial infections with fever complicating pregnancy or the puerperium

- Gonococcal septicaemia
- Gonococcal salpingitis (acute, purulent)
- Secondary syphilis (fever is unusual and low grade)
- Acute bacterial tonsillitis (streptococcal), rheumatic fever (Chapter 5)
- Streptococcal septicaemia
- Staphylococcal septicaemia
- Other septicaemia (Gram-negative rods)
- Listeriosis
- Tuberculosis (Chapter 1)
- Gas gangrene
- Tetanus
- Serious infections associated with the acquired immune deficiency syndrome (Chapter 17)

Although serious microbial disease is well controlled in the UK and the USA, mothers of young children, particularly of those at school, are exposed to the specific infectious diseases of childhood and in addition to the common upper respiratory tract infections: in this way they may contract mumps, chickenpox, measles, rubella, scarlet fever or acute bacterial tonsillitis, whooping cough, dysentery or viral or other bacterial diarrhoea. As young adults, they may contract poliomyelitis, or toxoplasmosis, and hepatitis A, B, or non-A, non-B may also occur [22]. Enterovirus and echovirus infections, together with those ascribable to herpes viruses, in particular, to cytomegalovirus and herpes simplex virus types I and II, are not uncommon, although few give rise to systemic disturbance. Virus infections of pregnancy, and their possible consequences are shown in Table 16.4. Fever may be marked in some of these infections, for example, in hepatitis, primary herpes or cytomegalovirus infections, influenza,

Table 16.2. Fungal diseases with fever (see also Chapter 1)

Disease	Geographical distribution	Remarks
Systemic candidosis	Worldwide	Rare during pregnancy, opportunistic infection
Cryptococcosis	Worldwide	Fever usually absent
North American blastomycosis	Southern, south-eastern mid-western USA	Fever often low grade
Paracoccidioidomycosis	South America	Fever often low grade
Coccidioidomycosis	South-western USA and Argentina	Half the infections are asymptomatic and afebrile – placental involvement is common in disseminated disease but congenital infection is not documented
Histoplasmosis	Americas, Africa, parts of Asia	Fever prolonged in severe cases
Phycomycosis	Worldwide	Opportunistic infection, rare
Aspergillosis	Worldwide	Fever lasts weeks or months in disseminated disease

mumps, measles and the meningoencephalitides, but it is often low grade and transitory. Their diagnosis is, however, important because of their known or reported deleterious effects on the fetus. Accounts of the clinical manifestations of the viral diseases commonly occurring during pregnancy are given by Hurley [20,21], Hanshaw and Dudgeon [18], Charles [9], Amstey [1] and Greenough *et al.* [17].

Most fevers presenting during pregnancy do not give rise to diagnostic difficulties, related as they are to disorders of the urinary or reproductive tracts, or to intercurrent infections that are common and frequent in the community. However, as in the non-pregnant, prolonged fever poses problems of investigation and diagnosis. With so many possible causes, it is not feasible to outline a scheme of investigation that is pertinent to every cause of fever. Clinical acumen, based on careful history-taking and accurate recording of the chronology of symptoms and signs, together with thorough clinical examination provide important leads. The place of residence, visits abroad, occupation and hobbies, keeping of pets, contact with known cases of infectious disease, localizing symptoms, skin rashes, heart murmurs, presence of masses, enlargement of spleen or liver, all give clues to the differential diagnosis.

Useful laboratory tests, particularly in prolonged fever, include the following:

1 cultures of blood or bone marrow (endocarditis, septicaemia, brucellosis, salmonellosis, listeriosis);
2 serum enzymes (hepatocellular disease);
3 blood counts and smears (blood dyscrasias, typhoid fever, parasitic infestation, lupus erythematosus, glandular fever, acute pyogenic infections);
4 tests for specific antibody (viral diseases, enteric fever, toxoplasmosis, venereal diseases);
5 immunological tests (connective tissue diseases);
6 cold agglutinins (mycoplasma infections).

During pregnancy, the urine should always be examined microbiologically, and physical examination may indicate that throat or vaginal swabs should be cultured. If specific lesions (e.g. herpetic vesicles) are present or there is reason to suspect viral infection, viriculture or electronmicroscopy is indicated, although diagnosis is usually established serologically. In the puerperium, specimens from throat, genital and urinary tracts, and a blood culture should always be examined. If there is any indi-

Table 16.3. Parasitic diseases with fever

Disease	Geographical distribution	Fever	Hazards to pregnancy
Fulminating amoebic dysentery	Worldwide	High	Pregnancy precipitates attack
Malaria	South and Central America, Africa, Asia	High relapsing	Anaemia, debility, cachexia of chronic or repeated infection more severe in pregnant women. Congenital disease. Hypoglycaemia with quinine treatment. Adventitious bacterial infection likely, and tuberculosis likely to extend and disseminate
Visceral leishmaniasis	Middle and Far East, Mediterranean, South and Central America	High irregular	
Trypanosomiasis	Mid, west and east Africa, Central and South America	High continuous or recurrent	
Toxoplasmosis	Worldwide	Usually absent	Risk of congenital transmission and congenital disease

cation of breast pathology, expressed breast milk should also be examined. The erythrocyte sedimentation rate, haemoglobin concentration, haemoglobin electrophoresis, blood smears and blood counts should be performed if the cause of fever remains obscure.

Infections associated with pregnancy and the puerperium

Associated infections

These are all acute infections, though recrudescence of chronic infection may occur. None is peculiar to pregnancy, but their incidence is increased in pregnant as compared with non-pregnant women.

Urinary tract infections (see also Chapter 7)

These are fully described by Brumfitt and Condie [6], Charles [9] and Gilstrap [14]. Infections of the urinary tract afflict some 6–7 per cent of pregnant women, occurring also with increased frequency during the puerperium. Much emphasis is placed on their early diagnosis and treatment. Any part of the renal tract may be involved and, with modern bacteriological techniques, infection by significant numbers of organisms can be detected before the onset of symptoms. The infections may be acute and primary, or recrudescences of chronic infection: they range from urethritis to acute pyelonephritis, which, in former days, was sometimes accompanied by blood stream infection ('catheter fever'). The usual causes during pregnancy are members of the *Enterobacteriaceae* and other Gram-negative rods, as well as the pathogenic Gram-positive cocci. The relationship of the less flagrant forms of urinary tract sepsis to abortion, prematurity, low birthweight and still-birth is not established with certainty.

Three major clinical syndromes are distinguishable: acute lower urinary tract infection, acute pyelonephritis, and chronic pyelonephritis. Infections of the lower urinary tract can be followed by acute pyelonephritis, but in adult women without obstruction, it is rare for the acute infection to become chronic. In any case, chronic pyelonephritis probably has several causes, of which infection is but one. The presenting symptoms include frequency of micturition, dysuria, strangury and suprapubic discomfort (urethral syndrome, cystitis), often with no fever or one of low grade. Although the infection may settle spontaneously within a few days, there is some danger of recurrence, and urinary reflux may result in ascending infection with acute pyelonephritis. About 5 per cent of pregnant women have significant bacteriuria (>100 000 organisms/ml) and some 40 per cent of these will develop overt urinary tract disease as pregnancy advances. Dilatation of the ureters and urinary stasis contribute to this outcome. Those with asymptomatic bacteriuria are usually given a week's course of antibiotic therapy (ampicillin cephalosporin or other).

The onset of acute pyelonephritis is usually sudden, with fever, shivering and rigors, malaise, pain in the loins, frequency and dysuria and tenderness in the renal angle. Pus appears in the urine and there is a leucocytosis. Bed rest is important, and the fluid intake should be at least 3 l/day. If the urine is acid, as it is with *Escherichia coli* infection, an alkaline mixture should be given. The results of bacteriological examination help in the choice of antibiotic to which the infecting microbe is sensitive. Nevertheless, treatment is usually started 'blind' with ampicillin or cephalosporin before the sensitivities are known. Single agent or combination therapy may be used. The urine should be cultured again, after apparent cure, to ensure that bacteriuria has not persisted.

Chronic pyelonephritis may present as chronic renal failure, sometimes preceded by symptomless proteinuria, or as a febrile illness, similar in presentation to the acute form. Eradication of infection, if demonstrated, may take many months of therapy, and antibiotics may have to be used in reduced dosage. The urine must be cultured at regular intervals.

Pyelonephritis, or 'pyelitis of pregnancy' was once the most frequent and important of the medical complications of pregnancy, with an incidence of just over 1 per cent and a maternal mortality of 3–4 per cent at the beginning of the antibiotic era. Fetal loss, from prematurity was 16–30 per cent. The complete clinical picture of frank pyelonephritis is seen far less frequently nowadays, almost certainly owing to early diagnosis and the prompt administration of antibiotics. Characteristically, the onset of the acute disease is about the fifth or sixth month of pregnancy or in the first week of the puerperium.

Most studies have shown that 4–7 per cent of women examined during pregnancy have significant bacteriuria, figures not unlike those recorded for the adult female population in general. Pregnancy itself need not cause any increase in prevalence of bacteriuria, though few would dispute the relationship of asymptomatic bacteriuria during early pregnancy to the subsequent development of symptoms referable to urinary tract infection. Acute pyelonephritis is particularly liable to develop in bacteriuric women, early treatment substantially reducing its incidence. For this reason, many antenatal clinics send urine to be screened for bacteriuria by quantitative methods. The term 'significant bacteriuria' implies that bacteria are multiplying in the bladder urine and, therefore, that infection as opposed to microbial contamination is present. Under the circumstances, the bacterial population, usually of known urinary pathogens, will ordinarily exceed 100 000/ml of urine. The specimen must be taken correctly and either processed promptly or stored at 4°C for examination later on the same day.

The principal route of infection is probably an ascending one, and the risk of introducing infection by catheterization has long been recognized. Much hospital-acquired infection, following catheterization or operations on the bladder, is associated with organisms that are being disseminated in the wards. Another route of infection is the lymphatic system, for the right kidney has a direct connection, via the lymphatics, with the ascending colon, to which it is directly related. Infection may be blood-borne and blood cultures are often positive in pyelonephritis. Experimentally, the intravenous injection of some urinary pathogens into laboratory animals causes localized disease of the kidney, but in the case of *E. coli*, the ureter must have been ligated or the kidney previously damaged, suggesting that local anatomical anomaly or malfunction is important in its genesis.

In the female, the proximity of the urethral orifice to the rectum, and the moist environment of the perineum, favour growth of microbes, including pathogens of the urinary tract. The distal 4 cm of the urethra is colonized by bacteria. Local minor trauma such as that occasioned by sexual intercourse may favour bacterial multiplication and, during pregnancy, increased concentrations of amino acids and lactose are believed to encourage growth of *E. coli* in the urine.

Mechanical factors, especially those that obstruct urinary flow, are important in promoting bacterial infection, and the immediate predisposing cause of urinary tract infections during pregnancy is stasis. Progesterone causes dilation of the ureters and oestrogens cause muscular hypertrophy at a time when changing anatomical relationships in the pelvis lead to a compression of the right ureter. Complete bladder emptying is important, for present evidence suggests that bacteria coming into contact with the mucosa are killed. Interference with normal micturition, such as may occur during delivery or in operations to repair the pelvic floor, promotes infection. Ureteric valve incompetence leading to reflux during pregnancy has been postulated but not demonstrated.

Most of the infections that occur sporadically in the population are caused by *E. coli* which is also most frequently isolated in obstetric and gynaecological practice. Organisms less frequently isolated include *Proteus* spp., *Streptococcus faecalis*, *Klebsiella* spp., staphylococci and *Pseudomonas aeruginosa*, micrococcus spp. and *Staphylococcus epidermidis* as well as *Enterobacteriaceae* carried in the introitus which are associated with the 'frequency dysuria' or 'urethral' syndrome, in which patients have symptoms suggestive of cystitis.

The bacteriological diagnosis of urinary tract infection depends on quantitative examination of freshly voided urine. Care must be taken in collection of specimens from women, and catheterization should be avoided. If the results of culture are equivocal or if there is persistent contamination, the urine may be sampled directly by suprapubic aspiration, which is quite safe in pregnant women. The presence of 100 000 organisms/ml is generally accepted as the criterion of infection within the urinary tract and special methods, including serotyping, may serve to distinguish relapse from re-infection.

Sulphonamides, amoxycillin, augmentin, oral cephalosporins, and nitrofurantoin are all used in treatment. Cotrimoxazole is also effective, though not generally recommended because of its potential toxicity for the fetus. 4-quinolones, such as norfloxacin and ciprofloxacin must be used with caution in pregnancy.

With early diagnosis and prompt and successful treatment, the long-term prognosis in terms of chronic infection and renal damage is good. However, it is prudent to follow the outcome in those who have responded slowly or only partially to treatment, and further urine examinations and intravenous pyelography — the latter carried out not less than 3 months post-partum — may be required.

Puerperal sepsis and wound infections

Puerperal sepsis includes a series of febrile disorders of the lying-in period that share the common aetiology of being wound infections of the genital tract. It may occur after delivery or abortion and is occasioned by several genera of pathogenic bacteria, of which the most notorious and dangerous are *Clostridium* and *Streptococcus*. In the great majority of fatal cases, the microbes are introduced from without, and such infections are preventable. In general, endogenous microbes, harboured in the vagina, such as *Enterobacteriaceae* and *Staphylococcus* cause less severe forms of sepsis.

Since the establishment of rigid schedules of asepsis and antisepsis in maternity units over the last century and since the introduction of chemotherapeutic agents and antibiotics, the aetiological pattern of serious puerperal sepsis has altered. Formerly, exogenous microbes accounted for the majority of fatal cases, being mainly Lancefield group A β haemolytic streptococci originating from the attendants, the patient's own body outside the genital tract, and from visitors; they spread to the parturient patient by droplet infection, infected dust, infected hands and contaminated fomites, such as instruments and dressings. Nowadays, aerobic non-haemolytic streptococci, anaerobic streptococci, members of the *Enterobacteriaceae*, occasionally staphylococci, *Clostridium perfringens*, *Streptococcus faecalis* (Lancefield group D) or haemolytic streptococci of other groups are encountered. As well as having extrinsic origins, all can be isolated from the vagina regularly. *Bacterioides*, *Mycoplasma* and other genera may be implicated in puerperal sepsis, as in other infections of the genital tract, but their causal relationship to disease therein and their relative frequency have been less thoroughly studied.

Puerperal sepsis is a wound infection which may involve any part of the parturient genital tract from infected episiotomies, perineal or cervical lacerations, metritis and endometritis, to involvement of the uterine appendages, with local or generalized peritonitis and invasion of the blood stream. Disease localized to the genital tract proper does not run a fatal course, but the prognosis is poor if peritonitis or blood stream infection supervenes as it is very likely to do if the causative agent is an unchecked streptococcus. The factors predisposing to infection include premature rupture of the membranes, repeated examination of the vagina, instrumentation and internal monitoring of labour, lacerations of the birth canal, episiotomy, manual rotation and forceps delivery. An increased rate of post-partum endometritis follows caesarean section. Factors tending to lower general resistance, such as malnutrition, intercurrent disease, anaemia, haemorrhage and maternal exhaustion also promote infection. The retention of blood clot, or of fragments of membrane or placenta encourages infection by providing a nidus in which bacteria may multiply. The basis of prevention is scrupulous hygiene, with a short labour and few vaginal examinations, followed by an uncomplicated vaginal delivery.

Fever is the cardinal sign of puerperal sepsis, and may arise before, during or after labour. Puerperal pyrexia occurring in the 48 hours succeeding delivery or abortion may also be caused by urinary tract infection, administration of contaminated intravenous infusions, aspiration pneumonia, or retained products of conception. Septic thrombophlebitis, 'third day fever', infection of an abdominal wound, breast engorgement with or without incipient mastitis or breast abscess, drug fevers, surgical misadventure with swabs or other foreign bodies, and fortuitous infection in sites remote from the genitourinary tract should all be considered, especially when fever arises later in the puerperium. Patients with streptococcal endometritis are acutely ill, with temperatures up to 39.5°C (104°F). The induration and purulent uterine discharge associated with less severe and more localized disease are usually absent, being replaced by diffuse slight pelvic tenderness and clear cervical discharge, in which Gram-positive cocci can be seen on staining. Treatment must be instituted without awaiting laboratory reports (see below). Low grade endometritis is characterized by diminution in the lochial flow before the onset of fever, uterine tenderness and a foul-smelling discharge from the endocervical canal.

The diagnosis of puerperal sepsis is made on clinical grounds, and the identity of the infecting microbes is established by the laboratory. Direct Gram-stained smears of exudate from the cervix or from within the uterus, are examined and the specimen is cultured. The nature and the sensitivity of the pathogen to antibiotics is usually established in less than 48 hours. The patient is treated with appropriate antibiotics, penicillin with an aminoglycoside used for incipient severe infection, and safe, broad spectrum antibiotics being used for low grade infections if the aetiological diagnosis is completely open. Surgical measures are used as indicated, and supportive therapy is given, including bed rest, fluids and oral hygiene.

Septic abortion and shock

The availability of contraceptive techniques and the legalization of abortion have led to diminution in the number of women with septic abortion, but the diagnosis should be suspected in every febrile woman who is bleeding in the first trimester of pregnancy. In the majority of cases the cervical os is open, and there is evidence of the passage of the products of conception. High, spiking fevers and the presence of hypotension are bad prognostic signs. Pelvic examination, with assessment of uterine size is important, for most serious infections follow attempts to terminate pregnancy in women beyond the 12th week of gestation. As in puerperal sepsis following delivery, extension of the infection beyond the uterus is attended by correspondingly grave risk for the patient. Plain X-rays of the abdomen with the patient both in the supine and the upright positions may demonstrate the presence of intraperitoneal or myometrial gas. Exploratory laparotomy may be required. Myometrial gas suggests *C. welchi* (*perfringens*) infection, and operative intervention may be required. Foreign bodies, such as an intrauterine contraceptive device, may require removal. Many patients respond successfully to curettage and antibiotic therapy or even antibiotic therapy alone (see Chapter 7). Many antibiotics have been used, but the most favoured regimen is a combination of intravenous penicillin and metronidazole with intramuscular aminoglycoside in high dosage. The blood pressure and urinary output should be measured at regular intervals, and aminoglycoside concentrations should be assayed.

The microbes causing septic abortion are similar to those causing post-delivery sepsis, but non-sporing anaerobes, such as *Bacteroides fragilis*, may be implicated more frequently and with Gram-negative aerobes, such as *E. coli* and *Klebsiella* spp. are related to endotoxic shock. The onset of bacteraemia is accompanied by fever, rigors, nausea, vomiting, diarrhoea and prostration. Tachycardia, tachypnoea, hypotension, usually with cool, pale extremities and often with peripheral cyanosis, oliguria and mental confusion are added to the development of septic shock.

The haematological manifestations of severe shock are considered in Chapter 3 and the renal problems in Chapter 7.

Listeriosis (see also Chapter 10)

There is probably only one common diagnostic pitfall in the investigation of fever during pregnancy and the puerperium. Though there are many forms of listeriosis, including superficial disease, characteristically in pregnant women listeriosis is associated with two or more febrile episodes [21]. The first, recognized only in retrospect as listeriosis, is associated with malaise, headache, fever, backache and abdominal or loin pain. Pharyngitis, conjunctivitis and diarrhoea are present in some cases. The condition is usually diagnosed as pyelonephritis, for the kidneys are involved in the listeric process, and often there seems to be a concomitant urinary tract infection with *E. coli* or other coliform. The patient is usually treated with antibiotics to which *Listeria monocytogenes* is susceptible and fever resolves only to return in 2–3 weeks, usually within 1–20 days of premature delivery of an infected child. The true nature of these episodes of fever will be recognized if the often slowly growing *Listeria* is actively sought in cultures of blood and other sites, such as the genital tract and urine and, after delivery, in the placenta and various sites in the sick newborn. If the child is born dead as often occurs [25], post-mortem cultures of heart blood, cerebrospinal fluid and viscera should be made. In about 40 per cent of cases of maternal listeriosis, fever is not marked and the patient presents with an influenza-like illness or even asymptomatically. Maternal and perinatal infections may require prolonged therapy (Box 16.5) and maternal infection can be severe resulting in adult respiratory distress syndrome (Chapter 1). Ampicillin should be given in high doses of at least 8 g/day in adults and 150 mg/kg/day in infants. Impairment of renal function reduces the rate of excretion of ampicillin and the dose can be reduced accordingly. Very high serum concentrations may be associated with cerebral irritation.

L. monocytogenes is ubiquitous in nature and has been recovered from soil, animal feeds, water and sewage, as well as infecting many species of birds and animals including man. Of the 13 serotypes I/IIa, I/IIb and IVb are those that are mainly associated with the food-borne infection in humans. The microbe can be transmitted transplacentally, and, although rare, congenital listeriosis is a well-recognized disease. Careful attention to food hygiene is important during pregnancy and certain high risk foods such as some of the soft cheeses and pâté should be avoided. In the UK the number of notifi-

Box 16.5. Treatment of listeriosis

- Ampicillin and gentamicin
- High doses parenterally (see above) e.g. ampicillin 200 mg/kg bodyweight/day, gentamicin 5–6 mg/kg/day
- Continue for 1 week after fever subsides
- Erythromycin or tetracycline for superficial disease

cations of pregnancy and neonatal listeriosis is declining, probably in consequence of these preventive measures. Pregnant women should each be given a copy of the Department of Health's booklet *While you are pregnant: safe eating and how to avoid infection from food and animals* [11].

Less common than listeriosis as a diagnostic problem, but equally important, is the occurrence of infective endocarditis, particularly when it occurs after prophylaxis with appropriate antibiotic [20]. The diagnosis is established by blood culture aided by echocardiography.

Toxoplasmosis

Toxoplasmosis is probably unique amongst the parasitic diseases of man in that its congenital form was recognized before that of postnatally acquired infection. The reported incidence of the congenital disease in the UK, though not so high as in France, exceeds that of congenital syphilis. There is little difference in the prevalence rates between sexes although, clearly, the disease is more important and more frequently diagnosed in women of childbearing age. There are few data from which to derive morbidity, mortality or case fatality rates.

Although placental transmission has been demonstrated in chronically infected mice, in humans congenital infection is believed to follow primary infection and the prognosis for subsequent pregnancies is good provided that there is no significant maternal immunosuppression as in patients with acquired immune deficiency syndrome (AIDS) (see Chapter 17). The risk to the fetus appears to be related to the gestational age at which primary maternal infection occurs, transmission being less likely in the first trimester, but resulting in more severe disease should it occur. Infection leading to still-birth or neonatal death, or to survival with ocular and cerebral involvement occurs only in the offspring of mothers who acquire and transmit infection in the first or second trimester.

Although transmission rates as high as 33 per cent have been reported following primary maternal infection, 72 per cent of the infected newborn were spared overt clinical infection. Such asymptomatic infants may suffer no serious consequences or they may later develop chorioretinitis, blindness, strabismus, hydrocephaly or microcephaly, cerebral calcification, psychomotor or mental retardation, epilepsy or deafness. Children known to have had congenital toxoplasmosis must, therefore, be kept under observation for months or years. The available data are insufficient to support or to refute the hypothesis that *Toxoplasma gondii* causes malformations during the period of organogenesis. The infected infant should be treated with spiramycin, or pyrimethamine/sulphonamide and folinic acid. There is some evidence that treatment of the mother who has an acute attack in pregnancy with spiramycin decreases the fetal risk.

Christie [10] gives an excellent general account of toxoplasmosis, while Lee [28] and Holliman [23] address the problems of diagnosis, management and treatment of toxoplasmosis during pregnancy. Remington and Desmonts [37] deal with congenital toxoplasmosis. Screening for toxoplasmosis during pregnancy is widely practised in continental Europe, but not in the UK where it is deemed ineffective [39] due in large part to differing prevalence on the two sides of the English Channel. In France, about 80 per cent of pregnant women will have had toxoplasmosis before pregnancy, whereas in the UK the figure is <20 per cent. Thus, in the UK over 80 per cent of the antenatal population would have to be tested repeatedly during pregnancy to detect evidence of primary infection by seroconversion, a logistically daunting task and one fraught with anxiety and scope for error. Although evidence extrapolated from selected studies indicates that 500 congenitally infected children could be born annually in the UK (50 with clinically apparent damage) fewer than 15 such children, not all of whom are damaged, are reported to the Communicable Disease Surveillance Centre.

If serological evidence of primary (seroconversion) or recent active infection (presence of specific toxoplasma IgM and other serological indicators) is detected, the fetus may be investigated by ultrasound examination and, if gestation is sufficiently early, by cordocentesis to provide fetal blood for laboratory investigation. Spiramycin 3 g daily in divided doses may be offered prophylactically. If fetal infection is established, treatment with sulphadiazine/pyrimethamine and vitamin supplements can be used to alternate at 3-weekly intervals with spiramycin. The maternal blood count should be monitored regularly if folate antagonists are used.

Forty-four children with congenital toxoplasmosis were enrolled over a 10-year period into The Chicago Collaborative Treatment Trial [30]; the standard regimen of therapy over 12 months, based on pyrimethamine, sulfadiazine and folinic acid, produced markedly more favourable outcomes than those previously reported for untreated children, or those treated only for 1 month. Spiramycin was not used in the majority of children.

Malaria

Plasmodium infection should be considered in any patient with fever and/or jaundice who has recently travelled through India, south-east Asia, Africa or South America. Patients with acute falciparum malaria may develop jaundice from haemolytic anaemia or hepatic congestion and deposition of haemosiderin.

Pregnant women have an increased prevalence of infection, and parasitaemia may be great [3] probably due to impaired host defences [16]. Haemolytic anaemia with jaundice may be severe in pregnancy, and hepatorenal syndrome is often the cause of death. Malaria may infect the placenta leading to spontaneous abortion, still-birth and low birthweight. Malaria parasites may cross the placenta, particularly in non-immune mothers [24]. Immune primagravidae are prone to relapse in the second trimester [40]. The placentae of patients treated for malaria in pregnancy should always be examined histologically for the presence of parasites. If these are present, the neonate is at risk and should be given prolonged antimalarial therapy.

Prophylaxis and treatment depend on the local area, the dominant plasmodium type and pattern of drug resistance. Chloroquine is the treatment of choice for severe infestation with *Plasmodium falciparum* in chloroquine-sensitive areas [26]; even though this drug has been suspected of causing neonatal deafness if used in the first trimester [40] it is not a major teratogen [43]. Quinine is less safe in pregnancy, although in a collaborative perinatal study of 106 women exposed to quinine in early pregnancy there was no increase in frequency of congenital malformation [19]. Quinine does not increase the risk of pre-term labour [29] but in pregnancy in particular, patients are at risk from quinine-induced hyperinsulinaemia [29] which has caused fatal hypoglycaemia [42]. Somatostatin analogues such as SMS 201−995 which inhibit insulin release are the treatment of choice for quinine-induced hypoglycaemia and may indeed be the only effective therapy [35].

In chloroquine-resistant areas, the combination of pyrimethamine and dapsone (Maloprim) has been used in pregnancy and is probably safe providing extra folate (10 mg/day) is given [5] (pyrimethamine and proguanil are folate antagonists). Pyrimethamine is excreted in breast milk but appears harmless to the breast-fed infant. The sulphone drug dapsone, and various sulphonamides, are often used in combination with trimethoprim or pyrimethamine or primaquine, but haemolysis may occur in neonates, and adults with glucose-6-phosphate dehydrogenase deficiency.

Patterns of resistance to antimalarials change so rapidly that expert advice should always be sought regarding treatment and prophylaxis. It is likely that proguanil and chloroquine are the safest drugs in pregnancy (PHLS Malaria Reference Laboratory 1984).

Malaria prophylaxis with chloroquine or proguanil should be continued through pregnancy and visitors to high risk (holoendemic areas) should continue with their prophylaxis for at least the last trimester and preferably until after delivery [4,27]. The crucial importance of compliance must be stressed and advice must be given on the avoidance of mosquito bites. Importation of malaria is increasing in the UK. Health advice for travellers outside the European Community is available in pamphlet form from the Department of Health, and is also accessible on Prestel.

Viral infections (see also Chapter 9 for hepatitis and Chapter 17 for HIV infection)

Nearly a fifth of all perinatal deaths are ascribed to congenital malformations, especially those of the central nervous system. Although the majority of maternal viral infections cause little harm, some may result in severe damage to the fetus. Very careful prospective studies performed on large cohort populations and other studies have failed to establish, unequivocally, teratogenic potential in viruses other than rubella virus and cytomegalovirus, although a strong case can be advanced linking varicella zoster infection with specific defect. There are many reports, retrospective analyses and partly controlled epidemiological studies attempting to link congenital malformations with maternal infection with mumps, influenza, varicella zoster, hepatitis virus, EB virus, herpes virus hominis, coxsackie A4 viruses and measles. There is also considerable evidence linking the cardiotropic coxsackie B3 and B4 viruses with fetal myocarditis, but the relationship to congenital heart disease cannot, as yet, be regarded as proven.

Leaving aside teratogenic effects (i.e. malformations consequent on infections blighting the fetus during the period of organogenesis), there is evidence of increased rates of abortion and stillbirth in intrauterine rubella and in cytomegalovirus infection, and fetal and perinatal death has been reported in the course of maternal herpes virus hominis infections, varicella zoster, hepatitis, mumps, poliomyelitis, variola or vaccinia, measles and influenza. Fetal wastage is not necessarily caused by viral invasion, but may be the result of maternal exhaustion and toxaemia. Because of the increased maternal morbidity and mortality from varicella zoster in pregnancy, pregnant women who come into close contact with cases and have been shown to be susceptible by lack of varicella antibody should receive zoster immunoglobulin (ZIG) as a prophylactic [33]. Patients who develop clinical varicella should be treated with parenteral acyclovir (see Chapter 1).

Neonatal illness and congenital infection may result following infection with rubella, cytomegalovirus, herpes virus, varicella zoster, variola or vaccinia, poliovirus, coxsackie B virus, the myxoviruses, and the hepatitis viruses. In general, neonatal infection is more likely to follow maternal infection at or about the time of delivery. Primary rubella is largely preventable through vaccination with live attenuated virus, and the high uptake of measles/mumps/rubella (MMR) vaccine since October 1988 in young children has interrupted the epidemic cycle and reduced the incidence to a low endemic level [31]. Reported infections during pregnancy fell to two in 1992 for England and Wales. Rubella re-infection, occasionally followed by congenital rubella, has been reported [38] in those vaccinated and this possibility should be borne in mind when investigating pregnant contacts. Screening for hepatitis B is widely practised antenatally in the UK. HBsAg carriage varies from $<0.5\%$ to 20 per cent in different parts of the world, being highest in the Far East. The risk of transmission to the child is highest in those who are HBeAg positive or who have acquired the acute infection at or about the time of delivery. Immunization, active and passive, is offered to children born to women who are HBsAg or HBeAg positive and is over 90 per cent effective. The emergence of vaccine-induced escape mutants [7] is worrying (see Chapter 9).

Diagnosis of congenital virus infection is based on serological tests that indicate primary infection in the mother, and active infection in the newborn. Viriculture is helpful.

Congenital infections are often grouped together under the apt, if unlovely, name of TORCH, or as some would have it, STORCH. The initials denote syphilis, toxoplasmosis, other viruses, rubella, cytomegalovirus and herpes virus hominis. A diagnostic laboratory, warned of the clinical possibility of congenital infection, will institute appropriate serological tests for these agents.

It has recently been realized that infection with human parvovirus may also affect the fetus, causing abortion, hydrops fetalis [2] and possibly aplastic anaemia [8]. Elevated maternal serum α fetoprotein seems to be a marker of putative fetal aplastic crisis [8]. The effect of infection in the mother is usually trivial, giving at most fever, a rash (erythema infectiosum) and mild arthropathy.

Genital herpes infection is of particular concern since the infant may become infected with the virus during vaginal delivery and since caesarean section has been advocated as a means of avoiding this risk. The risk appears to be confined to those who have proven herpetic lesions in the genital tract at the time of delivery and caesarean section should be reserved for such patients. Those who are asymptomatic and have had herpes infections in the past or earlier in pregnancy are at very low risk of producing an affected fetus [36].

Table 16.4. Viral infections during pregnancy implicated in fetal or neonatal disease

Virus	Potential effect on mother	Potential effect on fetus or newborn
Coxsackie A	Herpangina, hand–foot and mouth disease, cardiomyopathy	
A9		?Gastrointestinal defects
Coxsackie B	Often unnoticeable; aseptic meningitis; Bornholm disease	Myocarditis/meningoencephalitis; neonatal sepsis;
B2 and B4		?urogenital anomalies;
B3 and B4		?cardiovascular lesions
Cytomegalovirus	Usually asymptomatic but sometimes moderate to high fever in primary infection	Chronic infection; acute disease, late onset sequelae
ECHO virus	Rash of ECHO 9 may resemble rubella; maternal disease may mimic appendicitis or abruptio placentae, as in other enterovirus infections	Neonatal sepsis, fatal disseminated virus infection (hepatic necrosis)
Hepatitis A, B, C, E (Chapter 9)	Flu-like illness; chills and high fever, constitutional symptoms and jaundice, increased severity in pregnancy	Prematurity, neonatal hepatitis, vertical transmission of hepatitis B virus
Herpes simplex	Oral or genital infection more severe in pregnancy	?Abortion; ?prematurity; fatal disseminated infection (HSV-II > HSV-I); congenital malformations
HIV (see Chapter 17)	Asymptomatic; acceleration of disease; AIDS or PGL	Vertical transmission; infantile disease; ?CNS malformations
HTLV-1	Virus infection endemic in certain parts of the world	Vertical transmission; adult T cell leukaemia/ lymphoma may develop later in life
Influenza	Increased mortality in pandemics (see Chapter 1)	?Increased fetal mortality; ?congenital malformations; ?increase in childhood leukaemia
Lymphocytic choriomeningitis	Meningitis/ meningoencephalitis	Congenital disease
Measles	May be complicated by pneumonia and CCF; more severe and may be fatal	Probably increased fetal mortality; congenital measles
Mumps	No special effect	Increased fetal mortality; ?endocardial fibroelastosis
Parvovirus B19	Erythema infectiosum; no more severe in pregnancy	Abortion, hydrops fetalis; ?aplastic anaemia
Poliomyelitis	Increased severity and mortality	Fetal death; neonatal disease

Continued

Table 16.4. *(Continued)*

Virus	Potential effect on mother	Potential effect on fetus or newborn
Polyoma	Asymptomatic	?Increased risk of jaundice
Rubella	No special effect	Fetal death; chronic persisting infection; congenital malformations
Varicella zoster	Often more severe; maternal death (see text)	Neonatal chickenpox; probable specific congenital defect
Vaccinia and variola	Increased severity and mortality	Fetal death; intrauterine or neonatal disease
Venezuelan and Western equine encephalomyelitides	Meningoencephalitis	Neonatal encephalitis

References

1 Amstey MS. *Virus Infection in Pregnancy*. Grune & Stratton, New York, 1980.

2 Anand A, Gray ES, Brown T, Clewley JP & Cohen BJ. Human parvovirus infection in pregnancy and hydrops fetalis. *New England Journal of Medicine* 1987; **316**: 183–6.

3 Bray RS & Anderson MJ. Falciparum malaria and pregnancy. *Transactions of the Royal Society of Tropical Medicine and Hygiene* 1979; **73**: 427–31.

4 Bruce-Chwatt LJ. *Essential Malariology*. Heinemann Medical, London, 1980.

5 Bruce-Chwatt LJ. Malaria and pregnancy. *British Medical Journal* 1983; **286**: 1457–8.

6 Brumfitt W & Condie AP. Urinary infection. In: Philipp EE, Barnes J & Newton M (eds) *Scientific Foundations of Obstetrics and Gynaecology*. Heinemann Medical, London, 1977: 754–67.

7 Carman WF, Zanetti AR *et al*. Vaccine induced escape mutant of hepatitis B virus. *Lancet* 1990; **ii**: 325–9.

8 Carrington D, Gilmore DH *et al*. Maternal serum α-fetoprotein — a marker of fetal aplastic crisis during intrauterine human parvovirus infection. *Lancet* 1987; **i**: 433–5.

9 Charles D. *Infections in Obstetrics and Gynaecology*. WB Saunders, Philadelphia, 1980: 103–82.

10 Christie AB. *Infectious Diseases, Volume 2. Toxoplasmosis*. Churchill Livingstone, Edinburgh, 1987: 1253–74.

11 Department of Health and the Central Office of Information. *While you are pregnant: safe eating and how to avoid infection from food and animals* 1992: 4/92.

12 Dinarello CA & Wolff SM. Pathogenesis of fever in man. *New England Journal of Medicine* 1978; **298**: 607–712.

13 European Collaborative Study. Risk factors for mother to child transmission of HIV-1. *Lancet* 1992; **339**: 1007–12.

14 Gilstrap LC. Urinary tract infections in pregnancy. In: Gilstrap LC & Faro S (eds), *Infections in Pregnancy*. Wiley-Liss, New York, 1990: 15–27.

15 Gilstrap LC & Faro S. *Infections in Pregnancy*. Wiley-Liss, New York, 1990.

16 Gilles HM, Lawson JB *et al*. Malaria, anaemia and pregnancy. *Annals of Tropical Medicine and Parasitology* 1969; **63**: 245–63.

17 Greenough A, Osborne J & Sutherland S. *Congenital, Perinatal and Neonatal Infections*. Churchill Livingstone, Edinburgh, 1992.

18 Hanshaw JB & Dudgeon JA. *Viral Diseases of the Fetus and Newborn*. WB Saunders, Philadelphia, 1978.

19 Heinonen OP, Slone D & Shapiro S. *Birth Defects and Drugs in Pregnancy*. Publishing Sciences Group Inc, Littleton, Massachusetts: 1977.

20 Hurley R. Heart disease, parturition and antibiotic prophylaxis. In: Lewis PJ (ed), *Therapeutic Problems During Pregnancy*. MTP Press, Lancaster, 1977: 69–79.

21 Hurley R. Listeria. In: Weatherall DJ, Ledingham JGG, Warrell DA (eds), *Oxford Textbook of Medicine*, Volume 1. Oxford University Press, London, 1983: 5.329–31.

22 Hurley R (ed), *Viral Hepatitis: a Problem in Hospital Practice*. SOG Srl, Padua, 1983.

23 Holliman RE. *Toxoplasma gondii*. In: Greenough A, Osborne J & Sutherland S (eds), *Congenital, Perinatal and Neonatal Infections*. Churchill Livingstone, Edinburgh, 1992: 209–22.

24 Jelliffe EFP. Placental malaria and foetal growth failure. In: Aysen RN (ed), *Nutrition and Infection*. CIBA Foundation Study Group, No. 31, Churchill, London, 1967.

25 Khong TY, Frappell JM, Steel HM, Stewart CM & Burke

M. Perineal listeriosis. A report of six cases. *British Journal of Obstetrics and Gynaecology* 1986; **93**: 1083–7.

26 Lancet editorial. Malaria in pregnancy. *Lancet* 1983; **ii**: 84–5.

27 Lawson JB & Stewart DB. *Obstetrics and Gynaecology in the Tropics*. Edward Arnold, London, 1967: 52–9.

28 Lee RV. Parasites and pregnancy: the problems of malaria and toxoplasmosis. In: *Clinics in Perinatology: Infectious Complications of Pregnancy*. WB Saunders, London, 1988: 351–64.

29 Looareesuwan S, Phillips RE *et al*. Quinine and severe falciparum malaria in late pregnancy. *Lancet* 1985; **ii**: 4–7.

30 McAuley J, Boyer KM *et al*. Early and longitudinal evaluations of treated infants and children and untreated historical patients with congenital toxoplasmosis: the Chicago collaborative treatment trial. *Clinical Infectious Diseases* 1994; **18**: 38–72.

31 Miller E, Waight PA, Vurdien JE, Jones G, Tookey PA & Peckham CS. Rubella surveillance to December 1992: second joint report from the PHLS and National Congenital Rubella Surveillance Programme. *CDR Review. Communicable Disease Report*. Review, 1993, No. 3.

32 Monif GRG (ed), *Infectious Diseases in Obstetrics and Gynaecology*, 2nd edn. Harper & Row, Philadelphia, 1982.

33 Paryani SG & Arvin AM. Intrauterine infection with varicella-zoster virus after maternal varicella. *New England Journal of Medicine* 1986; **314**: 1542–6.

34 Petersdorf RG & Beeson PB. Fever of unexplained origin: report on 100 cases. *Medicine (Baltimore)* 1961; **40**: 1.

35 Phillips RE, Warrell DA *et al*. Effectiveness of SMS 201–995, a synthetic longacting somatostatin analogue, in treatment of quinine induced hyperinsulinaemia. *Lancet* 1986; **i**: 713–16.

36 Prober CG, Sullender WM, Yasukawa LL, Av DS, Yeager AS & Arvin AM. Low risk of herpes simplex virus infections in neonates exposed to the virus at the time of vaginal delivery to mothers with recurrent genital herpes simplex virus infections. *New England Journal of Medicine* 1987; **316**: 240–4.

37 Remington JS & Desmonts G. Toxoplasmosis in Remington JS & Klein JO (eds), *Infectious Diseases of the Fetus and Newborn Infant*, 3rd edn. WB Saunders, London, 1990: 89–195.

38 Ross R, Harvey DR & Hurley R. Reinfection and congenital rubella syndrome. *Practitioner* 1992; **236**: 246–51.

39 Royal College of Obstetricians and Gynaecologists: Multidisciplinary Working Group. *Prenatal Screening for Toxoplasma in the UK*. London, 1992.

40 Trusell RR & Beeley L. Infestations. In: *Clinics in Obstetrics and Gynaecology: Prescribing in Pregnancy*, Volume 8. WB Saunders, London, 1981: 333–40.

41 Weinstein L & Swartz MN. Host responses to infection. In: Sodeman WA & Sodeman TM (eds), *Pathology Physiology*, 6th edn. WB Saunders, Philadelphia, 1979: 545–9.

42 White NJ, Warrell DA *et al*. Severe hypoglycaemia and hyperinsulinaemia in falciparum malaria. *New England Journal of Medicine* 1983; **309**: 61–6.

43 Wolfe MS & Cordero JF. Safety of chloroquine in chemosuppression of malaria during pregnancy. *British Medical Journal* 1985; **290**: 1466–7.

Further reading

Barbara JAJ, Contreras M & Hewitt P. AIDS: a problem for the transfusion service? *British Journal of Hospital Medicine* 1986; **36**: 178–84.

Bennett IL & Beeson PB. The properties and biological effects of bacterial pyrogens. *Medicine* 1950; **29**: 365.

Boucher M, Yonekura ML, Wallace RJ & Phelan JP. Adult respiratory distress syndrome: A rare manifestation of *Listeria monocytogenes* infection in pregnancy. *American Journal of Obstetrics and Gynecology* 1984; **6**: 686–8.

Carne CA & Adler MW. Neurological manifestations of human immuno deficiency virus infection. *British Medical Journal* 1986; **293**: 462–3.

Centers for Disease Control Recommendations for assisting in the prevention of perinatal transmission of human T-lymphotropic virus type III/lymphadenopathy associated virus and acquired immunodeficiency syndrome. *Morbidity and Mortality Weekly Reports* 1985; **34**: 721–6, 731–2.

Curran JW, Morgan WM, Hardy AM, Jaffe HW, Darrow WW & Dowdle WR. The epidemiology of AIDS: current status and future prospects. *Science* 1985; **229**: 1352–7.

Cutting WAM. Breast feeding and HIV infection. *British Medical Journal* 1992; **305**: 788.

Department of Health and Social Security. *Acquired Immune Deficiency Syndrome, AIDS*. General information for doctors, May, London, 1985.

Department of Health and Social Security. *Acquired Immune Deficiency Syndrome, AIDS*. Information for Doctors concerning the introduction of the HTLV-III antibody test, October, 1985.

Department of Health and Social Security. *Acquired Immune Deficiency Syndrome, AIDS*. Guidance for Surgeons, Anaesthetists, Dentists and their Teams in Dealing with Patients Infected with HTLV-III, April, 1986.

Department of Health and Social Security. *Acquired Immune Deficiency Syndrome, AIDS*. Guidance for Doctors and AI Clinics Concerning AIDS and Artificial Insemination, July, 1986.

Hurley R. Viral diseases in pregnancy. In: Chamberlain GVP (ed), *Obstetrics and Gynaecology*. Northwood Publications, London, 1977; 68–82.

Hurley R. Virus infections in pregnancy and the puerperium. In: Waterson AP (ed), *Recent Advances in Clinical Virology*, Volume 3. Churchill Livingstone, Edinburgh, 1982.

Hurley R. Infection in pregnancy. In: Weatherall DJ, Ledingham JGG, Warrell DA (eds), *Oxford Textbook of Medicine*, Volume 1. Oxford University Press, London, 1983: 5484–9.

Jovaisas E, Koch MA, Schafer A, Stauber M & Lowenthal D. LAV/HTLV-III in 20-week fetus. *Lancet* 1985; **ii**: 1129.

Marion RW, Wiznia AA, Hutcheon RG & Rubinstein A. Human T-cell lymphotropic virus type III (HTLV-III) embryopathy. A new dysmorphic syndrome associated with intrauterine HTLV-III infection. *American Journal of Diseases of Children* 1986; **140**: 638–40.

Rowe PM. Resistance to HIV infection. *Lancet* 1993; **341**: 624.

Sprecher S, Soumenkoff G, Puissant F & Degueldre M. Vertical transmission of HIV in 15-week fetus. *Lancet* 1986; **ii**: 288.

Weber JN, Wadsworth J *et al*. Three year prospective study of HTLV-III/LAV infection in homosexual men. *Lancet* 1986; **i**: 1179.

17

Pregnancy Outcome and Management in HIV Infected Women

Frank D. Johnstone

Epidemiology, 568
HIV infection, 569
  Virology
  Pathogenesis and monitoring of disease progression
  Natural history
Testing and pregnancy, 571
  Counselling
  Selective testing
  Surveillance
Effect of pregnancy on HIV disease, 575
  Immune changes in pregnancy
  AIDS and subsequent prognosis
  Adverse effects of pregnancy on progression of HIV disease
Vertical transmission, 577
  Mode and timing of transmission
  Factors affecting vertical transmission
  Proportion of exposed babies infected
  Prognosis for the infected infant
Pregnancy outcome, 580
  Spontaneous abortion
  Congenital abnormality
  Induced abortion
  Obstetric complications
  Birthweight
  Delivery
HIV disease in pregnancy, 583
  Pneumocystis carinii pneumonia
  Candidiasis
  Tuberculosis
  Toxoplasmosis
  Cytomegalovirus
  Cryptococcosis
  Cervical neoplasia
  Other diseases
Prophylaxis in pregnancy, 585
  P. carinii
  Zidovudine
  Other antiretroviral drugs
  Other possible prophylaxis
Obstetric management, 587
  Antenatal
  Delivery
  Post-partum
Nosocomial transmission, 589
  Occupational transmission to health-care workers
  HIV infected health-care workers
  Infection control procedures
The future, 591

The human immunodeficiency virus (HIV) is a major world health concern, and is a common medical problem in pregnancy in many parts of the world. There are few purely obstetric issues, and pregnancy management is dominated by effective communication, up-to-date knowledge and expertise in the care of HIV disease. This chapter attempts to review briefly the main aspects of HIV infection which are relevant to pregnancy, and to suggest how these aspects relate to pregnancy management at the time of writing (December, 1992–September 1994).

Epidemiology

HIV has now been reported from countries throughout the world. It is estimated that one in 250 adults in the world is infected; that transmission occurs by heterosexual intercourse in 60 per cent of cases; and that 40 per cent of those infected are female. By the year AD 2000 World Health Organization (WHO) projections are that 30–40 million people will be infected, including 4–8 million children, and that 10–15 million children under the age of 15 years will have been orphaned as a result of parental HIV deaths.

In countries where HIV first spread by heterosexual intercourse (sub-Saharan Africa) the sex ratio is close to 1 : 1 and there has been little change with time. Where initial spread was amongst homosexual men and injection drug users (USA and Europe) many more men than women were infected early in the epidemic. However, the ratio of men to women in acquired immune deficiency syndrome (AIDS) cases is steadily decreasing, with a ratio in 1991 of 6.5 : 1 in Northern America and 5.2 : 1 in Europe. In addition, the increase in individuals reported to be infected by heterosexual contact shows no sign of slowing. It is therefore predicted that in industrialized countries also, women will form an increasing proportion of infected individuals, in the direction of parity with men.

As far as pregnancy is concerned, anonymous unlinked surveys have been used to give a clear picture of prevalence in several countries. In the USA (1989–90) the nationwide rate was approximately 1.5 per 1000 deliveries, with a range by state from 0 to 5.8 per 1000 [86]. In the UK, rates were highest in inner London, 1.6 per 1000 in 1991 [2] and Edinburgh, 2.5 per 1000 in 1990 [207]. Higher rates are reported from Italy, Spain and France. The rate amongst pregnant women in Paris was 2.8 per 1000 deliveries [46]. Several studies have shown a higher seroprevalence in women having induced abortion than in those having a term pregnancy [46,82]. Prevalence rates reported from antenatal clinic surveillance in Thailand have reached seven per 1000 [216]. Reported rates from sub-Saharan Africa have been 50 per 1000 pregnant women in 1989 in Kinshasa, Zaire [175], 130 per 1000 in 1991 in Nairobi, Kenya [209] and 120–310 per 1000 in rural and urban areas in Uganda [85].

In all countries HIV prevalence is increasing in pregnant women. HIV is already the leading cause of death in young adult women in many urban areas in sub-Saharan Africa and the USA. AIDS has therefore become the commonest cause of maternal mortality in large cities in the USA [148] and accounts for 90 per cent of deaths in childbearing, urban Rwandan women [131]. HIV infection is clearly becoming one of the major medical problems found in pregnancy in many parts of the world.

HIV infection

Virology

Within 2 years of the recognition of AIDS as a disease, the aetiological agent human immunodeficiency virus type 1 (HIV-1) had been discovered [10]. Since then its structure has been exposed to the full power of contemporary molecular biology. A separate, but related virus (HIV-2) was reported by Clavel *et al.* [38] and as these two viruses cause similar diseases they will be considered together. The virology of HIV has been extensively reviewed [89,146].

HIV contains two copies of a single-stranded RNA genome, and it is only with conversion of the genetic material into DNA that the viral genes can be transcribed and translated into proteins in the usual way. This is accomplished by a viral DNA polymerase with a ribonuclease (together called reverse transcriptase) and it is this reversal of the normal flow of genetic information which classifies HIV as a retrovirus. Once in the form of double-stranded DNA, the viral genetic information is spliced into the DNA of the host cell. It then serves as a template for viral gene transcription leading to production of new virus. Infection of that cell and its progeny is permanent.

The structure and functional organization of the HIV genome have been well described (Fig. 17.1) [89,113,146]. The envelope extracellular protein gp120 (a glycoprotein of 120 kDa) is crucial for the recognition and binding to the target cell receptor, CD4. At least three distinct regions of gp120 are necessary, and in the normal three-dimensional configuration they probably form a pocket to fit the binding site on CD4. Binding may alter the shape of the gp120 protein, revealing a part of another envelope protein, gp41, that is normally hidden. This part is hydrophobic and by interacting with the adjacent target cell membrane may induce the viral membrane and the cell membrane to fuse together, thus enabling HIV to be injected within the cell. Target cells have the CD4 receptor, a T cell surface glycoprotein which characterizes the T helper subset of lymphocytes. These cells interact with antigen presenting cells, which display antigen on their own cell membrane, together with class II major histocompatibility complex glycoproteins. Helper T cells then initiate an immune response against other cells bearing the antigen, and thus occupy a pivotal position in overall cell mediated immune response. However, although the CD4 lymphocyte is the main target, a proportion of peripheral monocytes (that mature to become macrophages), follicular dendritic cells, and Langerhans' cells express CD4 and can be infected by HIV. Microglial cells can also be infected and may produce very small amounts of CD4. These other cells do not seem to be destroyed by infection in the way that CD4 lymphocytes are, and may act as a reservoir of virus.

Early infection with HIV is characterized by very

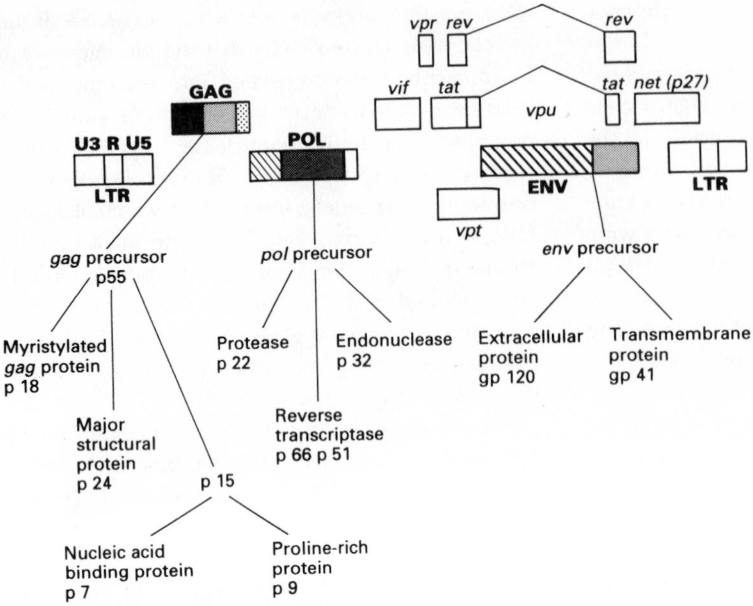

Fig. 17.1. Genetic organization of HIV [154, with permission].

high viral load. One study based on the polymerase chain reaction (PCR) technique showed a titre of PCR detectable virus in the plasma of nearly 10^5 particles/ml before seroconversion in an individual where fewer than 200 particles/ml were found subsequently [178]. Antibodies against the envelope and gag proteins are formed months after exposure to virus and viral load is then greatly reduced. Typically there is a long quiescent asymptomatic phase, but even in this phase most individuals show a steady loss of CD4 lymphocytes (about $60/mm^3$/year) and there are signs of 'activation' in response to HIV [20]. It has become clear that during this period the virus is not latent, but is chronically produced at a low level, and that this phase is characterized by interaction between HIV and the immune system. During this time there appears to be enormous diversity of viral species, and antigenic variation may be used by HIV to escape neutralization [211]. With time, the immune system gradually collapses, and this allows a higher viral load and also selection of more virulent 'fast' variants, that form high replicating, syncitium inducing isolates [211]. The CD4 lymphocyte population is then critically reduced, and major clinical disease supervenes.

Pathogenesis and monitoring of disease progression

Activation of lymphocytes is a consistent feature, even in early HIV infection. In addition, defects in HIV infection are not restricted to the pathognomonic depletion of CD4 T lymphocytes [211]. Throughout infection qualitative abnormalities have been demonstrated in B cells and monocytes [149]. There may also be early selective loss of antigen-primed T memory cells. The mechanisms of loss of CD4 cells are still being elucidated [146, 211].

Although early and subtle changes in function of the immune system may be important, at present monitoring is confined largely to quantitative studies of cell populations. Cohort studies have shown a loss of 60–100 CD4/lymphocytes mm^3/ year, and this surface marker remains the main predictor of disease progression. Increased lymphoid cell turnover is reflected in increased levels of β_2 microglobulin which is the short polypeptide chain located in the human histocompatibility complex, and neopterin, which is derived from guanosine triphosphate, produced by macrophages during activation of the cell mediated immune response. Both these markers reflect activation of the immune system, and have been shown to be independent predictors of disease progression [92,147]. Low levels of p24 antibodies correlate with disease progression, as does recurrence of p24 antigenaemia.

Natural history

The Centers for Disease Control (CDC) in Atlanta classified the effects of HIV infection (Table 17.1). Cohort studies have indicated that approximately 50 per cent of individuals with HIV infection will progress to AIDS after 10 years [163] but with more effective treatment the incubation period between infection and the development of AIDS is lengthening. At least in drug users, death from AIDS may greatly underestimate the number of deaths from HIV related disease. HIV infected individuals may die of tuberculosis, endocarditis or bacterial pneumonia without ever meeting the definition for AIDS. There is an established adverse effect on progression with increased age [23]. The effects of genetic factors and other infections are still being elaborated.

Table 17.1. Short, clinical classification of HIV infections [32]

Group I	Acute infection
Group II	Asymptomatic infection
Group III	Persistent generalized lymphadenopathy
Group IV	Other disease
A	Constitutional disease weight loss >10% bodyweight or >4.5 kg fevers >38°C diarrhoea >2 weeks
B	Neurological disease HIV encephalopathy Myelopathy Peripheral neuropathy
C	Secondary infectious disease • CI AIDS defining secondary infectious disease *Pneumocystis carinii* pneumonia Cerebral toxoplasmosis Cytomegalovirus retinitis • C2 Other specified secondary infectious Oral *Candida* Pulmonary tuberculosis Multidermatomal varicella zoster
D	Secondary cancers Kaposi's sarcoma Non-Hodgkin's lymphoma
E	Other conditions Lymphoid interstitial pneumonitis

Testing and pregnancy

There are now clear advantages to the individual in diagnosing HIV infection. Current evidence points to breakdown of the immune system as an active process from infection onwards, and in the future early treatment, before irreversible damage has resulted in collapse of the immune system, should become the optimal management. Nevertheless, current assessment of the value of early antiretroviral treatment, from the adequate follow-up provided by the large Concorde trial, has been disappointing [42].

In pregnancy — or preferably before pregnancy — knowledge of serostatus is particularly significant in allowing the woman to take an informed decision about childbearing, and in allowing her to take steps to protect her sexual partner(s). There are also precautions which can be taken during pregnancy which will avoid increasing the risk of vertical transmission, and treatment of the mother has been shown to reduce the chance of the baby being infected (see below). The infant can be monitored carefully and treated more readily for infection. The woman has an opportunity to develop a health-promoting lifestyle, and to start prophylaxis and antiretrovirals at the optimum time.

Public attitudes to testing change gradually, and the basic structure for testing should be in place before advances in treatment and prophylaxis mandate a universal offer of HIV testing. The principles of testing programmes have been extensively discussed [81,99,145,218].

Counselling

Counselling around HIV testing in pregnancy has been well described [93,197]. As Holman [93] has pointed out this has the function not only of testing HIV status, but also of providing specific information about the virus and its transmission ('education') and discussing means of reducing risks of acquiring or transmitting HIV ('prevention'). Topics which should be addressed in informing pregnant women about the HIV epidemic and the availability of HIV testing are highlighted in Box 17.1. Pre-test counselling itself also aims at ensuring informed consent. It needs to include the possible need for re-testing and awareness of equivocal results which have to be investigated further.

The structure for detailed discussion before HIV testing (shown in Box 17.1) is appropriate where a woman has a risk factor which puts her at very high risk, or comes from a geographical area with high prevalence. Particularly in an interactive discussion, it should be possible to ensure that the woman fully understands and wants testing. Where women do turn out to be seropositive, much of the ground has already been covered, and it is helpful in further counselling to be able to refer back to issues already covered in the previous discussion.

The situation is quite different in the case of women from populations with a low prevalence of infection, but where the prevalence is nevertheless appreciable enough to justify a universal offer of HIV testing. Antenatal care is already so complicated by explanations of routine tests, availability of prenatal diagnostic tests, health messages, explanation of antenatal care organization, relevant symptoms to report, etc., that patients are in danger of information overload. Where the chance of a woman being infected with HIV is very low, it seems unreasonable to carry out mandatory intensive counselling. Instead, written material should be available, and a brief discussion, covering the points in Box 17.1, with the midwife or obstetrician should take place. Questions from the patient may lead to a longer discussion, but my own belief is that women who want HIV testing should have access to this with fairly simple steps to ensure that they understand the test and give their consent. This opinion has support from ethical groups [25] and others [145].

Post-test counselling, where the woman is either seronegative or seropositive, is shown in Boxes 17.2 and 17.3.

Box 17.1. Issues covered in pre-test counselling (from [93] with permission)

Information

- Explanation of HIV infection and its relationship to AIDS
- Modes of HIV transmission
- Sexual and drug-related risk reduction behaviours
- The purpose of HIV antibody testing
- The meaning of HIV antibody test results
- The importance of knowing one's HIV antibody status, particularly with regard to treatment, pregnancy and perinatal transmission
- Documentation and reporting of test results

Assessment of patient

- Who are the supportive people in her life?
- If HIV positive, who could she confide in, who would be supportive and keep her confidence?
- How has she generally reacted to stressful situations?
- How does she think she might deal with a positive test result?

Selective testing

The most common screening programme in the West is probably targeted or selective testing. This means only offering testing to women who have risk features in their history and was the method advised by the Royal College of Obstetricians and Gynaecologists [184]. Recognized risk factors are shown in Box 17.4. This programme is effective in some situations, for example, where most infection is fuelled by injection drug use and where overall prevalence in the population is quite low. Thus studies in Paris [30] and Barcelona [40] suggested that careful targeting would identify most infected pregnant women. However, as the epidemic progresses, or in different social situations, selective testing may not be efficient. In the USA, three studies based on voluntary testing in antenatal clinics showed that only 13 of 60 seropositive women were identified [43,118,203] and only 20 per cent of seropositive pregnant women in London are thought to be recognized [1]. In general, it seems that as the pattern of the epidemic changes towards heterosexual transmission as the main source of spread, so selective testing becomes an

Box 17.2. HIV antibody negative counselling checklist (from [93] with permission). All items on this list should be discussed with the patient during the counselling session. The counsellor should initial each item

- Patient informed that her HIV antibody tests result is negative ________
- Reliability of test result. The HIV ELISA antibody test is >99% sensitive and specific ________
- Meaning of a negative test result:
  - (a) Indicates probable non-exposure to HIV ________
  - (b) If exposed to HIV within the past 6 months, antibody may not have developed ________
  - (c) If may have had exposure within the past 6 months, re-testing recommended ________
- Review of modes of HIV transmission:
  - (a) Sexual contact ________
  - (b) Direct blood or blood product injection ________
  - (c) Perinatal transmission ________
- Review of ways to avoid exposure to HIV:
  - (a) 'Safer sex' guidelines:
    - (i) Decreasing number of sexual partners decreases chance of exposure ________
    - (ii) If sexual partner is engaging in past or present risk behaviours, patient may be at continued risk of HIV exposure ________
    - (iii) Use of latex condoms and spermicide (spermicide to be used only when not pregnant) ________
    - (iv) HIV counselling and testing of sexual partner(s) discussed ________
  - (b) 'Safer use' guidelines, if appropriate:
    - (i) If using needles, *do not* share ________
    - (ii) Instructions on how to decontaminate needles — rinse twice with chlorine bleach, then rinse twice with water ________
- Patient informed that blood supply is tested for HIV and considered safe ________
- Literature for HIV negative results given to patient ________

Box 17.3. HIV antibody positive counselling checklist (from [93] with permission). All items below should be discussed with the patient during the counselling session(s). The counsellor should initial (and date items covered in subsequent sessions) each item. Asterisked items are considered essential to cover during the initial session

- Patient is informed that her HIV antibody test result is positive*
- Reliability of test result. A positive ELISA screening test is confirmed with a Western blot. False positives rarely occur* ________
- Meaning of a positive test result:
  - (a) Indicates infection with HIV* ________
  - (b) Duration of infection is considered lifelong* ________
  - (c) Patient at risk for developing AIDS related infections ________
- Explanation/review of HIV infection:
  - (a) Virus that attacks CD4 cells (part of the immune system) and, over time, destroys the body's ability to fight off certain 'opportunistic' infections* ________
  - (b) Spectrum of disease from asymptomatic stage to AIDS. Asymptomatic stage can last for several years; individual rate of disease development* ________
- Maintenance of health:
  - (a) Treatment options — ZDV and PCP prophylaxis as appropriate, based on CD4 cell counts* ________
  - (b) Nutrition ________
  - (c) Avoidance of drug use ________
  - (d) Importance of close medical follow-up ________
- Review of modes of HIV transmission*
  - (a) Sexual contact ________
  - (b) Direct blood or blood product injection ________
  - (c) Perinatal transmission ________
  - (d) Casual, household contact is *not* a mode of transmission ________
- Prevention of HIV transmission:
  - (a) 'Safer sex' guidelines*

Continued on page 574

Box 17.3. (*Continued*)

(i) Use of latex condoms and spermicide (spermicide to be used only when not pregnant) ________
(ii) Informing current/future sexual partner(s) ________
(b) 'Safer use' guidelines, if appropriate*
(i) If using needles, *do not* share ________
(ii) Instruction of how to decontaminate needles — rinse twice with chlorine bleach, then rinse twice with water ________
(c) Do not donate blood or organs ________
(d) Inform health-care personnel (e.g. dentists, clinicians at other facilities) of HIV status to receive appropriate health care ________
(e) Perinatal transmission is averted if pregnancy is avoided ________

- Confidentiality:
(a) Discussion of where HIV status is noted and who has access to the record* ________
(b) Discussion of who to share HIV test results with, why and in what circumstances (including, as applicable, sexual partners, relatives, friends, employers, health-care insurers, etc.) ________
- Perinatal/reproductive issues (as appropriate):
(a) Probabilities of perinatal transmission (based on current data) ________
(b) Spectrum of disease if child infected ________
(c) Option for termination of pregnancy, as available ________
(d) Breast-feeding discouraged if infant formula a suitable alternative ________
(e) Contraception/family planning issues discussed ________
(f) Risks of infant to other children or care-givers (HIV not casually transmitted) ________

Continued

Box 17.3 (*Continued*)

- Support systems:
(a) Patient identifies (if possible) support person(s) within social network ________
(b) Option of attending support group discussed ________
- Referred for evaluation of HIV status and ongoing medical care (as appropriate):
(a) Patient ________
(b) Other family members at risk for HIV (e.g. sexual partner, young children) ________
- Follow-up counselling appointment scheduled for*
Date ______ Time ______ Counsellor ________
- Literature for HIV positive results given to patient* ________
- Other patient questions/concerns discussed ________
- Comments (note referrals, specific patient concerns, etc.):

____
____
____

insufficient way of detecting HIV infected women in areas of high prevalence. It has also been argued that targeted testing discriminates against people and communities and leads to behavioural complacency in those not targeted [218]. Targeting by ethnic or sociodemographic criteria alone can contribute to labelling and stigmatizing groups of

Box 17.4. High risk groups for selective HIV testing in pregnant women. Not all these groups may readily be determined by direct questioning

- Sexual partners of men who have had sex with other men at any time since 1977
- Drug users or sexual partners of drug users who have injected themselves with drugs at any time since 1977
- Women who have had sex at any time since 1977 with people living in African countries except those on the Mediterranean, or who have sexual partners who have done so
- Sexual partners of haemophiliacs
- Women who are prostitutes

women and has the potential to lead to increased discrimination in already vulnerable groups of women [218]. Each geographical area therefore needs to define prevalence of infection in pregnancy, and also the proportion of infected women who will not be recognized by selective testing. With this information and consideration of costs, a decision can then be made about testing programmes. At present in the UK all women should have access to HIV testing in areas such as parts of inner London. In most areas of England outside London, where the prevalence is very low screening should continue to be selective; however, the trend should be towards informing all women about the HIV epidemic and HIV testing, and for all women to have access to testing if they so wish.

Information which became available in 1994 about the possible efficacy of Zidovudine and delivery by caesarean section in reducing vertical transmission (see below) means that screening policies need to be reassessed [9]; and such policies will need continuous reassessment in this rapidly developing field. Named testing for HIV in pregnancy must centre on benefits for the individual. With evidence building that vertical transmission may be considerably reduced by the above interventions, there are pressing reasons why women should know their serostatus. Each geographical area must therefore have a definite policy in the light of its prevalence of unknown cases of HIV in pregnancy. This remains a contentious area, but in my opinion, the time has come when, where resources allow, all pregnant women who want to have an HIV test should have access to this, and clinics with high prevalence should offer all pregnant women HIV testing.

Surveillance

HIV prevalence in pregnant women can be established easily and cheaply by unlinked anonymous testing of residual sera from specimens taken for clinical purposes other than HIV testing [74]. This is often done using neonatal screening cards, at a cost of £0.12 (sterling) for the reagent for each test [172] but using blood sent for grouping has the advantage of including women who have spontaneous or induced abortions. The ethical issues have been discussed [99]. Bayer [12] concluded that 'neither voluntariness nor privacy seemed threatened' and commented on the opposition to unlinked anonymous testing in the UK which prevented screening for some years. 'This represents a tragic misapplication of ethical principles in the face of the AIDS epidemic. There are no ethical grounds for opposing such studies. The rights of privacy do not preclude them; nor does the moral responsibility to warn the infected prevent the discovery of epidemiological patterns that are critical for the fashioning or broad public policy initiatives'.

More recently, many organizations in the UK have accepted that no fundamental ethical principles are breached by unlinked anonymous testing [74] and this was the conclusion of a committee examining ethical issues [25].

Surveillance data have a direct role in tempering take-up of testing. It is important that results are made available to the general public, and with this knowledge requests for named testing are likely to grow in response to higher prevalence. The information from surveillance testing is important in determining women's acceptance of testing.

Effect of pregnancy on HIV disease

Concern that pregnancy may adversely affect the course of HIV infection has been fuelled by a number of observations. Initially, women whose children developed AIDS were shown themselves to have a very high rate of progression [155,190]. Further concern has been raised by early case reports suggesting that the outcome of AIDS in pregnancy is poor [7,77,98,108,114,117,124,152,217]. Background theoretical factors are the widespread belief that pregnancy is associated with increased susceptibility to a number of infectious diseases [26,214]; and the fall in CD4 lymphocytes in peripheral blood which occurs in early pregnancy [106]. Finally, a number of studies have suggested a gender difference in prognosis from HIV, with women having a shorter survival time, and this has also focused attention on pregnancy as a possible co-factor.

As will be discussed, none of these arguments is compelling.

Immune changes in pregnancy

Normal pregnancy is accompanied by a reduction

of CD4 lymphocytes of about 100 cells/mm^3 in peripheral blood [106]. Acute falls in CD4 count associated with seroconversion illness have permitted opportunistic infection [36,44,96,173,212]. However, whether the fall in pregnancy has short- or long-term problems for HIV infected women is not clear-cut. Since CD4 lymphocytes have a half-life of months or years, the fall in peripheral blood in the early weeks of pregnancy presumably represents recompartmentalization, with concentration in tissues and lymph nodes. This may not necessarily alter the efficacy of the cell mediated immune response.

In HIV infected women, the correct studies to address CD4 lymphocyte loss in pregnancy have not been done. These would: (a) compare pregnant HIV infected women with non-pregnant HIV infected controls who are matched for risk group and immune status; (b) examine CD4 lymphocyte counts over the time period from before pregnancy to months or years post-partum; and (c) contrast the rate of depletion of CD4 cells over this time between the two groups. At present, some studies report a decline in CD4 count in pregnancy in HIV infected women [18,35] though others do not [37]. Biggar *et al.* [19] reported an increased loss of CD4 lymphocytes in pregnancy but the control group was not HIV infected and these data do not seem to support their claim. There is a need for better quality information in this area.

AIDS and subsequent prognosis

Whether susceptible women are more at risk of opportunistic infection during pregnancy, whether AIDS is more likely to be fatal in pregnancy, and whether the prognosis for survival is worse where AIDS occurs in pregnancy are all uncertain.

Early case reports of mortality may simply represent reporting bias [7,98,108,124,152,217]. Remarkably, the first report of survival following pneumocystic pneumonia (PCP) in pregnancy was as late as 1990 [90]. The only study comparing survival after AIDS in women according to whether or not they were pregnant was population based [103]. The women who developed PCP for the first time in pregnancy all survived this episode and the survival time did not differ between groups. However, the number of pregnant women was small (five).

Even if there is no biological reason for a poorer prognosis in pregnancy, there are ways in which pregnancy could increase the probability of an AIDS defining illness being fatal. There could be delay in diagnosis (because of a low index of suspicion or because symptoms of dyspnoea or tiredness were falsely ascribed to pregnancy) or there could be less aggressive investigation and treatment (because of concern about the fetus). Even if pregnancy has no major effect on opportunistic infections, women with poor prognostic markers or advanced HIV disease are at high risk of short-term deterioration, pregnant or not, and death around pregnancy carries the additional consequences for the fetus or child. Such women should therefore be discouraged from becoming pregnant.

Adverse effects of pregnancy on progression of HIV disease

Perhaps a more important issue, because it concerns a much larger number of women, is whether pregnancy has an effect on the natural history of HIV infection in women who are asymptomatic and who are not significantly immunocompromised. Early studies suggesting a very high rate of progression following pregnancy were biased because recruitment, for different reasons, targetted a subset at particularly high risk [77,155,190]. A similar more recent study has the same disadvantage of potential bias in enrolment, as well as lack of controls and a high loss to follow-up [76].

In controlled studies, there have been two reports of an adverse effect of pregnancy on progression of HIV disease. In a study of 290 HIV seropositive women in Paris [53] progression to CDC group 4 was greatest for the pregnant group, 15 per cent compared with 6 per cent in those who did not become pregnant. A study from Port au Prince, Haiti [54] reported a similar increase in progression to HIV related ill-health or AIDS in women who had a pregnancy with a mean of 21 months follow-up (47 per cent compared with 26 per cent in women who did not have a pregnancy).

By comparison, there have been several studies which have failed to show an adverse effect of pregnancy on the progression of HIV disease [14, 15,24,56,133,143,164,168,189].

All the above studies have methodological limitations. Common problems are that pregnant and non-pregnant groups have not been matched for important variables, particularly duration of disease which is usually not accurately known; there may be bias in recruitment from testing offered in pregnancy; there is implicit bias in that women who decided to have a pregnancy and who were able to conceive may have been less ill; there may be poor statistical power because of small numbers; length of follow-up is inevitably very variable but often quite short; and there may be a high (and potentially biased) loss to follow-up.

One further indirect piece of epidemiological evidence is the lack of any definite gender difference in HIV disease progression in natural history cohort studies. Perhaps the optimal design is an incident cohort including men and women. A group of 234 women and 422 men with accurate seroconversion dates have been enrolled in an Italian cohort [59]. So far no differences between men and women in rates of progression to AIDS have been found. Studies with prevalent cohorts controlled for CD4 counts at entry, have also not shown differences in overall progression rate [28,48,206] though one study did suggest more rapid progression in women than men in the subgroup with CD4 $<100/mm^3$ [48]. Patients who have acquired HIV infection through transfusion have also been studied and no differences attributable to gender have been found [22] [60]. Other studies suggesting that survival is shorter in women than men came from the USA, where HIV infected women may have poorer access to health care than do men [151]. Several studies showing a differential survival on univariate analysis no longer do so after more detailed analysis [8,94,127,162]. One study showed a higher proportion of women diagnosed at death, and no improvement for women since 1986, in contrast to the prognosis for men [8]. Women in another study presented with more advanced disease and more symptoms than men [180]. It therefore seems probable that access to medical care, which seems to be worse for infected women in the USA, because they may lack economic power, may be responsible for these differences rather than any gender effect.

Current evidence has been presented in some detail because this is an important issue as far as counselling about risk is concerned. Methodologically correct studies are difficult to conduct, and the effect of several possible co-factors needs to be considered. The overall impression from available evidence is that pregnancy has not been convincingly shown to accelerate progression. More carefully designed studies will clarify this in the future, and, as might be anticipated from theoretical considerations, some effect of pregnancy may well be demonstrated. However, on current evidence it seems unlikely that pregnancy will be a major adverse factor.

Vertical transmission

Most HIV infection in children is transmitted from the mother. This risk is a main concern of infected women, a major public health priority and a key target for prevention.

Mode and timing of transmission

The mode of transmission is uncertain [161]. Free virus or HIV infected maternal lymphocytes could be involved, and trophoblasts or macrophages (Hofbauer cells) could be infected in the placenta. *In vitro* studies show that trophoblast is readily infected by HIV [142,219] though there is dispute about whether this is by a pathway mediated by CD4 [142,219]. Lewis *et al.* [130] apparently located HIV antigen in villus trophoblast derivatives, villus mesenchymal cells and embryonic blood cell precursors in tissues from three out of three 8-week-old fetuses, and claimed that there is therefore a cytological pathway for transmission established by 8 weeks. One group detected HIV p24 antigen in villous Hofbauer cells and villous endothelium in four of nine placentas from HIV infected women [140]. Another group, studying term placenta from HIV infected women, localized HIV core antigen in stromal macrophages within chorionic villi, but not within the trophoblast layer [141].

The timing of transmission is of key interest. Whilst there is no doubt that transmission can occur *in utero* (transplacentally), intra-partum or postnatally (mainly through breast feeding) the proportions of all perinatal transmission which fall into these categories are not known.

Several early studies suggested that transmission of HIV could occur *in utero* [109,124,205]. Subsequently, successful culture of HIV was reported from four out of 14 second trimester fetuses [136,174] and HIV DNA sequence could be detected using PCR in 12 out of 41 fetuses [64,136,198,201]. In all these studies, precautions were taken to minimize the possibility of maternal cell contamination, but it is difficult to exclude this beyond all doubt. One study which seems to have done this used a polymorphic DNA sequence adjacent to the cystic fibrosis locus [45]. These authors examined only fetuses where the mother was heterozygous, and the fetus homozygous, for this sequence. In nine such fetuses, the maternal specific allele could not be detected, thus excluding maternal cell contamination, but HIV DNA sequences were detected in eight. This seems a suprisingly high rate of HIV detection in the light of known figures for transmission to the child, and raises the possibility that defective fragments of DNA are being identified rather than true infection. Isolated case reports of early HIV disease in the fetus or neonate also provide evidence of intrauterine infection [13,185].

Contact with infected blood and cervical secretions provides the potential for infection during vaginal delivery. Data which could offer support for intra-partum transmission have been those showing a low rate of identification of HIV at birth, but a higher rate weeks or months later [64,121]. However, this could be due to decreased sensitivity where small volumes of blood are used from newborns, or could relate to the fact that it is only with birth that the baby is subject to antigenic stimulation, and hence only then that significant HIV replication occurs. Further data, based on the International Registry of HIV Exposed Twins [78] showed that 44 per cent of first-borns, but only 21 per cent of second-born twins, were infected. This was held to mean that a substantial portion of HIV infection occurred because of the proximity of twin one to the cervix and hence perhaps occurred during passage through the birth canal. These studies have been influential in developing the current belief that most vertical transmission occurs around delivery (see below).

Most studies showing transmission apparently due to breast feeding have involved recent maternal seroconversion, when plasma viraemia will be very high [215,220]. The estimated risk in this situation is one in three [63]. However, detailed statistical review of the literature has concluded that even when the mother is infected before delivery, breast feeding poses an additional 14 per cent risk of transmitting HIV to the baby [63], and a relationship with duration of breast feeding has been reported [51].

Factors affecting vertical transmission

Few factors have consistently emerged as risk variables, and it seems likely that multiple factors relating to maternal infectivity, fetal resistance and placental state all interrelate in a complex arrangement.

Infectivity is generally believed to relate to viraemia, with high levels of virus and high infectivity at primary infection and in advanced disease. There is some support for this using clinical or immunological surrogates for high viral load [87, 186]. The large European Collaborative Study [67] examined risk factors using multivariate analysis, and showed a threefold increase in risk of vertical transmission when maternal CD4 count was <700 cells/mm^3. This is a high count, well within the normal range. One small study from Nairobi [120] claimed that transmission correlated with maternal viral load as assessed by quantitative PCR. More studies using new technology to quantitate viral load will clarify the issue.

The fetus is in an unusual situation as it already has antibody to HIV, passively transferred from the mother. This should be protective. The levels of antibody to epitopes on the hypervariable V_3 loop of gp120 or the principal neutralizing domain have been investigated by different research groups with conflicting results [3,17,55,79,88,119,120,167, 171,181,184,196]. Several studies suggested that antibody levels were highly predictive [60,85,127,192]. This has not been confirmed by others [3,17,88,119, 167,171,196] and certainly infection does seem to have occurred despite high maternal levels of antibodies. Any protective effect may be type specific rather than group specific [167]. An interesting finding in the European Collaborative Study [67] was that pre-term delivery before 34 weeks was associated with a doubling of the risk of transmission. This could be because HIV infection *per se* could lead to pre-term delivery, but perhaps more plausibly because such infants were more susceptible to infection because of low levels of passively transferred maternal antibodies.

As well as maternal factors, there are suggestions that placental damage may be associated with an increased risk of transmission. There is an association with chorioamnionitis [186]. The finding of a high transmission rate with maternal anaemia (though it could simply be a reflection of HIV disease activity) could result from malaria, which preferentially infects the placenta [58]. In addition, fetal genotype may be important. One small study found HLA-DR3 to be three times more common in infected infants [116] whilst another study reported that susceptibility to HIV infection was related to genetic variation in HLA immune response genes [110,111].

Finally, what obstetric factors could influence transmission? Invasive fetal procedures (cordocentesis, scalp sampling, application of scalp electrodes could result in micro-inoculation of the fetus with maternal blood and hence cause infection. Interestingly, the only fetal sample with maternal blood contamination in one study was the one where earlier cordocentesis had been performed [136]. Such procedures should therefore be avoided if possible, where the mother is infected. The role of caesarean section is unclear. In theory elective caesarean section could be protective by minimizing time spent by the baby exposed to cervical mucus and blood from cervical dilatation. The twin study referred to above [78] is compatible with this, and caesarean section was associated with a significant reduction in infection. However, infection of the baby has certainly occurred despite caesarean section being performed.

An important analysis of the effect of caesarean section, published in 1994, does not report on a randomized trial, but great efforts were made to assess confounding factors associated with transmission risk [68]. 1012 children from the European Collaborative Study were of known infection status. The odds of infection following caesarean section, relative to vaginal delivery, were 0.53 from within centre analysis, 0.55 including 5 other markers and 0.49 including also maternal CD4 count (largely by multiple imputation). The 95% CI were all less than 1. Surprisingly, whether caesarean section was done as an elective or emergency procedure made no difference (though from one subset, 60% of emergency operations were done with the mother's membranes remaining intact).

The situation is not straightforward, because caesarean section was not found to be protective in the French Perinatal Study, and meta-analysis of 11 prospective studies, heavily biased by the large European Collaborative Study, nevertheless showed only a 20% (95% CI 0%–37%) reduction in vertical transmission associated with caesarean section [62].

Keen for a definitive, randomized controlled trial, the authors of the European Study conclude appropriately as follows, 'Until randomised controlled trials evaluating both mode of delivery and anteretroviral therapy are completed, obstetricians are left in a dilemma. There is accumulating evidence that caesarean section is protective and a decision to continue with vaginal delivery could result in avoidable infections. On the other hand, the evidence is not conclusive and it would be undesirable if an ineffective procedure was to become routine practice'.

In 1994, important information became available about the effect of Zidovudine in reducing vertical transmission, as shown in the ACTG 076 trial. The striking results of this study replace the previous patchy information available [47,49,204] and are discussed below.

Further trials that are underway or under consideration are those using false receptors for the virus (soluble CD4), hyperimmunoglobulin [160], vaccines [176], passive immunotherapy using human anti-HIV monoclonal antibodies [221], nevirapine (a non-nucleoside reverse transcriptase inhibitor) and local anti-virals given intra-vaginally during labour. If most infection does occur around delivery, as currently believed, there are good grounds for the prevailing optimism that a large reduction in perinatal transmission should be achievable by such strategies.

Proportion of exposed babies infected

Transmission from mother to child has been estimated to vary between 13 and 32 per cent in developed countries and between 28 and 52 per cent in developing countries [50]. Some of the variation can be ascribed to methodological problems [66]. Thus some studies included younger children who were ill, hence inflating the numerator artificially. The definition proposed by the CDC [32] using persistence of antibody at 15 months as evidence of infection may overestimate transmission because a proportion of children who lose maternal antibody do so after 15 months. Other studies have a low follow-up rate, and one used virus culture in cord blood as an end point for infection. A standardized methodological approach to studies of mother to child transmission has been proposed [50]. Nevertheless, it seems likely that much of the variation in transmission is genuine and is related to population differences. These include particularly stages of HIV disease, but may also include other infections and breast feeding.

The largest, and methodologically correct, study is the European Collaborative Study [65,66]. The rate of vertical transmission, based on 721 children born to 701 mothers more than 18 months before the time of analysis, was 14.4 per cent (95 per cent CI 12–17.1 per cent). Maternal p24 antigenaemia and a CD4 count $<700/mm^3$ were associated with a higher risk of transmission. Delivery before 34 weeks was a risk factor (odds ratio 3.80, 95 per cent CI 1.62–8.91). This is an interesting finding, because it could mean that the fetal humoral response is a determining factor in the risk of infection following exposure. This would follow if the reason for susceptibility of the premature baby was the reduced accumulation of maternal specific IgG antibody.

Prognosis for the infected infant

There is some evidence of a bimodal age and clinical distribution of paediatric HIV infection. Approximately 30 per cent of infected children develop early onset AIDS or advanced HIV disease within the first year of life [22,66]. Other children have a more slowly progressive form of HIV disease, which allows some to survive into adolescence, though the majority are symptomatic. This pattern has been interpreted as suggesting that infection early in pregnancy could have devastating effects on the fetal immune system and result in severe early onset disease, whereas infection around the time of delivery could result in more prolonged survival [161].

Pregnancy outcome

Pregnancy wastage could result from interference with the fetomaternal immune relationship, a direct viral effect on trophoblast invasion or later placental development, early viral infection of the fetus, chorioamnionitis as a result of maternal immunosuppression, fetal damage due to recurrence of other infections, such as cytomegalovirus (CMV) or toxoplasmosis, or the general maternal effects of concurrent infections and poor nutritional status. In practice, at least for asymptomatic women in the developed world, such problems do not seem to be common.

Spontaneous abortion

A number of studies based on history of spontaneous abortion have suggested an increase in women infected with HIV [126,129,156,157]. In the largest prospective study to date [208] HIV antibody status was assessed in 195 women admitted to hospital in Kenya with abortion. Although there are methodological problems, particularly associated with selection of a control group, attempts were made to account for other variables and HIV was still statistically more common in the abortion group.

At present it is uncertain whether HIV is a direct cause of spontaneous abortion. Most published information suggests a trend in that direction, but the studies are either retrospective or there is doubt about whether the findings could be explained by a correlated variable, such as positive syphilis serology or other infectious disease. On theoretical and observational grounds an increased rate of abortion seems plausible, but the increase is likely to be small.

Congenital abnormality

A dysmorphic syndrome associated with HIV infection has been reported [137,138]. This syndrome included growth failure, microcephaly, flattened nasal bridge, oblique eyes, prominent forehead, triangular philtrum and patulous lips. Subsequent reports have not confirmed this finding [166,177] and an HIV dysmorphic syndrome was not seen in the large European Collaborative Study [67]. At present it seems doubtful that there is a specific syndrome, and the original observations may have been due to confounding from variables such as drug and alcohol use or ethnic group.

Most control studies have not specifically reported on structural congenital anomalies but where this has been done there was no association with HIV serostatus [27,129]. Prospective studies [5,21, 67,97,182] are uncontrolled but have not reported unusually high incidences of congenital abnormality. At present there seems to be no good evidence that HIV is specifically associated with congenital abnormality.

Induced abortion

An assumption has been made by health planners that women will seek induced abortion if they are discovered to be HIV seropositive. There is population support from this amongst non-infected women. In one study of pregnant women in France [159] the consensus about abortion for HIV infected women was strong, with 80 per cent of women in favour. Even if the estimated transmission rate of HIV was only 5 per cent a large proportion of women (46 per cent) remained in favour of termination of pregnancy.

The actual behaviour of HIV infected women appears discrepant from these expectations. In a study of methadone users in New York [192] 14 of 28 seropositive women and 16 of 36 seronegative women chose termination of pregnancy. The authors concluded that 'neither the perceived personal risk of perinatal transmission of HIV, nor the presence of concern about AIDS, was associated with an increased rate of pregnancy termination'.

A study from Edinburgh [102] compared seropositive and seronegative women tested for the same indications (mainly injection drug use). Of 69 seropositive women 31 chose termination (45 per cent) and 33 of 94 seronegative women did so (35 per cent). Interestingly, none of the 18 women first diagnosed as HIV seropositive in pregnancy at the antenatal clinic and counselled before 22 weeks accepted termination of pregnancy. Stated reasons were the desire for one child, current good health and local knowledge of infected mothers who were nevertheless well and had healthy, uninfected children. The significance of the problem was usually appreciated and many women had already identified a family member who was prepared to look after the child if the woman became too ill or died. Although not all reports agree, these two small studies may nevertheless be representative of choices made by HIV infected women. An understandable response for an asymptomatic woman who knows she has a lifelong infection with a potentially fatal disease must be to get on with her life, and this is likely to involve pregnancy.

Powerful factors motivate asymptomatic infected women with a wanted pregnancy to continue rather than accept induced abortion. Discussion about termination of pregnancy must be well informed and sensitive to the extremely difficult issues faced by the woman in making her decision. As much as possible, information should be specific and tailored to that individual woman based on social, clinical and laboratory assessment. The issues in this area have been very well described [191].

Obstetric complications

Adequately controlled studies from the West have shown no significant increase in pregnancy complications, except for infectious complications of the mother [16,104,153,194,195]. However, these studies are all small and lack statistical power to address the issue of relatively infrequent pregnancy complications.

In contrast, studies from Africa include 2249 infected mothers and 4308 HIV seronegative controls [27,31,85,91,112,125,186,209]. Whilst not completely consistent, several studies suggested that HIV seropositivity was associated with preterm delivery [85,186,209] and increased perinatal death [31,85,186].

A large and important case control study in Nairobi [210] focused on adverse pregnancy outcome: 373 women who delivered a pre-term baby, 324 who delivered a baby small for gestational age, 120 who had an intrauterine death, and 69 with an intra-partum death were compared for HIV status with 711 controls. HIV seropositivity was more common in the case groups but so were other, potentially confounding, features such as primiparity, lack of antenatal clinic attendance and maternal syphilis infection. However, linear logistic regression retained HIV status as a statistically significant associated outcome with modestly increased odds ratios of 2.1 (pre-term birth), 2.3 (small for gestational age), 2.7 (intrauterine death) and 2.9 (intra-partum death).

Whether the data from these studies can be assumed to relate causally, HIV infection with pregnancy outcome is neither straightforward nor clear-cut, and nor is the assumption that these findings apply equally in Europe and the USA. In these studies, control subjects are often loosely matched, and seropositive women differ from controls in other (though related) characteristics apart from HIV status [101]. In several studies attempts have been made to allow for these differences but not all potential confounders can be included.

Even if the increase in obstetric complications found in some studies in Africa does represent a genuine causal relationship, the findings may not apply equally in the West. Advanced HIV clinical disease may have been more common in the African studies [27,91,186]. Differences could have been due to the load of other infectious diseases, especially tuberculosis and malaria. Finally, there may be important nutritional differences, with women in Africa possibly more likely to enter pregnancy in a vulnerable nutritional state, and HIV disease in Africa more likely to have a weight losing pattern. Data from Africa relating pregnancy outcome and HIV disease together with maternal weight, weight gain and accompanying infections have not been reported.

The most likely probability on present evidence is that when women are asymptomatic and not significantly immune compromised, HIV infection *per se* does not have a major effect on pregnancy outcome. It is possible, from the African studies that even early disease may have a slight effect on birthweight, spontaneous abortion and pre-term labour. However, the major effect is likely to be due to advancing HIV disease, with the accompaniment of other infections (including chorioamnionitis) and deteriorating nutritional status. It seems inevitable that there will then be a detrimental effect on pregnancy, and there are data suggesting that this is so.

Birthweight

The contrast between data from the West and Africa, presented above, is seen even more clearly with regard to birthweight. None of the studies from Europe and the USA has suggested that HIV infection has any impact on birthweight [16,104,153,194,195] except for one preliminary study [105]. All studies from Africa are consistent in showing a decrease in birthweight in pregnancies from HIV infected mothers [27,31,85,91,112,125,129, 186,209]. There is some evidence that decrease in size is related to the stage of maternal disease [85,186]. An important and consistent observation is that birthweight seems unrelated to the infant's eventual HIV status [21,66,97,186].

The same caveats detailed above apply to these observations on birthweight. Any effect does not seem to be mediated through anticardiolipin antibodies. These antibodies are common in HIV infected women, but these infection-stimulated antibodies do not produce adverse pregnancy or thrombotic events (cf. the cardiolipin syndrome, Chapter 8) [103].

Delivery

There is little information about labour and delivery complications in HIV infected women. Nevertheless, labour ward management is likely to become more of a focus for critical review and interest, particularly as the birth process may be a significant time for transmission of HIV to the baby [78,121]. Other important issues are support to the mother around delivery, and the prevention of spread of HIV to health-care workers.

Two large studies of vertical transmission [97,

67], both reported a high caesarean section rate (23 and 26 per cent respectively). Both studies were uncontrolled and the reasons for caesarean section were not given. In controlled studies, there was no excess in caesarean sections found by Minkoff *et al.* [153]. In Edinburgh, comparing HIV seropositive and risk exposed seronegative women, there were no differences in any obstetric outcome. None of the large studies from Africa seem to have published on fetal distress in labour, labour complications or operative delivery.

It seems likely that there are no major differences in labour and delivery outcome attributable to HIV infection. In immunocompromised women, it is possible that premature rupture of the membranes may occur more frequently, and in such women the risk of chorioamnionitis may be increased. Similarly the risk of post-operative wound infection or post-partum endometritis is likely to be greater. The major factors which should mandate significant changes in practice would be convincing evidence that most vertical transmission occurs around delivery, that this could be significantly reduced by elective caesarian section, that other interventions were on their own not sufficiently effective, that there was no antagonism with other interventions or that protection offered by caesarian section did not extend only to the same patients, and that maternal risks were balanced with those of the fetus.

Even as more evidence accumulates, advice to patients may remain a matter of clinical judgement. Intuitively, the woman who has delivered easily and quickly before, and where the membranes can be conserved almost up to the point of delivery, may have little to gain from caesarian section. For the woman whose labour and delivery seem likely to be difficult and prolonged, on the other hand, caesarian section may be appropriate. The current clinical situation is probably as follows; caesarian section need not be advised for all HIV infected women; available data should be shared with HIV infected pregnant women, and they must be kept closely informed about further evidence as it accumulates; and HIV should be seen as a relative indication to be weighed with other clinical and patient preference considerations.

HIV disease in pregnancy

An important role for the obstetrician is to establish optimal linkage between the patient and physicians with expertise in HIV for both mother and child [176]. Where opportunistic infection does occur during pregnancy, management should be coordinated by a specialist in HIV disease. In view of the seriousness of these conditions, investigation and management should be optimal for the disease entity, and not unduly influenced by the fact that the woman is pregnant.

Assessment of illness is important in early pregnancy, and this includes CD4 lymphocyte count. This should comprise part of the framework within which the possibility of termination of pregnancy is discussed, and will be used to indicate PCP or retroviral prophylaxis. This measurement should be repeated each trimester.

Many early symptoms of HIV disease are non-specific and common in pregnancy (tiredness, dyspnoea, headache, anorexia, cough). In susceptible women, obstetricians must have a high index of suspicion, and a readiness to investigate and to consult with infectious disease colleagues. They should also explain to such women what symptoms may be significant and ask them to report these early.

Early assessment should also include baseline titres for CMV and toxoplasmosis because of the risks of recurrence during pregnancy. Screening for hepatitis B is essential because of the risks and preventability of perinatal infection [41]. As well as screening for syphilis, which is routine in most antenatal clinics, it may be advisable to screen for other sexually transmitted organisms, such as the *Gonococcus* and *Chlamydia*. Where tuberculosis is common, women should have Mantoux testing and unless they have had recent cervical screening, the opportunity should be taken to carry out cervical cytology or colposcopy. Medical management in pregnancy has been excellently described [188].

Pneumocystis carinii pneumonia

This has been the leading AIDS defining diagnosis for women (53 per cent) as well as for men (55 per cent) [71]. With routine prophylaxis for susceptible individuals it has become less common, and immediate mortality when PCP does occur has decreased markedly with improved expertise and earlier diagnosis.

PCP usually begins insidiously with gradual onset of shortness of breath, tiredness and a cough. Whilst chest X-ray may show diffuse interstitial infiltrates or perihilar infiltrates sparing the periphery it may be normal early in the course of disease. Similarly, arterial blood gases generally show hypoxaemia but may be normal in early disease. Diagnosis is usually with induced sputum after inhalation of hypertonic saline via an ultrasonic nebulizer, when the presence of *P. carinii* can be demonstrated.

First line treatment is usually trimethoprim/sulphamethoxazole. Although these drugs have theoretical risk, because trimethoprim is a folic acid inhibitor and sulphonamides may raise unconjugated bilirubin in the newborn, significant effects have not been reported [29] and the seriousness of PCP completely outweighs any possible theoretical fetal risk. Pentamidine is also effective, though, for reasons which are not understood, patients infected with HIV have an increased risk of serious side-effects from both drugs, so that nearly half of patients have to stop therapy because of adverse drug effects. Dapsone with trimethoprim has also been used to treat PCP effectively in those who fail first line drugs.

It is important to emphasize that similar clinical presentations can be found with viral, fungal, protozoal, mycobacterial or bacterial infections, all of which occur more frequently in HIV disease. Indeed bacterial infections are now one of the leading causes of HIV related death.

Candidiasis

Oesophageal candidiasis is a serious, AIDS defining condition, which may present with dysphagia, substernal chest pain and nausea [188]. It occurs at very low CD4 counts, but oropharyngeal candidiasis seems to occur at lesser degrees of immune compromise and chronic vaginal candidiasis appears common in HIV infected women, even those with relatively normal CD4 lymphocyte counts [95]. Treatment depends on the site, with antifungal pessaries for vaginal candidiasis and topical nystatin or cotrimoxazole for oropharyngeal candidiasis. Ketoconazole and fluconazole are not established as safe in pregnancy, but in some clinical situations will have to be used, despite the uncertainty about risk.

Tuberculosis

This is a major disease associated with HIV in Africa and in the eastern seaboard of the USA, where it is also associated with poverty and drug use. In this setting, prophylaxis is indicated where there is a positive tuberculin skin test or X-ray evidence of old tuberculosis. This prophylaxis is usually isoniazid, with pyridoxine to prevent peripheral neuropathy. Active tuberculosis may be difficult to diagnose in HIV infection with atypical presentations common and 72 per cent of cases extrapulmonary [193]. Treatment, usually with isoniazid, rifampicin and ethambutol, should be continued for at least 9 months. These drugs are recommended in pregnancy [4] (see Chapter 1).

Unfortunately, multidrug resistant tuberculosis is being increasingly reported in the USA and Africa. This is very difficult to treat and has a very high mortality.

Toxoplasmosis

T. gondii infection is not only important as a cause of morbidity and mortality in HIV infected women, but also as a cause of fetal damage.

Toxoplasmosis is generally a late manifestation of AIDS [188] and most commonly presents as encephalitis [144]. Symptoms include constant headache, seizures and hemiparesis, and diagnosis is most often based on history and computed tomography (CT) or nuclear magnetic resonance (NMR) brain scans. Treatment is usually with sulphadiazine and pyramethamine with folinic acid supplements.

As far as fetal infection is concerned, transmission in non-HIV infected pregnancy seems to occur almost exclusively during primary infection of the mother [179]. However, in HIV infected, immunocompromised individuals, re-activation of disease does occur in association with parasitaemia. Whether transplacental transmission of toxoplasma occurs in HIV infected women with latent or recurrent infection is not clear.

Cytomegalovirus (CMV)

CMV raises similar issues to those of toxoplasmosis. CMV disease tends to be a late HIV related illness, occurring in 7–20 per cent of AIDS illnesses [169] and most typically causing retinitis which can lead to blindness. However, many organ systems may be involved. CMV retinitis usually presents with the complaint of 'floaters' or loss of vision. Ganciclovir is the first line drug, but is only recommended for life- or sight-threatening disease. Animal studies have suggested teratogenicity and embryolethality at comparable doses to those used in humans [188]. Foscarnet is an alternative drug, also with evidence of teratogenicity in limited animal studies.

Unlike toxoplasmosis, fetal damage is well documented as occurring after re-activation of CMV infection in pregnancy [84]. In most pregnant populations the prevalence of immunity to CMV is 40–60 per cent [80] and therefore a high proportion of HIV infected pregnant women may be at risk. Data from transplant patients have shown that CMV shedding increases with worsening immunosuppression [80]. There do not appear to be published studies reporting the prevalence of CMV excretion in newborns in HIV infected pregnancy, and so far, severe congenital CMV infection does not seem to have been identified as a problem. Several ongoing studies should clarify this.

Cryptococcosis

This ubiquitous fungus rarely causes disease in the immunocompetent individual, but in immunocompromised women disease can develop from re-activation of previously contained infectious foci [188]. Presentation in AIDS is usually with central nervous system involvement or disseminated disease. Although very rare, congenital transmission has been reported [179].

Cervical neoplasia

There is good evidence that cervical intraepithelial neoplasia (CIN) is more common in women with HIV infection [69,134,135,187]. It also seems that CIN becomes more common at lower peripheral blood CD4 levels [135,139,188,200]. At an anecdotal level, rapid progression to invasive cervical carcinoma has been suggested to occur more frequently in HIV infected women, and vaginal and vulval intraepithelial neoplasia are also reported to occur more often.

All authors recommend more frequent surveillance of the cervix in HIV infected women, for example, twice yearly cervical cytology [122] or annual colposcopy [200]. As many women will attend infrequently, pregnancy may be an opportunity to offer cervical cytology or colposcopy.

Other diseases

In women with severe immunocompromise, protracted diarrhoea and precipitous weight loss (see Chapter 10), diffuse central nervous system dysfunction and focal neurological abnormality, may all have a large differential diagnosis. Specialist physicians have to be involved in the care of women whose immune state places them at risk of these conditions which may present considerable diagnostic and therapeutic problems.

Prophylaxis in pregnancy

As has been indicated above, discussion about pregnancy and pregnancy management should be specifically tailored to the needs of the individual woman. This means assessing the point she has reached in disease progression, and this in turn is largely dependent on the predictive markers CD4 lymphocyte count, p24 antigenaemia, p24 antibody index and β_2 microglobulin which all independently predict progression.

Where markers indicate advanced disease there are strong reasons for termination of pregnancy because of the risk of maternal opportunistic disease during pregnancy, the extra risk of vertical transmission and the short predicted lifespan of the woman. Where this is unacceptable, and the woman continues with the pregnancy, appropriate prophylaxis must be considered.

P. carinii

Although PCP has become less common with widespread prophylaxis, it still occurs in a majority of patients during the course of AIDS. Prophylaxis is therefore indicated as primary treatment where CD4 count is $<200/mm^3$ or there is stage IV disease. Prophylaxis is also mandatory as secondary treatment after resolution of PCP. These guidelines are well established, and even though there is a fall in peripheral blood CD4 count in pregnancy, the same guidelines should probably be adhered to in the pregnant woman.

The two main agents used for PCP prophylaxis are cotrimoxazole and pentamidine. The former drug is emerging as the first line drug with a lower recurrence risk in secondary prophylaxis. It is also effective in preventing the rare complication of extrapulmonary pneumocystis, may offer some protection against toxoplasma and bacterial infections, and is perhaps preferred to jet nebulizer pentamidine administration in late pregnancy where positioning may be uncomfortable. The recommended dosage of cotrimoxazole is 480 mg daily. Unfortunately, side-effects are common and cotrimoxazole may have to be stopped for this reason. There are also concerns about risks to the fetus, but although there are few data on long-term use of cotrimoxazole in pregnancy, there is no evidence of adverse fetal effects [29] and in the serious situation of an immunocompromised woman, the proven and likely benefits are thought to outweigh the possible risks to the fetus.

The standard pentamidine dose of 300 mg every 4 weeks administered through a jet nebulizer is known to be effective [128]. Although there are concerns about the safety of pentamidine in pregnancy, very little is absorbed systemically so that the amount reaching the fetus is likely to be very small. However, in addition to the disadvantages mentioned above, pneumothorax is a (relatively rare) risk of this treatment [115]. Nevertheless, this treatment is clearly indicated in pregnancy where the woman is at risk and either intolerant of cotrimoxazole or non-compliant with this regime. As with cotrimoxazole, side-effects will limit use of pentamidine in some women. For such women dapsone has been used as prophylaxis, but large-scale studies of its use have not yet been reported.

Zidovudine

Zidovudine (AZT, azidothymidine) is a nucleoside analogue which differs from thymidine in having an azido group (N_3) instead of a hydroxyl group at the 3 position on the ribose ring. After phosphorylation by cellular enzymes it inhibits transcription of viral RNA to DNA by competitive inhibition and chain termination.

Zidovudine is accepted as of proven efficacy in advanced HIV disease [70] and in early symptomatic patients [83] and some of the improvement in survival in recent years is attributed to the use of this drug. The situation is less clear in asymptomatic individuals. Studies have suggested short-term benefit to asymptomatic individuals with CD4 counts of $200-500/mm^3$ but questions remain about the long-term effectiveness of this approach, the benefit in terms of survival, and the optimal timing of initiation of treatment. Toxicity in terms of bone marrow suppression and gastrointestinal side-effects is common.

The risks and benefits of zidovudine treatment in pregnancy are still uncertain. Animal studies have not disclosed major adverse effects [188]. A review of 43 pregnancies where zidovudine was taken [204] was somewhat reassuring. Apart from mild anaemia in the babies, there were no consistent fetal adverse effects. However, only 11 women took zidovudine in the first trimester and as the authors state 'such data cannot be used to infer that zidovudine does not have some degree of teratogenicity'; they draw attention to isotretinoin, a well-established teratogen, which nevertheless is only associated with malformations in one pregnancy out of five.

There is great current interest in the (still unpublished in September 1994) ACTG 076 randomized, placebo-controlled trial of AZT [6,68,202]. This multicentre trial involved units in the US and France and had a target enrolment of 748 HIV infected women in their 14th–34th weeks of pregnancy who did not need AZT as part of their medical care. AZT was prescribed antenatally, (100 mg five times daily), intravenously in labour (loading dose of 2 mg/kg/hour for the first hour, then 1 mg/kg/hour until delivery) and given to the baby for 6 weeks (first dose within 24 hours and thereafter 2 mg/kg every 6 hours). Interim analysis on 364 pregnancies where at least one HIV culture test was available revealed a transmission rate of 8.3% in the AZT arm of the study and 25.3% among those receiving placebo. Both mothers and infants tolerated the AZT treatment well with no significant short-term side-effects other than reversible mild anaemia in some infants. On the basis of this interim analysis the study investigators stopped enrolment and offered AZT to the remaining currently enrolled pregnant women. Further data which have accumulated are consistent with these initial results.

The study has so far not been reported in full and follow-up of the infants for several years is planned. The long-term effects for the infant of exposure to AZT are unknown, and, assuming the lower transition rate is substantiated on more complete assessment, the decision to treat will depend for some time upon the perceived balance between known benefit and unknown risk.

Other antiretroviral drugs

Dideoxyinosine is a purine nucleoside analogue with pancreatitis and peripheral neuropathy as important side-effects, but efficacy demonstrated in terms of surrogate markers (CD4 cell levels and p24 antigenaemia). There are no data on use during human pregnancy, and this drug should only be used when clearly needed, and not as prophylaxis. The same applies to dideoxycytidine, a pyrimidine nucleoside analogue where again there are no data on use in pregnancy.

If prophylaxis and treatment move increasingly towards combination therapy, the issue of women entering pregnancy whilst taking these drugs may become more common.

Other possible prophylaxis

Other prophylactic strategies are aimed largely at prevention of vertical transmission. Under investigation or under consideration are maternal treatment with soluble CD4 (to reduce free virus with a false receptor), hyperimmunoglobulin (to reduce virus by antibody response) or active immunization (to achieve the same result) [160,176].

Obstetric management

There have been several reviews dealing with management in pregnancy [57,100,150,151,158]. One important principle is that care has to be supportive, and this often involves a multi-agency approach. The general practitioner, the community midwife, a physician with a special interest in HIV disease and the paediatrician who will follow-up the baby may all be involved as well as hospital obstetric staff. Social, drug and support group workers may also make a valuable contribution to the care of some patients. Whilst this skill mix offers many advantages and opportunities to the pregnant woman, it also carries the risk of conveying different, partially confusing messages and can involve duplication of effort. There is therefore an obligation on such a team to maintain effective communication with each other as well as with the patient.

Antenatal

Investigations which might be done at first contact in pregnancy, additional to routine antenatal tests, are shown in Box 17.5. These have all been previously discussed.

Obstetric care should involve a clear discussion of the information available about pregnancy and an explanation of the different risks involved. Where termination of pregnancy is an available option, this should be discussed and where the woman decides to continue the pregnancy, the plan of assessment and management should be discussed with her and related issues such as maintenance drug use, plans for drug reduction, PCP prophylaxis mode of delivery and antiretroviral therapy can be explored. Clearly these discussions have to be individualized to meet the particular situation of each patient.

Many difficult issues remain about different interventions, including the possibility that effects might be different in women with more advanced disease, that there might be synergy or antagonism between

Box 17.5. Investigations which may be appropriate depending on local laboratory facilities and local levels of disease (adapted from [101])

- Assessment of HIV disease
  - CD4+ lymphocyte count
  - p24 antigen
  - p24 antibody titre
  - β_2 microglobulin
  - Neopterin
- Baseline titres of conditions which may affect the fetus
  - Hepatitis B
  - Cytomegalovirus
  - Toxoplasmosis
- Screening for other related maternal disease
  - Mantoux test
  - Other sexually transmitted diseases
  - Cervical cytology/colposcopy

interventions, that future trials may be greatly constrained by existing beliefs, and that management plans for individuals, depending on multiple, effective interventions, all with some risks, will be problematic [165].

The situation at the moment is that this information needs to be discussed in detail with HIV infected women, so that a fully informed decision can be taken (see above) about AZT and mode of delivery. This all needs to be decided before the third trimester and a formal plan needs to be made about delivery in case of spontaneous premature rupture of the membranes.

As discussed above, in the West there is no evidence of major obstetric problems specifically associated with HIV, except for maternal infection. However, there are often associated factors, such as drug use, heavy cigarette smoking, and adverse living conditions which may predispose to pre-term delivery and intrauterine growth retardation. For this reason, careful obstetric surveillance, as well as medical surveillance is important.

Several invasive procedures have the potential to micro-innoculate maternal blood into the fetal compartment, and hence infect a fetus which might otherwise remain non-infected. Such procedures include chorion villus sampling, amniocentesis, cordocentesis and placental biopsy. How real a risk they pose is unknown but in one study of HIV transmission in the second trimester the only fetus where maternal cells were demonstrated was the only case where fetoscopy had been performed [136]. Because of the possible risks, it does not seem likely that techniques will become available for the prenatal diagnosis of HIV in the fetus. The uncertainty about when transmission occurs would also limit this approach. Instead, the hope is that with clearer evidence of the prognostic value of markers in the mother, more precise information in each individual case might allow more accurately based decisions to be made.

Delivery

As far as delivery is concerned, there are few substantial differences in obstetric management of the HIV infected woman. She has the same needs and should have access to the same care as other women. However, one important issue is the suggestion that a high proportion of vertical transmission may occur around the time of delivery, which has in turn raises the possibility of routine elective caesarean section or using antiretroviral vaginal treatment during labour. As presented above, the evidence for this is based largely on the collaborative twin study [78] and the European Collaborative Study [67] (see above).

Anaesthesia and surgery are known to induce important changes of the immune system so that surgery could have some effect on maternal disease in HIV infected women [72]. No work has been published on the use of antiretrovirals in the vagina. If much infection does occur around delivery this greatly increases the potential for prevention of transmission by the various suggested interventions.

During vaginal delivery, there are a number of precautions which can be taken which may minimize the risk of transmission. Application of scalp electrodes and fetal scalp sampling could create a portal of entry for maternal blood into the fetus. For this theoretical reason, it seems reasonable to avoid these procedures. There is some evidence for this advice, in that the European Collaborative Study [67] found HIV infection to be more common in babies where these procedures were done, though only in units where these procedures were not routine. Thus statistical significance was only reached within certain centres. Episiotomy, which may expose the fetus to much more maternal blood was also associated with an increased transmission risk under these same conditions. On theoretical grounds early artificial rupture of the membranes will also result in more prolonged exposure of the baby to maternal mucus and blood. With modern external monitoring techniques there can usually be adequate surveillance of the fetus without artificial rupture of the membranes, and this technique has not been shown to have clear advantages obstetrically [11]. It therefore seems preferable to leave the membranes intact for as long as possible. Other procedures which might be considered are early cord clamping which conceivably could reduce the risk of maternal cells gaining access to the fetal blood stream as the placenta detaches, and early bathing of the baby which minimizes the time of contact of maternal blood with the baby's body surface. Although it is unlikely that evidence of the value of early bathing of the baby will emerge, this intuitively seems correct care for the term baby.

Post-partum

The postnatal period is another time where further interactive discussion may be helpful. Women in developed countries where bottle feeding is relatively safe should be advised against breast feeding [63] but the balance of risk may be different in other situations, where breast feeding should continue to be promoted, as offering infants the optimum chance for survival. The mother should be encouraged to hug and kiss the baby in the knowledge that this will not transmit HIV infection. She may need to acquire confidence in her ability to care for the infant, and knowledge of which forms of physical contact may and may not be a possible risk to the baby. This is a useful time to re-state arrangements for follow-up of mother and baby, to answer questions about the baby and risk of HIV infection and to discuss contraception. Although to the obstetrician the delivery of the baby may be seen as the end of a process, to the mother, her general practitioner and the community carers it is the beginning. That is why it is so important that care during the pregnancy is supportive, multi-agency and largely based in the community.

Nosocomial transmission

Although the risk of nosocomial transmission of HIV is small, it is real, and awareness of this risk is resulting in substantial changes in infection control procedures. This subject has been excellently reviewed [39,107].

Occupational transmission to health-care workers

Most occupational transmission has occurred following needle-stick or other sharps injury, but there have been documented seroconversions after contamination of broken skin or mucous membranes [32,75].

Up to October 1992, seroconversion following a specific exposure incident had been reported in 51 cases, with a further 91 instances of presumed occupational source and four home-care transmissions [39]. Most of the documented exposures were needle-stick injuries and most of those involved a hollow needle containing infected blood. By August 1992 no seroconversion after an injury from a suture needle or other solid needle used in the operating theatre had been reported [107]. Most of the patients had CDC stage IV HIV disease. Although this will inevitably be a considerable underestimate of the total number of health-care workers infected by occupational risk, nevertheless the number is small in relation to the huge number of contacts between health-care workers and HIV infected individuals.

The risk of acquiring HIV from a single accidental exposure to HIV infected blood has been estimated at 0.38 per cent (95 per cent CI 0.18–0.70 per cent). This is based on 10 seroconversions in 2629 workers who sustained needle-stick injuries, and were included in follow-up studies [39]. The risk for non-parenteral exposure is thought to be much less, but no figure has been established.

Even at these low levels of risk the estimated lifetime risks to surgeons can be substantial, depending on local prevalence of HIV, number of operations being performed and needle-stick injury rate. Parenteral exposure occurs in 1–7 per cent of surgical procedures [73,170,213]. Glove perforation is commonplace [61] with a 55 per cent rate where the operator is performing caesarean section [199].

However, calculation of lifetime risk is dependent on estimates of seroconversion from blunt surgical needle trauma which may not be realistic. So far, studies of health-care workers have not indicated any major excess risk of HIV infection [33,34,132].

HIV infected health-care workers

The only report of transmission to a patient from a health-care worker is the single case of a Florida dentist with AIDS who may have transmitted HIV to five patients. The overall risk of such transfer is thought to be extremely low. Nevertheless, guidelines from the Department of Health and the Medical Defence Union are clear that HIV positive health workers should not perform vaginal or caesarean deliveries. In addition, the General Medical Council recommends that staff who think they have been at risk should be confidentially tested.

Infection control procedures

Basic precautions to avoid exposure to HIV are shown in Box 17.6. Particular issues in obstetrics have been dealt with in the Royal College of Obstetricians and Gynaecologists report [184]. Current opinion favours a high level of universal precautions in surgery or obstetrics, but with risk assessment and additional precautions for high risk patients and procedures. Recommendations for staff involved are shown in Box 17.7. The debate about whether particular precautions should be universal or selective will continue, though it seems clear that some intermediate position will be adopted by most health-care workers [107]. What is often not stressed is that the infected woman should not be subjected to any unnecessary and discriminatory infection control procedures which could isolate her or draw attention to her before other patients or relatives.

Box 17.6. Ways to avoid exposure to HIV and hepatitis in all departments (from [107] with permission)

- Apply basic hygienic practices with regular handwashing
- Cover existing wounds and skin lesions with waterproof dressings
- Take simple protective measures to avoid contamination of person and clothing with blood
- Protect mucous membrane of eyes, mouth and nose from blood splashes
- Take care to prevent wounds, cuts and abrasions in presence of blood
- Avoid use of sharps whenever possible
- Ensure safe handling and disposal of sharps
- Clear spillages of blood promptly and disinfect surfaces
- Ensure safe disposal of contaminated water

Box 17.7. Precautions recommended for staff (from [107] with permission)

- Invasive procedures in all patients
  - Have vaccination against hepatitis B
  - Cover all cuts and abrasions with waterproof dressings
  - Do not pass sharps hand to hand
  - Do not use hand needles
  - Do not guide needles with fingers
  - Do not re-sheath needles
  - Dispose of all sharps safely into approved containers
  - Put disposables and waste into yellow clinical waste bags for incineration
- Additional precautions when caring for known HIV and hepatitis B virus positive and high risk patients
  - Consider non-operative management
  - Remove unnecessary equipment from theatre
  - Observe highest level of theatre discipline
  - Have only experienced surgeons and health-care workers in theatre
  - Use: double glove, high efficiency masks, eye protection, boots, impervious gowns, closed wound drainage
  - Use disposable anaesthetic circuitry or appropriate method of decontamination
  - Disinfect theatre floor with hypochlorite (refer to local policies)

The future

There are likely to be important advances in treatment over the next few years, with results of trials of protease inhibitors, new antiretrovirals and vaccines becoming available. Prognostic indicators, for both maternal survival and vertical transmission, should become more precise. More information will become available about the possible protective effect of caesarean section on perinatal transmission, and also about how transmission may be modified by zidovudine, hyperimmunoglobulin local antivirals or soluble CD4. Increased identification of infected mothers and children, with improvement in organization of care, optimal timing of initiation of treatment, and advances in treatment should combine to ensure much longer survival, with a better quality of life.

Nevertheless there are uncertainties about related problems, such as multidrug resistant tuberculosis, and about health-care costs. How quickly the pandemic will continue to grow remains unclear. One important feature of HIV disease is that it predominantly targets young, productive adults in the prime of life. These are the individuals who normally have a low mortality and morbidity, and who provide much of the impetus to the national and domestic economy. The particular contribution of women, both in terms of the economy and the support of the young, old and infirm is critical, and the effect of widespread illness in young women may have profound effects on the economies of some countries and the support structure and stabilizing forces within the economy.

References

1 Ades AE, Parker S *et al*. Prevalence of maternal HIV-1 infection in Thames regions: results from anonymous unlinked neonatal testing. *Lancet* 1991; **337**: 1562–5.

2 Ades AE, Parker S *et al*. Two methods for assessing the risk factor composition of the HIV-1 epidemic in heterosexual women: South East England 1988–1991. *AIDS* 1992; **6**: 1031–6.

3 Allain JP, Mathews T *et al*. *Antibody to* V_3 *Loop Peptide does not Predict Vertical Transmission of HIV. Seventh International Conference on AIDS, Florence, June 1991*. Abstract WC3263.

4 American Thoracic Society and Centers for Disease Control. Treatment of tuberculosis and tuberculosis infection in adults and children. *American Review of Respiratory Disease* 1986; **134**: 355–63.

5 Andiman WA, Simpson BJ, Olson B, Dember L, Silva TJ & Miller G. Rate of transmission of human immunodeficiency virus 1 infection in infants: *in vitro* production of virus-specific antibody in lymphocytes. *Pediatric Infectious Disease Journal* 1990; **9**: 26–30.

6 Anonymous. Zidovudine for the prevention of HIV transmission from mother to infant. *Morbidity and Mortality Weekly Report* 1994, **43**: 285–7.

7 Antoine C, Morris M & Douglas D. Maternal and fetal mortality in acquired immunodeficiency syndrome. *New York State Journal of Medicine* 1986; **86**: 443–5.

8 Araneta MR, Lemp GJ *et al*. *Survival Trends among Women with AIDS in San Francisco. Seventh International Conference on AIDS, Florence, 1991*. Abstract MC 3122.

9 Banatvala JE, Chrystie IL. HIV screening in pregnancy: UK lags. *Lancet* 1994; **343**: 1113–14.

10 Barre-Sinoussi F, Cherma J-C *et al*. Isolation of a T lymphotropic retrovirus from a patient at risk from acquired immune deficiency syndrome (AIDS). *Science* 1983; **220**: 868–71.

11 Barrett JFR, Savage J, Phillipps K & Lilford RJ. Randomised trial of amniotomy in labour versus the intention to leave membranes intact until the second stage. *British Journal of Obstetrics and Gynaecology* 1992; **99**: 5–9.

12 Bayer R, Levine E & Wolf SM. HIV antibody screening: an ethical framework for evaluating proposal programmes. *Journal of the American Medical Association* 1986; **256**: 1768–74.

13 Beach RS, Garcia ER, Sosa R & Good RA. *Pneumocystis carinii* pneumonia in an HIV-1 infected neonate with theconium aspiration. *Pediatric Infectious Diseases Journal* 1991; **10**: 953–4.

14 Berrebi A, Kobuch WE, Puel J, Tricoire J, Herne P & Fournie A. *Effects of HIV Infection on Pregnancy. Fifth International Conference on AIDS, Montreal, 1989*. Abstract MBP25.

15 Berrebi A, Kobuch WE *et al*. Influence of pregnancy on human immunodeficiency virus disease. *European Journal of Obstetrics, Gynecology and Reproductive Biology* 1990; **37**: 211–17.

16 Berrebi A, Lahlov M *et al*. *Effects of HIV Infection on Pregnancy. Seventh International Conference on AIDS, Florence, June 1991*. Abstract WB2042.

17 Beyssen V, Meyohas MC *et al*. *Neutralization Titers in Sera from HIV-infected Pregnant Women, and their Correlation with Materno-fetal Transmission. Seventh International Conference on AIDS, Florence, June 1991*. Abstract WA1344.

18 Biedermann K, Rudin C *et al*. *Immune Parameters in HIV-positive Pregnant Women. Eighth International Conference on AIDS, Amsterdam, 1992*. Abstract PoC4725.

19 Biggar RJ, Pahwa S *et al*. Immunosuppression in

pregnant women infected with HIV. *American Journal of Obstetrics and Gynecology* 1989; **161**: 1239–44.

20 Bird AG. Monitoring of disease progression of HIV infection. In: Bird AG (ed), *Immunology of HIV Infection*. Kluwer Academic Publishers, London, 1992: 91–112.

21 Blanche S, Rouzioux C *et al*. A prospective study of infants born to women seropositive for human immunodeficiency virus type 1. HIV Infection in Newborns French Collaborative Study Group. *New England Journal of Medicine* 1989; **320**: 1643–8.

22 Blanche S, Tardieu M *et al*. Longitudinal study of 94 symptomatic infants with perinatally acquired human immunodeficiency virus infection. Evidence for a bimodal expression of clinical and biological symptoms. *American Journal of Diseases of Children* 1990; **144**: 1210–15.

23 Blaxhult A, Granath F, Lidman K & Giesecke J. The influence of age on the latency period to AIDS in people infected by HIV through blood transfusion. *AIDS* 1990; **4**: 125–9.

24 Bledsoe K, Olopoenia L, Barnes S, Delapenha R, Saxinger C & Frederick W. *Effect of Pregnancy on Progression of HIV Infection. Sixth International Conference on AIDS, San Francisco, 1990*. Abstract ThC652.

25 Boyd KM. HIV infection: the ethics of anonymised testing and of testing pregnant women. *Journal of Medical Ethics* 1990; **16**: 173–8.

26 Brabin BJ. Epidemiology of infection in pregnancy. *Review of Infectious Diseases* 1985; **7**: 579–603.

27 Braddick MR, Kreiss JK *et al*. Impact of maternal HIV infection on obstetrical and early neonatal outcome. *AIDS* 1990; **4**: 1001–5.

28 Brettle RP. Pregnancy and its effect on HIV/AIDS. Baillière's Clinical Obstetrics and Gynaecology. Baillière Tindall, London, 1992; **6**: 125–36.

29 Briggs GG, Freeman RK & Yaffe SJ (eds), *Drugs in Pregnancy and Lactation*. Williams and Wilkins, Baltimore, Maryland, 1986.

30 Brossard Y, Goudeau A *et al*. *A Sero-epidemiological Study of HIV in 15,465 Pregnant Women. Proceedings of the Fourth International Conference on AIDS, Stockholm, 1988*. 4632: 219.

31 Bulterys M, Chao A *et al*. *Maternal HIV Infection and Intrauterine Growth: A Prospective Cohort study in Butare, Rwanda. Seventh International Conference on AIDS, Florence, June 1991*. Abstract WC3224.

32 Centers for Disease Control. Classification system for human T-lymphotropic virus type III/lymphadenopathy-associated virus infections. *Morbidity and Mortality Weekly Reports* 1987; **36**: 334–9.

33 Centers for Disease Control. Preliminary analysis: HIV serosurvey of orthopedic surgeons, 1991. *Morbidity and Mortality Weekly Reports* 1991; **40**: 309–12.

34 Chamberland ME, Conely LJ *et al*. Health care workers with AIDS. *Journal of the American Medical Association* 1991; **266**: 3459–62.

35 Chiphangwi J, Nawrocki P, Dallabetta G, Hoover D, Odaka N & Saah A. *Post Partum T Lymphocyte Changes in HIV-1 Seropositive and Seronegative Malawian Women. Seventh International Conference on AIDS, Florence, 1991*. Abstract WC3233.

36 Cilla G, Trallero EP, Furundarena JR, Duadrado E, Iribarren JA & Neira F. Esophageal candidiasis and immunodeficiency associated with acute HIV infection. *AIDS* 1988; **2**: 399–400.

37 Ciraru-Vigneron N, Lefevre-Elbert V *et al*. *Evolution and Prognostic Value of Lymphocyte Count During Pregnancy in Healthy Women and HIV-infected Women. Eighth International Conference on AIDS, Amsterdam, 1992*. Abstract PoB3048.

38 Clavel F, Guetard B *et al*. Isolation of a new human retrovirus from West African patients with AIDS. *Science* 1986; **233**: 343–6.

39 Cockroft A. Nosocomial infection and infectious control procedures. In: Johnson M & Johnstone FD (eds) *HIV in Women*. Churchill Livingstone, Edinburgh, 1993: 273–84.

40 Coll O, Torne A *et al*. *Seroprevalence of HIV Antibodies in Barcelona's Obstetrical Population. Screening is not Justified in Non-risk Groups. Proceedings of the Seventh International Conference on AIDS, Florence, 1991*. WC3281, p 366.

41 Committee Report. Prevention of perinatal transmission of hepatitis B virus: prenatal screening of all pregnant women for hepatitis B surface antigen. *New York State Journal of Medicine* 1989; **89**: 352–4.

42 Concorde Coordinating Committee. Concorde: MRC/ANRS randomised double-blind controlled trial of immediate and deferred zidovudine in symptom-free HIV infection. *Lancet* 1994; **343**: 871–81.

43 Connor E, Goode L *et al*. *Seroprevalence of Human Immunodeficiency Virus (HIV) of Parturients at University Hospital, New Jersey, USA. Proceedings of the Fourth International Conference on AIDS, Stockholm, 1988*. Abstract 685: 375.

44 Cooper DA, Tindall B, Wilson EJ, Imrie AA & Penny R. Characterisation of T lymphocyte responses during primary infection with human immunodeficiency virus infection. *Journal of Infection* 1988; **157**: 889–96.

45 Courgnaud V, Laure F *et al*. Frequent and early in utero HIV-1 infection. *AIDS Research and Human Retroviruses* 1991; **7**: 337–41.

46 Couturier E, Brossard Y *et al*. HIV infection at outcome of pregnancy in the Paris area, France. *Lancet* 1992; **340**: 707–9.

47 Crane L, Schuman P *et al*. *Failure of Zidovudine (ZDV) to Prevent Vertical Transmission of HIV. Seventh International Conference on AIDS, Florence, June 1991*. Abstract MC3182.

48 Creagh T, Thompson M *et al*. *Gender Differences in the Spectrum of HIV Disease. Eighth International Conference on AIDS, Amsterdam, 1992*. Abstract MoC0032.

49 Crombleholme W, Wara D & Cambertoglio J. *Peri-*

natal HIV Transmission Despite Maternal/Infant AZT Therapy. Sixth International Conference on AIDS, San Francisco, 1990. Abstract ThC605.

50 Dabis F. *Methodological Issues in Mother-to-Child Transmission of HIV. Eighth International Conference on AIDS, Amsterdam 1992.* Abstract PoC4218.

51 de Martino M, Tovo P-A *et al.* HIV transmission through breast milk: appraisal of risk according to duration of feeding. *AIDS* 1992; **6**: 991–7.

52 Debouck C. The HIV-1 protease as a therapeutic target for AIDS. *AIDS Research and Human Retroviruses* 1992; **8**: 153–64.

53 Delfraissey JF, Pons JC *et al. Does Pregnancy Influence Disease Progression in HIV Positive Women. Fifth International Conference on AIDS, Montreal, 1989.* Abstract MBP34.

54 Deschamps M-M, Pape JW, Madhavan S & Johnson WD Jr. *Pregnancy and Acceleration of HIV Related Illness. Fifth International Conference on AIDS, Montreal, 1989.* Abstract MBP6.

55 Devash Y, Calvelli TA, Wood DG, Reagan KJ & Rubinstein A. Vertical transmission of human immunodeficiency virus is correlated with the absence of high affinity/avidity maternal antibodies to the gp120 principal neutralizing domain. *Proceedings of the National Academy of Science, USA* 1990; **87**: 3445–9.

56 Di Lenardo L, Truscia D, Giaquinto C & Grella PV. *A Prospective Study of HIV Pregnant Women. V International Conference on AIDS, Montreal, 1989.* Abstract MBP14.

57 Dinsmoor, MJ. HIV infection and pregnancy. *Medical Clinics of North America* 1989; **73**: 701–11.

58 Diro M & Beydoun SN. Malaria in pregnancy. *Southern Medical Journal* 1982; **75**: 959–62.

59 Dorrucci M, Rezza G *et al. Age Accelerates the Progression from HIV-Seroconversion to AIDS in Women. Eighth International Conference on AIDS, Amsterdam, 1992.* Abstract MoC0033.

60 Downs AM, Ancelle-Park RA & Brunet JB. Surveillance of AIDS in the European Community: recent trends and predictions to 1991. *AIDS* 1990; **4**: 1117–24.

61 Doyle PM, Alvi S & Johanson R. The effectiveness of double-gloving in obstetrics and gynaecology. *British Journal of Obstetrics and Gynaecology* 1992; **99**: 83–4.

62 Dunn DT, Newell ML, Mayaux MJ, Kind C, Hutto C, Goedert JJ, Andiman W. Perinatal AIDS Collaborative Transmission Studies. Mode of delivery and vertical transmission of HIV-1: a review of prospective studies. *Journal of AIDS* 1994 (in press).

63 Dunn DT, Newell ML, Aden AE & Peckham CS. Risk of human immunodeficiency virus type 1 transmission through breast feeding. *Lancet* 1992; **340**: 585–8.

64 Ehrnst A, Lindgren S *et al.* HIV in pregnant women and their offspring: Evidence for late transmission. *Lancet* 1991; **338**: 203–7.

65 European Collaborative Study. Mother to child transmission of HIV infection. *Lancet* 1988; **ii**: 1039–42.

66 European Collaborative Study. Children born to women with HIV-1 infection: natural history and risk of transmission. *Lancet* 1991; **337**: 253–8.

67 European Collaborative Study. Risk factors for mother-to-child transmission of HIV-1. *Lancet* 1992; **339**: 1007–12.

68 European Collaborative Study. Caesarean section and risk of vertical transmission of HIV-1 infection. *Lancet* 1994; **343**: 1464–67.

69 Feingold A, Vermund SH *et al.* Cervical cytologic abnormalities and papillomavirus in women infected with human immunodeficiency virus. *AIDS* 1990; **3**: 896–903.

70 Fischl MA, Richman DD *et al.* The efficacy of azidothymidine (AZT) in the treatment of patients with AIDS or AIDS related complex: a double-blind placebo-controlled trial. *New England Journal of Medicine* 1987; **317**: 185–91.

71 Fleming PL, Ciesieiski CA & Berkelman RL. *Sex-Specific Differences in the Prevalence of AIDS-Indicative Diagnoses. United States 1988–1989. Seventh International Conference on AIDS, Florence, 1991.* Abstract MC3210.

72 Fuith LC, Czarnecki M, Wachter H & Fuchs D. Mode of delivery in HIV-1 infected women (letter). *Lancet* 1992; **339**: 1603.

73 Geberding JL, Littell C *et al.* Risk of exposure of surgical personnel to patients' blood during surgery at San Francisco General Hospital. *New England Journal of Medicine* 1990; **322**: 1788–93.

74 Gill ON, Adler MW & Day NE. Monitoring the prevalence of HIV. *British Medical Journal* 1989; **299**: 1295–8.

75 Gioannini P, Sinicco A *et al.* HIV infection acquired by a nurse. *European Journal of Epidemiology* 1988; **4**: 119–20.

76 Gloeb DJ, Lai S, Efantis J & O'Sullivan MJ. Survival and disease progression in human immunodeficiency virus-infected women after an index delivery. *American Journal of Obstetrics and Gynecology* 1992; **167**: 152–7.

77 Gloeb DJ, O'Sullivan MJ & Efantis J. Human immunodeficiency virus infection in women 1. The effects of human immunodeficiency virus on pregnancy. *American Journal of Obstetrics and Gynecology* 1988; **159**: 756–61.

78 Goedert JJ, Duliege AM, Amos CI, Felton S & Biggar RJ. High risk of HIV-1 infection for first born twins. The International Registry of HIV-Exposed Twins. *Lancet* 1991; **338**: 1471–5.

79 Goedert JJ, Mendez H *et al.* Mother-to-infant transmission of human immunodeficiency virus type 1: association with prematurity or low anti-gp120. *Lancet* 1989; **ii**: 1351–4.

80 Gold E & Nankervis GA. Cytomegalovirus. In: Evans AS (ed), *Viral Infections in Humans*. Plenum Medical, New York, 1989: 175–89.

81 Goldberg D & Johnstone FD. HIV testing programmes in pregnancy. *Baillières Clinical Obstetrics and Gynaecology* 1992; **3**: 33–51.

82 Goldberg D, MacKinnon H *et al*. Prevalence of human immunodeficiency virus among childbearing women and those undergoing termination of pregnancy. *British Medical Journal* 1992; **304**: 1082–5.

83 Graham NMH, Zeger SL *et al*. Effect of zidovudine and *Pneumocystis carinii* pneumonia prophylaxis on progression of HIV-1 infection to AIDS. *Lancet* 1991; **338**: 265–9.

84 Griffiths PD, Baboonian C, Rutter D & Peckham C. Congenital and maternal cytomegalovirus infections in a London population. *British Journal of Obstetrics and Gynaecology* 1991; **98**: 135–40.

85 Guay L, Mmiro F *et al*. *Perinatal Outcome in HIV Infected Women in Uganda. Sixth International Conference on Aids, San Francisco, 1990*. Abstract ThC42.

86 Gwinn M, Pappaloanou M *et al*. Prevalence of HIV infection in child-bearing women in the United States. *Journal of the American Medical Association* 1991; **265**: 1704–8.

87 Hague RA, MacCallum L *et al*. Maternal factors in HIV transmission. *International Journal AIDS* 1993; **4**: 142–6.

88 Halsey NA, Markham R *et al*. *V_3 loop Peptide Antibodies in Haitian Women and Infant HIV-1 Infections. Seventh International Conference on AIDS, Florence, June 1991*. Abstract WA13.

89 Haseltine WA. Molecular biology of HIV-1. In: Dalgleish AG & Weiss R (eds), *AIDS and the New Viruses*. Academic Press, London, 1990: 11–40.

90 Hicks ML, Nolan GH, Maxwell SL & Mickle C. Acquired immunodeficiency syndrome and *Pneumocystis carinii* infection in a pregnant woman. *Obstetrics and Gynecology* 1990; **76**: 480–1.

91 Hira SK, Kamanga J *et al*. Perinatal transmission of HIV-1 in Zambia. *British Medical Journal* 1989; **299**: 1250–2.

92 Hofmann B, Wang Y, Cumberland WG, Detels R, Bozorgmerhri M & Fahey JL. Serum β_2-microglobulin level increases in HIV infection: related to seroconversion, CD4 T-cell fall and prognosis. *AIDS* 1990; **4**: 207–14.

93 Holman S. HIV counselling for women of reproductive age. *Baillières Clinical Obstetrics and Gynaecology* 1992; **6**: 53–68.

94 Horsburgh CR, Hanson D *et al*. *Predictors of Survival in HIV Infection Include CD4+ Cell Counts, AIDS-Defining Condition and Therapy but not Sex, Age, Race, or Risk Activity. Seventh International Conference on AIDS, Florence, 1991*. Abstract MC 3175.

95 Imam N, Carpenter CCJ *et al*. Hierarchical pattern of mucosal *Candida* infections in HIV-seropositive women. *American Journal of Medicine* 1990; **89**: 142–6.

96 Isaksson B, Albert J, Chiodi F, Furucrona A, Krook A & Putkonen P. AIDS two months after primary human immunodeficiency virus infection. *Journal of Infectious Diseases* 1988; **158**: 866–8.

97 Italian Multicentre Study. Epidemiology, clinical features and prognostic factors of paediatric HIV infection. *Lancet* 1988; **ii**: 1043–6.

98 Jensen N, O'Sullivan MJ, Gomez-del-Rio M. Acquired immunodeficiency (AIDS) in pregnancy. *American Journal of Obstetrics and Gynecology* 1984; **148**: 1145–6.

99 Johnstone FD. Antenatal screening for HIV: practical and ethical aspects. Review and case for anonymised unlinked studies. In: Templeton AA & Cusine DJ (eds), *Reproductive Medicine and the Law*. Churchill Livingstone, Edinburgh, 1990: 123–9.

100 Johnstone FD. Management of pregnancy in women with HIV infection. *British Journal of Hospital Medicine* 1992; **48**: 664–70.

101 Johnstone FD. Pregnancy outcome and pregnancy management in HIV infected women. In: Johnstone FD & Johnson MA (eds), *HIV and Women*. Churchill Livingstone, Edinburgh, 1993: 185–96.

102 Johnstone FD, Brettle RP *et al*. Women's knowledge of their HIV antibody state: its effect on their decision whether to continue the pregnancy. *British Medical Journal* 1990; **300**: 23–4.

103 Johnstone FD, Kilpatrick DC & Burns SM. Anticardiolipin antibodies and pregnancy outcome in women with human immunodeficiency virus infection. *Obstetrics and Gynecology* 1992; **80**: 92–6.

104 Johnstone FD, MacCallum L *et al*. Does infection with HIV affect the outcome of pregnancy? *British Medical Journal* 1988; **296**: 467.

105 Johnstone FD, MacCallum LR *et al*. *Population Based Controlled Study: Effects of HIV Infection on Pregnancy. Seventh International Conference on AIDS, Florence, June 1991*. Abstract WC3244.

106 Johnstone FD, Thong KJ, Bird AG, Whitelaw J. Lymphocyte subpopulations in early human pregnancy. *Obstetrics and Gynecology* 1994; **83**: 941–6.

107 Joint Working Party of the Hospital Infection Society and the Surgical Infection Study Group. Risks to surgeons and patients from HIV and hepatitis: guidelines on precautions and management of exposure to blood or body fluids. *British Medical Journal* 1992; **305**: 1337–43.

108 Joncas JM, Delage G *et al*. Acquired (or congenital) immunodeficiency syndrome in infants born of Haitian mothers. *New England Journal of Medicine* 1983; **308**: 842.

109 Jovaisas E, Koch MA *et al*. LAV/HTVL III in a 20 week fetus. *Lancet* 1985; **ii**: 1129.

110 Just J, Louie L *et al*. *Genetic Risk Factors for Perinatally Acquired HIV Infection. Seventh International Conference on AIDS, Florence, June 1991*. Abstract MC3044.

111 Just J, Louie L *et al*. *HLA Genotype and Risk of Vertical*

Transmission of HIV. Eighth International Conference on AIDS 1992, Amsterdam. Abstract POC 4225 PC282.

112 Kamenga M, Manzila T *et al*. *Maternal HIV Infection and Other Sexually Transmitted Diseases and Low Birth Weight in Zairian Children. Seventh International Conference on AIDS, Florence, June 1991*. Abstract WC3244.

113 Karn J. Control of HIV by tat, rev, ref and protease genes. *Current Opinion in Immunology* 1991; **3**: 526–36.

114 Kell PD, Barton SE *et al*. A maternal death caused by AIDS. Case Report. *British Journal of Obstetrics and Gynaecology* 1991; **98**: 725–7.

115 Kent A, Sepkowitz MD *et al*. Pneumothorax in AIDS. *Annals of Internal Medicine* 1991; **114**: 455–9.

116 Kilpatrick DS, Hague RA, Yap PL & Mok JYQ. HLA antigen frequencies in children born to HIV-infected mothers. *Disease Markers* 1991; **8**: 1–6.

117 Koonin LM, Ellerbrock TV *et al*. Pregnancy-associated deaths due to AIDS in the United States. *Journal of the American Medical Association* 1989; **261**: 1306–9.

118 Krasinski K, Borkowsky W, Bebenroth D & Moore T. Failure of voluntary testing for human immunodeficiency virus to identify infected parturient women in a high risk population. *New England Journal of Medicine* 1988; **318**: 185.

119 Krasinski K, Cao Y-Z *et al*. *Elevated Maternal Total and Neutralizing Anti-HIV-1 Antibody Does Not Prevent Perinatal HIV-1. Sixth International Conference on AIDS, San Francisco, June 1990*. Abstract ThC45.

120 Kreiss J, Datta P *et al*. *Vertical Transmission of HIV in Nairobi: Correlation with Maternal Viral Burden. Seventh International Conference on AIDS, Florence, June 1991*. Abstract MC3062.

121 Krivine A, Firtion G, Cao L, Francoval C, Henrion R & Lebon P. HIV replication during the first weeks of life. *Lancet* 1992; **339**: 1187–9.

122 LaGuardia KD. The other sexually transmitted disease: cervical intraepithelial neoplasia. In: Johnson MA, Johnstone FD (eds), *HIV Infection in Women*. Churchill Livingstone, Edinburgh, 1993: 247–61.

123 *Lancet* editorial. Zidovudine for mother, fetus and child: hope or poison? *Lancet* 1994; **344**: 207–9.

124 La Pointe N, Michaud J *et al*. Transplacental transmission of HTLV-III virus. *New England Journal of Medicine* 1985; **312**: 1325–6.

125 Lallemant M, Lallemant-LeCoeur S *et al*. Mother–child transmission of HIV-1 and infant survival in Brazzaville, Congo. *AIDS* 1989; **3**: 643–6.

126 Lasley-Bibbs V, Renzullo P *et al*. *Patterns of Pregnancy and Reproductive Morbidity Among HIV Infected Women in the US Army: A Retrospective Cohort Study. Sixth International Conference on AIDS, San Francisco, 1990*. Abstract ThC655.

127 Lemp GF, Payne SF *et al*. Survival trends for patients with AIDS. *Journal of the American Medical Association* 1990; **263**: 402–6.

128 Leoung GS, Feigl DW Jr *et al*. Aerosolized pentamidine for prophylaxis against *Pneumocystis carinii* pneumonitis – the San Francisco Community Prophylaxis Trial. *New England Journal of Medicine* 1990; **323**: 769–75.

129 Lepage P, Dabis F *et al*. Perinatal transmission of HIV-1: lack of impact of maternal HIV infection on characteristics of live births and on neonatal mortality in Kigali, Rwanda. *AIDS* 1991; **5**: 295–300.

130 Lewis SH, Reynolds-Kohler C, Fox HE & Nelson JA. HIV-1 in trophoblastic and villous Hofbauer cells, and haematological precursors in eight-week fetuses. *Lancet* 1990; **335**: 565–8.

131 Lindan CP, Allen S *et al*. Predictors of mortality among HIV-infected women in Kigali, Rwanda. *Annals of Internal Medicine* 1992; **116**: 320–8.

132 Lot F, Laporte A *et al*. *Differences Between Health Care Workers with AIDS and AIDS Patients? Seventh International Conference on AIDS, Florence 1991*. Abstract WD4152.

133 MacCallum LR, Cowan FM, Whitelaw J, Burns SM & Brettle RP. *Disease Progression Following Pregnancy in HIV Seropositive Women. Fifth International Conference on AIDS, Montreal 1989*. Abstract MBP3.

134 Maiman M, Fruchter RG *et al*. Human immunodeficiency virus infection and cervical neoplasia. *Gynecology and Oncology* 1990; **38**: 377–82.

135 Maiman M, Tarricone N *et al*. Colposcopic evaluation of human immunodeficiency virus-seropositive women. *Obstetrics and Gynecology* 1991; **78**: 84–8.

136 Mano H & Chermann J-C. Fetal human immunodeficiency virus type 1 infection of different organs in the second trimester. *AIDS Research and Human Retroviruses* 1991; **7**: 83–8.

137 Marion RW, Wiznia AA, Hutcheon G & Rubinstein A. Human T-cell lymphotrophic virus III (HTLV-111) embryopathy: a new dysmorphic syndrome associated with intra-uterine HTLV-111 infection. *American Journal of Diseases of Children* 1986; **140**: 638–40.

138 Marion RW, Wiznia AA, Hutcheon RG & Rubinstein A. Fetal AIDS syndrome score correlation between severity of dysmorphism and age at diagnosis of immunodeficiency. *American Journal of Diseases of Children* 1987; **141**: 429.

139 Marte C, Kelly P *et al*. Papanicolaou smear abnormalities in ambulatory care sites for women infected with human immunodeficiency virus. *American Journal of Obstetrics and Gynecology* 1992; **166**: 1232–7.

140 Martin AW, Brady K *et al*. Immunohistochemical localization of HIV p24 antigen in placental tissue. *Human Pathology* 1992; **23**: 411–14.

141 Mattern CFT, Murray K, Jensen A, Farzadegan H, Pang J & Modlin JF. Localization of HIV core antigen in term human placentas. *Pediatrics* 1992; **89**: 207–9.

142 Maury W, Potts BJ & Rabson AB. HIV-1 infection of first trimester and term human placental tissue: a possible mode of maternal-fetal transmission. *Journal of Infectious Diseases* 1989; **160**: 583–8.

143 Mazzarello G, Canessa A *et al. Influence of Pregnancy on HIV Disease Progression. Seventh International Conference on AIDS, Florence, 1991*. Abstract WC3235.
144 McCabe RE & Remington JS. *Toxoplasma gondii*. In: Mandell GL, Douglas JR & Bennett JE (eds), *Principles and Practice of Infectious Diseases*. Churchill Livingstone, New York, 1990: 2091–3.
145 McCarthy KH, Johnson MA & Studd JWW. Antenatal HIV testing. *British Journal of Obstetrics and Gynaecology* 1992; **99**: 867–8.
146 McClure MO & Dalgleish AG. Human immunodeficiency virus and the immunology of infection. *Baillières Clinical Obstetrics and Gynaecology*, 1992; **6**: 1–12.
147 Melmed RN, Taylor JM *et al*. Serum neoprotein changes in HIV-infected subjects: indicator of significant pathology, CD4 cell change, and the development of AIDS. *AIDS* 1989; **2**: 70–6.
148 Metz KJ, Parker AL & Halpin GJ. Pregnancy-related mortality in New Jersey, 1975–1989. *American Journal of Public Health* 1992; **82**: 595–9.
149 Miedema F, Petit AJC *et al*. Immunological abnormalities in human immunodeficiency virus (HIV) infected asymptomatic homosexual men. HIV affects the immune system before $CD4^+$ T helper cell depletion occurs. *Journal of Clinical Investigation* 1988; **82**: 1908–14.
150 Minkoff HL. AIDS in pregnancy. *Current Problems in Obstetrics, Gynecology and Fertility* 1989; **12**: 206–28.
151 Minkoff HL & Dehovitz JA. Care of women infected with the human immunodeficiency virus. *Journal of the American Medical Association* 1991; **266**: 2253–8.
152 Minkoff H, de Regt RH, Landesman S & Schwarz R. *Pneumocystis carinii* pneumonia associated with acquired immunodeficiency syndrome in pregnancy: a report of three maternal deaths. *Obstetrics and Gynecology* 1986; **67**: 284–7.
153 Minkoff HL, Henderson C *et al*. Pregnancy outcomes among mothers infected with human immunodeficiency virus and uninfected control subjects. *American Journal of Obstetrics and Gynecology* 1990; **163**: 1598–604.
154 Minkoff HL & Moreno JD. Drug prophylaxis for human immunodeficiency virus-infected pregnant women: ethical considerations. *American Journal of Obstetrics and Gynecology* 1990; **163**: 1111–14.
155 Minkoff HL, Nanda D *et al*. Follow-up of mothers of children with AIDS. *Obstetrics and Gynecology* 1987; **87**: 288–91.
156 Miotti PG, Dallabetta GA *et al*. A retrospective study of childhood mortality and spontaneous abortion in HIV-1 infected women in urban Malawi. *International Journal of Epidemiology* 1992; **21**: 792–9.
157 Miotti PG, Dallabetta GA *et al*. HIV-1 and pregnant women: associated factors, prevalence, estimate of incidence and role in fetal wastage in central Africa. *AIDS* 1990; **4**: 733–6.
158 Mitchell JL, Brown GM, Loftman P & Williams SB. HIV infection in pregnancy: detection, counselling and care. *Pediatric AIDS and HIV infection: Fetus to adolescent*. 1990; **1**: 78–82.
159 Moatti JP, Gales C *et al*. Social acceptability of HIV screening among pregnant women. *AIDS Care* 1990; **2**: 213–22.
160 Mofenson LM & Burns DN. Passive immunisation to prevent mother-infant transmission of human immunodeficiency virus: current issues and future directions. *Pediatric Infectious Disease Journal* 1991; **10**: 456–62.
161 Mok JYQ. Vertical transmission. In: Johnstone FD & Johnson M (eds), *HIV Infection in Women*. Churchill Livingstone, Edinburgh, 1993: 197–209.
162 Moore RD, Hidalgo J *et al*. Zidovudine and the natural history of AIDS. *New England Journal of Medicine* 1991; **324**: 1412–16.
163 Moss AR & Bacchetti P. Natural history of HIV infection. *AIDS* 1989; **3**: 55–61.
164 Nachman S. *HIV Infection During Pregnancy: A Longitudinal Study. Third International Conference on AIDS, Washington DC, 1987*. Abstract TP55.
165 Newell ML, Peckham CS. Working towards a European strategy for intervention to reduce vertical transmission of HIV. 1994; **101**: 192–6.
166 Nicolas S. Is there an HIV associated facial dysmorphism? *Pediatric Annals* 1988; **5**: 353.
167 Nsvami M, St Louis M *et al. Low Prevalence in HIV-Infected Zairian Mothers of Antibodies Against gp120 Neutralizing Epitopes of the MN HIV-1 Isolate Lack of Association with Perinatal HIV Transmission. Seventh International Conference on AIDS, Florence, June 1991*. Abstract MC3065.
168 Nzila N, Laga M, Brown C, Jingu M & Kivuvu M. *Does Pregnancy in HIV(+) Women Accelerate Progression to AIDS? Seventh International Conference on AIDS, Florence, 1991*. Abstract MC3149.
169 Palestine AG, Polis MA *et al*. A randomised, controlled trial of foscarnet in the treatment of cytomegalovirus retinitis in patients with AIDS. *Annals of Internal Medicine* 1991; **115**: 665–73.
170 Panlilio AL, Foy DR *et al*. Blood contacts during surgical procedures. *Journal of the American Medical Association* 1991; **265**: 1533–7.
171 Parekh BS, Shaffer N *et al*. Lack of correlation between maternal antibodies to V3 loop peptides of gp120 and perinatal HIV-1 transmission. *AIDS* 1991; **5**: 1179–84.
172 Peckham CS, Tedder RS *et al*. Prevalence of maternal HIV infection based on unlinked anonymous testing of newborn babies. *Lancet* 1990; **335**: 516–19.
173 Pedersen C, Gerstoft J, Lindhardt BO & Sindrup J. *Candida* oesophagitis associated with acute human immunodeficiency virus infection. *Journal of Infectious Diseases* 1987; **156**: 529–30.
174 Peutherer JF, Rebus S *et al. Detection of HIV in the fetus: A study of six cases. Fourth International Confer-*

ence on AIDS, Stockholm, June 1988. Abstract 7235.

175 Piot P, Laga M *et al*. The global epidemiology of HIV infection: continuity, heterogeneity, and change. *AIDS* 1990; **3**: 403–12.

176 Priolo L & Minkoff HL. HIV infection in women. *Baillière's Clinics in Obstetrics and Gynaecology* 1992; **6**: 617–28.

177 Quazi QH, Sheikh TM & Fikrig S. Lack of evidence for craniofacial dysmorphism in perinatal HIV infection. *Journal of Pediatrics* 1988; **112**: 7–11.

178 Qu Zhang L, Simmonds P, Ludlam CA & Leigh Brown AJ. Detection, quantification and sequencing of HIV-1 from the plasma of seropositive individuals and from factor VIII concentrates. *AIDS* 1991; **5**: 675–81.

179 Remington JS & Desmonts G. Toxoplasmosis. In: Remington JS & Klein JD (eds), *Infections for the Fetus and Newborn Infant*. WB Saunders, Philadelphia, 1990; 89–195.

180 Ribble D, Marte C, Tiersten A, Kelly J, Keyes C & Wolbert J. *Difference in Stage of Presentation and Presenting Symptoms Between Women and Men in a Primary Care AIDS Clinic. Fifth International Conference on AIDS, Monstreal, 1989*. Abstract WDP40: 749.

181 Robertson CA, Mok JYQ *et al*. Maternal antibodies to gp120 V_3 sequence do not correlate with protection against vertical transmission of human immunodeficiency virus. *Journal of Infectious Diseases* 1992; **166**: 704–9.

182 Rogers MF, Ou CY *et al*. Use of the polymerase chain reaction for early detection of the proviral sequences of human immunodeficiency virus in infants born to seropositive mothers. New York City Collaborative Study of Maternal HIV Transmission and Montefiore Medical Center HIV Perinatal Transmission Study Group. *New England Journal of Medicine* 1989; **320**: 1649–54.

183 Rossi P, Moschese V *et al*. Presence of maternal antibodies to human immunodeficiency virus 1 envelope glycoprotein gp120 epitopes correlates with the uninfected status of children born to seropositive mothers. *Proceedings of the National Academy of Sciences USA* 1989; **86**: 8055–8.

184 Royal College of Obstetricians and Gynaecologists. *HIV Infection in Maternity Care and Gynaecology—Revised Report of RCOG Subcommittee*. RCOG, London, 1990.

185 Rudin C, Meier D *et al*. *Intrauterine onset of symptomatic HIV disease. Eighth International Conference on AIDS, Amsterdam, 1992*. Abstract PoC4734.

186 Ryder RW, Nsa W *et al*. Perinatal transmission of the human immunodeficiency virus type 1 to infants of seropositive women in Zaire. *New England Journal of Medicine* 1989; **320**: 1637–42.

187 Schafer A, Friedman W, Mielke M, Schwartlander B & Koch MA. The increased frequency of cervical dysplasia-neoplasia in women infected with the human immunodeficiency virus is related to the degree of immunosuppression. *American Journal of Obstetrics and Gynecology* 1991; **164**: 593–9.

188 Schoenbaum EE, Davenny K & Holbrook K. The management of HIV disease in pregnancy. *Baillière's Clinical Obstetrics and Gynaecology* 1992; **6**: 101–24.

189 Schoenbaum EE, Davenny K, Selwyn PA, Hartel D & Rogers M. *The Effect of Pregnancy on Progression of HIV Related Disease. Fifth International Conference on AIDS, Montreal, 1989*. Abstract MBP8.

190 Scott GB, Fischl MA *et al*. Mothers of infants with the acquired immunodeficiency syndrome. Evidence for both symptomatic and asymptomatic carriers. *Journal of the American Medical Association* 1985; **253**: 363–6.

191 Selwyn PA & Antoniello P. Reproductive decision-making among women with HIV infection. In: Johnson M & Johnstone FD (eds), *HIV in Women*. Churchill Livingstone, Edinburgh 1993: 171–83.

192 Selwyn PA, Carter RJ *et al*. Knowledge of HIV antibody status and decision to continue or terminate pregnancy among intravenous drug users. *Journal of the American Medical Association* 1989; **261**: 3567–71.

193 Selwyn PA, Hartel D *et al*. A prospective study of the risk of tuberculosis among intravenous drug users with human immunodeficiency virus infection. *New England Journal of Medicine* 1989; **320**: 545–50.

194 Selwyn PA, Schoenbaum EE *et al*. Prospective study of human immunodeficiency virus infection and pregnancy outcomes in intravenous drug users. *Journal of the American Medical Association* 1989; **261**: 1289–94.

195 Semprini AE, Ravizza M *et al*. Perinatal outcome in HIV-infected pregnant women. *Gynecologic and Obstetric Investigation* 1990; **30**: 15–18.

196 Shaffer N, Parekh BS *et al*. *Maternal Antibodies to V_3 Loop Peptides of gp120 are Not Associated With Bulk of Perinatal HIV-1 Transmission. Seventh International Conference on AIDS, Florence, June 1991*. Abstract WC48.

197 Sher L. Counselling around HIV testing in women of reproductive age. In: Johnstone FD & Johnson M (eds), *HIV and Women*. Churchill Livingstone, Edinburgh, 1993: 17–35.

198 Siegel G, Schafer A *et al*. *HIV-1 in Fetal Organs and in Embryonic Placenta of HIV-1 Positive Mothers. Sixth International Conference on AIDS, San Francisco, June 1990*. Abstract FB445.

199 Smith JR & Grant JM. The incidence of glove puncture during caesarean section. *Journal of Obstetrics and Gynaecology* 1990; **10**: 316–18.

200 Smith JR, Kitchen VS *et al*. Is HIV infection associated with an increase in the prevalence of cervical neoplasia? *British Journal of Obstetrics and Gynaecology* 1993; **100**: 149–53.

201 Soeiro LR, Rashbaum WK *et al*. *The Incidence of Human Fetal HIV-1 Infection as Determined by the Presence of HIV-1 Infection as Determined by the Presence of HIV-1 DNA in Abortus Tissues. VII International Conference on*

AIDS, Florence, June 1991. Abstract WC3250.

202 Sperling RS. Prophylaxis and treatment during pregnancy. In: Johnstone FD & Johnson M (eds), *HIV in Women*. Churchill Livingstone, Edinburgh 1993: 211–19.

203 Sperling RS, Sacks HS *et al*. Umbilical cord serosurvey for human immunodeficiency virus in parturient women in a voluntary hospital in New York City. *Obstetrics and Gynecology* 1989; **73**: 179–81.

204 Sperling RS, Stratton P *et al*. A survey of zidovudine use in pregnant women with human immunodeficiency virus infection. *New England Journal of Medicine* 1992; **326**: 857–61.

205 Sprecher S, Soumenkoff G, Puissant F & Degueldre M. Vertical transmission of HIV in 15 week fetus. *Lancet* 1986; **ii**: 288–9.

206 Szabo S, Miller LH *et al*. *Gender Differences in the Natural History of HIV Infection. VIII International Conference on AIDS, Amsterdam, 1992*. Abstract MoC0030.

207 Tappin DM, Girdwood RWA *et al*. Prevalence of maternal HIV infection in Scotland based on unlinked anonymous testing of newborn babies. *Lancet* 1991; **337**: 1565–7.

208 Temmermann M, Lopita MI, Sanghvi HCG, Sinei SKF, Plummer FA & Piot P. Association of maternal HIV-1 infection with spontaneous abortion. *International Journal of STD and AIDS* 1992; **3**: 418–22.

209 Temmerman M, Mohamed Ali F *et al*. Rapid increase of both HIV-1 infection and syphilis among pregnant women in Nairobi, Kenya. *AIDS* 1992; **6**: 1181–5.

210 Temmermann M, Plummer FA *et al*. Infection with HIV as a risk factor for adverse obstetrical outcome. *AIDS* 1990; **4**: 1087–93.

211 Tersmette M. The role of HIV variability in the pathogenesis of AIDS. In: A Graham Bird (ed), *Immunology of HIV infection*. Kluwer Academic Publications, London, 1992: 31–43.

212 Tindall B, Hing M, Edwards P, Barnes T, Machie A & Cooper DA. Short communication: severe clinical manifestations of primary HIV infection. *AIDS* 1989; **3**: 747–9.

213 Tokars J, Bell D *et al*. *Percutaneous Injuries During Surgical Procedures. Proceedings of the Seventh International Conference on AIDS, Florence, June 1991*, **2**: 83.

214 Weinberg ED. Pregnancy-associated depression of cell-mediated immunity. *Review of Infectious Diseases* 1984; **6**: 814–31.

215 Weinbreck P, Loustaud V *et al*. Postnatal transmission of HIV infection. *Lancet* 1988; **i**: 482.

216 Weniger BG, Limpakarnjanarat K *et al*. AIDS in Thailand. *AIDS* 1991; **5**: 571–85.

217 Wetli CV, Roldan EO & Fujaco RM. Listeriosis as a cause of maternal death: an obstetric complication of the acquired immunodeficiency syndrome (AIDS). *American Journal of Obstetrics and Gynecology* 1983; **147**: 7–9.

218 Working Group on HIV testing of pregnant women and newborns. HIV infection, pregnant women and newborns. *Journal of the American Medical Association* 1990; **264**: 2416–20.

219 Zachar V, Noskov-Lauritsen N *et al*. Susceptibility of cultured human trophoblast to infection with human immunodeficiency virus type 1. *Journal of General Virology* 1991; **72**: 1253–60.

220 Ziegler JB, Cooper DA, Johnson RO & Gold J. Postnatal transmission of AIDS-associated retrovirus from mother to infant. *Lancet* 1985; **i**: 896–8.

221 Zolla-Pazner S & Gorny MK. Passive immunisation for the prevention and treatment of HIV infection. *AIDS* 1992; **6**: 1235–47.

Further reading

Bayer R. As the second decade of AIDS begins: an international perspective on the ethics of the epidemic. *AIDS* 1992; **6**: 527–32.

Berrebi A, Puel J, Tricoire, Herne H & Pontonnier G. *Influence of Gestation on HIV Infection. Sixth International Conference on AIDS, San Francisco, 1990*. Abstract ThC651.

Bisalinkumi E, Nawrocki P *et al*. *T-cell Subset Changes During the After Pregnancy in a Cohort of HIV-1 Seropositive and Seronegative African Mothers. Eighth International Conference on AIDS 1992, Amsterdam*. Abstract POA 2086 PA17.

Brettle RP, Richardson AM *et al*. *Survival Analysis by Gender and Risk Group for HIV in Edinburgh. Eighth International Conference on AIDS, Amsterdam, 1992*. Abstract MoC0066.

Bulfamante GP, Moneghini L, Viale G, Alfano RM, Ravizza M & Coggi G. *PCR-Southern Blotting Detection of HIV in Fetal Tissues. Eighth International Conference on AIDS 1992, Amsterdam*. Abstract POA 2466 PA80.

Carcassi C, Chiappe F *et al*. *A Study of 9 Infants Born from HIV-1 Positive Mothers who Continued Treatment with AZT During Pregnancy. Seventh International Conference on AIDS, Florence, June 1991*. Abstract WC3228.

Centers for Disease Control. Update: human immunodeficiency virus infection in health care workers exposed to blood of infected patients. *Morbidity and Mortality Weekly Reports* 1987; **36**: 285–9.

Clercq E De. HIV inhibitors targeted at the reverse transcriptase. *AIDS Research and Human Retroviruses* 1992; **8**: 119–34.

Ehrnst A, Sonnerborg A, Bergdahl S & Strannegard O. Efficient isolation of HIV from plasma during different stages of HIV infection. *Journal of Medical Virology* 1988; **26**: 23–32.

Feng T, Anderson J, Ofstead L, Defarrari E, Rocco L & Hutton N. *Obstetric and Perinatal Outcomes in HIV-infected Pregnant Women. Eighth International Conference on AIDS 1992, Amsterdam*. Abstract POB 3686. PB205.

Ferrazin A, Terragna A *et al*. *Zidovudine (ZDV) Therapy on*

HIV Infection During Pregnancy: Assessment of the Effect on the Newborns. VII International Conference on AIDS, Florence, June 1991. Abstract MC3023.

Johnstone FD, Willox L & Brettle RP. Survival time after AIDS in pregnancy. *British Journal of Obstetrics and Gynaecology* 1992; **99**: 633–6.

Leen CLS & Brettle RP. Natural history of HIV infection. In: Graham Bird A (ed), *Immunology of HIV Infection*. Kluwer Academic Publications, London, 1992: 1–30.

McBride G. Vaccines for HIV infected pregnant women? *British Medical Journal* 1991; **303**: 665.

Nixon D. Vaccines for HIV infected pregnant women? (letter) *British Medical Journal* 1991; **303**: 1061.

Nyongo A, Gichangi P, Temmermann M, Ndinya-Achola JO & Piot P. *HIV Infection as a Risk factor for chorioamnionitis in preterm birth. Eighth International Conference on AIDS 1992. Amsterdam*. Abstract POB 3469 PB165.

Rubinstein A, Calvelli T *et al*. *Correlation of Maternofetal (Abortus) HIV-1 Transmission with High Affinity/Avidity Antibodies to the Primary Neutralizing Domain (PND). Seventh International Conference on AIDS, Florence, June 1991*. Abstract MC3052.

Slade MS, Simmons RL *et al*. Immunodepression after major surgery in normal patients. *Surgery* 1975; **78**: 363–72.

Stevenson M, Bukrinsky M & Haggerty S. HIV-1 replication and potential targets for intervention. *AIDS Research and Human Retroviruses* 1992; **8**: 107–17.

Temmermann M, Koduoi T, Plummer FA, Ndinya-Achola JO & Piot P. *Maternal HIV Infection as a Risk Factor for Adverse Obstetrical Outcome. Eighth International Conference on AIDS 1992, Amsterdam*. Abstract POC 4232 PC283.

Vonesch B, Sturchio E *et al*. Detection of HIV-1 genome in leukocytes of human colistrum from anti-HIV-1 seropositive mothers. *AIDS Research and Human Retroviruses* 1992; **8**: 1283–7.

18

Substance Abuse

Michael de Swiet

Effect of opiate abuse on pregnancy and its outcome, 600
Neonatal withdrawal syndrome and other effects on children, 601
Management of pregnancy in the opiate-dependent woman, 602
Alcohol, 604
Cocaine, 605
Lysergic acid diethylamide, cannabis, phencyclidine, amphetamines, toluene, 606

The increase in the number of young people who abuse or are addicted to drugs has brought a corresponding increase in the number of women who abuse drugs during pregnancy. This is more of a problem in the USA from where most of the large series concerning drug abuse in pregnancy have been published; however, drug users are frequently seen in hospitals in the UK, particularly those catering for patients from the centres of large towns. Most of the following comments concern opiate cocaine and alcohol abuse, but since drug users usually abuse several different sorts of drugs, it is difficult to be certain that the effects ascribed to the above drugs are not due to other drugs taken in addition. In recent years the literature has been dominated by the wave of cocaine abuse which has swept over the USA and which has specific pregnancy problems (see below). Also, illicit drugs are so expensive that the drug addict is forced to adopt a very poor standard of living, often indulging in prostitution (with its associated risk of sexually transmitted disease) to pay for her drugs. These nutritional and social factors must also affect the outcome of pregnancy in drug addicts. For comprehensive reviews of the problem of drug abuse in pregnancy in the USA see Finnegan [26,27,28]. Human immunodeficiency virus (HIV) infection which is discussed in Chapter 17 has become the major problem in those who abuse drugs intravenously and in those who use prostitution to finance their drug habits, even if these do not involve needle sharing. For example in New York cocaine abuse increases the risk of the patient having HIV infection fivefold (and syphilis eightfold) [65].

Intravenous drug abuse obviously increases the risk of sepsis. An echocardiographic study from New York [46] showed abnormal valve structure in 21 of 23 intravenous drug abusers with heart murmurs even though they had no other signs or symptoms of heart disease. There should therefore be a much more liberal attitude towards echocardiography in intravenous drug abusers with heart murmurs in pregnancy than in other pregnant patients (see Chapter 5). Mycotic aneurysms [10], epidural abscess [89] and a marked increase in the risk of pneumonia [7] have also been reported.

In addition sharing of needles and syringes increases the risk of rhesus isoimmunization [11] presumably because rhesus negative women receive an innoculum of blood from syringes contaminated by other rhesus positive users.

Effect of opiate abuse on pregnancy and its outcome

Finnegan [27] quotes a number of obstetric complications of opiate abuse including abortion, abruption, breech presentation, previous caesarean section, etc., but she has not controlled for the social deprivation that we have already mentioned. From this point of view, a better series is that of Ostrea and Chavez [67] who studied 830 opiate-dependent mothers delivered in one hospital in Michigan, and compared them with 400 controls matched for social class and race (86 per cent black). The relative risks of meconium-stained amniotic fluid, anaemia, premature rupture of membranes, haemorrhage, multiple pregnancy and intrauterine growth retardation are shown in Table 18.1. It can be seen that the risk of these complications for the drug addict ranges between 1.5 and 5.5 times the risk in the control group. In addition, once born the infant has greater risk of jaundice, aspiration pneumonia (particularly meconium aspiration), transient tachypnoea and congenital abnormalities. The question of neonatal withdrawal is considered below. In contrast to earlier studies [34] the incidence of hyaline membrane disease in the pre-term drug-addicted group was the same as in the pre-term deliveries from the control group.

The congenital abnormalities found were varied; an excess risk has not been found in other studies [27]. At present, this should be considered a chance finding, but something to watch carefully.

It has been suggested that the frequent occurrence of meconium staining of the liquor, and hence of meconium aspiration is part of the fetal response to maternal drug withdrawal. Liu *et al.* [58] cite reports from mothers that increased fetal movements occur before subjective symptoms of withdrawal in the mother. Cardiotocographic findings, and falling maternal oestriol levels, also suggest fetal stress at the time of maternal withdrawal [58]. Experimental data in sheep [87] suggest that a fetal withdrawal syndrome can occur even within a few hours of maternal opiate administration and indicate that the fetus may be continually undergoing withdrawal because of fluctuating maternal opiate levels. In addition, fetal asphyxia may be precipitated by the increased oxygen consumption caused by excessive movement in an already compromised fetus [101].

The excess rate of multiple pregnancy has also been noted by Rementeria *et al.* [71] who found an overall multiple pregnancy rate of one in 32 pregnancies — about three times their usual rate. The excess was largely accounted for by dizygotic twins. Perhaps opiates stimulate the ovary to release an extra follicle, either directly or via the hypothalamus and gonadotrophin release.

Neonatal withdrawal syndrome and other effects on children

This will occur in 60–90 per cent of infants born to drug-dependent women [47,53,98], at between 4 hours and 2 weeks of age. The timing is related to the rate of metabolism of the opiate drugs. Heroin and morphia are metabolized rapidly, and infants

Table 18.1. Antenatal problems (%) and condition of infants at birth (%) in opiate abusers compared to controls* (from [38])

	Abuser ($n = 830$)	Controls ($n = 400$)	Relative risk (abuser/control)
Meconium staining	21.2	13.8	1.5
Anaemia†	13.4	8.2	1.6
Premature rupture of membranes	12.2	7.8	1.6
Haemorrhage (abruption and placenta praevia)	3.0	1.2	2.5
Multiple pregnancy	3.4	1.2	2.8
Premature delivery (<38 weeks)	18.5	9.8	1.9
Small for gestational age‡	16.5	3.0	5.5
Apgar <6 at 1 min	19.9	10.0	2.0
Perinatal mortality	2.7	1.0	2.7

* All differences were statistically significant $p < 0.05$.
† Haemoglobin <10 g/dl.
‡ Less than tenth percentile for weight in the Lubchenco curve.

will develop signs between 4 and 24 hours after delivery. Methadone is metabolized much more slowly, and signs do not occur until 1 day or even 1 week [15] or 2 weeks [27] after delivery.

The neonatal withdrawal syndrome is characterized by signs of central nervous hyperirritability (increased reflexes and tremor) with gastrointestinal dysfunction (continual finger sucking, with regurgitation of feeds and diarrhoea) and respiratory distress [27]. Paediatricians are undecided as to whether treatment should be with dilute opium solutions such as paregoric [26] or barbiturates [26]. In addition, chlorpromazine [15] and diazepam have also been used, but the latter causes a marked impairment in sucking [26].

Neonatal abstinence syndrome has also been reported with other non-narcotic drugs of addiction, such as barbiturates, pentazocine, ethyl alcohol and amphetamines [27].

Infants born to opiate-dependent mothers have an increased risk of dying unexpectedly from sudden infant death syndrome (SIDS). This risk varies from 1.6 per cent [43] to 21.4 per cent [70] compared to the overall population risk of 0.3 per cent [81]. The overall incidence of SIDS is declining; so in a more recent study in Los Angeles, Ward *et al.* [93] found a SIDS rate of 0.9 per cent in infants of substance abusing mothers, 0.1 per cent in infants of controls, still a substantially increased risk. Almost identical data were reported by Durand *et al.* [24] from Oakland also in California, where the SIDS rate was 0.9 per cent in infants of substance abusing mothers, 0.13 per cent in infants of controls. Although there must be social factors accounting, in part, for this increased incidence, it is of great theoretical importance, because of the possible interference by opiates with the normal development of cardiorespiratory control in the newborn infant, either directly or through maternal hypoventilation [64]. The fetuses of women on a methadone maintenance programme show decreased response to maternal carbon dioxide administration as judged by fetal breathing movements and when compared to controls. This response is decreased still further by acute methadone administration [72].

It is encouraging that Sardemann *et al.* [75] who studied 19 infants for 2 years after delivery from drug-addicted mothers in Denmark, did not find any evidence of behavioural disturbance, impaired intelligence, or growth retardation. However, most of the children have spent long periods in institutional care.

In another study opiate addicts were more likely to have been exposed to opiates during their birth than their non-addicted siblings [50]. The opiates were being given for therapeutic pain relief. So it is possible that opiate exposure *in utero* imprints the individual towards opiate addiction in later life.

Management of pregnancy in the opiate-dependent woman

The majority of problems that can occur in drug-dependent women during pregnancy are not specific to drug dependency and could, and do, occur in other women of low social class and poor health and nutrition. Specific problems for the attending doctor relate to the choice of which opiate should be used, and interactions between opiates and other drugs during pregnancy. One further practical problem is that drug addicts usually have very few patent, superficial veins. Indeed they may be the only people that can successfully perform venepuncture on themselves.

In 1973, Zelson *et al.* [98] published a study from New York which purported to show that heroin-exposed infants have a much better neonatal outcome than methadone-exposed infants, with less severe withdrawal symptoms and no cases of hyaline membrane disease despite their prematurity. For these reasons, they suggested that mothers should not be taken off a 'street' supply of heroin by changing them to a methadone maintenance programme. This bold suggestion made quite an impact at the time, but it was challenged, largely because the groups of methadone- and heroin-treated addicts were not necessarily comparable [66]. The general view now is that patients and their offspring are much better managed in a methadone maintenance programme, than trying to obtain heroin or other more rapidly acting opiates illegally. Such a programme will put the addict in contact with medical and social services, and this alone can improve her standard of living sufficiently to benefit her and her infant's health [73]. However, a recent study [25] indicates that although a methadone programme increases the number of prenatal visits in pregnancy, and reduces maternal anaemia, it does not necessarily affect the reduced birthweight or other adverse fetal outcomes in women who abuse opiates.

The reason for using methadone is that it is metabolized much more slowly than heroin (half-life 18–97 hours) and withdrawal symptoms do not occur until 72–96 hours after the last dose. The half-life of heroin is 4–10 hours, and withdrawal symptoms may occur within 24 hours after the last dose. Patients may be maintained on an oral methadone regime and they and their fetuses are much less likely to have withdrawal symptoms than when they are taking heroin. In addition, most countries have narcotics regulations which forbid the supply of heroin to addicts, but will legalize specific individuals to give methadone in cases of addiction. Unfortunately, patients may not like to change from heroin to methadone, because the latter does not produce the same feelings of pleasure. Nevertheless, for the reasons outlined above, all opiate addicts should be transferred to a methadone maintenance programme during pregnancy. The only exceptions are those that present in late pregnancy or during labour.

'Street' heroin is diluted to a varying extent with fillers such as lactose, making it difficult to know exactly how much heroin the addict has in fact been taking. Therefore, transfer to an adequate methadone regime takes time, because of the need to find the right dose and the longer duration of methadone action. There is therefore a risk of precipitating a withdrawal state during transfer, and, as indicated above, this may be particularly dangerous for the fetus. Indeed Liu *et al.* [58] have observed fetal distress in labour not due to recognized causes, which was relieved by administration of pethidine. For these reasons, it is best not to transfer to methadone the addict who presents late in pregnancy as an outpatient. Such patients should ideally be admitted and transferred to methadone with judicious use of short acting narcotics, to render them symptom free, and to prevent fetal distress and premature labour [32]. This is not an easy thing to do because of the manipulating, demanding characteristics of drug addicts, which cause considerable disruption in hospital routine, particularly in maternity hospitals, where the staff may not be experienced in managing such problems.

Analgesia during labour is best given by an epidural anaesthetic. If this is not possible, opiates such as pethidine can be given, but they will be less effective in an opiate addict. Because this effect is rather variable, it is better to give a standard dose, such as pethidine 100 mg intramuscularly more frequently, rather than a large (and possibly too large) dose at standard time intervals.

Pentazocine should not be used because it is a narcotic antagonist, and can precipitate a withdrawal reaction in an opiate addict [32]. Overdose of opiate should be treated with the specific antagonist naloxone which is given in an initial dose of 200 μg, followed by 100 μg every 2 min according to response. The dose given to the neonate is 5–10 μg/kg. Nalorphine should not be used because it causes respiratory depression, even though it is an opiate antagonist. All opiate antagonists may cause very severe withdrawal symptoms in the mother or her child. If necessary, these can be treated with further doses of opiate.

Narcotics interact dangerously with other drugs such as barbiturates, hypnotics, sedatives, general anaesthetics and tranquillizers causing central nervous system depression. These drugs should be given with great care, if at all, to drug addicts. In addition, muscle relaxants, such as D-tubocurarine can interact with opiates to cause severe respiratory depression.

Methadone is secreted in breast milk. The average concentration found by Blinick *et al.* [9] in a group of women taking an average of 52 mg/day was 0.27 μg/ml. This would be equivalent to a daily dose of 0.12 mg in an infant taking 450 ml of milk per day, or 0.04 mg/kg in a 3 kg infant. This is about one-twentieth of the maternal dose of 0.75 mg/kg for a 70 kg mother, and is clearly very little. Since there have been no reports of adverse effects of breast feeding by drug-dependent mothers, it would seem sensible to encourage breast feeding in these patients, particularly since it may be difficult for them to bond to their children. However, in a British series of heroin addicts [53], only four of 23 babies were breast fed successfully and only six were living in families that had a stable relationship. Note also the danger of transmission of HIV infection by breast feeding (see Chapter 17).

Alcohol

The fetal effects of other drugs of dependence are even harder to define than those of opiates, because their abusers do not form such a clear-cut group. However, it is indisputable that alcohol, if taken in sufficient quantities, will produce a specific fetal alcohol syndrome, first described by Jones and Smith [51]. The newborn child is growth retarded, with characteristic facies, narrow palpebral fissures, epicanthal folds, short nose and long philtrum. In addition, the children are often mentally retarded, and may have other major congenital abnormalities such as club foot [39] or chromosome abnormalities [33]. The craniofacial abnormalities may regress as the child grows up but the mental abnormalities do not. Persistent retardation has been documented at age 10 [82] and major social problems have been shown in adolescence [84].

By contrast one advantage of alcohol abuse is that it appears to reduce the risk of respiratory distress syndrome presumably by increasing lung maturation [49].

Although alcohol abuse has been considered to be very uncommon in the UK, Beattie *et al.* [6] have reported 40 cases from the west of Scotland, an area with a notoriously high incidence of alcoholism. Unfortunately measurement of mean corpuscular volume (MCV) and γ glutamyl transpeptidase (GTT) cannot be used very effectively [40] to screen for alcohol intake after the first trimester since both values decline to the normal range in heavy drinkers during the second trimester [5]. For example elevated GGT and elevated MCV predicts only 61 and 41 per cent of adverse fetal effects [97]. Furthermore the evidence from the Charing Cross study [96] is that modest alcohol consumption (1–2 glasses of wine per day) at the time of conception is associated with increased risk of low birthweight. Therefore screening in the antenatal clinic is not the answer. There must be greater awareness of the risk in the general population and in health-care professionals [95]. Although the overall incidence of alcohol consumption in pregnancy may be declining (from 32 per cent in 1985 to 20 per cent in 1988 in the USA [78]), this is not the case for smokers, the unmarried and younger less well-educated women [78].

It is not clear what the minimum daily alcohol intake is that affects the fetus, or the maximum daily intake that is safe. The majority of affected fetuses with full fetal alcohol syndrome has been born to mothers taking large quantities of alcohol: on average, 174 ml/day — the equivalent of at least 17 drinks [69]. However, growth retardation has been reported in patients taking much smaller quantities of alcohol, more than 100–400 ml/week [20] although corrections are not always made for important confounding variables such as smoking, social class [95] and paternal alcohol intake [57]. An intake of 100–140 ml/week is between one and two glasses of wine per day. No short-term detectable effects have been shown at levels of alcohol consumption <100 g per week [29,85].

Variation in the risk of developing fetal alcohol syndrome may relate to the metabolism of acetaldehyde, the first oxidation product of ethanol. Veghely [90] found that the blood level of acetaldehyde in mothers giving birth to a child with fetal alcohol syndrome was >40 μmol/l after a drink of alcohol whereas some heavy drinkers who had normal children had acetaldehyde levels <40 μmol/l. The validity of Veghely's measurements has been challenged [74]. The mechanism of intrauterine growth retardation is unknown. Deficiencies of zinc and copper which may cause growth retardation in other circumstances have been excluded [39].

It is very unlikely that the fetal alcohol syndrome is due to intercurrent consumption of other drugs, because the syndrome is specific to alcoholics, and those taking this quantity of alcohol do not, as a group, consistently abuse any other one drug. Acute intoxication of the infant at birth as would occur following unsuccessful treatment of pre-term labour with alcohol infusion, has been associated with impairment of intellectual development when assessed at 4–7 years [79]. It is postulated that the intoxicated infant does not bond satisfactorily with the mother who may also be intoxicated at birth [79]. The fetal heart trace also shows loss of beat-to-beat variation at maternal blood alcohol levels of 130–290 mg per 100 ml [41]. Such abnormalities should not be thought to indicate acute fetal distress or the necessity for immediate delivery [41].

Alcohol is secreted in breast milk where it achieves approximately the same concentration as in the maternal blood [54]. The dose of alcohol received by the baby will be small [54] but babies consume less milk if their mothers have been drinking [63] and there may be a minor impairment in motor though not mental development when the children are followed up at age 1 year [56]. Maternal alcohol intake also affects the flavour of milk [63]. So for all these reasons, mothers should not drink excessively when breast feeding.

Cocaine

Possible effects of cocaine in pregnancy are of considerable importance in view of the increasing popularity of this drug both in the USA and Europe. It is estimated that 5 million Americans use cocaine regularly and that each day 5000 use it for the first time [19]. Young women are particularly likely to use the drug because it is believed to enhance sexuality. Screening for cocaine and other substances of abuse either by routine testing of pregnant women's urine [61,80] or by testing meconium from her neonate [77] shows that the patient history seriously underestimates the size of the problem [18,61,62,77]. The overall prevalence of cocaine abuse was about 10 per cent in New York [61] and Pennsylvania [77], up to 25 per cent in Washington DC [76] and up to 30 per cent in Detroit [68] though <1 per cent in rural Missouri where alcohol was more of a problem [80].

Cocaine blocks the pre-synaptic uptake of noradrenaline producing excess transmitter and marked activation of the sympathetic nervous system. In the non-pregnant this has lead to myocardial infarction, arrhythmias, rupture of the aorta and cerebrovascular accidents [19]. In pregnancy mechanisms of adverse effect have been well reviewed by Volpe [92]. Congenital malformations reported have been sirenomelia [76], abnormalities of the genitourinary system [38,59] and limb–body abnormalities [88] possibly due to vasospasm in the fetal and uteroplacental circulation at a critical time in embryogenesis [91].

Chasnoff *et al.* [16] compared the offspring of a group of women who only abused marijuana in pregnancy with those who were also exposed to cocaine. Additional cocaine abuse was associated with an increased risk of intrauterine growth retardation; the marijuana-exposed group having reduced head size at birth alone. Several psychomotor indices remained impaired in the children at follow-up aged 2 years old [16]. This may well relate to the increased risk of cerebral infarction in the neonate of a cocaine-abusing mother shown by computed tomography (CT) scanning [45] and again thought to be due to cocaine-induced vasospasm [22].

The risks of pre-term delivery, intrauterine growth retardation and accidental haemorrhage are approximately doubled in those who 'ever' abuse cocaine in pregnancy [42]. Premature rupture of membranes and meconium staining of amniotic fluid are also more common [60]. However, it is possible that maternal cocaine abuse like maternal alcohol abuse (see above) may protect the pre-term neonate from developing respiratory distress syndrome [100].

Cocaine abuse does not shorten labour as is commonly believed [23] and indeed it has been associated with acute fetal distress in labour [86].

In Portland, Oregon neonatal cost for the infant of a cocaine-abusing mother averaged US$13 222 compared to US$1297 for the infant of a non-abusing mother [13]. These costs were largely due to the increased risk of prematurity. In another analysis [52] it was shown that between 1984 and 1988 there were an extra 4500 pre-term infants born in New York compared to what would have been expected from analysis of data between 1968 and 1988. The increase in prematurity was almost certainly due to cocaine abuse; the cost of caring for these extra pre-term infants was put at more than US$22 million at 1986 prices.

The most striking association between cocaine abuse and pregnancy is with accidental haemorrhage presumably related to hypertension induced by excess noradrenaline as described above. Several cases of abruption have been reported [2,17] all with large retroplacental clot and no evidence of coagulopathy, although additional thrombocytopenia has been recorded in one case [1].

In addition there is evidence of decreased uterine blood flow associated with noradrenaline release following cocaine administration to pregnant sheep

[12]. Although obstetricians should be aware that hypertension in a cocaine user may be due to the drug rather than any other pathology, it is more important for them to try to stop their patients using the drug in the first place.

Lysergic acid diethylamide (LSD), cannabis, phencyclidine, amphetamines, toluene

LSD may be teratogenic. There are several isolated reports of phocomelia [44] and other typical amniotic band lesions [4,14] which have been discussed by Blanc *et al.* [8]. The use of cannabis six or more times per week during pregnancy is associated with a reduction in gestation by about 1 week after allowing for confounding variables [31]. It also causes growth retardation [30,99]. Cannabis is secreted into breast milk [3], but there is no direct evidence of teratogenicity in humans [3]. It remains controversial whether these agents cause chromosomal damage in humans [44].

Phencyclidine (PCP or 'angel dust') is a hallucinogen which is widely used by the American adolescent population to alter body image. It is also used in pregnancy [35] and there have been reports of a dysmorphic fetus [36] and of neonatal withdrawal symptoms [83]. There are not sufficient data to state whether there are specific risks of phencyclidine abuse.

Amphetamine abuse has been studied in a group of 52 women [55]. The babies were growth retarded but no other abnormalities were significantly more frequent when compared to controls. Acute intravenous overdose has been implicated as a cause of intrauterine death [21].

Toluene which is inhaled in patients who sniff glue causes renal tubular acidosis. Fetuses born from women who are acidotic at the time of delivery are compromised and usually growth retarded [37,94]. In addition the mother is at risk from hypokalaemia, cardiac dysrhythmias and rhabdomyolysis which are excerbated by β sympathomimetic drugs given for pre-term labour to which the patients are also susceptible.

References

1 Abramowicz JS, Sherer DM & Woods JR Jr. Acute transient thrombocytopenia associated with cocaine abuse in pregnancy. *Obstetrics and Gynecology* 1991; **78**: 499–501.

2 Acker D, Sachs BP, Tracey KJ & Wise WE. Abruptio placentae associated with cocaine use. *American Journal of Obstetrics and Gynecology* 1983; **146**: 220–1.

3 Ashton CH. Cannabis: dangers and possible uses. *British Medical Journal* 1987; **294**: 141–2.

4 Assemany SR, Neu RL & Gardner LI. Deformities in a child whose mother took LSD. *Lancet* 1970; **i**: 1290.

5 Barrison IG, Wright TJ *et al.* Screening for alcohol abuse in pregnancy. *British Medical Journal* 1982; **285**: 1318.

6 Beattie J, Day R, Cockburn F & Garg RA. Alcohol and the fetus in the West of Scotland. *British Medical Journal* 1983; **287**: 17–20.

7 Berkowitz K & LaSala A. Risk factors associated with the increasing prevalence of pneumonia during pregnancy. *American Journal of Obstetrics and Gynecology* 1990; **163**: 981–5.

8 Blanc WA, Mattison DR, Kane R & Chauhan P. LSD, intrauterine amputations and amniotic-band syndrome. *Lancet* 1971; **ii**: 158–9.

9 Blinick G, Inturissi CE, Jerez E & Wallach RC. Methadone assays in pregnant women and their progeny. *American Journal of Obstetrics and Gynecology* 1975; **121**: 617–21.

10 Boike GM, Gove N *et al.* Mycotic aneurysms in pregnancy. *American Journal of Obstetrics and Gynecology* 1987; **157**: 340–1.

11 Bowman J, Harman C *et al.* Intravenous drug abuse causes Rh immunization. *Vox Sanguinis* 1991; **61**: 96–8.

12 Bunyon JP, Roubey R *et al.* Complete congenital heart block: Risk of occurrence and therapeutic approach to prevention. *Journal of Rheumatology* 1988; **15**: 1104–8.

13 Calhoun BC & Watson PT. The cost of maternal cocaine abuse: I. Perinatal cost. *Obstetrics and Gynecology* 1991; **78**: 731–4.

14 Carakushansky G, Neu KL & Gardner LI. Lysergide and cannabis as possible teratogens in man. *Lancet* 1969; **i**: 150–1.

15 Challis RE & Scopes JW. Late withdrawal symptoms in babies born to methadone addicts. *Lancet* 1977; **ii**: 1230.

16 Chasnoff IJ, Griffith DR, Freier C & Murray J. Cocaine/polydrug use in pregnancy: two-year follow-up. *Pediatrics* 1992; **89**: 284–9.

17 Chasnoff LJ, Burns WJ, Schnoll SH & Burns KA. Cocaine use in pregnancy. *New England Journal of Medicine* 1985; **313**: 666–7.

18 Colmorgen GH, Johnson C, Zazzarino MA & Durinzi K. Routine urine drug screening at the first prenatal visit. *American Journal of Obstetrics and Gynecology*

1992; **166**: 588–90.

19 Cregler LL & Mark H. Medical complications of cocaine abuse: special report. *New England Journal of Medicine* 1986; **23**: 1495–500.

20 Davis PJM, Partridge JW & Storrs CN. Alcohol consumption in pregnancy. How much is safe? *Archives of Disease in Childhood* 1982; **57**: 940–3.

21 Dearlove JC, Betteridge TJ & Henry JA. Stillbirth due to intravenous amphetamine. *British Medical Journal* 1992; **304**: 548.

22 Dixon SD & Bejar R. Echoencephalographic findings in neonates associated with maternal cocaine and methamphetamine use: incidence and clinical correlates. *Journal of Pediatrics* 1989; **155**: 770–8.

23 Dombrowski MP, Wolfe HM, Welch RA & Evans MI. Cocaine abuse is associated with abruptio placentae and decreased birthweight, but not shorter labour. *Obstetrics and Gynecology* 1991; **77**: 139–41.

24 Durand DJ, Espinoza AM & Nickerson BG. Association between prenatal cocaine exposure and sudden death infant syndrome. *Journal of Pediatrics* 1990; **117**: 909–11.

25 Edelin KC, Gurganious L, Golar K & Oellerich D. Methadone maintenance in pregnancy: consequences to care and outcome. *Obstetrics and Gynecology* 1988; **71**: 399–404.

26 Finnegan LP. Management of pregnant drug-dependent women. *Annals New York Academy of Sciences* 1978; **311**: 135–46.

27 Finnegan LP. Pathophysiological and behavioural effects of the transplacental transfer of narcotic drugs to the foetuses and neonates of narcotic-dependent mothers. *Bulletin on Narcotics* 1979; **31**: 1–59.

28 Finnegan LP (ed), *Drug Dependence in Pregnancy. Clinical Management of Mother and Child.* Castle House Publications, 1980.

29 Forrest F, de V Forey C *et al*. Reported social alcohol consumption during pregnancy and infants' development at 18 months. *British Medical Journal* 1991; **303**: 22–6.

30 Frank DA, Bauchner H & Parker S. Neonatal body proportionality and body composition after *in utero* exposure to cocaine and marijuana. *Journal of Pediatrics* 1990; **117**: 622–6.

31 Fried PA, Watkinson B & Willan A. Marijuana use during pregnancy and decreased length of gestation. *American Journal of Obstetrics and Gynecology* 1984; **150**: 23–7.

32 Fultz JM & Senay EC. Guidelines for the management of hospitalized narcotic addicts. *Annals of Internal Medicine* 1975; **82**: 815.

33 Gardner LI, Mitter N *et al*. Isochromosome 9q in an infant exposed to ethanol prenatally. *New England Journal of Medicine* 1985; **312**: 1521.

34 Glass L, Rajegowda BK & Evans HE. Absence of respiratory distress syndrome in premature infants of heroin addicted mothers. *Lancet* 1971; **ii**: 685–6.

35 Golden NL, Kuhnert BR *et al*. Phencyclidine use during pregnancy. *American Journal of Obstetrics and Gynecology* 1984; **148**: 254–9.

36 Golden NL, Sokol RJ & Rubin K. Angel dust: possible effects on the fetus. *Pediatrics* 1980; **65**: 16.

37 Goodwin TM. Toluene abuse and renal tubular acidosis in pregnancy. *Obstetrics and Gynecology* 1988; **71**: 715–18.

38 Greenfield SP, Rutigliano E, Steinhardt G & Elder JS. Genitourinary tract malformations and maternal cocaine abuse. *Urology* 1991; **37**: 455–9.

39 Halesmaki E, Raivo K & Ylikorkala O. A possible association between maternal drinking and fetal clubfoot. *New England Journal of Medicine* 1985; **312**: 790.

40 Halmesmaki E, Roine R & Salaspuro M. Gamma-glutamyl transferase, aspartate and alanine aminotransferases and their ratio, mean cell volume and urinary dolichol in pregnancy alcohol abusers. *British Journal of Obstetrics and Gynaecology*. 1992; **99**: 287–91.

41 Halmesmaki E & Ylikorkala O. The effect of maternal ethanol intoxication on fetal cardiotocography: a report of four cases. *British Journal of Obstetrics and Gynaecology* 1986; **93**: 203–5.

42 Handler A, Kirstin N, Davis F & Ferre C. Cocaine use during pregnancy: perinatal outcomes. *American Journal of Epidemiology* 1991; **133**: 818–25.

43 Harper G, Concepcion GS & Blenman S. Observations on the sudden death of infants born to addicted mother. *Proceedings Fifth National Conference on Methadone Treatment*. National Association for the Prevention of Addiction to Narcotics, New York, 1983: 1122.

44 Hecht F, Beals RK *et al*. Lysergic-acid-diethylamide and cannabis as possible teratogens in man. *Lancet* 1968; **ii**: 1087.

45 Heier LA, Carpanzano CR *et al*. Maternal cocaine abuse: the spectrum of radiologic abnormalities in the neonatal CNS. *American Journal of Neuroradiology* 1991; **12**: 951–6.

46 Henderson CE, Terribile S, Keefe D & Merkatz IR. Cardiac screening for pregnant intravenous drug abusers. *American Journal of Perinatology* 1989; **6**: 397–9.

47 Hill RM & Desmond MM. Management of the narcotic withdrawal syndrome in the neonate. *Pediatric Clinics in North America* 1963; **10**: 67–86.

48 Holmes RC & Black MM. Herpes gestationis. *Dermatologic Clinics* 1983; **1**: 195–203.

49 Ioffe S & Chernick V. Maternal alcohol ingestion and the incidence of respiratory distress syndrome. *American Journal of Obstetrics and Gynecology* 1987; **156**: 1231–5.

50 Jacobson B, Nyberg K *et al*. Opiate addiction in adult offspring through possible imprinting after obstetric treatment. *British Medical Journal* 1990; **301**: 1067–70.

51 Jones KL & Smith DW. Recognition of the fetal alcohol

syndrome in early infancy. *Lancet* 1973; **ii**: 999–1001.
52 Joyce T. The dramatic increase in the rate of low birthweight in New York city: an aggregate time-series analysis. *American Journal of Public Health* 1990; **80**: 682–4.
53 Klenka HM. Babies born in a district general hospital to mothers taking heroin. *British Medical Journal* 1986; **298**: 745–6.
54 Lawton ME. Alcohol in breast milk. *Australian and New Zealand Journal of Obstetrics and Gynaecology* 1985; **25**: 71–3.
55 Little BB, Snell LM & Gilstrap LC. Methamphetamine abuse during pregnancy: outcome and fetal effects. *Obstetrics and Gynecology* 1988; **72**: 541–4.
56 Little RE, Anderson KW *et al.* Maternal alcohol use during breast-feeding and infant mental and motor development at one year. *New England Journal of Medicine* 1989; **321**: 425–30.
57 Little RE & Sing CF. Association of father's drinking and infant's birth weight. *New England Journal of Medicine* 1986; **314**: 1644–5.
58 Liu DTY, Tylden E & Tukel SH. Fetal response to drug withdrawal. *Lancet* 1976; **ii**: 588.
59 Lutiger B, Graham K, Einarson TR & Koren G. Relationship between gestational cocaine use and pregnancy outcome: a meta-analysis. *Teratology* 1991; **44**: 405–14.
60 Mastrogiannis DS, Decavalas GO, Verma U & Tejani N. Perinatal outcome after recent cocaine usage. *Obstetrics and Gynecology* 1990; **76**: 8–11.
61 Matera C, Warren WB *et al.* Prevalence of use of cocaine and other substances in an obstetric population. *American Journal of Obstetrics and Gynecology* 1990; **163**: 797–801.
62 McCalla S, Minkoff HL *et al.* Predictors of cocaine use in pregnancy. *Obstetrics and Gynecology* 1992; **79**: 641–4.
63 Mennella JA & Beauchamp GK. The transfer of alcohol to human milk. *New England Journal of Medicine* 1991; **325**: 981–5.
64 Metcalfe J, Dunham MJ, Olsen GD & Krall MA. Respiratory and haemodynamic effects of methadone in pregnant women. *Respiration Physiology* 1980; **42**: 383–93.
65 Minkoff HL, McCalla S *et al.* The relationship of cocaine use to syphilis and human immunodeficiency virus infections among inner city parturient women. *American Journal of Obstetrics and Gynecology* 1990; **163**: 521–6.
66 O'Brien CP. Narcotic abuse during pregnancy. *New England Journal of Medicine* 1974; **291**: 311.
67 Ostrea EM & Chavez CJ. Perinatal problems (excluding neonatal withdrawal) in maternal drug addiction. A study of 830 cases. *Journal of Pediatrics* 1979; **94**: 292–4.
68 Ostrea EM, Brady M, Gause S, Raymundo AL & Stevens M. Drug screening of newborns by meconium analysis: a large-scale, prospective, epidemiological study. *Pediatrics* 1992; **89**: 107–13.
69 Ouellette EM, Rosett HL, Rosman P & Weiner L. Adverse effects on offspring of maternal alcohol abuse during pregnancy. *New England Journal of Medicine* 1977; **297**: 528–30.
70 Peirson PS, Howard P & Kleber HD. Sudden deaths in infants born to methadone-maintained addicts. *Journal of American Medical Association* 1972; **220**: 1733.
71 Rementeria JL, Janakammal S & Hollander M. Multiple births in drug-addicted women. *American Journal of Obstetrics and Gynecology* 1975; **122**: 958–60.
72 Richardson BS, O'Grady JP & Olsen GD. Fetal breathing movements and the response to carbon dioxide in patients on methadone maintenance. *American Journal of Obstetrics and Gynecology* 1984; **150**: 400–5.
73 Rosner MA, Keith L & Chasnoff I. North Western University Drug Dependence Program: The impact of intensive perinatal care on labour ad delivery outcomes. *American Journal of Obstetrics and Gynecology* 1982; **144**: 23–7.
74 Ryle PR & Thomson AD. Acetaldehyde and fetal alcohol syndrome. *Lancet* 1983; **ii**: 219–20.
75 Sardemann H, Madsen KS & Friis-Hansen B. Follow-up of children of drug-addicted mothers. *Archives of Disease in Childhood* 1976; **51**: 131–4.
76 Sarpong S & Headings V. Sirenomelia accompanying exposure of the embryo to cocaine. *Southern Medical Journal* 1992; **85**: 545–7.
77 Schutzman DL, Frankenfield Chernicoff M, Clatterbaugh HE & Singer J. Incidence of intrauterine cocaine exposure in a suburban setting. *Pediatrics* 1991; **88**: 825–7.
78 Serdula M, Williamson DF *et al.* Trends of alcohol consumption by pregnant women. *Journal of the American Medical Association* 1991; **265**: 876–9.
79 Sisenwein FE, Tejani NA, Boxer HS & DiGiuseppe R. Effects of methanol infusion during pregnancy on the growth and development of children at four to seven years of age. *American Journal of Obstetrics and Gynecology* 1983; **147**: 52–6.
80 Sloan LB, Gay JW, Snyder SW & Bales WR. Substance abuse during pregnancy in rural population. *Obstetrics and Gynecology* 1992; **79**: 245–8.
81 Southall DP, Richards JM *et al. Prospective Population Based Studies into Heart Rate and Breathing Patterns in Newborn Infants: Prediction of Infants at Risk of SIDS.* International Conference into SIDS, Baltimore, 1982.
82 Spohr HL, Willms J & Steinhausen HC. Prenatal alcohol exposure and long term developmental consequences. *Lancet* 1993; **341**: 907–10.
83 Strauss AA, Modanlou HD & Basu SK. Neonatal manifestations of maternal phencyclidine (PCP) abuse. *Pediatrics* 1981; **68**: 550.
84 Streissguth AP, Aase JM *et al.* Fetal alcohol syndrome in adolescents and adults. *Journal of the American Medical Association* 1991; **265**: 1961–7.

85 Sulaiman ND, du V Florey C, Taylor DJ & Ogston SA. Alcohol consumption in Dundee primigravidas and its effects on outcome of pregnancy. *British Medical Journal* 1988; **296**: 1500–3.

86 Sztulman L, Ducey JJ & Tancer ML. Intrapartum intranasal cocaine use and acute fetal distress. *Journal of Reproductive Medicine* 1990; **35**: 917–18.

87 Umans JG & Szeto HH. Precipitated opiate abstinence *in utero*. *American Journal of Obstetrics and Gynecology* 1983; **151**: 441–4.

88 Van Den Anker JN, Cohen Overbeek TE, Wladimiroff JW & Sauer PJJ. Prenatal diagnosis of limb-reduction defects due to maternal cocaine use. *Lancet* 1991; **338**: 1332.

89 Van Winter JT, Nielsen SN & Ogburn PL Jr. Epidural abscess associated with intravenous drug abuse in a pregnant patient. *Mayo Clinic Proceedings* 1991; **66**: 1036–9.

90 Veghely PV. Fetal abnormality and maternal ethanol metabolism. *Lancet* 1983; **ii**: 53–4.

91 Viscarello RR, Ferguson DD, Nores J & Hobbins JC. Limb–body wall complex associated with cocaine abuse: further evidence of cocaine's teratogenicity. *Obstetrics and Gynecology* 1992; **80**: 523–6.

92 Volpe JJ. Effect of cocaine use on the fetus. *New England Journal of Medicine* 1992; **327**: 399–407.

93 Ward SL, Bautista D *et al*. Sudden infant death syndrome in infants of substance abusing mothers. *Journal of Pediatrics* 1990; **117**: 876–81.

94 Wilkins Haug L & Gabow PA. Toluene abuse during pregnancy: obstetric complications and perinatal outcome. *Obstetrics and Gynecology* 1991; **77**: 504–9.

95 Wright JT & Toplis PJ. Alcohol in pregnancy. *British Journal of Obstetrics and Gynaecology* 1986; **93**: 201–2.

96 Wright JT, Waterson EJ *et al*. Alcohol consumption, pregnancy and low birth weight. *Lancet* 1983; **i**: 663–5.

97 Ylikorkala O, Stenman UH & Halmesmaki E. γ-Glutamyl transferase and mean cell volume reveal maternal alcohol abuse and fetal alcohol effects. *American Journal of Obstetrics and Gynecology* 1987; **157**: 344–8.

98 Zelson C, Lee SJ & Casalino M. Neonatal narcotic addiction. Comparative effects of maternal intake of heroin and methadone. *New England Journal of Medicine* 1973; **289**: 1216–20.

99 Zuckerman B, Frank DA *et al*. Effects of maternal marijuana and cocaine use on fetal growth. *New England Journal of Medicine* 1989; **320**: 762–8.

100 Zuckerman B, Maynard EC & Cabral H. A preliminary report of perinatal cocaine exposure and respiratory distress syndrome in premature infants. *American Journal of Diseases in Childhood* 1991; **145**: 696–8.

101 Zuspan FP, Gumpel JA *et al*. Fetal stress from methadone withdrawal. *American Journal of Obstetrics and Gynecology* 1975; **122**: 43–6.

19

Skin Diseases in Pregnancy

Martin M. Black & Susan C. Mayou

Physiological skin changes in pregnancy, 610
Pigmentation
Pruritus gravidarum (cholestasis of pregnancy)
Vascular changes
Purpura
Connective tissue and collagen
Glandular activity
Hair changes
Nails
Breasts and nipples
Dermatoses specific to pregnancy, 614
Pemphigoid (herpes) gestationis
Polymorphic eruption of pregnancy
Prurigo of pregnancy
Pruritic folliculitis of pregnancy
Papular dermatitis of pregnancy
Autoimmune progesterone dermatitis of pregnancy
The effect of pregnancy on other dermatoses, 619
Eczema
Acne vulgaris
Psoriasis and impetigo herpetiformis
Condylomata accuminata
Candidiasis
Leprosy
Pregnancy and collagen disease, 620
Pregnancy and inflammatory skin disease, 621
Erythema multiforme
Pregnancy and benign and malignant tumours, 621
Melanoma
Drug therapy during pregnancy, 621

Pregnancy is a period of profound temporary hormonal change which may affect the skin in numerous ways. Many are so common that they are not considered abnormal and are classified as 'physiological skin changes'. Other dermatoses occur less frequently and are specifically associated with the gravid state. Finally, pregnancy may modify pre-existing dermatological conditions. For other reviews see [13,23].

Physiological skin changes in pregnancy

There are a number of common skin changes in pregnancy which are thought to be related to hormonal changes.

Pigmentation

Hyperpigmentation is very common during pregnancy and occurs in up to 90 per cent of women [20]. It is one of the most commonly recognized signs of pregnancy and may be generalized or restricted to areas of normal hyperpigmentation such as nipples, areolae, perineum, vulva and perianal region. The linea alba, a tendinous median line on the anterior abdominal wall, frequently hyperpigments to become the linear nigra and may extend from the symphysis pubis to xiphisternum. Pigmentation increases in the first trimester particularly in dark-haired, dark-complexioned women and fades post-partum although it seldom returns to the pre-pregnancy level. Freckles and melanocytic naevi tend to darken and may increase in number. Recent scars may also hyperpigment.

Melasma

Irregular, sharply demarcated patches of facial pigmentation known as melasma develop in approximately 70 per cent of women during the second half of pregnancy [20,82]. It also occurs in up to 30 per cent of women taking oral contraceptives [58] and in essentially healthy women between early adulthood and the menopause [52]. The most common pattern is centrofacial, involving the forehead, cheeks, upper lip, nose and chin. The malar pattern is limited to cheeks and nose, and the mandibular type involves the ramus of the mandible [59]. Histologically, there are two patterns of pigmentation: the epidermal type, which occurs in 72 per cent of cases, in which the melanin is deposited mainly in the basal melanocytes, and the dermal type, which affects 13 per cent of patients, where the melanin is mainly in superficial and deep dermis [59]. Examination under Wood's light shows enhancement of colour contrast if melanin is primarily in the epidermis, and not if the melanin is located only in the dermis. Melasma can be categorized as epidermal, dermal, mixed or inapparent on Wood's light examination. In natural light, epidermal melasma appears light brown, dermal melasma blue–grey and the mixed type deep brown. The Wood's light inapparent category occurs in patients of dark complexion and in whom the pigment deposition is primarily dermal. There is no correlation between the clinical and histological patterns of Wood's light appearances [59].

Nearly 90 per cent of women with chloasma due to oral contraception have a past history of melasma of pregnancy [58].

PATHOGENESIS

Oestrogen and progesterone are known to be strong melanogenic stimulants [72] and these hormones may well be responsible for the hyperpigmentation of pregnancy. Serum and urinary melanocyte-stimulating hormone (MSH) levels have been reported as elevated during pregnancy with a rapid decrease post-partum [64]. Other work has however demonstrated no difference in β-MSH levels in the third trimester and after parturition [76]. Levels of β-MSH were higher than the mean level obtained from non-pregnant controls but were within the normal range and therefore thought unlikely to be responsible for the pigmentary changes [76].

The patterns of pigmentation may relate to differences in end-organ sensitivity or distribution of melanocytes. Sun exposure may also be relevant in the development of melasma.

TREATMENT

Treatment is unsatisfactory and consists of minimizing exposure to sunlight and subsequent avoidance of oral contraceptives. Sunscreens should be used and cosmetic camouflage with non-allergic products is helpful. Depigmenting agents may be effective and Kligman reports success in 14 out of 16 patients using twice daily application of 5 per cent hydroquinone, 0.1 per cent tretinoin and 0.1 per cent dexamethasone in ethanol and propylene glycol for 5–7 weeks [40]. Sanchez recommends the use of 2 per cent hydroquinone and 0.05 per cent tretinoin on the epidermal type of persistent melasma and believes that the dermal types respond poorly if at all to this therapy [59]. Depigmenting agents should always be used with caution as dermatitis, further hyperpigmentation or even hypopigmentation may ensue. Melasma usually fades within a year of delivery [25] although in one study 30 per cent of cases persisted after 10 years [64].

Pruritus gravidarum (cholestasis of pregnancy)

This term refers to intense pruritus which occurs as a manifestation of intrahepatic cholestasis of pregnancy, without any associated rash or clinical jaundice and usually in late pregnancy. Pruritus from all causes occurs in 17 per cent of pregnant women [20] and may be due to scabies, pediculosis, urticaria, atopic eczema, drug eruptions, candidiasis, trichomonal vaginitis or neurodermatitis. Once these underlying conditions have been excluded, a small group of patients remains whose pruritus is due to alteration in hepatic function. Pruritus gravidarum is considered to be a mild variant of recurrent cholestasis of pregnancy [2] (see Chapter 9). The incidence is between 0.02 and 2.4 per cent [11]. It usually begins in the third trimester with severe pruritus which may be generalized or confined to the abdomen.

Serum alkaline phosphatase and transaminases may be elevated and bilirubin normal or slightly raised. Liver biopsy reveals non-specific changes of cholestasis [1].

It is thought that in genetically susceptible women, physiological levels of oestrogen and progesterone interfere with hepatic excretion of the bile acids and that deposition of bile acid in the skin causes pruritus. Oestrogens act by interfering with the normal diffusion across the canalicular membrane [33] and progesterones by inhibiting hepatic glucuronyl transferase thus reducing oestrogen clearance [61].

Treatment

Mild forms of pruritus gravidarum may be treated with bland topical antipruritic creams such as calamine. More severe pruritus may respond to cholestyramine (Questran) 4 g three times a day. Antihistamines may be a useful adjunct. However, in some patients the pruritus may be so severe that pre-term delivery is necessary. If prematurity is a real hazard to the fetus, the use of dexamethasone [26] or ursodeoxycholic acid [54] should be considered to alleviate the cholestasis and therefore the pruritus and to allow pregnancy to continue.

Pruritus gravidarum usually settles rapidly post-partum but may recur with subsequent pregnancies and the oral contraceptive. The maternal and fetal prognosis is normal except in those patients with frank obstetric cholestasis (see Chapter 9).

Vascular changes

Oedema

Clinically apparent oedema of the face and hands occurs in approximately 50 per cent of pregnant women, whilst oedema of the legs not associated with pre-eclampsia develops in about 80 per cent [20]. It is usually non-pitting in nature and worse in the morning. It is probably due to several factors: increased fluid retention (approximately 2.5 l during pregnancy), increased vascular permeability, increased blood flow [35] and decreased colloid osmotic pressure of plasma.

Spider naevi

Vascular spiders develop between the second and fifth months of pregnancy and are present in about 57 per cent of white, and 10 per cent of black women by the third trimester [5]. This difference is probably due to difficulty in visualizing them on dark skin. In comparison, spider naevi are said to occur in 15 per cent of normal non-pregnant white women. They occur in the areas drained by the superior vena cava on the upper trunk and face, increase in size and number throughout pregnancy and fade post-partum. The majority (75 per cent) have disappeared by the seventh week after delivery [5]; the remainder persist and recurrence may occur at the same sites in subsequent pregnancies. Clinically they are indistinguishable from the spider naevi of chronic liver disease and consist of a central pulsating arteriole with radiating telangiectases. Treatment for persistent lesion is with cold point cautery or argon laser [52a].

Palmar erythema

Palmar erythema develops during pregnancy in 70 per cent of white, and 35 per cent of black, women [5]. Its onset is in the first trimester and it fades within 1 week of delivery. There are two clinical patterns: (a) diffuse mottling of the whole palm; and (b) erythema confined to the thenar and hypothenar eminences. The former is the more common. It frequently occurs within patients who also have spider naevi and both are thought to be due to high oestrogen levels. The rise in blood volume and blood flow are other possible factors.

Varices

Varices may affect as many as 40 per cent of pregnant women and may involve the saphenous system or small superficial vessels in the legs, as well as the haemorrhoidal and vulvar networks. They are due to several factors: increased venous pressure in femoral and pelvic vessels due to compression from the gravid uterus, increase in the blood volume, increased collagen fragility and a hereditary tendency to varicose veins. Varices tend to regress post-partum although not always completely.

Treatment is elevation of the legs and elastic support stockings. Thrombosis may occur in leg varices or haemorrhoids. Thromboembolism in pregnancy is considered in Chapter 4.

Haemangiomata

Haemangiomata develop on the head and neck in 5 per cent of pregnant women, appearing at the end of the first trimester and enlarging until term [25]. The 'pregnancy tumour' or telangiectatic epulis, is a similar lesion sited on oral mucosa or gingiva. It usually develops between 2 and 5 months gestation, affects 2 per cent of pregnant women and arises from interdental papillae on buccal or lingual surfaces of the gingiva. It is usually associated with extensive gingivitis and may bleed or ulcerate. All these lesions may be initiated by trauma and resemble pyogenic granulomata both clinically and histologically. Pre-existing haemangiomata may increase in size. High oestrogen levels are probably an aetiological factor. Surgical removal is the treatment for lesions which persist post-partum.

Purpura

This may occur on the legs during the second half of pregnancy due to increased capillary permeability and fragility [25]. Vasculitis and thrombocytopenia must be excluded.

Connective tissue and collagen

Striae (gravidarum and distensae)

Striae gravidarum develop during the second half of pregnancy in most women. They occur on the abdomen, breasts and thighs. Initially they are pink or violaceous linear wrinkles which develop perpendicular to skin tension lines. They become white and atrophic with time, although never disappear completely. They are identical to striae associated with puberty, obesity, Cushing's disease and steroid therapy.

The aetiology of striae is multifactorial: stretching is a localizing factor and striae do tend to occur more with overweight mothers or those carrying heavier babies or with multiple pregnancy [17]. There is also a familial tendency [45]. Rupture of collagen and elastic fibres [71], and increased adrenocortical activity have been considered important [17]. It has also been suggested that oestrogen and relaxin increase the collagen and sulphate-free mucopolysaccharides and that subsequent stretching leads to easier separation of collagen [45].

Histologically, striae consist of areas of broken and curled elastic fibres in the upper dermis with parallel bands of collagen and elastic fibres in the centre [55]. There is no specific treatment for striae and it is controversial as to whether emollient massage is effective in their prevention [17].

Skin tags or molluscum fibrosum gravidarum

Soft, fleshy, pendunculated, skin coloured or slightly pigmented papillomata may develop on the face, neck, upper anterior chest, axillae and under the breasts during the second half of pregnancy. They are about 1–5 mm in diameter and clinically and histologically identical to skin tags [16]. They are probably due to hormonal factors and regress post-partum. Persisting lesions may be removed by electrodesiccation.

Glandular activity

Sweat and apocrine glands

Eccrine sweating is increased during pregnancy [18] and may be associated with mila (due to occlusion of the sweat ducts) and intertrigo. Palmar eccrine sweating is, however, diminished [50]. Apocrine activity is also reduced with subsequent improvement of conditions such as Fox–Fordyce disease and hidradenitis suppurativa [20]. These may rebound post-partum.

Sebaceous glands

Sebaceous activity increases during the third trimester and acne occasionally develops during pregnancy. Sebaceous glands associated with lactiferous ducts on the areolae, hypertrophy as early as 6 weeks' gestation and appear as Montgomery's tubercles. They are one of the signs of early pregnancy.

Hair changes

Telogen effluvium

The proportion of hairs in anagen (the growing phase) increases during pregnancy [48]. Post-partum, the conversion from anagen hairs to telogen (resting) hairs is accelerated and post-partum hair loss or 'telogen effluvium' follows after 4–20 weeks [20]. Normally about 15 per cent of scalp hairs are in the telogen phase and in pregnancy this falls to 5 per cent, rising within a few months of delivery to 25 per cent. The hair loss is generally diffuse although may be more marked in the frontoparietal hairline in women with a tendency to male pattern baldness. Baldness seldom, if ever, occurs and spontaneous recovery usually takes place within 6 months of delivery [63], although it may take as long as 15 months [20]. Recovery is usually complete unless the telogen effluvium is severe, repeated in several pregnancies or associated with male pattern alopecia. With successive pregnancies hair loss tends to be less marked.

The diagnosis is made by finding large numbers of club hairs. Histologically, the follicles in telogen are normal. Increased adrenocorticosteroids and ovarian androgens probably account for the increase in anagen hairs and oestrogens prolong the anagen phase [82]. Telogen effluvium is probably caused by several factors including changes in endocrine balance, the stress of delivery, difficult labour and blood loss. No specific treatment is required apart from reassurance.

Some women develop male pattern hair loss in late pregnancy while in others the loss is diffuse. This is due to inhibition of anagen in some follicles and not due to increased loss [35]. The re-growth with the male pattern hair loss in unlikely to be complete.

There is no significant change in the anagen/telogen ratio of body hair [78].

Hirsutism

Hypertrichosis, most marked on face, arms and legs, is quite common in pregnancy but marked hirsutism is rare. It resolves post-partum but recurrence in subsequent pregnancies frequently occurs. Hirsutism may be accompanied by acne, deepening of the voice and clitoral enlargement and is probably due to increased adrenocorticosteroid and ovarian androgen secretion. Other causes of hirsutism, namely androgen-secreting ovarian tumours and polycystic ovaries, should be excluded. Treatment is with reassurance and cosmetic removal (depilatory creams and electrolysis).

Nails

Nail changes, consisting of transverse grooving, brittleness, distal onycholysis and subungual keratosis, may occur from the sixth week. The pathogenesis of these changes is not known. There is no effective treatment.

Breasts and nipples

Sore nipples with cracks and fissures commonly develop in the first few days of breast feeding. The soreness may limit sucking, and stasis, mastitis or breast abscess may follow. Nipple eczema may also develop and involve the breast. Secondary infection must be excluded. Fissures and eczema are avoided by gentle washing to remove saliva and milk and by use of emollients. The breasts should be left exposed if possible and secondary infection treated with antibiotics. Severely affected patients are often atopic.

Dermatoses specific to pregnancy

A number of dermatoses are specific to pregnancy, the puerperium or resulting from trophoblastic tumours. They have recently been reclassified into the following groups:

1 pemphigoid gestationis (herpes gestationis);
2 polymorphic eruption of pregnancy;
3 prurigo of pregnancy; and
4 pruritic folliculitis of pregnancy [9,28].

Pemphigoid (herpes) gestationis (PG)

PG is an intensely pruritic bullous eruption which occurs in one in 60 000 pregnancies [41] or in association with the trophoblastic tumours, choriocarcinoma [77] and hydatidiform mole [19]. The eruption initially consists of pruritic erythematous urticated papules and plaques, target lesions and annular wheals. Vesicles develop after a delay varying between a few days and a month and enlarge to become tense bullae (Fig. 19.1). In 90 per cent of patients the lesions begin in the peri-umbilical region and spread to involve thighs, breast, palms and soles (Fig. 19.1). The face and oral mucosa are only rarely involved. It may begin during the first or any subsequent pregnancy arising between 9 weeks gestation and 1 week post-partum [29]. In subsequent pregnancies recurrence usually occurs with an earlier onset and more severe disease. When PG develops during the mid-trimester, there is usually a period of relative remission in the last few weeks of pregnancy followed by an abrupt post-partum flare [35]. The bullous lesions tend to resolve within a month of delivery, but the urticated plaques may persist for over a year [29].

The aetiology of PG is unknown, but recent work highlights the immunopathological findings in this disease. Paternal histocompatibility antigens (HLA) were considered important following a study in which 50 per cent of the consorts were HLA-DR2 compared to 25 per cent of the controls [70]. However, this was not confirmed in another study in which the frequency of paternal HLA antigens was normal [31]. A paternal factor is likely as in some patients with pregnancies by several consorts, the onset of PG has coincided with a change in partner, and in one case a patient had PG in her first and second pregnancies and then had an unaffected pregnancy by a new consort [31].

Maternal HLA studies have revealed a significantly increased frequency of DR3 with DR4 [32]. DR3 and DR4 are associated with other diseases with an immune pathogenesis such as Graves' disease, rheumatoid arthritis and insulin-dependent diabetes mellitus, which suggests that their presence confers an increase in immune susceptibility in the patients with PG. A recent study has confirmed the association between PG and other autoimmune diseases, particularly Graves' disease [69]. The antigenic trigger is probably paternally derived as PG occurs not only in pregnancy but also in association with hydatidiform mole and choriocarcinoma, and in these trophoblastic tumours, the chromosomes are all paternally derived. There is also evidence that DR compatibility between mother and fetus favours a spared pregnancy [32]. Once initiated, PG is undoubtedly hormonally modulated.

Exacerbations may occur with ovulation or premenstrually suggesting that oestrogen is responsible. It tends to be in a phase of relative remission in late pregnancy and flares post-partum when the most significant hormonal change is a fall in progesterone. Progesterone has been shown to have immunosuppresive effects similar to glucocorticoids and may exert an inhibiting effect on PG [30]. Exacerbations, may also be induced by taking the contraceptive pill [47]. Holmes prescribed oral

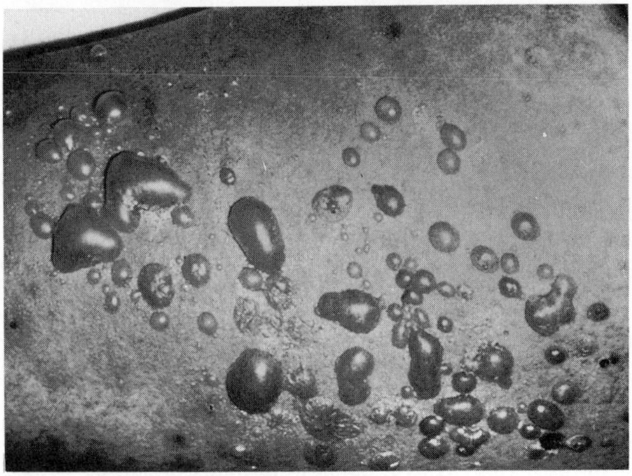

Fig. 19.1. Pemphigoid gestationis. Large tense bullae on the thigh.

contraceptives to eight patients and four experienced exacerbations; three were given combined oestrogen and progesterone, but the patient who flared most severely was given oestrogen alone. Two patients were given progesterone alone and their PG was unaffected. There is experimental evidence that at certain concentrations oestrogen may have immunoenhancing properties [39] and this may account for its effect in PG. Holmes *et al.* [32] also demonstrated that breast feeding was associated with a shorter and less severe post-partum illness suggesting that prolactin may have an immunosuppressant effect on the disease.

Fetal prognosis

It has been stated that PG is associated with an increased fetal and maternal risk [42] although other workers disagree and found that fetal prognosis was normal [67]. In a study of 50 infants from affected pregnancies, there was a significant increase in babies of low birthweight and small-for-dates babies which did not correlate with severity or duration of PG [43]. There were no stillbirths or maternal deaths and none of the four neonatal deaths were ascribed to PG. One infant developed a bullous eruption resembling PG which resolved within a week. A more recent study [68] has once again indicated a tendency for premature delivery to be associated with PG. As small-for-dates infants have a raised morbidity, it is essential that patients with PG are delivered in maternity units with access to special care facilities.

Pathology

Histologically, the early urticated lesions of PG show epidermal and papillary dermal oedema with occasional foci of eosinophilic spongiosis [62]. The bullae are subepidermal and contain numerous eosinophils. Ultrastructurally, the split occurs within the lamina lucida [62].

Direct immunofluorescence demonstrates C3 at the basement membrane zone in all patients with active PG [30]. Indirect immunofluorescence usually shows a C3 binding factor [56]. This PG factor is an IgG [36,38] and although it is only positive in 25 per cent of cases by conventional techniques, it can be demonstrated more reliably by immunoelectron microscopy [37].

Differential diagnosis

The main differential diagnosis is from the much more common polymorphic eruption of pregnancy (PEP), and bullous pemphigoid.

PEP usually affects primigravidae and the eruption starts in prominent striae. Urticarial plaques, weals and vesicles may occur in both disorders but only become frankly bullous in PG [30]. Histologically there are no features of early lesions to distinguish between the two, but on direct immunofluorescence, PEP is consistently negative [29,30] (see Table 19.1).

PG and bullous pemphigoid share several features. Both are characterized by pruritic, urticarial and bullous eruptions. Histological and immunofluorescent findings are also closely similar. However, the lesions of PG occur predominantly on the lower abdomen and thighs, whilst the distribution in bullous pemphigoid is more variable. The clinical

Table 19.1. Comparison of pemphigoid gestationis and polymorphic eruption of pregnancy (from [29])

	Pemphigoid gestationis	Polymorphic eruption of pregnancy
Incidence per 100 000 pregnancies	2	420
Morphology		
Urticarial lesions	+	+
Vesicles	+	+
Bullae	+	–
Prominent striae	3%	81%
Umbilical lesions	87%	12%
Post-partum exacerbations	75%	15%
Direct immunofluorescence	100%	0%
HLA-DR3	84%	46%
Associated autoimmune phenomena	+	–

activity of PG is affected by oestrogen and progesterone, but there is no evidence that these have any effect on bullous pemphigoid. Finally, the frequency of HLA antigens in bullous pemphigoid is normal. Nevertheless considerable similarities between PG and bullous pemphigoid led to the suggestion that 'pemphigoid' gestationis is a more appropriate term than 'herpes' gestationis [29,30].

Treatment

Mild cases of PG respond to treatment with antihistamines and topical fluorinated corticosteroids. Systemic steroids are indicated in more severe disease with bullae. Most cases respond to 40 mg daily of prednisolone and this can usually be reduced fairly rapidly to a daily maintenance dose of 10 mg. It should be increased again in anticipation of the post-partum flare which occurs so frequently. Plasmapheresis should be considered for severe cases [80]. Dapsone is best avoided as it can cause haemolytic disease of the newborn [27], although it has been given safely to treat leprosy during pregnancy [51]. A single case has recently been reported of complete remission of severe PG during treatment with ritodrine commenced for premature labour [49]. However, for the present systemic steroids remain the mainstay of treatment. Recently the use of new luteinizing hormone releasing hormone (LHRH) analogue, goserelin, led to a complete temporary remission in a long-standing case of PG [21].

Maternal prognosis

Once a patient has had an affected pregnancy, PG will usually recur in subsequent pregnancies [35] with an earlier onset and more severe disease. Thus many would caution against further pregnancy. However, occasional 'skipped' pregnancies can occur and some mothers are prepared to risk another pregnancy. HLA-DR3 typing may be a useful prognostic indicator as the absence of DR3 is associated with more mild disease.

Polymorphic eruption of pregnancy

This pruritic urticarial eruption develops in and around abdominal striae in approximately one in 240 pregnancies. It has previously been classified as pruritic urticarial papules and plaques of pregnancies [3,42], toxaemic rash of pregnancy [10] or late onset prurigo of pregnancy [15,53]. It has been suggested that these are all synonyms for the same eruption and PEP has been proposed [28]. Seventy-six per cent of patients are primigravidae and recurrence with subsequent pregnancies is rare [28]. PEP is significantly associated with increased abdominal skin distension and multiple pregnancies [12,14]. If a second episode does occur, it is much less severe than the first, which is in direct contrast to PG. The eruption usually begins in the last 5 weeks of pregnancy and rarely persists for more than a few weeks. It usually begins in prominent abdominal striae and may remain confined to the abdomen with relative sparing of the umbilicus (see Fig. 19.2). Sometimes it becomes widespread involving buttocks, shoulders and limbs.

The lesions consist of urticarial papules, plaques and polycyclic weals (Fig. 19.3). Vesicles occur in approximately 45 per cent and target lesions in 19 per cent, but the vesicles rarely enlarge beyond 2 mm [28] and thus bullous lesions as in PG are hardly ever seen.

Histology of the urticarial papules shows epidermal and upper dermal oedema with a perivascular infiltrate of lymphocytes, histiocytes and eosinophils. With the vesicular lesions, vesicular spongiosis occurs. Immunofluorescence is consistently negative [28].

Treatment is with antihistamines and mild topical steroids. Systemic corticosteroids have been effective in extensive disease [84]. In very severe cases elective delivery may be the only way to relieve pruritus [6].

Prurigo of pregnancy

This pruritic papular eruption affects one in 300 pregnancies [53] and begins earlier in pregnancy than PEP. It is also referred to as prurigo gestationis of Besnier and 'early onset prurigo of pregnancy'. The onset is usually between 25 and 30 weeks gestation and although the pruritus settles at delivery, the papules tend to persist for several months. The lesions consist of groups of excoriated papules

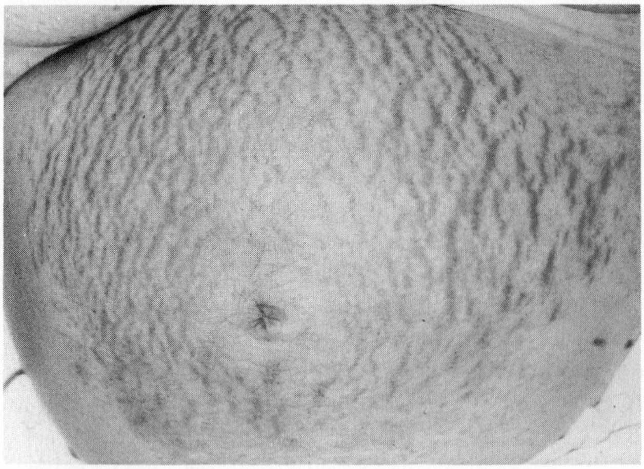

Fig. 19.2. Polymorphic eruption of pregnancy. Urticarial lesions in prominent abdominal striae.

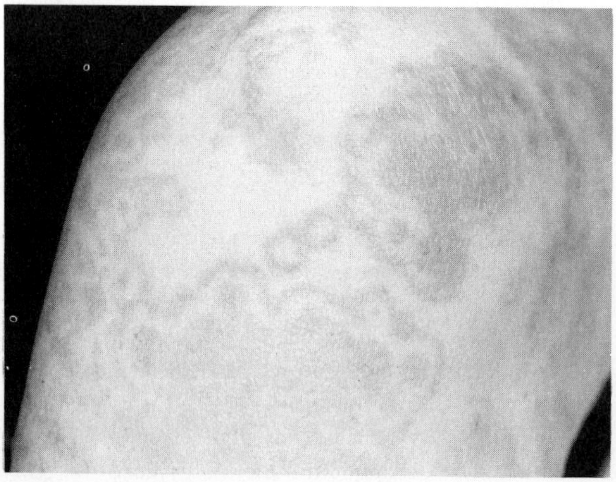

Fig. 19.3. Polymorphic eruption of pregnancy. Polycyclic weals on the knee.

on the extensor surface of limbs and abdomen, although they may become widespread.

Histology of the lesions demonstrates parakeratosis, acanthosis and perivascular lymphocytic infiltrate. Immunofluorescence is negative.

The cause is unknown, but many patients appear to be atopic. It has been suggested that prurigo of pregnancy may be the result of pruritus gravidarum developing in atopic individuals [29].

The rash may recur in subsequent pregnancies and there is no increased risk to mother or fetus. Treatment is symptomatic with antihistamines and topical corticosteroids.

Pruritic folliculitis of pregnancy

This is a pruritic folliculitis which begins between the fourth month of gestation and term and usually resolves by 2 weeks post-partum [85]. The eruption is acneiform with widespread follicular erythematous papules.

As the clinical appearance resembles the monomorphic type of acne seen in some patients taking systemic corticosteroids, it is possible that pruritic folliculitis may be a form of hormonally induced acne rather than a specific dermatosis of pregnancy. Histopathology demonstrates acute folliculitis with focal spongiosis and exocytosis of polymorphonuclear and mononuclear cells. In the dermis, there is oedema and a perivascular infiltrate. Direct immunofluorescence is negative. The maternal and fetal prognosis is normal. Treatment is with topical 10 per cent benzoyl peroxide and 1 per cent hydrocortisone.

Papular dermatitis of pregnancy

This was described as a distinct entity by Spangler *et al.* [73] as a widespread papular dermatitis associated with a significant fetal mortality of 30 per cent [73]. They found characteristic biochemical changes with urinary chorionic gonadotrophin levels in the last trimester raised and plasma cortisol and urinary oestriol reduced. Spangler *et al.* [73] felt that the clinical feature which distinguished those with papular dermatitis of pregnancy from those with prurigo of pregnancy was that the lesions were widespread rather than grouped on the extensor surfaces of limbs. Holmes and Black [28], however, suggested that these cases of Spangler *et al.* do not justify a separate classification and may simply represent more florid examples of prurigo of pregnancy or PEP [28]. It is important to point out that similar biochemical studies have not been performed in other specific dermatoses of pregnancy. Spangler *et al.* [73] claimed that administration of systemic steroids or diethylstilboestrol dramatically improved the fetal mortality to approximately 12 per cent.

The fetal mortality of 30 per cent which was reported [73], requires re-assessment. Spangler *et al.* [73] interpreted fetal deaths which occurred in pregnancies preceding the development of the papular eruption as related to the skin disorder which is hardly justified and grossly exaggerates the fetal risk. They also included spontaneous abortions in their data, but it would have been important to indicate their gestational age as first trimester spontaneous abortions are not uncommon in a normal population. In short, the fetal mortality in the cases of Spangler *et al.* was almost certainly overestimated and the way their mortality data were presented precludes a valid assessment. In our opinion papular dermatitis of pregnancy as defined by Spangler *et al.* [73] is a dubious entity in itself and the area still requires further study.

Autoimmune progesterone dermatitis of pregnancy

A single case of autoimmune progesterone dermatitis of pregnancy was described by Bierman [8]. It consisted of a non-pruritic acneiform eruption with papules, pustules and comedones on the fingers, arms, legs and buttocks. The eruption recurred in a subsequent pregnancy and both pregnancies terminated in spontaneous abortion. The striking histopathological features were of intense accumulation of eosinophils in hair follicles, epidermis, dermis and subcutis. Intradermal testing with aqueous progesterone produced a delayed hypersensitivity reaction and administration of an oral contraceptive containing norethindrone and mestranol resulted in a severe flare of the eruption. No premenstrual flares occurred. The dermatitis, which resolved rapidly on treatment with conjugated oestrogens, probably represents hypersensitivity to endogenous progesterone. No similar cases have since been reported.

The more common autoimmune progesterone dermatitis not associated with pregnancy is clinically distinct and consists of a polymorphic rash with urticaria, papulopustular vesicular or erythema multiforme-like lesions which recur on the trunk and extremities in the premenstrual period [22]. It is associated with previous use of progesterone-containing oral medication which appears to sensitize the body to endogenous progesterone [22]. There is usually a positive intradermal skin test to progesterone and treatment is with conjugated oestrogens or oophorectomy [65].

The effect of pregnancy on other dermatoses

The effect of pregnancy on other skin disorders is generally unpredictable although individual patients may react consistently.

Eczema

Atopic eczema frequently improves during pregnancy. However, if pruritus gravidarium develops, there may be exacerbation with development of prurigo.

Acne vulgaris

The effect of pregnancy on acne vulgaris is variable. Some patients improve whilst others develop acne for the first time. In these patients acne is often limited to the chin and may be associated with hirsutism. Tetracyclines and retinoids frequently prescribed for acne are contraindicated during pregnancy and their withdrawal may result in a flare.

Psoriasis and impetigo herpetiformis

Psoriasis may remain unchanged, clear or worsen and may also only manifest itself during pregnancy. Impetigo herpetiformis is a rare form of pustular psoriasis which can develop at any stage of gestation. The eruption consists of urticated erythema which begins in the flexures especially in the inguinal region. Superficial sterile pustules form at the margins of the lesions and the eruption may become widespread with involvement of mucosal surfaces. Fever, malaise, neutrophilia, hypocalcaemia and tetany are associated.

The histopathology is similar to that of pustular psoriasis with intraepidermal and subcorneal spongiform pustules of Kogoi and a perivascular infiltrate [44].

The disease usually remits at delivery but maternal and fetal mortality are high. Management requires intensive medical care with fluid and electrolyte replacement and correction of hypocalcaemia. Antibiotics are indicated for secondary infection and systemic corticosteroids may be helpful. Low dose methotrexate can be substituted post-partum to prevent rebound pustulation, but is contraindicated during pregnancy and lactation. Gonadotrophins are also reported to be helpful [57]. Fetal well-being should be carefully monitored and elective caesarean section performed if indicated to improve fetal morbidity [7].

Condylomata accuminata

Condylomata accuminata tend to grow rapidly during pregnancy even to the extent of interfering with delivery. Treatment with podophyllin is contraindicated but electrocoagulation and curettage may be effective.

Candidiasis

Candidiasis is 10–20 times more common in pregnancy when lowered vaginal pH and increased sweating create a favourable environment. It may be associated with pruritus vulvae and intertrigo. Infants born to affected mothers are increasingly prone to infection with *Candida*. Treatment is with topical nystatin or miconazole.

Leprosy

In general, patients with leprosy (Hansen's disease) do well in pregnancy. However, the subgroups of active lepromatous and dimorphous types have an increased incidence of obstetric complications and of Hansen's disease reactions. There is also an increased incidence of twins in lepromatous patients [51]. Although the sulphone drugs may be safely used as treatment during pregnancy [51], they have caused haemolytic disease of the newborn (HDN) [27] and dapsone has also caused HDN when transmitted through breast milk [60]. Patients with glucose-6-phosphate dehydrogenase deficiency are especially susceptible.

Pregnancy and collagen disease

(see Chapter 8)

Systemic lupus erythematosus (SLE) is no longer a contraindication to pregnancy, although it may precipitate a flare in up to 38 per cent of patients [20]. Women in complete clinical remission, irrespective of past manifestations of SLE, have the best chance of uncomplicated pregnancy and the highest incidence of fetal survival [24,46]. Exacerbation is more likely if the disease has been active in the preceding 6 years and may occur at any stage between early pregnancy and 8 weeks post-partum. Oral contraceptives may also induce exacerbations.

There is a higher fetal morbidity and mortality (see Chapter 8) and transient skin lesions clinically and histologically resembling those of SLE have been reported in the fetus [81].

Pregnancy has no consistent effect on discoid lupus erythematosus. The fetus is not affected. Dermatomyositis has been reported unchanged in 60 per cent, improved in 20 per cent and worsened in 20 per cent. Two patients first developed dermatomyositis during pregnancy. The fetal mortality is 46 per cent. Progesterone may aggravate dermatomyositis [78].

Systemic sclerosis and polyarteritis nodosa are discussed in Chapter 8.

Pregnancy and inflammatory skin disease

Urticaria may develop in late pregnancy and dermographism is also common. The specific dermatoses of pregnancy such as PG and prurigo of pregnancy may have an urticarial component. Treatment is with antihistamines.

Erythema multiforme

Erythema multiforme may also develop in successive pregnancies and can be differentiated histologically and on immunofluorescence from mild PG [35]. Drugs and viral infections, especially herpes simplex, are possible precipitating causes. Erythema nodosum and sarcoidosis are discussed in Chapter 1.

Pregnancy and benign and malignant tumours

Pregnancy usually has an adverse effect on neurofibromatosis (von Recklinghausen's disease). Lesions may appear for the first time or increase in size and number. Many patients have associated hypertension (see Chapter 6). Other complications include neuropathies associated with tumour growth and occasional sudden haemorrhage into neurofibromata.

Melanoma

Malignant melanoma accounts for nearly 50 per cent of metastases to the placenta and approximately 90 per cent involving the fetus. Stage 1 disease survival rates are unaffected by pregnancy but stage 2 survival rates are decreased [66]. Prognosis is also worse for those patients who have had previous pregnancies associated with growth or activation of a lesion subsequently diagnosed as melanoma. Pregnancy and oral contraception is best avoided in these and patients with stage 2 melanoma [66]. Treatment is as for melanoma in the non-pregnant state and termination of pregnancy appears to offer no appreciable maternal benefit.

Drug therapy during pregnancy

Ideally no drug should be prescribed for the first 3 months of pregnancy but potential guidelines for dermatological drug prescribing in pregnancy or the lactating period are now available [75]. Drugs of dermatological relevance that have already been considered and should not be given include methotrexate (psoriasis), tetracycline (see above, acne), podophyllin (see above, condylomata) and the vitamin A derivative isotretinoin and etretinate (see above, acne). Although cyclosporine remains contraindicated in pregnancy, recent experience indicates that there is no conclusive evidence of any teratogenic effect [83]. Furthermore there is still no evidence to suggest that PUVA is teratogenic when used to treat psoriasis. However, because PUVA is mutagenic, it is considered advisable to avoid PUVA treatments during pregnancy [74]. Those that should be given with caution include azathioprine, chloroquine, metronidazole and trimethoprim. In addition, thalidomide, now being advocated for the treatment of erythema nodosum, should not be used in pregnancy because of the well known risk of limb reduction defects and hydroxyurea and griseofulvin should not be used because of potential toxicity. Most of the commonly used antihistamines appear to be safe during pregnancy after the first trimester. The use of corticosteroids is discussed in Chapter 1.

Some antiviral agents such as idoxuridine are also contraindicated. Topical corticosteroids and tretinoin should be used sparingly in view of the risk of percutaneous absorption. Dithranol and tar appear to be safe.

All treatments should nevertheless be kept to a minimum, especially in the first trimester.

References

1 Aldercreutz H, Svanborg A & Anberg A. Recurrent jaundice in pregnancy. II A study of oestrogens and their conjugation in late pregnancy. *American Journal of Medicine* 1967; **42**: 341–7.

2 Aldercreutz H & Tenhunen R. Some aspects of the interaction between natural and synthetic female sex hormones and the liver. *American Journal of Medicine* 1970; **49**: 630–8.

3 Andersen B & Felding C. Pruritic urticarial papules and plaques of pregnancy. *Journal of Obstetrics and Gynaecology* 1992: **12**: 1–3.

4 Baxi LV, Ilovilam OP, Collins MH, Walther RR. Recurrent herpes gestationis with postpartum flare: A case report. *American Journal of Obstetrics and Gynecology* 1991; **164**: 778–80.

5 Bean WB, Cogswell R *et al*. Vascular changes in the skin in pregnancy. *Surgery, Gynaecology and Obstetrics* 1949; **88**: 739–52.

6 Beltrani VP & Beltrani VS. Pruritic urticarial papules and plaques of pregnancy: A severe case requiring early delivery from relief of symptoms. *Journal of the American Academy of Dermatology* 1992; **26**: 266–7.

7 Beveridge GW, Harkness RA & Livingstone JRB. Impetigo herpetiformis in two successive pregnancies. *British Journal of Dermatology* 1966; **78**: 106–12.

8 Bierman SM. Autoimmune dermatitis of pregnancy. *Archives of Dermatology* 1973; **107**: 896–901.

9 Black MM & Stephens CJM. The specific dermatoses of pregnancy: the British perspective. In: Callen JP, Dahl MV, Golitz LE, Greenway HT & Schachner LA (eds), *Advances in Dermatology*. Mosby Year Book, St Louis, 1992: 105–26.

10 Bourne G. Toxaemic rash of pregnancy. *Journal of the Royal Society of Medicine* 1962; **55**: 46212.

11 *British Medical Journal* editorial. *British Medical Journal* 1975; **iii**: 608.

12 Bunker CB, Erskine K *et al*. Severe polymorphic eruption of pregnancy occurring in twin pregnancies. *Clinical and Experimental Dermatology* 1990; **15**: 228–31.

13 Catanzarite V & Quirk SG. Papular dermatoses of pregnancy. *Clinical Obstetrics and Gynecology* 1990; **33**: 754–8.

14 Cohen LM, Capeless EL *et al*. Pruritic urticarial papules and plaques of pregnancy and its relationship to meternal-fetal weight gain and twin pregnancy. *Archives of Dermatology* 1989; **125**: 1534–6.

15 Cooper AJ & Fryer JA. Prurigo of late pregnancy. *Australasia Journal of Dermatology* 1980; **21**: 79–84.

16 Cummings K & Derbes VJ. Dermatoses associated with pregnancy. *Cutis* 1967; **3**: 120–6.

17 Davey CMH. Factors associated with the occurrence of striae gravidarum. *Journal of Obstetrics and Gynaecology of the British Commonwealth* 1972; **79**: 113.

18 Demis DB, Dobson RL & McGuire J. *Clinical Dermatology*. Harper & Row, New York, 1972.

19 Dupont C. Herpes gestationis with hydatidiform mole. *Transactions of St Johns Dermatological Society* 1974; **60**: 103.

20 Fitzpatrick TB, Eisen AZ & Wolff K. *Dermatology in General Medicine*. McGraw-Hill, New York, 1987: 2082.

21 Garvey MP, Handfield-Jones SE & Black MM. Pemphigoid gestationis response to chemical oophorectormy with goserelin. *Clinical and Experimental Dermatology* 1992; **17**: 443–5.

22 Hart RH. Autoimmune progesterone dermatitis. *Archives of Dermatology* 1977; **113**: 427–30.

23 Hayashi RH. Bullous dermatoses and prurigo of pregnancy. *Clinical Obstetrics and Gynecology* 1990; **33**: 746–53.

24 Hayslett JP & Reece EA. Systemic lupus erthematosus in pregnancy. *Clinical Perinatology* 1985; **12**: 539–50.

25 Hellreich PD. The skin changes of pregnancy. *Cutis* 1974; **13**: 82–6.

26 Hirvioja M, Tuimala R & Vuori J. The treatment of intrahepatic cholestasis of pregnancy by dexamethasone. *British Journal of Obstetrics and Gynaecology* 1992; **99**: 109–11.

27 Hocking DR. Neonatal haemolytic disease due to dapsone. *Medical Journal of Australia* 1968; **1**: 1130.

28 Holmes RC & Black MM. The specific dermatoses of pregnancy. A reappraisal with special emphasis on a proposed simplified classification. *Clinical and Experimental Dermatology* 1982; **7**: 65–73.

29 Holmes RC & Black MM. The specific dermatoses of pregnancy. *Journal of the American Academy of Dermatology* 1983; **8**: 405–12.

30 Holmes RC, Black MM *et al*. A comparative study of toxic erythema of pregnancy and herpes gestationis. *British Journal of Dermatology* 1982; **106**: 499–510.

31 Holmes RC, Black MM & James DCO. Paternal responsibility for herpes gestationis. In: MacDonald DM (ed), *Immunodermatology*. Butterworths, London, 1984: 251–3.

32 Holmes RC, Black MM *et al*. Clues to the aetiology and pathogenesis of herpes gestationis. *British Journal of Dermatology* 1983; **109**: 131–9.

33 Holzbach RT. Jaundice in pregnancy. *American Journal of Medicine* 1976; **61**: 367–76.

34 Hughes GRV. Connective tissue disease and the skin. *Clinical and Experimental Dermatology* 1984; **9**: 535–44.

35 Iffy L & Kaminetzky HA (eds). Skin diseases in Pregnancy. In: *Principles and Practice of Obstetrics and Perinatology*. John Wiley, Chichester, 1981: 1361–79.

36 Jordan RE, Heine KG *et al*. Immunopathology of herpes gestationis. Immunofluorescence studies and characterisation of 'HG factor'. *Journal of Clinical Investigation* 1976; **57**: 1426–33.

37 Jureka W, Holmes RC *et al*. An immunoelectron microscopy study of the relationship between herpes gestationis and polymorphic eruption of pregnancy. *British Journal of Dermatology* 1983; **108**: 147–51.

38 Katz SI, Hertz KC & Yaoita H. Herpes gestationis. Immunopathology and characterisation of the HG factor. *Journal of Clinical Investigation* 1976; **57**: 434–41.

39 Kenny JF, Pangburn PC & Trail G. Effect of oestradiol on immune competence: *in vivo* and *in vitro* studies. *Infection and Community* 1976; **13**: 448.

40 Kligman AM & Willis I. A new formula for depig-

menting human skin. *Archives of Dermatology* 1975; **111**: 540–7.
41 Kolodny RC. Herpes gestationis. A new assessment of incidence, diagnosis and foetal prognosis. *American Journal of Obstetrics and Gynecology* 1969; **104**: 39–45.
42 Lawley TJ, Hertz KC *et al*. Pruritic urticarial papules and plaques of pregnancy. *Journal of the American Medical Association* 1979; **241**: 1696–9.
43 Lawley TJ, Stingl G & Katz SI. Foetal and maternal risk factors in herpes gestationis. *Archives of Dermatology* 1978; **114**: 552–5.
44 Lever WF. *Histopathology of the Skin*. JB Lippincott, Philadelphia, 1985: 145.
45 Liu DTY. Striae gravidarum. *Lancet* 1974; **i**: 625.
46 Lundbert I & Hedfors E. Pregnancy outcome in patients with high titre anti-RNP antibodies: a retrospective study of 40 pregnancies. *Journal of Rheumatology* 1991; **18**: 359–62.
47 Lynch FN & Albrecht RJ. Hormonal factors in herpes gestationis. *Archives of Dermatology* 1966; **3**: 465–6.
48 Lyndfield YL. Effect of pregnancy on the human hair cycle. *Journal of Investigative Dermatology* 1960; **35**: 323–7.
49 MacDonald KJS & Raffle EJ. Ritodrine therapy associated with remission of pemphigoid gestationis. *British Journal of Dermatology* 1984; **111**: 630.
50 MacKinnon PCB & McKinnon IL. Palmar sweating in pregnancy. *Journal of Obstetrics and Gynaecology of the British Empire* 1955; **62**: 298–9.
51 Maurus JN. Hansen's disease in pregnancy. *Obstetrics and Gynecology* 1978; **52**: 22–5.
52 Newcomer VD, Linberg MC & Sternberg TH. A melanosis of the face 'cholasma'. *Archives of Dermatology* 1961; **83**: 284–97.
52a Newton JA & McGibbon DH. Cutaneous telangiectasia treated with the argon laser. *British Journal of Dermatology* 1985; **113** (suppl) 29–36.
53 Nurse DS. Prurigo of pregnancy. *Australasia Journal of Dermatology* 1968; **9**: 258–67.
54 Palma J, Reyes H, Rivalta J, Ighesions J & Gonzalez M. Management of intrahepatic cholestasis in pregnancy. *Lancet* 1992; **339**: 1478.
55 Pinkus H, Keech MK & Mehregan AH. Histopathology of striae distensae with special reference to striae and wound healing in the Marfan syndrome. *Journal of Investigative in Dermatology* 1966; **46**: 293–9.
56 Provost TT & Tomasi TB. Evidence of complement activiation via the alternative pathway in skin diseases I. Herpes gestationis, systemic lupus erythematosus and bullous pemphigoid. *Journal of Clinical Investigation* 1973; **52**: 1779–87.
57 Rasmussen KA & Ehrenskjold MI. Impetigo herpetiformis. A case in a pregnant women treated with antex. *Acta Obstetricia et Gynaecologica Scandinavica* 1965; **44**: 563.
58 Resnick S. Melasma induced by oral contraceptive drugs. *Journal of the American Medical Association* 1967; **199**: 601–5.
59 Sanchez NP, Pathak MA *et al*. Melasma; a clinical, light microscopic, ultrastructural and immunofluorescence study. *Journal of the American Academy of Dermatology* 1981; **4**: 698–710.
60 Sanders SW, Zone JJ *et al*. Haemolytic anaemia transmitted through breast milk. *Annals of Internal Medicine* 1982; **96**: 485–6.
61 Sasseville D, Wilkinson RD & Schnader JY. Dermatoses of pregnancy. *International Journal of Dermatology* 1981; **20**: 223–41.
62 Schaumberg-Lever G, Saffold OE *et al*. Herpes gestationis. Histology and ultrastructure. *Archives of Dermatology* 1973; **107**: 888.
63 Schiff BL, Pawtucket RI & Kern AB. Study of postpartum alopecia. *Archives of Dermatology* 1963; **87**: 609–11.
64 Schizume K & Lerner AB. Determination of melanocyte-stimulating hormone in urine and blood. *Journal of Clinical Endocrinology and Metabolism* 1954; **14**: 1491.
65 Shelley WB, Preucel RW & Spoont SS. Autoimmune progesterone dermatitis. Cure by oophorectomy. *Journal of the American Medical Association* 1964; **190**: 35.
66 Shiu MA, Schottenfeld D *et al*. Adverse effect of pregnancy on melanoma. A reappraisal, *Cancer* 1976; **37**: 181–7.
67 Shornick JK, Bangert JL *et al*. Herpes gestationis. Clinical and histologic features of twenty eight cases. *Journal of the American Academy of Dermatology* 1983; **8**: 214.
68 Shornick JK & Black MM. Fetal risks in herpes gestationis. *Journal of the American Academy of Dermatology* 1992; **26**: 63–8.
69 Shornick JK & Black MM. Secondary auto-immune diseases in herpes gestationis (pemphigoid gestationis). *Journal of the American Academy of Dermatology* 1992; **26**: 563–6.
70 Shornick JK, Stastny P & Gilliam JN. High frequency of histocompatibility antigens HLA-DR3 and DR4 in herpes gestationis. *Journal of Clinical Investigation* 1981; **68**: 553–5.
71 Shuster S. The cause of striae distense. *Acta Dermatovenereologica Supplementum (Stockholm)* 1979; **59**: 161–9.
72 Snell R. The pigmentary changes occurring in breast skin during pregnancy and following oestrogen treatment. *Journal of Investigative Dermatology* 1964; **43**: 181–6.
73 Spangler AS, Reddy W *et al*. Papular dermatitis of pregnancy. *Journal of the American Medical Association* 1962; **181**: 577–81.
74 Stern RS & Lange R. Outcomes of pregnancies among women and partners of men with a history of exposure to methoxsalen photochemotherapy (PUVA) for the treatment of psoriasis. *Archives of Dermatology* 1991; **127**: 347–400.
75 Stockton DL & Paller AS. Drug administration to the

pregnant or lactating woman: A reference guide for dermatologists. *Journal of the American Academy of Dermatology* 1990; **23**: 87–103.

76 Thody AJ, Plummer NA *et al*. Plasma SS-melanocyte-stimulating hormone levels in pregnancy. *Journal of Obstetrics and Gynaecology of the British Commonwealth* 1974; **81**: 875–7.

77 Tillman WG. Herpes gestationis with hydatidiform mole and chorion epithelioma. *British Medical Journal* 1950; **i**: 1471.

78 Trotter M. The activity of hair follicles with reference to pregnancy. *Surgery, Gynaecology and Obstetrics* 1935; **60**: 1092–5.

79 Tsai A, Lindheimer MD *et al*. Dermatomyositis complicating pregnancy. *Obstetrics and Gynecology* 1973; **41**: 570–3.

80 Van Der Wiel A, Hart H *et al*. Plasma exchange in herpes gestationis. *British Medical Journal* 1980; **281**: 1041.

81 Vonderheid EC, Koblenzer PJ *et al*. Neonatal lupus erythematosus. *Archives of Dermatology* 1976; **112**: 698–705.

82 Wade TR, Wade SL & Jones HE. Skin changes and diseases associated with pregnancy. *Obstetrics and Gynecology* 1978; **52**: 233–42.

83 Wright S, Glover M & Baker H. Psoriasis, cyclosporine, and pregnancy. *Archives of Dermatology* 1991; **127**: 426.

84 Yancey KB, Hall RB & Lawley T. Pruritic urticarial papules and plaques of pregnancy. *Journal of the American Academy of Dermatology* 1984; **10**: 473–80.

85 Zoberman E & Farmer ER. Pruritic folliculitis of pregnancy. *Archives of Dermatology* 1981; **117**: 20–2.

Further reading

Beckett MA & Goldberg NS. Pruritic urticarial plaques and papules of pregnancy and skin distension. *Archives of Dermatology* 1991; **127**: 125–6.

Gillis M, Mortel R & McGavron MH. Maternal malignant melanoma metastatic to the products of conception. Report of a case. *Gynaecology and Oncology* 1976; **4**: 38.

Holmes RC & Black MM. Herpes gestationis. *Dermatologic Clinics* 1983; **1**: 195–203.

Holmes RC & Black MM. The fetal prognosis in pemphigoid gestationis. *British Journal of Dermatology* 1984; **110**: 67–72.

Kreek MJ, Weser E *et al*. Recurrent cholestatic jaundice of pregnancy with demonstrated oestrogen sensitivity. *American Journal of Medicine* 1967; **43**: 795–803.

Reid R, Ivey KJ *et al*. Foetal complications of obstetric cholestasis. *British Medical Journal* 1976; **i**: 870–2.

Salvatore MA & Lynch PJ. Erythema nodosum, oestrogens and pregnancy. *Archives in Dermatology* 1980; **116**: 557–8.

Schatz M, Patterson R *et al*. Corticosteroid therapy for the pregnant asthmatic patient. *Journal of the American Medical Association* 1975; **233**: 804–7.

Sherlock S. Jaudice in pregnancy. *British Medical Bulletin* 1968; **24**: 39–43.

Wise R. Prescribing in pregnancy: antibiotics. *British Medical Journal* 1987; **294**: 42–6.

Wong RC & Ellis CN. Physiologic skin changes in pregnancy. *Journal of the American Academy of Dermatology* 1984; **10**: 929–38.

20

Psychiatry in Pregnancy

Peter F. Liddle

Pharmacological treatment, 625
Psychological treatment, 626
Social issues in management, 626
Antenatal psychiatric disorder, 627
Depression during pregnancy
Anxiety during pregnancy
Obsessional ruminations and phobias
Pre-existing psychiatric disorders, 630
Chronic depression
Manic depressive psychosis
Schizophrenia
Disorders in the post-partum period, 634
Puerperal psychosis
Postnatal depression

Psychiatric disorders in pregnancy and the puerperium reflect a complex interplay between the physiological, psychological and social aspects of conceiving, carrying, delivering and nurturing a baby, and the pre-existing psychological adjustment of the woman. To a large extent, the signs and symptoms of psychiatric disorders in pregnancy and the puerperium resemble the signs and symptoms of psychiatric disorders occurring at other times, but precipitating factors are shaped by circumstances unique to childbearing. Furthermore, the need on the one hand to achieve relatively rapid resolution of symptoms threatening the well-being of the mother and her child, whilst on the other hand avoiding unnecessary pharmacological treatment in pregnancy, presents unique challenges in the planning of treatment.

The most common disorders presenting during pregnancy are depression, anxiety and various specific phobias. Furthermore, the optimum management of pre-existing psychiatric disorder during pregnancy requires careful planning. In the puerperium, the majority of women experience the transient mood disturbance known as the blues. A smaller proportion develop postnatal depression which is more sustained and can be associated with substantial adverse effects on the woman, her baby and her partner. The most serious disorder of the puerperium is post-partum psychosis which is rare but has a potentially devastating effect on the woman and her family. Before considering each of these clinical conditions in detail, we should briefly consider some general issues regarding management of psychiatric disorder in relation to pregnancy.

Pharmacological treatment

During pregnancy, planning pharmacological treatment entails balancing of benefits against risks. For the long-established exemplars of all the major classes of psychotrophic medication, the available evidence indicates that overt developmental abnormalites following exposure *in utero* are very unlikely, except possibly in the case of lithium and, perhaps also of carbamazepine (see Chapter 15). However, there is also a theoretical possibility, as yet neither confirmed nor refuted by evidence, that exposure to psychotrophic medication might produce subtle alterations in the development of the central nervous system influencing behaviour later in life. Furthermore, many psychotrophic drugs can produce toxic effects such as excitation or depression of the central nervous system, extra-pyramidal motor signs and anticholinergic effects that might be harmful in the neonate.

The risks of marked fetal malformation are greatest in the first trimester, but the neural architecture of the brain takes shape throughout intrauterine development, so potential influences on central nervous system development might not be confined to the first trimester. Thus, whilst it is most important to minimize drug exposure in the first trimester, caution is required throughout the pregnancy, and in the final weeks, risks of adverse influence on labour and the physiology of the newborn infant must be taken into account. When psychological treatment alone might be successful, as is the case in mild depression and simple anxiety states, it is clearly preferable to avoid pharmacological treatment. However, it is important not to underestimate the consequences for both mother and child, including the dangers of disrupted antenatal care, self-neglect or self-harm, likely to result if mental disorder in pregnancy is not treated adequately. Therefore for severe depression, disabling anxiety and for active psychotic disorders, pharmacological treatment is justified. The question of prophylaxis in cases of prior psychotic illness demands a careful evaluation of the likelihood of relapse.

Most psychotrophic medications, including antipsychotic medication as well as antidepressants and anxiolytics, are excreted in breast milk, though in many instances a breast-feeding infant is likely to receive a very small dose. In cases of serious mental disorder in the post-partum period, such as psychosis or severe depression, pharmacological treatment is almost always essential because the dangers of inadequately treating such disorders include risk of maternal suicide and a non-negligible risk of injury to the infant. For treatments with a substantial potential for toxicity, such as lithium and high doses of antipsychotic medication, the balance of risk indicates that the mother should not breast feed. For tricyclic antidepressant medication, for benzodiazepine anxiolytics, and for low doses of antipsychotic medication, there is little evidence of substantial risk to the breast-feeding infant, and the balance between the risks and benefits of breast feeding are not clear-cut. Therefore, if the mother wishes to breast feed while taking such medication, she should be told that the available evidence suggests low risk, but if the baby shows unexpected drowsiness, irritability or twitchiness after feeding, she should seek medical advice. If at that stage there is convincing evidence of such effects on the baby, discontinuation of breast feeding should be recommended. Some clinicians have argued that it is valuable to perform measurements of levels of the psychotrophic medication in the infant serum, but this is not a routine practice in the UK.

Psychological treatment

Usually, the major goal of treatment of mental disorder in pregnancy and the puerperium is control of symptoms over a time scale of months. For such purposes, short-term, goal-orientated psychotherapies such as behavioural therapy, cognitive therapy and cognitive–analytic therapy are especially useful. The strategies and techniques required are similar to those required in other settings, but in addition, there are several features specific to pregnancy and the puerperium that demand recognition.

The worries encountered in pregnancy and the puerperium frequently reveal distorted beliefs about pregnancy and motherhood, which are fostered by cultural myths. For a woman who experiences in the second trimester a disconcerting sense that control of her life has been taken from her and who is unsure how she will cope with motherhood, the expectation of her family and friends that she should by this stage be serene and content, reinforces her sense of inadequacy. It is less easy for her to confide in friends and there is danger of a vicious cycle driven by negative self-evaluation. For the primiparous mother of a 2-month-old infant who only encounters other young mothers in public settings where they manage to maintain a competent facade, her own awareness of her fragile competence at home reinforces the growing realization that she is failing to achieve the image of motherhood that had been inculcated in her since childhood. Again there is a risk of a vicious cycle in which low self-esteem creates a depressed mood that further diminishes self-esteem. In such situations, there is need for education, and for simple psychological strategies to help restore a balanced perspective.

Social issues in management

For the economically deprived, pregnancy and parenthood present severe challenges and major stresses that can either precipitate or maintain mental illness. The clinician often needs to adopt the role of advocate exerting influence to obtain social services for the patient. Even amongst those who are relatively well-off, for many young couples the struggle for economic security places pressure on both partners to work. Hence, when pregnancy and motherhood makes this impossible, practical economic difficulties (often compounded by the covert pressures arising from society's conflicting attitudes towards combining work and motherhood) place substantial pressures on the woman and on her relationship with her partner.

Antenatal psychiatric disorder

The antenatal period is not a time of increased risk of psychiatric disorder for the majority of women. Indeed, it is probable that for many, the happiness and hope associated with pregnancy helps enhance self-esteem and affords some protection against mental illness. However, the absence of a statistical increase in mental disorder in pregnancy conceals a more complex picture. For women in adverse social circumstances, and for those who suffered difficulty in conceiving, or who have faced persisting threat of miscarriage, pregnancy can be fraught with worry. Even in benign circumstances, the potentially destabilizing influence of rapidly increasing hormone levels and the tiring physiological demands of pregnancy can lead to changeable mood and irritability. Thus, attention to emotional health is an important aspect of antenatal care.

Depression during pregnancy

The evidence suggests that the first trimester is the time of highest risk for depression in pregnancy. Approximately 10 per cent of women suffer depression during that time [18]. This is similar to the expected prevalence of depression in non-pregnant women, and there is no reason to propose that the pathophysiology of depression arising in pregnancy differs from that of depression at other times. However, the nature of the stresses that precipitate the episode of depression tend to reflect the specific psychosocial stressors associated with pregnancy.

As in other types of depression, the cardinal clinical feature is low mood, often accompanied by anxiety. The low mood is usually associated with low self-esteem, pessimism, loss of interest and of capacity for enjoyment. There is usually impairment of concentration, and disturbance of sleep and appetite. Suicide is rare, but the clinician must always perform an assessment of potential suicide risk. There is a substantial overlap between the features of depression and anxiety. It is not uncommon for depression to be associated with agoraphobia. Untreated, antenatal depression tends to persist for many months, and in some cases, it is a precursor of postnatal depression.

Treatment

In mild cases, the most appropriate treatment is usually cognitive therapy. In more severe cases, such as those characterized by marked early morning wakening and or suicidal ideas, treatment with a tricyclic antidepressant such as amitriptyline, imipramine or lofepramine, is warranted. Although more recently developed antidepressants, such as the serotonin re-uptake inhibitors, offer the potential advantages of fewer anticholinergic side-effects and less risk of death from overdose, less information is available about potential risk to the fetus, so it is probably best to avoid these newer drugs unless marked problems with side-effects or high risk of self-harm provide a specific reason for avoiding the longer established tricyclics in an individual case.

With regard to the tricyclic antidepressants, the evidence suggests that the risk to the fetus is low. In 1972, McBride reported congenital limb deformity in the child of a mother who had taken imipramine during pregnancy [20], but a systematic large-scale survey failed to confirm an association between tricyclic antidepressants and limb deformity [1]. There is thus very slight evidence that tricyclic antidepressants might be harmful in the first trimester, and this risk should not preclude their use in cases of severe depression. In view of the substantial anticholinergic effects of amitryptiline and imipramine, the neonate is at risk of neuromuscular irritability and of disturbance of visceral function if the mother has a substantial serum level at the time of delivery. Therefore, in the final weeks of pregnancy it is desirable to reduce the dose and then withdraw the drug entirely prior to delivery if possible.

Anxiety during pregnancy

Pregnancy is associated with risk and a degree of concern about possible dangers is natural and appropriate. Normal concerns are usually best dealt with by straightforward explanation of the issues, avoiding unwarranted reassurance as this is liable to undermine the trust that is essential for a reasonably confident approach to the pregnancy.

In cases where the worry is clearly disproportionate to the circumstances, and is accompanied by other characteristic symptoms of anxiety such that ability to function becomes impaired, the condition has crossed the boundary of normal reaction and should be regarded as an illness. The symptoms of an anxiety disorder include a subjective sense of anxiety; somatic symptoms such as tachycardia, dyspnoea, tremor and gastrointestinal disturbance; sleep disturbance and impaired concentration. In pregnancy, gastrointestinal symptoms, especially nausea and vomiting are a frequently encountered feature of anxiety, presumably because the normal physiological events of pregnancy predispose to such gastrointestinal disturbances.

Sometimes the anxiety occurs in discrete episodes of panic in which there is sudden onset of somatic symptoms of anxiety, often accompanied by fears of perceived catastrophe, such as a fear of heart attack, fainting in embarrassing circumstances or going mad. Such episodes of panic can be appear to arise 'out of the blue' without obvious precipitants, but in other cases are clearly related to specific precipitating circumstances, such as travelling in public transport or being in a public place such as a supermarket. In instances where there is a specific precipitant, the patient tends to avoid the precipitating situation, thereby reinforcing a phobic fear of that situation. Specific phobias are discussed below, but it is important to note that phobic fears, especially agoraphobia, are commonly encountered in association with more generalized anxiety.

Anxiety states are also frequently accompanied by low mood and other features of depression. It is probable that there is an intrinsic overlap between the pathophysiology of anxiety and depression, such that at least in milder cases, there is often little point in attempting to distinguish between the two conditions.

The treatment of anxiety states in pregnancy might entail either psychological treatments alone, or a combination of pharmacological and psychological treatment. In relatively mild cases, psychological treatment is usually to be preferred. The principal psychological techniques for anxiety management are derived from behaviour therapy and cognitive therapy. Two cardinal behavioural strategies are learning to relax in anxiety provoking situations, and planning activities that deflect the person away from pre-occupation with worrying thoughts. However, it should be noted that avoidance of a feared situation is in itself likely to enhance the fear by reinforcing the belief that avoidance is the only way of alleviating the symptoms. Cognitive techniques entail learning to recognize the distorted thinking processes that underlie disproportionate fear, and then weighing up the evidence with the object of putting the situation in a reasonable perspective. Psychological management of anxiety is as successful as pharmacological management in mild to moderate cases, especially when the source of the fears can be identified readily.

In severe anxiety disorders, such as cases where there is a persistent generalized anxiety which is disabling, or there are frequent panic attacks which are not clearly related to a specific precipitant, it is usually preferable to employ pharmacological treatment. Benzodiazepine anxiolytics, such as diazepam, can provide effective relief of symptoms, at least in the short term, but present a risk of dependence if used for more than a few weeks. Although early studies suggested a possible relationship between cleft lip and palate, and exposure to diazepam *in utero*, a large case controlled study found no evidence for such an association [32]. Because of risk of depression of respiration in the neonate, and of muscular hypotonia, it is necessary to minimize use of benzodiazepines in the final weeks of the pregnancy. Tricyclic antidepressants are also effective anxiolytics, and in some circumstances are to be preferred to benzodiazepines. Treatment with a tricyclic is preferable when the anxiety is accompanied by features of depression.

Case illustration. A woman who had had six terminations of pregnancy on the grounds of severe hyperemesis was referred for psychiatric assessment during the first trimester of her seventh pregnancy. She had been admitted to hospital because of intractable vomiting. She was pale and weak. Although she reported that both she and her husband were eager to have a baby, she was convinced that she could not possibly tolerate the vomiting any longer. She had enjoyed a very sheltered childhood, and had never acquired any confidence that she could withstand demanding situations. Despite being adamant that the vomiting was a purely physical disorder, she was prepared to accept that anxiety about the continuation of the vomiting might itself generate tension that would act to perpetuate the vomiting, and willingly accepted help to develop psychological strategies for coping.

After several sessions directed at building her confidence so that she could reduce the severity of the vomiting by recognizing when she was being drawn into distorted catastrophic thoughts about her ability to cope, the vomiting did indeed abate. She was discharged from hospital, and at follow-up several weeks later, was no longer troubled by vomiting. However, she was wracked by indecision about whether or not she wanted to have a baby. She was appalled by the thought that motherhood would annihilate her image of herself as a care-free young wife, cherished by and giving delight to her husband. By 20 weeks' gestation, she had decided to continue with the pregnancy, but felt trapped by the circumstances. On the one hand, she did not want to disappoint her husband in his wish for a child, but on the other, she was convinced that she had destroyed the happiness that they had previously shared as a care-free couple. She was dismayed by her own selfishness in wanting to avoid the responsibility of motherhood. As her resentment grew, so too did her sense of guilt. The vomiting recommenced, now clearly triggered by negative thoughts about the pregnancy. She began to contemplate suicide.

By 22 weeks she was showing overt evidence of depression. She was tearful, hopeless and sleeping poorly. Treatment with a tricyclic antidepressant led to an improvement in her pattern of sleep, but the negative thoughts about the pregnancy persisted. In subsequent weeks, she became preoccupied by fears that she would not cope with the delivery. She was tormented by the fear that when she saw the baby she would hate it vehemently. She was also horrified by the prospect of her facade of self-control disintegrating in a state of uncontrolled screaming during labour. Thoughts of suicide persisted. Diazepam was added to the antidepressant in an attempt to control the mounting anxiety, and a combination of cognitive and behavioural techniques employed to build up her ability to cope when the dose of medication was reduced in the final weeks of the pregnancy.

This case demonstrates not only the overlap between physical symptoms, anxiety and depression, but also the need to employ a variety of treatment strategies, pharmacological and psychological, to control her various symptoms whilst attempting to overcome her almost total inability to perceive herself as capable of taking responsibility, which lay at the heart of her problem.

Obsessional ruminations and phobias

Obsessional ruminations are distressing recurrent fears which the patient recognizes are unreasonable, but which intrude insistently into everyday mental activity. Phobias are unreasonable fears of specific situations or objects. Obsessions and phobias can arise in a context of more wide-ranging anxiety as in the case presented above of the young woman whose overwhelming anxiety about her ability to bear the responsibilities of motherhood led to obsessional ruminations about the delivery. They can also occur as a part of a primary depressive disorder. In other instances, a specific obsession or phobia occurs in relative isolation, with other symptoms such as depressed mood or generalized anxiety either absent or forming only a very minor component of the clinical picture.

The major component of treatment for phobias is a combination of cognitive and behavioural therapy. Simple phobias, in which the subject has a well-focused fear of a particular situation usually respond well to a behavioural approach directed at achieving exposure of the patient to the feared situation, thereby demonstrating to the patient that her irrational fears do not come to fruition. Behavioural techniques such as progressive muscular relaxation, and cognitive techniques which encourage the patient to evaluate the evidence about the fears in a balanced manner, are used to facilitate the goal of exposure.

Obsessional ruminations respond less well to behavioural techniques. Although cognitive therapy is sometimes effective, it is often necessary to combine cognitive therapy with pharmacological therapy. When a brief course of anxiolytic medication is required to break a vicious cycle between worrying thoughts and symptoms of anxiety, a benzodiazepine is preferred. Diazepam is appropriate when the anxiety is likely at any time of the day, and the shorter acting temazepam when the anxiety is likely to be encountered at predictable times. If benzodiazepines are used regularly over a period of several weeks, withdrawal symptoms on cessation of treatment become a problem. Therefore, when a longer period of treatment is anticipated, it is sometimes preferable to use a tricyclic antidepressant. Clomipramine has been demonstrated to be especially effective for treating obsessive–compulsive disorders [13].

Case illustration. A 28-year-old woman who was successful in her professional career, developed a pattern of nausea and vomiting that was worse in the evening during the mid-trimester of her first pregnancy. She recognized that the nausea was associated with the prospect of eating the evening meal with her husband. The marriage was happy, and both partners wanted the baby. She reported that she had suffered from a similar problem with vomiting during a traumatic relationship with her first serious boyfriend a decade previously. When this pattern recurred during the pregnancy she became obsessed with the fear that her relationship with her husband might disintegrate, and developed a phobia concerning eating the evening meal with her husband. A careful examination of her feelings revealed no grounds for suspecting any intrinsic problem in the relationship. In the circumstances, the most credible explanation appeared to be that the normal physiological disturbances of gastrointestinal function in the first trimester had re-activated memories of the way in which previous relationship difficulties had been expressed in gastrointestinal symptoms, and created a vicious circle in which the fear of the implications of the vomiting itself reinforced the disturbed autonomic activity that maintained the gastrointestinal upset.

Weekly sessions of cognitive therapy directed at dealing with the cognitions associated with the anxiety that began to build as the evening approached achieved some improvement, but after 6 weeks the problem persisted. At that stage, addition of temazepam, 10 mg taken in the late afternoon, broke the vicious cycle in which somatic symptoms of anxiety fuelled her worries about her marital relationship. The temazepam was then gradually withdrawn by setting a decreasing target for the number of days per week on which she would take the temazepam. In the latter stages of pregnancy, she was seen intermittently for supportive sessions.

Pre-existing psychiatric disorders

In circumstances where a woman receiving long-term treatment for psychiatric disorder is considering having a baby, it is important that she and her partner are encouraged to take account of the potential interaction between childbearing and the illness, and in particular, to consider the question of a carefully monitored reduction or discontinuation of psychotrophic medication prior to conception.

Chronic depression

Depression is prevalent in the general population, and in a substantial proportion of cases it runs a very chronic course. In many instances, pre-existing chronic depression has shown at best an equivocal response to prior treatment with antidepressant medication. Hence, if the patient is taking antidepressant medication prior to, or at the time of, conception, it is usually preferable to institute a trial withdrawal of this medication, replacing pharmacotherapy with supportive psychotherapy. The goal is to contain symptoms throughout the pregnancy and help the patients find pragmatic solutions to the specific psychosocial problems they encounter. If trial withdrawal of antidepressant medication leads to a substantial exacerbation of the depression, antidepressant medication should be re-instated, though if possible, recommencement should be delayed until after the end of the first trimester.

Manic depressive psychosis

The lifetime risk of suffering manic depressive psychosis is approximately 1–2 per cent. It is a condition characterized by episodes of acute illness interspersed with periods of relatively normal psychological function. Prophylactic medication, such as lithium carbonate helps maintain stability of mood. Carbamazepine is of similar efficacy as a prophylactic agent, though less widely used. Antipsychotics, which include phenothiazines such as chlorpromazine and trifluoperazine, and butyrophenones such as haloperidol, are also used as prophylaxis, but the main role of these drugs is in the treatment of acute episodes.

The major issues facing a woman with manic depressive illness who wishes to have a baby are: (a) the risk that the child will inherit manic depressive illness; (b) the risk of psychotic relapse if prophylactic medication is discontinued during pregnancy; (c) the high risk of a psychotic relapse in the post-partum period; and (d) the risk of damage to the fetus if either lithium or carbamazepine is taken in the first trimester of pregnancy.

The risk that the child will suffer manic depressive illness lies in the range 10–15 per cent, and the risk that the mother will suffer a psychotic episode in the post-partum period is as high as 50 per cent if no precautions are taken. If the woman and her partner decide that they nonetheless wish to have a child, it is important to plan the management of the illness throughout pregnancy and in the post-partum period with great care, to minimize the risk of the woman suffering a psychotic relapse.

Prophylactic treatment during pregnancy

Maternal treatment with lithium carbonate is associated with maldevelopment of the heart and great vessels, especially with Ebstein's anomaly which is a maldevelopment of the tricuspid valve [24]. The severity of this abnormality ranges from incompatibility with live birth to relative minor impairment of cardiac function. Data based on an international register of lithium-exposed pregnancies suggested that the risk of significant congenital abnormality when the mother takes lithium in the first trimester was about 10 per cent, including 8 per cent with cardiovascular malformation of whom half suffered Ebstein's anomaly [21]. However, a recent multicentre prospective study [14] of 138 pregnancies in which lithium was taken in the first trimester found the prevalence of major congenital abnormality was only 2.8 per cent, with one case of Ebstein's anomaly. In the control group, the prevalence of major abnormality was 2.4 per cent, with no cases of Ebstein's anomaly. Thus, the risk associated with lithium exposure is probably lower than had hitherto been accepted.

Until the late 1980s, the available information suggested that carbamazepine was a potentially useful alternative to lithium for prophylaxis against manic depressive illness in pregnancy, but more recent evidence raises the possibility of risk of harm to the developing fetus. A prospective study of 35 children of women taking carbamazepine (for epilepsy in all but one case) who expressed concern about the risk during the pregnancy, found minor craniofacial defects in 11 per cent, fingernail hypoplasia in 26 per cent and a degree of developmental delay in 20 per cent [15]. The study employed several criteria for developmental delay, of which the least stringent was a score of 1 SD below the population average. Sixteen per cent of a normal population would be expected to have a score below such a criterion. Furthermore, in the absence of a control group suffering from epilepsy, observed abnormalities cannot necessarily be attributed to treatment with carbamazepine, especially as epilepsy can be associated with fetal abnormality unrelated to medication [34]. Thus the question of the risk associated with carbamazepine remains controversial.

There are no clearly established teratogenic effects attributable to the principal long-established antipsychotic medications, but some studies have raised the possibility of such effects. A retrospective study of 315 infants whose mothers had been exposed to phenothiazines, mainly aliphatic phenothiazines similar to chlorpromazine, found congenital malformation in 3.5 per cent compared with a frequency of 1.6 per cent in a control group of 12764 women [33]. The initial reports from a large epidemiological study of the children of women treated with phenothiazines for hyperemesis, 80 per cent of whom received prochlorperazine (a phenothiazine with a piperazine side chain that is used mainly as antiemetic) indicated no significant excess of congenital abnormalities. However, a careful re-analysis taking account of the stage of pregnancy at which exposure to medication occurred, revealed a trend for an increase in abnormalites when the mother had taken the phenothiazine between the sixth and 10th week of gestation [6]. On the basis of these data, it is possible to conclude with 90 per cent confidence that any excess of abnormalities associated with exposure to such medication lies in the range between −0.1 and 5 per cent. Furthermore, there is a report of two cases of severe limb deformity in the children of women treated with prochlorperazine for hyperemesis [31].

Several other studies, including one of 472 women treated for nausea and vomiting in early pregnancy with trifluoperazine, which also belongs to the piperazine class of phenothiazines, found no excess of congenital abnormality [22]. Overall, with regard to phenothiazines, there is slight evidence that aliphatic phenothiazines and also the piperazine phenothiazine, prochlorperazine, might be associated with a small increase in the risk of congenital abnormalities, but there is no evidence of such risk with trifluoperazine. With regard to the butyrophenones, a study of pregnancies in which there was exposure to haloperidol revealed no increase in congenital abnormalities [36], but the mean dose was only 1.2 mg/day, which is barely one tenth of the dose required for maximal antipsychotic effect.

Antipsychotics present a risk of acute toxicity in the infant, especially of extrapyramidal signs and anticholinergic effects. A 7-year follow-up study of children exposed to antipsychotic medication *in utero* found that 21.2 per cent of the 80 children exposed for >2 months exhibited abnormal motor activity at 36–60 hours after birth, compared with 11.8 per cent of the 76 exposed for <2 months and 9.6 per cent of 115 control children who were not exposed to medication [30].

Benzodiazepines such as diazepam can play a useful role in controlling the prodromal anxiety and sleep disturbance that can evolve into a manic relapse, with little risk of teratogenic effects. Alprazolam possibly also has a specific antimanic effect.

Whilst the role of prophylactic medication is a major factor in reducing the risk of psychotic episodes, the potential role of psychosocial factors should not be underestimated. Stressful life events, and also sustained tension, play a substantial role in precipitating psychotic episodes. Hence, advice about planning life in a way that minimizes the risk of stressful events, and the use of cognitive and/or behavioural anxiety management techniques to reduce the impact of unavoidable stresses, can reduce the risk of psychotic relapse.

For the majority of women with a history of manic depressive illness, the most appropriate management in the first trimester is a combination of psychological coping strategies with the intermittent use of either anxiolytic medication such as diazepam, or antipsychotic medication such as trifluoperazine, at the first sign of the non-specific symptoms, such as agitation and sleep disturbance, that can herald the onset of a psychotic episode. However, close vigilance and a preparedness to utilize medication when required is essential, since florid psychotic relapse is likely to result in potentially irresponsible and/or dangerous behaviour and the need for large doses of medication. Furthermore, as a manic episode develops, insight is often lost, leading to great difficulty in maintaining collaboration with treatment, and to the possibility that compulsory hospital treatment will become necessary.

In the second trimester, prophylactic lithium carbonate might be re-commenced if past history indicates a substantial risk of relapse. If on the other hand, the history indicates a low risk of relapse, it is preferable to continue to utilize psychological coping strategies augmented by anxiolytic or antipsychotic medication at times when non-specific symptoms occur. In the final few weeks of pregnancy, all medication should be minimized. Stillbirth has been reported in women taking lithium in the final weeks of pregnancy [35], and it is preferable to discontinue lithium treatment in the final few weeks, re-commencing on the first day post-partum. Because of shifts in body fluid distribution in the immediate post-partum period, the serum level should be monitored very closely. It is not advisable to breast feed while taking lithium. The management of psychotic illness in the post-partum period is discussed in the section on post-partum disorders.

Treatment of acute episodes

In the event of an acute manic relapse, antipsychotic medication such as trifluoperazine, haloperidol or chlorpromazine should be used as required to control symptoms. The evidence regarding congenital malformations considered above slightly favours use of high potency phenothiazines such as trifluoperazine in preference to lower potency phenothiazines such as chlorpromazine, but in circumstances where a marked sedative effect is required, chlorpromazine might be preferable. In cases of depressive relapse, tricyclic antidepressants are likely to be beneficial, but at least in severe cases, electroconvulsive therapy (ECT) should be considered, as the evidence indicates that it is both a safe and effective treatment in pregnancy [25].

Schizophrenia

The lifetime risk of suffering schizophrenia is approximately 1 per cent and the majority of cases begin in young adult life, but perhaps because of the reduced fertility associated with this chronically disabling disorder, pregnant schizophrenic patients present much less frequently than pregnant women with a history of manic depressive psychosis. The issues facing a woman suffering from schizophrenia who wishes to become pregnant are: (a) the risk that the child will inherit schizophrenia; (b) the pressures that caring for a child will put on a schizophrenic mother; (c) the balance between benefits and harm from antipsychotic medication during the pregnancy; and (d) the risk of psychotic relapse in the post-partum period.

Long-term risks

The risk that the child of a schizophrenic mother will suffer from schizophrenia is approximately 12 per cent. With regard to the long-term well-being of the mother and child, estimation of the difficulties is made complex by the variability of the illness. In a small minority, the time course resembles that of manic depressive psychosis, with periods of virtually normal psychological function between psychotic episodes. In the majority, there is a degree of residual disability between episodes of acute disturbance that ranges from mildly impaired ability to deal with stressful situations, to a markedly reduced ability to organize life in a coherent manner. Thus each case must be assessed taking account of the clinical features of that case and the individual's wishes and social circumstances. Nonetheless, for the majority of cases it is likely that the demands of parenthood would present serious problems for a woman with schizophrenia.

Stabilization of the mental state in pregnancy

The role of antipsychotic medication in reducing the risk of schizophrenic relapse is well established. Many recent studies in non-pregnant women (reviewed in [12]) have tested strategies for minimizing the usage of long-term medication, such as reduction in dosage or targetted treatment administered only at times when prodromal symptoms emerge. However, in all of these studies, the strategy intended to reduce exposure to medication resulted in a significantly increased rate of relapse. Nonetheless, most of these studies found that relapse was rare in the first few months after reducing or stopping the medication, raising the possibility that such strategies might be useful in pregnancy.

As mentioned in the discussion of manic depressive illness, there is equivocal evidence that antipsychotic medication in pregnancy is associated with congenital abnormality in the fetus, and in addition some risk of acute toxicity in the neonate. On balance, the evidence suggests that in cases where the illness is severe, with persisting symptoms that tend to be exacerbated by reduction in medication, it is probably best to continue antipsychotic medication throughout the pregnancy, with a cautious reduction in dose in the final few weeks. In less severe cases, it is reasonable to consider withdrawal of medication during the first trimester and then to use either a low to medium dose of medication (e.g. 25 mg fluphenazine decanoate every 4 weeks), or a targeted treatment strategy, for the remainder of the pregnancy. A typical targeted treatment strategy might entail use of 5 mg haloperidol or trifluoperazine twice daily or perhaps chlorpromazine 50 mg twice daily whenever non-specific prodromal symptoms occur.

In the event of psychotic relapse during pregnancy, doses of an oral antipsychotic medication such as trifluoperazine, chlorpromazine or haloperidol adequate to control symptoms, should be given. Immediately after delivery, normal dose antipsychotic medication should be resumed in all cases. Antipsychotic medication is excreted in the breast milk. If the dose is substantial or there is any evidence of exprapyramidal side-effects in the infant, it is preferable to advise against breast feeding.

Psychosocial management also has a major part to play throughout the pregnancy and in the post-partum period. Sustained support, usually by a community psychiatric nurse, is essential to help resolve practical problems and to facilitate collaboration with the proposed medication strategy.

In this account of the treatment of pre-existing psychotic illness in pregnancy, schizophrenia has been considered separately from manic depressive illness. However, whilst typical cases of schizophrenia and of manic depressive psychosis are quite distinct, these two illnesses lie at the ends of a spectrum of disorders exhibiting mixed clinical features. Those cases lying near the midpoint of this spectrum are described as schizoaffective. The management programme for each case must be tailored for the individual. To the extent that the clinical picture is dominated by relatively poor psychological function even during stable phases of the illness, the management programme will place emphasis on the use of maintenance antipsychotic medication and close supervision by a community psychiatric nurse. On the other hand, if the dominant clinical feature is episodic disturbance, the most appropriate management programme is likely to include a combination of cognitive strategies to cope with stress; benzodiazepines or low doses of antipsychotics at times of non-specific symptoms; and the use of prophylactic lithium carbonate, at least in the post-partum period.

Disorders in the post-partum period

The post-partum period is a time of psychological vulnerability. Approximately 60 per cent of women suffer from transient disturbance of mood known as the blues during the first post-partum week [29]. The blues typically occur on the fifth post-partum day, and last for 24–36 hours. Although tearfulness is the most common sign, the mood is characteristically labile. In some instances, there is a period of unnaturally elevated mood, perhaps accompanied by irritability, which is known as the highs. This period of elevated mood typically begins on the third post-partum day. Both the blues and the highs are associated with increased risk of depression at 6 weeks post-partum [8,9]. The other early onset disorder, much more serious in its implications, is post-partum psychosis. It is probable that the physiological changes of the first post-partum week, especially the rapid changes in cortisol, oestrogen and progesterone levels, play a part in these early onset disorders.

Puerperal psychosis

Puerperal psychosis, which occurs in approximately one in 500 births [16], usually begins with an abrupt onset in the first 2 weeks after delivery. In the majority of cases the clinical features resemble those of manic depressive psychosis. There is a marked disturbance of mood which is usually labile, fluctuating between abnormal elation, irritability and depression. This mood disturbance is accompanied by delusions and hallucinations. The content of the delusions varies greatly between cases. Grandiose or religious themes are quite common, but delusions of guilt and abnormality in the infant can also occur, especially in cases in which the mood is predominantly depressed. In clinical assessment, it is important to identify any delusional beliefs focused on the infant, as such delusions might indicate risk of harm. Hallucinations are usually auditory, but in some cases are visual. Attention is seriously impaired and in some cases there is disorientation. Sleep is usually seriously disturbed, the patient often paces about in an agitated manner, and behaviour may be disinhibited. There is a risk of suicide or infanticide.

Aetiology

Since the majority of cases exhibit manic depressive features, and furthermore, individuals with a past history of manic depressive episodes are at very high risk of developing a psychotic episode in the puerperal period, it is reasonable to assume that the majority of cases reflect the interaction of a manic depressive predisposition with the physiological and psychological events of childbirth. This proposal is supported by the finding of Wieck *et al.* of an oestrogen-related dopamine receptor sensitivity in those who become psychotic [38]. However, this requires confirmation in a larger sample of patients.

In a small minority of cases that might be described as overtly organic psychoses, the aetiology involves disturbance of brain physiology secondary to systemic metabolic disorder, infection, cardiovascular or respiratory disease, drug toxicity or drug withdrawal. Hence the assessment of post-partum psychosis must include a history of the use of both therapeutic drugs and drugs of abuse, and an assessment of cardiovascular, respiratory, hepatic and renal function. The clinical features of psychosis with an overtly organic cause can be similar to those of idiopathic post-partum psychosis, but disorientation and/or visual hallucinations are more common and should alert the clinician to the need for an especially thorough general medical examination.

Treatment

Close supervision and support are essential because the woman's ability to care for herself and her baby are severely impaired. In virtually all cases, hospital admission is indicated because of behavioural disturbance and the risk of suicide or infanticide. If possible, admission should be to a mother and baby unit with the facilities and expertise to meet the needs of mother and baby whilst minimizing the need for separation of the mother from her baby. If the mother is unwilling to accept hospital admission, the need for compulsory admission under the Mental Health Act should be assessed.

The florid psychotic symptoms should be treated with antipsychotic medication such as chlorpromazine or haloperidol. ECT is likely to provide the most certain and safe resolution of symptoms, and should be considered if florid disturbance persists or presents severe management problems.

The evidence suggests that for women who have suffered from previous post-partum psychosis, or who have had repeated episodes of psychosis at any time, prophylactic treatment with lithium from the first post-partum day reduces the risk [35] though larger studies of the value of this treatment are required.

Postnatal depression

Whilst the occurrence of depression in the post-partum period is undeniable, the question of whether or not postnatal depression should be regarded as distinct from other forms of depression still remains a subject of controversy. The best available evidence regarding prevalence, from a recent study of 232 post-partum women by Cox *et al.* [4], indicates that there is no significant increase in prevalence of depression during the first 6 months post-partum, in comparison with the prevalence in an equivalent time interval in a group of women from the same geographical area matched for age, marital status and number of children. In the postnatal group, the point prevalence at 6 months post-partum was 9.1 per cent and the period prevalence in the 6 months since delivery was 13.8 per cent. In the control group, the point prevalence at assessment 6 months after an index date was 8.2 per cent and the period prevalence in the intervening 6 months was 13.4 per cent.

However, there was evidence for a clustering of dates of onset of depression in the weeks shortly after delivery. In the group with postnatal depression, half had onset in the 5 weeks following delivery, one tenth had onset during pregnancy and one tenth had had the onset prior to becoming pregnant. In the control group, one sixth of the cases with depression had onset in the 5 weeks after the index date, approximately one tenth had onset in the 40 weeks prior to the index date and a little over one quarter had onset more than 40 weeks prior to the index date. Thus, the post-partum group were less likely than the controls to have had long-standing depression, but did show evidence of an excess number having onset in the first 5 weeks post-partum.

Although there is some evidence of a temporal

relationship between childbirth and onset of depression, it remains unknown whether or not post-partum depression has a specific pathophysiology or merely reflects the interaction between the stresses of childbirth and predisposition to depression acting through a mechanism similar to that mediating the relationship between other types of stressors and depression.

Clinical features

The principal clinical features of post-partum depression, as in depression arising in other circumstances, are depressed or anxious mood, irritability, loss of ability to enjoy activities, self-depreciation, guilty or pessimistic pre-occupations, and somatic disturbances such as poor appetite and disturbed sleep. It can be difficult to distinguish the pathological sleep disorder of depression from the disturbance due to the demands of the infant, but inability to sleep even when the baby is settled, and waking earlier than is necessary, are indicative of depression.

Features that are relatively specific to post-partum depression include pre-occupation with inadequacy as a mother, undue anxiety about the infant, and in severe cases, hopelessness about the future of the infant. These negative cognitions can in extreme cases lead to suicide or even infanticide. Whilst such serious sequelae are rare in non-psychotic depression, it is nonetheless essential for the clinician to be alert to the possibility because failure to detect the risk can have such terrible consequences.

Prognosis

The illness usually persists for many months, and often for more than a year [28], especially if untreated. Pre-menstrual mood disturbance can become a dominant feature that lingers on long after the postnatal depression has resolved in some cases [37]. There is evidence for adverse effects on the baby and on the relationship with the partner. Murray *et al.* [23] have reviewed the evidence of effects on the child and conclude that there can be delayed development that remains detectable at age 4 years. Many studies have shown a relationship between postnatal depression and poor marital relationships [26] though the direction of causation is unclear.

Aetiology

Whilst a full account of the aetiology is unlikely until the pathophysiology of the condition has been more clearly delineated, it is possible to identify many of the contributing factors in a way that provides a foundation for a rational approach to early detection of the illness and to the formulation of a management programme. It is helpful to classify these various factors as predisposing factors, precipitating factors and maintaining factors.

PREDISPOSING FACTORS

A previous history of depression, either following previous childbirth or at other times predisposes to postnatal depression [27]. This indicates that the pathophysiology of postnatal depression has at least some overlap with that of other depressive illnesses. In individual cases, it is sometimes clear that social disadvantage and pre-existing marital disharmony have played a predisposing role, though it is difficult to obtain reliable statistical support for the role of any specific psychosocial stressor. It is likely that any one of a wide variety of different forms of pre-existing chronic psychosocial stress might play a role in predisposing to depression.

PRECIPITATING FACTORS

Precipitating factors include both the events associated with the delivery itself, especially with caesarean section [9,27], and the subsequent stresses of caring for a young infant. It is probable that the psychological response to the event of delivery can precipitate depression just as various types of major life events can precipitate depression in other circumstances. In the months following childbirth the mother experiences not only the physically exhausting demands of caring for a young baby, but in addition is vulnerable to insidious negative self-evaluation. One source of negative self-evaluation that can play a role in precipitating depression is the discrepancy between the expectations of motherhood and the reality of coping with an infant, especially if the baby's sleeping pattern or feeding proves difficult, and/or there is inadequate support from partner or family.

The role of the physiological processes of childbirth in precipitating depression is less clear. Although the puerperium is a time of rapid hormonal change, there is no clear, consistent evidence of abnormal levels of either oestrogen or progesterone in those who become depressed. Harris *et al.* [10] found that low levels of progesterone (measured in saliva) were associated with depression in women who were breast feeding, whilst there was a positive correlation between progesterone level and depression in those who were bottle feeding. Mild thyroiditis occurs after about 5 per cent of births [7], often associated with hyperthyroidism followed by hypothyroidism which is usually transient (see Chapter 12). As both hyper- and hypothyroidism can be associated with depression, it is possible that thyroid disturbance contributes to postnatal depression.

MAINTAINING FACTORS

The vicious cycle established between the mood and lack of energy, and negative evaluation of one's role as a mother can be a potent factor in the maintenance of depression. The problem can be compounded if the partner becomes demoralized or feels rejected, leading to escalating tension within the relationship.

Treatment

The optimum balance between social, psychological and pharmacological management depends on individual circumstances, but in most cases of moderate or greater severity, all three approaches are usually required. The first issue to be addressed in formulating a management programme is ensuring there is an adequate network of support for the mother and her child, from family, friends, voluntary services or statutory services. Providing information about the nature of postnatal depression to both the woman and to her partner can itself help reduce the demoralizing sense of inadequacy. Cognitive therapy is the form of individual psychotherapy which lends itself most readily to the needs of women with postnatal depression. It can break the vicious cycle between mood and negative evaluation of self that tends to maintain the depression.

There have been no adequate trials to determine which type of pharmacological therapy is best. In depression in general, treatment with tricyclic antidepressants is associated with substantial improvement in about 70 per cent of cases, and clinical experience suggests a similar level of efficacy in postnatal depression. Lofepramine has a lower incidence of anticholinergic side-effects than the longer established tricyclics such as imipramine and amitryptiline, and is somewhat safer in overdose [19]. The more recently developed serotonin re-uptake inhibitors, such as paroxetine and sertraline are even safer in overdose, and produce gastrointestinal side-effects such as nausea but no anticholinergic effects.

The more recently a drug has been introduced, the greater the uncertainty about its safety in breast-feeding mothers, though the risk to the breast-feeding infant is probably low for both the tricyclics and the newer serotonin re-uptake inhibitors. For tricyclic antidepressants the data suggest that the infant dose per unit of bodyweight is less than one-hundredth of the maternal dose per unit of bodyweight [2], and the available data indicate similarly low infant doses for the serotonin re-uptake inhibitors, fluoxetine and fluvoxamine [39].

On the basis of an uncontrolled trial, Dalton [5] proposed that treatment with progesterone, starting with injections for the first 5 days and then continuing with suppositories until the re-establishment of regular menstruation, is effective in preventing post-partum depression but there is no evidence from controlled trials to support this. If the findings of Harris *et al.* [10] regarding differing relationships between depression and progesterone levels in breast-feeding and bottle-feeding mothers prove to be robust, progesterone treatment would be expected to relieve depression in breast-feeding mothers and to exacerbate it in bottle-feeding mothers, but on balance, use of progesterone to treat postnatal depression cannot yet be recommended.

There is somewhat stronger evidence suggesting that oestrogen has a therapeutic effect. The available evidence indicates that oestrogen can be used to treat depression that is not related to childbirth [17]. Furthermore, a small double-blind placebo-controlled study in women with postnatal depression found that oestrogen patches produce a significant benefit [11]. One issue that must be addressed is the risk of thrombosis, especially in light of the evidence that combined oral contraceptive (OC) pills containing synthetic oestrogen are associated with increased risk. The risks of thrombosis with oestrogen patch therapy for postnatal depression have not yet been clearly established, but are probably substantially lower than with OC. The synthetic oestrogens used in OC are several times more potent than the natural oestrogens in the oestrogen patch in inducing the liver enzymes that produce clotting factors [3].

At this stage it is difficult to draw definitive conclusions about the optimum pharmacological treatment for postnatal depression. The tricyclic antidepressants are the most firmly established, mainly on the grounds of their efficacy for treating depression in other circumstances, but recent evidence suggests that treatment with oestrogen patches might also be effective. It is not clear whether or not there is a specific subgroup of cases in which hormonal factors play a more substantial role, and for which hormonal treatment might therefore offer the most rational approach.

Case illustration. A woman who considered that she had not coped well with the labour in each of her first three pregnancies was very concerned that in this, her fourth and intended final pregnancy, the delivery should be a wonderful experience. She was quite anxious when admitted to hospital but was unable to convince her busy midwife that she was in labour until evidence of a rapidly progressing second stage precipitated a hurried transfer to the delivery suite. The baby was born as she was wheeled along the corridor. In the following weeks, she was distressed and angry. After about 4 weeks she developed a clear-cut depression characterized by tearfulness, difficulty in sleeping, poor appetite and loss of ability to obtain pleasure from any experiences. She was pre-occupied with painful and angry memories about the experience of the delivery, but her anger was compounded by a tendency to blame herself as well as the hospital.

She was treated with lofepramine, but when there was little evidence of response after 4 weeks at a dose of 140 mg daily, the dose was increased to 210 mg daily. In the following weeks there was some improvement in sleep and appetite, and a small improvement in mood. However, the angry and guilty pre-occupations continued, and were further enhanced by a feeling of anger and disappointment that this time which should have been joyful was being ruined by depression. A series of cognitive therapy sessions attempted to address these issues, while treatment with lofepramine was continued. Slowly, over a period of several months her mood improved, although she experienced more severe pre-menstrual mood disturbance than before the pregnancy. Even a year later she found that visits to the hospital re-opened the painful wounds of her former experience, and it was not until more than 18 months after the birth that she was fully recovered.

Such clinical experiences illustrate the complex interaction between predisposing, precipitating and maintaining factors in maternal mental disorder, and the severity of the distress and disruption that can persist for many months after the birth.

References

1 Australian Drug Evaluation Committee. Tricyclic antidepressants and limb reduction deformities. *Medical Journal of Australia* 1973; **1**: 768–9.
2 Buist A, Norman TR & Dennerstein L. Breast-feeding and the use of psychotrophic medication: a review. *Journal of Affective Disorders* 1990; **19**: 197–206.
3 Campbell S. Potency and hepatocellular effects of oestrogens after oral, percutaneous and subcutaneous administration. In: VanKeep PA, Utian WH & Vermeulan A (eds), *The Controversial Climacteric*. MTP Press, Lancaster, 1982: 103.
4 Cox JL, Murray D & Chapman G. A controlled study of the onset, duration and prevalence of post-natal depression. *British Journal of Psychiatry* 1993; **163**: 27–31.
5 Dalton K. Progesterone prophylaxis used successfully in postnatal depression. *Practitioner* 1985; **229**: 507–8.
6 Edlund MJ & Craig TJ. Antipsychotic drug use and birth defects: an epidemiologic re-assessment. *Comprehensive Psychiatry* 1984; **25**: 32–7.
7 Gerstein HC. How common is post partum thyroiditis? *Archives of Internal Medicine* 1990; **150**: 1397–400.
8 Glover V, Liddle P, Taylor A, Adams D & Sandler M. Mild hypomania (the highs) can be a feature of the first

postpartum week: association with later depression. *British Journal of Psychiatry* 1994; **164**: 517–21.

9 Hannah P, Adams D, Lee A, Glover V & Sandler M. Links between early post-partum mood and post-natal depression. *British Journal of Psychiatry* 1992; **160**: 777–80.

10 Harris B, Johns S *et al*. The hormonal environment of post-natal depression. *British Journal of Psychiatry* 1989; **154**: 660–7.

11 Henderson AF, Gregoire AJP, Kumar R & Studd JWW. The treatment of severe post-natal depression with oestradiol skin patches. *Lancet* 1991; **ii**: 816.

12 Hirsch S. Pharmacological and psychosocial long-term treatment of schizophrenia. In: Brunello N, Mendelewicz J & Racagni J (eds), *New Generation of Antipsychotic Drugs: Novel Mechanisms of Action*. Karger, Basel, 1993: 77–8.

13 Insel TR, Mueller EA, Gilin JC, Siever L & Murphy DL. Tricyclic response in obsessive compulsive disorder. *Progress in Neuropsychopharmacology and Biological Psychiatry* 1984; **9**: 25–31.

14 Jacobson SJ, Jones K *et al*. Prospective multicentre study of pregnancy outcome after lithium exposure during the first trimester. *Lancet* 1992; **339**: 530–3.

15 Jones KL, Lacro RV, Johnson KA & Adams J. Pattern of malformations in the children of woman treated with carbamazepine during pregnancy. *New England Journal of Medicine* 1989; **320**: 1661–6.

16 Kendell RE, Chalmers JC & Platz C. Epidemiology of puerperal psychosis. *British Journal of Psychiatry* 1987; **150**: 662–73.

17 Klaiber EL, Broverman DM, Vogal W & Kobabayashi Y. Estrogen replacement therapy for severe persistent depression in women. *Archives of General Psychiatry* 1979; **36**: 550–4.

18 Kumar R & Robson KM. A prospective study of emotional disorders in childbearing women. *British Journal of Psychiatry* 1984; **144**: 35–47.

19 Lancaster SG & Gonzales JP. Lofepramine: a review of its pharmacodynamic and pharmacokinetic properties, and therapeutic efficacy in depressive illness. *Drugs* 1989; **37**: 123–40.

20 McBride WG. Limb deformities associated with iminodibenzyl hydrochloride. *Medical Journal of Australia* 1972; **1**: 49.

21 McElhatten P. *Review of the Use of Lithium in Human Pregnancy*. Guy's Hospital Teratology Information Service, London, 1990.

22 Moriarty AJ & Nance NR. Trifluoperazine and pregnancy. *Canadian Medical Association Journal* 1963; **88**: 375–6.

23 Murray L, Cooper PJ & Stein A. Post natal depression and infant development. *British Medical Journal* 1991; **302**: 978–9.

24 Nora JJ, Nora HA & Toews WH. Lithium, Ebstein's anomaly and other congenital heart defects. *Lancet* 1974; **ii**: 594–5.

25 Nurnberg HG. An overview of somatic treatment of psychosis during pregnancy and post-partum. *General Hospital Psychiatry* 1989; **11**: 328–38.

26 O'Hara MW & Zekowski EM. Post-partum depression: a comprehensive review. In: Kumar R & Brockington F (eds), *Motherhood and Mental Illness, Volume 2. Causes and Consequences*. Wright, London, 1988.

27 O'Neill T, Murphy P, Greene VT. Postnatal depression: aetiological factors. *Irish Medical Journal* 1990; **83**: 17–18.

28 Pitt B. Atypical depression following childbirth. *British Journal of Psychiatry* 1968; **114**: 1325–35.

29 Pitt B. Maternity blues. *British Journal of Psychiatry* 1973; **122**: 431–5.

30 Platt JE, Friedhoff AJ, Broman SH, Bond R, Laska E & Lin SP. Effects of prenatal neuroleptic drug exposure on motor performance in children. *Human Psychopharmacology* 1989; **4**: 205–13.

31 Rafla N. Limb deformities associated with prochlorperazine. *American Journal of Obstetrics and Gynecology* 1987; **156**: 1557.

32 Rosenberg L, Mitchell AA, Parsells JL, Pashayan H, Louik C & Shapiro S. Lack of relation of oral clefts to diazepam use during pregnancy. *New England Journal of Medicine* 1983; **309**: 1282–5.

33 Rumeau-Rouquette J, Goujard J & Huel G. Possible teratogenic effect of phenothiazines in human beings. *Teratology* 1977; **15**: 57–64.

34 Scialli AR & Lione A. The teratogenic effects of carbamazepine. *New England Journal of Medicine* 1989; **321**: 1480.

35 Stewart DE, Klompenhouwer JL, Kendell RE & van Hulst AM. Prophylactic lithium in puerperal psychosis. The experience of three centres. *British Journal of Psychiatry* 1991; **158**: 393–7.

36 Van Waes A & Van de Velde EJ. Safety evaluation of haloperidol in the treatment of hyperemesis gravidarum. *Journal of Clinical Pharmacology* 1969; **9**: 224–6.

37 Warner P, Bancroft J, Dixson A & Hampson M. The relationship between premenstrual depressive mood and depressive illness. *Journal of Affective Disorders* 1991; **23**: 9–23.

38 Wieck A, Kumar R, Hirst AD, Marks MN, Campbell IC & Checkley SA. Increased sensitivity of dopamine receptors and recurrence of affective psychosis after childbirth. *British Medical Journal* 1990; **303**: 613–16.

39 Wright S, Dawling S & Ashford JJ. Excretion of fluvoxamine in breast milk. *British Journal of Clinical Pharmacology* 1991; **31**: 209.

Index

Abdominal malignancy 404
Abortion, spontaneous
acute renal failure 279
anticoagulant therapy association 162
artificial heart valves 156
cirrhosis 353
coeliac disease 389
cyanotic congenital heart disease, maternal 147
diabetes mellitus 430
folate deficiency 44
HIV infection 580–1
homocystinuria 521
hypopituitarism 493
hypothyroidism 466
inflammatory bowel disease (IBD) 398
leukaemia 61
listeriosis 394
malaria 562
paroxysmal nocturnal haemoglobinuria (PNH) 60
phenylketonuria 523
prolactin-secreting pituitary tumour 486
puerperal sepsis/wound infection 558, 559
recurrent
anticardiolipin antibodies 310
dysfibrinogenaemia, hereditary 107
factor XIII (fibrin stabilizing factor) deficiency 107
hypofibrinogenaemia, hereditary 107
lupus anticoagulant association 96
subclinical autoimmune disease 310
renal transplant patients 263, 264
sickle cell disease (HbSS) 52
systemic lupus erythematosus (SLE) 307, 308, 309
cardiolipin syndrome 309, 310
lupus anticoagulant/cardiolipin antibodies 309
thrombocythaemia 59
viral infections 563
Abruptio placentae 85
adult respiratory distress syndrome/shock lung 20
antifibrinolytic agents 85
blood volume restoration 85
chronic hypertension in pregnancy (CHT) 209
cocaine abuse 605
disseminated intravascular coagulation (DIC) 78, 84–6
rapid screening tests 85
dysfibrinogenaemia, hereditary 107
heparin therapy 85
homocystinuria 521
hypofibrinogenaemia, hereditary 107
post-partum haemorrhage 85
pre-eclampsia/eclampsia 190
renal cortical necrosis 286
Accelerated whole blood clotting time 79
Acetylcholine
gestational vomiting 384
lower oesophageal sphincter pressure (LOSP) 381
Acetylsalicylic acid 285
Achondroplasia 20, 520–1
cardiorespiratory compromise 520
prenatal diagnosis 520
Acne 613, 614
drug treatment in pregnancy 621
effect of pregnancy 620
Acrodermatitis enteropathica 390
Acromegaly 487–8
diagnosis 488
hyperglycaemia management 488
pregnancy-associated tumour expansion 488
treatment 488
ACTH etopic secretion, Cushing's syndrome 489, 490
ACTH plasma levels
Addison's disease 495
congenital adrenal hyperplasia 496
intrauterine suppressive treatment 496
Cushing's syndrome 489–90
normal pregnancy 489, 490
ACTH-secreting pituitary tumour 483
Cushing's syndrome 488, 489, 490
imaging 491
treatment 491
Acyclovir
herpes simplex rectal/perianal ulcers 409
herpes virus hepatitis
HIV infection/AIDS, gastrointestinal infections 391
safety in pregnancy 391
varicella in pregnancy 17, 563
Adaptation to pregnancy, physiological
glucose homeostasis 425
respiratory system 1–4
Addison's disease 495
clinical features 495
diagnosis 495
fetal complications 495
labour management 495
persistent vomiting 384
steroid replacement therapy 495
Adenosine, tachyarrythmias management 155
Adenovirus infection 16
gastroenteritis 397
Adrenal carcinoma 491
Adrenal cortical tumour
Cushing's syndrome 212, 489, 490
surgery 491
hypertension 491
imaging 490–1
medical therapy 491
pulmonary oedema 491
Adrenal failure, acute 495–8
Adrenal gland disease 495–8
Adrenal haemorrhage/necrosis 191
Adrenal hyperplasia, congenital 496–8
carrier detection 496
desmolase deficiency 498
diagnosis 496
effects on pregnancy 497–8
fertility 497
genetic aspects 496
hypertension 498
labour 497, 498
masculinization of female fetal genitalia 496, 497
pregnancy following 497
pregnancy management/outcome 498
prenatal diagnosis 496
treatment 496
17-hydroxyprogesterone monitoring 496, 498

Adrenal hyperplasia, congenital *Cont.*
intrauterine ACTH
suppression 11, 496
Adrenaline teratogenicity 9
Adrenocortical insufficiency
maternal renal transplant 270, 274
neonatal with Cushing's
syndrome 491
overwhelming neonatal
infection 270
Sheehan's syndrome 492
Adrenocorticotrophic hormone *see* ACTH
Adult respiratory distress syndrome
(ARDS) 20–1
acute pyelonephritis 20, 258
listeriosis 560
management 21
mortality 21
pancreatitis 364, 365
Aeromonas hydrophilia diarrhoea 391
Afibrinogenaemia, hereditary 107
Agoraphobia, antenatal 627, 628
AIDS *see* HIV infection/AIDS
Air embolism 539
Air travel, thromboembolism risk 117
Airways resistance 4
Airways conductance 4
Albendazole 395
Albumin
calcium binding 506
serum level 322
see also Hypoalbuminaemia
thyroxine (T_4) binding 460
Albuminoids
adverse reactions 81
haemorrhage management 81
Alcohol abuse 600, 604–5
antenatal screening 604
breast feeding 605
fetal alcohol syndrome 604
fetal lung maturation 604
intrauterine growth retardation 604
neonatal abstinence syndrome 602
pancreatitis 364
Alcohol consumption, safety in
pregnancy 604
Aldosterone 212
Alginic-acid antacids 382
Alkaline phosphatase serum level 321, 322
acute fatty liver of pregnancy 327
Budd–Chiari syndrome 357
common bile duct stones with
pancreatitis 364
intrahepatic cholestasis of pregnancy
(IHCP) 332
osteoblast activity marker 506
osteomalacia 513
primary biliary cirrhosis 356
pruritus gravidarum (cholestasis of
pregnancy) 611
Alkylating agents, fetal effects 15
Alloimmune thrombocytopenia, fetal
(AIT) 96–7
fetal blood sampling 97
incidence 96
intrauterine intracranial haemorrhage
96, 97
management 97
pathogenesis 96
platelet-specific antibody 96
Aloe 407
Alpha$_1$ antitrypsin deficiency 19 20
prenatal diagnosis 20
Alpha$_2$ plasmin inhibitor 117
Alpha adrenergic blocking agents 211
Alpha fetoprotein assay
human parvovirus infection 563
hydrocephalus, maternal
shunt-treated 545
maternal diabetes mellitus 446
neural tube defect prenatal
diagnosis 537
primary liver cancer 360
Alport's syndrome 246
prenatal diagnosis 251
Alprazolam 632
Altitude effects, $PaCO_2/PaO_2$ 2
Aluminium hydroxide 382
Aluminium silicate, hydrated 392
Aluminium-containing antacids 382
Alverine 408
Amanita phalloides poisoning 350
Ambulatory peritoneal dialysis, chronic
(CAPO) 276
Aminocaproic acid 126
Aminoglycosides
cystic fibrosis 19
gram negative sepsis 259
puerperal sepsis/wound
infection 559
septic abortion 560
urinary tract infection (UTI) 259
Aminophylline 153
bronchial asthma 8, 9
intravenous administration 9
slow-release preparation 9
side effects 9
toxicity in neonate 10
5-Aminosalicylic acid (5-ASA) 398, 400
inflammatory bowel disease
(IBD) 400
mode of action 401
Amiodarone 153, 155
breast feeding contraindication 155
fetal/maternal thyroid effects 155
Amitriptyline
antenatal depression 627
muscle contraction headache 546
neonatal side effects 627
Amniocentesis
congenital adrenal hyperplasia 497
haemoglobinopathy 55, 56
HIV infection vertical
transmission 588
thyrotoxicosis 473
Amniotic fluid embolism 122, 539
adult respiratory distress syndrome/
shock lung 20
differential diagnosis 86
disseminated intravascular
coagulation (DIC) 78, 86–7
rapid fluid infusion 86, 87
Amniotic fluid volume assessment 152
Amoebiasis 396
congenital/neonatal infection 395, 396
with inflammatory bowel disease
(IBD) 400
intestinal disease 396, 554
liver involvement 396
hepatic rupture/infarction 325
liver abscess 359
travellers' diarrhoea 391
treatment prior to delivery 395
Amoxycillin 16, 17
listeriosis 394
typhoid/paratyphoid fever 394
Amphetamine abuse 606
neonatal abstinence syndrome 602
Amphotericin B 17
Ampicillin 16, 159
acute pyelonephritis 557
asymptomatic bacteriuria 257, 557
Campylobacter infection 393
clearance in pregnancy 17
dosage 17
Gram negative sepsis 259
listeriosis 394, 560
pseudomembranous colitis 392
renal transplant patients, labour
management 268
urinary tract infection (UTI) 259, 558
Amylase serum levels 363
acute renal failure 279
pancreatitis 363, 364
Amyloidosis
haematuria 260
nephrotic syndrome 252
Anaemia
haemodialysis patients 275
heart failure risk with heart
disease 152
paraplegia 549
septicaemia with acute renal
failure 282
thromboembolism risk 118
Anaesthesia 22–3
achondroplasia 520
bronchial asthma 11
diabetes mellitus 443
emergency, antacid use 382–3
inhalation of gastric contents
adult respiratory distress
syndrome/ shock lung 20
maternal mortality 22–3
preventative guidelines 23
lower oesophageal sphincter pressure
(LOSP) 381
myasthenia gravis 548
myotonic muscular dystrophy 548
opiate interactions in addicts 603
pre-eclampsia 207
scleroderma 315
Anaesthesia
sickle cell disease (HbSS) 53
see also Regional
Anal sphincter injuries 408
Anaphylaxis 20

Anaphylotoxins (C_{3a}/C_{5a}) 324
Androgen therapy 525
Angiography
  cerebral venous thrombosis 540
  late post-partum eclampsia 542
  stroke, ischaemic 539
  subarachnoid haemorrhage 541
Angioneurotic oedema, hereditary 525–6
  breast feeding 526
  C1-esterase inhibitor defect 525
  delivery 525
  effects of pregnancy 525
Angiotensin II (AII)
  arterial refractoriness 183
  renal responsivity 229
Angiotensin-converting enzyme (ACE) inhibitors 165, 240
  chronic hypertension in pregnancy (CHT) 210
  pulmonary oedema management 153
  safety in pregnancy 210, 213, 248
Ankylostoma duodenale see Hookworm
Anogenital warts 409
Anorectal disorders 408–10
Antacids 382
  breast feeding 382
  dietary phosphate binding 506
  emergency anaesthesia 382–3
  gastric aspiration prevention in labour 22, 23
  peptic ulcer disease 388
  renal bone disease 517
  safety in pregnancy 382
  self-medication 379
Antenatal diagnosis *see* prenatal diagnosis
Ante-partum haemorrhage
  acute renal failure 280
  cocaine abuse 605
  folate deficiency 44
  hypertrophic obstructive cardiomyopathy 164
Anthraquinone laxatives 407
Antibasement membrane nephritis 253
Antibiotic prophylaxis
  heart disease, labour management 150, 159
  hydrocephalus, maternal shunt-treated 545
  renal transplant patients
    intrauterine contraceptive device (IUD) insertion 271
    labour management 268
Antibiotic therapy
  acute pyelonephritis 259, 557
  asymptomatic bacteriuria 257, 557
  bacterial peritonitis with cirrhosis 355
  chronic pyelonephritis 557
  cystic fibrosis 19
  gallstones 362
  impetigo herpetiformis 620
  intrauterine infection 88
  listeriosis 394, 560
  puerperal sepsis/wound infection 559
  septic abortion/septic shock 283–4, 560
  shigellosis 394
  toxoplasmosis 561
  travellers' diarrhoea 392
  typhoid/paratyphoid fever 394
  upper respiratory tract infection 16
  urinary tract infection (UTI) 558
Anticholinergic agents
  bronchial asthma 10
  fetal adverse effects 401
  pancreatitis 364
  in proprietary antacids 382
Anticholinesterase agents 548
Anticoagulant therapy
  artificial heart valves 161–2
    replacement 155–6
  breast feeding 156
  cerebral venous thrombosis 540
  Eisenmenger's syndrome 167
  fetal adverse effects 162
  heart disease 155–7
  myocardial infarction 164
  paroxysmal nocturnal haemoglobinuria (PNH) 61
  polycythaemia rubra vera (PRV) 59
  pre-eclampsia 205
  puerperal cardiomyopathy 165
  stroke 540
Anticoagulants, naturally occurring in haemostasis 74–5
Anticonvulsants
  acute liver failure 350
  breast milk levels 539
  cerebral venous thrombosis 540
  congenital malformations 45, 537, 538
    monotherapy 538
    pathogenesis 537–8
  eclampsia prevention/treatment 202–4, 543
  epilepsy 538–9
    blood level monitoring 538
  folate deficiency 45–6, 536, 538
  neonatal coagulopathy 45, 537
  oral contraceptive interaction 536
  osteomalacia 517–18
  post-partum dosage 539
  pre-eclampsia 208
  pregnancy-induced changes in metabolism 536
Antidiarrhoeal agents
  contraindication in pregnancy 408
  self-medication 379
Antidiuretic hormone (AVP)
  metabolic clearance rate (MCR) 231
  osmotic threshold for release 231
Anti-DNA antibodies 306, 307
Antidysrhythmic drugs 154–5
  long-term prophylaxis 155
Anti-emetic drug therapy 385
  hyperemesis gravidarum 385
  safety 385–6
  self-medication 379
Antifibrinolytic agents 85–6
Antihistamines
  anti-emetics 385
  pemphigoid (herpes) gestationis 617
  polymorphic eruption of pregnancy 617
  prurigo of pregnancy 618
  pruritus gravidarum 612
  safety in pregnancy 621
  urticaria 621
Antihypertensive drugs 212–13
  chronic hypertension in pregnancy (CHT) 209, 210, 211, 240
  coarctation of aorta 169
  eclamptic hypertensive encephalopathy 543
  Marfan's syndrome 170
  pre-eclampsia 199–200, 208
    escape from blood pressure control 202
    extreme hypertension 199–200
    longer-term hypertension control 201–2
    prevention 205–6
  uteroplacental perfusion effects 200, 201
Anti-inhibitor coagulation complex (Autoplex) 100
Anti-La antibodies 308
Antimalarial drugs
  breast feeding 312
  malaria prophylaxis/treatment 562
  neonatal therapy 562
  rheumatoid arthritis 314
  systemic lupus erythematosus (SLE) 307, 311, 312
Antimotility agents 401
Anti-nuclear factor 306, 307
Antiplasminogens 76
Antiplasmins 76
Antiplatelet agents
  pre-eclampsia prevention 206–7
  thromboprophylaxis 131–2
Antipsychotic medication
  breast feeding contraindication 626, 634
  manic depressive psychosis 631
    acute relapse 633
  neonatal acute toxicity 632
  puerperal psychosis 635
  safety in pregnancy 631–2, 633
  schizoaffective disorders 634
  schizophrenia 633
Antipyretic drugs 553
Anti-Ro antibodies 308, 309
Antispasmodic agents 408
Antithrombin III (ATIII) 75
  acute fatty liver of pregnancy 89, 327
  pre-eclampsia 98, 191, 197
  thromboembolism risk prediction 132
Antithrombin III (ATIII) concentrate 133
  acute fatty liver of pregnancy 89
  haemolytic uraemic syndrome (HUS) 286
  hypertension-associated hepatic disorders 330

Antithrombin III (ATIII)
deficiency 132–4
acquired following Fontan procedure 171
antithrombin III concentrate therapy 133
Budd–Chiari syndrome 357
genetic aspects 132, 133
labour/delivery management 133
neonate management 133–4
pre-pregnancy counselling 133
recurrent thromboembolism 129
subcutaneous heparin prophylaxis 133
thromboembolism 133
prophylaxis 131, 133
thrombosis treatment 133
venography 133
warfarin prophylaxis 133
Antithyroid drugs
agranulocytosis 470
breast feeding contraindication 471
fetal goitre/hypothyroidism 469
screening 468
post-partum thyroiditis 474
thyroid crisis (thyroid storm) 472
thyrotoxicosis 469–70
fetal thyrotoxicosis management 473
monitoring 469, 471
neonatal 471, 474
supplementary T4 replacement therapy 470, 473
transplacental passage 463
potential goitrogens 463, 464
Antituberculous drugs 12–13
teratogenicity 13
Antiviral agents
acute liver failure 351
hepatitis B 343
Anuria 279
septic shock 284
Anxiety 625
antenatal 628–9
treatment 628
associated agoraphobia 628
associated depression 627, 628
bronchial asthma 7
clinical features 628
panic attacks 628
pharmacological treatment 626
pre-eclamptic hypertension 204
Aortic dissection
coarctation of aorta 169
cocaine abuse 605
Marfan's syndrome 170
Aortic regurgitation
incidence 145
pulmonary oedema 161
Aortic stenosis
incidence 145
maternal death 161
risk of recurrence 147
surgery/valvuloplasty 161
syncope 148
systolic murmur 149
Aortic valve disease 145, 161
Aortic valve replacement 151, 162
Aortic valvuloplasty 151
Aortocaval compression
labour with heart disease 157
supine position 183
Apex heart beat 149
Aphthous stomatitis 380
associated disorders 380
management 380
Aplastic anaemia 58
hereditary 101
pure red cell asplasia 58
Apocrine gland changes 613
Appendicitis 403–4
appendectomy 404
intestinal obstruction 404
persistent vomiting 384
pregnancy outcome 403
ultrasound diagnosis 404
Aprotinin (Trasylol) 76, 126
abruptio placentae 85–6
Arbovirus infection 350
Arginine vasopression (AVP)
renal vascular responses II 230
see also DDAVP
Arrhythmias 145
cocaine abuse 605
Arterial blood gas measurement 2
breathlessness 5
cystic fibrosis 19
pulmonary embolus 121
sampling in sitting position 121
Arteriovenous malformation (AVM), subarachnoid haemorrhage 541
Artificial heart valve replacement 161
anticoagulant therapy 155–6
thromboembolism risk 155
Artificial heart valves 127, 161–3
antibiotic prophylaxis in labour 159
anticoagulant therapy 161–2
fetal adverse effects 162
Ascaris lumbricoides see roundworm
Ascites
Budd–Chiari syndrome 357, 358
cirrhosis 355
pancreatitis 364, 365
pre-eclampsia 190
Aspartate amino transferase (AST) 321
acute fatty liver of pregnancy 327
HELLP syndrome 324
hepatic rupture/infarction 325
hyperemesis gravidarum 323
hypertension-associated hepatic disease 323
intrahepatic cholestasis of pregnancy (IHCP) 332
Aspergillus infection 266
Aspirin 59, 98, 103
migraine prophylaxis 546
myocardial infarction 164
pre-eclampsia prevention 206–7, 208
rheumatoid arthritis 313
safety in pregnancy 311
systemic lupus erythematosus (SLE) 307, 311
heparin combination 312
prednisone combination 312
recurrent early pregnancy loss 312
thromboembolism prophylaxis 131, 132
homocystinuria 522
thyroid crisis (thyroid storm) 472
Asplenia syndrome 126
Astrovirus gastroenteritis 397
Atenolol 154
fetal growth retardation 154
pre-eclampsia 202
Atopic eczema 619
Atrial fibrillation 152, 153
anticoagulant therapy 155
thyroid crisis (thyroid storm) 472
Atrial natriuretic factor (ANF) 230
Atrial septal defect, maternal 145, 146
Atrophic thyroiditis 468
Atropine
bronchial asthma 10
fetal adverse effects 10, 401
inflammatory bowel disease 400, 401
lower oesophageal sphincter pressure (LOSP) 381
Autoimmune chronic active hepatitis 353
fertility 353
management 355
Autoimmune haemolytic anaemia (AIHA) 58
Autoimmune progesterone dermatitis of pregnancy 619
Autoimmune thrombocytopenic purpura (AITP) 89–96
delivery 93, 94–5
diagnosis 90–1
fetal blood sampling 93–4
fetal thrombocytopenia 89, 90–1, 92, 93, 95
intracranial haemorrhage at delivery 94
platelet count assessment 93
HIV-associated 95–6
incidence 89
management 91–2
antenatal interventions 91
corticosteroid therapy 91–2
intravenous IgG 91, 92
medical therapies 92–3
splenectomy 91, 92, 93
neonatal management 95
neonatal thrombocytopenia 94, 95
perinatal mortality 91, 95
platelet surface antigen autoantibodies 90
Autoimmune thyroid disease
fetal hypothyroidism 468
post-partum hypothyroidism 475
sporadic goitre 465, 466
thyroid hormone replacement therapy 466
thyrotoxicosis 469
Azathioprine 58, 93, 165, 248
breast feeding 272
chronic active hepatitis 353
Crohn's disease 401
fertility impairment 272

fetal effects 267, 270, 621
chromosomal aberrations 272, 311
long-term use 401
inflammatory bowel disease (IBD) 398
liver transplantation 352
red cell 6-thioguanine monitoring 267
renal transplant patients 261, 264, 267
rheumatoid arthritis 314
systemic lupus erythematosus (SLE) 307, 311 312

Bacterial overgrowth 394
Bacteriuria, asymptomatic (covert) 227, 254–9, 557
acute infection following 255–6, 557
antenatal screening 255, 557
benefits of eradication 256
chronic renal disease 238
diabetes mellitus 248
diagnosis 254–5
incidence 255
long-term follow-up 257–8
natural history 256
post-partum intravenous urography (IVU) 258
pregnancy outcome 256–7
relapse/re-infection 257
renal (upper tract) infection 256
site of infection localization 255
source of infection 255
treatment 257
antibiotic therapy 257, 557
duration of therapy 257
urine collection 254–5
urine examination 254–5
Bacteroides
puerperal sepsis/wound infection 559
septic abortion 560
Balantidium coli diarrhoea 391
Balsalazide 401
Barbiturates 7
fetal adverse effects 401
neonatal abstinence syndrome 602
opiate interactions 603
Basilar artery migraine 546
Beclomethasone
bronchial asthma 10
side effects 10
Bed rest
acute pyelonephritis 557
acute rheumatic fever 161
gallstones 362
heart disease 152
hypertension-associated hepatic disorders 330
inflammatory bowel disease (IBD) 400
pre-eclampsia 198–9
thromboembolism risk 117, 129
Behaviour therapy 626
antenatal anxiety 628, 629
obsessional ruminations 630
phobias 629
Behçet's syndrome 380
Bell's palsy 546
Bendectin/Debendox, safety in pregnancy 385–6
Benign familial haematuria syndrome 247
Bentall composite graft 170
Benzodiazepines
antenatal anxiety 628
breast feeding 539, 626
dependence 628, 630
manic depressive psychosis 632
obsessional ruminations 630
schizoaffective disorders 634
Benzoyl peroxide 619
Bephenium 395
Bernard–Soulier syndrome 101
Berry aneurysm rupture 541
Beta adrenergic antagonists (beta blockers) 154
chronic hypertension in pregnancy (CHT) 210, 212–13
cirrhosis with portal hypertension 355
hydralazine combined treatment 200
hypertrophic obstructive cardiomyopathy 164
Marfan's syndrome 170
phaeochromocytoma 211
post-partum hypertension 208
post-partum thyroiditis 474
pre-eclampsia 202, 212
safety in pregnancy, 154, 210
thyrotoxicosis 471
Beta human chorionic gonadotrophin (bHCG)
gestational trophoblastic disease 360
cerebral metastases 544
gestational vomiting/hyperemesis gravidarum 384
primary liver cancer 360
Beta sympathomimetic drugs
bronchial asthma inhalation therapy 7, 8–9, 11
contraindications 160
criteria for stopping therapy 160
drug interactions 160
Eisenmenger's syndrome 169
ergometrine interaction 159–60
heart disease patients 160
metabolic effects 160
premature labour 159, 160
diabetes mellitus 448
myocardial infarction 163
oxygen saturation monitoring 160
side effects 8, 9
cardiovascular/pulmonary oedema 159–60
hyperglycaemia in diabetic pregnancy 9
Beta thromboglobulin
deep vein thrombosis 119
pre-eclampsia 190
Betamethasone 91, 159
bronchial asthma inhalation
therapy 8
fetal therapeutic effects 11
Bile acid plasma level 322
intrahepatic cholestasis of pregnancy (IHCP) 332, 333
Bile salt metabolism 362
Biliary cirrhosis, primary 356
differential diagnosis 356
impact of pregnancy 354
maternal/fetal outcome 356
vitamin D supplements 517
Biliary tract disease 361–3
Biliary tract obstruction
common bile duct stones 363
fever 553
Bilirubin
congenital metabolic disorders 358
fetal levels 322
HELLP syndrome 324
maternal metabolism 322
Biophysical profile, maternal diabetes mellitus 448
Bisacodyl 407
Bjork–Shiley prosthetic valve 162
thrombosis during pregnancy 156
Bladder catheterization 169
Blastomycosis 554
lung infection 17
Blood count
acute renal failure 279
fever diagnosis 555, 556
renal transplant patients 263
Blood culture 555
Blood group O, thromboembolism risk reduction 118
Blood pressure
measurement 186–7
direct/indirect 184
errors 184–5
Korotkoff sounds 184, 185, 186–7
normal pregnancy 183, 185
pre-eclampsia 188, 196
variability/sampling errors 185
Blood sugar
acute renal failure 279, 282
septic shock 282
Blood transfusion
abruptio placentae 85
haemodialysis patients 275
haemorrhage management 82–3
infections transmitted in fresh blood 82
iron deficiency anaemia correction 39
paraplegia 549
paroxysmal nocturnal haemoglobinuria (PNH) 60
pre-eclampsia 207
pure red cell aplasia 58
renal disease 242, 286
screening 82
sickle cell disease (HbSS) 52
complications 52
exchange transfusion regime 53
α thalassaemia 48
β thalassaemia 49

Blood volume 33–6
benefits of hypervolaemia 35
delivery 34–5
plasma volume 33–4
puerperium 34–5
red cell mass 34
Body temperature 552
Bone 505–13
cellular remodelling 505, 509
effect of pregnancy on mineral content 512–13
hormonal regulation of calcium/phosphate 506–9
calcitonin 509
1,25-dihydroxyvitamin D 508
parathyroid hormone (PTH) 509
metabolism 505
mineralization 505–6, 508
Bone cells 505
Bone diseases 505
Bone dysplasias 520
Bone loss
breast feeding 512–13, 519
pregnancy 512–13
Bone marrow iron 38–9
Bone matrix 505
composition 505
mineralization 505–6
Bowel habit, changes in pregnancy 406
Brain tumour 543–4
headache 546
Breast abscess 614
puerperium 553
pyrexia 559
Breast feeding
alcohol consumption 605
amiodarone contraindication 155
amoebiasis 396
anticoagulant therapy 156
antihelminthics contraindication 395, 396
antithyroid drugs contraindication 471
antituberculous drugs 14
benzodiazepines 626
bone loss 512–13, 519
bronchial asthma 11
calcium absorption 510
calcium demand 509
calcium supplements 515
Campylobacter infection 393
coeliac disease onset prevention 388
Cushing's syndrome 491
cystic fibrosis 19
diabetes insipidus 494
diabetes mellitus 444
dindevan contraindication 156
epilepsy 536
folate deficiency 43
hepatitis B 343
hereditary angioneurotic oedema 526
HIV infection 577, 578, 589, 604
hypothyroidism 468
indomethacin contraindication 314
iodine-containing expectorants contraindication 7
lithium contraindication 626, 633
nipple soreness 614
opiate addicts 603
phenindione contraindication 127
phenolphthalein contraindication 407
phenylketonuria 524
prolactin-secreting pituitary tumour 487
psychotropic drugs 626
puerperal cardiomyopathy 166
pyrimethamine 563
quinacrine 395
quinolones contraindication 394
radioisotope scanning
iodine contraindication 119
lung scan 121
renal transplant patients 272
salazopyrine 401
schistosomiasis therapy contraindication 396
schizophrenia 634
shigellosis 394
steroid therapy 400
subcutaneous heparin therapy 128
systemic lupus erythematosus (SLE) 312
non-steroidal anti-inflammatory drugs 312
tricyclic antidepressants 626
typhoid/paratyphoid fever 394
vitamin D supplements 515
warfarin anticoagulation 127, 128
Breast milk, drug content
aminophylline 9
antacids 382
anticonvulsants 539
antidysrhythmic drugs 154
antipsychotic medication 634
antithyroid drugs 471
antituberculous drugs 14
azathioprine 272
bronchial asthma treatment 11
cannabis 606
ciprofloxacin 394
cyclosporin 272
cyproheptidine 491
digoxin 153
folic acid 43
H_2 antagonists 382
immunosuppressive steroid therapy 272
methadone 603
metoclopramide 386
phenolphthalein 407
psychotrophic drugs 626
pyrimethamine 562
quinolones 394
serotonin re-uptake inhibitors 637
spironolactone 355
tricyclic antidepressants 637
Breathlessness 5
heart disease 143, 148
Bretylium tosylate 154
Bromocriptine 118
growth hormone-secreting pituitary tumour 488
prolactin-secreting pituitary tumour 484, 485, 486, 544
large tumours 486
tumour expansion management in pregnancy 487
tumour-related complications 485
safety in pregnancy 485, 486
vaginal administration 485
Bronchial asthma 1, 6–12
acute severe (status asthmaticus) 8
intravenous beta-sympathomimetic drugs 9
oxygen therapy 8
theophylline infusion 9
aminophylline, oral slow release 8
anaesthesia/analgesia 11
anticholinergic drugs 10
anxiety management 7
beta$_2$ sympathomimetic drugs
inhaled 7, 8–9, 11
oral 8
breast feeding 11
chest infection treatment 7, 8
desensitization therapy 7
diabetic patients 9
disodium cromoglycate 10
effect of pregnancy 6
epidemiology 6
exercise-induced 8
genetic counselling 11–12
hospital admission 8
labour 11, 495
management 7–11
peak expiratory flow home monitoring 7
pneumothorax/pneumomediastinum 21
prostaglandin therapy 6, 11
risk to fetus 6–7
salbutamol 11
steroid therapy 6, 10–11, 495
inhaled prophylactic treatment 8
oral 8
theophyllines 9–10
Bronchiectasis 19–20
Bronchitis
acute 16
chronic 19–20
Brucellosis 555
Budd–Chiari syndrome 357–8
aetiology 357
diagnosis 357–8
haematological features 357–8
liver transplantation 352
oral contraceptive contraindication 352
pregnancy management/outcome 358
Bupivacaine 169
Butyrophenones
manic depressive psychosis 631
safety in pregnancy 631, 632

C reactive protein
acute rheumatic fever 161
deep vein thrombosis 119

C1 esterase inhibitor concentrates 525
Caesarean section
abruptio placentae 85
achondroplasia 520
amniotic fluid embolism 86
arteriovenous malformation (AVM) 541
autoimmune thrombocytopenic purpura (AITP) 90, 93, 94–5
blood loss 34
caecal volvulus complicating 404
cirrhosis 355
coarctation of aorta 170
colonic pseudo-obstruction complicating 404
condyloma acuminata 409
congenital adrenal hyperplasia 498
congenital heart block with SLE 313
deep vein thrombosis 119
diabetes mellitus 448, 449, 450
Eisenmenger's syndrome 167
endolaryngeal intubation pressor response attenuation 200
epidural anaesthesia 23
heart disease 158
epilepsy 536
gastric aspiration prevention 23
haemodialysis patients 276
HELLP syndrome 325
hepatic rupture/infarction 326
herpes simplex virus (HSV) genital infection 348, 563
HIV infection 583, 588, 591
transmission to health-care workers 589–90
vertical transmission 579, 580, 583
hydrocephalus, maternal shunt-treated 545
hypertension-associated hepatic disorders 331
ileostomy 403
impetigo herpetiformis 620
intracranial mass lesion 544
intrapartum lumbosacral plexopathy 547
kyphoscoliosis 20
Marfan's syndrome 170
maternal cardiopulmonary arrest 155
osteogenesis imperfecta tarda 520
permanent urinary diversion 250
polycythaemia rubra vera (PRV) 59
post-partum endometritis 559
postnatal depression 636
pre-eclampsia 207
thromboembolism risk following bed rest 117
prosthetic valve thrombosis 156
puerperal cardiomyopathy 166
renal transplant patients 268–9, 273
septic pelvic thrombophlebitis 134
thromboembolism risk 118
prophylaxis 129
Calamine 612
Calcitonin 507
calcium/phosphate regulation 509
neonatal level 512
pregnancy-associated elevation 512
Calcitonin gene-related peptide 144
Calcitonin therapy 520
Calcium 506
absorption 508
in pregnancy 509, 510
albumin binding 506
bone 505, 506
mineralization 506, 508
mobilization 509
dietary intake 506
extracellular fluid 506
fetal accumulation 509
free ionized concentration 506
homeostasis 505
changes in pregnancy 509–13
hormonal regulation 506–9
calcitonin 509
1,25-dihydroxyvitamin D 508
parathyroid hormone (PTH) 509
vitamin D 506, 507–9
lactation losses 515
lactation-associated demand 509
placental active transport 511–12
renal excretion 231
in pregnancy 510
renal tubular reabsorption 506, 508, 509
requirement in pregnancy 509
serum level 506
osteomalacia 513, 514–15
in pregnancy 510–11
renal transplant patients 263, 267
vitamin D metabolism 507, 508
Calcium channel blockers
magnesium sulphate interaction 200
migraine prophylaxis 546
pre-eclamptic hypertension 199, 200–1
Calcium deficiency
coeliac disease 388
dental caries 381
intestinal malabsorption disorders 515–16
total parenteral nutrition 405
Calcium supplements
hypertension-associated hepatic disorders 330
hypoparathyroidism 519
lactation 515
osteogenesis imperfecta tarda 520
pre-eclampsia prevention 206
renal bone disease 517
renal transplant patients 264
Calcium-containing antacids 382
Campylobacter fetus (C. intestinalis) 392
Campylobacter infection 392–3
adverse fetal outcome 392–3
delivery 393
diagnosis 392
HIV infection/AIDS 391
management 392
microbial surveillance of neonate 393
neonatal 393
preventive dietary advice 393
travellers' diarrhoea 391
Campylobacter jejuni (C. coli) 392
Campylobacter pylori see Helicobacter pylori
Candidiasis 620
aphthous stomatitis 380, 391
HIV infection 391, 584
treatment 584
oesophageal 584
dysphagia 391, 584
oropharyngeal 584
vaginal 584
Cannabis 606
Captopril 153
scleroderma 315
Carbamazepine
birth defects with polytherapy 538
diabetes insipidus 494
epilepsy, blood level monitoring 538
folate malabsorption 538
manic depressive psychosis 631
neural tube defects 537
post-partum dosage 539
safety in pregnancy 537, 625, 631
vitamin D deficiency 517
Carbimazole
fetal thyroid function 470
neonatal scalp defects 470
side effects 470
thyrotoxicosis 469
neonatal 474
Carbon tetrachloride, acute liver failure 350
Carcinoembryonic antigen (CEA)
colorectal carcinoma 409
primary liver cancer 360
Cardiac arrest
high dose prostaglandin E_2 157
management 155
pulmonary embolus 121
Cardiac output 5, 143, 182
adult respiratory distress syndrome/shock lung 21
distribution 35
dye dilution measurement technique 144
epidural anaesthesia 158
fall in late pregnancy 143–4
heart disease 144, 157
labour 144, 157
multiple pregnancy 152
pre-eclampsia 188
prostaglandin E2 effect 157
vasoactive mediators 144
Cardiolipin antibodies
fetal risk association in SLE 308, 309, 310–311
congenital heart block 308
platelet antibodies/maternal thrombocytopenia 311
HIV infection 582
hypertension association 310
recurrent early abortion *see* cardiolipin syndrome
thromboembolism risk 118, 129, 131, 310
Cardiolipin syndrome 132, 311
clinical features 310
fetal loss 134, 308, 309, 310

Cardiomyopathy 164–6
congestive 166
electrocardiography 150
hypertrophic obstructive 164–5
puerperal (peripartum/pregnancy) cardiomyopathy 165–6
cerebral ischaemia/stroke 539
Cardiopulmonary bypass 151
aortic dissection in Marfan's syndrome 170
prosthetic valve thrombosis 156
Cardiotocography
intrahepatic cholestasis of pregnancy (IHCP) 333
maternal heart disease 152
systemic lupus erythematosus (SLE) 313
Cardiovascular changes of pregnancy 182–3
Carnitine deficiency 358
Carotid artery dissection 539
Carpal tunnel syndrome 547
Castor oil 407
Caudal anaesthesia 19
Caudal regression syndromes, maternal diabetes mellitus 429, 446
Cefoxitin 392
Central pontine myelinosis 385
Central venous pressure (CVP)
acute renal failure 279, 284
amniotic fluid embolism 86
labour management
chronic renal disease 242
heart disease 157
septic shock 284
Cephalexin 558
Cephalosporins 16, 17
acute pyelonephritis 557
asymptomatic bacteriuria 257, 557
Campylobacter infection 393
gram negative sepsis 259
listeriosis 394
pseudomembranous (antibiotic-associated) colitis 392
septic shock 284
urinary tract infection (UTI) 259, 558
Cerebral aneurysm rupture 539, 541
Cerebral angiography 536
Cerebral arterial thrombosis 313
Cerebral embolus 165
Cerebral haemorrhage
coarctation of aorta 169
pre-eclampsia/eclampsia 189, 202, 205
Cerebral ischaemia 539
Cerebral oedema
acute liver failure 351
eclampsia 192, 542, 543
Cerebral venous thrombosis 539, 540–1
clinical features 540
diagnosis/neuroimaging 540
headache 546
post-partum 540
recurrence 541
treatment 540–1
Cerebrospinal fluid (CSF)
examination 535
eclamptic hypertensive encephalopathy 192–3, 542
pesudotumour cerebri 545
Cerebrovascular disease 539–43
Cervical condylomata 409
Cervical neoplasia
with HIV infection 585
intraepithelial neoplasia 409
Charcot–Marie–Tooth disease 1
Chenodeoxycholic acid serum level 322
intrahepatic cholestasis of pregnancy (IHCP) 332
Chenodeoxycholic acid therapy 363
Chest X-ray
heart disease 149
pericardial disease 167
puerperal (peripartum/pregnancy) cardiomyopathy 165
pulmonary embolus 120–1
routine 12
Chickenpox *see* Varicella zoster virus (VZV)
Chlamydia infection
HIV infection 583
pneumonia 16
Chloramphenicol 393
Chlormethiazole 204, 543
Chloroquine
Plasmodium falciparum malaria 562
rheumatoid arthritis 314
safety in pregnancy 314, 562, 621
systemic lupus erythematosus (SLE) 311
effects of withdrawal 311
Chlorpromazine
fetal/neonatal effects 386
manic depressive psychosis 631
acute relapse 633
neonatal opiate withdrawal syndrome 602
puerperal psychosis 635
schizophrenia 634
thyroid crisis (thyroid storm) 472
Chlorpropamide 441
diabetes insipidus 494
fetal hyperinsulinaemia 441
safety in pregnancy 494
Cholangiocarcinoma 360
biliary obstruction 363
inflammatory bowel disease 358
Cholecystectomy 363
Cholecystokinin 509
Cholera 391, 554
Cholesterol lithiasis 362
Cholesterol plasma level 322
Cholestryramine
primary biliary cirrhosis 356
pruritus gravidarum 612
pruritus with IHCP 333
vitamin K_1 supplements 333
vitamins binding 356
Cholic acid serum levels 322
intrahepatic cholestasis of pregnancy (IHCP) 332
Chondrodysplasia punctata 126, 127, 155
Chondrodystrophies 20
Chorea gravidarum 307
Choriocarcinoma 544
cerebral ischaemia/stroke 539
cerebral metastases 544
subarachnoid haemorrhage 541
treatment 544
clinical features 544
pemphigoid (herpes) gestationis 614, 615
primary 361
thyrotoxicosis 461, 469
see also Trophoblastic disease, gestational
Chorionic villus sampling 250
cogenital adrenal hyperplasia 496
fetal limb reduction abnormalities 57
fetal loss 57
haemoglobinopathy 55, 56–7
haemophilias 106
HIV infection vertical transmission 588
transcervical/transabdominal method 57
Chromium deficiency 398
Chromosomal aberrations
azathioprine therapy 272, 311
maternal renal transplant 270
Cimetidine 23
anti-androgenic effects 382
obstetrical anaesthesia preparation 383
peptic ulcer disease 388
safety in pregnancy 382
Ciprofloxacin
safety in pregnancy 394, 558
urinary tract infection (UTI) 558
Cirrhosis 353–356
abstinence from alcohol 354, 355
antithrombin III (ATIII) activity 75
ascites 355
bacterial peritonitis 355
chronic active hepatitis 353
delivery 355
fertility 353
fetal outcome 353
hepatitis B 338, 342
impact of pregnancy 353–4
bleeding oesophageal varices 354, 355
management in pregnancy 354
portal hypertension 354, 355, 356
medical management 355
post-partum complications 354
primary liver cancer 360
termination of pregnancy 355
Cleft lip/palate 46, 91
maternal epilepsy/anticonvulsant therapy 537
Clindamycin 392
Clonidine 210
Clonorchis sinensis 363, 396
Closing volume 4
Clostridial antitoxin 283
Clostridial infection
acute renal failure 282
puerperal sepsis/wound infection 559

treatment 284
Clostridium difficile
pseudomembranous colitis 392
travellers' diarrhoea 391
Clostridium welchi (perfringens)
puerperal sepsis/wound infection 558
septic abortion 560
Clotting factor concentrates
bleeding oesophageal varices 355
hypertension-associated hepatic disorders 330
Clotting factors 71, 74
inhibitors 74–5
CO_2 production 2, 4
Coagulation disorders 71–108
acute renal failure 278, 279
Budd–Chiari syndrome 357, 358
clinical manifestations 100
hypertension-associated hepatic disorders 330
inherited disorders 101–8
maternal anticonvulsant therapy 537, 538
nephritis, hereditary 246
pre-eclampsia 97–8, 190–1, 197–8
superimposed on chronic hypertension in pregnancy (CHT) 209
treatment 205
septic shock 284
subarachnoid haemorrhage 541
thromboembolism risk 117
Coagulation system 73–4
cascade activation 73, 74
extrinsic mechanism 73, 74
intrinsic mechanism (contact system) 73, 74
local fibrin plug formation 73
Coarctation of aorta 145, 169–70
aortic dissection 169, 211
cerebral haemorrhage 169
chronic hypertension in pregnancy (CHT) 211
fetal outcome 147
management 169–70
maternal mortality 169
surgery 152
Cocaine abuse 600, 605–6
antenatal haemorrhage 605
associated HIV infection 600
berry aneurysm/AVM rupture 541
cardiovascular adverse effects 605
incidence 605
neonatal cerebral infarction 605
pregnancy outcome 605
Coccidioidomycosis 17, 554
Codeine phosphate
inflammatory bowel disease 401
muscle contraction headache 546
Coeliac disease 388–90
antacids 382
aphthous stomatitis 380
clinical features 388–9
diagnosis 390
differential diagnosis 390
epidemiology 388
fetal outcome 389
impact of pregnancy 389
infertility 389
investigations 379
management in pregnancy 390
monitoring/follow-up 390
oesophageal malignancy 390
vitamin D malabsorption 516
Cognitive therapy 626
antenatal anxiety 628, 629
antenatal depression 627
obsessional ruminations 630
phobias 629, 630
postnatal depression 637, 638
schizoaffective disorders 634
Cognitive–analytic therapy 626
Cold sores 553
Colectomy
inflammatory bowel disease (IBD) 402, 403
pregnancy outcome 403
Colitis, non-specific 397
Collagen disease *see* Connective tissue disease
Collapse in pregnancy 122–3
Colonic carcinoma 409
Colonic motility 406
Colonic pseudo-obstruction (Ogilvie's syndrome) 404
Colorectal carcinoma 409–10
surgery 409
Colostomy, inflammatory bowel disease (IBD) 399, 402–3
Coma, hyperammonaemic 526
Common bile duct stones 362
diagnosis 362
pancreatitis 364
Common bile duct, pregnancy-associated changes 361
Computerized tomography (CT)
acute fatty liver of pregnancy 330
Campylobacter neonatal infection 393
cerebral venous thrombosis 540
eclamptic cerebral pathology 192, 542
gastrointestinal tract disorders 379
head and neck, fetal radiation exposure 536
hepatic rupture/infarction 325
hypopituitarism/Sheehan's syndrome 493
liver metastases 361
prolactin-secreting pituitary tumour
bromocriptine therapy monitoring 485
tumour-related symptoms in pregnancy 486
pseudotumour cerebri 545
septic pelvic thrombophlebitis 135
toxoplasmosis encephalitis 584
Condylomata acuminata 409, 620
Congestive cardiac failure
diuretic therapy 153
thromboembolism risk 118
Congestive cardiomyopathy 166
Connective tissue disease 315
chronic renal disease 247, 254
effect of pregnancy 620–1
heart block in newborn 308, 309
laboratory tests 555
overlap syndrome 307
proteinuria with active urinary sediment 239
respiratory failure 1
Conn's syndrome 212
Constipation 406–7
idiopathic slow transit 406
incidence 406
inflammatory bowel disease 402
management 402, 407
dietary fibre intake 407
laxatives 407
stool bulking agents 407
small intestinal/colonic transit time 406
Constrictive pericarditis 167
Contraception
diabetes mellitus 450–1
nephropathy 439
haemodialysis patients 274
liver transplant patients 352
paroxysmal nocturnal haemoglobinuria (PNH) 60
renal transplant patients 271–2
Coproporphyria, hereditary (HC) 526
Cor pulmonale 168–9
maternal mortality 146
Cordae tendinae rupture 161
Coronary arteriography 164
Coronary artery anomalous origin 163
Coronary artery disease 145
Coronary artery dissection 164
Coronavirus gastroenteritis 397
Cortical necrosis, acute 279, 280
differential diagnosis 280
septic abortion 284
Corticosteroid therapy *see* Steroid therapy
Corticotrophin releasing hormone (CRH) 488–9
placental secretion 489
Cortisol plasma levels 211
Addison's disease 495
Cushing's syndrome 488, 489–90
normal pregnancy 489, 490
Cotrimoxazole 16
candidiasis with HIV infection 584
Pneumocystis carinii pneumonia prophylaxis 586
side effects 586
urinary tract infection (UTI) 558
Coxsackie virus infection 563, 564
neonatal illness/congenital infection 563
Craniopharyngioma
diabetes insipidus 494
pressure effects/hypopituitarism 492
Craniosynostosis 473
Creatinine clearance 227–8
acute liver failure 351
chronic renal disease 238
renal function assessment in pregnancy 239
renal transplant patients 263

Creatinine clearance *Cont.*
serial surveillance 264
timing of blood sample 240
Creatinine plasma level 230, 232
acute liver failure 351
acute renal failure 279
HELLP syndrome 324
levels jeopardizing pregnancy 234, 237
nephron population relationship 234
pre-eclampsia 197, 201
renal function assessment in pregnancy 239
renal transplant patients 263
Cretinism 465
Crohn's disease 397
cholesterol lithiasis 362
effects of pregnancy 399, 400
fertility 398, 400
fetal outcome 399
incidence 397
liver involvement 358
metabolic bone disease 516
nutritional deficiency correction 401
perianal fistulae 408
resective surgery 402
spontaneous abortion 398, 400
vitamin D/calcium malabsorption 516
Cryoprecipitate
factor VIII deficiency (haemophilia A) 105
volume replacement in haemorrhage management 82
von Willebrand's disease 103, 104
Cryosupernatant 99
Cryptococcosis
congenital transmission 585
HIV infection 585
liver involvement 349
lung infection 17
Cryptosporidium
HIV infection/AIDS
liver involvement 349
small bowel infection 391
travellers' diarrhoea 391
Crystalloids
SAG–mannitol blood 83
volume replacement in haemorrhage management 81
Cushing's disease 488, 489
Cushing's syndrome 488–93
adrenal tumour imaging 490–1
adrenal tumour resection 491
bilateral adrenalectomy 491
breast feeding 491
causes 488–9
ACTH-secreting pituitary tumour 490
adrenal cortical tumour 489, 490
ectopic ACTH 489, 490
pituitary gland pathology (Cushing's disease) 488, 489
chronic hypertension in pregnancy (CHT) 211–212, 491
clinical features 489
diagnosis 211, 489
ACTH dependency 490
biochemical investigation 489–90
dexamethasone suppression test 211, 490
exogenous CRH response 490
hypercortisolism 488, 489–90
fetal outcome 491
incidence in pregnancy 489
neonatal adrenal insufficiency 491
pituitary surgery 491
pituitary tumour imaging 490–1
treatment 491
CV205–502 485
Cycling peritoneal dialysis, chronic (CCPO) 276
Cyclizine, safety in pregnancy 385, 386
Cyclophosphamide 93, 248
teratogenicity 15
Wegener's granulomatosis 15
Cyclosporin A
blood level monitoring 352
breast feeding 272
liver transplantation 352
nephrotoxicity 267, 352
oral contraceptive interaction 352
renal transplant patients 261, 264, 267–8, 270
fetal exposure 273
intrauterine growth retardation 273
safety in pregnancy 270, 621
side effects 268, 352
Cyproheptadine 491
Cystic fibrosis 17–19, 365
antibiotic therapy in pregnancy 19
breast feeding 19
carrier screening 18
genetic aspects 17, 18
labour management 19
patient counselling 18–19
pneumothorax 21
post-anaesthetic atelectasis 19
pregnancy outcome 18
prenatal diagnosis 18
prognosis 17, 18
vitamin D malabsorption 516
Cystinosis 250
Cystinuria 249
drug treatment 357
Cystitis, acute 258
Cytomegalovirus (CMV) 554, 564
fetal damage 348–9, 563, 585
fetal loss 563
fever 554
hepatitis 334, 347, 348–9
HIV infection/AIDS 580, 583, 585
biliary tract involvement 349
dysphagia 391
retinitis 585
neonatal illness/congenital infection 270, 271, 563, 585
passive immunization 349
reactivation in pregnancy 348
renal transplant patients 266
congenital infection 270, 271
screening 263
serological diagnosis 349
TORCH (STORCH) infections 563
transmission in transfused blood 82
Cytomegalovirus (CMV) immunoglobulin 271
Cytosine arabinoside 61
Cytotoxic drug therapy
leukaemia 61
systemic lupus erythematosus (SLE) 311
teratogenicity 61

Danazol 92
hereditary angioneurotic oedema 525
masculinization of female fetus 525
Danthron 407
Dapsone
haemolytic disease of newborn 617, 620
malaria prophylaxis/treatment 562
pemphigoid (herpes) gestationis 617
Pneumocystis carinii pneumonia prophylaxis/treatment 584, 586
trimethoprim combination 584
DC conversion 155
DDAVP
diabetes insipidus 494
factor VIII deficiency (haemophilia A) 105
von Willebrand's disease 103, 104
DDAVP response test 494
risk in late pregnancy 494
D-dimer 191
HELLP syndrome 324
de Quervain's thyroiditis 475
thyrotoxicosis 469
Deep vein thrombosis 116
caesarean section 118
diagnosis 119–20
beta thromboglobulin 119
blood flow measurement 119
C reactive protein 119
calf vein thrombosis 120
Doppler flow studies 119, 120
light reflective rheography 120
liquid crystal thermography 119
plethysmography 119–20
proximal thrombosis 119, 120
ultrasound 119, 120
venography 119, 120
following past thromboembolism 130
incidence 116
with pulmonary embolus 121
skin ulceration 116
thrombectomy 126
thrombolytic therapy 125
venous stasis 117
warfarin treatment 128–9
see also Thromboembolism
Dehydration
cerebral venous thrombosis 540
neonatal body temeperature elevation 552
renal transplant patients 265
reversible renal function deterioration 240

thromboembolism risk 118
Delivery
antithrombin III (ATIII) deficiency 133
autoimmune thrombocytopenic purpura (AITP) 93, 94–5
blood loss 345
Campylobacter infection 393
chronic renal disease 240, 241
cirrhosis 355
diabetes mellitus 449–50
haemodialysis patients 276
haemostasis 77
hereditary angioneurotic oedema 525
herpes simplex virus (HSV) genital infection 271, 563
HIV infection/AIDS 583, 588
hypertension-associated hepatic disorder 331
myocardial infarction 164
oesophageal varices, bleeding 355
osteogenesis imperfecta tarda 520
permanent urinary diversion 250
pneumothorax/pneumomediastinum 22
pre-eclampsia *see* Pre-eclampsia
puerperal (peripartum/pregnancy) cardiomyopathy 166
pulmonary vascular disease 169
renal transplant patients 266, 268–9, 273
von Willebrand's disease 104
Dengue 350
Dental caries 381
Depigmenting agents 611
Depression 625
antenatal 627–8
associated agoraphobia 627
associated anxiety 627, 628
chronic 630–1
clinical features 628
postnatal *see* Postnatal depression
treatment 626, 627–8
Dermatological drug prescribing 621
Dermatomyositis 315
fetal outcome 621
impact of pregnancy 620
Dermatoses 614–20
effects of pregnancy 619–20
specific to pregnancy 614–19
Dermographism 621
Desensitization therapy 7
Desmolase deficiency 498
Dexamethasone 91
eclamptic hypertensive encephalopathy 543
fetal therapeutic effects 11
congenital adrenal hyperplasia 496
hyperpigmentation/melasma 611
prolactin-secreting pituitary tumour 487
pruritus gravidarum 612
systemic lupus erythematosus (SLE) 313
thyroid crisis (thyroid storm) 472
Dexamethasone suppression test 490
Dextrans 129
adverse reactions 81, 129
volume replacement in haemorrhage management 81
Diabetes insipidus 493–4
breast feeding 494
causes 493
clinical features 494
DDAVP treatment 494
deterioration in pregnancy 494
diagnosis 492–3, 494
DDAVP response 494
pituitary dependent/nephrogenic 492
hypopituitarism/Sheehan's syndrome 492
incidence 494
labour 494
pituitary tumour 544
expansion 493
prolactin-secreting 486, 487
post-partum haemorrhage 492
prenatal diagnosis of congenital form 251
transient in pregnancy 494
Diabetes mellitus 423–51
with acromegaly 488
antenatal screening 437–8
autonomic neuropathy 445
bacteriuria 248
blood glucose monitoring/home measurement 440, 446
breast feeding 444
bronchial asthma management 9
cerebral dysfunction/intellectual development in offspring 430
cholesterol lithiasis 362
congenital malformations 423, 429–30, 439, 446
contraception 450–1
delivery 449–50
diagnosis in pregnancy 436–7
dietary restrictive treatment 439, 446
dietary fibre 441, 442
dietary restriction alone 441–2
hypocaloric diets 441
ketonaemia 441–2
plus insulin 442–3
established (pre-gestational) 425
fetal acid-base balance 432
fetal biophysical profile 448
fetal effects 429–36, 439, 445, 446
of ketoacidosis 432
poor diabetic control association 429, 430, 434
of toxaemia/pyelonephritis 448
unexplained death *in utero* 431–2
fetal haematology 428
fetal heart rate (FHR) monitoring 447–8
fetal hyperglycaemic hyperinsulism (Pederson hypothesis) 427, 433–4, 435
pancreatic beta cell hypertrophy 427–8
fetal outcome 248, 423, 430–1
fetal plasma glucose level 426–7
fetal well-being indices 447–8
glucose tolerance test (GTT) 424, 425, 437, 438
glycosuria 437
glycosylated haemoglobin 428–9, 430, 433, 437–8, 439, 440, 446
glycosylated plasma proteins 429, 437–8, 440
hypertension 248, 446, 448
haemodialysis patients 276
hypertrophic cardiomyopathy in neonate 435
insulin therapy 439
dosage adjustment 439, 440
effect of daily events 440
intrauterine growth retardation 445, 446
ultrasound 447
joint pregnancy diabetic clinic 439
ketoacidosis 432
labour
blood glucose control 443
early intervention policy 449
intrapartum monitoring 450
intravenous glucose/insulin 443
operative procedures 443
spontaneous 449
macrosomia 443–4, 446
ultrasound monitoring 447
vaginal delivery 434
maternal hazards 248
medical management 438–45
inpatient versus outpatient care 440
treatment principles 439–40
neonatal morbidity 432–7
hypocalcaemia 435
hypoglycaemia 434, 436
hypomagnesaemia 435
jaundice 435
polycythaemia 434–5
poor diabetic control association 434, 435–6
neonatal respiratory distress syndrome 434
nephropathy see Diabetic nephropathy
normoglycaemia as treatment aim 423, 439, 440
obstetric management 445–50
first trimester 446
renal function tests 446
second trimester 446
third trimester 446
oral hypoglycaemic agents 439, 441, 444
peripheral oedema 248
peritoneal dialysis 276
intraperitoneal insulin 276
pituitary infarction 492
placental oxygen transfer 431–2
placental perfusion 431
postnatal management 443–4
potential diabetes 424, 437, 438
pre-eclampsia 248
pre-pregnancy care 438–9
pre-term labour 448–9

Diabetes mellitus *Cont.*
  renal transplant patients 263
    with pancreatic transplant 263
  retinopathy *see* Diabetic retinopathy
  septic shock with acute renal failure 282
  specialist diabetic midwife/nurse 439
  stroke 539
  terminology 424–5
  transient of pregnancy 232
  transient tachypnoea of newborn 434
  type 1 insulin dependent (IDDM) 425
    continuous subcutaneous insulin infusion (CSII) 441
    insulin therapy 440–1
    maximum tolerated dose insulin therapy 441
    pregnancy in prodromal stage 426
  type 2 non-insulin dependent (NIDDM) 425
  White classification 425
  see also Gestational diabetes mellitus (GDM)
Diabetic liaison nurse 438, 439
Diabetic nephropathy 243, 248, 444–5
  contraceptive counselling 439
  fetal surveillance 445
  microalbuminuria monitoring 248
  nephrotic syndrome 248, 252
  pregnancy outcome 245, 445
  pre-pregnancy counselling 439
  termination of pregnancy 451
  transient nephrotic syndrome 445
Diabetic retinopathy 439, 445
  termination of pregnancy 451
Dialysis
  acute renal failure 281, 287
    pre-eclampsia/eclampsia 285
    septic abortion 283
  adult respiratory distress syndrome 21
  haemolytic uraemic syndrome (HUS) 285
  uterine activity 287
Diaphragm level 3
Diaphragmatic hernia 126
Diarrhoea
  infectious 554
  investigations 379, 392
  management 392
Diazepam
  antenatal anxiety 628, 629
  bronchial asthma 7
  dependence 628
  eclampsia prevention/treatment 203, 204, 543
  manic depressive psychosis 632
  neonatal opiate withdrawal syndrome 602
  neonatal side effects 203
  obsessional ruminations 630
  safety in pregnancy 628
Diazoxide 199, 200
Diclofenac 312
Dicyclomine
  in Bendectin/Debendox 385, 386
  irritable bowel syndrome 408
Dideoxycytidine 587
Dideoxyinosine 587
Dietary cravings 380
Dietary fibre 406, 407
  constipation management 407
  diabetes mellitus management 441, 442
Diethylstilboestrol 387, 619
Diet, pregnancy-associated changes 380
Digitalis intoxication 154
Digitoxin
  toxicity 153
  transplacental passage 153
Digoxin 154
  heart disease 152–3
    labour management 153, 157
  neonatal thyrotoxicosis 474
  pericardial disease 167
  secretion in breast milk 153
  septic shock with acute renal failure 284
  thyroid crisis (thyroid storm) 472
  transplacental passage 153
1,25-Dihydroxyvitamin D (1,25-OHD) 507–8
  actions 508
  bone mineralization regulation 508
  fetal production 511–12
  neonatal levels 510
  placental synthesis 510
  pre-eclampsia 190
  pregnancy-associated elevation 510
  puerperal level 510
  renal calcium/phosphate reabsorption 508
  renal 1α-hydrolase control of synthesis 508–9
  small intestinal calcium/phosphate absorption 508, 510
  target organs 508
Di-iodotyrosine (DIT) 459, 460
Diltiazem 154
Dimenhydrinate 385, 386
Dindevan 156
Diphenhydramine 386
Diphenoxylate 392
  inflammatory bowel disease 401
Dipyridamole
  haemolytic uraemic syndrome (HUS) 285
  pre-eclampsia prevention 206
  thromboprophylaxis 132
    artificial heart valves 156
Disodium azodisalicylate 401
Disodium cromoglycate
  bronchial asthma 10
  isoprenaline combination 10
Disopyramide 154
Disseminated intravascular coagulation (DIC) 71, 77–8
  abruptio placentae 84–6
  acute cortical necrosis 280
  acute fatty liver of pregnancy (AFLP) 88–9
  acute liver failure 349
  adult respiratory distress syndrome/shock lung 20, 21
  amniotic fluid embolism 86–7
  antithrombin III (ATIII) activity 75
  associated obstetric conditions 78
  factor VIII measurement 84
  fibrin degradation products (FDPs) 80, 84
  fibrinopeptide A 84
  haemorrhage management 78–83
  HELLP syndrome 324
  hepatic subcapsular haemorrhages 325
  induced abortion 88
  intrauterine infection 88
  low grade, *in vitro* tests 83–4
  pancreatitis 365
pre-eclampsia 191, 197, 198, 205, 324
    liver damage 191
    post-partum 205
  purpura fulminans 88
  rapid screening tests 79, 80, 85
    fibrinogen estimation 80
    thrombin time 80
  retained dead fetus 87
  septicaemia with acute renal failure 282, 284
  severity of clinical manifestations 77–8
  soluble fibrin complexes 84
  thrombocytopenia 89
  trigger mechanisms 77
  vaginal delivery/caesarean section 83
Dithranol, safety in pregnancy 621
Diuretic therapy 233
  acute renal failure 280
  adult repiratory distress syndrome/shock lung 21
  chronic hypertension in pregnancy (CHT) 210, 213
  cirrhosis 355
  indications 241
  neonatal thyrotoxicosis 474
  nephrotic syndrome 252
  pericardial disease 167
  pre-eclampsia 204, 205, 212, 241
    laryngeal oedema 207
  prerenal failure (vasomotor nephropathy) 280
  reversible renal function deterioration 240
  thyroid crisis (thyroid storm) 472
Domperidone 382
  safety in pregnancy 385
Dopamine 168
  gestational vomiting 384
  septic shock with acute renal failure 284
Doppler flow studies
  Budd–Chiari syndrome 357
  deep vein thrombosis 119, 120
  heart valve regurgitant flow 150
  placental perfusion
    diabetes mellitus 431
    maternal heart disease 152

post-partum eclamptic encephalopathy 542
umbilical blood flow
congenital heart block with SLE 313
diabetes mellitus 447
Dorbanex 407
Down's syndrome 446, 498
Doxycycline 385, 386
D-penicillamine
cystinuria 249
fetal effects 357
Wilson's disease 355, 356
Droperidol 386
Drug abuse *see* Substance abuse
D-tubocurarine, opiate interactions 603
Dubin Johnson syndrome 358
Duodenal biopsy 390
Dwarf tapeworm (*Hymenolepsis nana*) 395
Dysentery, bacterial 554
Dsyfibrinogenaemia, hereditary 107
Dyspepsia 381, 382
Dysrhythmias 122
chest pain 148
electrocardiography 150
ischaemic heart disease 154
puerperal (peripartum/pregnancy) cardiomyopathy 165
syncope 148
treatment 152–5

Ebstein's anomaly 171
lithium teratogenesis 631
Echocardiography
Doppler flow studies 150
Ebstein's malformation 171
heart disease 150
heart murmurs in intravenous drug abusers 600
hypertrophic cardiomyopathy 164
maternal diabetes mellitus 435
Marfan's syndrome 170
pericardial disease 167
puerperal (peripartum/pregnancy) cardiomyopathy 165
stroke 539
transoesophageal 150
Echovirus infection 554, 564
Eclampsia 188, 192, 195, 541–3
acute adrenal failure 495
acute renal failure 284
adult respiratory distress syndrome 20
anticonvulsant drugs 202–4, 208
antihypertensive treatment 543
blood pressure measurement errors 185
cerebral haemorrhage 189
cerebral pathology 192, 539, 541–3
chonic renal disease 241
convulsions 192
characteristics 541
pathogenesis 192–3
cortical blindness 192
CSF pressure 192–3
disseminated intravascular coagulation (DIC) 78, 191
hepatic subcapsular haemorrhages 325
hypertension 192, 542
post-partum 208
incidence 192
intracerebral haematoma 542
late post-partum 542
long-term sequelae 212
management 543
maternal mortality 189, 191, 192
neurodiagnostic studies 542
prevention/treatment 202–4
proteinuria 192
Ectopic beats 148
Ectopic kidney 251
Ectopic pregnancy
disseminated intravascular coagulation (DIC) 88
primary choriocarcinoma 361
renal transplant patients 264, 272
rupture 384
tubal, abdominal complications 405
Eczema 619
Ehlers–Danlos syndrome 146
Eisenmenger's syndrome 146, 167–9
epidural anaesthesia contraindication 158
haemodynamics 167, 168
heart–lung transplantation 167
hypertensive pregnancy 167
management 167
labour 167–9
pulmonary vasodilators 168
maternal mortality 146, 167
syncope 148
termination of pregnancy 150
Ejection systolic murmur 143, 149
Electrocardiography (ECG)
acute renal failure 279
acute rheumatic fever 161
heart disease 149–50
myocardial infarction 163
puerperal (peripartum/pregnancy) cardiomyopathy 165
pulmonary embolus 121
Electroconvulsive therapy (ECT)
manic depressive psychosis 633
puerperal psychosis 635
Electroencephalography (EEG) 535
eclamptic hypertensive encephalopathy 542
Electrolyte imbalance
acute renal failure 281
pancreatitis 365
resective surgery for IBD 402
reversible renal function deterioration 240
Electromyography (EMG) 535
Elemental diets 401
Emphysema 19–20
pneumothorax 21
Enalapril 153
Endocarditis
cerebral ischaemia/stroke 539
heart disease 158–9
antibiotic prophylaxis in labour 158–9
laboratory tests 555
Listeria monocytogenes 561
maternal mortality 158, 159
mitral regurgitation 161
prophylaxis 161
subarachnoid haemorrhage 541
Endometriosis
haematuria 260
intestinal obstruction 404
Endomyocardial fibrosis 166
neonatal lupus syndrome 308
Endoscopic retrograde cholecystopancreatography 363
Endoscopic sclerotherapy 355–6
Endothelial derived relaxing factor (EDRF)
guanosine monophosphate (cGMP) second messenger 230
haemolytic uraemic syndrome (HUS) 285
hypertension in pregnancy 253
pre-eclampsia 72
renal vasodilatation of pregnancy 230
Endothelial dysfunction
haemolytic uraemic syndrome (HUS) 285
pre-eclampsia 193, 324
systemic lupus erythematosus (SLE) 307
Endothelium, role in haemostasis 72
Endotoxic shock
adult respiratory distress syndrome 20
clinical features 559
disseminated intravascular coagulation (DIC) 88
septic abortion 559
Endotoxin, bacterial 552
Endotracheal intubation
achondroplasia 520
acute liver failure 351
hereditary angioneurotic oedema 525, 526
pre-eclampsia 207
scleroderma 315
Enflurane 381
Enoxparine 125, 132
Entamoeba histolytica see Amoebiasis
Enteric fevers 554
laboratory tests 555
Enterobateriaceae
puerperal sepsis/wound infection 558
urinary tract infection (UTI) 556, 558
Enterobius vermicularis see Threadworm
Enterovirus infection 554
Eosinophilic granuloma 492
Ephedrine 9
Epidural abscess, intravenous drug abusers 600
Epidural anaesthesia
achondroplasia 520
autoimmune thrombocytopenic

Epidural anaesthesia *Cont.*
purpura (AITP) 94
bronchial asthma 11
caesarean section 23
cardiac output 158
cirrhosis 355
cystic fibrosis 19
Eisenmenger's syndrome 167–8
heart disease 158
contraindications 158
hereditary angioneurotic oedema 525
hypertension-associated hepatic disorders 331
hypertrophic obstructive cardiomyopathy 164–5
kyphoscoliosis 20
multiple sclerosis 546
myocardial infarction 164
opiate addicts 603
osteogenesis imperfecta tarda 520
pre-eclampsia 207
primary pulmonary hypertension 169
puerperal (peripartum/pregnancy) cardiomyopathy 166
severe respiratory impairment 23
sickle cell disease (HbSS) 53
with subcutaneous heparin therapy 128
urolithiasis management 249
Epilepsy 536–9
anticonvulsant therapy 536, 537, 538–9
blood level monitoring 536, 538
folate deficiency 536, 538
neonatal coagulopathy 537, 538
post-partum 539
vitamin K1 prophylaxis 538–9
birth defects 537–8
dysmorphic features and digital hypoplasia 537
monotherapy 538
neural tube defects 537
orofacial clefts 537
pathogenesis 537–8
prevention 538
breast feeding 536
effect of pregnancy 536
family history 537
fetal effects of convulsions 537
folate supplements 45, 538
incidence 536
labour 536
oral contraception 536
pre-pregnancy counselling 537, 538
status epilepticus 537
Episiotomy
anal sphincter injuries 408
blood loss at delivery 35
HIV infection vertical transmission 589
puerperal sepsis/wound infection 559
renal transplant patients 268
ureterosigmoid anastomosis 250
Epsilon aminocaproic acid (EACA) 76
abruptio placentae 85
hereditary angioneurotic oedema 525
pancreatitis 364
Epstein–Barr virus (EBV) 563
hepatitis 334, 347
transmission in transfused blood 82
Ergocalciferol 515
Ergometrine 164, 169
beta sympathomimetic drug interaction 159–60
bronchial asthma 11
heart disease 158
pre-eclampsia, labour management 207
Ergot alkaloids 546
Erythema multiforme 621
Erythema nodosum 15
Erythromycin 16
Campylobacter infection 393
listeriosis 394
pneumonia 17
pseudomembranous colitis 392
Erythropoietin
maternal diabetes mellitus 428, 435
red cell production increase 34
Escherichia coli
haemolytic uraemic syndrome (HUS) 285
peritonitis with cirrhosis 355
septic abortion 282, 560
travellers' diarrhoea 391
urinary tract infection 255, 257, 259, 557
acute pyelonephritis 557
cyclosporin A nephrotoxicity susceptibility 268
Ethacrynic acid 153
Ethambutol
fetal effects 13
tuberculosis 13
with HIV infection 584
Etiocholanolone 552
Etretinate 621
Exchange transfusion
haemolytic uraemic syndrome (HUS) 286
jaundice with maternal diabetes mellitus 435
neonatal thyrotoxicosis 474
Exercise
beneficial effects 5
capacity 4–5
Extracellular space body fluid increase 233

Fabry's disease, prenatal diagnosis 251
Factor I *see* Fibrinogen
Factor II (prothrombin) 117
Factor II (prothrombin) deficiency 108
Factor V 117
protein C inhibition 75
Factor V deficiency 108
Factor VII 73, 74, 117
phospholipid complex formation 117
pre-eclampsia 191
Factor VII deficiency 108
Factor VIII 74, 117
compensated DIC 84
complex with von Willebrand's factor (vWF) 102
post-partum activity 104
pre-eclampsia 98, 191
protein C inhibition 75
thromboembolism risk prediction 132
Factor VIII antibody 99–100
aetiology 99
autoimmune disorders association 99
clinical manifestations 99–100
management 100
Factor VIII concentrate 104
Factor VIII deficiency (haemophilia A) 104
carrier detection 106
clinical manifestations 105
genetic aspects 105
incidence 104
management in pregnancy 105
molecular aspects 102
preconceptional investigations 105, 106
prenatal diagnosis 106
risks of pregnancy for carriers 105
Factor VIII-related antigen (VIIIRAg) *see* von Willebrand's factor (vWF)
Factor IX 117
Factor IX antibody 99
Factor IX concentrate 105, 106
Factor IX deficiency (haemophilia B) 104
carrier detection 106
clinical manifestations 105
genetic aspects 105
incidence 105
management in pregnancy 105–6
preconceptional investigations 105, 106
prenatal diagnosis 106
risks of pregnancy for carriers 105
Factor X 73, 74, 117
antithrombin III inhibition 75
Factor X deficiency 108
Factor XI concentrate 107
Factor XI deficiency (plasma thromboplastin antecedent (PTA) deficiency) 106–7
clinical manifestations 107
genetic aspects 107
management 107
Factor XII 73
Factor XIII (fibrin stabilizing factor) deficiency 107–8
clot solubility test 108
genetic aspects 107
Fallot's tetralogy
fetal outcome 147
corrected cases 147
maternal mortality 146
open heart surgery 152
phenylketonuria 523
pregnancy 145

risk of recurrence 147
syncope 148
Familial polyposis 410
Fanconi's anaemia 101
Fatty acid metabolism, congenital disorders 358
Fatty liver of pregnancy, acute (AFLP) 192, 323, 326–31
aetiology 329
antithrombin III deficiency 89
blood films 89
clinical features 327, 328
diabetes insipidus 494
diagnosis 326–7, 328
differential diagnosis 327–8
disseminated intravascular coagulation (DIC) 88–9
early delivery 331
incidence 326
laboratory findings 327
liver transplantation 352
microvesicular steatosis 327, 238
morality, maternal/fetal 326
neonatal abnormalities 330
pancreatitis 364
pathology 327
persistent vomiting 384
portal hypertension 356
pregnancy-induced hypertension/HELLP syndrome overlap 329–30
recurrence 331
renal failure 285, 286
Fenoterol
bronchial asthma 9
side effects 8, 159
Fentanyl 169, 383
Ferritin 38
iron deficiency 41–2
Fetal alcohol syndrome 604
Fetal anticonvulsant syndrome 537–8
Fetal blood sampling
autoimmune thrombocytopenic purpura (AITP) 93–4, 95
calcium/phosphate serum level 511
congenital heart block with SLE 313
cytotoxic drug therapy for leukaemia 62
diabetic nephropathy 445
fetal alloimmune thrombocytopenia (AIT) 97
fetal thyroid function 468
haemoglobinopathy 55
HIV infection vertical transmission 588
maternal heart disease 152
platelet function abnormalities, hereditary 101
protein C deficiency 134
thrombocytopenia, hereditary disorders 101
thyrotoxicosis 473
toxoplasmosis 561
Fetal heart rate (FHR) monitoring
diabetes mellitus 447–8
intrapartum 450
thyrotoxicosis 473
see also Cardiotocography
Fetal hypoxia
bronchial asthma 7
hypertension-associated hepatic disorders 330
Fetal monitoring
chronic renal disease 241
diabetic nephropathy 445
intrahepatic cholestasis of pregnancy (IHCP) 333
maternal heart disease 152
renal transplant patients 268
Fetal scalp blood sampling
autoimmune thrombocytopenic purpura (AITP) 93
HIV infection vertical transmission 588
renal transplant patients 268
FEV_1 4
bronchial asthma 6, 7
epidural anaesthesia for caesarean section 23
Fever 552–6
causes 553
clinical features 553
diagnosis 555
endogenous pyrogen 552
epidemic infections 554
fungal diseases 555
infectious diseases 553
laboratory tests 555–6
non-infectious diseases 553, 554
non-specific bacterial infections 553, 554, 556–7, 558–9
parasitic diseases 556
pattern of febrile response 552–3
periodic 552
puerperal sepsis/wound infection 559
rigors 552, 553
septic abortion 559
special bacterial infections 555
of unknown origin (FUO) 553
virus infections 554
Fibrin
breakdown by plasmin 76
deposition in pre-eclampsia 191
placental/spiral artery deposition 77
Fibrin degradation products (FDPs) 76
abruptio placentae 85
acute fatty liver of pregnancy 327
blood sampling artefacts 79
clearance with blood volume restoration 81, 85
disseminated interavascular coagulation (DIC) 78, 80
low grade compensated 84
haemorrhage 79–80, 81
HELLP syndrome 324
pre-eclampsia 98, 191
diagnosis 197
Fibrin monomers/polymers 84
Fibrin plug formation 73
Fibrin stabilizing factor deficiency *see* Factor XIII deficiency
Fibrinogen 71, 73, 74, 117
abnormal forms 134
recurrent thromboembolism 129
breakdown by plasmin 76
genetic disorders 107
thrombin breakdown products 84
Fibrinogen concentrate 82
Fibrinogen estimation
abruptio placentae 85
haemorrhage, rapid screening tests 79, 80
pre-eclampsia 191
thromboembolism risk prediction 132
Fibrinolysis 71, 75–6
disseminated intravascular coagulation (DIC) 78
inherited abnormalities 132
inhibitors 76
thromboembolism risk 117
Fibrinopeptide A 84
compensated DIC 84
placental separation 117
pre-eclampsia 98, 191
thromboembolism risk prediction 132
Fibrinopeptide B 84
Fibromuscular dysplasia
cerebral ischaemia/stroke 539
hepatic rupture/infarction 325
Fibronectin 193, 197
Fibrosing alveolitis 5
Filtration fraction (FF) 227
Fish oil supplements 206
Fissure in ano 408
Flecainide 153
Fluconazole 584
Flucytosine 17
Fludrocortisone 498
Fluid balance
acute renal failure 279, 281
Addison's disease 495
pancreatitis 365
Fluoxetine 637
Fluphenazine decanoate 663–4
Flurbiprofen 312
Fluvoxamine 637
Focal glomerular sclerosis 235
Folic acid 42–3
absorption 42, 44
in breast milk 43
dietary sources 44
metabolism 42
multiple pregnancy 42
plasma level 42
post-partum 43
red cell 43
requirement 44
with anticonvulsant therapy 45
disorders affecting 45
neonate/young infant 46
in pregnancy 42
Folic acid deficiency
with anticonvulsant therapy 45, 536, 538
aphthous stomatitis 380
associated obstetric complications 44
cleft lip/palate 46

Folic acid deficiency *Cont.*
coeliac disease 389, 390
diagnosis 43
formiminoglutamic acid excretion (FIGLU test) 43
interpretation of investigations 43
intestinal malabsorption 42
lactation 43
megaloblastic anaemia 43–5
multiple pregnancy 44
neural tube defects 46
periconceptional 46
pre-term infant 46
Folic acid supplements 44, 45
acute liver failure 351
anticonvulsant therapy/epilepsy 45, 538
antimalarials treatment 563
coeliac disease 390
daily requirements 390
Gaucher's disease 524
HbH disease 48
inflammatory bowel disease 403
intestinal parasite infestation 395
iron supplement combinations 39, 45
neural tube defect prevention 46, 390
pre-pregnancy 46
routine prophylaxis 45
salazopyrine therapy 401
sulphadiazine/pyramethamine therapy 584
α thalassaemia 48
β thalassaemia 50
total parenteral nutrition 405
toxoplasmosis 561
Fontan procedure 170–1
Footdrop 547
Forbe's disease 525
Forced expiratory volume in 1 second *see* FEV_1
Forceps delivery
cirrhosis 355
cystic fibrosis 19
ileostomy 403
myocardial infarction 164
pneumothorax/pneumomediastinum 22
prolactin-secreting pituitary tumour 487
puerperal sepsis/wound infection 559
severe respiratory impairment 23
thromboembolism risk 118
Formiminoglutamic acid excretion (FIGLU) test 43
Foscarnet 585
Fox–Fordyce disease 613
Fraxiparin 125
Free erythrocyte protoporphyrin (FEP) 38
Free fatty acids, total parenteral nutrition 405
Free ionized calcium 506
Free T_4 index (FTI) 461, 462
hypothyroidism 467
thyrotoxicosis 469
Fresh frozen plasma (FFP)
abruptio placentae 85
acute liver failure 351
amniotic fluid embolism 87
antithrombin III replacement 133
bleeding oesophageal varices 355
factor IX deficiency (haemophilia B) 105
factor XIII (fibrin stabilizing factor) deficiency 108
haemorrhage management 82, 83
induced abortion 88
hereditary angioneurotic oedema 525, 526
hypertension-associated hepatic disorders 330
septic shock with acute renal failure 284
von Willebrand's disease 103, 104
Frusemide 153, 158
acute renal failure 280
FSH secreting pituitary tumour 483
Fungal infection 554
aphthous stomatitis 380
haematuria 259
lungs 17
renal transplant patients 266
Furazolidone 397

Galactosaemia 407
Gallbladder disease 361–3
oral contraceptives association 361
Gallbladder, pregnancy-associated changes 361
Gallstones 363
bile acid therapy contraindication 363
cholesterol 362
clinical features 362
intrahepatic cholestasis of pregnancy (IHCP) 332
lithotripsy contraindication 363
management 362–3
maternal/fetal outcome 363
oral contraceptives association 361
pancreatitis 363, 364, 365
in pregnancy 362–3
Gamma glutamyl transpeptidase
common bile duct stones with pancreatitis 364
primary biliary cirrhosis 356
Ganciclovir 585
Gastrointestinal disorders 387–90
Gastric acid secretion 387
Gastric contents aspiration 122, 382
adult respiratory distress syndrome 20
management 22
maternal mortality 22, 23
Mendelson's syndrome 382
preventive measures in labour 22
antacid administration 22, 23
guidelines 23
starvation 22, 23
preventive obstetrical anaesthesia preparation 383
puerperal pyrexia 559
Gastric emptying 379
Gastric lesions investigation 379
Gastric malignancy, primary 409
Gastrin
calcitonin stimulation 509
serum level 387
Gastroenteritis, viral 397
Gastrointestinal haemorrhage
acute liver failure 351
bleeding oesophageal varices 354, 355–6
hypertension-associated hepatic disorders 330
peptic ulcer disease 387, 388
pseudoxanthoma elasticum 522
Gastrointestinal infection/infestation 390–7
bacterial infections 391–4
with HIV infection/AIDS 391–2
intestinal parasites 395–7
viral gastroenteritis 397
Gastrointestinal malignancy 409–10
Gastrointestinal tract 379–410
anorectal/perineal disorders 408–10
diagnostic techniques 379
gastrointestinal disorders 387–90
gastro-oesophageal disorders 381–7
oral cavity disorders 380–1
self-medication 379
Gastro-oesophageal disorders 381–2
Gastro-oesophageal reflux 381
hiatus hernia 381
investigations 379
management 381–2
antacids 382
oesophagitis 381
pathophysiology 381
Gaucher's disease 524–5
carrier detection 524
enzyme therapy 524
gene therapy 524
portal hypertension 356
prenatal diagnosis 524
splenectomy 524
Gaviscon 382
Gelatin solutions 81
Genetic counselling
bronchial asthma 11–12
Gaucher's disease 524
polycystic kidney disease (PKD) 250
renal diesease, inherited 250
Gentamicin 159
Campylobacter infection 393
cystic fibrosis 19
septic shock 284
urinary tract infection (UTI) 259
Geophagia 380
Gestational diabetes mellitus (GDM) 424–5
diagnosis 436
early delivery policy 449
fetal macrosomia 434
first trimester counselling 446
Forbe's disease 525
insulin therapy 439–40
management 441

postnatal 444
neonatal polycythaemia 435
oral contraceptive use 450
pancreatic beta cell insufficiency 426
perinatal mortality 432
restrictive dietary advice 439
terminology 437
type 2 diabetes mellitus (NIDDM) development 444
see also Gestational impaired glucose tolerance (GIGT)
Gestational hypertension 187
Gestational impaired glucose tolerance (GIGT) 425, 437
labour 443
management 441
postnatal 443, 444
perinatal mortality 432
type 2 diabetes mellitus (NIDDM) development 444
Gestosis *see* pre-eclampsia
Giardiasis 396–7
clinical features 397
congenital/neonatal infection 395
transmission 397
travellers' diarrhoea 391
treatment prior to delivery 395
Gilbert's disease 358
Ginger anti-emetic therapy 385
Gingivitis, hyperplastic 380–1
Glandular fever 555
Glanzmann's disease *see* Thrombasthenia
Glioma, malignant 544
Globin gene analysis 55–6
Globulin lysis time 117
Globulins, serum level 322
see also immunoglobulins
Glomerular blood pressure (P_{GC}) 228
Glomerular filtration rate (GFR) 227, 228, 230
chronic renal disease, perinatal outcome relationship 235
effects of hyperperfusion of pregnancy 232, 233
estimation in pregnancy 240
nephron population relationship 234
vasoactive hormone responses 229
Glomerular plasma flow 228
Glomerulonephritis, acute 243
Glomerulonephritis, antibasement membrane 253
Glomerulonephritis, chronic 243, 245
hypertension 245
superimposed pre-eclampsia 245
Glomerulonephritis, diffuse proliferative (DPGN) 245, 246
Glomerulonephritis, familial *see* Nephritis, hereditary
Glomerulonephritis, focal (FGN) 242, 244, 245, 246, 254
Glomerulonephritis, immune-complex-associated 342
Glomerulonephritis, membranoproliferative (MPGN) 244, 245, 246, 254
impact of pregnancy 235
nephrotic syndrome 252
Glomerulonephritis, membranous 244, 245, 246
Heymann nephritis animal model 253
Glomerulonephritis, proliferative 244
nephrotic syndrome 252
Glomerulonephritis, rapidly progressive 239
Glucagon therapy 364
Glucose homeostasis
fetal 426–8
maternal 425
abnormalities 425–6
Glucose tolerance test (GTT)
antenatal screening 437
gestational diabetes mellitus (GDM) 424, 425, 436–7
postnatal management 443, 444
normal pregnancy 425
Glucose-6-phosphate dehydrogenase deficiency 620
Gluten-free diet 390
Glycogen storage disease 524–5
Glycosuria 232
diabetes mellitus 437
post-urinary tract infection 254
Goitre 462
endemic 459, 463–5
cretinism 465
fetal wastage 465
fetal
maternal antithyroid drug treatment 463, 464
maternal thyrotoxicosis 473
hypothyroidism 466
non-toxic 465
post-partum thyroiditis 474, 475
pregnancy-associated 461
sporadic 465–6
thyrotoxicosis 469, 470, 471, 473
Goitrogens 463, 464
cretinism 465
Gold therapy 314
Goserelin 617
Granisetron 386
Graves' disease 469
antithyroid drug treatment 470
supplementary T_4 470
fetal thyrotoxicosis screening 473
neonatal thyrotoxicosis 472
thyroid status fluctuations 469, 470
TSH receptor binding inhibiting antibodies (TBII) 473
see also Thyrotoxicosis
Greenfield filter 129
Griseofulvin 621
Growth hormone
calcium/phosphate homeostasis 506
isolated deficiency (sexual ateliosis) 488
levels in pregnancy 488
placental secretion 488
renal 1α-hydrolase activation 509, 510
Growth hormone-secreting pituitary tumour 483
acromegaly *see* Acromegaly
Guillain–Barré syndrome 1, 546, 547
Guthrie test 522, 523

H_2 antagonists
acute liver failure 351
gastric aspiration prevention in labour 23, 383
obstetrical anaesthesia preparation 383
pancreatitis 364
safety in pregnancy 382
Haemaccel 81
Haemangiomata 613
Haematemesis 388
Haematuria 259
asymptomatic microscopic 239
Haemodialysis 274–6
acute renal failure 281, 287
contraception counseling 274
heparinization 287
pregnancy counselling 274
pregnancy management 274–6
anaemia 275–6
delivery 276
dialysis strategy 275
dialysis-induced uterine contractions 275
dietary counselling 276
early assessment 274–5
hypertension 276
objectives 275
pregnancy outcome 275
Haemoglobin
structural aspects 47
variants 47, 50–4
Haemoglobin concentration
iron deficiency 37
normal levels 37
pre-eclampsia 40
Haemoglobinopathies 47–58
folate supplements 45
prenatal diagnosis 47, 55–7
amnitoic fluid fibroblasts 55, 56
chorion villus sampling 55, 56–7
fetal blood sampling 55
globin gene analysis 55–6
screening 54–5
pre-pregnancy 57–8
rationale 57
Haemolytic anaemia
folate supplements 45
haemolytic uraemic syndrome (HUS) 285
HELLP syndrome 324
malaria 562
neonatal lupus syndrome 308
pre-eclampsia 97
specific to pregnancy 58
Haemolytic uraemic syndrome (HUS) 98–9, 285–6
clinical features 285
outcome 285
pathophysiology 285
post-partum renal failure 284, 285
prostacyclin (PGI_2) deficiency 72

Haemolytic uraemic syndrome (HUS) *Cont.*
  renal disease 98
  SLE renal-flare comparison 307
  treatment 99, 285–6
Haemophilia A *see* Factor VIII deficiency
Haemophilia B *see* Factor IX deficiency
Haemophilias 104–8
Haemophilus influenzae 16
Haemorrhage
  abruptio placentae 85
  acute renal failure 279
  disseminated intravascular coagulation (DIC) 77, 78, 88
  Ehlers–Danlos syndrome 146
  factor VIII antibody 99, 100
  fibrin degradation products (FDPs) 79–80, 81
  fluid replacement 81–3
    fresh frozen plasma (FFP) 82
    plasma component therapy 82
    plasma substitutes 81
    red cell transfusion 82–3
    SAG-mannitol blood 83
    whole fresh blood 81–2
  induced abortion 88
  intra-abdominal 123
  leukaemia 61
  management 78–83
    rapid screening tests 79–80
    venous blood sampling 79
  placental separation 71
  pseudoxanthoma elasticum 522
  purpura fulminans 88
  thromboembolism risk 118
  see also post-partum haemorrhage
Haemorrhoidectomy 408
Haemorrhoids 408, 612
Haemostasis 71–7
  acquired primary defects 89–96
  clotting factor inhibitors 74–5
  inherited disorders 100–8
    coagulation disorders 101–8
    history taking 100–1
    platelet abnormalities 101
    preconceptional investigations 100
    prenatal diagnosis 100
  placental separation 77
  platelets 72–3
  post-traumatic arrest of bleeding 73
  local response 73
  platelet activation/aggregation 73
  pregnancy/delivery-associated changes 76–7
  vascular integrity 71–2
  role of endothelium 72
Hair changes 614
Haloperidol
  manic depressive psychosis 631
    acute relapse 633
  puerperal psychosis 635
  safety in pregnancy 632
  schizophrenia 634
Halothane
  acute liver failure 350
  bronchial asthma 11
  lower oesophageal sphincter pressure (LOSP) 381
Hand-Schueller-Christian disease 492
Hashimoto's thyroiditis 475
  fetal hypothyroidism 468
HbBarts 48
HbH disease 48
HBIG immunoprophylaxis
  contacts of patient 352
  hepatitis B 343–4, 345–6
    vaccine poor responders 347
  re-infection prevention following liver transplantation 352
HBsAg hyperimmunoglobulin 271
Headache 546
  muscle contraction 546
Heart block, congenital 170
  anti-Ro/anti-La antibody association 308–9, 312
  rheumatoid arthritis, 308, 313
  systemic lupus erythematosus (SLE) 307, 308, 312
    diagnosis before delivery 313
Heart chamber size 150
Heart disease 143–71
  acquired 160–7
  antenatal care 152
  anticoagulant therapy 155–7
  atrial fibrillation 152, 153
  bed rest 152
  beta sympathomimetic drugs 160
    contraindications 160
    side effects 159–60
  breathlessness 148
  cardiopulmonary arrest management 155
  chest pain 148
    clinical management 150–2
  congenital 167–71
    anticoagulant therapy 155
    fetal outcome 147
    lithium teratogenesis 631
    maternal diabetes mellitus 429, 446
    open heart surgery 151, 152
    phenylketonuria 523, 524
    pregnancy 145
    risk of recurrence in offspring 147
  digoxin 152–3
  diuretic therapy 153–4
  dysrhythmias treatment 154–5
    DC conversion 155
    drugs 154–5
    long-term prophylaxis 155
  endocarditis 158–9
  fetal monitoring 152
  fetal outcome 147
  heart failure
    risk factors 152
    treatment 152–3
  history taking 148
  hospital admission 152
  incidence 143, 144–5
  investigations 149–50
    chest radiography 149
    echocardiography 150
    electrocardiography 149–50
  labour 157–8
    antibiotic prophylaxis 150, 158–9
    aortocaval compression 157
    cardiac output 157
    epidural anaesthesia 158
    third stage 158
  left atrial pressure measurement 144
  management in pregnancy 147–60
    obstetric/cardiac combined clinic 147
  maternal mortality 143, 145–6
    New York Heart Association (NYHA) classification 148
  oxytocic drugs 158
  physical signs 148–9
  physiological aspects 143–4
  post-partum haemorrhage 158
  pulmonary oedema 153, 159–60
  regional block 158
  surgery 150–2
    aortic valvuloplasty 151
    cardiopulmonary bypass 151
    mitral valvotomy 151
    mitral valvuloplasty 151
    open heart surgery 151
  syncope 148
  termination of pregnancy 150
Heart failure
  management 152–8
  oxytocics contraindication 158
  pleural effusion 22
  puerperal (peripartum/pregnancy) cardiomyopathy 165, 166
Heart rate 144
Heart sounds 149
  ejection systolic sound 143, 149
  intravenous drug abusers 600
  systolic murmurs 149
Heart transplantation 166
  pregnancy management 171
  puerperal cardiomyopathy 171
Heartburn 381
Heart–lung transplantation 167
Helicobacter pylori 387
HELLP syndrome 191, 285, 323, 324–5
  acute fatty liver of pregnancy 329–30
  diagnosis 324
  hepatic rupture/infarction 325
  liver transplantation 352
  periportal fibrin deposition 324
  persistent vomiting 384
  post-partum recovery 325
  pre-emptive delivery 324–5
  recurrence 331
Helminthic infestations 395–6
Hemiplegic migraine 546
Heparin
  abruptio placentae 85
  amniotic fluid embolism 87
  antithrombin III (ATIII) enhancement 75
  antithrombin III deficiency 133
  assay 127, 128, 156
  cerebral venous thrombosis 540
  contamination of venous blood samples 79
  continuous intravenous 129, 156,

157, 162, 163
labour management 156
monitoring 156
Eisenmenger's syndrome 167
haemodialysis 275, 287
haemolytic uraemic syndrome (HUS) 285
long-term intravenous 129
pre-eclampsia 128, 205
protamine sulphate
neutralization dose 124
neutralization test 156
protein C deficiency 134
purpura fulminans 88
recurrent thromboembolism 129
retained dead fetus 87
reversal of therapy 124
septic abortion 88
side effects 124
bone demineralization 130–1, 133, 156, 519
of chlorobutol preservative 124
prolonged therapy 130–1, 133
thrombocytopenia 131
subcutaneous 127, 130, 131, 134, 155, 156, 157, 171, 312–5
continuous infusion 129
self-administration 128
thromboembolism chronic phase monitoring 127–8
systemic lupus erythematosus (SLE) 312
aspirin combination 312
thromboembolism prophylaxis 312
thromboembolism
acute phase treatment 121, 124–5
chronic phase treatment 127–9
emergency resuscitation 121
high dose intravenous therapy 124–5
subcutaneous fixed dose therapy 125
thrombolytic therapy comparison 125
treatment monitoring 124
thromboprophylaxis 75, 129, 130, 131, 134, 312
artificial heart valves 156, 157, 162, 163
Fontan procedure 171
homocystinuria 522
paroxysmal nocturnal haemoglobinuria (PNH) 61
polycythaemia rubra vera (PRV) 59
safety of regimes 130
transient ischaemic attacks (TIA) 540
see also low molecular weight heparins
Heparin-induced osteopenia 130–1, 133, 519
Heparin-induced thrombocytopenia 131
Hepatic abscess 359
Hepatic adenoma
oral contraceptive association 359
primary liver cancer association 360
rupture 359
Hepatic arteriography
hepatic rupture/infarction 326
liver metastases of trophoblastic disease 361
Hepatic blood flow 321
Hepatic encephalopathy 349
cirrhosis 355
pancreatitis 365
paracetamol overdose 350
viral hepatitis 350
Hepatic fibrosis, congenital 356
Hepatic focal nodular hyperplasia 359
primary liver cancer association 360
Hepatic metastases of trophoblastic disease 360
Hepatic rupture/infarction 323, 325–6
clinical features 325
fetal/maternal outcome 326
hepatic resection 326
obstetric intervention 326
pathogenic mechanisms 325
post-partum 325, 331
prognosis 325
transcatheter embolization 326
Hepatic vein thrombosis 61
Hepatic venous catheterization 357
Hepatitis A 333, 334, 335–6, 554, 564
acute liver failure 350
clinical features 335
immunoglobulin immunoprophylaxis 336
contacts of patient 352
incubation period 335
management 335
serological diagnosis 334, 335
transmission 335, 336
to newborn 335, 336
vaccine 336
Hepatitis B 333, 334, 338–47, 554, 564
acute infection 338, 342
acute liver failure 338, 350, 351
antenatal screening 342–3, 563
antiviral therapies 343, 351
blood transfusion screening 82
breast feeding 343
chronic active hepatitis 342, 353
chronic carriage (HBsAg positivity) 338, 342
risk factors 338
chronic persistent hepatitis 338, 352
cirrhosis 338, 342
core antigen (HBcAg) 339, 340, 343
e antigen (HbeAg) 339, 340, 341, 342
hepatitis D co-infection 347
high risk groups 343, 347
immunization 344, 563
administration schedules 344, 346
failures 346
health care personnel 345
maternal 344–5
neonatal 345–6
neonatal transmission prevention 343
immunoprophylaxis, passive (HBIG) 338, 340, 343–4, 345, 352
contacts of patient 352
neonatal 342, 343
incidence 338
liver transplantation 352
neonatal infection 270–1
acute neonatal hepatitis 341
carrier state prevention 271
chronic carrier state 340, 341
immune-complex-associated glomerulonephritis 342
maternal renal transplant 270–1
outcome 340
prevention 343
pre-term delivery 338
primary liver cancer 338, 342
renal transplant patients 266, 270–1
serological diagnosis 334, 338, 339
serological responses 338–9
serum HBsAg 339, 340, 342–3
chronic carriage 341
cord blood 340
serum viral DNA 339, 340, 342
sperm donor screening 342
transmission 338, 339–40, 341, 342
in early childhood 338
ethnic differences 339
horizontal 338, 340, 341, 342
vertical 338, 339–40, 343
vaccine-induced escape mutants 563
Hepatitis C 334, 337, 564
acute liver failure 350
antiviral therapies 337
chronic hepatitis/cirrhosis 337, 352
liver transplant reinfection 352
serological diagnosis 334, 337
transmission 337
neonatal 337
Hepatitis D 334
fulminant liver failure 351
immunoprophylaxis 347
liver transplant reinfection 352
serological diagnosis 334, 347
vertical transmission 347
Hepatitis E 333, 334, 335, 336–7, 564
acute liver failure 350
incubation period 336
management 337
severity in pregnancy 336–7
transmission 337
Hepatitis, chronic 352–9
active 353
obstetric outcome 353
cirrhosis 353–6
fertility 353
persistent 352–5
Hepatitis, viral 333–347, 554, 563
acute liver failure 350
antiviral agents 351
delivery 351
chronic active hepatitis 353
clinical features 333
differential diagnosis 333
fever 554
maternal/fetal outcome 334, 563
neonatal infection 563
screening contacts 352
serological diagnosis 333, 334, 350

Hepatitis, viral *Cont.*
severity in pregnancy 333–4
transmission 334
Hepatocellular carcinoma *see* Liver cancer, primary
Hepatoma *see* Liver cancer, primary
Heroin
breast feeding 603
neonatal withdrawal syndrome 601, 603
pregnancy outcome 602
Herpes hominis virus (HHV) 563
fetal/perinatal loss 563
renal transplant patient screening 263
TORCH (STORCH) infections 563
Herpes simplex virus (HSV) 554, 564
diagnosis 334, 348
erythema multiforme association 621
genital infection 391
delivery 271, 563
hepatitis 334, 347
HIV infection/AIDS 391
laboratory tests 555
maternal renal transplant 271
neonatal infection 271, 348
oral ulcers 391
primary infection 554
rectal/perianal ulcers 408–9
renal transplant patients 266
type II reactivation 348
Herpes viruses
hepatitis 333, 334, 347–8
neonatal infection 563
Heymann nephritis 253
Hiatus hernia 381
Hickman line 129, 157
Hidradenitis suppurativa 613
Hirsutism 614, 620
Histamine
gestational vomiting 384
lower oesophageal sphincter pressure (LOSP) 381
Histiocytosis X 492
Histoplasmosis 554
liver involvement in AIDS 349
HIV infection/AIDS 564, 568–91
antigenic variation 570
aphthous stomatitis 380, 391
asymptomatic phase 570
autoimmune thrombocytopenic purpura (AITP) 95–6
biliary tract disease 363
blood transfusion screening 82
breast feeding 589
CD4 lymphocyte count in monitoring 583, 585, 586, 588
CD4 lymphocyte infection 569
CD4 lymphocyte population reduction 570
CD4 lymphocyte pregnancy-associated reduction 575
cervical cytology/colposcopy 583–5
cervical neoplasia 585
classification of infections 571
counselling 571–4, 577
disease in pregnancy 583–5
assessment/screening 583, 585
disease progression monitoring 570–1
beta microglobulin marker 570, 585, 588
neopterin marker 571, 588
p24 antibody/antigenaemia marker 571, 585, 588
in drug abusers 600
dysphagia 391
effect of pregnancy 575–7
AIDS prognosis 576
disease progression 575, 576–7
immune changes 575–6
epidemiology 568–9
gender difference in disease progression 577
pregnant women 569, 575
surveillance 575
gastrointestinal tract malignancy 391–2
in health care workers 590
occupational transmission 590
hepatitis B immunization failure 346
heterosexual transmission 568, 572
infection control procedures 590
liver involvement 349
natural history 571
nosocomial transmission 589–90
obstetric management 587–9
antenatal care 587–8
delivery 583, 588
neonatal management 589
post-partum care 589
opportunistic infection 349, 576, 583
antenatal screening 583
Campylobacter diarrhoea 393
candidiasis 584
cryptococcosis 585
cytomegalovirus (CMV) 580, 583, 585
gastrointestinal infection 391–2, 394
hepatitis B 583
hepatitis C 337
intestinal parasites 395
listeriosis 393, 394
Pneumocystis carinii pneumonia 17, 576, 583, 584, 586
pneumonia 16, 17
prophylaxis 583
toxoplasmosis 561, 580, 583, 584–6
treatment 584, 585
tuberculosis 12, 14, 583, 584
typhoid fever 394
oral manifestations 391
platelet immune destruction 95–6
pregnancy outcome 580–2
birthweight 582, 588
congenital malformations 581
obstetric complications 581–2
spontaneous abortion 580–1
pre-term delivery 579, 580, 582, 588
prevalence in pregnancy 569, 575
retroviral prophylaxis 583, 586–7
intrapartum vaginal use 588
in pregnancy 585–7
risk factors 572, 574
target cells 569
termination of pregnancy 581, 583, 585, 587
testing 571–5
advantages 571
informed consent 572
post-test antibody negative counselling 572, 573
post-test antibody positive counselling 572, 573–4
pre-test counselling 571–2
screening policies 575
selective 572, 574–5
unlinked anonymous 575
vertical transmission 571, 575, 577–80, 588
breast feeding 577, 578, 604
caesarean section 579, 580, 583
fetal HIV antibody 578
fetal HLA genotype 579
information for patients 583, 588
intrapartum 577, 578, 588–9
invasive fetal procedures 579, 588
placental factors 579
preventive therapeutic strategies 579–80, 587
prognosis for infant 580
rate 580
risk factors 578–9
transplacental infection 577
virology 569–71
zidovudine 579, 586–7
vertical transmission prophylaxis 586–7
Hodgkin's disease 62–3, 553
effects of pregnancy 62
HIV infection, gastrointestinal tract involvement 393
treatment 62
long-term effects on offspring 63
Homocystinuria 521–2
cerebral venous thrombosis 540
clinical features 521
osteoporosis 521, 522
pregnancy outcome 521
pyridoxine therapy 118–19, 521, 522
recurrent thromboembolism 118–19, 129, 521
treatment 521
Hookworm 395
Hospital admission
chronic hypertension 240
chronic renal disease 238
diabetes mellitus 440, 446
pre-eclampsia 198, 199, 240
puerperal psychosis 635
HTLV-1 infection 564
Human chorionic gonadotrophin (HCG)
sporadic goitre stimulation 465
thyroid gland hypertrophy 461
TSH suppression 462
Human immunodeficiency virus *see* HIV infection/AIDS
Human papilloma virus (HPV) 409
Human parvovirus 558, 563
Human placental lactogen (HPL) 488

renal 1α-hydrolase activation 509, 510
Hycanthone 396
Hydatid liver disease 359
Hydatiform mole
adult respiratory distress syndrome (ARDS) 20
disseminated intravascular coagulation (DIC) 78
hyperthyroidism 461
liver metastases 360
pemphigoid (herpes) gestationis 614, 615
pre-eclampsia 194, 198
renal transplant patients 264
thyrotoxicosis 469
Hydralazine 153, 159
adrenergic blocking agent combined treatment 200
fetal monitoring/fetal distress 200, 201
hypertension-associated hepatic disorders 331
methyldopa combined treatment 200, 202
noradrenaline release stimulation 199, 200
pre-eclamptic hypertension 199–200
side effects 199
Hydrocephalus, maternal shunt-treated 545
Hydrocortisone 91, 94
Addison's disease 495
congenital adrenal hyperplasia
labour management 498
treatment in utero 496
cover for labour
bronchial asthma 11
renal transplant patients 268
systemic lupus erythematosus (SLE) 311
prolactin-secreting pituitary tumour 487
pruritic folliculitis of pregnancy 619
replacement therapy
adrenal cortical tumour surgery 491
anterior pituitary deficiency 493
safety in pregnancy 498
Hydronephrosis
acute 260
acute renal failure 276
normal pregnancy 227
Hydrops fetalis 198
Hydroquinone 611
Hydroureter 260
Hydroxychloroquine 307
25-Hydroxycholcalciferol (25-OHD) 507
fetal/maternal levels 512
osteomalacia 514
plasma level in pregnancy 512
renal metabolism 507
serum level 507
11-Hydroxylase deficiency 496
17-Hydroxylase deficiency 496
21-Hydroxylase deficiency 496, 497
Hydroxyproline plasma/urine levels
bone matrix metabolic destruction 509
osteomalacia 514
3β-Hydroxysteroid dehydrogenase deficiency 496
17-Hydroxysteroids 211
5-Hydroxytryptamine
gestational vomiting 384
lower oesophageal sphincter pressure (LOSP) 381
Hydroxyurea 621
Hymenolepsis nana see Dwarf tapeworm
Hyoscine
fetal adverse effects 401
irritable bowel syndrome 408
Hyperalimentation *see* total parenteral nutrition
Hyperbaric oxygen 284
Hyperbilirubinaemia 322–3
congenital disorders 358
intrahepatic cholestasis of pregnancy (IHCP) 332
Hypercholesterolaemia 322
Hypercoagulable state
antithrombin III (ATIII) activity 75
cerebral ischaemia/stroke 539
cerebral venous thrombosis 540
chronic glomerulonephritis 245
paroxysmal nocturnal haemoglobinuria (PNH) 60
polycythaemia rubra vera (PRV) 59
protein C/protein S deficiency 75
thrombocythaemia *see* Thrombocythaemia
Hyperemesis gravidarum 383
acute renal failure 279
anti-emetic drug therapy 385
fetal damage 632
complications 385
fetal outcome 386–7
hepatic dysfunction 323
management 385
mechanism 384
risk factors 383
thyrotoxicosis 469
total parenteral nutrition 385
Hyperglycaemia 123
Cushing's syndrome 491
fetal acid-base balance 432
fetal limits 427
Hyperglycinaemia 524
Hyperoxaluria
primary, prenatal diagnosis 251
resective surgery for IBD 402
Hyperparathyroidism
hypercalciuria 509
hypophosphataemia/hyperphosphaturia 509
metabolic acidosis 509
physiological in pregnancy 510
primary 518
bone disease 518
hypercalcaemial crisis in pregnancy 518
medical management 518
neonatal hypocalcaemia 518
pancreatitis 364, 518
pregnancy outcome 518
surgery 518
secondary
chronic renal disease 517
type I rickets/osteomalacia 513
tertiary 267
Hyperpigmentation 610
pathogenesis 611
Hyperprolactinaemia 483–7
drug-induced 483
see also Prolactin-secreting pituitary tumour
Hypertension in pregnancy 182–213
abruptio placentae 209
acromegaly 488
acute episode management 241
acute porphyria 526
adrenal cortical tumour 491
asymptomatic bacteriuria association 256
chronic glomerulonephritis 245
chronic renal disease 233, 235, 237, 240, 254
antenatal monitoring 238
connective tissue disease 247, 248
elective delivery 241
polycystic kidney disease (PKD) 250
reflux nephropathy 249
rodent models 253
specific renal diseases 246
superimposed pre-eclampsia 240
treatment 240
coarctation of aorta 211
cocaine abuse 605, 606
congenital adrenal hyperplasia 498
Conn's syndrome 212
Cushing's syndrome 211–12, 491
definitions 183, 185–7
diabetes mellitus 248, 446
diabetic nephropathy 444–5
encephalopathy 192, 193
eclamptic 542, 543
essential 187
haemodialysis patients 276
haemolytic uraemic syndrome (HUS) 285
heart failure risk with heart disease 152
hepatic disorders *see* hypertension–associated hepatic disorders
hospital admission 241
long-term sequelae 212
lupus anticoagulant/cardiolipin antibodies 309
oral contraceptive use 212
patient characteristics 208
perinatal outcome 208, 209
phaeochromocytoma 211
plasma urate 197
post-partum 208
pre-eclampsia see Pre-eclampsia
pseudoxanthoma elasticum 522
renal transplant patients 273
third trimester 266–8

Hypertension in pregnancy *Cont.*
superimposed pre-eclampsia 187, 209, 210, 212, 266
prevention/treatment 240–1
signs 209
systemic lupus erythematosus (SLE) 307–8, 312
third trimester presentation 209, 266–8
treatment 209–10
angiotensin-converting enzyme (ACE) inhibitors 210
antihypertensive drugs 209, 210, 211, 240
beta adrenergic blocking agents 210
diuretics 210, 241
see also pre-eclampsia
Hypertension-associated hepatic disorders 323–31
acute fatty liver of pregnancy 326–31
clinical features 323
differential diagnosis 323
HELLP syndrome 324–5
hepatic rupture/infarction 325–6
management 330–1
early delivery 331
neonatal problems 330
post-partum problems 331
pre-eclampsia 191–2, 201, 323–4
Hyperthyroidism
hydatiform mole/choriocarcinoma association 461
incidence 459
osteomalacia 514
physiological in neonate 462
post-partum 474
supraventricular tachycardia 154
thyroid stimulating hormone (TSH) levels 460
see also Thyrotoxicosis
Hypertrichosis 614
Hypertrophic obstructive cardiomyopathy 164–5
diagnosis 164
epidural anaesthesia contraindication 158
familial form 164
labour 164–5
management 164–5
pathological features 164
syncope 148
Hypertyrosinaemia 524
Hyperventilation
acute asthma attack 7
altitude effects 2
cystic fibrosis 18
progesterone effects 3
Hypervolaemia, physiological 233
Hyperxanthinuria 524
Hypoalbuminaemia
neonatal 330
pre-eclampsia 190
septic shock 282
Hypocalcaemia
hypoparathyroidism 519
neonatal
maternal Crohn's disease 516
maternal diabetes mellitus 435
maternal hyperparathroidism 518
maternal osteomalacia 514–15
maternal renal transplant 270
pseudohypoparathyroidism 519
septicaemia with acute renal failure 282
Hypofibrinogenaemia, hereditary 107
Hypoglycaemia 123
acute fatty liver of pregnancy 327, 330
acute liver failure 351, 352
differential diagnosis 493
hypertension-associated hepatic disorders 330, 331
post-partum 331
neonatal
maternal diabetes mellitus 423, 434
maternal renal transplant 270
Hypoparathyroidism 519
Hypopituitarism 492–3
hormone replacement therapy 493
indices of pituitary function in pregnancy 493
lymphocytic hypophysitis 544
post-partum haemorrhage 492
pregnancy outcome 493
provocative tests 492
Hypotension
acute renal failure 278
postural 35
Hypothyroidism 466–8
anovulation/amenorrhoea 466
body temperature reduction 552
breast feeding 468
clinical features 466, 467
congenital malformations 466
constipation 407
fetal 468
cretinism 465
treatment *in utero* 468
hyperprolactinaemia 483
incidence 459, 466
maternal antithyroid drug treatment 463
neonatal
maternal thyrotoxicosis 470, 471
screening 468
thyroid function tests 468
post-partum 474
pre-eclampsia 467
pregnancy outcome 466
Sheehan's syndrome 492
thyroid function tests 467
thyroid hormone replacement therapy 466, 467–8
dosage monitoring 468
thyroid stimulating hormone (TSH) levels 460
TSH immunoradiometric assay (IRMA) 462
Hysterectomy, abdominal 284

Ibuprofen 312
Idoxuridine 621
IgA nephropathy 242, 245, 246, 254
hereditary transmission 246
HLA Bw35 association 246
impact of pregnancy 235
Ileal conduit 250
Ileal pouch–anal anastomosis 403
Ileostomy
inflammatory bowel disease (IBD) 399, 402–3
pregnancy outcome 403
intestinal obstruction 404
Ileus, postoperative 405
Iliac vein surgical interruption 129
Imipramine
antenatal depression 627
muscle contraction headache 546
neonatal side effects 627
Immune thrombocytopenic purpura (ITP) 58
Immunodeficiency
aphthous stomatitis 380
intestinal parasite infestation 395
listeriosis 393, 394
pneumonia 16
Immunoglobulin immunoprophylaxis
hepatitis A 336, 343
contacts of patient 352
hepatitis B 343–5
hepatitis D 347
HIV vertical transmission prevention 579
safety 344
Immunoglobulin infusion
autoimmune thrombocytopenic purpura (AITP) 91, 92, 95
fetal alloimmune thrombocytopenia (AIT) 97
Guillain–Barré syndrome 547
neonatal thrombocytopenia 94
systemic lupus erythematosus (SLE) 312
transplacental effect 92
Immunoglobulin serum levels 322
Immunosuppressive therapy
autoimmune conditions 58
autoimmune thrombocytopenic purpura (AITP) 93
factor VIII antibody 100
haemolytic uraemic syndrome (HUS) 285
heart transplantation 171
puerperal (peripartum/pregnancy) cardiomyopathy 165
renal transplant patients 261, 267
breast feeding 272
neonatal problems 270
rheumatoid arthritis 314
systemic lupus erythematosus (SLE) 96, 311
Impetigo herpetiformis 620
Incompatible blood transfusion 270
Indomethacin
breast feeding 314
rheumatoid arthritis 314
safety in pregnancy 311
Induced labour
Eisenmenger's syndrome 167

heart disease 157
Infection
acute renal failure 278
fever 553, 554
heart failute risk with heart disease 152
non-specific bacterial 553, 554, 556–7, 558–62
Infectious disease 552–65
bacterial 555
epidemic 554
fever 552–6
diagnosis/laboratory test 555–6
fungal 554, 555
viral infections 554, 562–3, 564–5
Inferior vena cava surgical interruption 129
Inflammatory bowel disease (IBD) 403
active disease at conception 398–9
anorectal/perineal disorders 408
aphthous stomatitis 380
colonic carcinoma 409, 410
colostomy 339, 402–3
effects of pregnancy 339
effects on pregnancy 398, 400
emergency surgery 402–3
delivery 402
maternal/fetal outcome 402
fertility 397–8, 399–400
drug therapy 398
following surgery 399, 400
fetal outcome 398, 400
haematuria 260
ileal pouch/anal anastomoisis 403
ileostomy 399, 402–3
incidence 397
intestinal obstruction 403, 404
investigations 379
liver involvement 358–9
monitoring 380
nutritional status assessment 403
pregnancy management 400–3
acute severe disease 400
chronic disease 401–2
drug therapies 400–1
total parenteral nutrition 401
presentation in pregnancy/puerperium 399
spontaneous abortion 398, 400
total parenteral nutrition 402, 405
vitamin D/calcium malabsorption 516
Inflammatory skin disease 621
Influenza 554, 563, 564
fetal/perinatal loss 563
fever 554
pneumonia 16, 17
Insulin
fetal levels 427
maternal glucose homeostasis 425
Insulin resistance
glucose homeostasis abnormalities 425, 426
pregnancy-induced 425
Insulin therapy
combined dietary restrictive regimes 442–3
continuous subcutaneous insulin infusion (CSII) 441
gestational diabetes mellitus (GDM) 441
gestational impaired glucose tolerance (GIGT) 441
labour management 443
maximum tolerated dose method 441
postnatal 443
tocolytic drugs/steroid therapy for diabetic pre-term labour 448
type 1 insulin dependent diabetes mellitus (IDDM) 440–1
Insulin-glucagon infusion 351
Insulinoma, pancreatic 365
Interferon therapy
hepatitis B 343
hepatitis C 338
leukaemia 62
thrombocythaemia 59
viral hepatitis with acute liver failure 351
Intermittent porphyria, acute (AIP) 526
Interstitial fluid 233
Intertrigo 613
Intestinal obstruction 404
differential diagnosis 404
incidence 404
inflammatory bowel disease (IBD) 403
management 404, 405
persistent vomiting 384
Intestinal parasite infestation 395–7
congenital/neonatal infection 395
effects of pregnancy 395
fetal outcome 395
incidence 395
treatment 395
Intracranial haemorrhage 123
factor XIII (fibrin stabilizing factor) deficiency 108
fetal alloimmune thrombocytopenia (AIT) 96, 97
fetal thrombocytopenia 94
maternal renal transplant 268
Intracranial hypertension, benign *see* Pseudotumour cerebri
Intracranial pressure, raised
cerebral venous thrombosis 540
persistent vomiting 384
pituitary tumour 486, 488
Intragastric pressure 381
Intrahepatic cholestasis of pregnancy (IhCP) 331–3
clinical features 331
fetal distress/fetal outcome 332–3
gallstones 332
genetic predisposition 332
incidence 331
jaundice 331–2, 333
management 332–3
oral contraceptives 332, 333
pre-term labour 332–3
pruritus 331, 332
recurrence 333
Intrapartum lumbosacral plexopathy 547
Intrauterine contraceptive device (IUCD) 560
diabetes mellitus 451
renal transplant patients 271
Intrauterine growth retardation
acromegaly 488
acute pyelonephritis 258
Addison's disease 495
alcohol abuse 604
antidysrhythmic drugs 154
bronchial asthma 6–7
bronchiectasis 19
chronic renal disease 241
coarctation of aorta 147
cocaine abuse 605
cyanotic congenital heart disease 147
diabetes mellitus 445, 446
ultrasound 447
diabetic nephropathy 445
heart disease, fetal monitoring 152
HELLP syndrome 325
HIV infection 582, 588
hyperemesis gravidarum 386
intestinal parasite infestation 395
phenylketonuria 523, 524
placental pathology 194
platelet count 73
pre-eclampsia 190
reflux nephropathy 249
renal transplant patients 269, 273
systemic lupus erythematosus (SLE) 312
tetralogy of Fallot 147
thyrotoxicosis 473
zinc deficiency 41
Intravenous urography (IVU)
asymptomatic bacteriuria 258
renal transplant patients 269
urolithiasis 249
Iodine
secretion in breast milk 11
thyroid storage 460
thyroid uptake/metabolism 459
effect of pregnancy 461
transplacental passage 463
Iodine administration
neonatal thyrotoxicosis 474
neurological cretinism 465
pre-pregnancy treatment 465
prophylactic 459, 461
Iodine deficiency
cretinism 459, 465
endemic goitre 459, 463
fetal/neonatal hypothyroidism 465
sporadic goitre 465–6
Iodine-containing cough medicine 7, 16, 463
Iodized salt 461, 465, 466
Ipratropium bromide 10
Ipsalazide 401
Iron deficiency
anaemia 36, 41–2
colorectal carcinoma 409
developing countries 40, 41
geophagia 380
management 39
pre-term birth association 37

Iron deficiency *Cont.*
prevention 36
aphthous stomatitis 380
coeliac disease 388, 390
ferritin 38, 41
free erythrocyte protoporphyrin (FEP) 38
haemoglobin concentration 37
marrow iron 38–9
multigravidae 40
non-haematological effects 36–7
adult hypertension 37
CNS abnormalities 36–7
mitochondrial function 36
temperature maintenance 36
prevention *see* Iron supplements
red cell indices 37
serum iron 37–8
storage iron status 41
total iron binding capacity (TIBC) 37–8
total parenteral nutrition 405
Iron dextran 39
Iron metabolism 35
absorption 35, 36, 41
haem iron 36
dietary source availability 35, 36, 41
total iron requirement 35
transport to fetus 35
Iron serum levels 37–8
Iron sorbitol citrate 39
Iron status assessment 35
Iron supplements
anaemia prevention 36, 39, 40–2
chelating agent interactions 356
ferritin 38
folic acid combinations 39, 45
anticonvulsants interactions 45
Gaucher's disease 524
inflammatory bowel disease 401
intestinal parasite infestation 395
intramuscular 39
iron absorption 36
paroxysmal nocturnal haemoglobinuria (PNH) 60
red cell mass increase 34
serum iron 38
side effects 39
α thalassaemia 48
β thalassaemia minor 50
zinc bioavailability 41
Iron, dietary 35, 36
Irritable bowel syndrome 407–8
Ischaemic heart disease 148
dysrhythmias 154
Isoniazid
fetal abnormalities 13
pyridoxine supplements 13, 584
tuberculosis
HIV infection 584
treatment of neonate 14
Isoprenaline
bronchial asthma 8–9
disodium cromoglycate combination 10
septic shock 284
side effects 8
Isospora 391
Isotretinoin 621
Isoxsuprine 159
Ispaghula 407

Jaundice
congenital bilirubin metabolism disorders 358
hepatitis A 335
intrahepatic cholestasis of pregnancy (IHCP) 331, 332, 333
malaria 562
maternal diabetes mellitus 423, 435
maternal opiate addiction 601
neonatal hypothyroidism 465
pancreatitis 365
pre-eclampsia 191
septicaemia with acute renal failure 282
viral hepatitis 333
Jejunal biopsy 390
Jejuno-ileal bypass 405–6
vitamin D deficiency 516
Jugular venous pressure 149

Kanamycin 259
Kaolin cephalin clotting time 124
Kaolin preparations 392
Kaposi's sarcoma
dysphagia 391
gastrointestinal tract involvement 393
HIV infection/AIDS 391, 393
Kawasaki's disease 163
Kernicterus 323
Ketoconazole 584
17-Ketosteroids 211
Kidney 227–33
normal anatomical changes 227
overdistension syndrome 227
size 227
Klebsiella
pneumonia 16
septic abortion 284, 560
urinary tract infection 255, 558
Korotkoff sounds 184, 185, 186–7
Korsakow's psychosis 385, 405
^{81m}kryptom lung scan 121
Kwashiorkor 323
Kyphoscoliosis 20

Labetalol
post-partum hypertension 208
pre-eclampsia 199, 200, 202, 210
general anaesthesia management 207
Labour
cardiac output 144
gastric aspiration prevention 22
guidelines 23
heart disease 157–8
antibiotic prophylaxis 150, 158–9
third stage 158
Lactation suppression 118
Lactic acid dehydrogenase (LDH)
HELLP syndrome 324
hepatic rupture/infarction 325
serum level 321–2
Lactobacillus acidophilus 381
Lactose intolerance 407
Lactulose 354
constipation management 407
inflammatory bowel disease 402
safety in pregnancy 407
Large bowel malignancy 409
Laryngeal oedema 190, 207, 241
Laryngeal papillomata, neonatal 409
Laryngoscopy 207
Late onset prurigo of pregnancy *see* Polymorphic eruption of pregnancy
Laxatives
constipation management 402, 407
intestinal parasite purgation 395
self-medication 379
Left atrial myxoma 161
Left atrial pressure measurement 144
Leg purpura 613
Leg varices 612, 613
Legionella pneumophilia pneumonia 16, 17
Leprosy 620
Leucopenia, neonatal
maternal renal transplant 270, 274
neonatal lupus syndrome 308
Leucoplakia 260
Leukaemia 61–2
Levamisole 401
LH secreting pituitary tumour 483
Light reflective rheography 120
Lignocaine 548
Lincomycin 392
Lipase, serum level 363
Lipid nephrosis 252
Liquid crystal thermography 119
Liquid paraffin 407
Listeria monocytoneges 560
infective endocarditis 560
listeriosis *see* Listeriosis
renal transplant patients 266
susceptibility with SLE/steroid therapy 312
Listeriosis 393–4, 560–1
adult respiratory distress syndrome (ARDS) 560
antibiotic therapy 560
clinical features 560
diagnosis 394, 555, 560
fever 553, 560
management 394, 560
neonatal infection 560
preventive dietary advice 394, 561
transmission 560
Lithium 171
breast feeding contraindication 626, 633
fetal damage 625, 631
manic depressive psychosis 631, 632
late pregnancy management 632–3
puerperal psychosis prophylaxis 635

schizoaffective disorders 634
Lithotripsy 363
Liver biopsy, percutaneous 322
acute fatty liver of pregnancy 330
AIDS opportunistic infection 349
Budd–Chiari syndrome 357
chronic hepatitis 352
cirrhosis with gastrointestinal haemorrhage 355
cytomegalovirus (CMV) infection 349
intrahepatic cholestasis of pregnancy (IHCP) 332
pruritus gravidarum (cholestasis of pregnancy) 611
Liver cancer, primary 359–60
cirrhosis 360
differential diagnosis 360
hepatitis B 338, 342
hepatitis C 337
oral contraceptives association 360
prognosis 360
Liver disease 323–61
antithromboin III (ATIII) activity 75
cholesterol lithiasis 362
hyperprolactinaemia 483
incidental to pregnancy 333–61
laboratory tests 555
peculiar to pregnancy 323–33
hypertension-associated *see* Hypertension-associated hepatic disorders
vitamin D malabsorption 517
Liver failure, acute 349, 350
clinical features 349
delivery 351
differential diagnosis 350
fetal outcome 352
haematological features 349
liver transplantation 349, 350, 352
management 350–2
microbial infection 351
obstetric outcome 350
persistent vomiting 384
prognosic indicators 351
renal function impairment/monitoring 351
Liver failure, fulminant (FHF) 349
Liver failure, late onset (subacute hepatic necrosis) 349
Liver function tests 321, 322
acute renal failure 279
pre-eclampsia 191, 195
renal transplant patients 266
Liver metabolism 321–2
drug/toxins clearance 321
Liver position, third trimester 322
Liver transplantation 325, 331
acute liver failure 350, 352
Budd–Chiari syndrome 358
pregnancy/contraception counselling 352
viral hepatitis 352
Wilson's disease 357
Liver tumours 359–61
oral contraceptive steroids 359
Lofepramine 627, 637, 638
Logiparin 125
Long QT syndrome 154
Long-acting thyroid stimulator (LATS) 473
Low molecular weight heparins 131, 540
bone demineralization 132
prophylactic use 131, 132
thromboembolism management 125
Lower oesophageal sphincter pressure (LOSP) 381
drug effects 382
gastro-oesophageal reflux 381
Lown–Ganong–Levine syndrome 154, 160
Lumbosacral plexopathy, intrapartum 547
Lung cancer 22
Lung compliance 4
Lung scan 121
Lupus anticoagulant 132
Budd–Chiari syndrome 357–8
cerebral ischaemia/stroke 539
cerebral venous thrombosis 540
fetal risk association in SLE 309, 310, 311
hypertension association 310
recurrent fetal loss assocation 96
thromboembolism association 96, 118, 129, 131, 309, 311
Lupus nephropathy 247, 307–8
impact of pregnancy 325
nephrotic syndrome 252
renal biopsy 239
Lyme disease 546
Lymphocytic choriomeningitis 564
Lymphocytic hypophysitis 544
Lysergic acid diethylamide (LSD) 606

Macrosomia
acromegaly 488
Cushing's syndrome 491
maternal diabetes mellitus 423, 433–4
vaginal delivery 434
Magnesium hydroxide 382
constipation management 407
inflammatory bowel disease 402
Magnesium sulphate
calcium channel blocker interaction 200
contraindication with myasthenia gravis 548
eclampsia prevention/treatment 203–4, 543
intraperitoneal administration 276
side effects 204
Magnesium trisilicate 22, 382
Magnesium-containing antacids 382
Magnetic resonance imaging (MRI)
acute fatty liver of pregnancy 330
adrenal cortical tumour 490
Campylobacter neonatal infection 393
cerebral venous thrombosis 540
eclamptic cerebral pathology 192, 542
gastrointestinal tract disorders 379
hepatic rupture/infarction 325
hypopituitarism/Sheehan's syndrome 493
pituitary tumours 484
bromocriptine therapy monitoring 485
tumour-related symptoms in pregnancy 486
pseudotumour cerebri 545
spinal examination 536
toxoplasmosis encephalitis 584
Malaria 562
cold sores 553
fever 553
Plasmodium falciparum 562
post-partum placental examination 562
prophylaxis/treatment 562
neonatal antimalarial therapy 562
prior to delivery 395
quinine-induced hypoglycaemia 493
Male pattern hair loss 614
Malformation, congenital
antipsychotic medication 631–2
cocaine abuse 605
cytotoxic drug therapy 61, 62
diabetes mellitus 423, 429–30, 446
poor diabetic control association 429
epilepsy 537–8
folate deficiency 44
immunosuppressive drugs/renal transplant patients 270
lithium teratogenesis 631
maternal viral infection 562–3
opiates addiction 601
radiation exposure, diagnostic 535–6
thyroid disease 466, 469
Wilson's disease 357
Malignant disease
renal transplant patients 272
thromboembolism risk 118
Mallory–Weiss oesophageal tear 385
Maloprim 562
Manic depressive psychosis 631–3
acute episodes 633
genetic aspects 631
post-partum relapse 631, 635
prophylactic treatment 631–633
Mannitol
acute liver failure 351
eclamptic hypertensive encephalopathy 543
oliguria differential diagnosis 280
prerenal failure (vasomotor nephropathy) 280
Marfan's syndrome 520
antihypertensive treatment 170
aortic dissection 170
Bentall composite graft surgery 170
cardiological aspects 170
formes frustes 170
molecular aspects 170, 521
prenatal diagnosis 170, 521

Marfan's syndrome *Cont.*
uterine inversion, spontaneous 170, 521
valve replacement surgery 152
Massive gut resection 405
Mastitis 553, 614
puerperal pyrexia 559
May–Heggelin anomaly 101
MCH
iron status 37
α thalassaemia 48
β thalassaemia minor 50
MCHC
iron status 37
α thalassaemia 48
β thalassaemia minor 50
MCV
iron status 37
α thalassaemia 48
β thalassaemia minor 50
Measles 554, 563, 564
fetal/perinatal loss 563
fever 555
Measles/mumps/rubella (MMR) vaccine 563
Mebendazole 395
Mebeverine 408
Mechanical contraceptive methods 451
Meclozine 385, 386
Megakaryocytic aplasia, hereditary 101
Megaloblastic anaemia 43–5
coeliac disease 388, 389
folate deficiency 43–5
incidence 44
neonate/pre-term infant 46
puerperium 45
thrombocytopenia 89
vitamin B_{12} deficiency 46
Melanocyte stimulating hormone (MSH) 611
Melanoma, malignant 621
Melasma 610–11
Mendelson's syndrome 382
hyperemesis gravidarum 385
Meningococcal septicaemia 553
Meningoencephalitis, viral 555
Mental retardation
cretinism 465
fetal alcohol syndrome 604
maternal hyperglycinaemia 524
phenylketonuria 523
Meralgia paraesthetica 547
6-Mercaptopurine
Crohn's disease 401
reproductive performance effects 272
Mesalazine 401
Metabolic acidosis
acute fatty liver of pregnancy 327
beta-sympathomimetic drug-associated 9
diabetes mellitus fetal effects 432
hyperparathyroidism 509
septic shock 282
Metabolic bone disease 513–20
pre-pregnancy counselling 513
Metastatic malignancy
adult respiratory distress syndrome 20
portal hypertension 356
Methadone
breast feeding 603
fetal cardiorespiratory control 602
neonatal withdrawal syndrome 602
pregnancy outcome 602–3
Methimazole
breast milk levels 471
fetal thyroid function 470
neonatal scalp defects 470
thyroid crisis (thyroid storm) 472
thyrotoxicosis 469, 474
Methotrexate
impetigo herpetiformis 620
teratogenicity 61, 621
Methoxamine 168
Methyl cellulose 407
Methyldopa 159
chronic active hepatitis 353
chronic hypertension in pregnancy (CHT) 210, 212
hyperprolactinaemia 483
post-partum hypertension 208
pre-eclampsia 201–2, 212
hydralazine combined treatment 200, 202
Metoclopramide 382, 383, 386
gastric aspiration prevention in labour 23
hormonal side effects 386
hyperemesis gravidarum 385
mode of action 386
safety in pregnancy 385, 386
Metrizamide 133
Metronidazole
amoebiasis 396
liver abscess 359
giardiasis 397
inflammatory bowel disease (IBD) 401
renal transplant patients, labour management 268
safety in pregnancy 396, 401, 621
septic abortion 284, 560
Metyrapone
adrenal cortical tumour 491
hypopituitarism/Sheehan's syndrome investigation 492, 493
Mexiletine 154
Miconazole 620
Microcephaly
phenylketonuria 523, 524
warfarin teratogenesis 127
Micrococcus sp. 558
Middle cerebral artery migraine 546
Midstream urine specimen (MSU) 254, 258, 261
acute renal failure 279
renal transplant patients 263
Migraine, classic 546
Milia 613
Mineral oil lubricants 407
Minimal change nephrotic syndrome (MCNS) 246
Minute ventilation 5
Misoprostol 382
Mitotane 491
Mitral regurgitation 161
endocarditis 161
incidence 145
systolic murmur 149
Mitral stenosis 160, 161
incidence 145
labour 153, 157, 158, 161
pulmonary oedema 153, 161
surgery 151, 161
fetal outcome 151
symptoms in pregnancy 148
Mitral valve disease 127, 161
cardiac output 144
congenital in pregnancy 145
cordae tendinae rupture 161
digoxin 153
left atrial pressure following delivery 144
Mitral valve prolapse
cerebral ischaemia/stroke 539
congenital in pregnancy 150
pseudoxanthoma elasticum 522
systolic murmur 149
Mitral valve replacement 162
Mitral valvotomy 151
Mitral valvuloplasty 151
Molluscum fibrosum gravidarum 613
Monoiodotyrosine (MIT) 459, 460
Montgomery's tubercles 613
Morphine 153
intrathecal 169
neonatal withdrawal syndrome 601
Mortality, maternal
acute fatty liver of pregnancy 326
acute pancreatitis 363
acute renal failure 278
AIDS 569, 576
aortic stenosis 161
bleeding oesophageal varices 354
brain tumours 543
cerebrovascular disease 539, 541
coarctation of aorta 169, 211
eclampsia/pre-eclampsia 189, 191, 192, 542
Eisenmenger's syndrome 167
endocarditis 158, 159
fever of infectious origin 553
heart disease 143, 145–6
hepatic adenoma rupture 359
myocardial infarction 163
phaeochromocytoma 211
puerperal (peripartum/pregnancy) cardiomyopathy 165, 166
pulmonary embolus 116
pulmonary vascular disease 169
renal transplant patients 262, 263, 271
subarachnoid haemorrhage 541
systemic lupus erythematosus (SLE) 307
Motilin
lower oesophageal sphincter pressure (LOSP) 381
small bowel transit time 406
Moya moya disease 539
Multiple pregnancy
acute fatty liver of pregnancy 327
blood loss at delivery 34
cardiac output 152

folic acid 42, 44
heart failure risk with heart disease 152
heart transplant patient 171
intestinal obstruction 404
leprosy 620
maternal opiates addiction 601
plasma volume 34, 190
pre-eclampsia 198
puerperal (peripartum/pregnancy) cardiomyopathy 165
red cell mass 34
retained dead fetus with living twin 87
vitamin B_{12} 46
Multiple sclerosis 545–6
effect of pregnancy 545
post-partum exacerbation 545
Mumps 554, 563, 564
fetal/perinatal loss 563
fever 555
pancreatitis 364
Muscle contraction headache 546
Mushroom poisoning 350
Myasthenia gravis 547–8
myasthenic crisis 548
neonatal 548
obstetric analgesia/anaesthesia 548
post-partum exacerbation 548
Mycobacterium avium intracellulare 391
Mycoplasma infection
laboratory tests 555
pneumonia 16, 17
puerperal sepsis/wound infection 559
Mycotic aneurysm
hepatic rupture/infarction 325
intravenous drug abusers 600
Myelography, lumbar 536
Myocardial infarction 122, 163–4
causes 163
cocaine abuse 605
delivery 164
diagnosis 163–4
incidence 163
left atrial pressure measurement 144
left ventricular aneurysm 163
management 164
mortality 163
with normal coronary arteries 163
pre-eclampsia 163
Myotonic muscular dystrophy 548
Myxoviruses 563

N-acetyl cysteine 350
Nail changes 614
Nalorphine 603
Naloxone 603
Nausea *see* Vomiting/nausea
Necator americanus see Hookworm
Necrotizing enterocolitis 435
Neonatal *Campylobacter* meningitis 392, 393
Neonatal lupus syndrome 307, 308–9
Neonatal respiratory distress syndrome
alcohol abuse 604
cocaine abuse 605
diabetes mellitus 434
maternal renal transplant 274
Nephrectomy
pregnancy following 243, 252
unilateral, animal models 252–3
Nephritis, hereditary 246–7, 250
nephrotic syndrome 252
Nephroblastoma (Wilms' tumour) 252
Nephronophthisis 250
Nephrotic syndrome 252
causes 252
diabetes mellitus 248
Finnish congenital, prenatal diagnosis 251
pre-eclampsia 189, 252
renal biopsy 239
steroid therapy 239
Neural tube defects
diabetes mellitus 429, 446
folate deficiency 46
folate supplements in prevention 390
hydrocephalus, maternal shunt-treated 545
maternal epilepsy 537
prenatal diagnosis 537
valproic acid 538
zinc deficiency 390
Neurofibromatosis (von Recklinghausen's disease) 621
Neurological disorders 535–49
acute porphyria 526
coeliac disease 388
diagnostic tests 535–6
hyperemesis gravidarum 385
Neuropathy 546–7
Neuroradiological examination 535
Nevirapine 579
Niclosamide 395
Nifedipine
magnesium sulphate interaction 200
post-partum hypertension 208
pre-eclamptic hypertension 200–1, 202
side effects 200
Nimodipine 201
Nipple eczema 614
Nipple soreness/fissures 614
Niridazole 396
Nitrates
cirrhosis with oesophageal varices 355
pulmonary oedema management 153
Nitric oxide (NO) *see* Endothelial derived relaxing factor (EDRF)
Nitrofurantion
asymptomatic bacteriuria 257
neonatal hemolytic anaemia 257
urinary tract infection (UTI) 558
Nitroglycerine 164
endolaryngeal intubation pressor response attenuation 200
pre-eclampsia 199, 200
general anaesthesia management 207
Nitroprusside 168
NO synthase 230
Nocardiosis pneumonia 17
Non-steroidal anti-inflammatory drugs
acute liver failure 350
rheumatoid arthritis 314
systemic lupus erythematosus (SLE) 311, 312
breast feeding 311
Noradrenaline 168
lower oesophageal sphincter pressure (LOSP) 381
renal vascular responses 230
Norfloxacin 558
Norwalk-like virus gastroenteritis 391, 397
Nulacin 382
Nutritional status assessment 403
Nystatin 584, 620

Obesity
blood pressure measurement errors 184
heart failure risk with heart disease 152
pseudotumour cerebri 545
thromboembolism risk 118, 129
type 2 diabetes mellitus (NIDDM) development 444
Obsessional ruminations 629–30
treatment 630
Occulocerebrorenal syndrome of Lowe 251
Oedema 149, 612
diabetes mellitus 248
heart disease 149
nephrotic syndrome 252
physiologic/volume homeostasis 197, 241
pre-eclampsia 190, 195, 241
diagnostic value 197
management 204–5
Oesophageal disorders, *see also* Gastro-oesophageal disorders
Oesophageal malignancy 390
Oesophageal rupture 21
Oesophageal varices, bleeding
cirrhosis 354
delivery 355
management 355–6
endoscopic sclerotherapy 355–6
portal pressure reduction 355
maternal mortality 354
Oesophageal varices, transient 321, 354
Oesophagitis 381–2
antacids 382
upper endoscopy 388
Oesophagogastroduodenoscopy *see* Upper endoscopy
Oestrogen
arteriovenous shunt dilatation 541
bile acid/bile salt metabolism 362, 612
brain tumour enlargement 484, 543
gallbladder disease 361
gestational vomiting/hyperemesis gravidarum 384
haemodynamic effects 144
lower oesophageal sphincter pressure (LOSP) 381

Oestrogen *Cont.*
peptic ulcer healing 387
pigmentation changes 611
pituitary tumour enlargement 484
renal 1α-hydrolase activation 510
T_4 binding globulin (TBG) stimulation 461, 462
urinary tract effects 558
Oestrogen therapy
postnatal depression 637–8
suppression of lactation 118
thromboembolism risk 118, 638
Ogilvie's syndrome *see* Colonic pseudo-obstruction
Oliguria 279
differential diagnosis 278
Olsalazine 401
Omeprazole 382
Ondansetron 386
Open heart surgery 151
congenital heart disease 151, 152
perinatal mortality 151
Opiates
bronchial asthma 11
lower oesophageal sphincter pressure (LOSP) 381
pulmonary oedema management 153
Opiates addiction 600–4
drug interactions 603
effects on children 602
multiple pregnancy 601
neonatal withrawal syndrome 601–2
pregnancy management 602–4
analgesia for labour 603
methadone maintenance programme 602–3
opiate overdose management 603
pregnancy outcome 600–1
sudden infant death syndrome (SIDS) 602
Optic atrophy 155, 156
Oral cavity disorders 380–81
coeliac disease 389
HIV infection/AIDS 391
Oral contraceptive 60
anticonvulsant interaction 536
antithrombin III (ATIII) activity reduction 75
antithrombin III deficiency 133
Budd–Chiari syndrome 357, 358
cerebral venous thrombosis 540
diabetes mellitus 450–1
epilepsy 536
gallbladder effects/disease 361
cholesterol lithiasis 362
hypertension 212
intrahepatic cholestasis of pregnancy (IHCP) 332, 333
liver lesions 359
liver transplant patients 352
lower oesophageal sphincter pressure (LOSP) 381
malignant melanoma 621
melasma 610
pemphigoid (herpes) gestationis 615
primary liver cancer 360
prolactin-secreting pituitary tumours 484, 487
pruritus gravidarum 612
renal transplant patients 271
sickle cell syndromes 51–2
stroke/transient ischaemic attacks (TIA) 539
systemic lupus erythematosus (SLE) 620
thromboembolism 130, 451
viral hepatitis susceptibility 334
Oral hypoglycaemic agents 439, 441
breast feeding contraindication 444
Ornithine carbamoyltransferase deficiency 526–7
carrier screening 527
diagnosis 527
treatment 527
Osmolarity, plasma 231
Osmoregulation 231
Osteoblasts 505
alkaline phosphatase 506
bone mineralization 506
bone remodelling 505
parathyroid hormone (PTH) stimulation 509
Osteoclasts 505
bone remodelling 505
parathyroid hormone (PTH) stimulation 509
Osteocytes 505
Osteogenesis imperfecta congenita 520
Osteogenesis imperfecta tarda 520
Osteomalacia
anticonvulsants-associated 517–8
chronic renal disease 517
classification 513, 514
cultural lack of sunlight exposure 515
gastrointestinal/hepatic 515–17
histopathological features 513
neonatal hypocalcaemia 514–15
nutritional 513–15
renal tubular acidosis 517
secondary hyperthyroidism 514
serum calcium levels 514
vitamin D supplements 515
Osteopenia, drug-induced 517
see also Heparin-induced osteopenia
Osteoporosis
homocystinuria 521
of pregnancy 519–20
Oxamniquine 396
Oxprenolol 154
fetal growth effect 210
post-partum hypertension 208
pre-eclampsia 202
Oxygen consumption 1–2, 5
Oxygen therapy 168
Oxyphenacetin 407
Oxytocin
diabetes mellitus 443
heart disease 158
heart failure 158
myotonic muscular dystrophy 548
pre-eclampsia 207
Oxytocinase *see* Vasopressinase
P-50 2
Packed cell volume (PCV) 37
Packed red cell transfusion
amniotic fluid embolism 87
induced abortion with haemorrhage 88
$Pa{CO_2}$ 2
bronchial asthma 6
Palmar erythema 322, 612
Pancreatic disease 363–5
Pancreatic islet beta cell insufficiency 425, 426
Pancreatic malignancy 365
Pancreatic transplant patients 261, 264
Pancreatitis 363–5
amylase levels 363, 364
clinical features 364
differential diagnosis 364
gallstone disease 363, 364, 365
haemorrhagic 364
hypertension-associated hepatic disorders 330
post-partum 331
management 364–5
maternal/fetal outcome 363
persistent vomiting 384
primary hyperparathyroidism 518
total parenteral nutrition 364–5, 405
$Pa{O_2}$ 1–2
Papular dermatitis of pregnancy 619
Para-aminosalicylic acid (PAS) 13
Paracervical block 548
Paracetamol 16, 17
liver failure with overdose 350
muscle contraction headache 546
N-acetyl cysteine antidote 350
rheumatoid arthritis 313
systemic lupus erythematosus (SLE) 311
Parainfluenzavirus 16
Paramethadione 538
Paraplegia 548–9
Parasitic infestation 554
fever 556
intestinal 395–7
laboratory tests 555
Parathyroid adenoma 518
Parathyroid carcinoma 364
Parathyroid disease 518–19
Parathyroid hormone (PTH)
actions on bone 509
calcium transplacental transport 512
calcium/phosphate homeostasis 506, 509
osteomalacia 514
pregnancy-associated elevation 510
in puerperium 510
renal actions 509
bicarbonate handling 509
1α-hydrolase activation 508, 509
Paratyphoid fever 394
Parenteral nutrition 281
see also total parenteral nutrition
Paromomycin
giardiasis 397
Paroxetine 637
Paroxysmal atrial tachycardia 154

Paroxysmal nocturnal haemoglobinuria (PNH) 60–1
  Budd–Chiari syndrome 357, 358
  cerebral venous thrombosis 540
  management 60
  red cell defect 60
  thromboembolism risk 60,119
Partial thromboplastin time
  factor VIII antibody 100
  haemorrhage, rapid screening tests 79
  heparin treatment monitoring 124, 157
Parvovirus B19 564
Patent ductus arteriosus
  in pregnancy 145
    corrected cases 145
Peak expiratory flow 4
  home monitoring in ashtmatics 7
Pectin preparations 392
Pel–Ebstein fever 553
Pelvic kidney 243
Pemphigoid (herpes) gestationis 614–17
  clinical features 615
  differential diagnosis 615–17
  HLA antigens in aetiology 615
  oestrogen-associated exacerbation 616
  pathology 616
  polymorphic eruption of pregnancy comparison 616
  post-partum flare 615
  pregnancy outcome 616
  prognosis 617
  recurrence 615, 617
  treatment 617
Penicillamine 314
Penicillin allergy 7
Penicillins 161
  cystic fibrosis 19
  inflammatory bowel disease (IBD) 401
  pneumonia 17
  puerperal sepsis/wound infection 559
  septic abortion 560
  urinary tract infection (UTI) 259
Pentamidine
  Pneumocystis carinii pneumonia 584
    prophylaxis 586
  safety in pregnancy 586
  side effects with HIV infection 584, 586
Pentazocine
  contraindication in opiate addicts 603
  neonatal abstinence syndrome 602
Peppermint oil 408
Pepsinogen serum level 387
Peptic ulcer disease 387–8
  acute presentation 387
  diagnosis 379, 387
  haemorrhage/perforation 387, 388
  healing in pregnancy 387
  management 388
    drug therapy 382, 388
  prevalence 387
Percutaneous nephrostomy 249
Percutaneous transhepatic cholecystography 362
Pergolide 485
Periarteritis nodosa 243
  hypertension 248
  renal involvement 248
Pericardial disease 166–7
  management 167
  pulmonary oedema 167
Pericardiectomy 167
Perineal disorders 408–10
Peripartum cardiomyopathy *see* puerperal cardiomyopathy
Peripheral pulmonary stenosis 169
Peripheral vascular resistance 144, 183
Periportal hepatic necrosis 191
Peritoneal dialysis 276–7
  acute renal failure 281, 287
Peritonitis
  cirrhosis 355
  pancreatitis 365
Persistent atrial tachycardia 154
Pethidine
  bronchial asthma 11
  opiate addict management 603
Phaeochromocytoma
  chronic hypertension 211
  von Hipple–Lindau disease 251
pH, arterial 2–3
Pharyngolaryngeal oedema 241
Phencyclidine 606
Phenindione 127
Phenobarbitone
  birth defects with polytherapy 538
  breast milk levels 539
  eclamptic hypertensive encephalopathy 543
  folate malabsorption 538
  neonatal coagulopathy 537, 538
  osteomalacia 517
  post-partum dosage 539
  pre-eclampsia 204
  pruritus with IHCP 333
Phenolphthalein 407
Phenothiazines
  manic depressive psychosis 631
    acute relapse 633
  safety in pregnancy 385, 386, 631–2
Phentolamine 168
  septic shock 284
Phenylbutazone 314
Phenylephrine 168
Phenylketonuria 522–4
  breast feeding 524
  dietary treatment 522
    re-introduction in pregnancy 523
  dietary tyrosine supplementation 523
  gene therapy 524
  maternal hyperphenylalaninaemia 523
    fetal damage 523
    routine screening 523–4
  metabolic defect 522
  neonatal screening (Guthrie test) 522
Phenytoin 154
  birth defects
    distal digital hypoplasia and hypertelorism 537
    orofacial clefts 537
    pathogenesis 538
  eclampsia prevention/treatment 203, 543
  epilepsy, blood level monitoring 538
  folate malabsorption 538
  neonatal coagulopathy 537, 538
  osteomalacia 517
  post-partum dosage 539
Phlebotomy 59
Phobias, specific 625
  antenatal 629–30
  treatment 629
Phosphate 506
  bone mineralization 506, 508
  bone mobilization 509
  dietary intake 506
  gut absorption 508
    antacid therapy 506
  homeostasis 505
    changes in pregnancy 509–15
    renal 506
  hormonal regulation 506–9
    calcitonin 509
    parathyroid hormone 509
    vitamin D 506, 507–9
  placental active transport 511
  renal 1α-hydrolase regulation 510
  renal tubular reabsorption 506, 508, 509
  serum level 506
    osteomalacia 513
    in pregnancy 510–11
    renal transplant patients 263, 267
Pica 380
Piperazine 395
Pituitary apoplexy 486, 487, 544
Pituitary gland disorders 483–94
Pituitary tumours 483, 544
  diabetes insipidus 494, 544
  diagnosis 483–4
  hormone secretion 483
  hyperprolactinaemia 483–4
  pituitary apoplexy 486, 487, 544
  pregnancy-associated enlargement 544
  pressure effects/hypopituitarism 492
  visual field defects 544
Placenta accreta 78
Placenta separation
  factors reducing risk of haemorrhage 71
  haemostasis 71, 77, 117
Plague 554
Plasma exchange
  haemolytic uraemic syndrome (HUS) 98, 99
  hypertension-associated hepatic disorders 330
  systemic lupus erythematosus (SLE) 312
  thrombotic thrombocytopenic purpura (TTP) 98, 99

Plasma protein fraction (PPF)
haemorrhage management 81
septic shock 284
Plasma substitutes 81
Plasma thromboplastin antecedent (PTA) deficiency *see* factor XI deficiency
Plasma volume 33–4, 190, 233
benefits of hypervolaemia 35
multigravidae 34
multiple pregnancy 34
pre-eclampsia 40, 190, 195
puerperium 34
Plasma volume expansion 229
pre-eclampsia 204–5
Plasmapheresis
Guillain–Barré syndrome 547
haemolytic uraemic syndrome (HUS) 285
myasthenia gravis 548
pemphigoid (herpes) gestationis 617
platelet function abnormalities, hereditary 101
systemic lupus erythematosus (SLE) 312
Plasmin 75
fibrin/fibrinogen breakdown 76
inhibition 76
Plasminogen 75
aberrant forms 134
inhibition 76
Plasminogen activator 75
tissue activity 75–76
Plasminogen activator inhibitor 76
HELLP syndrome 324
pre-eclampsia 193
Platelet count 72, 73
abruptio placentae 85
autoimmune thrombocytopenic purpura (AITP) 89
fetal assessment 93, 94, 95
neonatal assessment 94
fetal assessment 93
fetal blood sampling 93–4
maternal renal transplant 268
haemorrhage management 79, 82
pre-eclampsia 97, 98, 190, 191, 197, 201
labour management 207
prospective serial counts 197
renal transplant patients 266
Platelet factor 4 190
Platelet function abnormality
clinical manifestations 100
inherited disorders 101
Platelet HpA1 grouping 96
Platelet transfusion
abruptio placentae 85
autoimmune thrombocytopenic purpura (AITP) 91, 94, 95
bleeding oesophageal varices 355
fetal alloimmune thrombocytopenia (AIT) 97
haemorrhage management 82
hypertension-associated hepatic disorders 330
May–Heggelin anomaly 101
neonatal thrombocytopenia 94
platelet function abnormalities, hereditary 101
septic shock 284
Platelets
activation/aggregation 73
adhesion
basement membrane collagen 73
von Willebrand's factor (vWF) 102
ADP release 73
fate 72
haemostasis 72–3
HIV-associated immune destruction 95–6
local fibrin plug formation 73
maternal sensitization to fetal antigen 96
origin 72
turnover in pregnancy 72–3
vascular integrity 71, 72
von Willebrand's disease 102
Platelet-specific antibodies 96
Plesiomonas shigelloides 391
Plethysmography 119–20
Pleural effusion 22
amoebic liver abscess 359
pancreatitis 364, 365
post-partum 22
Plumbism, congenital 380
Pneumococcal infection 553
Pneumocystis carinii
AIDS patients 17, 349, 576, 584, 586
liver dysfunction 349
pneumonia 17, 576, 584
prophylaxis 586
treatment 584
renal transplant patients 266
Pneumomediastinum 21–2, 123
malignant mediastinum 22
treatment 22
Pneumonia 16–17
fungal 17
hospital-acquired 16, 17
intravenous drug abusers 600
maternal mortality 17
pleural effusion 22
post-operative in puerperum 553
risks to fetus 17
therapy 17
viral 16, 17
Pneumopericardium 21
Pneumothorax 21–2, 123
tension 22
treatment 22
Podophyllin 409
contraindication in pregnancy 620, 621
Poliomyelitis 554, 564
fetal/perinatal loss 563
neonatal infection 563
Polyarteritis nodosa 315
hepatic rupture/infarction 325
termination of pregnancy 315
Poly-ASA 401
Polycystic kidney disease (PKD) 251
antenatal diagnosis 250
genetic aspects 250
genetic counselling 250
hypertension 250
liver cysts 250
pregnancy outcome 245
renal insufficiency 250
Polycystic liver disease 359
portal hypertension 356
Polycythaemia rubra vera (PRV) 59
Budd–Chiari syndrome 357, 358
prognosis 59
Polymorphic eruption of pregnancy 617–18
lesion characteristics 617
pemphigoid gestationis comparison 616
treatment 618
Polymyositis 547
Polyoma virus 565
Polyphenolic laxatives 407
Porcine xenografts 162
Porencephaly 97
Porphyria 359, 526
Portal hypertension
cirrhosis 354, 355, 356
non-cirrhotic causes 356
Portal vein pressure 231
Position effects
aortic compression 183
arterial blood gas measurements 2
blood pressure measurement 184
cardiac output measurement 182
plasma volume measurement 33
Positive end expiratory pressure (PEEP) 21
Post-partum angiopathy 542
Post-partum blues/highs 634
Post-partum convulsions, differential diagnosis 542
Post-partum haemorrhage
abruptio placentae 85
acute adrenal failure 495
adult respiratory distress syndrome 20
diabetes insipidus 492
heart disease 158
hypertension-associated hepatic disorders 330
hypertrophic obstructive cardiomyopathy 164
hypopituitarism/Sheehan's syndrome 492
intrahepatic cholestasis of pregnancy (IHCP) 333
pre-eclampsia 205
prostaglandin E2 treatment 157
von Willebrand's disease 104
Post-partum hypothyroidism 475
Post-partum psychiatric disorders 634–8
Post-partum psychosis 625
Post-partum stroke 539
Post-partum thyroiditis 474–5
cytomegalovirus (CMV) 348
hepatitis C *see* hepatitis C
Postnatal depression 625, 635–8
clinical features 636
maintaining factors 637

precipitating factors 363
prevalence 635
prognosis 636
treatment 637–8
Poststreptococcal glomerulonephritis, acute 243
Praziquantel 396
Prazosin 210
Prednisolone 91
autoimmune hepatitis 353
breast feeding 312, 400
inflammatory bowel disease (IBD) 400
pemphigoid (herpes) gestationis 617
safety in pregnancy 498
Prednisone 60, 97, 165
Bell's palsy 546
bronchial asthma 8, 10
change to inhaled steroid 10
fetal effects 11, 267
oestriol level effects 10–11
pseudotumour cerebri 545
renal transplant patients 261, 267
side effects 267, 312
systemic lupus erythematosus (SLE) 307, 312
aspirin combination 312
Wegener's granulomatosis 15
Pre-eclampsia 212
abruptio placentae 84
acute fatty liver of pregnancy 327, 329–30
acute renal failure 190, 278, 279, 284
adult respiratory distress syndrome 20
anticoagulant therapy 205
anticonvulsant therapy 202–4, 208
antihypertensive therapy 199–201, 208
escape from blood pressure control 202, 241
longer-term control 201–2
prophylactic 205–7
uteroplacental perfusion effects 200, 201
antiplatelet agents, prophylactic 206
ascites 190
bed rest 117, 198–9
blood pressure measurements 188
calcium supplements in prevention 206
cardiac output 188
cardiovascular system involvement 188–9
cerebral haemorrhage 189, 199, 202, 205
clinical presentation 187–8
coagulation disturbance 97–8, 190–1, 197–8
treatment 205
complications 195
cortical blindness 192
definition 187, 188
delivery 208
deferral 201
early elective 198, 199, 201, 202, 205, 241
pre-term birth management 206
diabetes mellitus 248
diagnosis 194–8
differentiation from renal disease 238, 254
signs of maternal syndrome 195
1, 25-dihydroxyvitamin D 190
disseminated intravascular coagulation (DIC) 78, 191, 197, 198, 205, 324
HELLP syndrome 191
liver damage 191
diuretic therapy 204, 205, 241
'dry' form 190
endothelial damage in pathogenesis 72, 193, 324
epidural anaesthesia 207
fetal predisposing factors 198
fetal syndrome 194, 195
signs 195
fibrin degradation products (FDPs) 98, 197
fibrinopeptide A 98
fish oil supplements in prevention 206
gallbladder wall thickening 362
general anaesthesia management 207
haemoglobin concentration 40
heparin metabolism 128
hepatic involvement 191–2, 196, 323–4
subcapsular haemorrhages 325
hospital admission 198, 199
hydatiform mole 194
hypertension 187, 188, 189, 192, 194, 195, 196–7, 198
complications 189, 199
post-partum 208
third trimester escape of blood pressure 202, 241
hypoalbuminaemia 190
hypocalciuria 190
hypothyroidism 467
incidence 188
inherited predisposition 198
intrauterine growth retardation 190
labour management 207
laryngeal oedema 190
intubation 207
long-term sequelae 212
management 198–202, 204–5
conservative, severe symptoms 201
treatment summary 208
maternal mortality 189, 192
microangiopathic haemolysis 97, 191
monitoring of maternal condition 198, 199, 201
myocardial infarction 163
nervous system involvement 192–3
see also Eclampsia
oedema 188, 190, 195, 197, 204–5, 241
plasma volume expansion 204–5
oral contraceptive use 212
patient characteristics 208
placental pathology 194
hyperplacentosis 198
plasma creatinine 197
plasma urate 189, 195, 197, 232
plasma volume 40, 190, 195
platelet count 197, 207
platelets 97–8
lifespan 73
post-partum pleural effusion 22
prevention 205–6
progression to eclampsia 188
prostacyclin (PGI2) in pathogenesis 72
proteinuria 187, 188, 189, 192, 195
pulmonary oedema 190, 204, 207
renal cortical necrosis 286
renal involvement 189–90, 197
complications 190
glomerular pathology 189
nephrotic syndrome 252
renal function impairment 189
renal transplant patients 266–8, 273
risk factors 198
salt restriction 204, 205
screening 198
sedatives 204
soluble fibrin complexes 84, 98
superimposed on chronic hypertension 187, 209, 210, 212, 266
acute episode management 241
with chronic renal disease 240, 241
prevention/treatment 240–1
signs 209
Swan–Ganz catheterization 144
systemic disturbance 188
systemic lupus erythematosus (SLE) 311
α thalassaemia hydropic fetus 49, 56
thrombocytopenia 97, 191, 192, 195
thromboembolism 117, 118
urine testing 187–8
vascular catecholamine/angiotensin II responsiveness 188
ventilation-perfusion imbalance 4
vitamin E in prevention 206
weight gain
dietary restriction 206
excessive 197
weight as risk factor 198
Pregnancy cardiomyopathy *see* puerperal cardiomyopathy
Pregnancy counselling
haemodialysis patients 274
liver transplantation 352
Pregnancy-induced hypertension (PIH) 187
Prenatal diagnosis
achondroplasia 520
$alpha_1$ antitrypsin deficiency 20
congenital adrenal hyperplasia 496
cystic fibrosis 18
Gaucher's disease 524
haemoglobinopathy 47, 55–7
haemophilias 106
haemostasis defects, hereditary 100
Marfan's syndrome 170, 521
neural tube defects 537

Prenatel diagnosis *Cont.*
osteogenesis imperfecta congenita 520
platelet function abnormalities, hereditary 101
polycystic kidney disease (PKD) 250
protein C deficiency 134
renal disease, hereditary 251
sickle cell syndrome 54, 55
β thalassaemia 49, 57
thrombocytopenia, hereditary 101
von Willebrand's disease 103
Pre-pregnancy counselling
antithrombin III deficiency 133
chronic renal disease 234
diabetes mellitus 438–9
epilepsy 538
heart disease 150
metabolic bone disease 513
recurrent thromboembolism 129
renal transplant patients 271, 273
Prerenal failure (vasomotor nephropathy) 278, 280
differential diagnosis 280
management 280
Pre-term labour
alcohol infusion tocolysis 604
beta sympathomimetic drug tocolysis 9, 160
cardiovascular side effects 159, 160
criteria for stopping therapy 160
oxygen saturation monitoring 160
bronchial asthma 6
cocaine abuse 605
diabetes mellitus 448–9
folate deficiency 44, 46
haemodialysis patients 276
HIV infection 579, 582, 588
hypertension-associated hepatic disorders 330
intrahepatic cholestasis of pregnancy (IHCP) 332–3
iron deficiency anaemia 37
listeriosis 394
paraplegia 548
pneumonia 17
pre-eclampsia 207
renal transplant patients 268, 269–70, 273
sickle cell disease (HbSS) 52
systemic lupus erythematosus (SLE) 308
thrombolytic therapy 125
total parenteral nutrition 405
Primidone
neonatal coagulopathy 537, 538
neonatal withdrawal symptoms 539
Procainamide 153
Procaine 548
Prochlorperazine
anti-emetic therapy 386
safety in pregnancy 632
Proctitis, non-specific 397
Proctocolectomy 408
Progesterone
bile acid/bile salt metabolism 362, 612
brain tumour enlargement 543
bronchial asthma 6
lower oesophageal sphincter pressure (LOSP) 381
pigmentation changes 611
postnatal depression 637
red cell carbonic anhydrase 3
respiratory stimulant effect 3, 4
small bowel transit time 406
urinary tract effects 558
Progesterone therapy
postnatal depression 637
pulmonary lymphangioleiomyomatosis 16
Proguanil 562
Prolactin
renal 1α-hydrolase activation 509, 510
serum levels 484
Prolactin-secreting pituitary tumour 483–7, 544
anovulation/amenorrhoea treatment 484
breast feeding 487
bromocriptine treatment 484–5, 486, 544
contraception 487
diabetes insipidus 486, 487
diagnosis 483–4
effect of pregnancy 484–5
gonadotrophin treatment 484
labour 487
macroadenomas 484, 485, 486, 544
microadenomas 484, 485, 486, 544
pituitary apoplexy 486, 487
pregnancy management 486–7
prolactin levels 484, 486–7
radiotherapy 485
raised intracranial pressure 486, 487
spontaneous abortion 486
surgery 485, 487, 544
termination of pregnancy 487
tumour expansion 484–5, 486
management in pregnancy 487
tumour-related pregnancy complications 486
visual field defects 484, 485, 486, 487
visual field monitoring 486
Promazine 383
Promethazine 383
safety in pregnancy 386
Propranolol 153, 154, 170
fetal effects 471
migraine prophylaxis 546
post-partum thyroiditis 474
side effects 471
thyroid crisis (thyroid storm) 472
thyrotoxicosis 471
neonatal 474
Propylthiouracil
breast milk levels 471
fetal thyroid function 470
side effects 470
thyroid crisis (thyroid storm) 472
thyrotoxicosis 469, 474
neonatal 474
Prostacyclin (PGI2) 71–2
deficiency in platelet consumption syndromes 72
haemodynamic effects 144
pre-eclampsia 72
renal vascular responses 229
thrombus formation prevention 71
vessel wall production 72
Prostacyclin (PGI_2) infusion
acute renal failure 285
Eisenmenger's syndrome 168
haemolytic uraemic syndrome (HUS) 286
pre-eclampsia 205, 284
Prostacyclin synthase 72
Prostaglandin E_1 therapy 351
Prostaglandin E_2 therapy 157
Prostaglandin synthase inhibitors 311
Prostaglandin therapy
hypertension-associated hepatic disorders 330
pancreatitis 364
Prostaglandins
bronchial asthma 6
haemodynamic effects 144
lower oesophageal sphincter pressure (LOSP) 381
renal vascular responses 229
Protamine sulphate
heparin therapy reversal 124
neutralization test 129, 156
heparin treatment monitoring 124
Protein C 75, 134
HELLP syndrome 324
inhibition with lupus anticoagulant 311
pre-eclampsia 191
Protein C concentrate 134
Protein C deficiency 132
acquired following Fontan procedure 171
cerebral venous thrombosis 540
genetic aspects 134
heparin therapy/prophylaxis 134
incidence 134
poor obstetric outcome 134
prenatal diagnosis 134
purpura fulminans neonatalis 75, 134
recurrent thromboembolism 75, 129, 134
thromboembolism prophylaxis 134
warfarin therapy-associated skin necrosis 134
Protein S 75, 134
Protein S deficiency 132
acquired following Fontan procedure 171
purpura fulminans in neonate 134
recurrent thromboembolism 75, 129, 134
warfarin therapy-associated skin necrosis 134
Protein-calorie malnutrition 405
Proteinuria 231, 232
with active urinary sediment 239
acute renal failure 279
chronic renal disease
antenatal monitoring 238

preserved function/mild impairment 235
specific renal diseases 246
pre-eclampsia 187, 188, 189, 192, 195
superimposed on chronic hypertension 209
renal transplant patients 265, 266
third trimester 266
systemic lupus erythematosus (SLE) 306
Proteus
septic shock 284
urinary tract infection 255, 558
Prothrombin *see* factor II
Prothrombin ratio 325
Prothrombin time
acute liver failure 351
haemorrhage, rapid screeninig tests 79
Prurigo gestationis of Besnier *see* Prurigo of pregnancy
Prurigo of pregnancy 617–18
Late onset *see* Polymorphic eruption of pregnancy
Pruritic folliculitis of pregnancy 618–19
treatment 619
Pruritic urticarial papules and plaques of pregnancy (PUPPP) *see* Polymorphic eruption of pregnancy
Pruritus
hepatitis A 335
intrahepatic cholestasis of pregnancy (IHCP) 331, 332, 333
viral hepatitis 333
Pruritus gracidarum (cholestasis of pregnancy) 331, 611–12
atopic eczema exacerbation 619
incidence 611
treatment 612
Pseudo von Willebrand's disease 103
Pseudohypoparathyroidism 519
Pseudomembranous (antibiotic-associated) colitis 392
Pseudomonas
septic shock 284
urinary tract infection 255, 558
Pseudotumour cerebri 545
headache 546
Pseudoxanthoma elasticum 522
Psoriasis 620
drug treatment in pregnancy 621
PUVA treatment 621
Psychiatric disorders 625–38
antenatal 627–30
pharmacological treatment 625–6
post-partum 634–8
pre-existing 630–4
psychological treatments 626
social issues 626–7
Psychiatric drug prescribing 625–6
Psychotrophic drugs
excretion in breast milk 626
safety in pregnancy 625
Ptyalism 383
Pudendal block
cirrhosis 355
myasthenia gravis 548
Puerperal (peripartum/pregnancy) cardiomyopathy 165–6
cardiac transplantation 166
delivery 166
diagnosis 165
heart transplantation 171
incidence 165
management 165–6
mortality 166
pathogenesis 166
risk factors 165
Puerperal psychosis 634–5
aetiology 635
clinical features 634
treatment 635
Puerperal pyrexia 559
causes 559
Puerperal sepsis 559
acute renal failure 281
clinical features 559
diagnosis 559
pathogenic bacteria 558–9
prognosis 559
treatment 559
Puerperal wound infection 559
Puerperium
blood volume 34–5
cerebral venous thrombosis 540
clotting factor changes 117
eclamptic convulsions 192
fever diagnosis 555
infections 553, 554
megaloblastic anaemia 45
myocardial infarction 163
pre-eclampsia 187, 188
subcutaneous heparin therapy 128
thromboembolism 117
paroxysmal nocturnal haemoglobinuria (PNH) 60
prophylaxis 129
warfarin therapy 128, 129
target INR 128
Pulmonary angiography 126
Pulmonary artery pressure
adult respiratory distress syndrome 21
assessment of risk of pregnancy 150
cystic fibrosis 19
Pulmonary aspiration syndrome *see* Gastric contents aspiration
Pulmonary capillary wedge pressure (PCWP) 283
Pulmonary diffusing capacity 4
Pulmonary embolectomy 126
Pulmonary embolus 116, 122
abortion 118
anticoagulation 121
arterial blood gases 2, 121
chest radiograph 120–1
clinical manifestations 120
deep vein thrombosis 121
diagnosis 120–1
differential diagnosis 7
electrocardiogram 121
embolectomy 126
following past thromboembolism 130
heparin, subcutaneous 155
incidence 116
lung function following 116
lung scans 121
paroxysmal nocturnal haemoglobinuria (PNH) 61
puerperal (peripartum/pregnancy) cardiomyopathy 165
pulmonary angiography, clot fragmentation 126
pulmonary hypertension following 116
sickle cell disease (HbSS) 54, 118
stroke, ischaemic 540
thrombolytic therapy versus heparin 125
treatment
acute phase 121
chronic phase 121
emergency resuscitation 121
warfarin therapy 155
see also Thromboembolism
Pulmonary eosinophilic granuloma 15
Pulmonary gas transfer 4
Pulmonary hypertension
anticoagulant therapy 155
assessment of risk of pregnancy 150
maternal congenital heart disease 146
primary 146, 150, 168–9
termination of pregnancy 150
Pulmonary lymphangioleiomyomatosis 15–16
differential diagnosis 16
Pulmonary oedema
adrenal cortical tumour 491
aortic regurgitation 161
beta-sympathomimetic drug-association 9, 159–60
heart disease 153, 159–60
mitral stenosis 161
pancreatitis 365
pericardial disease 167
pre-eclampsia 190, 204, 207
Pulmonary stenosis
in pregnancy 145
systolic murmur 149
Pulmonary vascular disease 167–70
Pulmonary veno-occlusive disease
maternal mortality 146
termination of pregnancy 150
Pure red cell aplasia 58
Purpura 613
Purpura fulminans 75, 88
protein C/protein S deficiency in neonate 134
PUVA treatment 621
Pyelonephritis, acute 227, 242, 258, 556
acute renal failure 281, 285
adult respiratory distress syndrome 20, 259
antibiotic therapy 557
clinical features 557
fetal outcome 258
gram negative sepsis 259
persistent vomiting 384

Pyelonephritis, chronic 556
  antibiotic therapy 557
  clinical features 248, 557
Pyogenic infection, acute 555
Pyramethamine
  folinic acid supplements 584
  toxoplasmosis with HIV infection 584
Pyrantel pamoate 395–7
Pyrexia of unknown origin (PUO) 553
Pyridoxine (vitamin B6) therapy
  anti-emetic therapy 385
  Bendectin/Debendox 385, 386
  homocystinuria 118–9, 521, 522
  with isoniazid therapy 584
  Wilson's disease 356
Pyrimethamine
  malaria prophylaxis/treatment 562
  toxoplasmosis 561
Pyrizinamide 13
Pyrogen, endogenous 552

Quinacrine
  breast feeding 395
  giardiasis 397
  Taenia solium treatment 395
Quinidine 154
Quinine
  associated hypoglycaemia 562
  malaria prophylaxis/treatment 562
  safety in pregnancy 562
Quinolones
  breast feeding contraindication 394
  safety in pregnancy 558
  urinary tract infection (UTI) 558

Radiation enteritis 405
Radiation exposure, fetal damage 535–6
Radiactive iodine treatment 471
Radiography of gastrointestinal tract disorders 379
Radioisotope scanning
  fetal radiation exposure 121
  iodine contraindication 119
  pulmonary embolus diagnosis 121
  venography 119
Radiotherapy
  acromegaly 488
  long-term effects on offspring 63
Ranitidine 23
  obstetrical anaesthesia preparation 383
  safety in pregnancy 382
Rat-bite fever 553
Raynaud's phenomenon 314
Recombinant human erythropoietin (rHuEpo) 274
  haemodialysis patients 275
Rectal carcinoma 393
Red cell carbonic anhydrase 3
Red cell count (RBC) 37
Red cell indices
  iron deficiency 37
  sickle cell syndromes 54
  α thalassaemia 48
  β thalassaemia minor 50
Red cell mass 34
  iron requirement 35
  multiple pregnancy 34
  oxygen requirement relationship 35
Reflux nephropathy 242, 248–9, 254
  hereditary transmission 249
  hypertension 249
  impact of pregnancy 235
  pregnancy outcome 245
  renal dysfunction 248–9
Regional anaesthesia
  abruptio placentae 85
  heart disease 158
  myasthenia gravis 548
  myotonic muscular dystrophy 548
  polycythaemia rubra vera (PRV) 59
  scleroderma 315
  severe respiratory impairment 23
  sickle cell disease (HbSS) 53
  see also Epidural anaesthesia; Spinal anaesthesia
Reiter's syndrome 380
Relapsing fever 553
Relapsing polychondritis 315
Relaxin 144
Renal artery stenosis 238, 243
Renal biopsy 189, 238–9, 245, 445
  acute cortical necrosis 280
  acute renal failure 280
  antepartum indications 239
  pre-biopsy evaluation 239
  renal transplant rejection 266
Renal blood flow
  autoregulation 229
  vasoactive hormone responses 229–30
  vasodilatation of pregnancy 228
    additional vasodilatory responsivity 229–30
    endothelial derived relaxing factor (EDRF) system 230
Renal cortical necrosis
  bilateral (BRCN) 286
  pre-eclampsia 191
Renal disease, chronic 233–61
  anaemia 58
  antenatal care 237–8
  antenatal renal function monitoring 240
  antithrombin III (ATIII) activity 75
  collagen disorders 247–8
  counselling 226
    pre-pregnancy 234
  delivery
    blood replacement 242
    elective 240, 241
    pre-term 241, 242
  deterioration of renal function 235, 236–7, 252
    reversible causes 240
  diagnosis in pregnancy 238–40
    renal biopsy 238–9
  fetal surveillance 241
  haemodialysis patients *see* Haemodialysis patients
  hospital admission 238
  hypertension 233, 235, 237, 238, 240, 241, 250, 254
    rodent models 252–3
    treatment 240
  impact of pregnancy 234–7, 254
    animal models 252–3
    long-term effects 252–3
    moderate impairment 236–7
    preserved function/mild impairment 235–6
    severe impairment 237
  management in pregnancy 238
  osteomalacia/congenital rickets 517
  pathophysiology 233–4
  perinatal outcome 235, 237
  peritoneal dialysis 276–8
  specific renal diseases 242–54
  systemic lupus erythematosus (SLE) 307–8
Renal disease, inherited 250–1
  prenatal diagnosis 251
Renal failure, acute 276–82
  acute cortical necrosis 279, 280
  acute fatty liver of pregnancy 327
  acute pyelonephritis 285
  acute tubular necrosis 278, 280
  causes 277, 278, 286
  dialysis 281
  differential diagnosis 279–80
    intravenous mannitol trial 280
    urine sodium concentration 278, 280
    urine specific gravity 280
    urine/plasma (U:P) osmolality ratio 278, 279, 280
  diuretics 280
  electrolyte replacement 281
  fetal salvage 280
  fluid volume balance 281
  incidence 276, 278
  investigation 279–80
  management 280–1
  maternal mortality 278
  oliguria 279
    differential diagnosis 278
  parenteral carbohydrate/essential L-aminoacids 281
  pathology 278–9
    renal ischaemia 278, 279
  phases 279
  polyuria 279
  pre-eclampsia/eclampsia 190, 284
  prerenal failure (vasomotor nephropathy) 278, 279, 280
  recovery phase 279
  renal biopsy 280
  septic shock *see* septic shock
  treatment 286–7
Renal function
  assessment in pregnancy 239–40
  changes in indices 231
  clinical aspects 231–2
  deterioration, antepartum 232–3
    reversible causes 240
  haemodynamic changes 227–33
    causes 229

ultrasound assessment 228
vascular autoregulation 229
osmoregulation (osmotic threshold changes) 231
pre-eclampsia 189–90, 197
volume homeostasis 233
Renal 1α-hydrolase
1,25-dihydroxyvitamin D synthesis control 508–9
pregnancy-associated activation 510
Renal metabolism 1, 35
Renal osteodystrophy, delivery management 269
Renal plasma flow (RPF) 227, 228
Renal rupture
non-traumatic 261
traumatic 259
Renal sodium retention 229
Renal transplant patients 261–74
allograft function 264–5
allograft rejection 266
allograft survival 262–3
antenatal care 263
breast feeding 272
contraception counselling 261, 271
delivery 266, 268–9, 273
pre-term 269–70, 273
diabetes mellitus 263
dietary counselling 264
dyspepsia management 266
gynaecological problems 272
haemolytic uraemic syndrome (HUS) 286
hypertension 273
third trimester 266
immunosuppressive therapy 266–7
long-term paediatric problems 272–3
malignancy association 272
impact of pregnancy 273
infections management 266
labour management 268
long-term maternal follow-up 271
long-term medical problems 263
mortality 262, 263, 271
obstetric outcome 263, 264, 266, 273
early pregnancy problems 264
paediatric management 269–70, 274
congenital abnormalities 271
viral infections 270–1
parathyroid dysfunction 266–7
pelvic osteodystrophy 269
postnatal assessment 270–2
pre-eclampsia 266–8, 273
pregnancy counselling 261
guidelines 261
pregnancy management 263–4
pre-pregnancy assessment 261
pre-pregnancy counselling 271, 273
renal function deterioration, reversible causes 265
rhesus (Rh) antibody screening 264
therapeutic termination 264, 273
Renal tubular acidosis 517
Renal vascular resistance (RVR) 227, 228
Renal vein thrombosis
maternal diabetes mellitus 435
nephrotic syndrome 252
Renin/angiotensin II (AII) system 229
Reserpine 483
Residual volume 2, 4
bronchial asthma 6
cystic fibrosis 18
Respiratory adaptation to pregnancy 1–4
airway resistance 4
CO_2 production 2, 4
diaphragm level 3
gas transfer (pulmonary diffusing capacity) 4
hyperventilation 3
oxygen consumption 1–2
P-50 2
$Paco_2$ 2
Pao_2 1–2
pH, arterial 2–3
residual volume 2, 4
tidal volume 2, 4
ventilatory equivalent 2
vital capacity 3
Respiratory system disorders 5–23
Respiratory tract infection 16–17
bronchial asthma exacerbation 7, 8
Retained dead fetus
adult respiratory distress syndrome 20
disseminated intravascular coagulation (DIC) 78, 87
with living twin 87
management 87
renal cortical necrosis 285
soluble fibrin complexes 84
Retinal haemorrhage 385
Retinoids 620
Reye's syndrome 328, 329
Rhesus isoimmunization
intravenous drug abusers 600
pre-eclampsia 198
renal transplant patient screening 263
Rheumatic fever, acute 161
diagnosis 161
treatment 161
Rheumatic heart disease
aortic valve disease 161
atrial fibrillation 145
chronic 160–1
digoxin 153
endocarditis 161
fetal outcome 147
incidence 144, 145
long-term survival, effect of pregnancies 146
maternal mortality 146
mitral valve cordae tendinae rupture 161
mitral valve disease 161
symptoms in pregnancy 148
tricuspid valve 161
Rheumatoid arthritis 313–14
congenital heart block 308, 313
drug treatment 313–14, 357
pregnancy-associated α3-glycoprotein 313
puerperal exacerbations 313
Rhinovirus infection 16
Rickets 515
chronic renal disease 517
classification 513, 514
histopathological features 513
maternal hypoparathyroidism 519
pelvic diameter reduction 515
renal tubular phosphate reabsorption impairment 513
type I 513
type II 513
Rifampicin
fetal abnormalities 13
tuberculosis 13
HIV infection 584
Rift Valley fever 350
Right atrial pressure 149
acute renal failure 279, 284
labour in heart disease patients 157
septic shock 284
Right ventricular output assessment 282–3
Rigors 552, 553
Ristocetin cofactor assay 102
Ritodrine
cardiovascular side effects/pulmonary oedema 159
pemphigoid (herpes) gestationis 617
Rotavirus gastroenteritis 391, 397
Rotor's syndrome 358
Roundworm (*Ascaris lumbricoides*) 395
congenital/neonatal infection 395, 396
obstetric deaths 395
treatment 395
Rubella 554, 565
immunity status 439
neonatal illness/congenital infection 563
cardiac malformations 147
fetal loss 563
TORCH (STORCH) infections 563
vaccination 563
re-infection following 563
Rubidomycin 61

Sacral agenesis, diabetes mellitus 429, 446
S-adenosyl-L-methionine 332, 333
Salazopyrine
active metabolites 400
breast feeding 401
folic acid metabolism 401
inflammatory bowel disease (IBD) 400
chronic disease 402
infertility 398
levels in fetus 401
rectal preparations 401
rheumatoid arthritis 314
safety in pregnancy 401
side effects 401

Salbutamol
  bronchial asthma 7, 8–9, 11
  side effects 8, 9, 159
Salicylates 161
  breast feeding 312
  systemic lupus erythematosus (SLE) 312
Salmeterol 9
Salmonella
  antibiotic resistance 394
  delivery of symptomless carriers 394
  HIV infection/AIDS 391
  laboratory tests 555
  traveller's diarrhoea 391
Salmonella typhi vaccination 394
Salt restriction 233
  pre-eclampsia 204, 205
Sanarelli–Schwartzman reaction 286
Sarcoidosis 14–15
  bilateral hilar lymphadenopathy 14
  differential diagnosis 14
  diffuse lung infiltration 14
  management 14–15
  portal hypertension 356
  vitamin D sensitivity 15
Scarlet fever 554
Schistosoma haematobiu 396
Schistosoma japonicum 396
Schistosoma mansonii 396
Schistosomiasis 396
  drug therapy 396
  gastrointestinal tract involvement 396
  liver involvement 356, 396
Schizoaffective disorders 634
Schizophrenia 633–4
  breast feeding 634
  course 633
  genetic aspects 633
  medication during pregnancy 633–4
  post-partum management 634
  psychosocial management 634
  relapse management 634
Schwangerschafts protein (SP1) 384
Scleroderma 243, 314–15
  abdominal wall compliance 247
  anaesthetic problems 315
  diffuse cutaneous form 314
  fetal outcome 315
  localized cutaneous form 314
  prognosis 314–315
  proteinuria with active urinary sediment 239
  Raynaud's phenomenon 314
  SCL-70 antibodies 314
  see also Systemic sclerosis
Sclerosing cholangitis 358
Sebaceous gland changes 613
Sedatives
  bronchial asthma 7
  cirrhosis 355
  opiate interactions 603
  pre-eclampsia 204
Selective termination 87
Senokot 407
Septic abortion 559–60
  acute renal failure 278, 281
  antibiotic therapy 283
  diagnosis 282, 283
  disseminated intravascular coagulation (DIC) 78, 88, 282
  endotoxic shock 560
  see also Septic shock
  management 560
  pathogens 560
  prognosis 559–60
  surgical intervention 283
Septic pelvic thrombophlebitis 134–5
Septic shock 281–4, 559–60
  acid-base status 282
  acute renal failure 281–2
  antibiotic therapy 283–4
  disseminated intravascular coagulation (DIC) 284
  haemodynamic evaluation 282–3
  investigations 282
  management 283
  pathology 281–2
  peripheral perfusion inadequacy 282
  presentation 282
  surgical intervention 283
  Swan–Ganz catheterization 144
  volume replacement 283–4
Septicaemia 123
  acute renal failure 281
  Campylobacter infection 392, 393
  hypertension-associated hepatic disorders 330
  laboratory tests 555
  rigors 553
Serotoinin re-uptake inhibitors 627
  breast feeding 637
  postnatal depression 637
Sertraline 637
Sex hormone binding globulin (SHBG) 468
Sex steroids
  calcium/phosphate homeostasis 506
  renal 1α-hydrolase activation 509
SGOT 321
  HELLP syndrome 324
  hepatic rupture/infarction 325
  hypertension-associated hepatic disease 323
Sheehan's syndrome 492, 539
  pre-eclampsia 191
Shigellosis 392, 394
  antibiotic resistance 394
  delivery of symptomless carriers 394
  HIV infection/AIDS 391
  management 394
  travellers' diarrhoea 391
Shock
  amniotic fluid embolism 86
  blood pressure measurement errors 185
  disseminated intravascular coagulation (DIC) 78
  purpura fulminans 88
  see also Septic shock
Shock lung *see* Adult respiratory distress syndrome (ARDS)
Sickle cell disease (HbSS) 51–4
  blood transfusion in pregnancy
    management 52
    complications 52
    exchange transfusion regime 53
  Central African Republic (CAR) haplotype 51
  cerebral ischaemia/stroke 539
  clinical expression 51
  contraception 51–2
  folate supplements 45
  general/regional anaesthesia 53
  genetic control of prognosis 51
  perioperative pulmonary complications 53
  pregnancy 52
  prenatal diagnosis 54, 55
    globin gene analysis 56
  pulmonary embolus 118
  risks to fetus 52
  sickling crises 51, 53
  subarachnoid haemorrhage 541
Sickle cell haemoglobin (HbS) 50
  detection 54
  sickling process 50
Sickle cell thalassaemia 50
  diagnosis 54
Sickle cell trait (HbAS) 50, 51–2
  pregnancy 53
Sickle cell/HbC disease (HbSC) 50
  sickling crises in pregnancy/puerperium 51
Sigmoidoscopy
  amoebiasis 396
  gastrointestinal tract disorders 379
  pseudomembranous colitis 392
  schistosomiasis 396
Single nephron glomerular filtration rate (SNGFR) 228
Single photon emission computed tomography (SPECT) 542
Single ventricle 171
  maternal mortality 146
Sjögren's syndrome 308
Skin disorders 610–21
  breast/nipples 614
  coeliac disease 389
  collagen disease 613, 620–1
  dermatoses 614–20
  glandular activity 613
  hair 614
  melasma 610–11
  nails 614
  pigmentation disorders 610
  pregnancy-associated 610–12
  pruritus gravidarum (cholestasis of pregnancy) 611–12
  vascular 612–13
Skin metabolism 35
Skin tags 613
Small bowel resection
  cholesterol lithiasis 362
  vitamin B_{12} supplements 401
Small bowel transit time 406
Small for dates infant
  coeliac disease 389
  hyperemesis gravidarum 386
  hypertension-associated hepatic disorders 330

nephrotic syndrome 252
pancreatic beta cell reduction 428
plasma volume 190
pre-eclampsia 195
renal transplant patients 270
SMS 201–995 562
Soap enemas 407
Sodium bicarbonate antacids 382
Sodium citrate 23, 382, 383
Sodium nitroprusside 199, 200
Sodium restriction 355
Sodium retention 233
Solitary kidney 243, 251
animal models 252
Soluble fibrin complexes 98, 190
Somatostatin analogues
growth hormone-secreting pituitary tumour 488
quinine-induced hypoglycaemia 562
Sperm donor screening 342
Spherocytosis, hereditary 45
Spider naevi 322, 612
Spinal anaesthesia 546
Spinal osteoporosis, post-pregnancy 519
Spinal X-ray 536
Spiral arteries
fibrin deposition 77
lesions in pre-eclampsia 194
Spiramycin 561
Spironolactone
ascites 355, 358
breast feeding contraindication 355
Splenectomy 91, 92, 93
Spontaneously hypertensive rat (SHR) 253
Sporotrichosis 17
Staphylococcus
pneumonia 16
puerperal sepsis/wound infection 558
travellers' diarrhoea 391
urinary tract infection 255, 558
Staphylococcus epidermidis 558
Starr–Edwards prosthetic valve 156
Status asthmaticus *see* Bronchial asthma, acute severe
Status epilepticus 537
Sterculia 407
Steroid therapy
acute liver failure 351
acute renal failure 279
acute rheumatic fever 161
Addisonian collapse on withdrawal 10
in labour 11
Addison's disease 495
adult respiratory distress syndrome 21
alternate day 10, 15
aphthous stomatitis 380
autoimmune chronic active hepatitis 355
autoimmune thrombocytopenic purpura (AITP) 91–2, 95
Bell's palsy 546
breast feeding 272
bronchial asthma 6, 7, 8, 10–11, 495
change from oral to inhaled steroid 10
chronic active hepatitis 353
congenital adrenal hyperplasia 496, 498
Cushing's syndrome 489
eclamptic hypertensive encephalopathy 543
factor VIII antibody 100
fetal alloimmune thrombocytopenia (AIT) 97
fetal lung maturation 11, 207, 448, 449
haemolytic uraemic syndrome (HUS) 99, 285
hyperemesis gravidarum 385
hypothalamo-pituitary–adrenal axis of fetus 11
impetigo herpetiformis 620
inflammatory bowel disease (IBD) 398, 400
metabolic bone disease 516
labour management 268, 311, 495
liver transplantation 352
nephrotic syndrome 239
oestriol level effects 10–11
pancreatitis 364
papular dermatitis of pregnancy 619
pemphigoid (herpes) gestationis 617
polymorphic eruption of pregnancy 617
prurigo of pregnancy 618
pseudotumour cerebri 545
renal transplant patients 268, 270
rheumatoid arthritis 313
safety in pregnancy 10, 270, 400, 498
septic shock with acute renal failure 283
side effects 91
systemic lupus erythematosus (SLE) 311, 495
C_3 complement level monitoring of disease 311
puerperium 247, 312
thrombotic thrombocytopenic purpura (TTP) 99
viral hepatitis 353
Stool bulking agents
constipation 407
irritable bowel syndrome 408
STORCH infections *see* TORCH infections
Streptococcus
acute rheumatic fever 161
cold sores 554
endocarditis 158
pneumonia 16
puerperal sepsis/wound infection 558, 559
Streptococcus faecalis
puerperal sepsis/wound infection 559
urinary tract infection 558
Streptococcus mutans 381
Streptococcus pneumoniae pneumonia 16, 17
Streptokinase
deep vein thrombosis 125
haemolytic uraemic syndrome (HUS) 285
pulmonary embolus 125
thromboembolism 121, 125
Streptomycin 13
Striae gravidarum 613
Stroke volume 144
Stroke, ischaemic 539–40
causes 539
post-partum 539
prognosis 540
treatment 540
Strongyloides stercoralis
HIV infection/AIDS 391
inflammatory bowel disease (IBD) 400
traveller's diarrhoea 391
Subacute hepatic necrosis *see* Liver failure, late onset
Subacute thyroiditis 475
sporadic goitre 465
Subaortic stenosis see Hypertrophic obstructive cardiomyopathy (HOCM)
Subarachnoid haemorrhage 541
headache 546
labour 541
polycystic kidney disease (PKD) 250
Substance abuse 600–6
heart murmurs in pregnancy 600
hepatitis B chronic carriage (HBsAg positivity) 338
hepatitis B risk 343, 344
hepatitis C 337
nutritional/social factors 600
Succinylcholine 154
Sudden infant death syndrome (SIDS) 602
Suicide, maternal 626, 627, 634, 635, 636
Sulfamethoxazole 392
Sulphadiazine
folinic acid supplements 584
toxoplasmosis 561
with HIV infection 584
Sulphapyridine 400
Sulphasalazine *see* Salazopyrine
Sulphonamides
asymptomatic bacteriuria 257
fetal hyperbilirubinaemia 257
toxoplasmosis 561
urinary tract infection 259, 558
Supine hypotension 183
Suprapubic aspiration urine collection 254, 558
Supratentorial astrocytoma 544
Supraventricular tachycardia 155
fetal 152
hyperthyroidism 154
Surfactant, pulmonary
diabetes mellitus 434, 449
phosphatidyl glycerol measurement 449
Swan–Ganz catheterization 144, 150
adult respiratory distress syndrome 21

Swan–Ganz catheterization *Cont.*
hypertension-associated hepatic disorders 330
labour in heart disease patients 157, 161
pulmonary vascular disease 169
Sweat gland changes 613
Syncope 148
heart disease 148
hypertrophic obstructive cardiomyopathy 164
ventricular tachycardia 155
Syntocinon 164
bronchial asthma 11
heart disease 158
pre-eclampsia 207
Syphilis
blood transfusion screening 82
cerebral ischaemia/stroke 539
nephrotic syndrome 252
TORCH (STORCH) infections 563
Systemic lupus erythematosus (SLE) 58, 243, 247, 306–15, 620
abortion 307, 308, 309
drug treatment 312
recurrent 96, 312
anticardiolipin antibodies 309
false positive Wasserman reaction 310
suppression 312
chorea gravidarum 307
congenital heart block 307, 308–9, 312
anti-Ro antibodies 312
diagnosis before delivery 313
ydropic fetus 313
preventive drug therapy 313, 313
diagnostic criteria 306
differentiation from pre-eclampsia 306–7
drug treatment 307, 311
C_3 complement level monitoring of disease 311
puerperal exacerbations 312
effect of pregnancy 307
fetal outcome 312, 620
fever 555
hypertension 307–8
immunosuppressive therapy 96
labour 495
fetal blood gas monitoring 313
steroid cover 311
lupus anticoagulant 96, 309
suppression 312
maternal mortality 307
mitral valve cordae tendinae rupture 161
myocardial infarction 163
neonatal lupus syndrome 307, 308–9
cardiac defects 307, 308–9
cardiolipin antibodies 309
haematological abnormalities 308
perinatal death 309
skin lesions 309
transplacental maternal antibodies 308
nephropathy *see* Lupus nephropathy
oral contraceptive use 620
overlap syndrome 307
pregnancy management 311–13
cardiotocography 313
pregnancy outcome 245, 308–11
pregnancy-associated flare 620
prevalence 306
prognosis 307
relapse in puerperium/post-partum syndrome 247
renal 'flare' management 307
steroid therapy 495
thrombocytopenia 96
thromboembolism prophylaxis 312
Systemic sclerosis 247
hypertension 248
pulmonary fibrosis 5
renal involvement 247

T_3 resin uptake (RU) 461, 462
hypothyroidism 467
thyrotoxicosis 469
T_4 binding globulin (TBG) 460
effect of pregnancy 461
fetal levels 462
Taenia saginata 395
Taenia solium 395
Takayasu's arteritis 147
Tamoxifen 16
Tapeworm 395
Tar preparations 621
Technetium99 HIDA scan 362
^{99}mTechnetium scan
fetal radiation exposure 121
lung scan 121
secretion in breast milk 121
venography 119
Teicoplanin 159
Telangiectatic epulis 613
Telogen effluvium 614
Temazepam 630
Tension pneumothorax 22
Tepid sponging 17
Terbutaline
bronchial asthma 7, 8–9
side effects 8, 159
Termination of pregnancy
acute severe asthma (status asthmaticus) 8
adrenal carcinoma 491
aortic coarctation 169, 211
aplastic anaemia 58
cirrhosis 355
cystic fibrosis 18
diabetic nephropathy/retinopathy 445, 451
disseminated intravascular coagulation (DIC) 88
Eisenmenger's syndrome 167
heart disease 147, 150, 152
HIV infection 581, 583, 586, 587
leukaemia 62
Marfan's syndrome 170
periarteritis nodosa 248
platelet function abnormalities, hereditary 101
polyarteritis nodosa 315
polycystic kidney disease (PKD) 250
prolactin-secreting pituitary tumour 487
pulmonary vascular disease 169
renal transplant patients 264, 273
selective termination 87
Wegener's granulomatosis 15
Tetany, neonatal 518
Tetracycline
acne 620
acute fatty liver of pregnancy 328, 329
contraindication in pregnancy 8, 16, 257, 621
pseudomembranous colitis 392
secretion in breast milk 11
Thalassaemia major *see* β Thalassaemia
Thalassaemia syndromes 47–50
folate supplements 45
α Thalassaemia 47–9
genetic aspects 47–8
HbBarts 48
HbH disease 48
hydropic fetus 49
obstetric complications 49, 56
major 48
management 48–9
prenatal diagnosis
amniotic fluid fibroblasts 56
globin gene analysis 56
α thalassaemia hydrops 56
red cell indices 48
sickle cell gene interactions 51
β thalassaemia 47, 49–50
genetic counselling 49
incidence 49
major 49, 57
prognosis 50
treatment 50
minor 50
pregnancy management 50
prenatal diagnosis 49, 55, 57
globin gene analysis 56
oligonucleotide DNA probes 56
Thalidomide 385
contraindication in pregnancy 621
erythema nodosum treatment 621
Theophyllines
bronchial asthma 8, 9–10
toxicity in neonate 10
Thiabendazole 395
Thiazide diuretics 153
cirrhosis 355
pancreatitis 364
pre-eclampsia 204
Thioguanine 61
Thiopentone 381
Thirst 231
Threadworm (*Enterobius vermicularis*) 395
Throat swabs 555
Thrombasthenia (Glanzmann's disease) 101
Thrombectomy 126
Thrombin
antithrombin III (ATIII) inhibition

75, 132
fibrinogen breakdown 84
local fibrin plug formation 73
Thrombin time
abruptio placentae 85
chronic heparin therapy monitoring 128
haemorrhage, rapid screening tests 79, 80
Thrombin-antithrombin III complexes 117
Thrombocytopenia 59, 73, 89
aspirin treatment 59
autoimmune thrombocytopenic purpura (AITP) 89–96
clinical manifestations 100
fetal
maternal diabetes mellitus 428, 432
maternal renal transplant 268, 274
Gaucher's disease 524
HELLP syndrome 324
heparin-associated 131
hereditary disorders 101
IgG infusion 92
neonatal
hypertension-associated hepatic disorders 330
lupus syndrome 308
pre-eclampsia 97, 191, 192, 195
septic shock 282
systemic lupus erythematosus (SLE) 96, 306, 308
Thrombocytopenia with absent radii (TAR syndrome) 101
Thrombocytosis *see* Thrombocythaemia
Thromboembolism 116–35
acute phase treatment 121, 124–6
high dose intravenous heparin 124–5
subcutaneous fixed dose heparin 125
surgery 125, 126
thrombolytic therapy 125–6
age-associated risk 118, 129
anaemia 118
antithrombin III deficiency 133
artificial heart valves 155–6
atypical sites 118
bed rest 117, 129
blood group O influence 118
cardiolipin antibodies 118, 129
chronic phase treatment 121, 126–9
heparin 127–9
labour management 128
puerperium 128–9
clotting factor alterations 117
congestive heart failure 118
dehydration 118
diagnosis 119–21
emergency resuscitation 121
ethnic differences 118
Fontan procedure 171
haemorrhoids 612
homocystinuria 118–19, 521
incidence 116–17
post-partum 117
leg varices 612
lupus anticoagulant association 96, 118, 129, 309, 311
obesity 118
oestrogen patch therapy 638
operative delivery 117–18, 129
oral contraceptive association 450
parity 118, 129
paroxysmal nocturnal haemoglobinuria 60, 119
polycythaemia rubra vera (PRV) 59
prophylaxis 129–32
following past thromboembolism 129, 130, 131
heparin 75
high-risk patients 131
low-risk patients 131
prediction of women at risk 132
protein C deficiency, familial 75
protein S deficiency, familial 75
recurrent 129
pre-pregnancy counselling 129
screening tests 129
risk factors 117–19
septic pelvic thrombophlebitis 134–5
sickle cell disease 118
systemic lupus erythematosus (SLE) 312
thrombophilia 132–4
treatment 121, 124–9
venous stasis 117
Thrombolytic therapy
antithrombin III deficiency 133
cerebral venous thrombosis 540
myocardial infarction 164
premature labour association 125
reversal 126
thromboembolism 121, 125–6
heparin comparison 125
Thrombomodulin 75
Thrombophilia 132–4
Thrombophlebitis
incidence 116
puerperum 553
septic 559
Thromboplastin 73, 74
Thrombotic thrombocytopenic purpura (TTP) 98–9, 285
cerebral ischaemia stroke 539
clinical manifestations 98
management 98–9
prostacyclin (PGI2) deficiency 72
Thromboxane 72
Thromboxane synthetase inhibitors 330
Thrombus formation 72
Thymic atrophy 270
Thyroid biopsy 475
Thyroid crisis (throid storm) 469, 472
Thyroid disease 459–76
Thryoid function tests 461–4
hypothyroidism 467
neonatal screening 468
solitary thyroid nodule 475
thyrotoxicosis 469
Thyroid gland
calcitonin secretion 507–509
effect of pregnancy 461–4
fetal function 462–3
hypertrophy 461
see also Goitre
normal physiology 459–61
pituitary feedback control 460
maternal/fetal relationship 463
Thyroid hormone replacement therapy
anterior pituitary deficiency 493
hypothyroidism 466, 467–8
dosage monitoring 468
fetal treatment *in utero* 468
post-partum 475
neurological cretinism 465
sporadic goitre 466
supplementary to antithyroid drugs 470
fetal thyrotoxicosis 473
thyroid malignancy 475
Thyroid malignancy 475, 509
Thyroid nodule 475
Thyroid solitary toxic adenoma 469
Thyroid stimulating antibodies (TSAb) 472–3
assay 473
long-acting thyroid stimulator (LATS) 473
neonatal thyrotoxicosis 474
Thyroid stimulating hormone (TSH) 460
fetal levels 462
neonatal surge 462–3
thyroid gland hypertrophy 461
endemic goitre 465
Thyroid stimulating hormone (TSH) assay
hypothyroidism 467
immunoradiometric assay (IRMA) 461–4
thyrotoxicosis 469
antithyroid drugs monitoring 469
Thyroid stimulating hormone (TSH) secreting pituitary tumour 483
Thyroiditis
post-partum 474–5
postnatal depression 637
Thyrotoxicosis 468–74
anovulation/amenorrhoea 469
antithyroid drugs 469–70
fetal outcome 471
monitoring 471
beta adrenergic blocking drugs 471
body temperature elevation 552
clinical features 469
congenital malformations 469
fetal 472–3
adverse outcome 473
thyroid-stimulating antibodies (TSAb) 472–3
fetal mortality 469
gestational vomiting/hyperemesis gravidarum 384
incidence 469
neonatal 472–4
clinical features 474
mortality 474

Thyrotoxicosis *Cont.*
onset 474
thyroid-stimulating antibodies (TSAb) 472–3, 474
treatment 474
TSH receptor binding inhibiting antibodies (TBII) measurement 473
radioactive iodine treatment 471–2
surgery 471
thyroid crisis (thyroid storm) 469, 472
thyroid function tests 469
TSH immunoradiometric assay (IRMA) 462
Thyrotrophin *see* Thyroid stimulating hormone (TSH)
Thyrotrophin-releasing hormone (TRH) 460
placental form 461
Thyroxine (T4) 459
control of synthesis 460
fetal levels 462
gestational vomiting/hyperemesis gravidarum 384
levels in pregnancy 461
neonatal levels 462, 463
peripheral deiodination 459, 460
physiological role 460–1
plasma protein binding 460
release 460
synthesis 459
endemic goitre 465
transplacental passage 463
Ticlopidine 98
Tidal volume 2, 4
Tinidazole
amoebiasis 396
giardiasis 397
Tissue heart valves 162–3
Tissue plasminogen activator 117
inhibition with lupus anticoagulant 311
Tocolytic therapy
cardiovascular side effects 159
diabetes mellitus 448–9
Tolazline 168
Toluene abuse 606
Tonsillitis, acute bacterial 554
TORCH (STORCH) infections 563
Total haemoglobin 35
Total iron binding capacity (TIBC) 37–8
Total parenteral nutrition 405
fetal outcome 405
hyperemesis gravidarum 385
inflammatory bowel disease (IBD) 401, 402
jejuno-ileal bypass 406
lipid emulsions 405
maternal monitoring 405
pancreatitis 364–5
Total serum calcium 506
Total thyroxine (T4) 461, 462
hypothyroidism 467
thyrotoxicosis 469
antithyroid drugs monitoring 469
Toxaemia *see* Pre-eclampsia
Toxaemic rash of pregnancy *see* Polymorphic eruption of pregnancy
Toxic erythema of pregnancy *see* Polymorphic eruption of pregnancy
Toxoplasmosis 380, 554, 561–2
antenatal investigation of primary infection 561
antibiotic therapy 561
congenital disease 561
follow-up 561
treatment of infant 561
fetal damage 561, 584–5
HIV infection 580, 583, 584–5, 586
encephalitis 584
treatment 584
laboratory tests 555
screening in pregnancy 561
TORCH (STORCH) infections 563
Tranexamic acid (AMCA) 76
Transcutaneous oxygen saturation measurement 5
Transfer factor 4
breathlessness 5
pulmonary lymphangioleiomyomatosis 16
Transferrin 35
Transient hip osteoporosis of pregnancy 519
Transient hypertension of pregnancy 187
Transient ischaemic attacks (TIA) 539
anticoagulant therapy 540
Transient tachypnoea of newborn
diabetes mellitus 434
maternal opiates addiction 601
Transposition of great arteries 171
Travellers' diarrhoea 391
antimicrobial therapy 392
management 392
Trematode infestation 396
Tretinoin
hyperpigmentation/melasma 611
safety in pregnancy 621
Trichuris trichiura see Whipworm
Tricuspid atresia 170
fetal outcome 170
Fontan procedure 170–1
acquired thrombotic state 171
thromboprophylaxis 171
maternal outcome 170
Tricuspid regurgitation 149
systolic murmur 149
Tricuspid valve disease 161
Tricyclic antidepressants
antenatal anxiety 628
antenatal depression 619, 627
breast feeding 626, 637
lower oesophageal sphincter pressure (LOSP) 381
manic depressive psychosis 633
migraine prophylaxis 546
muscle contraction headache 546
obsessional ruminations 630
postnatal depression 637, 638
safety in pregnancy 627
Triethylene tetramine dihydrochloride (trientine) 356
Trifluoperazine
manic depressive psychosis 631
acute relapse 633
safety in pregnancy 632
schizophrenia 634
Triglyceride plasma level 322
pancreatitis 363, 364
Tri-iodothyronine (T4) 459
fetal levels 462
levels in pregnancy 461
neonatal levels 462, 463
physiological role 460–1
plasma protein binding 460
release 460
synthesis 459
control 460
endemic goitre 465
Trimethadione 538
Trimethobenzamide 386
Trimethoprim
safety in pregnancy 257, 392, 621
travellers' diarrhoea 392
urinary tract infection (UTI) 259
Trimethoprim/sulphamethoxazol
Pneumocystis carinii pneumonia 584
side effects with HIV infection 584
Triploid fetus 198
Trisomic fetus 198
Trophoblastic disease, gestational
liver metastases 360
pemphigoid (herpes) gestationis 614, 615
Tropical sprue 394
vitamin B_{12} deficiency 46
Trypanosomiasis 395
Trypsin inhibitors 364
TSH receptor binding inhibiting antibodies (TBII) assay 473
Tubal pregnancy, abdominal complications 405
Tuberculosis 12–14, 553
adrenal gland destruction/ Addison's disease 495
antituberculous drugs 12–13
fetal effects 13
congenital 12
constrictive pericarditis 167
diagnosis 12
effect of pregnancy 12
extrapulmonary 13–14
HIV infection 583, 584
prophylaxis 584
treatment 584
neonatal BCG vaccination 14
pleural effusion 22
pneumothorax 21
portal hypertension 356
pregnancy outcome 12
renal transplant patients 266
susceptibility with SLE/steroid therapy 312
Tuberous sclerosis 250
Tubular necrosis, acute 278–9, 280
differential diagnosis 280

septic abortion 284
Typhoid fever 394
laboratory tests 555
management 394
Typhoid vaccination 394, 552

Ulcerative colitis
effects of pregnancy 399
fertility 397–398, 400
fetal outcome 399
incidence 397
liver involvement 358
proctocolectomy 408
resective surgery 402
spontaneous abortion 398, 400
Ultrasound
achondroplasia 521
acute fatty liver of pregnancy 330
adrenal cortical tumour 490
amoebic liver abscess 359
appendicitis 404
common bile duct stones 362, 363
congenital heart block with SLE 313
congenital heart disease 147, 152
deep vein thrombosis 119, 120
diabetes mellitus
fetal monitoring 447
pregnancy management 446
fetal thyrotoxicosis 473
gallstones in pregnancy 362
gastric contents volume estimation 383
gastrointestinal tract disorders 379
hepatic rupture/infarction 325, 326
intrahepatic cholestasis of pregnancy (IHCP) 332
liver metastases 361
maternal hydrocephalus, shunt-treated 545
neural tube defects 537
osteogenesis imperfecta 520
phenylketonuria 524
renal transplant rejection 266
solitary thyroid nodule 475
toxoplasmosis 561
Umbilical blood flow
congenital heart block with SLE 313
diabetes mellitus 447
Upper endoscopy
cirrhosis with gastrointestinal haemorrhage 355–6
duodenal biopsy for coeliac disease 390
gastrointestinal tract disorders 379
peptic ulcer disease 387–8
Upper respiratory tract infection 16
Urate plasma level 231
acute fatty liver of pregnancy 327
pre-eclampsia 189–90, 195, 197, 232
renal transplant patients 266
superimposed on chronic hypertension 209
urolithiasis 249
Urea plasma level 231, 232
acute renal failure 279
haemodialysis patients 275
levels jeopardizing pregnancy 234
renal transplant patients 263
Ureter
normal dilatation 227
urinary stasis 227
Ureteral tube/stent placement 249
Ureteric obstruction 553
Ureterosigmoid anastomosis 250
Urethral syndrome 558
Urethritis 556
Urinary catheterization 556, 557
Urinary diversion, permanent 250
Urinary free cortisol
Cushing's syndrome 489–90
normal pregnancy 489, 490
Urinary stasis
normal pregnancy 227
urinary tract infection 255, 558
Urinary stone composition 249
Urinary tract dilatation 227, 260
Urinary tract infection (UTI) 258–9, 553, 556–8
acute 556
antibiotic therapy 259, 558
duration 259
asymptomatic bacteriuria relationship 255, 256, 557
chronic renal disease, antenatal detection 238
clinical features 557
diagnostic criteria 558
follow-up 558
following previous urinary tract infection 255, 256
glycosuria following 254
gram negative sepsis 259
haematuria 259
heart failure risk with heart disease 152
incidence 556
lower tract (cystitis) 258, 259
paraplegia 549
pathogens 558
permanent urinary diversion 250
puerperal pyrexia 559
renal transplant patients 264, 266
reversible renal function deterioration 240
routes of infection 557, 558
solitary kidney 251
sudden unexpected postperinatal death association 257
upper tract (acute pyelonephritis) 258, 259
urine samples for diagnosis 558
urolithiasis 249
Urinary tract neoplasm 259
Urinary tract obstruction
acute renal failure 276, 278
reversible renal function deterioration 240
Urinary tract overdistension syndrome 260
Urinary tract rupture, non-traumatic 260
Urinary tract surgery 243
Urine culture 557
Urine examination
acute renal failure 279, 280
fever diagnosis 555
pre-eclampsia 187–8
Urine sodium concentration 278, 280
Urine specific gravity 280
Urine/plasma (U : P) osmolality ratio 278, 280
Urokinase 125
Urolithiasis 243, 249–50
epidural block in management 249
haematuria 259
internal ureteral tube/stent placement 249
intravenous urography (IVU) 249–250
percutaneous nephrostomy 250
stone composition 249
Ursocholic acid therapy 363
Ursodeoxycholic acid 612
Urticaria 621
Uterine atony 35

Vaccinia 563, 565
Vaginal swabs 555
Valproic acid
birth defects with polytherapy 538
epilepsy 538
folate malabsorption 538
neural tube defects 537, 538
Vancomycin 159
pseudomembranous colitis 392
Varicella zoster virus 554, 565
fetal/perinatal loss 563
hepatitis 334, 347
neonatal illness/congenital infection 563
pneumonia 17
teratogenic potential 563
treatment in pregnancy 17, 563
zoster immunoglobulin (ZIG) prophylaxis 17, 563
Varices 612
Variegate porphyria (VP) 526
Variola 563, 565
Vasculitis
cerebral ischaemia/stroke 539
subarachnoid haemorrhage 541
Vasomotor nephropathy *see* Prerenal failure
Vasopressinase (oxytocinase) 231
Vegetarians
iron absorption 36
iron status 41
vitamin B_{12} levels 46, 47
Vegetations, bacterial 150
Venezuelan encephalomyelitis 565
Veno-occlusive disease 168–9
Venography
antithrombin III deficiency 133
deep vein thrombosis diagnosis 119, 120
radiation exposure 119, 120
septic pelvic thrombophlebitis 135
Venous stasis 117

Venous thrombosis
pancreatitis 365
paroxysmal nocturnal haemoglobinuria (PNH) 60
Ventilation, mechanical
acute liver failure 351
acute severe asthma (status asthmaticus) 8
adult respiratory distress syndrome 21
amniotic fluid embolism 87
pulmonary oedema management 154
Ventilatory equivalent 2
Ventricular dysrhythmia, autosomal dominant 154
Ventricular septal defect
in pregnancy 145
systolic murmur 149
Ventricular tachycardia 154
prophylaxis 155
syncope 155
Verapamil 153, 154
Vesicoureteric/intrarenal reflux 248
Vibrio cholerae 391, 554
Vincristine 93
Viral infection 554–5, 562–3, 564–5
congenital malformations 563
fever 554
laboratory tests 555
renal transplant patients 266
congenital infection 270–1
Visual field defects
Cushing's syndrome 491
growth hormone-secreting pituitary tumour 488
hypopituitarism/Sheehan's syndrome 493
pituitary adenoma 544
prolactin-secreting pituitary tumours 484, 485, 486, 487
pregnancy monitoring 486
pseudotumour cerebri 545
Vital capacity 3
cystic fibrosis 18
kyphoscoliosis 20
Vitamin B_1 deficiency 385
Vitamin B_6 (pyridoxine) deficiency
coeliac disease 388
total parenteral nutrition 405
Vitamin B_{12}
absorption 46
dietary intake 46–7
multiple pregnancy 46
Vitamin B_{12} deficiency 46–7
aphthous stomatitis 380
coeliac disease 388, 390
folate supplement effects 45
megaloblastic anaemia 46
resective surgery for IBD 402
Vitamin B_{12} supplements
Crohn's disease 401
ileal resection 401
Vitamin D
anticonvulsant effects on metabolism 517–18
calcium /phosphate homeostasis 506, 507–9
dietary sources 507
1α hydrolase enzyme
placental 507
renal 507
25-hydroxycholcalciferol (25–OHD) 507
in pregnancy 512
renal metabolism 507
serum level 507
liver metabolism 507
skin-derived 507, 512
small intestinal absorption 507
status assessment in pregnancy 512
see also 1,25-Dihydroxyvitamin D
Vitamin D binding globulin 507
Vitamin D deficiency
Crohn's disease 401
cultural lack of sunlight exposure 515
1,25-dihydroxyvitamin D (1,25–OHD) 508
intestinal malabsorption disorders 515–16
jejuno-ileal bypass 516
neonatal/infant morbidity 515
osteomalacia 513, 515
renal bone disease 517
rickets 513
Vitamin D malabsorption 388, 515, 516
Vitamin D supplements
anticonvulsant therapy 517, 518
contraindication in sarcoidosis 15
Crohn's disease 516
cystic fibrosis 516
haemodialysis patients 275, 276
hypoparathyroidism 519
jejuno-ileal bypass 516
osteomalacia 515
primary biliary cirrhosis 517
renal bone disease 517
renal transplant patients 264
rickets 515
routine administration 515
Vitamin deficiencies
aphthous stomatitis 380
resective surgery for IBD 402
total parenteral nutrition 405
Vitamin E 206
Vitamin K, protein C/protein S dependence 75
Vitamin K deficiency
hyperemesis gravidarum 385
hypertension-associated hepatic disorders 330
intrahepatic cholestasis of pregnancy (IHCP) 332, 333
Vitamin K_1 therapy
acute liver failure 351
anticonvulsant therapy sol epilepsy 45, 538–9
bleeding oesophageal varices 355
intrahepatic cholestasis of pregnancy (IHCP) 333
primary biliary cirrhosis 356
Volume replacement
adult respiratory distress syndrome 21
haemorrhage 81–3
prerenal failure (vasomotor nephropathy) 280
septic shock 283–4
Volvulus 404
Vomiting/nausea 379, 380, 383–7
Addison's disease 495
differential diagnosis 404
disease associations 384
epidemiology 383–4
fetal outcome 386–8
gastric contents aspiration 382
hyperemesis gravidarum 383
management 384–5
anti-emetic drug therapy 385
morning sickness 384–5
mechanisms 384
oesophagitis 381
risk factors 383, 384
total parenteral nutrition 405
von Gierke's disease 525
von Hipple–Lindau disease
prenatal diagnosis 251
renal involvement 251
von Recklinghausen's disease *see* Neurofibromatosis
von Willebrand's disease 101–4
clinical manifestations 103
delivery, haemorrhagic risk 104
genetic aspects 102
incidence 101–2
molecular aspects 102–3
platelet aggregation 102
pregnancy 104
prenatal diagnosis 103
ristocetin cofactor assay 102
subtypes 103
management 104
severe bleeding disorders 103
treatment 103–4
DDAVP (L-diamino-8-arginine-vasopressin) 103, 104
substitution therapy 103–4
von Willebrand's factor (vWF)
factor VIII complex 102
platelet adhesion 102
pre-eclampsia 193, 197
ristocetin cofactor assay 102
thrombotic thrombocytopenic purpura (TTP) 98, 99
Vulval squamous cell carcinoma 409

Warfarin
atrial fibrillation 152
intracerebral fetal haemorrhage 126, 127
pre-eclampsia 205
in puerperium 127, 128, 129, 156
target INR 128
skin necrosis with protein C/protein S deficiency 134
teratogenesis 126, 127, 156–7, 162, 163
asplenia syndrome 126
chondrodysplasia punctata 126, 127
diaphragmatic hernia 126

thromboembolism chronic phase treatment 121, 126–7
thromboembolism prophylaxis 130, 131
antithrombin III deficiency 133
artificial heart valves 155, 156–7
homocystinuria 522
protein C deficiency 134
treatment monitoring 128
use in pregnancy 126, 127
vitamin K reversal 156
Wedge pressure (indirect left atrial pressure) 157, 158, 161
Wegener's granulomatosis 15, 243, 247–8, 315
hypertension/proteinuria 247
Weight gain
haemodialysis patients 275
pre-eclampsia 197, 206
total body water 233
Wernicke–Korsakoff syndrome
hyperemesis gravidarum 385
total parenteral nutrition 405
Western equine encephalomyelitis 565
Whipple's disease (*Tropheryma whippelii*) 394
Whipworm (*Trichuris trichiura*) 395
Whole fresh blood
acute liver failure 351
haemorrhage management 81–2
hypertension-associated hepatic disorders 330
Whooping cough 554
Wilson's disease 356–7
acute liver failure 356
chronic active hepatitis 353
congenital abnormalities 357
diagnosis 356
fertility 353, 356
impact of pregnancy 354
management 355
pregnancy outcome 356
Wiskott–Aldrich syndrome 101
Wolff–Parkinson–White syndrome 154, 160
Wound infection, puerperal 553, 559
clinical features 559
diagnosis 559
fever 559
pathogenic bacteria 558
predisposing factors 558
prognosis 558
treatment 559
X-linked familial hypophosphataemia 508
X-ray pelvimetry 269

Yttrium^{90} implants 487

Zidovudine 575, 586–7
HIV infection
ACTG 076 trial 586–7
prophylaxis 586–7
vertical transmission 579, 586–7
safety in pregnancy 586
side effects 586
Zinc bioavailability 41
Zinc deficiency
acrodermatitis enteropathica 390
coeliac disease 390
congenital anomalies 390
inflammatory bowel disease (IBD) 398
neural tube defect 390
Zoster immunoglobulin (ZIG) 17, 563